Cellular and Molecular Immunology

EIGHTH EDITION

Abul K. Abbas, MBBS

Distinguished Professor in Pathology
Chair, Department of Pathology
University of California San Francisco
San Francisco, California

Andrew H. Lichtman, MD, PhD

Professor of Pathology
Harvard Medical School
Brigham and Women's Hospital
Boston, Massachusetts

Shiv Pillai, MBBS, PhD

Professor of Medicine and Health Sciences and Technology
Harvard Medical School
Massachusetts General Hospital
Boston, Massachusetts

Illustrations by
David L. Baker, MA
Alexandra Baker, MS, CMI
DNA Illustrations, Inc.

ELSEVIER
SAUNDERS

1600 John F. Kennedy Blvd.
Ste 1800
Philadelphia, PA 19103-2899

CELLULAR AND MOLECULAR IMMUNOLOGY
International Edition

ISBN: 978-0-323-22275-4
ISBN: 978-0-323-31614-9

Notices

Knowledge and best practice in this field are constantly changing. As new research and experience broaden our understanding, changes in research methods, professional practices, or medical treatment may become necessary.

Practitioners and researchers must always rely on their own experience and knowledge in evaluating and using any information, methods, compounds, or experiments described herein. In using such information or methods they should be mindful of their own safety and the safety of others, including parties for whom they have a professional responsibility.

With respect to any drug or pharmaceutical products identified, readers are advised to check the most current information provided (i) on procedures featured or (ii) by the manufacturer of each product to be administered, to verify the recommended dose or formula, the method and duration of administration, and contraindications. It is the responsibility of practitioners, relying on their own experience and knowledge of their patients, to make diagnoses, to determine dosages and the best treatment for each individual patient, and to take all appropriate safety precautions.

To the fullest extent of the law, neither the Publisher nor the authors, contributors, or editors assume any liability for any injury and/or damage to persons or property as a matter of products liability, negligence or otherwise, or from any use or operation of any methods, products, instructions, or ideas contained in the material herein.

Library of Congress Cataloging-in-Publication Data

Abbas, Abul K., author.
  Cellular and molecular immunology / Abul K. Abbas, Andrew H. Lichtman, Shiv Pillai ; illustrations by David L. Baker, Alexandra Baker. -- Eighth edition.
    p. ; cm.
  Includes bibliographical references and index.
  ISBN 978-0-323-22275-4 (pbk. : alk. paper)
  I. Lichtman, Andrew H., author. II. Pillai, Shiv., author. III. Title.
  [DNLM: 1. Immunity, Cellular. 2. Antibody Formation--immunology. 3. Antigens--immunology. 4. Immune System Diseases--immunology. 5. Lymphocytes--immunology. QW 568]
  QR185.5
  616.07'97--dc23
                                                                            2014014817

Senior Content Strategist: James Merritt
Senior Content Development Manager: Rebecca Gruliow
Publishing Services Manager: Jeff Patterson
Project Manager: Clay S. Broeker
Design Direction: Louis Forgione

Printed in Canada

Last digit is the print number: 9 8 7 6 5 4 3 2 1

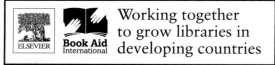

Dedication

To Our Students, Our Colleagues, and Our Families

PREFACE

This eighth edition of *Cellular and Molecular Immunology* includes substantial additions and revisions, which we made to keep the textbook current with scientific advances and, at the same time, maintain the clear and readable style that has been typical of past editions. Whenever we have added new information, we have focused primarily on important concepts and have not increased the length of the book. We have also rewritten many sections for increased clarity, accuracy, and completeness.

Among the major changes is a reorganization of the chapters dealing with T lymphocyte responses in order to more clearly describe early T cell activation events, differentiation and functions of subsets of CD4+ helper T cells, and functions of CD8+ cytotoxic T cells. In addition, the entire book has been updated to include important recent advances in immunology. Some of the topics that have been significantly revised are innate lymphoid cells, the developmental pathways of macrophages and dendritic cells, and immune checkpoints in tumor immunity. It is remarkable and fascinating to us that new principles continue to emerge from analyses of the complex systems that underlie immune responses. Perhaps one of the most satisfying developments for students of human disease is that basic principles of immunology are now laying the foundation for rational development of new immunologic therapies. Throughout the book, we have tried to emphasize these new therapeutics and the fundamental concepts on which they are based.

We have also continued to improve our illustration program. New figures have been added, and previously used figures have been reviewed and often changed for accuracy and clarity. We have kept design features such as the use of bold italic text to highlight "take-home messages" to make the book easy to read. The lists of suggested readings continue to emphasize recent review articles that provide in-depth coverage of particular topics for the interested reader. We have divided the lists into sections based on themes to help readers find the most useful articles for their needs.

Individuals who have helped us with specific topics are (in alphabetical order) Drs. Jonathan Abbas, Mark Anderson, Homer Boushey, Andrew Gross, Stephen Hauser, Miriam Merad, Michael Rosenblum, Wayne Shreffler, and Catherine Wu; all were generous with advice and comments. We thank Dr. Hiroshi Kawamoto for the cover illustration. Our illustrators, David and Alexandra Baker of DNA Illustrations, remain full partners in the book and provide invaluable suggestions for clarity and accuracy. Several members of the Elsevier staff played critical roles. Our editor, James Merritt, has been a source of support and encouragement. Our managing editor, Rebecca Gruliow, shepherded the book through its preparation and into Production. Lou Forgione was responsible for managing the design, and Clay Broeker was in charge of the production stage. We also owe a debt of gratitude to our families for their unflagging support and their tolerance of our absences. Finally, our students were the original inspiration for the first edition of this book, and we remain continually grateful to them, because from them we learn how to think about the science of immunology and how to communicate knowledge in the clearest and most meaningful way.

ABUL K. ABBAS

ANDREW H. LICHTMAN

SHIV PILLAI

CONTENTS

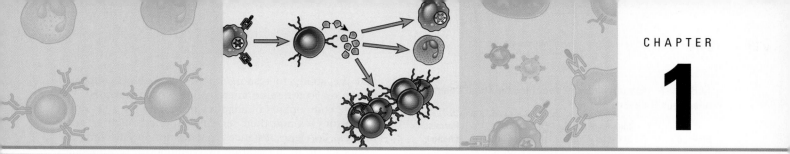

Properties and Overview of Immune Responses

The term *immunity* is derived from the Latin word *immunitas,* which referred to the protection from legal prosecution offered to Roman senators during their tenures in office. Historically, immunity meant protection from disease and, more specifically, infectious disease. The cells and molecules responsible for immunity constitute the **immune system**, and their collective and coordinated response to the introduction of foreign substances is called the **immune response**.

The physiologic function of the immune system is defense against infectious microbes. However, even noninfectious foreign substances can elicit immune responses. Furthermore, mechanisms that normally protect individuals from infection and eliminate foreign substances also are capable of causing tissue injury and disease in some situations. Therefore, a more inclusive definition of the immune response is a reaction to components of microbes as well as to macromolecules, such as proteins and polysaccharides, and small chemicals that are recognized as foreign, regardless of the physiologic or pathologic consequence of such a reaction. Under some situations, even self molecules can elicit immune responses (so-called autoimmune responses). Immunology is the study of immune responses in this broader sense and of the cellular and molecular events that occur after an organism encounters microbes and other foreign macromolecules.

Historians often credit Thucydides, in the fifth century BC in Athens, as having first mentioned immunity to an infection that he called plague (but that was probably not the bubonic plague we recognize today). The concept of protective immunity may have existed long before, as suggested by the ancient Chinese custom of making children resistant to smallpox by having them inhale powders made from the skin lesions of patients recovering from the disease. Immunology, in its modern form, is an experimental science in which explanations of immunologic phenomena are based on experimental observations and the conclusions drawn from them. The evolution of immunology as an experimental discipline has depended on our ability to manipulate the function of the immune system under controlled conditions. Historically, the first clear example of this manipulation, and one that remains among the most dramatic ever recorded, was Edward Jenner's successful vaccination against smallpox. Jenner, an English physician, noticed that milkmaids who had recovered from cowpox never contracted the more serious smallpox. On the basis of this observation, he injected the material from a cowpox pustule into the arm of an 8-year-old boy. When this boy was later intentionally inoculated with smallpox, the disease did not develop. Jenner's landmark treatise on **vaccination** (Latin *vaccinus,* of or from cows) was published in 1798. It led to the widespread acceptance of this method for inducing immunity to infectious diseases, and vaccination remains the most effective method for preventing infections (Table 1-1). An eloquent testament to the importance of immunology was the announcement by the World Health Organization in 1980 that smallpox was the first disease that had been eradicated worldwide by a program of vaccination.

Since the 1960s, there has been a remarkable transformation in our understanding of the immune system and its functions. Advances in cell culture techniques (including monoclonal antibody production), immunochemistry, recombinant DNA methodology, x-ray crystallography, and creation of genetically altered animals (especially transgenic and knockout mice) have changed immunology from a largely descriptive science into one in which diverse immune phenomena can be explained in structural and biochemical terms. In this chapter, we outline the general features of immune responses and introduce the concepts that form the cornerstones of modern immunology and that recur throughout this book.

TABLE 1-1　Effectiveness of Vaccines for Some Common Infectious Diseases

Disease	Maximum Number of Cases (Year)	Number of Cases in 2009	Percentage Change
Diphtheria	206,939 (1921)	0	−99.99
Measles	894,134 (1941)	61	−99.99
Mumps	152,209 (1968)	982	−99.35
Pertussis	265,269 (1934)	13,506	−94.72
Polio (paralytic)	21,269 (1952)	0	−100.0
Rubella	57,686 (1969)	4	−99.99
Tetanus	1,560 (1923)	14	−99.10
Haemophilus influenzae type B	~20,000 (1984)	25	−99.88
Hepatitis B	26,611 (1985)	3,020	−87.66

This table illustrates the striking decrease in the incidence of selected infectious diseases in the United States for which effective vaccines have been developed. Data from Orenstein WA, Hinman AR, Bart KJ, Hadler SC: Immunization. In Mandell GL, Bennett JE, Dolin R (eds.): *Principles and practices of infectious diseases*, 4th ed. New York, 1995, Churchill Livingstone; and *Morbidity and Mortality Weekly Report* 58:1458–1469, 2010.

INNATE AND ADAPTIVE IMMUNITY

Defense against microbes is mediated by the early reactions of innate immunity and the later responses of adaptive immunity (Fig. 1-1 and Table 1-2). **Innate immunity** (also called **natural** or **native immunity**) provides the early line of defense against microbes. It consists of cellular and biochemical defense mechanisms that are in place even before infection and are poised to respond rapidly to infections. These mechanisms react to products of microbes and injured cells, and they respond in essentially the same way to repeated exposures. The mechanisms of innate immunity are specific for structures that are common to groups of related microbes and may not distinguish fine differences between microbes. The principal components of innate immunity are (1) physical and chemical barriers, such as epithelia and antimicrobial chemicals produced at epithelial surfaces; (2) phagocytic cells (neutrophils, macrophages), dendritic cells, and natural killer (NK) cells and other innate lymphoid cells; and (3) blood proteins, including members of the complement system and other mediators of inflammation.

In contrast to innate immunity, there are other immune responses that are stimulated by exposure to infectious agents and increase in magnitude and defensive capabilities with each successive exposure to a particular microbe. Because this form of immunity develops as a response to infection and adapts to the infection, it is called **adaptive immunity** (also called **specific** or **acquired immunity**). The adaptive immune system recognizes and reacts to a large number of microbial and nonmicrobial substances. The defining characteristics of adaptive immunity are the ability to distinguish different substances, called **specificity**, and the ability to respond more vigorously to repeated exposures to the same microbe, known as **memory**. The unique components of adaptive immunity are cells called **lymphocytes** and their secreted products, such as **antibodies**. Foreign substances that induce specific immune responses or are recognized by lymphocytes or antibodies are called **antigens**.

Cytokines are a large group of secreted proteins with diverse structures and functions, which regulate and coordinate many activities of the cells of innate and adaptive immunity. All cells of the immune system secrete at least some cytokines and express specific signaling receptors for several cytokines. The nomenclature for cytokines is inconsistent, with some named *Interleukin* followed by a number, and others named for a biological activity first attributed to them, such as tumor necrosis factor (TNF) or interferon. Among the many functions of cytokines we will discuss throughout this book are growth and differentiation of all immune cells, activation of effector functions of lymphocytes and phagocytes, and directed movement of immune cells from blood into tissues and within tissues. The large subset of structurally related cytokines that regulate cell migration and movement are called **chemokines**. Some of the most effective drugs developed recently to treat immunologic diseases target cytokines, which reflects the importance of these proteins in immune responses.

Mechanisms for defending the host against microbes are present in all multicellular organisms. The phylogenetically oldest mechanisms of host defense are those of innate immunity, which are present even in plants and insects. About 500 million years ago, jawless fish, such as lampreys and hagfish, developed an immune system containing lymphocyte-like cells that may function like lymphocytes in more advanced species and even respond to immunization. The antigen receptors on these cells are variable leucine-rich receptors that are capable of recognizing many antigens but are distinct from the antibodies and T cell receptors that appeared later in evolution. The more specialized defense mechanisms that constitute adaptive immunity are found in vertebrates only. Most of the components of the adaptive immune system, including lymphocytes with highly diverse antigen receptors, antibodies, and specialized lymphoid tissues, evolved coordinately within a short time in jawed vertebrates (e.g., sharks) about 360 million years ago.

Innate and adaptive immune responses are components of an integrated system of host defense in which numerous cells and molecules function cooperatively. The mechanisms of innate immunity provide effective initial defense against infections. However, many pathogenic microbes have evolved to resist innate immunity, and their elimination requires the more powerful mechanisms of adaptive immunity. There are numerous connections between the innate and adaptive immune systems. The innate immune response to microbes stimulates adaptive immune responses and influences the nature of the adaptive responses. Conversely, adaptive immune responses often work by enhancing the protective mechanisms of innate immunity, making them more capable of effectively combating pathogenic microbes.

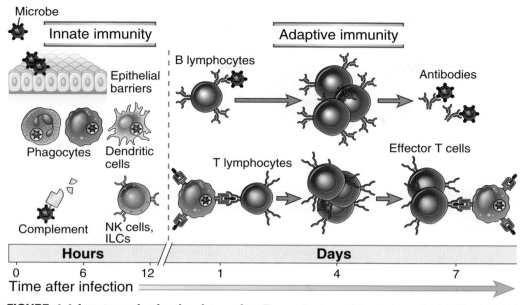

FIGURE 1-1 Innate and adaptive immunity. The mechanisms of innate immunity provide the initial defense against infections. Adaptive immune responses develop later and require the activation of lymphocytes. The kinetics of the innate and adaptive immune responses are approximations and may vary in different infections. *ILC*, innate lymphoid cell; *NK*, natural killer.

TYPES OF ADAPTIVE IMMUNE RESPONSES

There are two types of adaptive immune responses, called humoral immunity and cell-mediated immunity, that are mediated by different components of the immune system and function to eliminate different types of microbes (Fig. 1-2). **Humoral immunity** is mediated by molecules in the blood and mucosal secretions, called **antibodies**, which are produced by cells called **B lymphocytes** (also called **B cells**). Antibodies recognize microbial antigens, neutralize the infectivity of the microbes, and target microbes for elimination by various effector mechanisms. Humoral immunity is the principal defense mechanism against extracellular microbes and their toxins because secreted antibodies can bind to these microbes and toxins and assist in their elimination. Antibodies themselves are specialized and may activate different mechanisms to combat microbes (**effector mechanisms**). For example, different types of antibodies promote the ingestion of microbes by host cells (phagocytosis), bind to and trigger the release of inflammatory mediators from cells, and are actively transported into the lumens of mucosal organs and through the placenta to provide defense against ingested and inhaled microbes and against infections of the newborn, respectively.

Cell-mediated immunity, also called **cellular immunity**, is mediated by **T lymphocytes** (also called **T cells**). Intracellular microbes, such as viruses and some bacteria, survive and proliferate inside phagocytes and other host cells, where they are inaccessible to circulating antibodies. Defense against such infections is a function of cell-mediated immunity, which promotes the destruction of microbes residing in phagocytes or the killing of infected cells to eliminate reservoirs of infection. Some T lymphocytes also contribute to eradication of extracellular microbes by recruiting leukocytes that destroy

TABLE 1-2   Features of Innate and Adaptive Immunity

	Innate	Adaptive
Characteristics		
Specificity	For molecules shared by groups of related microbes and molecules produced by damaged host cells	For microbial and non-microbial antigens
Diversity	Limited; germline encoded	Very large; receptors are produced by somatic recombination of gene segments
Memory	None	Yes
Nonreactivity to self	Yes	Yes
Components		
Cellular and chemical barriers	Skin, mucosal epithelia; antimicrobial molecules	Lymphocytes in epithelia; antibodies secreted at epithelial surfaces
Blood proteins	Complement, others	Antibodies
Cells	Phagocytes (macrophages, neutrophils), natural killer cells, innate lymphoid cells	Lymphocytes

these pathogens and by helping B cells make effective antibodies.

Protective immunity against a microbe is usually induced by the host's response to the microbe (Fig. 1-3). The form of immunity that is induced by exposure to a foreign antigen is called **active immunity** because the immunized individual plays an active role in responding

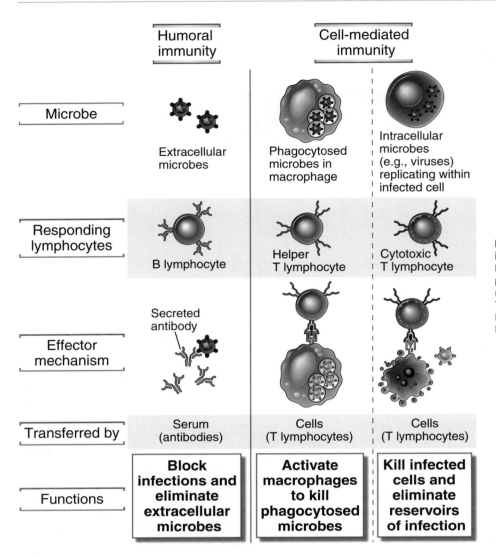

Humoral immunity	Cell-mediated immunity	
Microbe		
Extracellular microbes	Phagocytosed microbes in macrophage	Intracellular microbes (e.g., viruses) replicating within infected cell
Responding lymphocytes		
B lymphocyte	Helper T lymphocyte	Cytotoxic T lymphocyte
Effector mechanism		
Secreted antibody		
Transferred by		
Serum (antibodies)	Cells (T lymphocytes)	Cells (T lymphocytes)
Functions		
Block infections and eliminate extracellular microbes	**Activate macrophages to kill phagocytosed microbes**	**Kill infected cells and eliminate reservoirs of infection**

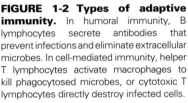

FIGURE 1-2 Types of adaptive immunity. In humoral immunity, B lymphocytes secrete antibodies that prevent infections and eliminate extracellular microbes. In cell-mediated immunity, helper T lymphocytes activate macrophages to kill phagocytosed microbes, or cytotoxic T lymphocytes directly destroy infected cells.

to the antigen. Individuals and lymphocytes that have not encountered a particular antigen are said to be *naive*, implying that they are immunologically inexperienced. Individuals who have responded to a microbial antigen and are protected from subsequent exposures to that microbe are said to be immune.

Immunity can also be conferred on an individual by transferring serum or lymphocytes from a specifically immunized individual in experimental situations, a process known as adoptive transfer (see Fig. 1-3). The recipient of such a transfer becomes immune to the particular antigen without ever having been exposed to or having responded to that antigen. Therefore, this form of immunity is called **passive immunity**. Passive immunization is a useful method for conferring resistance rapidly, without having to wait for an active immune response to develop. A physiologically important example of passive immunity is the transfer of maternal antibodies through the placenta to the fetus, which enables newborns to combat infections before they develop the ability to produce antibodies themselves. Passive immunization against toxins by the administration of antibodies from immunized

animals is a lifesaving treatment for potentially lethal infections, such as rabies, and snake bites. The technique of adoptive transfer has also made it possible to define the various cells and molecules that are responsible for mediating specific immunity. In fact, humoral immunity was originally defined as the type of immunity that could be transferred to unimmunized, or naive, individuals with antibody-containing cell-free portions of the blood (i.e., plasma or serum) obtained from previously immunized individuals. Similarly, cell-mediated immunity was defined as the type of immunity that could be transferred to naive animals with cells (T lymphocytes) from immunized animals, but not with plasma or serum.

The first experimental demonstration of humoral immunity was provided by Emil von Behring and Shibasaburo Kitasato in 1890. They showed that if serum from animals that had been immunized with an attenuated form of diphtheria toxin was transferred to naive animals, the recipients became specifically resistant to diphtheria infection. The active components of the serum were called antitoxins because they neutralized the pathologic effects of the diphtheria toxin. This result led to the treatment of

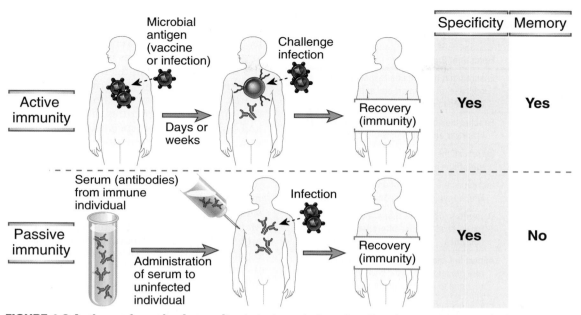

FIGURE 1-3 Active and passive immunity. Active immunity is conferred by a host response to a microbe or microbial antigen, whereas passive immunity is conferred by adoptive transfer of antibodies or T lymphocytes specific for the microbe. Both forms of immunity provide resistance to infection and are specific for microbial antigens, but only active immune responses generate immunologic memory. Therapeutic passive transfer of antibodies, but not lymphocytes, is done routinely and also occurs during pregnancy (from mother to fetus).

otherwise lethal diphtheria infection by the administration of antitoxin, an achievement that was recognized by the award of the first Nobel Prize in Physiology or Medicine to von Behring. In the 1890s, Paul Ehrlich postulated that immune cells use receptors, which he called side chains, to recognize microbial toxins and, subsequently, secrete these receptors to combat microbes. He also coined the term *antibodies* (*antikörper* in German) for the serum proteins that bound toxins, and substances that generated antibodies were called *antigens*. The modern definition of antigens includes substances that bind to specific lymphocyte receptors, whether or not they stimulate immune responses. According to strict definitions, substances that stimulate immune responses are called **immunogens**, but the term antigen is often used interchangeably with immunogen. The properties of antibodies and antigens are described in Chapter 5. Ehrlich's concepts are a remarkably prescient model for the function of B cells in humoral immunity. This early emphasis on antibodies led to the general acceptance of the humoral theory of immunity, according to which host defense against infections is mediated by substances present in body fluids (once called humors).

Elie Metchnikoff initially championed the cellular theory of immunity, which stated that host cells are the principal mediators of immunity. His demonstration of phagocytes surrounding a thorn stuck into a translucent starfish larva, published in 1883, was perhaps the first experimental evidence that cells respond to foreign invaders. Ehrlich and Metchnikoff shared the Nobel Prize in 1908, in recognition of their contributions to establishing these fundamental principles of immunity. Sir Almroth Wright's observation in the early 1900s that factors in immune serum enhanced the phagocytosis of bacteria by coating the bacteria, a process known as **opsonization**, lent support to the belief that antibodies prepare

microbes for ingestion by phagocytes. These early cellularists were unable to prove that specific immunity to microbes could be mediated by cells. The cellular theory of immunity became firmly established in the 1950s, when it was shown that resistance to an intracellular bacterium, *Listeria monocytogenes,* could be transferred to animals with cells but not with serum. We now know that the specificity of cell-mediated immunity is due to lymphocytes, which often function in concert with other cells, such as phagocytes, to eliminate microbes.

In the clinical setting, immunity to a previously encountered microbe is measured indirectly, either by assaying for the presence of products of immune responses (such as serum antibodies specific for microbial antigens) or by administering substances purified from the microbe and measuring reactions to these substances. A reaction to an antigen is detectable only in individuals who have previously encountered the antigen; these individuals are said to be *sensitized* to the antigen, and the reaction is an indication of *sensitivity*. Such a reaction to a microbial antigen implies that the sensitized individual is capable of mounting a protective immune response to the microbe.

CARDINAL FEATURES OF ADAPTIVE IMMUNE RESPONSES

All humoral and cell-mediated immune responses to foreign antigens have a number of fundamental properties that reflect the properties of the lymphocytes that mediate these responses (Table 1-3).

- *Specificity and diversity.* Immune responses are specific for distinct antigens and, in fact, for different portions of a single complex protein, polysaccharide,

TABLE 1-3   Cardinal Features of Adaptive Immune Responses

Feature	Functional Significance
Specificity	Ensures that the immune response to a microbe (or nonmicrobial antigen) is targeted to that microbe (or antigen)
Diversity	Enables the immune system to respond to a large variety of antigens
Memory	Increases the ability to combat repeat infections by the same microbe
Clonal expansion	Increases the number of antigen-specific lymphocytes to keep pace with microbes
Specialization	Generates responses that are optimal for defense against different types of microbes
Contraction and homeostasis	Allows the immune system to recover from one response so that it can effectively respond to newly encountered antigens
Nonreactivity to self	Prevents injury to the host during responses to foreign antigens

or other macromolecule (Fig. 1-4). The parts of such antigens that are specifically recognized by individual lymphocytes are called **determinants** or **epitopes.** This fine specificity exists because individual lymphocytes express membrane receptors that can distinguish subtle differences in structure between distinct epitopes. Clones of lymphocytes with different specificities are present in unimmunized individuals and are able to recognize and respond to foreign antigens. This concept is the basic tenet of the clonal selection hypothesis, which is discussed in more detail later in this chapter.

The total number of antigenic specificities of the lymphocytes in an individual, called the lymphocyte repertoire, is extremely large. It is estimated that the immune system of an individual can discriminate 10^7 to 10^9 distinct antigenic determinants. This ability of the lymphocyte repertoire to recognize a very large number of antigens is the result of variability in the structures of the antigen-binding sites of lymphocyte receptors for antigens, called **diversity**. In other words, there are many different clones of lymphocytes that differ in the structures of their antigen receptors and therefore in their specificity for antigens, contributing to a total repertoire that is extremely diverse. The expression of different antigen receptors in different clones of T and B cells is the reason that these receptors are said to be clonally distributed. The molecular mechanisms that generate such diverse antigen receptors are discussed in Chapter 8.

- *Memory.* Exposure of the immune system to a foreign antigen enhances its ability to respond again to that antigen. Responses to second and subsequent exposures to the same antigen, called secondary immune responses, are usually more rapid, larger, and often qualitatively different from the first, or primary, immune response to that antigen (see Fig. 1-4). Immunologic memory occurs because each exposure to an antigen generates long-lived memory cells specific for the antigen, which are more numerous than the naive lymphocytes specific for the antigen that exist before antigen exposure. In addition, memory cells have special characteristics that make them more efficient at responding to and eliminating the antigen than are naive lymphocytes that have not previously been exposed to the antigen. For instance, memory B lymphocytes produce antibodies that bind antigens with higher affinities than do antibodies produced in primary immune responses, and memory T cells react much more rapidly and vigorously to antigen challenge than do naive T cells.

- *Clonal expansion.* Lymphocytes specific for an antigen undergo considerable proliferation after exposure to that antigen. The term *clonal expansion* refers to an

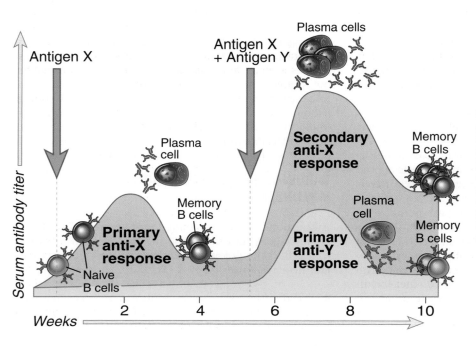

FIGURE 1-4 Specificity, memory, and contraction of adaptive immune responses. Antigens X and Y induce the production of different antibodies (specificity). The secondary response to antigen X is more rapid and larger than the primary response (memory). Antibody levels decline with time after each immunization (contraction, the process that maintains homeostasis). The same features are seen in cell-mediated immune responses.

increase in the number of cells that express identical receptors for the antigen and thus belong to a clone. This increase in antigen-specific cells enables the adaptive immune response to keep pace with rapidly dividing infectious pathogens.

- *Specialization.* As we have already noted, the immune system responds in distinct and special ways to different microbes, maximizing the effectiveness of antimicrobial defense mechanisms. Thus, humoral immunity and cell-mediated immunity are elicited by different classes of microbes or by the same microbe at different stages of infection (extracellular and intracellular), and each type of immune response protects the host against that class of microbe. Even within humoral or cell-mediated immune responses, the nature of the antibodies or T lymphocytes that are generated may vary from one class of microbe to another. We will return to the mechanisms and functional significance of such specialization in later chapters.

- *Contraction and homeostasis.* All normal immune responses wane with time after antigen stimulation, thus returning the immune system to its resting basal state, a state called **homeostasis** (see Fig. 1-4). This contraction of immune responses occurs largely because responses that are triggered by antigens function to eliminate the antigens, thus eliminating an essential stimulus for lymphocyte survival and activation. Lymphocytes (other than memory cells) that are deprived of these stimuli die by apoptosis.

- *Nonreactivity to self.* One of the most remarkable properties of every normal individual's immune system is its ability to recognize, respond to, and eliminate many foreign (non-self) antigens while not reacting harmfully to that individual's own (self) antigenic substances. Immunologic unresponsiveness is also called **tolerance.** Tolerance to self antigens, or self-tolerance, is maintained by several mechanisms. These include eliminating lymphocytes that express receptors specific for some self antigens, inactivating self-reactive lymphocytes, or suppressing these cells by the actions of other (regulatory) cells. Abnormalities in the induction or maintenance of self-tolerance lead to immune responses against self (autologous) antigens, which may result in disorders called **autoimmune diseases.** The mechanisms of self-tolerance and its failure are discussed in Chapter 15.

These features of adaptive immunity are necessary if the immune system is to perform its normal function of host defense (see Table 1-3). Specificity and memory enable the immune system to mount heightened responses to persistent or recurring exposure to the same antigen and thus to combat infections that are prolonged or occur repeatedly. Diversity is essential if the immune system is to defend individuals against the many potential pathogens in the environment. Specialization enables the host to "custom design" responses to best combat different types of microbes. Contraction of the response allows the system to return to a state of rest after it eliminates each foreign antigen and to be prepared to respond to other antigens. Self-tolerance is vital for preventing harmful reactions against one's own cells and tissues while maintaining a diverse repertoire of lymphocytes specific for foreign antigens.

Immune responses are regulated by a system of positive feedback loops that amplify the reaction and by control mechanisms that prevent inappropriate or pathologic reactions. When lymphocytes are activated, they trigger mechanisms that further increase the magnitude of the response. This positive feedback is important to enable the small number of lymphocytes that are specific for any microbe to generate the response needed to eradicate that infection. Many control mechanisms become active in immune responses to prevent excessive activation of lymphocytes, which may cause collateral damage to normal tissues, and to avoid responses against self antigens. In fact, a balance between activating and inhibitory signals is characteristic of all immune responses. We will mention specific examples of these fundamental features of the immune system throughout this book.

CELLULAR COMPONENTS OF THE ADAPTIVE IMMUNE SYSTEM

The principal cells of the adaptive immune system are lymphocytes, antigen-presenting cells, and effector cells. Lymphocytes are the cells that specifically recognize and respond to foreign antigens and are therefore the mediators of humoral and cellular immunity. There are distinct subpopulations of lymphocytes that differ in how they recognize antigens and in their functions (Fig. 1-5). **B lymphocytes** are the only cells capable of producing antibodies. They recognize extracellular soluble and cell surface antigens, and they differentiate into antibody-secreting plasma cells, thus functioning as the mediators of humoral immunity. **T lymphocytes**, the cells of cell-mediated immunity, recognize the antigens of intracellular microbes and the T cells either help phagocytes to destroy these microbes or they kill the infected cells. T cells do not produce antibody molecules. Their antigen receptors are membrane molecules distinct from but structurally related to antibodies (see Chapter 7). T lymphocytes have a restricted specificity for antigens; they recognize peptides derived from foreign proteins that are bound to host proteins called **major histocompatibility complex** (MHC) molecules, which are expressed on the surfaces of other cells. As a result, these T cells recognize and respond to cell surface–associated but not soluble antigens (see Chapter 6).

T lymphocytes consist of functionally distinct populations, the best defined of which are **helper T cells** and **cytotoxic** (or **cytolytic**) **T lymphocytes** (CTLs). In response to antigenic stimulation, helper T cells secrete cytokines, which are responsible for many of the cellular responses of innate and adaptive immunity and thus function as the "messenger molecules" of the immune system. The cytokines secreted by helper T lymphocytes stimulate the proliferation and differentiation of the T cells themselves and activate other cells, including B cells, macrophages, and other leukocytes. CTLs kill cells that produce foreign antigens, such as cells infected by viruses and other intracellular microbes. Some T lymphocytes, which are called **regulatory T cells**, function mainly to inhibit immune responses. A small population of T lymphocytes that express some cell surface proteins found on NK cells are called **NKT cells;** their specificities and role

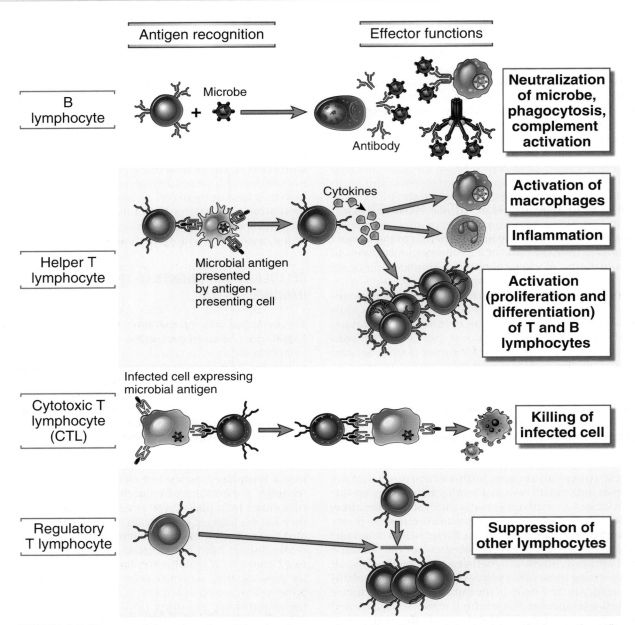

FIGURE 1-5 Classes of lymphocytes. B lymphocytes recognize soluble antigens and develop into antibody-secreting cells. Helper T lymphocytes recognize antigens on the surfaces of antigen-presenting cells and secrete cytokines, which stimulate different mechanisms of immunity and inflammation. Cytotoxic T lymphocytes recognize antigens on infected cells and kill these cells. Regulatory T cells suppress and prevent immune responses (e.g., to self antigens).

in host defense are not well understood. We will return to a more detailed discussion of the properties of lymphocytes in Chapter 2 and in later chapters. Different classes of lymphocytes can be distinguished by the expression of surface proteins that are named CD molecules and numbered (see Chapter 2).

The initiation and development of adaptive immune responses require that antigens be captured and displayed to specific lymphocytes. The cells that serve this role are called **antigen-presenting cells** (APCs). The most specialized APCs are **dendritic cells**, which capture microbial antigens that enter from the external environment, transport these antigens to lymphoid organs, and present the antigens to naive T lymphocytes to initiate immune

responses. Other cell types function as APCs at different stages of cell-mediated and humoral immune responses. We will describe the functions of APCs in Chapter 6.

The activation of lymphocytes by antigen leads to the generation of numerous mechanisms that function to eliminate the antigen. Antigen elimination often requires the participation of cells that are called **effector cells** because they mediate the final effect of the immune response, which is to get rid of the microbes. Activated T lymphocytes, mononuclear phagocytes, and other leukocytes function as effector cells in different immune responses.

Lymphocytes and APCs are concentrated in anatomically discrete lymphoid organs, where they interact with one another to initiate immune responses. Lymphocytes are also present in the blood; from the blood, they can recirculate through lymphoid tissues and home to peripheral tissue sites of antigen exposure to eliminate the antigen (see Chapter 3).

The cells of the immune system interact with one another and with other host cells during the initiation and effector stages of innate and adaptive immune responses. Many of these interactions are mediated by cytokines. We will describe the functions of individual cytokines when we discuss immune responses in which these proteins play important roles.

OVERVIEW OF IMMUNE RESPONSES TO MICROBES

Now that we have introduced the major components of the immune system and their properties, it is useful to summarize the principles of immune responses to different types of microbes. Such a summary will be a foundation for the topics that are discussed throughout this book. The immune system has to combat many diverse microbes. As we will see shortly, immune responses to all infectious pathogens share some common features, and responses to different classes of these microbes may also have unique features. How these adaptive immune reactions are initiated, orchestrated, and controlled are the fundamental questions of immunology. We start with a discussion of the innate immune response.

The Early Innate Immune Response to Microbes

The innate immune system blocks the entry of microbes and eliminates or limits the growth of many microbes that are able to colonize tissues. The main sites of interaction between individuals and their environment—the skin, lungs, and gastrointestinal and respiratory tracts—are lined by continuous epithelia, which serve as barriers to prevent the entry of microbes from the external environment. If microbes successfully breach the epithelial barriers, they encounter other cells of innate immunity. The cellular innate immune response to microbes consists of two main types of reactions—inflammation and antiviral defense. **Inflammation** is the process of recruitment of leukocytes and plasma proteins from the blood, their accumulation in tissues, and their activation to destroy the microbes. Many of these reactions involve cytokines that are produced by dendritic cells, macrophages, and other types of cells during innate immune reactions. The major leukocytes that are recruited in inflammation are the phagocytes, neutrophils (which have short life spans in tissues) and monocytes (which develop into tissue macrophages). Phagocytes ingest microbes and dead cells and destroy these in intracellular vesicles. **Antiviral defense** consists of a cytokine-mediated reaction in which cells acquire resistance to viral infection and killing of virus-infected cells by specialized cells of the innate immune system, natural killer (NK) cells.

Microbes that are able to withstand these defense reactions in the tissues may enter the blood, where they are recognized by the circulating proteins of innate immunity. Among the most important plasma proteins of innate immunity are components of the complement system. When complement proteins are activated by microbial surfaces, proteolytic cleavage products are generated that mediate inflammatory responses, coat (opsonize) the microbes for enhanced phagocytosis, and directly lyse microbes. Other plasma proteins enter sites of infection during inflammatory reactions and help combat microbes in extravascular tissues.

The reactions of innate immunity are effective at controlling and even eradicating infections. However, as mentioned earlier, many pathogenic microbes have evolved to resist innate immunity. Defense against these pathogens requires the more powerful and specialized mechanisms of adaptive immunity.

The Adaptive Immune Response

The adaptive immune system uses three main strategies to combat most microbes.

- *Antibodies.* Secreted antibodies bind to extracellular microbes, block their ability to infect host cells, and promote their ingestion and subsequent destruction by phagocytes.
- *Phagocytosis.* Phagocytes ingest microbes and kill them, and antibodies and helper T cells enhance the microbicidal abilities of the phagocytes.
- *Cell killing.* Cytotoxic T lymphocytes (CTLs) destroy cells infected by microbes that are inaccessible to antibodies and phagocytic destruction.

The goal of the adaptive response is to activate one or more of these defense mechanisms against diverse microbes that may be in different anatomic locations, such as the intestines or airways, the circulation, or inside cells.

All adaptive immune responses develop in sequential steps, each of which corresponds to particular reactions of lymphocytes (Fig. 1-6). We start this overview of adaptive immunity with the first step, which is the recognition of antigens.

The Capture and Display of Microbial Antigens

Because the number of naive lymphocytes specific for any antigen is very small (on the order of 1 in 10^5 or 10^6 lymphocytes) and the quantity of the available antigen may also be small, special mechanisms are needed to capture microbes, to concentrate their antigens in the correct location, and to deliver the antigens to specific lymphocytes. Dendritic cells located in epithelia and connective tissues capture microbes, digest their proteins into fragments, and express on their surface microbial peptides bound to MHC molecules, which are the specialized peptide display molecules of the adaptive immune system. Dendritic cells carry their antigenic cargo to draining lymph nodes through which naive T lymphocytes continuously recirculate. Thus, the chance of a T cell with receptors for a particular antigen finding that antigen is greatly increased by concentrating many antigens and T cells in the same anatomic location. Dendritic cells also display microbial peptides in the spleen.

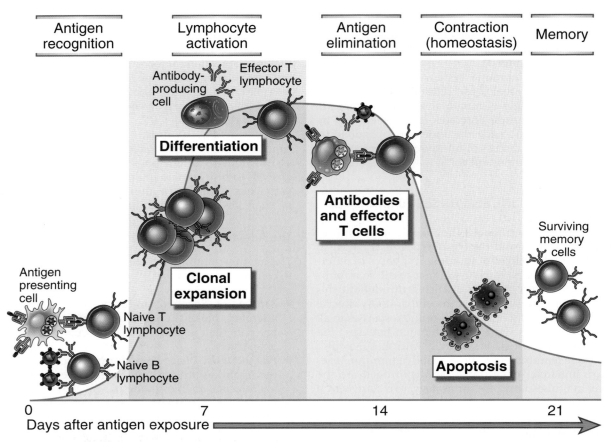

FIGURE 1-6 Phases of adaptive immune responses. Adaptive immune responses consist of distinct phases, the first three being the recognition of antigen, the activation of lymphocytes, and the elimination of antigen (the effector phase). The response contracts (declines) as antigen-stimulated lymphocytes die by apoptosis, restoring homeostasis, and the antigen-specific cells that survive are responsible for memory. The duration of each phase may vary in different immune responses. The y-axis represents an arbitrary measure of the magnitude of the response. These principles apply to humoral immunity (mediated by B lymphocytes) and cell-mediated immunity (mediated by T lymphocytes).

Intact microbes or microbial antigens that enter lymph nodes and spleen are recognized in unprocessed (native) form by specific B lymphocytes. Antigens may also be displayed to B lymphocytes by certain APCs in lymphoid organs.

Antigen Recognition by Lymphocytes

Lymphocytes specific for a large number of antigens exist before exposure to the antigen, and when an antigen enters a secondary lymphoid organ, it binds to (selects) the antigen-specific cells and activates them (Fig. 1-7). This fundamental concept is called the **clonal selection hypothesis**. It was suggested by Niels Jerne in 1955, and most clearly enunciated by Macfarlane Burnet in 1957, as a hypothesis to explain how the immune system could respond to a large number and variety of antigens. According to this hypothesis, antigen-specific clones of lymphocytes develop before and independent of exposure to antigen. A *clone* refers to a lymphocyte of one specificity and its progeny. A characteristic of the immune system is that a very large number of clones is generated during the maturation of lymphocytes, thus maximizing the potential for recognizing diverse microbes.

The activation of naive T lymphocytes requires recognition of peptide-MHC complexes presented on dendritic cells. Because T cell receptors are specific for MHC-associated peptides, these lymphocytes can interact only with cell-associated antigens (because MHC molecules are cell surface proteins) and not with free antigen. This feature is necessary because all the functions of T lymphocytes are dependent on their physical interactions with other cells. To respond, the T cells need to recognize not only antigens but also other molecules, called **costimulators**, which are induced on the APCs by microbes. Antigen recognition provides specificity to the immune response, and the need for costimulation ensures that T cells respond to microbes (the inducers of costimulatory molecules) and not to harmless substances.

B lymphocytes use their antigen receptors (membrane-bound antibody molecules) to recognize antigens of many different chemical types.

Engagement of antigen receptors and other signals trigger lymphocyte proliferation and differentiation. The reactions and functions of T and B lymphocytes differ in important ways and are best considered separately.

Cell-Mediated Immunity: Activation of T Lymphocytes and Elimination of Intracellular Microbes

Activated CD4⁺ helper T lymphocytes proliferate and differentiate into effector cells whose functions are

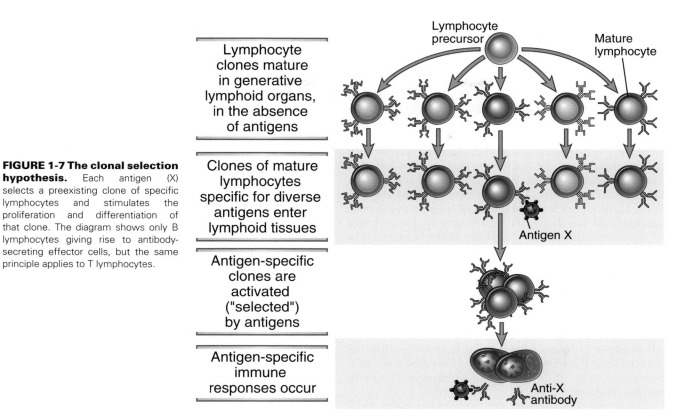

Lymphocyte clones mature in generative lymphoid organs, in the absence of antigens

Clones of mature lymphocytes specific for diverse antigens enter lymphoid tissues

Antigen-specific clones are activated ("selected") by antigens

Antigen-specific immune responses occur

Lymphocyte precursor

Mature lymphocyte

Antigen X

Anti-X antibody

FIGURE 1-7 The clonal selection hypothesis. Each antigen (X) selects a preexisting clone of specific lymphocytes and stimulates the proliferation and differentiation of that clone. The diagram shows only B lymphocytes giving rise to antibody-secreting effector cells, but the same principle applies to T lymphocytes.

mediated largely by secreted cytokines. When naive CD4+ T cells are activated by antigen, they secrete the cytokine interleukin-2 (IL-2), which is a growth factor that stimulates the proliferation (clonal expansion) of the antigen-specific T cells. Some of the progeny of these activated lymphocytes differentiate into effector cells that can secrete different sets of cytokines and thus perform different functions. Many of the effector cells leave the lymphoid organs where they were generated and migrate to sites of infection and accompanying inflammation. When these differentiated effector T cells again encounter cell-associated microbes, they are activated to perform the functions that are responsible for elimination of the microbes. Some CD4+ helper T cells secrete cytokines that recruit leukocytes and stimulate production of microbicidal substances in phagocytes. Thus, these T cells help phagocytes to kill the infectious pathogens. Other CD4+ helper T cells secrete cytokines that help B cells produce a type of antibody called immunoglobulin E (IgE) and activate leukocytes called eosinophils, which are able to kill parasites that may be too large to be phagocytosed. As we discuss later, some CD4+ helper T cells stay in the lymphoid organs and stimulate B cell responses.

Activated CD8+ lymphocytes proliferate and differentiate into CTLs that kill cells harboring microbes in the cytoplasm. These microbes may be viruses that infect many cell types or bacteria that are ingested by macrophages but escape from phagocytic vesicles into the cytoplasm (where they are inaccessible to the killing machinery of phagocytes, which is largely confined to vesicles). By destroying the infected cells, CTLs eliminate the reservoirs of infection.

Humoral Immunity: Activation of B Lymphocytes and Elimination of Extracellular Microbes

On activation by antigen, B lymphocytes proliferate and differentiate into cells that secrete different classes of antibodies with distinct functions. The response of B cells to protein antigens requires activating signals (help) from CD4+ T cells (which is the historical reason for calling these T cells *helper* cells). B cells can respond to many nonprotein antigens without the participation of helper T cells.

Some of the progeny of the expanded B cell clones differentiate into antibody-secreting **plasma cells**. Each plasma cell secretes antibodies that have the same antigen-binding site as the cell surface antibodies (B cell receptors) that first recognized the antigen. Polysaccharides and lipids stimulate secretion mainly of the antibody class called IgM. Protein antigens induce the production of antibodies of functionally different classes (IgG, IgA, IgE) from a single clone of B cells. The production of these classes of antibodies with different functions is called class switching. The process requires the action of helper T cells. It provides plasticity in the antibody response, enabling it to serve many functions. Helper T cells also stimulate the production of antibodies with increased affinity for the antigen. This process, called affinity maturation, improves the quality of the humoral immune response.

The humoral immune response combats microbes in many ways. Antibodies bind to microbes and prevent them from infecting cells, thus neutralizing the microbes. In fact, antibodies are the only mechanisms of adaptive immunity that prevent an infection from becoming established; this is why eliciting the production of potent antibodies is a key goal of vaccination. IgG antibodies coat microbes and target them for phagocytosis because phagocytes (neutrophils and macrophages) express receptors for parts of IgG molecules. IgG and IgM activate the complement system, and complement products promote phagocytosis and destruction of microbes. Some antibodies serve special roles at particular anatomic sites. IgA is secreted from mucosal epithelia and neutralizes microbes in the lumens of mucosal tissues, such as the respiratory and gastrointestinal tracts. Maternal IgG is actively transported across the placenta and protects the newborn until the baby's immune system becomes mature. Most antibodies have half-lives of a few days, but most IgG antibodies have half-lives of about 3 weeks. Some antibody-secreting plasma cells migrate to the bone marrow and live for years, continuing to produce low levels of antibodies. The antibodies that are secreted by these long-lived plasma cells provide immediate protection if the microbe returns to infect the individual. More effective protection is provided by memory cells that are activated by the microbe and rapidly differentiate to generate large numbers of plasma cells.

Immunologic Memory

An effective immune response eliminates the microbes that initiated the response. This is followed by a contraction phase, in which the expanded lymphocyte clones die and homeostasis is restored.

The initial activation of lymphocytes generates long-lived **memory cells**, which may survive for years after the infection. Memory cells are more effective in combating microbes than are naive lymphocytes because, as mentioned earlier, memory cells represent an expanded pool of antigen-specific lymphocytes (more numerous than naive cells specific for the antigen) and respond faster and more effectively against the antigen than do naive cells. This is why generating memory responses is another important goal of vaccination. We will discuss the properties of memory lymphocytes in later chapters.

In the remainder of the book, we describe in detail the recognition, activation, regulation, and effector phases of innate and adaptive immune responses. The principles introduced in this chapter recur throughout this book.

SUMMARY

* Protective immunity against microbes is mediated by the early reactions of innate immunity and the later responses of adaptive immunity. Innate immune responses are stimulated by molecular structures shared by groups of microbes and by molecules expressed by damaged host cells. Adaptive immunity is specific for different microbial and nonmicrobial antigens and is increased by repeated exposures to antigen (immunologic memory).

* Humoral immunity is mediated by B lymphocytes and their secreted products, such as antibodies, and is the mechanism of defense against extracellular microbes. Cell-mediated immunity is mediated by T lymphocytes and their products, such as cytokines, and is important for defense against intracellular microbes.

* Immunity may be acquired by a response to antigen (active immunity) or conferred by transfer of antibodies or effector cells (passive immunity).

* Many features of the immune system are of fundamental importance for its normal functions. These include specificity for different antigens, a diverse repertoire capable of recognizing a wide variety of antigens, memory of antigen exposure, the capacity for rapid expansion of clones of antigen-specific lymphocytes in response to the antigen, specialized responses to different microbes, maintenance of homeostasis, and the ability to discriminate between foreign antigens and self antigens.

* Lymphocytes are the only cells capable of specifically recognizing antigens and are thus the principal cells of adaptive immunity. The total population of lymphocytes consists of many clones, each with a unique antigen receptor and specificity. The two major subsets of lymphocytes are B cells and T cells, and they differ in their antigen receptors and functions. Specialized antigen-presenting cells capture microbial antigens and display these antigens for recognition by lymphocytes. The elimination of antigens often requires the participation of various effector cells.

* The adaptive immune response is initiated by the recognition of foreign antigens by specific lymphocytes. Lymphocytes respond by proliferating and by differentiating into effector cells, whose function is to eliminate the antigen, and into memory cells, which show enhanced responses on subsequent encounters with the antigen. The activation of lymphocytes requires antigen and additional signals that may be provided by microbes or by innate immune responses to microbes.

* CD4+ helper T lymphocytes help macrophages to eliminate ingested microbes and help B cells to produce antibodies. CD8+ CTLs kill cells harboring intracellular pathogens, thus eliminating reservoirs of infection.

* Antibodies, the products of B lymphocytes, neutralize the infectivity of microbes and promote the elimination of microbes by phagocytes and by activation of the complement system.

SELECTED READINGS

Burnet FM: A modification of Jerne's theory of antibody production using the concept of clonal selection, *Australian Journal of Science* 20:67–69, 1957.

Jerne NK: The natural-selection theory of antibody formation, *Proceedings of the National Academy of Sciences USA* 41: 849–857, 1955.

Litman GW, Rast JP, Fugmann SD: The origins of vertebrate adaptive immunity, *Nature Reviews Immunology* 10:543–553, 2010.

Silverstein AM: *Paul Erlich's receptor immunology: the magnificent obsession*, New York, 2001, Academic Press.

Silverstein AM: Cellular versus humoral immunology: a century-long dispute, *Nature Immunology* 4:425–428, 2003.

Travis J: On the origins of the immune system, *Science* 324: 580–582, 2009.

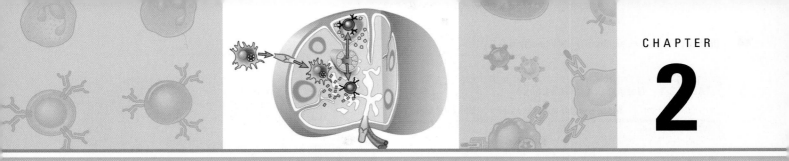

Cells and Tissues of the Immune System

The cells of the innate and adaptive immune system are normally present as circulating cells in the blood and lymph, as anatomically defined collections in lymphoid organs, and as scattered cells in virtually all tissues. The anatomic organization of these cells and their ability to circulate and exchange among blood, lymph, and tissues are of critical importance for the generation of immune responses. The immune system faces numerous challenges to generate effective protective responses against infectious pathogens. First, the system must be able to respond rapidly to small numbers of many different microbes that may be introduced at any site in the body. Second, in the adaptive immune response, very few naive lymphocytes specifically recognize and respond to any one antigen. Third, the effector mechanisms of the adaptive immune system (antibodies and effector T cells) may have to locate and destroy microbes at sites that are distant from the site where the immune response was induced. The ability of the immune system to meet these challenges and to optimally perform its protective functions is dependent on the remarkably rapid and varied responses of immune cells and the way these cells are

organized in lymphoid tissues yet are capable of migrating from one tissue to another.

This chapter describes the cells and tissues that compose the immune system. In Chapter 3, we describe the traffic patterns of lymphocytes throughout the body and the mechanisms of migration of lymphocytes and other leukocytes.

CELLS OF THE IMMUNE SYSTEM

The cells that serve specialized roles in innate and adaptive immune responses are phagocytes, dendritic cells, antigen-specific lymphocytes, and various other leukocytes that function to eliminate antigens. These cells were introduced briefly in Chapter 1. Here we describe the morphology and functional characteristics of the cells of the immune system and how they are organized in lymphoid tissues. The numbers of some of these cell types in the blood are listed in Table 2-1. Although most of these cells are found in the blood, their responses to microbes usually occur in lymphoid and other tissues and therefore may not be reflected by changes in their numbers in the circulation.

Phagocytes

Phagocytes, including neutrophils and macrophages, are cells whose primary function is to ingest and destroy microbes and get rid of damaged tissues. The functional responses of phagocytes in host defense consist of sequential steps: recruitment of the cells to the sites of infection, recognition of and activation by microbes, ingestion of the microbes by the process of phagocytosis, and destruction of ingested microbes. In addition, through direct contact and by secreting cytokines, phagocytes communicate with other cells in ways that promote or regulate immune responses. These functions of phagocytes are important in innate immunity, as we will discuss in Chapter 4, and also in the effector phase of some adaptive immune responses, as we will discuss in Chapter 10. As a prelude to more detailed discussions of the role of phagocytes in immune responses in later chapters, we will now describe the morphologic features

TABLE 2-1	Normal Blood Cell Counts	
	Mean Number per Microliter	Normal Range
White blood cells (leukocytes)	7400	4500–11,000
Neutrophils	4400	1800–7700
Eosinophils	200	0–450
Basophils	40	0–200
Lymphocytes	2500	1000–4800
Monocytes	300	0–800

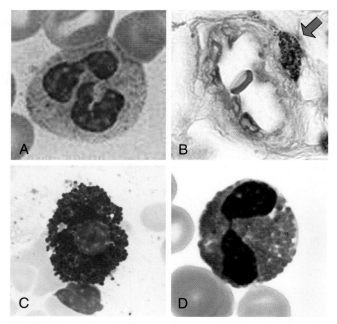

FIGURE 2-1 Morphology of neutrophils, mast cells, basophils, and eosinophils. A, The light micrograph of a Wright-Giemsa–stained blood neutrophil shows the multilobed nucleus, because of which these cells are also called polymorphonuclear leukocytes, and the faint cytoplasmic granules. **B,** The light micrograph of a Wright-Giemsa–stained section of skin shows a mast cell *(arrow)* adjacent to a small blood vessel, identifiable by the red blood cell in the lumen. The cytoplasmic granules in the mast cell, which are stained purple, are filled with histamine and other mediators that act on adjacent blood vessels to promote increased blood flow and delivery of plasma proteins and leukocytes into the tissue. *(Courtesy of Dr. George Murphy, Department of Pathology, Brigham and Women's Hospital, Boston, Massachusetts.)* **C,** The light micrograph of a Wright-Giemsa–stained blood basophil shows the characteristic blue-staining cytoplasmic granules. *(Courtesy of Dr. Jonathan Hecht, Department of Pathology, Brigham and Women's Hospital, Boston, Massachusetts.)* **D,** The light micrograph of a Wright-Giemsa–stained blood eosinophil shows the characteristic segmented nucleus and red staining of the cytoplasmic granules.

of neutrophils and macrophages and briefly introduce their functional responses.

Neutrophils

Neutrophils, also called polymorphonuclear leukocytes, are the most abundant population of circulating white blood cells and mediate the earliest phases of inflammatory reactions. Neutrophils circulate as spherical cells about 12 to 15 μm in diameter with numerous membranous projections. The nucleus of a neutrophil is segmented into three to five connected lobules, hence the synonym *polymorphonuclear leukocyte* (Fig. 2-1, *A*). The cytoplasm contains granules of two types. The majority, called specific granules, are filled with enzymes such as lysozyme, collagenase, and elastase. These granules do not stain strongly with either basic or acidic dyes (hematoxylin and eosin, respectively), which distinguishes neutrophil granules from those of two other types of circulating granulocytes, called **basophils** and **eosinophils**. The remainder of the granules of neutrophils, called azurophilic granules, are lysosomes that contain enzymes and other microbicidal substances, including defensins and cathelicidins, which we will discuss in Chapter 4. Neutrophils are produced in the bone marrow and arise from precursors that also give rise to mononuclear phagocytes. Production of neutrophils is stimulated by granulocyte colony-stimulating factor (G-CSF). An adult human produces more than 1×10^{11} neutrophils per day, each of which circulates in the blood for hours or a few days. Neutrophils may migrate to sites of infection rapidly after the entry of microbes. After entering tissues, neutrophils function only for 1 to 2 days and then die.

Mononuclear Phagocytes

The mononuclear phagocyte system includes circulating cells called monocytes and tissue resident cells called macrophages. Macrophages, which are widely distributed in organs and connective tissue, play central roles in innate and adaptive immunity. Many tissues are populated with long-lived resident macrophages derived from yolk sac or fetal liver precursors during fetal development, and they assume specialized phenotypes depending on the organ (Fig. 2-2). Examples are Kupffer cells lining the sinusoids in the liver, sinusoidal macrophages in the spleen, alveolar macrophages in the lung, and microglial cells in the brain. In adults, cells of the macrophage lineage arise from committed precursor cells in the bone marrow, driven by a protein called monocyte (or macrophage) colony-stimulating

factor (M-CSF). These precursors mature into monocytes, which enter and circulate in the blood (see Fig. 2-2), and then migrate into tissues, especially during inflammatory reactions, where they further mature into macrophages.

Monocytes are 10 to 15 μm in diameter, and they have bean-shaped nuclei and finely granular cytoplasm containing lysosomes, phagocytic vacuoles, and cytoskeletal filaments (Fig. 2-3). Monocytes are heterogeneous and consist of different subsets distinguishable by cell surface markers and functions. In both humans and mice, the most numerous monocytes, sometimes called classical monocytes, produce abundant inflammatory mediators and are rapidly recruited to sites of infection or tissue injury. In humans, these monocytes are identifiable by high cell surface expression of CD14 and lack of expression of CD16 (CD14++CD16−), and in mice the equivalent subset is identifiable as Ly6high. Non-classical monocytes, which make up a minority of blood monocytes, are CD14+CD16++ in humans and Ly6clow in mice. These cells contribute to tissue repair after injury, and are known to crawl along endothelial surfaces (described as *patrolling*). An intermediate human subset has also been described (CD14++CD16+).

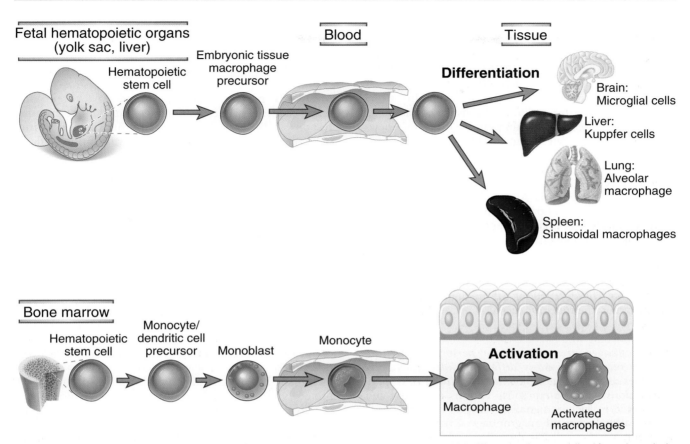

FIGURE 2-2 Maturation of mononuclear phagocytes. Tissue resident macrophages, which differentiate into specialized forms in particular organs, are derived from precursors in the yolk sac and fetal liver during fetal life. Monocytes arise from a precursor cell of the myeloid lineage in the bone marrow, circulate in the blood, and are recruited into tissues in inflammatory reactions, where they further mature into macrophages. Subsets of blood monocytes exist, which have distinct inflammatory or reparative functions (not shown).

Tissue macrophages perform several important functions in innate and adaptive immunity.

- A major function of macrophages in host defense is to ingest and kill microbes. The mechanisms of killing, which we will discuss in Chapter 4, include the enzymatic generation of reactive oxygen and nitrogen species that are toxic to microbes, and proteolytic digestion.

- In addition to ingesting microbes, macrophages also ingest dead host cells, including cells that die in tissues because of trauma or interrupted blood supply and neutrophils that accumulate at sites of infection. This is part of the cleaning up process after infection or sterile tissue injury. Macrophages also recognize and engulf apoptotic cells before the dead cells can release their contents and induce inflammatory responses.

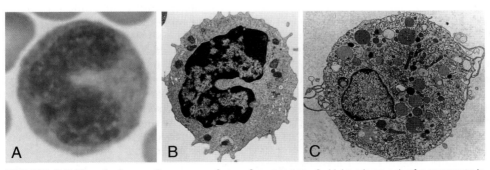

FIGURE 2-3 Morphology of mononuclear phagocytes. A, Light micrograph of a monocyte in a peripheral blood smear. **B,** Electron micrograph of a peripheral blood monocyte. *(Courtesy of Dr. Noel Weidner, Department of Pathology, University of California, San Diego.)* **C,** Electron micrograph of an activated tissue macrophage showing numerous phagocytic vacuoles and cytoplasmic organelles. *(From Fawcett DW: Bloom and Fawcett: a textbook of histology, 12th ed, New York, 1994, Chapman & Hall. With kind permission of Springer Science and Business Media.)*

Throughout the body and throughout the life of an individual, unwanted cells die by apoptosis as part of many physiologic processes, such as development, growth, and renewal of healthy tissues, and the dead cells are eliminated by macrophages.

- Activated macrophages secrete several different cytokines that act on endothelial cells lining blood vessels to enhance the recruitment of more monocytes and other leukocytes from the blood into sites of infections, thereby amplifying the protective response against the microbes. Some important macrophage-derived cytokines are discussed in Chapter 4.
- Macrophages serve as APCs that display antigens to and activate T lymphocytes. This function is important in the effector phase of T cell–mediated immune responses (see Chapter 10).
- Macrophages promote the repair of damaged tissues by stimulating new blood vessel growth (angiogenesis) and synthesis of collagen-rich extracellular matrix (fibrosis). These functions are mediated by cytokines secreted by the macrophages that act on various tissue cells.

Macrophages are activated to perform their functions by recognizing many different kinds of microbial molecules as well as host molecules produced in response to infections and injury. These various activating molecules bind to specific signaling receptors located on the surface of or inside the macrophage. Examples of these receptors are the Toll-like receptors, which are of central importance in innate immunity and will be discussed in detail in Chapter 4. Macrophages are also activated when receptors on their plasma membrane bind opsonins on the surface of microbes. Opsonins are substances that coat particles for phagocytosis. Examples of opsonin receptors are complement receptors and antibody Fc receptors, discussed in Chapter 13. In adaptive immunity, macrophages are activated by secreted cytokines and by membrane proteins on T lymphocytes, which we will discuss in Chapter 10.

Macrophages can acquire distinct functional capabilities, depending on the types of activating stimuli they are exposed to. The clearest example of this is the response of macrophages to different cytokines made by subsets of T cells. Some of these cytokines activate macrophages to become efficient at killing microbes, called **classical activation.** Other cytokines activate macrophages to promote tissue remodeling and repair, called **alternative activation**. These different pathways of activation and the cytokines involved are discussed in Chapter 10. Macrophages may also assume different morphologic forms after activation by external stimuli, such as microbes. Some develop abundant cytoplasm and are called epithelioid cells because of their resemblance to epithelial cells of the skin. Activated macrophages can fuse to form multinucleated giant cells.

Macrophages typically respond to microbes nearly as rapidly as neutrophils do, but macrophages survive much longer at sites of inflammation. Unlike neutrophils, macrophages are not terminally differentiated and can undergo cell division at an inflammatory site. Therefore, macrophages are the dominant effector cells of the later stages in the innate immune response, several days after an infection begins.

Mast Cells, Basophils, and Eosinophils

Mast cells, basophils, and eosinophils are three additional cells that play roles in innate and adaptive immune responses. All three cell types share the common feature of having cytoplasmic granules filled with various inflammatory and antimicrobial mediators. Another common feature of these cells is their involvement in immune responses that protect against helminths and reactions that cause allergic diseases. We will introduce the features of these cells in this section and discuss their functions in more detail in Chapter 20.

Mast Cells

Mast cells are bone marrow–derived cells present in the skin and mucosal epithelia, which contain abundant cytoplasmic granules filled with histamine and other mediators. The cytokine stem cell factor (also called c-Kit ligand) is essential for mast cell development. Normally, mature mast cells are not found in the circulation but are present in tissues, usually adjacent to small blood vessels and nerves (Fig. 2-1, *B*). Their cytoplasm contains numerous membrane-bound granules, which are filled with acidic proteoglycans that bind basic dyes. Mast cells express high-affinity plasma membrane receptors for a type of antibody called IgE and are usually coated with these antibodies. When the antibodies on the mast cell surface bind antigen, signaling events are induced that lead to release of the cytoplasmic granule contents into the extracellular space. The released granule contents, including histamine, promote changes in the blood vessels that cause inflammation. Mast cells function as sentinels in tissues, where they recognize microbial products and respond by producing cytokines and other mediators that induce inflammation. These cells provide defense against helminths and other microbes, but are also responsible for symptoms of allergic diseases (see Chapter 20).

Basophils

Basophils are blood granulocytes with many structural and functional similarities to mast cells. Like other granulocytes, basophils are derived from bone marrow progenitors (a lineage different from that of mast cells), mature in the bone marrow, and circulate in the blood. Basophils constitute less than 1% of blood leukocytes (see Table 2-1). Although they are normally not present in tissues, basophils may be recruited to some inflammatory sites. Basophils contain granules that bind basic dyes (Fig. 2-1, *C*), and they are capable of synthesizing many of the same mediators as mast cells. Like mast cells, basophils express IgE receptors, bind IgE, and can be triggered by antigen binding to the IgE. Because basophil numbers are low in tissues, their importance in host defense and allergic reactions is uncertain.

Eosinophils

Eosinophils are blood granulocytes that express cytoplasmic granules containing enzymes that are harmful to the cell walls of parasites but can also damage host tissues. Eosinophil granules contain basic proteins that bind acidic dyes such as eosin (Fig. 2-1, *D*). Like neutrophils and basophils, eosinophils are bone marrow–derived. The cytokines GM-CSF, IL-3, and IL-5 promote eosinophil maturation from myeloid precursors. Some eosinophils are normally present in peripheral tissues, especially in mucosal linings of the respiratory, gastrointestinal, and genitourinary tracts, and their numbers can increase by recruitment from the blood in the setting of inflammation.

Antigen-Presenting Cells

Antigen-presenting cells (APCs) are cells that capture microbial and other antigens, display them to lymphocytes, and provide signals that stimulate the proliferation and differentiation of the lymphocytes. By convention, APC usually refers to a cell that displays antigens to T lymphocytes. The major type of APC that is involved in initiating T cell responses is the **dendritic cell**. Macrophages and B cells present antigens to T lymphocytes in cell-mediated and humoral immune responses, respectively. A specialized cell type called the **follicular dendritic cell** displays antigens to B lymphocytes during particular phases of humoral immune responses. Many APCs, such as dendritic cells and macrophages, also recognize and respond to microbes during innate immune reactions and thus link innate immune reactions to responses of the adaptive immune system. In addition to the introduction presented here, APC function is described in more detail in Chapter 6.

Dendritic Cells

Dendritic cells are the most important APCs for activating naive T cells, and they play major roles in innate responses to infections and in linking innate and adaptive immune responses. They have long membranous projections and phagocytic capabilities and are widely distributed in lymphoid tissues, mucosal epithelium, and organ parenchyma. Most dendritic cells are part of the myeloid lineage of hematopoietic cells and arise from a precursor that can also differentiate into monocytes but not granulocytes (Fig. 2-4). Maturation of dendritic cells is dependent on a cytokine called Flt3 ligand, which binds to the Flt3 tyrosine kinase receptor on the precursor cells. Similar to macrophages, dendritic cells express receptors that recognize molecules typically made by microbes and not mammalian cells, and they respond to the microbes by secreting cytokines.

The majority of dendritic cells in skin, mucosa, and organ parenchyma, which are called **classical** (or **conventional**) **dendritic cells**, respond to microbes by migrating to lymph nodes, where they display microbial protein antigens to T lymphocytes. One subpopulation of dendritic cells, called **plasmacytoid dendritic cells**, are early cellular responders to viral infection. They recognize nucleic acids of intracellular viruses and produce soluble proteins called type I interferons, which have potent antiviral activities. Populations of dendritic cells may also be derived from embryonic precursors and, during inflammation, from monocytes. We will discuss the

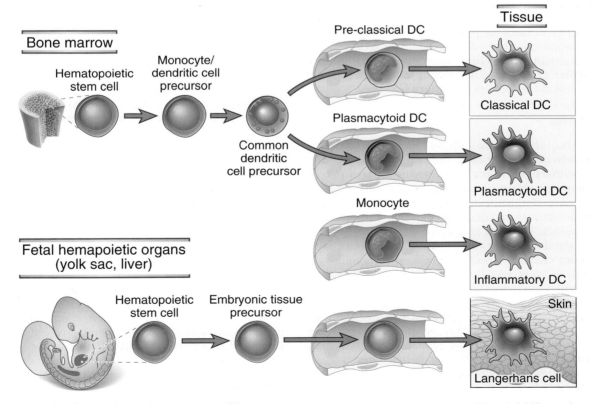

FIGURE 2-4 Maturation of dendritic cells. Dendritic cells arise from a common precursor cell of the myeloid lineage in the bone marrow and further differentiate into subsets, the major ones being classical dendritic cells and plasmacytoid dendritic cells. Inflammatory dendritic cells may arise from monocytes in inflamed tissues, and some tissue-resident dendritic cells, such as Langerhans cells in the skin, may develop from embryonic precursors.

role of dendritic cells as mediators of innate immunity and as APCs in Chapters 4 and 6, respectively.

Other Antigen-Presenting Cells

In addition to dendritic cells, macrophages and B lymphocytes are important antigen-presenting cells for CD4+ helper T cells. Macrophages present antigens to helper T lymphocytes at the sites of infection, which leads to helper T cell activation and production of molecules that further activate the macrophages. This process is important for the eradication of microbes that are ingested by the phagocytes but resist killing; in these cases, helper T cells greatly enhance the microbicidal activities of the macrophages. B cells present antigens to helper T cells, which is a key step in the cooperation of helper T cells with B cells for antibody responses to protein antigens. We will discuss these antigen presenting functions of macrophages and B cells in Chapters 10 and 12, respectively.

Cytotoxic T lymphocytes (CTLs) are effector CD8+ T cells that can recognize antigens on any type of nucleated cell and become activated to kill the cell. Therefore, all nucleated cells are potentially APCs for CTLs.

Follicular Dendritic Cells

Follicular dendritic cells (FDCs) are cells with membranous projections that are found intermingled in collections of activated B cells in the lymphoid follicles of lymph nodes, spleen, and mucosal lymphoid tissues. FDCs are not derived from precursors in the bone marrow and are unrelated to the dendritic cells that present antigens to T lymphocytes. FDCs bind and display protein antigens on their surfaces for recognition by B lymphocytes. This is important for the selection of B lymphocytes that express antibodies that bind antigens with high affinity (see Chapter 12). FDCs also contribute to the structural organization of the follicles (see later).

Lymphocytes

Lymphocytes, the unique cells of adaptive immunity, are the only cells in the body that express clonally distributed antigen receptors, each specific for a different antigenic determinant. Each clone of T and B lymphocytes expresses antigen receptors with a single specificity, which is different from the specificities of the receptors in all other clones. Thus, the antigen receptors of these lymphocytes are clonally distributed. As we shall discuss here and in later chapters, there are millions of lymphocyte clones in the body, enabling the organism to recognize and respond to millions of foreign antigens.

The role of lymphocytes in mediating adaptive immunity was established by several lines of evidence accumulated over decades of research. One of the earliest clues came from the observation that humans with congenital and acquired immune deficiency states had reduced numbers of lymphocytes in the peripheral circulation and in lymphoid tissues. Experiments done mainly with mice showed that protective immunity to microbes can be adoptively transferred from immunized to naive animals only by lymphocytes or their secreted products. In vitro experiments established that stimulation of lymphocytes

with antigens leads to responses that show many of the characteristics of immune responses induced under more physiologic conditions in vivo. Following the identification of lymphocytes as the mediators of humoral and cellular immunity, many discoveries were made at a rapid pace about different types of lymphocytes, their origins in the bone marrow and thymus, their roles in various immune responses, and the consequences of their absence. Among the most important findings was that clonally distributed, highly diverse and specific receptors for antigens are produced by lymphocytes but not by any other types of cells. During the past three decades, an enormous amount of information has accumulated about lymphocyte genes, proteins, and functions. We probably now know more about lymphocytes than about any other cells in all of biology.

One of the most interesting questions about lymphocytes has been how the extremely diverse repertoire of antigen receptors with different specificities is generated from the small number of genes for these receptors that are present in the germline. It is now known that the genes encoding the antigen receptors of lymphocytes are formed by recombination of DNA segments during the maturation of these cells. There is a random aspect to these somatic recombination events that results in the generation of millions of different receptor genes and a highly diverse repertoire of antigen specificities among different clones of lymphocytes (see Chapter 8).

The total number of lymphocytes in a healthy adult is about 5×10^{11}. Of these, ~2% are in the blood, ~4% in the skin, ~10% in the bone marrow, ~15% in the mucosal lymphoid tissues of the gastrointestinal and respiratory tracts, and ~65% in lymphoid organs (mainly the spleen and lymph nodes). We first describe the properties of these cells and then their organization in various lymphoid tissues.

Subsets of Lymphocytes

Lymphocytes consist of distinct subsets that are different in their functions and protein products (Table 2-2). The major classes of lymphocytes were introduced in Chapter 1 (see Fig. 1-5). Morphologically, all lymphocytes are similar, and their appearance does not reflect their heterogeneity or their diverse functions. **B lymphocytes**, the cells that produce antibodies, were so called because in birds they were found to mature in an organ called the bursa of Fabricius. In mammals, no anatomic equivalent of the bursa exists, and the early stages of B cell maturation occur in the bone marrow. Thus, *B lymphocytes* now refer to bone marrow–derived lymphocytes. **T lymphocytes**, the mediators of cellular immunity, arise in the bone marrow, and migrate to and mature in the thymus; *T lymphocytes* refer to thymus-derived lymphocytes.

Subsets of B and T lymphocytes exist with distinct phenotypic and functional characteristics. The major subsets of B cells are follicular B cells, marginal zone B cells, and B-1 cells, each of which is found in distinct anatomic locations within lymphoid tissues. Follicular B cells express highly diverse, clonally distributed sets of antibodies that serve as cell surface antigen receptors and as the key secreted effector molecules of adaptive humoral immunity. In contrast, B-1 and marginal-zone B cells produce antibodies with very limited diversity.

TABLE 2-2 Lymphocyte Classes

Class	Functions	Antigen Receptor and Specificity	Selected Phenotype Markers	Percentage of Total Lymphocytes*		
				Blood	Lymph Node	Spleen
αβ T Lymphocytes						
CD4+ helper T lymphocytes	B cell differentiation (humoral immunity) Macrophage activation (cell-mediated immunity) Stimulation of inflammation	αβ heterodimers Diverse specificities for peptide–class II MHC complexes	CD3+, CD4+, CD8−	35-60†	50–60	50–60
CD8+ cytotoxic T lymphocytes	Killing of cells infected with viruses or intracellular bacteria	αβ heterodimers Diverse specificities for peptide–class I MHC complexes	CD3+, CD4−, CD8+	15-40	15–20	10–15
Regulatory T cells	Suppress function of other T cells (regulation of immune responses, maintenance of self-tolerance)	αβ heterodimers Specific for self and some foreign antigens (peptide-class II MHC complexes)	CD3+, CD4+, CD25+ FoxP3+ (most common, but other phenotypes as well)	Rare	10	10
NKT cells	Suppress or activate innate and adaptive immune responses	αβ heterodimers Limited specificity for glycolipid-CD1 complexes	CD56, CD16 (Fc receptor for IgG), CD3	5-30	Rare	10
γδ T lymphocytes	Helper and cytotoxic functions (innate immunity)	γδ heterodimers Limited specificities for peptide and nonpeptide antigens	CD3+, CD4 and CD8 variable	Rare	Rare	Rare
B Lymphocytes						
Follicular B cells	Antibody production (humoral immunity)	Surface Ig Diverse specificities for many types of molecules	Fc receptors, class II MHC, CD19, CD23	5-20	20–25	40–45
Marginal zone B cells	Antibody production (humoral immunity)	Surface Ig Limited specificities for a restricted set of molecules	IgM, CD27	2–3	3–5	7–10

This table summarizes the major properties of the lymphocytes of the adaptive immune system. Not included are NK cells and other innate lymphoid cells, which are discussed in Chapter 4.
*The percentages are approximations, based on data from human peripheral blood and mouse lymphoid organs.
†In most cases, the ratio of CD4+CD8− to CD8+CD4− is about 2:1.
Ig, immunoglobulin; MHC, major histocompatibility complex.

The two major T cell subsets are CD4+ helper T lymphocytes and CD8+ CTLs, which express antigen receptors called αβ T cell receptors (TCRs), and function as the mediators of cellular immunity. CD4+ regulatory T cells are a third subset of T cells expressing αβ receptors; their function is to inhibit immune responses. In addition, NKT cells and γδ T cells are two numerically smaller subsets of T cells that express TCRs with limited diversity, analogous to the antibodies made by B-1 cells. The functions of these classes of B and T cells will be discussed in later chapters.

The expression of various membrane proteins is used to distinguish distinct populations of lymphocytes (see Table 2-2). For instance, most helper T cells express a surface protein called CD4, and most CTLs express a different surface protein called CD8. These and many other surface proteins are often called markers because they identify and discriminate between (mark) different cell populations. These markers not only delineate the different classes of lymphocytes but also have many functions in the cell types in which they are expressed. The most common way to determine if a surface phenotypic marker is expressed on a cell is to test if antibodies specific for the marker bind to the cell. In this context, the antibodies are used by investigators or clinicians as analytical tools. There are available hundreds of different pure antibody preparations, called monoclonal antibodies, each specific for a different molecule and labeled with probes that can be readily detected on cell surfaces by use of appropriate instruments. (Monoclonal antibodies are described in Chapter 5, and methods to detect labeled antibodies bound to cells are discussed in Appendix IV.) The cluster of differentiation (CD) nomenclature is a widely adopted uniform method for naming cell surface molecules that

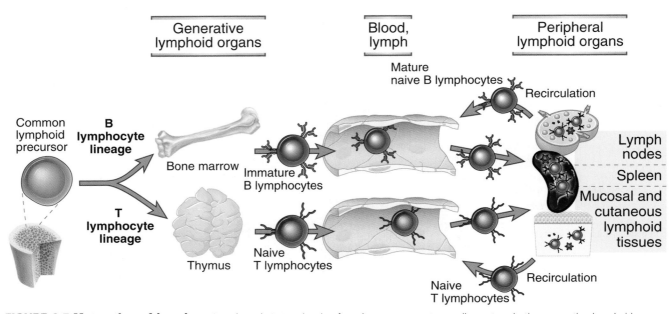

FIGURE 2-5 Maturation of lymphocytes. Lymphocytes develop from bone marrow stem cells, mature in the generative lymphoid organs (bone marrow and thymus for B and T cells, respectively), and then circulate through the blood to secondary lymphoid organs (lymph nodes, spleen, regional lymphoid tissues such as mucosa-associated lymphoid tissues). Fully mature T cells leave the thymus, but immature B cells leave the bone marrow and complete their maturation in secondary lymphoid organs. Naive lymphocytes may respond to foreign antigens in these secondary lymphoid tissues or return by lymphatic drainage to the blood and recirculate through other secondary lymphoid organs.

are characteristic of a particular cell lineage or differentiation stage, have a defined structure, and are recognized by a group (cluster) of monoclonal antibodies. Thus, all structurally defined cell surface molecules are given a CD number designation (e.g., CD1, CD2). Although originally devised to define leukocyte subtypes, CD markers are found on all cell types in the body. Appendix III provides a current list of leukocyte CD markers that are mentioned in this book.

Development of Lymphocytes

After birth, lymphocytes, like all blood cells, arise from stem cells in the bone marrow. The origin of lymphocytes from bone marrow progenitors was first demonstrated by experiments with radiation-induced bone marrow chimeras. Lymphocytes and their precursors are radiosensitive and are killed by high doses of γ-irradiation. If a mouse of one inbred strain is irradiated and then injected with bone marrow cells or small numbers of hematopoietic stem cells of another strain that can be distinguished from the host, all the lymphocytes that develop subsequently are derived from the bone marrow cells or hematopoietic stem cells of the donor. Such approaches have proved useful for examining the maturation of lymphocytes and other blood cells.

All lymphocytes go through complex maturation stages during which they express antigen receptors and acquire the functional and phenotypic characteristics of mature cells (Fig. 2-5). The anatomic sites where the major steps in lymphocyte development occur are called the generative lymphoid organs. These include the bone marrow, where precursors of all lymphocytes arise and B cells mature, and the thymus, where T cells mature. We will discuss the processes of B and T lymphocyte maturation

in much more detail in Chapter 8. These mature B and T cells are called **naive lymphocytes**. Naive lymphocytes are functionally quiescent, but after activation by antigen, they proliferate and go through dramatic changes in phenotype and functional activity.

Populations of Lymphocytes Distinguished by History of Antigen Exposure

Naive lymphocytes that emerge from the bone marrow or thymus migrate into peripheral lymphoid organs, where they are activated by antigens to proliferate and differentiate into effector and memory cells, some of which then migrate into tissues (Fig. 2-6 and Table 2-3). The activation of lymphocytes follows a series of sequential steps beginning with the synthesis of new proteins, such as cytokine receptors and cytokines, which are required for many of the subsequent changes. The naive cells then undergo proliferation, resulting in increased size of the antigen-specific clones, a process called **clonal expansion**. In some infections, the numbers of microbe-specific T cells may increase more than 50,000-fold, and the numbers of specific B cells may increase up to 5000-fold. This rapid clonal expansion of microbe-specific lymphocytes is needed to keep pace with the ability of microbes to rapidly replicate. Concurrently with clonal expansion, antigen-stimulated lymphocytes differentiate into **effector cells** whose function is to eliminate the antigen. Other progeny of antigen-stimulated B and T lymphocytes differentiate into long-lived **memory cells**, whose function is to mediate rapid and enhanced (i.e., secondary) responses to subsequent exposures to antigens. Mixtures of naive, effector, and memory lymphocytes are always present in various sites throughout the body, and these populations can be distinguished by several functional and phenotypic criteria (Table 2-3).

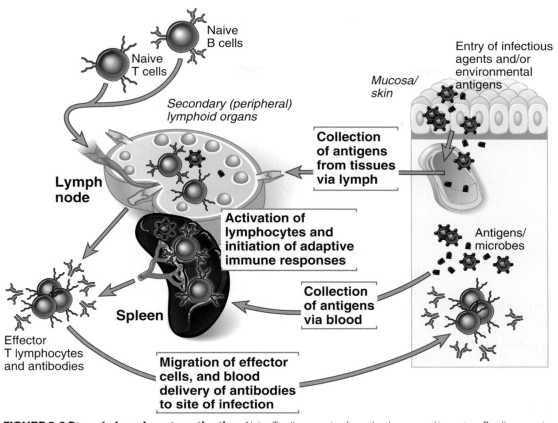

FIGURE 2-6 Steps in lymphocyte activation. Naive T cells emerging from the thymus and immature B cells emerging from the bone marrow migrate into secondary lymphoid organs, including lymph nodes and spleen. In these locations, B cells complete their maturation; naive B and T cells activated by antigens differentiate into effector and memory lymphocytes. Some effector and memory lymphocytes migrate into peripheral tissue sites of infection. Antibodies secreted by effector B cells in lymph node, spleen, and bone marrow (not shown) enter the blood and are delivered to sites of infection.

The details of lymphocyte activation and differentiation as well as the functions of each of these populations will be addressed later in this book. Here we will summarize the phenotypic characteristics of each population.

Naive Lymphocytes

Naive lymphocytes are mature T or B cells that are found in the peripheral lymphoid organs and circulation and have never encountered foreign antigen. (The term *naive* refers to the idea that these cells are immunologically inexperienced because they have not encountered antigen.) Naive lymphocytes typically die after 1 to 3 months if they do not recognize antigens. Naive and memory lymphocytes are both called resting lymphocytes because they are not actively dividing, nor are they performing effector functions. Naive (and memory) B and T lymphocytes cannot be readily distinguished morphologically, and both are often called small lymphocytes when observed in blood smears. A small lymphocyte is 8 to 10 μm in diameter and has a large nucleus with dense heterochromatin and a thin rim of cytoplasm that contains a few mitochondria, ribosomes, and lysosomes but no visible specialized organelles (Fig. 2-7). Before antigenic stimulation, naive lymphocytes are in a state of rest, or in the G_0 stage of the cell cycle. In response to stimulation, they enter the G_1 stage of the cell cycle before going on

to divide. Activated lymphocytes are larger (10 to 12 μm in diameter), have more cytoplasm and organelles and increased amounts of cytoplasmic RNA, and are called large lymphocytes or lymphoblasts (see Fig. 2-7).

The survival of naive lymphocytes depends on signals generated by antigen receptors and cytokines. It is postulated that the antigen receptor of naive B cells generates survival signals even in the absence of antigen. Naive T lymphocytes recognize various self antigens weakly, enough to generate survival signals but without triggering the stronger signals that are needed to initiate clonal expansion and differentiation into effector cells. The need for antigen receptor expression to maintain the pool of naive lymphocytes in peripheral lymphoid organs was demonstrated in studies with mice in which the genes that encode the antigen receptors of B cells or T cells were deleted after the lymphocytes matured. In these studies, naive lymphocytes that lost their antigen receptors died within 2 or 3 weeks.

Cytokines are also essential for the survival of naive lymphocytes, and naive B and T cells express receptors for these cytokines. The most important of these cytokines are interleukin-7 (IL-7), which promotes survival and, perhaps, low-level cycling of naive T cells, and B cell–activating factor (BAFF), a cytokine belonging to the TNF family, which is required for naive B cell survival.

TABLE 2-3   Characteristics of Naive, Effector, and Memory Lymphocytes

Cell type	Stage		
	Naive	Activated or effector	Memory
Helper T lymphocytes			
B lymphocytes			

	Naive	Activated or Effector	Memory
T Lymphocytes			
Migration	Preferentially to secondary lymphoid organs	Preferentially to inflamed tissues	Preferentially to inflamed tissues, mucosal tissues
Frequency of cells responsive to particular antigen	Very low	High	Low
Effector functions	None	Cytokine secretion; cytotoxic activity	None
Cell cycling	No	Yes	+/−
Surface protein expression			
IL-2R (CD25)	Low	High	Low
L-selectin (CD62L)	High	Low	Variable
IL-7R (CD127)	Moderately high	Low	High
Adhesion molecules: integrins, CD44	Low	High	High
Chemokine receptor: CCR7	High	Low	Variable
Major CD45 isoform (humans only)	CD45RA	CD45RO	CD45RO; variable
Morphology	Small; scant cytoplasm	Large; more cytoplasm	Small
B Lymphocytes			
Membrane immunoglobulin (Ig) isotype	IgM and IgD	Frequently IgG, IgA, IgE	Frequently IgG, IgA, IgE
Affinity of Ig produced	Relatively low	Increases during immune response	Relatively high
Effector function	None	Antibody secretion	None
Morphology	Small; scant cytoplasm	Large; more cytoplasm; plasma cell	Small
Surface protein expression			
Chemokine receptor: CXCR5	High	Low	?
CD27	Low	High	High

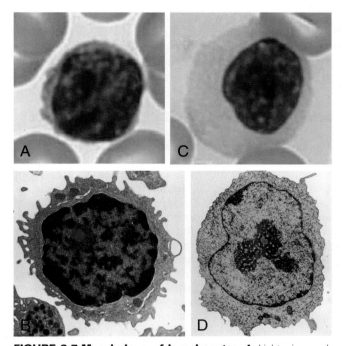

FIGURE 2-7 Morphology of lymphocytes. A, Light micrograph of a lymphocyte in a peripheral blood smear. *(Courtesy of Jean Shafer, Department of Pathology, University of California, San Diego. Copyright 1995-2008, Carden Jennings Publishing Co., Ltd.)* **B,** Electron micrograph of a small lymphocyte. *(Courtesy of Dr. Noel Weidner, Department of Pathology, University of California, San Diego.)* **C,** Light micrograph of a large lymphocyte (lymphoblast). *(Courtesy of Jean Shafer, Department of Pathology, University of California, San Diego. Copyright 1995–2008, Carden Jennings Publishing Co., Ltd.)* **D,** Electron micrograph of a large lymphocyte (lymphoblast). *(From Fawcett DW:* Bloom and Fawcett: a textbook of histology, *12th ed, New York, 1994, Chapman & Hall. With kind permission of Springer Science and Business Media.)*

In the steady state, the pool of naive lymphocytes is maintained at a fairly constant number because of a balance between spontaneous death of these cells and the production of new cells in the generative lymphoid organs. Any loss of lymphocytes leads to a compensatory proliferation of the remaining ones and increased output from the generative organs. A demonstration of the ability of the lymphocyte population to fill the available space is the phenomenon of homeostatic proliferation. If naive cells are transferred into a host that is deficient in lymphocytes (said to be lymphopenic), the transferred lymphocytes begin to proliferate and increase in number until they reach roughly the numbers of lymphocytes in normal animals. This process occurs in the clinical situation of hematopoietic stem cell transplantation for the treatment of certain malignancies and genetic diseases. Homeostatic proliferation appears to be driven by the same signals—weak recognition of some self antigens and cytokines, mainly IL-7—that are required for the maintenance of naive lymphocytes.

Effector Lymphocytes

After naive lymphocytes are activated, they become larger and begin to proliferate. Some of these cells differentiate into effector lymphocytes that have the ability to produce molecules capable of eliminating foreign antigens. Effector T lymphocytes include helper cells and CTLs, and effector

B lymphocytes are antibody-secreting cells, including plasma cells. Helper T cells, which are usually CD4+, express surface molecules such as CD40 ligand (CD154) and secrete cytokines that bind to receptors on macrophages and B lymphocytes, leading to their activation. CTLs have cytoplasmic granules filled with proteins that, when released, kill the cells that the CTLs recognize, which are usually virus-infected and tumor cells. Both CD4+ and CD8+ effector T cells usually express surface proteins indicative of recent activation, including CD25 (a component of the receptor for the T cell growth factor IL-2), and altered patterns of adhesion molecules (selectins and integrins, discussed in Chapter 3). The majority of differentiated effector T lymphocytes are short-lived and not self-renewing.

Many antibody-secreting B cells are morphologically identifiable as **plasma cells**. They have characteristic nuclei placed eccentrically in the cell and with the chromatin distributed around the nuclear membrane in a cartwheel pattern; abundant cytoplasm containing dense, rough endoplasmic reticulum that is the site where antibodies (and other secreted and membrane proteins) are synthesized; and distinct perinuclear Golgi complexes, where antibody molecules are converted to their final forms and packaged for secretion (Fig. 2-8). It is estimated that half or more of the messenger RNA in these cells codes for antibody proteins and a single plasma cell can secrete thousands of antibody molecules per second. Plasma cells develop in lymphoid organs and at sites of immune responses, and some of them migrate to the bone marrow, where they may live and secrete antibodies for long periods after the immune response is induced and even after the antigen is eliminated. **Plasmablasts**, which are circulating precursors of long-lived tissue plasma cells, can be found in low numbers in the blood.

Memory Lymphocytes

Memory cells may survive in a functionally quiescent or slowly cycling state for months or years without a need for stimulation by antigen and presumably after the antigen is eliminated. They can be identified by their expression of surface proteins that distinguish them from naive

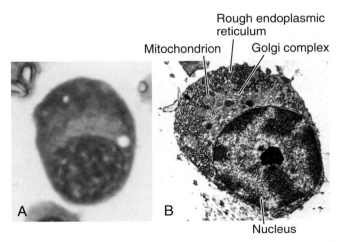

FIGURE 2-8 Morphology of plasma cells. A, Light micrograph of a plasma cell in tissue. **B,** Electron micrograph of a plasma cell. *(Courtesy of Dr. Noel Weidner, Department of Pathology, University of California, San Diego.)*

and recently activated effector lymphocytes, although it is still not clear which of these surface proteins are definitive markers of memory populations (see Table 2-3). Memory T cells, like naive but not effector T cells, express high levels of the IL-7 receptor (CD127). Memory T cells also express surface molecules that promote their migration into sites of infection anywhere in the body (see Chapter 3). In humans, most naive T cells express a 200-kD isoform of a surface molecule called CD45 that contains a segment encoded by an exon designated A and is therefore called CD45RA (for restricted A). In contrast, most activated and memory T cells express a 180-kD isoform of CD45 in which the A exon RNA has been spliced out; this isoform is called CD45RO. However, this way of distinguishing naive from memory T cells is not perfect, and interconversion between CD45RA$^+$ and CD45RO$^+$ populations has been documented.

Memory B lymphocytes may express certain classes (isotypes) of membrane Ig, such as IgG, IgE, or IgA, as a result of isotype switching, whereas naive B cells express only IgM and IgD (see Chapters 5 and 12). In humans, CD27 expression is a marker for memory B cells.

Memory cells appear to be heterogeneous, and there are subsets that differ especially with respect to their location and migratory properties. Memory T and B cells will be discussed further in Chapters 9 and 12, respectively.

The distinguishing features of naive, effector, and memory lymphocytes reflect different programs of gene expression that are regulated by transcription factors and by stable epigenetic changes, including histone methylation and acetylation and chromatin remodeling. For example, a transcription factor called Kruppel-like factor 2 (KLF-2) is required for maintenance of the naive T cell phenotype. The phenotypes of functionally different types of CD4$^+$ effector T cells, called T$_H$1, T$_H$2, and T$_H$17 cells, depend on transcription factors T-bet, GATA-3, and RORγT, respectively, as well as epigenetic changes in cytokine gene loci (see Chapter 10). Other transcription factors are required for maintaining the phenotypes of memory B and T cells. Our understanding of the molecular determinants of lymphocyte phenotype is still incomplete and evolving.

Innate Lymphoid Cells

Innate lymphoid cells (ILCs) include several developmentally related subsets of bone marrow–derived cells with lymphoid morphology and effector functions similar to those of T cells, but lacking T cell antigen receptors. The major functions of ILCs are to provide early defense against infectious pathogens, to recognize stressed and damaged host cells and help to eliminate these cells, and to influence the nature of the subsequent adaptive immune response.

The first and best characterized innate lymphoid cells are natural killer (NK) cells, which secrete the cytokine IFNγ and kill infected and damaged cells and secrete IFNγ, a cytokine also produced by the T$_H$1 subset of CD4$^+$ effector T cells. We will describe NK cells in more detail in Chapter 4. Other subsets of innate lymphoid cells secrete cytokines that are also produced by certain subsets of CD4$^+$ helper T cells, including IL-5, IL-13, IL-17, and IL-22. The functions of these cytokines are described

in Chapter 10, when we discuss the effector functions of CD4$^+$ T cells. Lymphoid tissue–inducer cells are a subset of ILCs that produce the cytokines lymphotoxin and TNF, and are essential for the formation of organized secondary lymphoid tissues, described later in this chapter.

ANATOMY AND FUNCTIONS OF LYMPHOID TISSUES

To optimize the cellular interactions necessary for antigen recognition and lymphocyte activation in adaptive immune responses, lymphocytes and APCs are localized and concentrated in anatomically defined tissues or organs, which are also the sites where foreign antigens are transported and concentrated. Such anatomic compartmentalization is not fixed because, as we will discuss in Chapter 3, many lymphocytes constantly recirculate and exchange between the circulation and the tissues.

Lymphoid tissues are classified as generative organs, also called primary or central lymphoid organs, where lymphocytes first express antigen receptors and attain phenotypic and functional maturity, and peripheral organs, also called secondary lymphoid organs, where lymphocyte responses to foreign antigens are initiated and develop (see Fig. 2-5). Included in the generative lymphoid organs of adult mammals are the bone marrow and the thymus, the sites of maturation of B cells and T cells, respectively. B lymphocytes partially mature in the bone marrow, enter the circulation, then populate secondary lymphoid organs, including spleen and lymph nodes, and complete their maturation mainly in the spleen. T lymphocytes mature in the thymus, and then enter the circulation and populate peripheral lymphoid organs and tissues. Two important functions shared by the generative organs are to provide growth factors and other molecular signals needed for lymphocyte maturation and to present self antigens for recognition and selection of maturing lymphocytes (see Chapter 8).

The peripheral lymphoid tissues include the lymph nodes, spleen, cutaneous immune system, and mucosal immune system. In addition, poorly defined aggregates of lymphocytes are found in connective tissues and in most organs. All peripheral lymphoid organs also share common functions, including the delivery of antigens and responding naive lymphocytes to the same location so that adaptive immune responses can be initiated, and an anatomic organization that allows T cells and B cells to interact cooperatively.

Bone Marrow

The bone marrow is the site of generation of most mature circulating blood cells, including red blood cells, granulocytes, and monocytes, and the site of early events in B cell maturation. The generation of all blood cells, called **hematopoiesis** (Fig. 2-9), occurs initially during fetal development in blood islands of the yolk sac and the para-aortic mesenchyme, then shifts to the liver between the third and fourth months of gestation, and finally shifts to the bone marrow. At birth, hematopoiesis takes place mainly in the bones throughout the skeleton, but it becomes increasingly restricted to the marrow of the

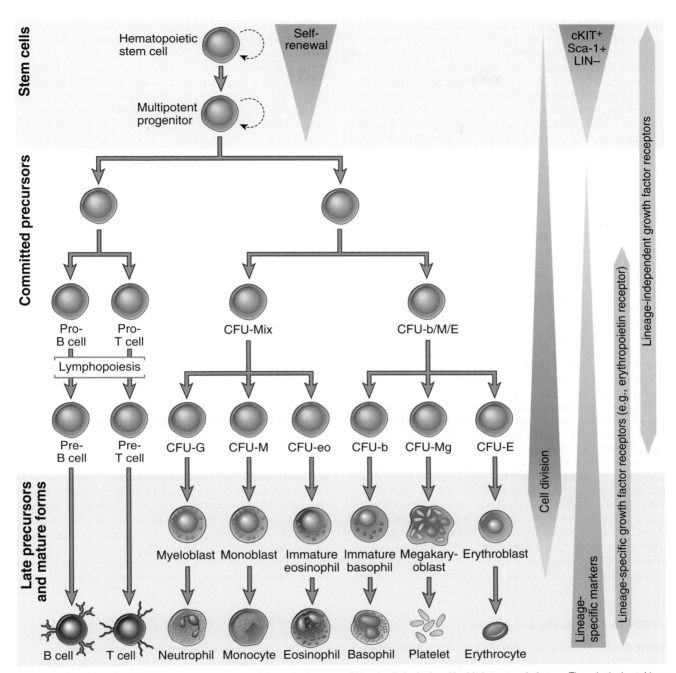

FIGURE 2-9 Hematopoiesis. The development of the major lineages of blood cells is depicted in this hematopoietic tree. The principal cytokines that drive the maturation of different lineages are described in Table 2-4. The development of lymphocytes is described later in this chapter and in Figure 8-2. Most dendritic cells are also derived from the same common myeloid precursor that monocytes are derived from *(not shown)*. Mast cells, NK cells, and other innate lymphoid cells *(not shown)* are also derived from committed progenitors in the bone marrow.

flat bones, so that by puberty, hematopoiesis occurs mostly in the sternum, vertebrae, iliac bones, and ribs. The red marrow that is found in these bones consists of a sponge-like reticular framework located between long bony trabeculae. The spaces in this framework contain a network of blood-filled sinusoids lined by endothelial cells attached to a discontinuous basement membrane. Outside the sinusoids are clusters of the precursors of blood cells in various stages of development as well as mature fat cells. The blood cell precursors mature and

migrate through the sinusoidal basement membrane and between endothelial cells to enter the vascular circulation. When the bone marrow is injured or when an exceptional demand for production of new blood cells occurs, the liver and spleen often become sites of extramedullary hematopoiesis.

Red blood cells, granulocytes, monocytes, dendritic cells, platelets, B and T lymphocytes, and NK cells all originate from a common hematopoietic stem cell (HSC) in the bone marrow (see Fig. 2-9). HSCs are pluripotent, meaning that a single HSC can generate all different types of mature blood cells. HSCs are also self-renewing because each time they divide, at least one daughter cell maintains the properties of a stem cell while the other can differentiate along a particular lineage (called asymmetric division). HSCs can be identified by the presence of surface markers, including the proteins CD34 and c-Kit, and the absence of lineage-specific markers that are expressed in mature cells. HSCs are maintained within specialized microscopic anatomic niches in the bone marrow. In these locations, nonhematopoietic stromal cells provide contact-dependent signals and soluble factors required for continuous cycling of the HSCs. HSCs give rise to two kinds of multipotent progenitor cells, one that generates lymphoid and some myeloid cells and another that produces more myeloid cells, erythrocytes, and platelets. The common myeloid-lymphoid progenitor gives rise to committed precursors of T cell, B cell, or innate lymphoid cell lineages, as well as to some myeloid cells. The common myeloid-megakaryocyte-erythroid progenitors give rise to committed precursors of the erythroid, megakaryocytic, granulocytic, and monocytic lineages, which give rise, respectively, to mature red blood cells, platelets, granulocytes (neutrophils, eosinophils, basophils), and monocytes. Most dendritic cells arise from a branch of the monocytic lineage.

The proliferation and maturation of precursor cells in the bone marrow are stimulated by cytokines. Many of these cytokines are called **colony-stimulating factors** because they were originally assayed by their ability to stimulate the growth and development of various leukocytic or erythroid colonies from marrow cells. Hematopoietic cytokines are produced by stromal cells and macrophages in the bone marrow, thus providing the local environment for hematopoiesis. They are also produced by antigen-stimulated T lymphocytes and cytokine-activated or microbe-activated macrophages, providing a mechanism for replenishing leukocytes that may be consumed during

immune and inflammatory reactions. The names and properties of the major hematopoietic cytokines are listed in Table 2-4.

In addition to self-renewing stem cells and their differentiating progeny, the marrow contains numerous long-lived antibody-secreting plasma cells. These cells are generated in peripheral lymphoid tissues as a consequence of antigenic stimulation of B cells and then migrate to the bone marrow. The marrow also contains recirculating mature follicular B cells that may respond there to blood borne microbes. In addition, some long-lived memory T lymphocytes migrate to and may reside in the bone marrow.

Thymus

The thymus is the site of T cell maturation. The thymus is a bilobed organ situated in the anterior mediastinum. Each lobe is divided into multiple lobules by fibrous septa, and each lobule consists of an outer cortex and an inner medulla (Fig. 2-10). The cortex contains a dense collection of T lymphocytes, and the lighter-staining medulla is more sparsely populated with lymphocytes. Bone marrow–derived macrophages and dendritic cells are found almost exclusively in the medulla. Scattered throughout the thymus are nonlymphoid epithelial cells, which have abundant cytoplasm. Thymic **cortical epithelial cells** produce IL-7, which is required early in T cell development. A different subset of epithelial cells found only in the medulla, called **medullary thymic epithelial cells** (MTEC), plays a special role in presenting self antigens to developing T cells and causing their deletion. This is one mechanism of ensuring that the immune system remains tolerant to self, and is discussed in detail in Chapter 15. In the medulla there are structures called Hassall's corpuscles, which are composed of tightly packed whorls of epithelial cells that may be remnants of degenerating cells. The thymus has a rich vascular supply and efferent lymphatic vessels that drain into

TABLE 2-4	Hematopoietic Cytokines			
Cytokine	**Size**	**Principal Cellular Sources**	**Principal Immature Cell Targets**	**Principal Cell Populations Induced**
Stem cell factor (c-Kit ligand)	24 kD	Bone marrow stromal cells	Hematopoietic stem cells	All
Interleukin-7 (IL-7)	25 kD	Fibroblasts, bone marrow stromal cells	Immature lymphoid progenitors	T lymphocytes
Interleukin-3 (IL-3)	20–26 kD	T cells	Immature progenitors	All
Granulocyte-monocyte colony-stimulating factor (GM-CSF)	18–22 kD	T cells, macrophages, endothelial cells, fibroblasts	Immature and committed myeloid progenitors, mature macrophages	Granulocytes and monocytes, macrophage activation
Monocyte colony-stimulating factor (M-CSF)	Dimer of 70–90 kD; 40-kD subunits	Macrophages, endothelial cells, bone marrow cells, fibroblasts	Committed progenitors	Monocytes
Granulocyte colony-stimulating factor (G-CSF)	19 kD	Macrophages, fibroblasts, endothelial cells	Committed granulocyte progenitors	Granulocytes
Flt-3 ligand	30kD	Bone marrow stromal cells	Hematopoietic stem cells, dendritic cell and B cell progenitors	Classical and plasmacytoid dendritic cells, B cells

mediastinal lymph nodes. The epithelial component of the thymus is derived from invaginations of the ectoderm in the developing neck and chest of the embryo, forming structures called branchial pouches. Dendritic cells, macrophages, and lymphocyte precursors are derived from the bone marrow.

Humans with DiGeorge syndrome suffer from T cell deficiency because of a chromosomal deletion that eliminates genes required for thymus development (see Chapter 21). In the nude mouse strain, which has been widely used in immunology research, a mutation in the gene encoding a transcription factor causes a failure of differentiation of certain types of epithelial cells that are required for normal development of the thymus and hair follicles. Consequently, these mice lack T cells and hair.

The lymphocytes in the thymus, also called **thymocytes**, are T lymphocytes at various stages of maturation. The most immature cells enter the thymus, and their maturation begins in the cortex. As thymocytes mature, they migrate toward the medulla, so that the medulla contains mostly mature T cells. Only mature naïve T cells exit the thymus and enter the blood and peripheral

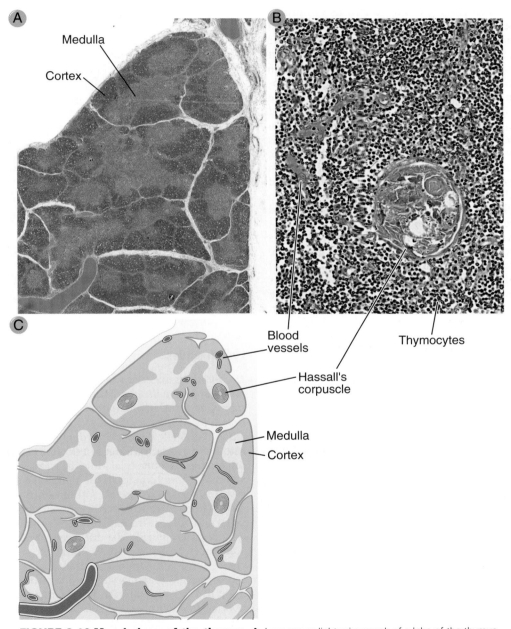

FIGURE 2-10 Morphology of the thymus. A, Low-power light micrograph of a lobe of the thymus showing the cortex and medulla. The darker blue-stained outer cortex and paler blue inner medulla are apparent. **B,** High-power light micrograph of the thymic medulla. The numerous small blue-staining cells are developing T cells called *thymocytes*, and the larger pink structure is Hassall's corpuscle, uniquely characteristic of the thymic medulla but whose function is poorly understood. **C,** Schematic diagram of the thymus illustrating a portion of a lobe divided into multiple lobules by fibrous trabeculae.

lymphoid tissues. The details of thymocyte maturation are described in Chapter 8.

The Lymphatic System

The lymphatic system consists of specialized vessels that drain fluid from tissues into and out of lymph nodes and then into the blood (Fig. 2-11). It is essential for tissue fluid homeostasis and for immune responses. Interstitial fluid is constantly formed in all vascularized tissues by movement of a filtrate of plasma out of capillaries, and the rate of local formation can increase dramatically when tissue is injured or infected. The skin, epithelia, and parenchymal organs contain numerous lymphatic capillaries that absorb this fluid from spaces between tissue cells. Lymphatic capillaries are blind-ended vascular channels lined by overlapping endothelial cells without the tight intercellular junctions or basement membrane that are typical of blood vessels. These lymphatic capillaries permit free uptake of interstitial fluid, and the overlapping arrangement of the endothelial cells and one-way valves within their lumens prevent backflow of the fluid. The absorbed fluid, called **lymph**, is pumped into convergent, progressively larger lymphatic vessels by the contraction of perilymphatic smooth muscle cells and the pressure exerted by movement of the musculoskeletal tissues. These vessels merge into afferent lymphatics that drain into lymph nodes, and the lymph drains out of the nodes through efferent lymphatics. Because lymph nodes are connected in series by lymphatics, an efferent lymphatic exiting one node may serve as the afferent vessel for another. The efferent lymph vessel at the end of a lymph node chain joins other lymph vessels, eventually culminating in a large lymphatic vessel called the thoracic duct. Lymph from the thoracic duct is emptied into the superior vena cava, thus returning the fluid to the blood stream. Lymphatics from the right upper trunk, right arm, and right side of the head drain into the right lymphatic duct, which also drains into the superior vena cava. About two liters of lymph are normally returned to the circulation each day, and disruption of the lymphatic system by tumors or some parasitic infections may lead to severe tissue swelling.

The lymphatic system collects microbial antigens from their portals of entry and delivers them to lymph nodes, where they can stimulate adaptive immune responses. Microbes enter the body most often through the skin and the gastrointestinal and respiratory tracts. All of these tissues are lined by epithelia that contain dendritic cells, and all are drained by lymphatic vessels. The dendritic cells capture microbial antigens and enter lymphatic vessels. Other microbes and soluble antigens may enter lymphatics independently of dendritic cells. In addition, soluble inflammatory mediators, such as chemokines, that are produced at sites of infection enter the lymphatics. The lymph nodes are interposed along lymphatic vessels and act as filters that sample the soluble and dendritic cell–associated antigens in the lymph before it reaches the blood. The captured antigens can then be seen by cells of the adaptive immune system. This process is described in Chapter 6.

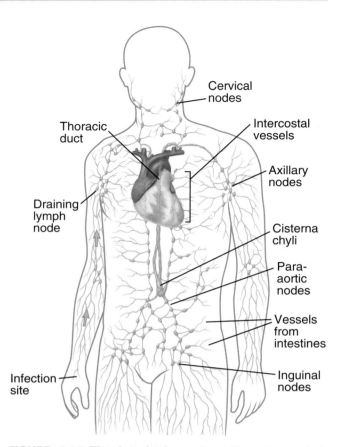

FIGURE 2-11 The lymphatic system. The major lymphatic vessels, which drain into the inferior vena cava (and superior vena cava, not shown), and collections of lymph nodes are illustrated. Antigens are captured from a site of infection and the draining lymph node to which these antigens are transported and where the immune response is initiated.

Lymph Nodes

Lymph nodes are encapsulated, vascularized secondary lymphoid organs with anatomic features that favor the initiation of adaptive immune responses to antigens carried from tissues by lymphatics (Fig. 2-12). Lymph nodes are situated along lymphatic channels throughout the body and therefore have access to antigens encountered at epithelia and originating in interstitial fluid in most tissues. There are about 500 lymph nodes in the human body. A lymph node is surrounded by a fibrous capsule, beneath which is a sinus system lined by reticular cells, cross-bridged by fibrils of collagen and other extracellular matrix proteins and filled with lymph, macrophages, dendritic cells, and other cell types. Afferent lymphatics empty into the subcapsular (marginal) sinus, and lymph may drain from there directly into the connected medullary sinus and then out of the lymph node through the efferent lymphatics. Beneath the inner floor of the subcapsular sinus is the lymphocyte-rich cortex. The outer cortex contains aggregates of cells called **follicles**. Some follicles contain central areas called **germinal centers**, which stain lightly with commonly used histologic stains. Each germinal center consists of a dark zone packed with proliferating B cells called centroblasts, and a light zone containing cells called centrocytes that have stopped

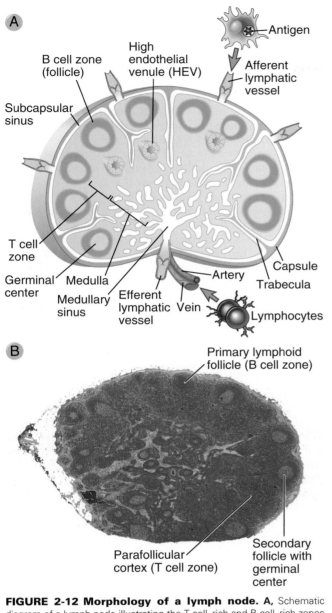

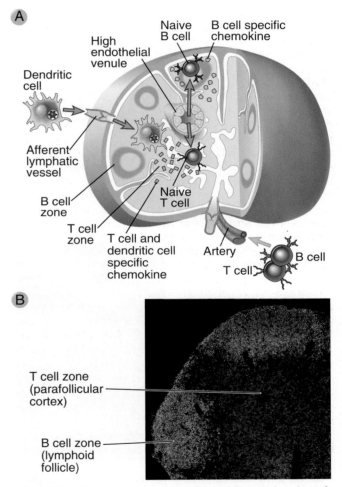

unique architecture of reticular fibers and stromal cells (Fig. 2-13). Follicles are the B cell zones. They are located in the lymph node cortex and are organized around FDCs, which have processes that interdigitate to form a dense reticular network. Primary follicles contain mostly mature, naive B lymphocytes. Germinal centers develop in response to antigenic stimulation. They are sites of remarkable B cell proliferation, selection of B cells producing high-affinity antibodies, and generation of memory B cells and long-lived plasma cells.

The T lymphocytes are located mainly beneath and more central to the follicles, in the paracortical cords.

FIGURE 2-12 Morphology of a lymph node. A, Schematic diagram of a lymph node illustrating the T cell–rich and B cell–rich zones and the routes of entry of lymphocytes and antigen (shown captured by a dendritic cell). **B,** Light micrograph of a lymph node illustrating the T cell and B cell zones. *(Courtesy of Dr. James Gulizia, Department of Pathology, Brigham and Women's Hospital, Boston, Massachusetts.)*

FIGURE 2-13 Segregation of B cells and T cells in a lymph node. A, The schematic diagram illustrates the path by which naive T and B lymphocytes migrate to different areas of a lymph node. The naive lymphocytes enter the node through an artery, leave the circulation by moving across the wall of the high endothelial venule, and then the B and T cells migrate to different zones of the lymph node drawn by chemokines that are produced in these areas and bind selectively to either cell type. Also shown is the migration of dendritic cells, which pick up antigens from the sites of antigen entry, enter through afferent lymphatic vessels, and migrate to the T cell–rich areas of the node. **B,** In this section of a lymph node, the B lymphocytes, located in the follicles, are stained green; the T cells, in the parafollicular cortex, are red. The method used to stain these cells is called *immunofluorescence* (see Appendix IV for details). *(Courtesy of Drs. Kathryn Pape and Jennifer Walter, University of Minnesota School of Medicine, Minneapolis.)* The anatomic segregation of T and B cells is also seen in the spleen (see Fig. 2-15).

proliferating and are being selected to survive and differentiate further. The germinal center reaction during humoral immune responses is described in Chapter 12. Follicles without germinal centers are called primary follicles, and those with germinal centers are called secondary follicles. The cortex around the follicles is called the parafollicular cortex or paracortex and is organized into cords, which are regions with a complex microanatomy of matrix proteins, fibers, lymphocytes, dendritic cells, and mononuclear phagocytes.

Anatomic Organization of B and T Lymphocytes

B and T lymphocytes are sequestered in distinct regions of the cortex of lymph nodes, each region with its own

These T cell–rich zones, often called the paracortex, contain a network of **fibroblastic reticular cells** (FRCs), many of which form the outer layer of tube-like structures called FRC conduits (Fig. 2-14). The conduits range in diameter from 0.2 to 3 μm and contain organized arrays of extracellular matrix molecules, including parallel bundles of collagen fibers embedded in a meshwork of fibrillin microfibers, all tightly surrounded by a basement membrane produced by a sleeve of FRCs. These conduits begin at the subcapsular sinus and extend to both medullary sinus lymphatic vessels and cortical blood vessels, called **high endothelial venules** (HEVs). Naive T cells

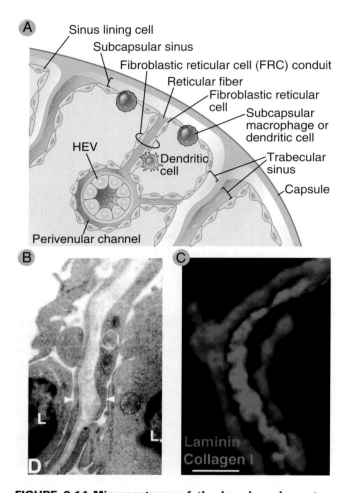

FIGURE 2-14 Microanatomy of the lymph node cortex. A, Schematic of the microanatomy of a lymph node depicting the route of lymph drainage from the subcapsular sinus, through fibroreticular cell conduits, to the perivenular channel around the high endothelial venule (HEV). **B,** Transmission electron micrograph of an FRC conduit surrounded by fibroblast reticular cells (arrowheads) and adjacent lymphocytes (L). *(From Gretz JE, Norbury CC, Anderson AO, Proudfoot AEI, Shaw S: Lymph-borne chemokines and other low molecular weight molecules reach high endothelial venules via specialized conduits while a functional barrier limits access to the lymphocyte microenvironments in lymph node cortex,* The Journal of Experimental Medicine *192:1425–1439, 2000.)* **C,** Immunofluorescent stain of an FRC conduit formed of the basement membrane protein laminin (red) and collagen fibrils (green). *(From Sixt M, Nobuo K, Selg M, Samson T, Roos G, Reinhardt DP, Pabst R, Lutz M, Sorokin L: The conduit system transports soluble antigens from the afferent lymph to resident dendritic cells in the T cell area of the lymph node,* Immunity *22:19-29, 2006. Copyright © 2005 by Elsevier Inc.)*

enter the T cell zones through the HEVs, as described in detail in Chapter 3. T cells are densely packed around the conduits in the lymph node cortex. Most (~70%) of the cortical T cells are CD4[+] helper T cells, intermingled with relatively sparse CD8[+] cells. These proportions can change dramatically during the course of an infection. For example, during a viral infection, there may be a marked increase in CD8[+] T cells. Dendritic cells are also concentrated in the paracortex of the lymph nodes, many of which are closely associated with the FRC conduits.

The anatomic segregation of B and T lymphocytes in distinct areas of the node is dependent on cytokines that are secreted by lymph node stromal cells in each area and that direct the migration of the lymphocytes (see Fig. 2-13). Naive T and B lymphocytes are delivered to a node through an artery and leave the circulation and enter the stroma of the node through the HEVs, which are located in the center of the cortical cords. The type of cytokines that determine where B and T cells reside in the node are called **chemokines** (chemoattractant cytokines), which bind to chemokine receptors on the lymphocytes. Chemokines include a large family of 8- to 10-kD cytokines that are involved in a wide variety of cell motility functions in development, maintenance of tissue architecture, and immune and inflammatory responses. We will discuss the properties of chemokines and their receptors in Chapter 3. Naive T cells express a receptor called CCR7 that binds the chemokines CCL19 and CCL21 produced by stromal cells in the T cell zones of the lymph node. These chemokines promote naive T cell movement from the blood, through the wall of the HEVs, into the T cell zone. Dendritic cells that are activated by microbes and enter the node through lymphatics also express CCR7, and this is why they migrate to the same area of the node as do naive T cells (see Chapter 6). Naive B cells express low levels of CCR7 and higher levels of another chemokine receptor, CXCR5, which recognizes a chemokine, CXCL13, produced only in follicles by FDCs. Thus, circulating naive B cells also enter lymph nodes through HEVs and are then attracted into the follicles. Another cytokine called lymphotoxin (which is not a chemokine) plays a role in stimulating CXCL13 production, especially in the follicles. The functions of chemokines and other cytokines in regulating where lymphocytes are located in lymphoid organs and in the formation of these organs have been established by numerous studies in mice. For example, CXCR5 knockout mice lack B cell–containing follicles in lymph nodes and spleen, and CCR7 knockout mice lack T cell zones.

The development of lymph nodes as well as of other peripheral lymphoid organs depends on lymphoid tissue–inducer cells and the coordinated actions of several cytokines, chemokines, and transcription factors. During fetal life, lymphoid tissue–inducer cells, which are a subset of innate lymphoid cells discussed earlier, stimulate the development of lymph nodes and other secondary lymphoid organs. This function is mediated by various proteins expressed by the inducer cells, the most thoroughly studied being the cytokines lymphotoxin-α (LTα) and lymphotoxin-β (LTβ). Knockout mice lacking either of these cytokines do not develop lymph nodes or secondary lymphoid tissues in the gut. Splenic white pulp development is also disorganized in these mice. The LTβ produced by the inducer cells stimulates stromal cells in different locations of a developing secondary lymphoid organ to secrete chemokines that help organize the structure of the lymphoid organs. FDCs are activated by LTβ to produce the chemokine CXCL13, which serves to recruit B cells and organize the developing follicle. Fibroblastic reticular cells (FRCs, mentioned earlier), are activated to produce CCL19 and CCL21, which recruit T cells and dendritic cells and form the T cell zone.

The anatomic segregation of B and T cells ensures that each lymphocyte population is in close contact with the appropriate APCs, that is, B cells with FDCs and T cells with dendritic cells. Furthermore, because of this precise segregation, B and T lymphocyte populations are kept apart until it is time for them to interact in a functional way. As we will see in Chapters 9 and 12, after stimulation by antigens, B and T cells change their expression of chemokine receptors, and begin to migrate toward one another in response to signals from chemokines and other mediators. Activated T cells either migrate toward follicles to help B cells or exit the node and enter the circulation. Activated B cells migrate into germinal centers and, after differentiation into plasma cells, may home to the bone marrow.

Antigen Transport Through Lymph Nodes

Lymph-borne substances that enter the subcapsular sinus of the lymph node are sorted by molecular size and delivered to different cell types to initiate various immune responses. The floor of the subcapsular sinus is constructed in a way that permits cells in the sinus to contact or migrate into the underlying cortex but does not allow soluble molecules in the lymph to freely pass into the cortex. Microbes and high–molecular-weight antigens are taken up by sinus macrophages and presented to cortical B lymphocytes just beneath the sinus. This is the first step in antibody responses to these antigens. Low–molecular-weight soluble antigens are transported out of the sinus through the FRC conduits and passed to resident cortical dendritic cells located adjacent to the conduits. The resident dendritic cells extend processes between the cells lining the conduits and into the lumen and capture and pinocytose the soluble antigens inside the conduits. The contribution of this pathway of antigen delivery may be important for initial T cell immune responses to some microbial antigens, but larger and sustained responses require delivery of antigens to the node by tissue dendritic cells, as discussed in Chapter 6. In addition to antigens, there is evidence that soluble inflammatory mediators, such as chemokines and other cytokines, are transported in the lymph that flows through the conduits; some of these may act on the adjacent dendritic cells, and others may be delivered to HEVs into which the conduits drain. This is a possible way in which tissue inflammation can be sensed in the lymph node and thereby influence recruitment and activation of lymphocytes in the node.

Spleen

The spleen is a highly vascularized organ whose major functions are to remove aging and damaged blood cells and particles (such as immune complexes and opsonized microbes) from the circulation and to initiate adaptive immune responses to blood-borne antigens. The spleen weighs about 150g in adults and is located in the left upper quadrant of the abdomen. The splenic parenchyma is anatomically and functionally divided into red pulp, which is composed mainly of blood-filled vascular sinusoids, and lymphocyte-rich white pulp. Blood enters the spleen through a single splenic artery that pierces the capsule at the hilum and divides into progressively smaller branches that remain surrounded by protective and supporting fibrous trabeculae (Fig. 2-15). Some of the arteriolar branches of the splenic artery end in extensive vascular sinusoids that are filled with large numbers of erythrocytes and are lined by macrophages and other cells. The sinusoids end in venules that drain into the splenic vein, which carries blood out of the spleen and into the portal circulation. The red pulp macrophages serve as an important filter for the blood, removing microbes, damaged cells, and antibody-coated (opsonized) cells and microbes. Individuals lacking a spleen are susceptible to disseminated infections with encapsulated bacteria such as pneumococci and meningococci. This may be because such organisms are normally cleared by opsonization and phagocytosis, and this function is defective in the absence of the spleen.

The white pulp contains the cells that mediate adaptive immune responses to blood-borne antigens. In the white pulp are many collections of densely packed lymphocytes, which appear as white nodules against the background of the red pulp. The white pulp is organized around central arteries, which are branches of the splenic artery distinct from the branches that form the vascular sinusoids. Several smaller branches of each central artery pass through the lymphocyte-rich area and drain into a marginal sinus. A region of specialized cells surrounding the marginal sinus, called the **marginal zone**, forms the boundary between the red pulp and white pulp. The architecture of the white pulp is analogous to the organization of lymph nodes, with segregated T cell and B cell zones. In the mouse spleen, the central arteries are surrounded by cuffs of lymphocytes, most of which are T cells. Because of their anatomic location, morphologists call these T cell zones **periarteriolar lymphoid sheaths**. B cell–rich follicles occupy the space between the marginal sinus and the periarteriolar sheath. As in lymph nodes, the T cell areas in the spleen contain a network of complex conduits composed of matrix proteins lined by FRC-like cells. The marginal zone just outside the marginal sinus is a distinct region populated by B cells and specialized macrophages. The B cells in the marginal zone, known as marginal zone B cells, are functionally distinct from follicular B cells and have a limited repertoire of antigen specificities. The architecture of the white pulp is more complex in humans than in mice, with both inner and outer marginal zones and a perifollicular zone. Antigens in the blood are delivered into the marginal sinus by circulating dendritic cells or are sampled by the macrophages in the marginal zone.

The anatomic arrangements of the APCs, B cells, and T cells in the splenic white pulp promote the interactions required for the efficient development of humoral

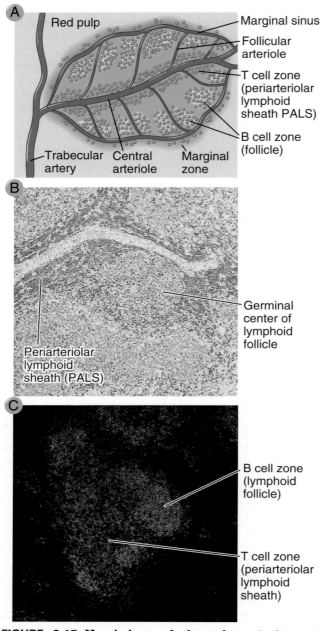

FIGURE 2-15 Morphology of the spleen. A, Schematic diagram of the spleen illustrating T cell and B cell zones, which make up the white pulp. **B,** Photomicrograph of a section of human spleen showing a trabecular artery with adjacent periarteriolar lymphoid sheath and a lymphoid follicle with a germinal center. Surrounding these areas is the red pulp, rich in vascular sinusoids. **C,** Immunohistochemical demonstration of T cell and B cell zones in the spleen, shown in a cross-section of the region around an arteriole. T cells in the periarteriolar lymphoid sheath are stained red, and B cells in the follicle are stained green. *(Courtesy of Drs. Kathryn Pape and Jennifer Walter, University of Minnesota School of Medicine, Minneapolis.)*

immune responses, as we will discuss in Chapter 12. The segregation of T lymphocytes in the periarteriolar lymphoid sheaths and B cells in follicles and marginal zones is a highly regulated process, dependent on the production of different cytokines and chemokines by the stromal cells in these different areas, analogous to the case for lymph nodes. The chemokine CXCL13 and its receptor CXCR5 are required for B cell migration into the follicles, and CCL19 and CCL21 and their receptor CCR7 are required for naive T cell migration into the periarteriolar sheath. The production of these chemokines by nonlymphoid stromal cells is stimulated by the cytokine lymphotoxin.

Regional Immune Systems

All major epithelial barriers of the body, including the skin, gastrointestinal mucosa, and bronchial mucosa, have their own system of lymph nodes, nonencapsulated lymphoid structures, and diffusely distributed immune cells, which work in coordinated ways to provide specialized immune responses against the pathogens that enter at those barriers. The skin-associated immune system has evolved to respond to a wide variety of environmental microbes. The components of the immune systems associated with the gastrointestinal and bronchial mucosa are called the mucosa-associated lymphoid tissue (MALT) and are involved in immune responses to ingested and inhaled antigens and microbes. The skin and MALT contain a large proportion of the cells of the innate and adaptive immune systems. We will discuss the special features of these regional immune systems in Chapter 14.

SUMMARY

* The anatomic organization of the cells and tissues of the immune system is of critical importance for the generation of effective innate and adaptive immune responses. This organization permits the rapid delivery of innate immune cells, including neutrophils and monocytes, to sites of infection and permits a small number of lymphocytes specific for any one antigen to locate and respond effectively to that antigen regardless of where in the body the antigen is introduced.

* The cells that perform the majority of effector functions of innate and adaptive immunity are phagocytes (including neutrophils and macrophages), APCs (including macrophages and dendritic cells), and lymphocytes.

* Neutrophils, the most abundant blood leukocyte with a distinctive multilobed segmented nucleus and abundant cytoplasmic lysosomal granules, are rapidly recruited to sites of infection and tissue injury, where they perform phagocytic functions.

* Monocytes are the circulating precursors of tissue macrophages. All tissues contain resident macrophages, which are phagocytic cells that ingest and kill microbes and dead host cells and secrete cytokines and chemokines that promote the recruitment of leukocytes from the blood and initiate the repair of damaged tissues.

* APCs function to display antigens for recognition by lymphocytes and to promote the activation of lymphocytes. APCs include dendritic cells, mononuclear phagocytes, and FDCs.

* B and T lymphocytes express highly diverse and specific antigen receptors and are the cells responsible for the specificity and memory of adaptive immune responses. Many surface molecules are differentially expressed on different subsets of lymphocytes as well as on other leukocytes, and these are named according to the CD nomenclature.

* Innate lymphoid cells are effector cells of the innate immune system, some of which perform similar functions to CD4+ or CD8+ effector T cells. These cells, which include NK cells, do not express highly diverse, clonally distributed antigen receptors.

* Both B and T lymphocytes arise from a common precursor in the bone marrow. B cell development proceeds in the bone marrow, whereas T cell precursors migrate to and mature in the thymus. After maturing, B and T cells leave the bone marrow and thymus, enter the circulation, and populate peripheral lymphoid organs.

* Naive B and T cells are mature lymphocytes that have not been stimulated by antigen. When they encounter antigen, they proliferate, and differentiate into effector lymphocytes that have functions in protective immune responses. Effector B lymphocytes are antibody-secreting plasma cells. Effector T cells include cytokine-secreting CD4+ helper T cells and CD8+ cytotoxic T lymphocytes.

* Some of the progeny of antigen-activated B and T lymphocytes differentiate into memory cells that survive for long periods in a quiescent state. These memory cells are responsible for the rapid and enhanced responses to subsequent exposures to antigen.

* The organs of the immune system may be divided into the generative, or primary, lymphoid organs (bone marrow and thymus), where lymphocytes mature, and the peripheral, or secondary, organs (lymph nodes, spleen, and mucosal and cutaneous immune systems), where naive lymphocytes are activated by antigens.

* Bone marrow contains the stem cells for all blood cells, including lymphocytes, and is the site of maturation of all of these cell types except T cells, which mature in the thymus.

* Extracellular fluid (lymph) is constantly drained from tissues through lymphatics into lymph nodes and eventually into the blood. Microbial antigens are carried in soluble form and within dendritic cells in the lymph to lymph nodes, where they are recognized by lymphocytes.

* Lymph nodes are encapsulated secondary lymphoid organs located throughout the body along lymphatics, where naive B and T cells respond to antigens that are collected by the lymph from peripheral tissues. The spleen is an encapsulated organ in the abdominal cavity where senescent or opsonized blood cells are removed from the circulation, and in which lymphocytes respond to blood-borne antigens.

* Lymph nodes and the white pulp of the spleen are organized into B cell zones (the follicles) and T cell zones. The T cell areas are also the sites of residence of mature dendritic cells, which are APCs specialized for the activation of naive T cells. FDCs reside in the B cell areas and serve to activate B cells during humoral immune responses to protein antigens. The development of secondary lymphoid tissues depends on cytokines and lymphoid tissue inducer cells.

SELECTED READINGS

Cells of the Immune System

Chow A, Brown BD, Merad M: Studying the mononuclear phagocyte system in the molecular age, *Nature Reviews Immunology* 11:788–798, 2011.

Davies LC, Jenkins SJ, Allen JE, Taylor PR: Tissue-resident macrophages, *Nature Immunology* 14:986–995, 2013.

Farber DL, Yudanin NA, Restifo NP: Human memory T cells: generation, compartmentalization and homeostasis, *Nature Reviews Immunology* 14:24–35, 2014.

Geissmann F, Manz MG, Jung S, Sieweke MH, Merad M, Ley K: Development of monocytes, macrophages, and dendritic cells, *Science* 327:656–661, 2010.

Surh CD, Sprent J: Homeostasis of naive and memory T cells, *Immunity* 29:848–862, 2008.

Wynn TA, Chawla A, Pollard JW: Macrophage biology in development, homeostasis, and disease, *Nature* 496:445–455, 2013.

Tissues of the Immune System

Bronte V, Pittet MJ: The spleen in local and systemic regulation of immunity, *Immunity* 39:806–818, 2013.

Lane P, Kim M-Y, Withers D, Gaspal F, Bekiaris V, Desanti G, Khan M, McConnell F, Anderson G: Lymphoid tissue inducer cells in adaptive CD4 T cell dependent responses, *Seminars in Immunology* 20:159–163, 2008.

Mueller SN, Germain RN: Stromal cell contributions to the homeostasis and functionality of the immune system, *Nature Reviews Immunology* 9:618–629, 2009.

Ruddle NH, Akirav EM: Secondary lymphoid organs: responding to genetic and environmental cues in ontogeny and the immune response, *Journal of Immunology* 183:2205–2212, 2009.

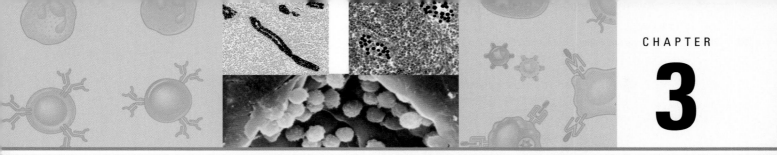

Leukocyte Circulation and Migration into Tissues

A unique property of the immune system that distinguishes it from all other tissue systems in the body is the constant and highly regulated movement of its major cellular components through the blood, into tissues, and often back into the blood again. This movement accomplishes three main functions (Fig. 3-1):

- Delivery of leukocytes of myeloid lineage (mainly neutrophils and monocytes) from the circulation into tissue sites of infection or injury, where the cells perform their protective functions of eliminating infectious pathogens, clearing dead tissues, and repairing the damage.
- Delivery of lymphocytes from their sites of maturation (bone marrow or thymus) to secondary lymphoid organs, where they recognize antigens and differentiate into effector lymphocytes.

- Delivery of effector lymphocytes from the secondary lymphoid organs in which they were produced to sites of infection in any tissue, where they perform their protective functions.

The migration of a leukocyte out of the blood and into a particular tissue, or to a site of an infection or injury, is often called leukocyte **homing**, and the general process of leukocyte movement from blood into tissues is called **migration** or **recruitment**. The ability of lymphocytes to repeatedly home to secondary lymphoid organs, reside there transiently, and return to the blood is called **recirculation**. The recruitment of leukocytes and plasma proteins from the blood to sites of infection and tissue injury is a major part of the process of **inflammation**. Inflammation is triggered by recognition of microbes and dead tissues in innate immune responses and is refined and prolonged during adaptive immune responses. The inflammatory response delivers the cells and molecules of host defense to the sites where offending agents need to be combated. The same process is responsible for causing tissue damage and underlies many important diseases. We will return to inflammation in the context of innate immunity in Chapter 4 and in the discussion of inflammatory diseases in Chapter 19.

OVERVIEW OF LEUKOCYTE MIGRATION

Leukocyte homing and recruitment to any tissue are governed by some common principles.

- Naive lymphocytes continuously migrate mainly into secondary lymphoid tissues, and not into other tissues whether or not there is infection or injury, while lymphocytes that have been previously activated by antigen (e.g., effector lymphocytes) as well as myeloid leukocytes preferentially home into tissues where there is infection or tissue injury.
- Leukocyte homing and recruitment require the temporary adhesion of the leukocyte to the endothelial lining of blood vessels, a process that involves molecules on the surfaces of both the leukocytes (homing receptors and chemokine receptors) and endothelial cells (addressins and chemokines).
- Endothelial cells at sites of infection and tissue injury are activated by cytokines secreted by macrophages and

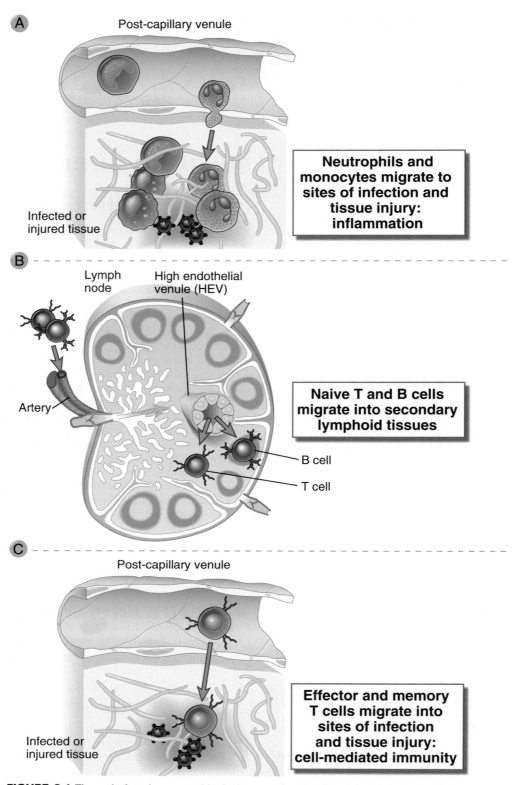

FIGURE 3-1 The main functions served by leukocyte migration from blood into tissues. **A,** Neutrophils and monocytes that arise in the bone marrow, circulate in the blood, and are recruited into tissue sites of infection or injury, where they eliminate infectious pathogens, clear dead tissues, and repair the damage. **B,** Naive lymphocytes that arise in bone marrow or thymus home to secondary lymphoid organs, such as lymph nodes (or spleen, not shown), where they become activated by antigens and differentiate into effector lymphocytes. **C,** Effector lymphocytes that develop in secondary lymphoid organs migrate into tissue sites of infection, where they participate in microbial defense.

other tissue cells at these sites, resulting in increased expression of adhesion molecules and chemokines. The consequence is increased adhesiveness of the endothelial cells for circulating myeloid leukocytes and previously activated lymphocytes.

Because the expression of the molecules that mediate leukocyte-endothelial adhesion is typically dependent on the activation of the cells involved, leukocytes migrate through endothelium mainly when they need to, following encounter with microbes and necrotic tissues. These are the most common stimuli for activating leukocytes and endothelial cells.

Leukocyte recruitment from the blood into tissues requires adhesion of the leukocytes to the endothelial lining of post-capillary venules and then movement through the endothelium and vessel wall into the extravascular tissue. This is a multistep process in which each step is orchestrated by different types of molecules, including chemokines and adhesion molecules. The same basic process occurs for different types of leukocytes (neutrophils, monocytes, and naive and effector lymphocytes) homing to different types of tissues (secondary lymphoid organs, infected tissues), although the specific chemokines and adhesion molecules vary in ways that result in different migration properties for each cell type. Before describing the process, we will discuss the properties and functions of the adhesion molecules and chemokines that are involved in leukocyte recruitment.

ADHESION MOLECULES ON LEUKOCYTES AND ENDOTHELIAL CELLS INVOLVED IN LEUKOCYTE RECRUITMENT

Adhesion of circulating leukocytes to vascular endothelial cells is mediated by two classes of molecules, called **selectins** and **integrins**, and their ligands. The expression of these molecules varies among different types of

leukocytes and in blood vessels at different locations, and these differences influence which cell types migrate preferentially into which tissues.

Selectins and Selectin Ligands

Selectins are plasma membrane carbohydrate-binding adhesion molecules that mediate an initial step of low-affinity adhesion of circulating leukocytes to endothelial cells lining post-capillary venules (Table 3-1). The extracellular domains of selectins are similar to C-type lectins, so called because they bind carbohydrate structures (the definition of *lectins*) in a calcium-dependent manner. Selectins and their ligands are expressed on leukocytes and endothelial cells.

Endothelial cells express two types of selectins, called **P-selectin** (CD62P) and **E-selectin** (CD62E). P-selectin, so called because it was first found in platelets, is stored in cytoplasmic granules of endothelial cells and is rapidly redistributed to the lumenal surface in response to histamine from mast cells and thrombin generated during blood coagulation. E-selectin is synthesized and expressed on the endothelial cell surface within 1 to 2 hours in response to the cytokines interleukin-1 (IL-1) and tumor necrosis factor (TNF), which are produced by tissue macrophages in response to infection. Microbial products such as lipopolysaccharide (LPS) also stimulate E-selectin expression on endothelial cells. We will describe IL-1, TNF, and LPS in our discussion of inflammation in Chapter 4.

The ligands on leukocytes that bind to E-selectin and P-selectin on endothelial cells are complex sialylated carbohydrate groups related to the Lewis X or Lewis A family. These chemical structures are present on various surface glycoproteins of granulocytes, monocytes, and some previously activated effector and memory T cells. The best defined of these is the tetrasaccharide sialyl Lewis X (sLeX). A leukocyte membrane glycoprotein called P-selectin glycoprotein ligand 1 (PSGL-1) is post-translationally

TABLE 3-1	**Major Leukocyte-Endothelial Adhesion Molecules**		
Family	**Molecule**	**Distribution**	**Ligand (molecule; cell type)**
Selectin	P-selectin (CD62P)	Endothelium activated by histamine or thrombin	Sialyl Lewis X on PSGL-1 and other glycoproteins; neutrophils, monocytes, T cells (effector, memory)
	E-selectin (CD62E)	Endothelium activated by cytokines (TNF, IL-1)	Sialyl Lewis X (e.g., CLA-1) on glycoproteins; neutrophils, monocytes, T cells (effector, memory)
	L-selectin (CD62L)	Neutrophils, monocytes, T cells (naive and central memory), B cells (naive)	Sialyl Lewis X/PNAd on GlyCAM-1, CD34, MadCAM-1, others; endothelium (HEV)
Integrin	LFA-1 (CD11aCD18)	Neutrophils, monocytes, T cells (naive, effector, memory), B cells (naive)	ICAM-1 (CD54), ICAM-2 (CD102); endothelium (upregulated when cytokine activated)
	Mac-1 (CD11bCD18)	Neutrophils, monocytes, dendritic cells	ICAM-1 (CD54), ICAM-2 (CD102); endothelium (upregulated when cytokine activated)
	VLA-4 (CD49aCD29)	Monocytes, T cells (naive, effector, memory)	VCAM-1 (CD106); endothelium (upregulated when cytokine activated)
	$\alpha_4\beta_7$ (CD49dCD29)	Monocytes, T cells (gut homing, naive, effector, memory), B cells (gut homing)	VCAM-1 (CD106), MadCAM-1; endothelium in gut and gut-associated lymphoid tissues

CLA-1, cutaneous lymphocyte antigen 1; *GlyCAM-1*, glycan-bearing cell adhesion molecule 1; *HEV*, high endothelial venule; *ICAM-1*, intracellular adhesion molecule 1; *IL-1*, interleukin-1; *LFA-1*, leukocyte function–associated antigen 1; *MadCAM-1*, mucosal addressin cell adhesion molecule 1; *PNAd*, peripheral node addressin; *PSGL-1*, P-selectin glycoprotein ligand 1; *TNF*, tumor necrosis factor; *VCAM-1*, vascular cell adhesion molecule 1; *VLA-4*, very late antigen 4.

modified to display the carbohydrate ligands for P-selectin. Several different molecules may display the carbohydrate ligands for E-selectin, including the glycoproteins PSGL-1 and E-selectin ligand-1 and some glycolipids.

A third selectin, called **L-selectin** (CD62L), is expressed on leukocytes and not on endothelial cells. The ligands for L-selectin are sialomucins on endothelial cells, whose expression is increased by cytokine activation of the cells. A major recognition determinant that L-selectin binds to on these sialomucins is sialyl 6-sulfo Lewis X. L-selectin on neutrophils promotes the adhesion of these cells to endothelial cells that are activated by IL-1, TNF, and other cytokines produced at sites of inflammation. In adaptive immunity, L-selectin is important for naive T and B lymphocytes to home into lymph nodes through specialized blood vessels called **high endothelial venules**. The sialomucin ligands on high endothelial venules that bind to L-selectin on naive lymphocytes are collectively called peripheral node addressin (PNAd). Leukocytes express L-selectin or the carbohydrate ligands for P-selectin and E-selectin at the tips of their microvilli, facilitating interactions with molecules on the endothelial cell surface.

Integrins and Integrin Ligands

Integrins are heterodimeric cell surface proteins composed of two noncovalently linked polypeptide chains that mediate adhesion of cells to other cells or to extracellular matrix, through specific binding interactions with various ligands. There are more than 30 different integrins, all with the same basic structure, containing one of more than 15 types of α chains and one of seven types of β chains. The extracellular globular heads of both chains contribute to interchain linking and to divalent cation-dependent ligand binding. The cytoplasmic domains of the integrins interact with cytoskeletal components (including vinculin, talin, actin, α-actinin, and tropomyosin). The name *integrin* for this family of proteins derives from the idea that these proteins coordinate (i.e., integrate) signals triggered by extracellular ligands with cytoskeleton-dependent motility, shape change, and phagocytic responses.

In the immune system, two important integrins that are expressed on leukocytes are **LFA-1** (leukocyte function–associated antigen 1, more precisely named $\alpha_L\beta_2$ or CD11aCD18) and **VLA-4** (very late antigen 4, or $\alpha_4\beta_1$ or CD49dCD29) (see Table 3-1). One important ligand for LFA-1 is intercellular adhesion molecule 1 (**ICAM-1,** CD54), a membrane glycoprotein expressed on cytokine-activated endothelial cells and on a variety of other cell types, including lymphocytes, dendritic cells, macrophages, fibroblasts, and keratinocytes. The extracellular portion of ICAM-1 is composed of globular domains, called immunoglobulin (Ig) domains, which share sequence homology and structural features with domains found in Ig molecules. Many proteins in the immune system contain Ig domains and belong to the Ig superfamily (see Chapter 5). LFA-1 binding to ICAM-1 is important for leukocyte-endothelial interactions (discussed later) and T cell interactions with antigen-presenting cells (see Chapter 6). Two other Ig superfamily ligands for LFA-1 are ICAM-2,

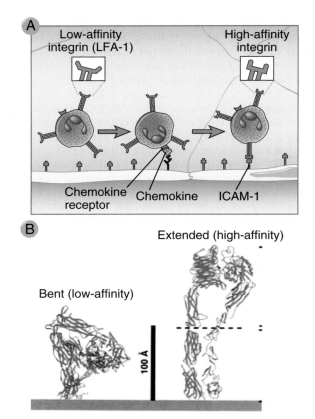

FIGURE 3-2 Integrin activation. A, The integrins on blood leukocytes are normally in a low-affinity state. If a leukocyte comes close to endothelial cells, such as when selectin-dependent rolling of leukocytes occurs, then chemokines displayed on the endothelial surface can bind chemokine receptors on the leukocyte. Chemokine receptor signaling then occurs, which activates the leukocyte integrins, increasing their affinity for their ligands on the endothelial cells. **B,** Ribbon diagrams are shown of bent and extended conformations of a leukocyte integrin, corresponding to low- and high-affinity states, respectively. *(**B,** From Takagi J, Springer TA: Integrin activation and structural rearrangement,* Immunological Reviews *186:141–163, 2002.)*

which is expressed on endothelial cells, and ICAM-3, which is expressed on lymphocytes. VLA-4 binds to vascular cell adhesion molecule 1 (**VCAM-1,** CD106), an Ig superfamily protein expressed on cytokine-activated endothelial cells in some tissues. Other integrins also play roles in innate and adaptive immune responses. For example, Mac-1 ($\alpha_M\beta_2$, CD11bCD18) on circulating monocytes binds to ICAM-1 and mediates adhesion to endothelium. Mac-1 also functions as a complement receptor, binding particles opsonized with a product of complement activation called the inactivated C3b (iC3b) fragment (discussed in Chapters 4 and 13), and thereby enhances phagocytosis of microbes.

An important feature of integrins is their ability to respond to intracellular signals by rapidly increasing their affinity for their ligands (Fig. 3-2). This is referred to as integrin activation and occurs in all leukocytes in response to chemokine binding to chemokine receptors and in T cells when antigen binds to antigen receptors. Chemokine and antigen receptor engagement in cells induces biochemical signals that involve GTP-binding proteins (described in more detail in Chapter 7), eventually leading to the association of RAP family molecules and cytoskeleton-interacting proteins with the cytoplasmic tails of the integrin proteins. This results in conformational changes in the extracellular domains of the integrins that lead to increased affinity. In the low-affinity state, the stalks of the extracellular domains of each integrin subunit are bent over, and the ligand-binding globular heads are close to the membrane. In response to alterations in the cytoplasmic tail, the stalks extend, bringing the globular heads away from the membrane to a position where they more effectively interact with their ligands (see Fig. 3-2). The process by which intracellular signals, generated in response to chemokines or antigen, alter the binding functions of the extracellular domain of integrins is called inside-out signaling.

Chemokines also induce membrane clustering of integrins. This results in increased local concentration of integrins on the cell surface, leading to increased avidity of integrin interactions with ligands on the endothelial cells, and therefore tighter binding of the leukocytes to the endothelium.

CHEMOKINES AND CHEMOKINE RECEPTORS

Chemokines are a large family of structurally homologous cytokines that stimulate leukocyte movement and regulate the migration of leukocytes from the blood to tissues. The name *chemokine* is a contraction of chemotactic cytokine. We referred to the role of chemokines in the organization of lymphoid tissues in Chapter 2, and now we will describe the general properties of this family of cytokines and their multiple functions in innate and adaptive immunity. Table 3-2 summarizes the major features of individual chemokines and their receptors.

Chemokine Structure, Production, and Receptors

There are about 50 human chemokines, all of which are 8- to 10-kD polypeptides that contain two internal disulfide loops. Chemokines are classified into four families on the basis of the number and location of N-terminal cysteine residues. The two major families are the CC (also called β) chemokines, in which the two defining cysteine residues are adjacent, and the CXC (or α) family, in which these residues are separated by one amino acid. These differences correlate with the organization of the subfamilies into separate gene clusters. A few additional chemokines have either a single cysteine (C family) or two cysteines separated by three amino acids (CX_3C). Chemokines were originally named on the basis of how they were identified and what responses they triggered, but a standard nomenclature has been adopted, based in part on which receptors the chemokines bind to (see Table 3-2). Although there are exceptions, recruitment of neutrophils is mainly mediated by CXC chemokines, monocyte recruitment is more dependent on CC chemokines, and lymphocyte recruitment is mediated by both CXC and CC chemokines.

The chemokines of the CC and CXC subfamilies are produced by leukocytes and by several types of tissue cells, such as endothelial cells, epithelial cells, and fibroblasts. In many of these cells, secretion of chemokines is induced by recognition of microbes through various cellular receptors of the innate immune system, discussed in Chapter 4. In addition, inflammatory cytokines, including TNF, IL-1, and IL-17, induce chemokine production. Several CC chemokines are also produced by activated T cells, providing a link between adaptive immunity and recruitment of inflammatory leukocytes.

The receptors for chemokines belong to the seven-transmembrane, guanosine triphosphate (GTP)–binding (G) protein–coupled receptor (GPCR) superfamily. These receptors initiate intracellular responses through associated trimeric G proteins. The G proteins stimulate cytoskeletal changes and polymerization of actin and myosin filaments, resulting in increased cell motility. As previously discussed, these signals also change the conformation of cell surface integrins and increase the affinity of the integrins for their ligands. Chemokine receptors may be rapidly downregulated by exposure to the chemokine, and this is a likely mechanism for termination of responses.

Different combinations of chemokine receptors are expressed on different types of leukocytes, which result in distinct patterns of migration of the leukocytes. There are 10 distinct receptors for CC chemokines (called CCR1 through CCR10), six for CXC chemokines (called CXCR1 through CXCR6), and one for CX_3CL1 (called CX_3CR1) (see Table 3-2). Chemokine receptors are expressed on all leukocytes, with the greatest number and diversity seen on T cells. The receptors exhibit overlapping specificity for chemokines within each family, and the pattern of cellular expression of the receptors determines which cell types respond to which chemokines. Certain chemokine receptors, notably CCR5 and CXCR4, act as coreceptors for the human immunodeficiency virus (HIV) (see Chapter 21).

Biologic Actions of Chemokines

Some chemokines are produced by cells in response to external stimuli and are involved in inflammatory reactions, and other chemokines are produced constitutively in tissues and play a role in tissue organization. The main actions of chemokines are enhancing adhesion of circulating leukocytes to endothelium through integrin activation and stimulating directed leukocyte movement in tissues by chemoattraction.

- ***Chemokines are essential for the recruitment of circulating leukocytes from blood vessels into extravascular sites.*** Leukocyte recruitment from blood into tissues is regulated by the actions of several chemokines. Different chemokines act on different cells and, in coordination with the types of adhesion molecules expressed, thus control the nature of the inflammatory infiltrate. Chemokines play two roles in inflammation.
  - ○ ***Increased adhesion of leukocytes to endothelium.*** Chemokines produced in the tissues bind to heparan sulfate proteoglycans on endothelial cells that line post-capillary venules. The bound chemokines are displayed in this way to circulating leukocytes that are attached to the endothelial surfaces through adhesion molecule interactions. Endothelial display

TABLE 3-2　Chemokines and Chemokine Receptors

Chemokine	Original Name	Chemokine Receptor	Major Function
CC Chemokines			
CCL1	I-309	CCR8	Monocyte recruitment and endothelial cell migration
CCL2	MCP-1	CCR2	Mixed leukocyte recruitment
CCL3	MIP-1α	CCR1, CCR5	Mixed leukocyte recruitment
CCL4	MIP-1β	CCR5	T cell, dendritic cell, monocyte, and NK recruitment; HIV coreceptor
CCL5	RANTES	CCR1, CCR3, CCR5	Mixed leukocyte recruitment
CCL7	MCP-3	CCR1, CCR2, CCR3	Mixed leukocyte recruitment
CCL8	MCP-2	CCR3, CCR5	Mixed leukocyte recruitment
CCL9	MIP-1γ	CCR1	DC recruitment, osteoclast differentiation
CCL11	Eotaxin	CCR3	Eosinophil, basophil, and T_H2 recruitment
CCL12	MCP-5	CCR2	Mixed leukocyte recruitment
CCL13	MCP-4	CCR2, CCR3	Mixed leukocyte recruitment
CCL14	HHC-1	CCR1, CCR5	
CCL15	MIP-1δ	CCR1, CCR3	Mixed leukocyte recruitment
CCL16	HHC-4	CCR1, CCR2	Lymphocyte and monocyte recruitment
CCL17	TARC	CCR4	T cell recruitment
CCL18	DC-CK1	CCR8	Lymphocyte and dendritic cell homing
CCL19	MIP-3β/ELC	CCR7	T cell and dendritic cell migration into parafollicular zones of lymph nodes
CCL20	MIP-3α	CCR6	Th17 recruitment, DC positioning in tissue
CCL21	SLC	CCR7	T cell and dendritic cell migration into parafollicular zones of lymph nodes
CCL22	MDC	CCR4	NK cell, T cell recruitment
CCL23	MPIF-1	CCR1	Monocyte, neutrophil, T cell migration
CCL24	Eotaxin-2	CCR3	Eosinophil, basophil, and T_H2 recruitment
CCL25	TECK	CCR9	Lymphocyte recruitment into intestine
CCL26	Eotaxin-3	CCR3	Eosinophil, basophil, and T_H2 recruitment
CCL27	CTACK	CCR10	T cell recruitment into skin
CCL28	MEC	CCR10	T and B cell homing to mucosa
CXC Chemokines			
CXCL1	GROα	CXCR2	Neutrophil recruitment
CXCL2	GROβ	CXCR2	Neutrophil recruitment
CXCL3	GROγ	CXCR2	Neutrophil recruitment
CXCL4	PF4	CXCR3B	Platelet aggregation
CXCL5	ENA-78	CXCR2	Neutrophil recruitment
CXCL6	GCP-2	CXCR1, CXCR2	Neutrophil recruitment
CXCL7	NAP-2	CXCR2	Neutrophil recruitment
CXCL8	IL-8	CXCR1, CXCR-2	Neutrophil recruitment
CXCL9	Mig	CXCR3	Effector T cell recruitment
CXCL10	IP-10	CXCR3, CXCR3B	Effector T cell recruitment
CXCL11	I-TAC	CXCR3, CXCR7	Effector T cell recruitment
CXCL12	SDF-1$\alpha\beta$	CXCR4	Mixed leukocyte recruitment; HIV coreceptor
CXCL13	BCA-1	CXCR5	B cell migration into follicles; T follicular helper cell migration into follicles
CXCL14	BRAK		Monocyte and dendritic cell migration
CXCL16	—	CXCR6	Macrophage scavenger receptor
C Chemokines			
XCL1	Lymphotactin	XCR1	T cell and NK cell recruitment
XCL2	SCM-1β	XCL1	
CX$_3$C Chemokines			
CX$_3$CL1	Fractalkine	CX$_3$CR1	T cell, NK cell, and monocyte recruitment; CTL and NK cell activation

provides a high local concentration of chemokines, enabling them to bind to chemokine receptors on the leukocytes. Signals from chemokine receptors lead to enhanced integrin affinity, which results in firm adhesion of the leukocyte, a critical step for migration of leukocytes out of blood vessels into extravascular tissue.

○ *Migration of leukocytes to site of infection or tissue damage*. Chemokines produced in the extravascular tissues act on leukocytes that have exited the circulation and stimulate movement of leukocytes along the concentration gradient of the secreted protein toward its source, a process called chemokinesis. Thus, leukocytes migrate toward infected and damaged cells in tissues.

● *Chemokines are involved in the development of lymphoid organs, and they regulate the traffic of lymphocytes and other leukocytes through different regions of peripheral lymphoid tissues.* We discussed the function of chemokines in the anatomic organization of lymphoid tissues in Chapter 2.

● *Chemokines are required for the migration of dendritic cells from sites of infection into draining lymph nodes.* Dendritic cells are activated by microbes in peripheral tissues, and they then migrate to lymph nodes to inform T lymphocytes of the presence of infection (discussed in Chapter 6). This migration depends on expression of

a chemokine receptor, CCR7, which is induced when the dendritic cell encounters microbes. CCR7 binds a chemokine produced by lymphatic endothelial cells in tissues, thus promoting the movement of the dendritic cell into the lymphatic vessels that drain into lymph nodes. Once in a lymph node, the dendritic cells are attracted by the same chemokines produced in the interfollicular zones, where naive T cells also migrate in response to these chemokines. This explains how dendritic cells and naive T cells localize to the same place in lymph nodes, enabling the dendritic cells to present antigen to the T cells.

LEUKOCYTE-ENDOTHELIAL INTERACTIONS AND LEUKOCYTE RECRUITMENT INTO TISSUES

Selectins, integrins, and chemokines work in concert to regulate the migration of leukocytes into tissues. Studies of these interactions in vitro under conditions that mimic flowing blood, and in vivo using intravital microscopic techniques, have established a sequence of events common to migration of most leukocytes into most tissues (Fig. 3-3). These events include the following.

● *Selectin-mediated rolling of leukocytes on endothelium.* Endothelial cells lining postcapillary venules are

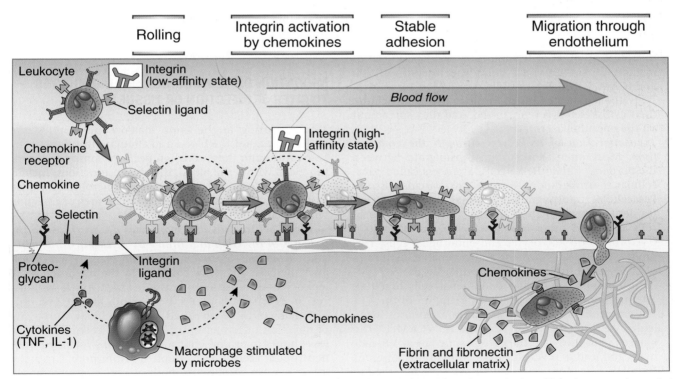

FIGURE 3-3 Multistep leukocyte-endothelial interactions mediating leukocyte recruitment into tissues. At sites of infection, macrophages that have encountered microbes produce cytokines (such as TNF and IL-1) that activate the endothelial cells of nearby venules to produce selectins, ligands for integrins, and chemokines. Selectins mediate weak tethering of blood leukocytes on the endothelium, and the shear force of blood flow causes the leukocytes to roll along the endothelial surface. Chemokines produced in the surrounding infected tissues or by the endothelial cells are displayed on the endothelial surface and bind to receptors on the rolling leukocytes, which results in activation of the leukocyte integrins to a high-affinity binding state. The activated integrins bind to their Ig superfamily ligands on the endothelial cells, and this mediates firm adhesion of leukocytes. The leukocytes then crawl to junctions between endothelial cells and migrate through the venular wall. Neutrophils, monocytes, and T lymphocytes use essentially the same mechanisms to migrate out of the blood.

activated in response to microbes, cytokines (including TNF and IL-1) produced by macrophages and other tissue cells that encounter the microbes, and other mediators such as histamine and thrombin that may be produced during various inflammatory reactions. Cytokines stimulate endothelial expression of E-selectin and other mediators induce surface expression of P-selectin. At sites of inflammation, blood vessels dilate and blood flow slows. As a result, leukocytes, being larger than red cells, tend to move away from the central axial flow and closer to the vessel lining, a process known as margination. This allows the ligands for E- and P-selectins expressed on the microvilli of the leukocytes to bind to the selectins on the endothelial cells. Because selectin-selectin ligand interactions are of low affinity (K_d ~100 μm) with a fast off-rate, they are easily disrupted by the shear force of the flowing blood. As a result, the leukocytes repetitively detach and bind again and thus roll along the endothelial surface. This slowing of leukocytes on the endothelium allows the next set of stimuli in the multistep process to act on the leukocytes.

- *Chemokine-mediated increase in affinity of integrins.* Chemokines displayed on endothelial cells of post-capillary venules at an infection site bind to their receptors on the rolling leukocytes. As discussed before, this results in stronger binding of leukocyte integrins to their ligands on the endothelial surface.
- *Stable integrin-mediated adhesion of leukocytes to endothelium.* In parallel with the activation of integrins, the expression of their ligands on the endothelial cells is upregulated by inflammatory cytokines and microbial products at the infection site. These ligands include VCAM-1, which binds the integrin VLA-4, and ICAM-1, which binds LFA-1 and Mac-1 integrins. Thus, the leukocytes attach firmly to the endothelium, their cytoskeleton is reorganized, and they spread out on the endothelial surface.
- *Transmigration of leukocytes through the endothelium.* Most often, leukocytes transmigrate between the borders of endothelial cells, a process called paracellular transmigration, to reach extravascular tissues. Paracellular transmigration depends on integrins on the leukocytes and their ligands on the endothelial cells as well as other proteins, notably CD31, which is expressed on leukocytes and endothelial cells. This process requires a transient and reversible disruption of adherens junction proteins, primarily the VE-cadherin complex, that hold endothelial cells together. The mechanism responsible for disruption of the VE-cadherin complex involves activation of kinases when leukocyte integrins bind ICAM-1 or VCAM-1. The kinases phosphorylate the cytoplasmic tail of VE-cadherin and lead to reversible disruption of the adherens complex. Less often, leukocytes have been observed to move through endothelial cells rather than between them, by a poorly understood process called transcellular migration.

These basic steps are seen in the migration of all leukocytes through the endothelium. However, neutrophils, monocytes, and different subsets of lymphocytes differ in which tissues they migrate into and when they do so in inflammatory reactions and the steady state. This specificity in leukocyte migration is based on the expression of distinct combinations of adhesion molecule and chemokine receptors, as we will discuss in more detail later.

Evidence for the essential role of selectins, integrins and chemokines in leukocyte migration has come from gene knockout mice and rare inherited human diseases called *leukocyte adhesion deficiencies*. For example, mice lacking fucosyltransferases, which are enzymes required to synthesize the carbohydrate ligands that bind to selectins, have marked defects in leukocyte migration and immune responses. Humans who lack the Golgi fucose transporter needed to express the carbohydrate ligands for E-selectin and P-selectin on neutrophils have similar problems, resulting in a syndrome called type 2 leukocyte adhesion deficiency (LAD-2) (see Chapter 21). Similarly, an autosomal recessive inherited deficiency in the *CD18* gene, which encodes the β subunit of LFA-1 and Mac-1, is the cause of an immune deficiency disease called type 1 leukocyte adhesion deficiency (LAD-1). These disorders are characterized by recurrent bacterial and fungal infections, lack of neutrophil accumulation at sites of infection, and defects in adherence-dependent lymphocyte functions. Rare human mutations in the signaling pathways linking chemokine receptors to integrin activation also result in impaired leukocyte adhesion and recruitment into tissues and therefore ineffective leukocyte defense against infections, a syndrome called type 3 leukocyte adhesion deficiency (LAD-3).

MIGRATION OF NEUTROPHILS AND MONOCYTES TO SITES OF INFECTION OR TISSUE INJURY

After maturing in the bone marrow, neutrophils and monocytes enter the blood and circulate throughout the body. Although these cells can perform some phagocytic functions within the blood, their main functions, including phagocytosis and destruction of microbes and dead tissue cells, take place in extravascular sites of infection virtually anywhere in the body.

Blood neutrophils and monocytes are recruited to tissue sites of infection and injury by a selectin-, integrin-, and chemokine-dependent multistep process, which follows the basic sequence common to the migration of all leukocytes into tissues, discussed earlier. As we will discuss in detail in Chapter 4, neutrophils are the first type of leukocyte to be recruited from the blood into a site of infection or tissue injury. Monocyte recruitment follows hours later and continues, perhaps for days, after neutrophil recruitment stops. Furthermore, in some inflammatory sites, neutrophils are not recruited at all, but monocytes are. These different migratory behaviors likely reflect variations in relative expression of adhesion molecules and chemokine receptors on neutrophils versus monocytes. Neutrophils express CXCR1 and CXCR2, which bind multiple GRO family chemokines including CXCL8 (IL-8), the major chemokine supporting neutrophil migration into tissues (see Table 3-2).

Early neutrophil recruitment is a consequence of early and abundant CXCL8 production by tissue resident macrophages in response to infections. In contrast to neutrophils, classical monocytes, which are the main type of monocyte recruited to inflammatory sites, express CCR2. This receptor binds several chemokines, the most important one for monocyte recruitment being CCL2 (MCP-1). Thus, monocyte recruitment occurs when resident tissue cells express CCL2 in response to infection. Nonclassical monocytes lack CCR2 but express CX_3CR1. The ligand for this receptor, CX_3CL1 (also called fractalkine), is expressed both in soluble form and as a membrane-bound molecule that can support adhesion of monocytes to endothelium.

MIGRATION AND RECIRCULATION OF T LYMPHOCYTES

Lymphocytes are continuously moving through the blood, lymphatic vessels, secondary lymphoid tissues, and peripheral nonlymphoid tissues, and distinct populations of lymphocytes show different trafficking patterns through these sites (Fig. 3-4). When a mature naive T cell emerges from the thymus and enters the blood, it homes to lymph nodes, spleen, or mucosal lymphoid tissues and migrates into the T cell zones of these secondary lymphoid tissues. If the T cell does not recognize antigen in these sites, it remains naive and leaves the nodes or mucosal tissue through lymphatics and eventually drains

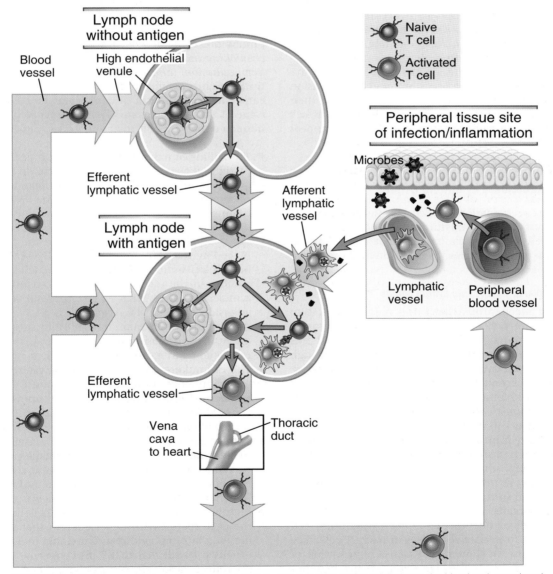

FIGURE 3-4 Pathways of T lymphocyte recirculation. Naive T cells preferentially leave the blood and enter lymph nodes across the high endothelial venules. Dendritic cells bearing antigen enter the lymph nodes through lymphatic vessels. If the T cells recognize antigen, they are activated, and they return to the circulation through the efferent lymphatics and the thoracic duct, which empties into the superior vena cava, then into the heart, and ultimately into the arterial circulation. Effector and memory T cells preferentially leave the blood and enter peripheral tissues through venules at sites of inflammation. Recirculation through peripheral lymphoid organs other than lymph nodes is not shown.

back into the blood stream. Once back in the blood, a naive T cell repeats its cycle of homing to secondary lymphoid tissues. This trafficking pattern of naive lymphocytes, called **lymphocyte recirculation**, maximizes the chances that the small number of naive lymphocytes that are specific for a particular foreign antigen will encounter that antigen if it shows up anywhere in the body. Lymphocytes that have recognized and become activated by antigen within secondary lymphoid tissues proliferate and differentiate to produce thousands of effector and memory cells. The effector and memory lymphocytes may move back into the blood stream and then migrate into sites of infection or inflammation in peripheral (non-lymphoid) tissues.

Some effector lymphocyte subsets preferentially home to a particular tissue, such as skin or gut (see Chapter 14). The existence of different homing patterns ensures that different subsets of lymphocytes are delivered to the tissue microenvironments where they are required to combat different types of microbes and not, wastefully, to places where they would serve no purpose. In the following section, we describe the mechanisms and pathways of lymphocyte recirculation and homing. Our discussion emphasizes T cells because more is known about their movement through tissues than is known about B cell recirculation, but many of the same mechanisms appear to apply to both cell types.

Recirculation of Naive T Lymphocytes Between Blood and Secondary Lymphoid Organs

T lymphocyte recirculation depends on mechanisms that control entry of naive T cells from the blood into lymph nodes as well as molecular signals that control when naive T cells exit the nodes. We will discuss these two mechanisms separately.

Migration of Naive T Cells into Lymph Nodes

The homing mechanisms that bring naive T cells into lymph nodes are very efficient, resulting in a net flux of lymphocytes through lymph nodes of up to 25×10^9 cells each day. On average, each lymphocyte goes through one node once a day. Peripheral tissue inflammation, which usually accompanies infections, causes a significant increase of blood flow into lymph nodes and consequently an increase in T cell influx into lymph nodes draining the site of inflammation. At the same time, egress of the T cells into efferent lymphatics is transiently reduced by mechanisms we will discuss later, so that T cells stay in lymph nodes that drain sites of inflammation longer than in other lymph nodes. Protein antigens are concentrated in the lymph nodes and other secondary lymphoid organs, where they are presented to T cells by dendritic cells, the type of antigen-presenting cell that is best able to initiate responses of naive T cells (see Chapter 6). Thus, movement and transient retention of naive T cells in the secondary lymphoid organs, together with capture and concentration of antigen, maximize the chances of T cell activation and initiation of an adaptive immune response.

Homing of naive T cells into lymph nodes and mucosa-associated lymphoid tissues occurs through specialized post-capillary venules called high endothelial venules (HEVs) located in the T cell zones. Naive T lymphocytes are delivered to secondary lymphoid tissues through arterial blood flow, and they leave the circulation and migrate into the stroma of lymph nodes through HEVs. These vessels are lined with plump endothelial cells and not the flat endothelial cells that are typical of other venules (Fig. 3-5). HEVs are also present in mucosal lymphoid tissues, such as Peyer's patches in the gut, but not in the spleen. The endothelial cells of HEVs are specialized to display certain adhesion molecules and chemokines on their surfaces, discussed later, which support the selective homing of only certain populations of lymphocytes. Certain cytokines, such as lymphotoxin, are required for HEV development. In fact, HEVs may develop in extralymphoid sites of chronic inflammation where such cytokines are produced for prolonged periods.

Naive T cell migration out of the blood through the HEVs into the lymph node parenchyma is a multistep process consisting of selectin-mediated rolling of the cells, chemokine-induced integrin activation, integrin-mediated firm adhesion, and transmigration through the vessel wall. This process includes the sequential events described earlier for migration of all leukocytes (see Fig. 3-3), but some of the molecules involved are relatively specific for homing of naive T cells to lymph nodes (Fig. 3-6).

- The rolling of naive T cells on HEVs in peripheral lymphoid organs is mediated by L-selectin on the lymphocytes binding to its carbohydrate ligand, peripheral node addressin (PNAd), on HEVs. The PNAd carbohydrate groups that bind L-selectin may be attached to different sialomucins on the HEV in different tissues. For example, on lymph node HEVs, the PNAd is displayed by two sialomucins, called GlyCAM-1 (glycan-bearing cell adhesion molecule 1) and CD34. In Peyer's patches in the intestinal wall, the L-selectin ligand is a molecule called MadCAM-1 (mucosal addressin cell adhesion molecule 1).

- As with leukocyte migration in other sites, the subsequent firm adhesion of the naive T cells to the HEVs is mediated by integrins, mainly LFA-1.

- The chemokines that activate the naive T cell integrins to a high-affinity state are CCL19 and CCL21, which are uniquely involved in leukocyte homing to T cell zones of lymphoid tissues (see Chapter 2). The main source of CCL19 and CCL21 is fibroblast reticular cells within the T cell zone, and CCL19 is also constitutively produced by HEVs. These chemokines are displayed on the surface of the HEV and recognized by rolling lymphocytes. Both these chemokines bind to the chemokine receptor CCR7, which is expressed at high levels on naive lymphocytes. This interaction of the chemokines with CCR7 ensures that naive T cells increase integrin avidity and are able to adhere firmly to HEVs. Recall that CCR7 also governs dendritic cell migration via lymphatics into lymph nodes.

The important role for L-selectin and chemokines in naive T cell homing to secondary lymphoid tissues is supported by many different experimental observations. Lymphocytes from L-selectin knockout mice do

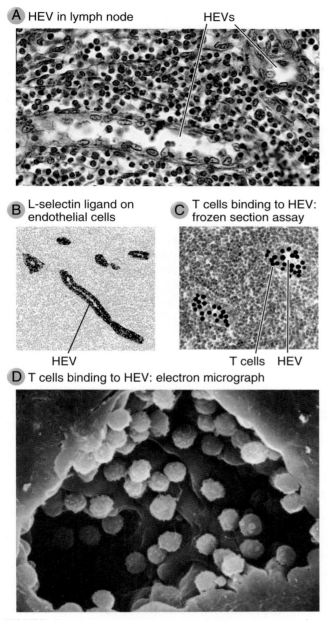

A HEV in lymph node   HEVs

B L-selectin ligand on endothelial cells

C T cells binding to HEV: frozen section assay

HEV

T cells   HEV

D T cells binding to HEV: electron micrograph

FIGURE 3-5 High endothelial venules. **A,** Light micrograph of an HEV in a lymph node illustrating the tall endothelial cells. *(Courtesy of Dr. Steve Rosen, Department of Anatomy, University of California, San Francisco.)* **B,** Expression of L-selectin ligand on HEVs, stained with a specific antibody by the immunoperoxidase technique. (The location of the antibody is revealed by a brown reaction product of peroxidase, which is coupled to the antibody; see Appendix IV for details.) The HEVs are abundant in the T cell zone of the lymph node. *(Courtesy of Drs. Steve Rosen and Akio Kikuta, Department of Anatomy, University of California, San Francisco.)* **C,** A binding assay in which lymphocytes are incubated with frozen sections of a lymph node. The lymphocytes (stained dark blue) bind selectively to HEVs. *(Courtesy of Dr. Steve Rosen, Department of Anatomy, University of California, San Francisco.)* **D,** Scanning electron micrograph of an HEV with lymphocytes attached to the luminal surface of the endothelial cells. *(Courtesy of J. Emerson and T. Yednock, University of California, San Francisco, School of Medicine. From Rosen SD, Stoolman LM: Potential role of cell surface lectin in lymphocyte recirculation. In Olden K, Parent J [Eds.]: Vertebrate lectins. New York, 1987, Van Nostrand Reinhold.)*

not bind to peripheral lymph node HEVs, and the mice have a marked reduction in the number of lymphocytes in peripheral lymph nodes. There are very few naive T cells in the lymph nodes of mice with genetic deficiencies in CCL19 and CCL21, or CCR7.

Exit of T Cells from Lymph Nodes

Naive T cells that have homed into lymph nodes but fail to recognize antigen and are not activated will eventually return to the blood stream. This return to the blood completes one recirculation loop and provides the naive T cells another chance to enter secondary lymphoid tissues and search for the antigens they can recognize. The major route of reentry into the blood is through the efferent lymphatics, perhaps via other lymph nodes in the same chain, then through the lymphatic vasculature to the thoracic or right lymphatic ducts, and finally into the superior vena cava or right subclavian vein.

The exit of naive T cells from lymph nodes is dependent on a lipid chemoattractant called sphingosine 1-phosphate (S1P), which binds to a signaling receptor on T cells called sphingosine 1-phosphate receptor 1 (S1PR1) (Fig. 3-7). S1P is present at higher concentrations in the blood and lymph than in tissues. This concentration gradient is maintained because an S1P-degrading enzyme, S1P lyase, is present in most tissues, so the lipid is catabolized in tissues more than in the lymph and blood. S1PR1 is a G protein–coupled receptor. Signals generated by S1P binding to S1PR1 on naive T cells stimulate directed movement of the cells along the S1P concentration gradient out of the lymph node parenchyma. Circulating naive T cells have very little surface S1PR1 because the high blood concentration of S1P causes internalization of the receptor. After a naive T cell enters a lymph node, where S1P concentrations are low, the surface S1PR1 is reexpressed over a period of several hours. This time lag allows a naive T cell to interact with antigen-presenting cells. Once the S1PR1 receptor is expressed, the T cell leaves the lymph node and is directed down the S1P concentration gradient into the efferent lymphatic.

If a naive T cell is activated by antigen in the lymph node, the reexpression of S1PR1 is suppressed for several days, and therefore the ability of the cells to leave the lymphoid tissue in response to an S1P gradient is delayed. This suppression of S1PR1 is controlled in part by cytokines called type I interferons that are expressed during innate immune responses to infections, as we will discuss in Chapter 4. Antigenic stimulation and interferons together increase the expression of a T cell membrane protein called CD69, which binds to S1PR1 and reduces its cell surface expression. Thus, the activated T cell becomes transiently insensitive to the S1P gradient. This allows the antigen-activated T cells to remain in the lymphoid organ and undergo clonal expansion and differentiation into effector T cells, a process that may take several days. When differentiation into effector cells is complete, the cells lose CD69, reexpress S1PR1, and therefore become responsive to the concentration gradient of S1P, which mediates the exit of the cells from the lymph node.

S1P and the S1PR1 are also required for mature naive T cell egress from the thymus and migration of antibody-secreting B cells from secondary lymphoid organs.

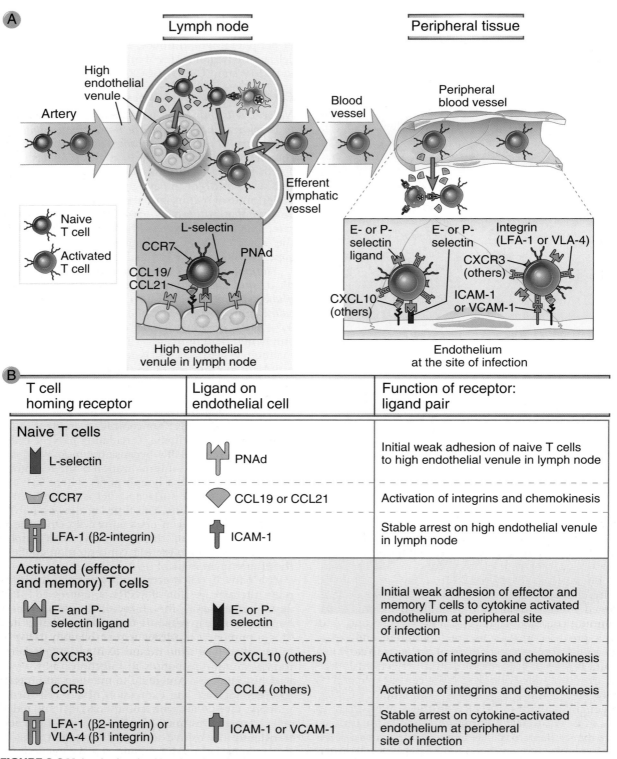

T cell homing receptor	Ligand on endothelial cell	Function of receptor: ligand pair
Naive T cells		
L-selectin	PNAd	Initial weak adhesion of naive T cells to high endothelial venule in lymph node
CCR7	CCL19 or CCL21	Activation of integrins and chemokinesis
LFA-1 (β2-integrin)	ICAM-1	Stable arrest on high endothelial venule in lymph node
Activated (effector and memory) T cells		
E- and P-selectin ligand	E- or P-selectin	Initial weak adhesion of effector and memory T cells to cytokine activated endothelium at peripheral site of infection
CXCR3	CXCL10 (others)	Activation of integrins and chemokinesis
CCR5	CCL4 (others)	Activation of integrins and chemokinesis
LFA-1 (β2-integrin) or VLA-4 (β1 integrin)	ICAM-1 or VCAM-1	Stable arrest on cytokine-activated endothelium at peripheral site of infection

FIGURE 3-6 Molecules involved in migration of naive and effector T lymphocytes. **A,** Naive T lymphocytes home to lymph nodes as a result of L-selectin binding to peripheral lymph node addressin (PNAd) on high endothelial venules, which are present only in secondary lymphoid organs, and as a result of binding chemokines (CCL19 and CCL21) displayed on the surface of the high endothelial venule. Activated T lymphocytes, including effector cells, home to sites of infection in peripheral tissues, and this migration is mediated by E-selectin and P-selectin, integrins, and chemokines that are produced at sites of infection. Additional chemokines and chemokine receptors, besides the ones shown, are involved in effector/memory T cell migration. **B,** The adhesion molecules, chemokines, and chemokine receptors involved in naive and effector/memory T cell migration are described.

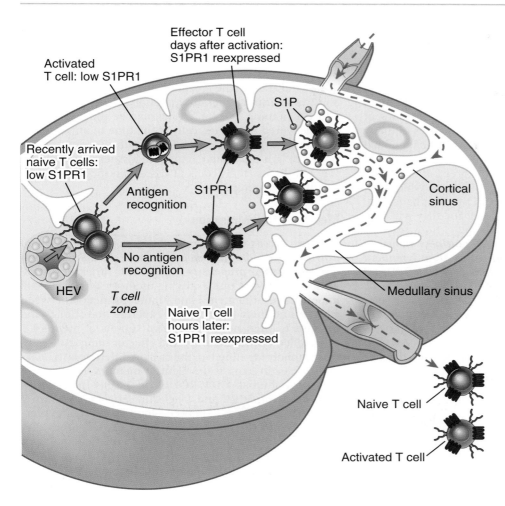

FIGURE 3-7 Mechanism of egress of lymphocytes from lymphoid organs. Circulating naive T cells have low levels of S1PR1 because the receptor is internalized after binding S1P in the blood. Therefore, naive T cells that have recently entered a lymph node cannot sense the S1P concentration gradient between the T cell zone of the node and the lymph in the medullary sinus and efferent lymphatics, and these T cells cannot exit the node. After activation of a naive T cell by antigen, S1PR1 is not reexpressed for several days, and the activated cells also will not leave the node. After several hours for naive T cells or days for activated and differentiated effector T cells, S1PR1 is reexpressed, and these cells can then sense the S1P gradient and exit the node.

Our understanding of the role of S1P and S1PR1 in T cell trafficking is based in large part on studies of a drug called fingolimod (FTY720), which binds to S1PR1 and causes its down-modulation from the cell surface. Fingolimod blocks T cell egress from lymphoid organs and thereby acts as an immunosuppressive drug. It is approved for the treatment of multiple sclerosis, an autoimmune disease of the central nervous system, and there is great interest in use of fingolimod and other drugs with a similar mechanism of action to treat various autoimmune diseases and graft rejection. Additional experimental evidence for the central role of S1P in naive T cell trafficking comes from studies of mice with genetic ablation of S1PR1. In these mice, there is failure of T cells to leave the thymus and populate secondary lymphoid organs. If naive T cells from S1PR1 knockout mice are injected into the circulation of other mice, the cells enter the lymph nodes but are unable to exit.

Recirculation of T Cells Through Other Lymphoid Tissues

Naive T cell homing into gut-associated lymphoid tissues, including Peyer's patches and mesenteric lymph nodes, is fundamentally similar to homing to other lymph nodes and relies on interactions of the T cells with HEVs. As in other tissues, these interactions are mediated by selectins, integrins, and chemokines. One particular feature of naive T cell homing to mesenteric lymph nodes and Peyer's patches is the contribution of the Ig superfamily molecule MadCAM-1 (mucosal addressin cell adhesion molecule 1), which is expressed on HEVs in these sites but not typically elsewhere in the body. Naive T cells express two ligands that bind to MadCAM-1, L-selectin and the integrin $\alpha_4\beta_7$, and both contribute to the rolling step of naive T cell homing into gut-associated lymphoid tissues.

Naive T cell migration into the spleen is not as finely regulated as homing into lymph nodes. The spleen does not contain HEVs, and it appears that naive T cells are delivered to the marginal zone and red pulp sinuses by mechanisms that do not involve selectins, integrins, or chemokines. However, CCR7-binding chemokines do participate in directing the naive T cells into the white pulp. Even though homing of naive T cells to the spleen appears to be less tightly regulated than homing into lymph nodes, the rate of lymphocyte passage through the spleen is very high, about half the total circulating lymphocyte population every 24 hours.

Migration of Effector T Lymphocytes to Sites of Infection

Effector T cells that have been generated by antigen-induced activation of naive T cells exit secondary lymphoid tissues through lymphatic drainage and return to the circulating blood. Many of the protective antimicrobial functions of effector T cells must be performed locally at sites of infections, therefore these cells must be able to leave lymphoid tissues. During differentiation of naive T cells into effector cells, the cells undergo a change in expression of S1PR1, chemokine receptors, and adhesion molecules, which promote egress from lymph nodes. From the lymphatics, the effector T cells will drain into the blood, and they will then be able to circulate throughout the body.

Circulating effector T cells preferentially home to peripheral tissue sites of infection rather than lymphoid tissues, because of a change in adhesion molecule and chemokine receptor expression. The process of effector lymphocyte homing into infected tissues occurs in postcapillary venules and is mediated by the same multistep selectin-, integrin-, and chemokine-dependent process described for other leukocytes (see Fig. 3-6). As with neutrophils and monocytes, effector T cells in the circulation, but not naive T cells, express selectin ligands, integrins, and chemokine receptors, which bind to the types of selectins, integrin ligands, and chemokines, respectively, that are expressed in activated endothelium (see Fig. 3-6). Conversely, the two molecules needed for selective entry of naive T cells into secondary lymphoid organs through HEV (CCR7 and L-selectin) are reduced on effector T cells, therefore these cells do not readily reenter lymphoid tissues.

Antigen-induced activation of effector T cells in inflamed tissues and the continued presence of chemokines keep the integrins on these cells in high-affinity states, and this favors retention of the effector T cells at these sites. Most effector cells that enter a site of infection eventually die at these sites after performing their effector functions.

Different subsets of effector T cells exist, each with distinct functions, and these subsets have different although often overlapping patterns of migration. Effector T cells include CD8+ cytotoxic T cells and CD4+ helper T cells. Helper T cells include T_H1, T_H2, and T_H17 subsets, each of which expresses different types of cytokines and protects against different types of microbes. The characteristics and functions of these subsets will be discussed in detail in Chapter 10. For now, it is sufficient to know that the migration of these subsets shows some differences. This is because the array of chemokine receptors and adhesion molecules expressed by each subset differs in ways that result in preferential recruitment of each subset into inflammatory sites elicited by different types of infections.

Some effector cells have a propensity to migrate to particular types of tissues. This selective migration capacity is acquired during the differentiation of the effector T cells from naive precursors in secondary lymphoid tissues. By enabling distinct groups of effector T cells to migrate to different sites, the adaptive immune system directs cells with specialized effector functions to the locations where they are best suited to deal with particular types of infections. The clearest examples of populations of effector T cells that specifically home to different tissues are skin-homing and gut-homing T cells, whose migration patterns reflect the expression of different adhesion molecules and chemokine receptors on each subset. Remarkably, these distinct migratory phenotypes of skin-homing and gut-homing effector T cells may be induced by signals delivered to naive T cells at the time of antigen presentation by dendritic cells in either subcutaneous lymph nodes or gut-associated lymphoid tissues, respectively. We will discuss the details of tissue-specific lymphocyte homing in Chapter 14.

Memory T Cell Migration

Memory T cells are heterogeneous in their patterns of expression of adhesion molecules and chemokine receptors and in their propensity to migrate to different tissues. Because the ways of identifying memory T cells are still imperfect (see Chapters 2 and 9), the distinction between effector and memory T cells in experimental studies and humans is often not precise. Two subsets of memory T cells, called central memory and effector memory T cells, were initially identified on the basis of differences in CCR7 and L-selectin expression. Central memory T cells were defined as human CD45RO+ blood T cells that express high levels of CCR7 and L-selectin; effector memory T cells were defined as CD45RO+ blood T cells that express low levels of CCR7 and L-selectin but express other chemokine receptors that bind inflammatory chemokines. These phenotypes suggest that central memory T cells home to secondary lymphoid organs, whereas effector memory T cells home to peripheral tissues. Although central and effector memory T cell populations can also be detected in mice, experimental studies have indicated that CCR7 expression is not a definitive marker to distinguish these memory T cell subpopulations. Nonetheless, it is clear that some memory T cells either remain in or tend to home to secondary lymphoid organs, whereas others migrate into peripheral tissues, especially mucosal tissues. In general, the peripheral tissue–homing effector memory T cells respond to antigenic stimulation by rapidly producing effector cytokines, whereas the lymphoid tissue–based central memory cells tend to proliferate more, providing a pool of cells for recall responses.

MIGRATION OF B LYMPHOCYTES

Naive B cells use the same basic mechanisms as do naive T cells to home to secondary lymphoid tissues throughout the body, which enhances their likelihood of responding to microbial antigens in different sites. Immature B cells leave the bone marrow through the blood, enter the red pulp of the spleen, and migrate to the periphery of the white pulp. As they mature further, the B cells express the chemokine receptor CXCR5, which promotes their movement into the white pulp in response to a chemokine called CXCL13. Once the maturation is completed within the white pulp, naive follicular B cells reenter the circulation and home to lymph nodes and mucosal lymphoid tissues. Homing of naive B cells from the blood into lymph nodes involves rolling interactions on HEVs, chemokine activation of integrins, and stable arrest, as described earlier for naive T cells. This process requires the chemokine receptors CXCR4 and CCR7 on naive B cells and their respective ligands CXCL12 and CCL19/CCL21. Once naive B cells enter the stroma of secondary lymphoid organs, they migrate into follicles, the site where they may encounter antigen and become activated. This migration of naive B cells into follicles is mediated by CXCL13, which is produced in follicles by non-hematopoietic stromal cells called follicular dendritic cells, and binds to the CXCR5 receptor on naive B cells. CXCL13 is displayed on fibroblastic reticular cell conduits in the T-cell zone and follicular dendritic cell conduits in follicles, both of which serve to guide the directional movement of the B cells. Homing of naive B cells into Peyer's patches involves CXCR5 and the integrin $\alpha_4\beta_7$, which binds to MadCAM-1. During the course of B cell responses to protein antigens, B cells and helper T cells must directly interact, and this is made possible by highly regulated movements of both cell types within the secondary lymphoid organs. These local migratory events, and the chemokines that orchestrate them, will be discussed in detail in Chapter 12.

Egress of B cells from secondary lymphoid organs depends on S1P. This has been shown for differentiated antibody-secreting plasma cells in lymph nodes and spleen, which leave these secondary lymphoid organs in which they were generated from naive B cells by antigen activation and home to bone marrow or tissue sites. Follicular B cells in the spleen migrate to the marginal zone and then are carried by fluid through the red pulp and into the circulation. S1PR1-deficient follicular B cells have diminished ability to leave the spleen. Presumably, naive follicular B cells that have entered secondary lymphoid tissues but do not become activated by antigen reenter the circulation, as naive T cells do, but it is not clear how this process is controlled. Splenic marginal zone B cells shuttle back and forth between the marginal zone and follicles, but do not egress into the circulation in rodents. In humans, these cells circulate and are also found surrounding follicles in lymph nodes.

Subsets of B cells committed to producing particular types of antibodies migrate from secondary lymphoid organs into specific tissues. As we will describe in later chapters, different populations of activated B cells may secrete different types of antibodies, called isotypes, each of which performs a distinct set of effector functions. Many antibody-producing plasma cells migrate to the bone marrow, where they secrete antibodies for long periods. Most bone marrow–homing plasma cells produce IgG antibodies, which are then distributed throughout the body via the blood stream. B cells within mucosa-associated lymphoid tissues usually become committed to expression of the IgA isotype of antibody, and these committed cells may home specifically to epithelium-lined mucosal tissues. This homing pattern, combined with the local differentiation within the mucosa of B cells into IgA-secreting plasma cells, serves to optimize IgA responses to mucosal infections as well as to ensure basal IgA protection at mucosal barriers. As we will discuss in more detail in Chapter 14, IgA is efficiently secreted into the lumen of tissues lined by mucosal epithelia, such as the gut and respiratory tract.

The mechanisms by which different B cell populations migrate to different tissues are, not surprisingly, similar to the mechanisms we described for tissue-specific migration of effector T cells, and depend on expression of distinct combinations of adhesion molecules and chemokine receptors on each B cell subset. For example, bone marrow–homing IgG-secreting plasma cells express VLA-4 and CXCR4, which bind respectively to VCAM-1 and CXCL12 expressed on bone marrow sinusoidal endothelial cells. In contrast, mucosa-homing IgA-secreting plasma cells express $\alpha_4\beta_7$, CCR9, and CCR10, which bind respectively to MadCAM-1, CCL25, and CCL28, expressed or displayed on mucosal endothelial cells. IgG-secreting B cells are also recruited to chronic inflammatory sites in various tissues, and this homing pattern can be attributed to CXCR3 and VLA-4 on these B cells binding to VCAM-1, CXCL9, and CXCL10, which are often found on the endothelial surface at sites of chronic inflammation.

SUMMARY

* Leukocyte migration from blood into tissues occurs through post-capillary venules and depends on adhesion molecules expressed on the leukocytes and vascular endothelial cells as well as chemokines.
* Selectins are carbohydrate-binding adhesion molecules that mediate low-affinity interaction of leukocytes with endothelial cells, the first step in leukocyte migration from blood into tissues. E-selectin and P-selectin are expressed on cytokine-activated endothelial cells and bind to selectin ligands on leukocytes, and L-selectin is expressed on leukocytes and binds ligands on endothelial cells.
* Integrins are a large family of adhesion molecules, some of which mediate tight adhesion of leukocytes with activated endothelium, a critical step in leukocyte migration from blood into tissues. The important leukocyte integrins include LFA-1 and VLA-4, which bind to ICAM-1 and VCAM-1, respectively, on endothelial cells. Chemokines and other signals at sites of infection increase the affinity of integrins on leukocytes, and various cytokines (TNF, IL-1) increase the expression of integrin ligands on endothelium.
* Migration of leukocytes from blood into tissues involves a series of sequential interactions with endothelial cells, starting with low-affinity leukocyte binding to and rolling along the endothelial surface (mediated by selectins and selectin ligands). Next, the leukocytes become firmly bound to the endothelium through interactions of leukocyte integrins binding to Ig superfamily ligands on the endothelium.
* Lymphocyte recirculation is the process by which naive lymphocytes continuously migrate from the blood into the secondary lymphoid organs

Continued

through HEVs, back into the blood through lymphatics, and into other secondary lymphoid organs. This process maximizes the chance of naive T cell encounter with the antigen it recognizes and is critical for the initiation of immune responses.

* Naive B and T cells migrate preferentially to lymph nodes; this process is mediated by binding of L-selectin on lymphocytes to peripheral lymph node addressin on HEVs in lymph nodes and by binding of the CCR7 receptor on lymphocytes to the chemokines CCL19 and CCL21, which are produced in lymph nodes.

* The effector and memory lymphocytes that are generated by antigen stimulation of naive cells exit the lymph node by a process dependent on the sphingosine-1 phosphate receptor on the lymphocytes and a gradient of sphingosine-1 phosphate. Effector T cells have decreased expression of L-selectin and CCR7 but increased expression of integrins and E-selectin and P-selectin ligands, and these molecules mediate binding to endothelium at peripheral inflammatory sites. Effector and memory lymphocytes also express receptors for chemokines that are produced in infected peripheral tissues.

SELECTED READINGS

Adhesion Molecules

Hogg N, Patzak I, Willenbrock F: The insider's guide to leukocyte integrin signalling and function, *Nature Reviews Immunology* 11:416–426, 2011.

Kolaczkowska E, Kubes P: Neutrophil recruitment and function in health and inflammation, *Nature Reviews Immunology* 13:159–175, 2013.

Ley K, Laudanna C, Cybulsky MI, Nourshargh S: Getting to the site of inflammation: the leukocyte adhesion cascade updated, *Nature Reviews Immunology* 7:678–689, 2007.

Muller WA: Mechanisms of leukocyte transendothelial migration, *Annual Review of Pathology* 6:323–344, 2011.

Chemokines

Griffith JW, Sokol CL, Luster AD: Chemokines and chemokine receptors: positioning cells for host defense and immunity, *Annual Review of Immunology* 32:659–702, 2014.

Sallusto F, Baggiolini M: Chemokines and leukocyte traffic, *Nature Immunology* 9:949–952, 2008.

Zlotnik A, Yoshie O: The chemokine superfamily revisited, *Immunity* 36:705–716, 2012.

Lymphocyte Migration Through Lymphoid Tissues

Bajénoff M, Egen JG, Qi H, Huang AY, Castellino F, Germain RN: Highways, byways and breadcrumbs: directing lymphocyte traffic in the lymph node, *Trends in Immunology* 28:346–352, 2007.

Cyster JG, Schwab SR: Sphingosine-1-phosphate and lymphocyte egress from lymphoid organs, *Annual Review of Immunology* 30:69–94, 2012.

Masopust D, Schenkel JM: The integration of T cell migration, differentiation and function, *Nature Reviews Immunology* 13:309–320, 2013.

Sigmundsdottir H, Butcher EC: Environmental cues, dendritic cells and the programming of tissue-selective lymphocyte trafficking, *Nature Immunology* 9:981–987, 2008.

Weninger W, Biro M, Jain R: Leukocyte migration in the interstitial space of non-lymphoid organs, *Nature Reviews Immunology* 14, 2014, in press.

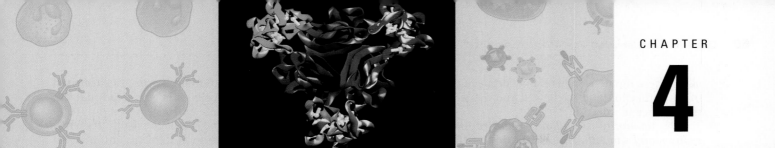

Innate Immunity

OVERVIEW OF INNATE IMMUNITY

The innate immune system, which was briefly introduced in Chapter 1, consists of many cell types and soluble molecules in tissues and the blood that constantly prevent microbes from invading and establishing infections. If microbes do establish a foothold, innate immune responses provide early defense, before adaptive immune responses can develop (see Fig. 1-1). In this chapter, we will describe in more detail the components, specificity, and anti-microbial mechanisms of the innate immune system. Although the focus of much of this book is on the role of the adaptive immune response in host defense and disease, throughout we will discuss the impact of the innate immune system on adaptive immune responses and how the innate immune system contributes to protection against infections.

Functions and Reactions of Innate Immune Responses

Innate immunity serves three essential functions that protect us against microbes and tissue injury.

- *Innate immunity is the initial response to microbes that prevents, controls, or eliminates infection of the host by many pathogens.* The importance of innate immunity in host defense is illustrated by clinical observations and experimental studies showing that deficiencies, inhibition, or elimination of any of several mechanisms of innate immunity markedly increases susceptibility to infections, even when the adaptive immune system is intact and functional. Many pathogenic microbes have evolved strategies to resist innate immunity, and these strategies are crucial for the virulence of the microbes. Innate immune responses to such microbes may keep the infection in check until more specialized adaptive immune responses are activated. Adaptive immune responses, often being more potent and specialized, are able to eliminate microbes that resist the defense mechanisms of innate immunity.
- *Innate immune mechanisms eliminate damaged cells and initiate the process of tissue repair.* These mechanisms recognize and respond to host molecules that are produced by, released from, or accumulate in stressed, damaged, and dead host cells. The injury that

elicits these innate responses may occur in the context of both infection and sterile cell and tissue damage in the absence of infection.

- *Innate immunity stimulates adaptive immune responses and can influence the nature of the adaptive responses to make them optimally effective against different types of microbes.* Thus, innate immunity not only serves defensive functions early after infection but also provides the danger signals that alert the adaptive immune system to respond. Moreover, different components of the innate immune response often react in distinct ways to different microbes (e.g., bacteria versus viruses) and thereby influence the type of adaptive immune response that develops. We will return to this concept at the end of the chapter.

The two major types of responses of the innate immune system that protect against microbes are inflammation and antiviral defense. Inflammation is the process by which circulating leukocytes and plasma proteins are brought into sites of infection in the tissues and are activated to destroy and eliminate the offending agents. Inflammation is also the major reaction to damaged or dead cells and to accumulations of abnormal substances in cells and tissues. Antiviral defense consists of changes in cells that prevent virus replication and increase susceptibility to killing by lymphocytes, thus eliminating reservoirs of viral infection.

In addition to active inflammation and anti-viral response to infections, the innate immune system includes physical and chemical defenses at epithelial barriers such as the skin and lining of the gastrointestinal and respiratory tracts, which function at all times to block microbial entry. In addition, the innate immune system includes several circulating cells, such as neutrophils, and proteins, such as complement, that can help eliminate microbes in the blood.

Comparative Features of Innate and Adaptive Immunity

In order to understand how innate and adaptive immunity complement each other to protect against pathogens, it is instructive to highlight their important differences.

- Innate immune responses to a microbe are immediate and do not require prior exposure to the microbe. In other words, innate immune effector cells and molecules are either fully functional even before infection or rapidly activated by microbes to prevent, control, or eliminate infections. In contrast, effective adaptive immune responses to a newly introduced microbe develop over several days as clones of lymphocytes undergo expansion and differentiate into functional effector cells.
- There is no appreciable change in the quality or magnitude of the innate immune response to a microbe upon repeated exposure, that is, there is little or no memory. In contrast, repeated exposure to a microbe enhances the rapidity, magnitude, and effectiveness of adaptive immune responses.
- The innate immune response is activated by recognition of a relatively limited set of molecular structures that are either products of microbes or are expressed by injured or dead host cells. It is estimated that the innate immune system recognizes only about 1000 products of microbes and damaged cells. By contrast, the adaptive immune system potentially can recognize millions of different molecular structures of microbes, and can also recognize nonmicrobial environmental antigens as well as self antigens that are normally present in healthy tissues. The various types of receptors that account for the different specificities of the innate and adaptive immune systems are described later in this chapter and in subsequent chapters.

Evolution of Innate Immunity

Innate immunity, the first line of defense against infections, is phylogenetically the oldest part of the immune system. It coevolved with microbes to protect all multicellular organisms from infections. Some components of the mammalian innate immune system are remarkably similar to components in plants and insects, suggesting that these appeared in common ancestors long ago in evolution. For example, peptides that are toxic to bacteria and fungi, called defensins, are found in plants and mammals and have essentially the same tertiary structure in both life forms. A family of receptors that we will discuss in detail later in this chapter, called Toll-like receptors, recognize pathogenic microbes and activate antimicrobial defense mechanisms. Toll-like receptors are found in every life form in the evolutionary tree from insects up to mammals. The major signal transduction pathway that Toll-like receptors engage to activate cells, called the NF-κB pathway in mammals, also shows remarkable evolutionary conservation. In fact, most of the mechanisms of innate immune defense that we will discuss in this chapter appeared very early in evolution, when the first multicellular organisms evolved, about 750 million years ago. An adaptive immune system, in contrast, is clearly recognizable only in vertebrates that appeared about 350 to 500 million years ago.

We begin our discussion of innate immunity by describing how the innate immune system recognizes microbes and damaged host cells. We will then proceed to the individual components of innate immunity and their functions in host defense.

RECOGNITION OF MICROBES AND DAMAGED SELF BY THE INNATE IMMUNE SYSTEM

The specificities of innate immune recognition have evolved to combat microbes and are different from the specificities of the adaptive immune system in several respects (Table 4-1).

The innate immune system recognizes molecular structures that are produced by microbial pathogens. The microbial substances that stimulate innate immunity are often shared by classes of microbes and are called **pathogen-associated molecular patterns (PAMPs)**. Different types of microbes (e.g., viruses,

TABLE 4-1   Specificity of Innate and Adaptive Immunity

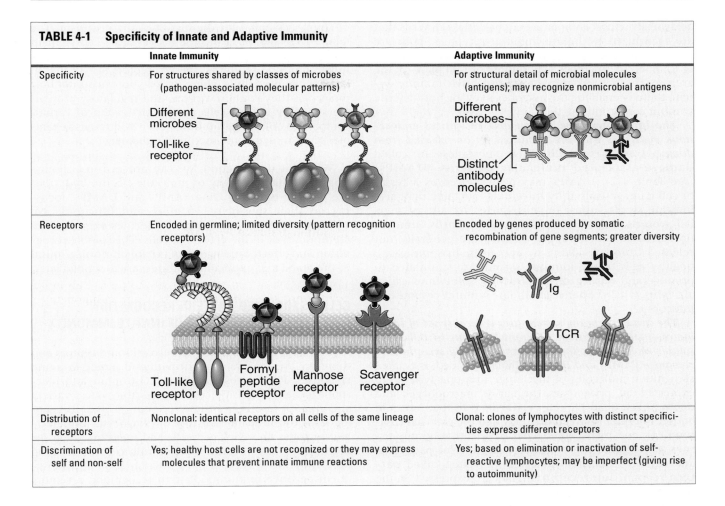

	Innate Immunity	Adaptive Immunity
Specificity	For structures shared by classes of microbes (pathogen-associated molecular patterns)	For structural detail of microbial molecules (antigens); may recognize nonmicrobial antigens
Receptors	Encoded in germline; limited diversity (pattern recognition receptors)	Encoded by genes produced by somatic recombination of gene segments; greater diversity
Distribution of receptors	Nonclonal: identical receptors on all cells of the same lineage	Clonal: clones of lymphocytes with distinct specificities express different receptors
Discrimination of self and non-self	Yes; healthy host cells are not recognized or they may express molecules that prevent innate immune reactions	Yes; based on elimination or inactivation of self-reactive lymphocytes; may be imperfect (giving rise to autoimmunity)

gram-negative bacteria, gram-positive bacteria, fungi) express different PAMPs. These structures include: nucleic acids that are unique to microbes, such as double-stranded RNA found in replicating viruses and unmethylated CpG DNA sequences found in bacteria; features of proteins that are found in microbes, such as initiation by *N*-formylmethionine, which is typical of bacterial proteins; and complex lipids and carbohydrates that are synthesized by microbes but not by mammalian cells, such as lipopolysaccharide (LPS) in gram-negative bacteria, lipoteichoic acid in gram-positive bacteria, and oligosaccharides with terminal mannose residues found in microbial but not in mammalian glycoproteins (Table 4-2). Whereas the innate immune system has evolved to recognize only a limited number of molecules that are unique to microbes, the adaptive immune system is capable of recognizing many more diverse foreign substances whether or not they are products of microbes.

The innate immune system recognizes microbial products that are often essential for survival of the microbes. This feature of innate immune recognition is important because it ensures that the targets of innate immunity cannot be discarded by microbes in an effort to evade recognition by the host. An example of a target of innate immunity that is indispensable for microbes is double-stranded viral RNA, which is an essential intermediate in the life cycle of many viruses. Similarly, LPS and lipoteichoic

TABLE 4-2   Examples of PAMPs and DAMPs

Pathogen-Associated Molecular Patterns		Microbe Type
Nucleic acids	ssRNA	Virus
	dsRNA	Virus
	CpG	Virus, bacteria
Proteins	Pilin	Bacteria
	Flagellin	Bacteria
Cell wall lipids	LPS	Gram-negative bacteria
	Lipoteichoic acid	Gram-positive bacteria
Carbohydrates	Mannan	Fungi, bacteria
	Glucans	Fungi
Damage-Associated Molecular Patterns		
Stress-induced proteins	HSPs	
Crystals	Monosodium urate	
Nuclear proteins	HMGB1	

CpG, cytosine-guanine–rich oligonucleotide *dsRNA*, double-stranded RNA; *HMGB1*, high-mobility group box 1; *HSP*, heat shock protein; *LPS*, lipopolysaccharide; *ssRNA*, single-stranded RNA.

acid are structural components of bacterial cell walls that are recognized by innate immune receptors; both are required for bacterial survival. In contrast, as we will see in Chapter 16, microbes may mutate or lose many of the antigens that are recognized by the adaptive immune system, thereby enabling the microbes to evade host defense without compromising their own survival.

The innate immune system also recognizes endogenous molecules that are produced by or released from damaged and dying cells. These substances are called **damage-associated molecular patterns (DAMPs)** (see Table 4-2). DAMPs may be produced as a result of cell damage caused by infections, but they may also indicate sterile injury to cells caused by any of myriad reasons, such as chemical toxins, burns, trauma, or decreased blood supply. DAMPs are generally not released from cells dying by apoptosis. In some cases, healthy cells of the immune system are stimulated to produce and release certain DAMPs, sometimes called alarmins, which enhance the innate immune response to infections.

The innate immune system uses several types of cellular receptors, present in different locations in cells, and soluble molecules in the blood and mucosal secretions to recognize PAMPs and DAMPs (Table 4-3). Cell-associated recognition molecules of the innate immune system are expressed by phagocytes (primarily macrophages and neutrophils), dendritic cells, epithelial cells that form the barrier interface between the body and the external environment, and many other types of cells that occupy tissues and organs. These cellular receptors for pathogens and damage-associated molecules are often called **pattern recognition receptors**. They are expressed on the surface, in phagocytic vesicles, and in the cytosol of various cell types, all of which are locations where microbes may be present (Fig. 4-1). When these cell-associated pattern recognition receptors bind to PAMPs and DAMPs, they activate signal transduction pathways that promote the antimicrobial and proinflammatory functions of the cells in which they are expressed. In addition, there are many proteins present in the blood and extracellular fluids that recognize PAMPs (see Table 4-3). These soluble molecules are responsible for facilitating the clearance of microbes from blood and extracellular fluids by enhancing uptake into phagocytes or by activating extracellular killing mechanisms.

The receptors of the innate immune system are encoded by inherited (germline) genes, whereas the genes encoding receptors of adaptive immunity are generated by somatic recombination of gene segments in the precursors of mature lymphocytes. As a result, the diversity of innate immune system receptors, and the range of their specificities, are small compared with those of B and T cells of the adaptive immune system. Furthermore, whereas the adaptive immune system can distinguish between antigens of different microbes of the same class and even different antigens of one microbe, innate immunity can distinguish only classes of microbes, or only damaged cells from healthy cells, but not particular species of microbes or cell types.

The innate immune system does not react against normal, healthy cells and tissues. This characteristic is, of course, essential for the health of the organism. The failure to recognize healthy self is because of three main mechanisms—normal cells do not produce ligands for innate immune receptors, these receptors are located in cellular compartments where they do not encounter host molecules they could recognize, and regulatory proteins expressed by normal cells prevent activation of various components of innate immunity. We will discuss examples of such regulation later in this chapter.

With this introduction, we can proceed to a discussion of the large variety of molecules in the body that are capable of recognizing PAMPs and DAMPs, focusing on their specificity, location, and functions. We will begin with cell-associated molecules expressed on membranes or in the cytosol of cells. The soluble recognition and effector molecules of innate immunity, found in the blood and extracellular fluids, are described later.

CELL-ASSOCIATED PATTERN RECOGNITION RECEPTORS AND SENSORS OF INNATE IMMUNITY

Most cell types express pattern recognition receptors and therefore are capable of participating in innate immune responses. Phagocytes, including neutrophils and macrophages, and dendritic cells express the widest variety and greatest number of these receptors. This is in keeping with the fundamental role of phagocytes in detecting microbes and damaged cells and ingesting them for destruction, and the role of dendritic cells in reacting to microbes in ways that elicit inflammation and subsequent adaptive immunity. Pattern recognition receptors are linked to intracellular signal transduction pathways that activate various cellular responses, including the production of molecules that promote inflammation and destroy microbes.

We will organize our discussion around several distinct classes of cellular pattern recognition receptors that differ in their structure and specificity for various types of microbes.

Toll-Like Receptors

Toll-like receptors (TLRs) are an evolutionarily conserved family of pattern recognition receptors expressed on many cell types that recognize products of a wide variety of microbes as well as molecules expressed or released by stressed and dying cells. Toll was originally identified as a *Drosophila* gene involved in establishing the dorsal-ventral axis during embryogenesis of the fruit fly, but subsequently it was discovered that the Toll protein also mediated antimicrobial responses in these organisms. Furthermore, the cytoplasmic domain of Toll was found to be similar to the cytoplasmic region of the receptor for the innate immune cytokine interleukin-1 (IL-1). These discoveries led to the identification of mammalian homologues of Toll, which were named *Toll-like receptors*. There are nine different functional TLRs in humans, named TLR1 through TLR9 (Fig. 4-2).

The TLRs are type I integral membrane glycoproteins that contain leucine-rich repeats flanked by characteristic

TABLE 4-3 Pattern Recognition Molecules of the Innate Immune System

Pattern Recognition Receptors	Location	Specific Examples	PAMP/DAMP Ligands
Cell-Associated			
Toll-like receptors (TLRs)	Plasma membrane and endosomal membranes of dendritic cells, phagocytes, B cells, endothelial cells, and many other cell types	TLRs 1-9	Various microbial molecules including bacterial LPS and peptidoglycans, viral nucleic acids
NOD-like receptors (NLRs)	Cytosol of phagocytes, epithelial cells, and other cells	NOD1/2	Bacterial cell wall peptidoglycans
		NLRP family (inflammasomes)	Intracellular crystals (urate, silica); changes in cytosolic ATP and ion concentrations; lysosomal damage
RIG-like receptors (RLRs)	Cytosol of phagocytes and other cells	RIG-1, MDA-5	Viral RNA
Cytosolic DNA sensors (CDSs)	Cytosol of many cell types	AIM2; STING-associated CDSs	Bacterial and viral DNA
C-type lectin–like receptors (CLRs)	Plasma membranes of phagocytes	Mannose receptor	Microbial surface carbohydrates with terminal mannose and fructose
		Dectin	Glucans present in fungal cell walls
Scavenger receptors	Plasma membranes of phagocytes	CD36	Microbial diacylglycerides
N-Formyl met-leu-phe receptors	Plasma membranes of phagocytes	FPR and FPRL1	Peptides containing N-formylmethionyl residues
Soluble			
Pentraxins	Plasma	C-reactive protein	Microbial phosphorylcholine and phosphatidylethanolamine
Collectins	Plasma	Mannose-binding lectin	Carbohydrates with terminal mannose and fructose
	Alveoli	Surfactant proteins SP-A and SP-D	Various microbial structures
Ficolins	Plasma	Ficolin	N-Acetylglucosamine and lipoteichoic acid components of the cell walls of gram-positive bacteria
Complement	Plasma	Various complement proteins	Microbial surfaces

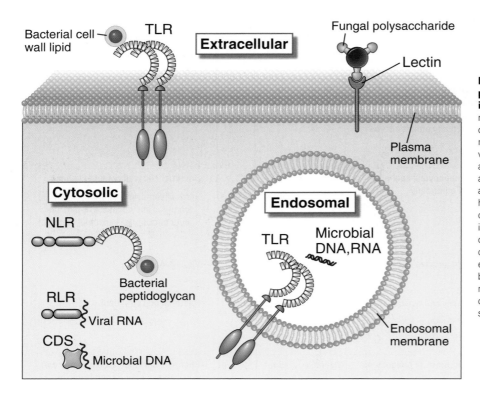

FIGURE 4-1 Cellular locations of pattern recognition receptors of the innate immune system. Some pattern recognition molecules, including members of the TLR family (see Fig. 4-2) and lectin receptors, are expressed on the cell surface, where they may bind extracellular pathogen-associated molecular patterns. Other TLRs are expressed on endosomal membranes and recognize nucleic acids of microbes that have been phagocytosed by cells. Cells also contain cytosolic sensors of microbial infection, including the NOD-like receptor (NLR) family of receptors, RIG-like receptors (RLRs), and cytosolic DNA sensors (CDS). Only selected examples of microbial PAMPs recognized by these receptors are shown. Cytosolic receptors that recognize products of damaged cells (DAMPs) as well as some microbes are shown in Figure 4-4.

cysteine-rich motifs in their extracellular regions, which are involved in ligand binding, and a Toll/IL-1 receptor (TIR) homology domain in their cytoplasmic tails, which is essential for signaling. TIR domains are also found in the cytoplasmic tails of the receptors for the cytokines IL-1 and IL-18, and similar signaling pathways are engaged by TLRs, IL-1, and IL-18.

Mammalian TLRs are involved in responses to a wide variety of molecules that are expressed by microbial but not by healthy mammalian cells. The ligands that the different TLRs recognize are structurally diverse and include products of all classes of microorganisms (see Fig. 4-2). Examples of bacterial products that bind to TLRs are LPS and lipoteichoic acid, which are constituents of the cell walls of gram-negative bacteria and gram-positive bacteria, respectively, and flagellin, the protein subunit component of the flagella of motile bacteria. Examples of nucleic acids that are TLR ligands are double-stranded RNAs, which make up the genomes of some viruses and are generated during the life cycle of most RNA viruses but are not produced by eukaryotic cells; single-stranded RNAs, which are distinguished from cellular cytoplasmic single-stranded RNA transcripts by their location within endosomes and by their high guanosine and uridine content; and unmethylated CpG dinucleotides, which are common in prokaryotes but rare in vertebrate genomes.

TLRs are also involved in response to endogenous molecules whose expression or location indicates cell damage. Examples of host molecules that engage TLRs include heat shock proteins (HSPs), which are chaperones induced in response to various cell stresses, and high-mobility group box 1 (HMGB1), an abundant DNA-binding protein involved in transcription and DNA repair. Both HSPs and HMGB1 are normally intracellular but may become extracellular when

released from injured or dying cells. From their extracellular location, they activate TLR2 and TLR4 signaling in dendritic cells, macrophages, and other cell types.

The structural basis of TLR specificities resides in the multiple extracellular leucine-rich modules of these receptors, which bind directly to PAMPs or to adaptor molecules that bind the PAMPs. There are between 16 and 28 leucine-rich repeats in TLRs, and each of these modules is composed of 20 to 30 amino acids that include conserved LxxLxLxxN motifs (where L is leucine, x is any amino acid, and N is asparagine) and amino acid residues that vary between different TLRs. The ligand-binding variable residues of the modules are on the convex surface formed by α helices and β turns or loops. These repeats contribute to the ability of some TLRs to bind hydrophobic molecules such as bacterial LPS. Ligand binding to the leucine-rich domains causes physical interactions between TLR molecules and the formation of TLR dimers. The repertoire of specificities of the TLR system is extended by the ability of TLRs to heterodimerize with one another. For example, dimers of TLR2 and TLR6 are required for responses to peptidoglycan.

Specificities of the TLRs are also influenced by various non-TLR accessory molecules. This is best defined for the TLR4 response to LPS. LPS first binds to soluble LPS-binding protein in the blood or extracellular fluid, and this complex serves to facilitate delivery of the LPS to the surface of the responding cell. An extracellular protein called MD2 (myeloid differentiation protein 2) binds to the lipid A component of LPS, forming a complex that then interacts with TLR4 and initiates signaling. Another protein called CD14 is also required for efficient LPS-induced signaling. CD14 is expressed by most cells (except endothelial cells) as a soluble protein or as a glycophosphatidylinositol-linked membrane

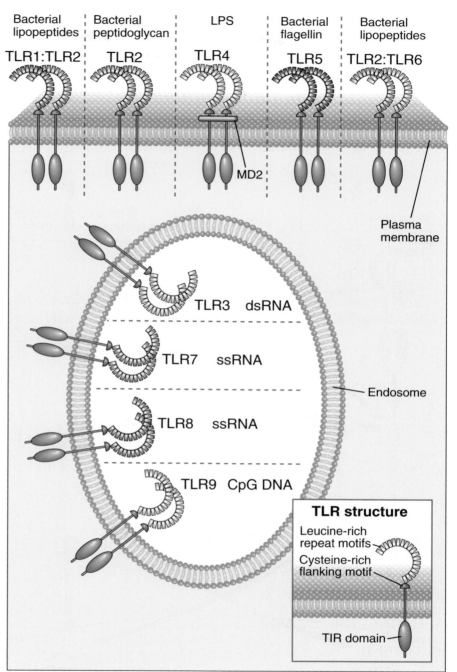

FIGURE 4-2 Structure, location, and specificities of mammalian TLRs. Note that some TLRs are expressed on the cell surface and others in endosomes. TLRs may form homodimers or heterodimers.

protein. Both CD14 and MD2 can also associate with other TLRs. Thus, different combinations of accessory molecules in TLR complexes may serve to broaden the range of microbial products that can induce innate immune responses.

TLRs are found on the cell surface and on intracellular membranes and are thus able to recognize microbes in different cellular locations (see Fig. 4-2). TLRs 1, 2, 4, 5, and 6 are expressed on the plasma membrane, where they recognize various PAMPs in the extracellular environment. Some of the most potent microbial stimuli for innate immune responses bind to these plasma membrane TLRs, such as bacterial LPS and lipoteichoic acid,

which are recognized by TLRs 4 and 2, respectively. In contrast, TLRs 3, 7, 8, and 9 are mainly expressed inside cells on endoplasmic reticulum and endosomal membranes, where they detect several different nucleic acid ligands that are typical of microbes but not mammals, as discussed earlier (see Fig. 4-2). These include double-stranded RNA, which binds to TLR3, and unmethylated CpG motifs, which bind to TLR9. TLR7 and TLR8 recognize single-stranded RNA, and TLR9 recognizes single- or double-stranded DNA; these nucleic acid ligands are not unique to microbes, but their location in endosomes likely reflects origin from microbes. This is because host cell RNA and DNA are not normally present in endosomes, but microbial RNA and DNA may end up in endosomes of neutrophils, macrophages, or dendritic cells when the microbes are phagocytosed by these cells. Thus, the endosomal TLRs may distinguish nucleic acids of normal cells from microbial nucelic acids on the basis of the cellular location of these molecules. A protein in the endoplasmic reticulum called UNC-93B is required for the endosomal localization and proper function of TLRs 3, 7, 8 and 9. Genetic deficiency in UNC-93B

leads to susceptibility to certain viral infections, especially herpes simplex virus encephalitis, demonstrating the importance of the endosomal location of TLRs for innate defense against viruses.

TLR recognition of microbial ligands results in the activation of several signaling pathways and ultimately transcription factors, which induce the expression of genes whose products are important for inflammatory and antiviral responses (Fig. 4-3). The signaling pathways are

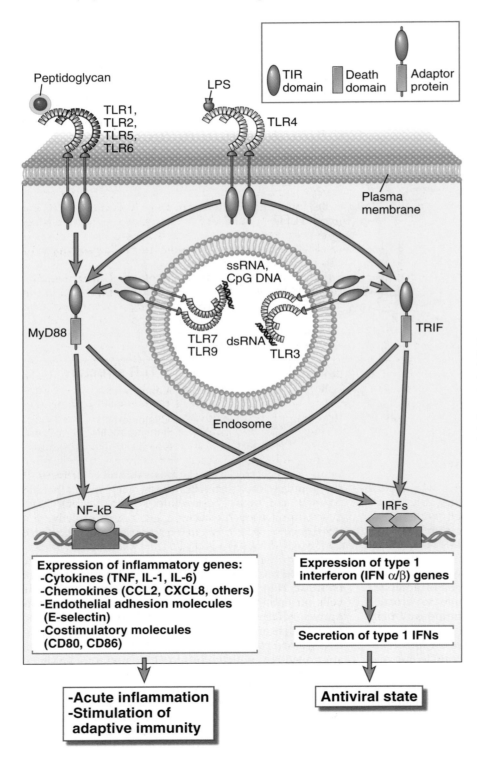

FIGURE 4-3 Signaling pathways and functions of TLRs. TLRs 1, 2, 5, and 6 use the adaptor protein MyD88 and activate the transcription factors NF-κB and AP-1. TLR3 uses the adaptor protein TRIF and activates the IRF3 and IRF7 transcription factors. TLR4 can activate both pathways. TLRs 7 and 9 in the endosome use MyD88 and activate both NF-κB and IRF7.

initiated by ligand binding to the TLR at the cell surface or in the endoplasmic reticulum or endosomes, leading to dimerization of the TLR proteins. Ligand-induced TLR dimerization is predicted to bring the TIR domains of the cytoplasmic tails of each protein close to one another. This is followed by recruitment of TIR domain–containing adaptor proteins, which facilitate the recruitment and activation of various protein kinases, leading to the activation of different transcription factors. The major transcription factors that are activated by TLR signaling pathways are nuclear factor κB (NF-κB), activation protein 1 (AP-1), interferon response factor 3 (IRF3), and IRF7. NF-κB and AP-1 stimulate the expression of genes encoding many of the molecules required for inflammatory responses, including inflammatory cytokines (such as TNF and IL-1), chemokines (e.g., CCL2 and CXCL8), and endothelial adhesion molecules (e.g., E-selectin) (discussed later). IRF3 and IRF7 promote production of type I interferons (IFN-α and IFN-β), which are important for anti-viral innate immune responses.

Different combinations of adaptors and signaling intermediates are used by different TLRs, accounting for the common and unique downstream effects of the TLRs. For example, cell surface TLRs that engage the adaptor MyD88 lead to NF-κB activation, and TLR signaling that uses the adaptor called TRIF (TIR domain–containing adaptor inducing IFN-β) leads to IRF3 activation. All TLRs except TLR3 signal through MyD88 and are therefore capable of activating NF-κB and inducing an inflammatory response. TLR3 signals through TRIF and therefore activates IRF3 and induces expression of type I interferons. TLR4 signals through both MyD88 and TRIF and is able to induce both types of responses. The endosomal TLRs 7 and 9, which are most highly expressed in plasmacytoid dendritic cells (see Chapter 6), signal through a MyD88-dependent, TRIF-independent pathway that activates both NF-κB and IRFs. Therefore, TLR7 and TLR9, like TLR4, induce both inflammatory and antiviral responses. We will discuss the details of NF-κB activation in Chapter 7.

Cytosolic Receptors for PAMPs and DAMPs

In addition to the membrane-bound TLRs, which sense pathogens outside cells or in endosomes, the innate immune system has evolved to equip cells with pattern recognition receptors that detect infection or cell damage in the cytosol (see Fig. 4-1 and Table 4-3). Three major classes of these cytosolic receptors are NOD-like receptors, RIG-like receptors, and cytosolic DNA sensors. These cytosolic receptors, similar to the TLRs, are linked to signal transduction pathways that promote inflammation or type I interferon production. The ability of the innate immune system to detect infection in the cytosol is important because parts of the normal life cycles of some microbes, such as viral gene translation and viral particle assembly, take place in the cytosol. Some bacteria and parasites have mechanisms that enable them to escape from phagocytic vesicles into the cytosol. Microbes can produce toxins that create pores in host cell plasma membranes, including endosomal membranes, through which microbial molecules can enter the cytosol. These pores also can

result in changes in the concentration of endogenous molecules, such as ions, in the cytoplasm, which are reliable signs of infection and damage and are detected by the cytosolic receptors.

NOD-Like Receptors

NOD-like receptors (NLRs) are a family of more than 20 different cytosolic proteins, some of which recognize PAMPs and DAMPs and recruit other proteins to form signaling complexes that promote inflammation. This family of proteins is named after NOD (nucleotide oligomerization domain–containing protein). Typical NLR proteins contain at least three different domains with distinct structures and functions. These include a leucine-rich repeat domain that senses the presence of ligand, similar to the leucine-rich repeats of TLRs; a NACHT (neuronal apoptosis inhibitory protein [NAIP], CIITA, HET-E, and TP1) domain, which allows NLRs to bind to one another and form oligomers; and an effector domain, which recruits other proteins to form signaling complexes. There are three NLR subfamilies, the members of which use different effector domains to initiate signaling. The three effector domains are called CARD (caspase recruitment domain), Pyrin domain, and BIR domain. NLRs are found in a wide variety of cell types, although some NLRs have restricted tissue distributions. Some of the best studied NLRs are found in immune and inflammatory cells and in barrier epithelial cells.

NOD1 and NOD2, members of the CARD domain–containing NOD subfamily of NLRs, are expressed in the cytosol of several cell types including mucosal epithelial cells and phagocytes, and they respond to bacterial cell wall peptidoglycans. NOD2 is highly expressed in intestinal Paneth cells in the intestine, where it stimulates expression of antimicrobial substances called defensins in response to pathogens. NOD1 recognizes diaminopimelic acid (DAP) derived mainly from gram-negative bacterial peptidoglycan, whereas NOD2 recognizes a distinct molecule called muramyl dipeptide derived from both gram-negative and gram-positive peptidoglycans. These peptides are released from intracellular or extracellular bacteria; in the latter case, their presence in the cytosol requires specialized bacterial mechanisms of delivery of the peptides into host cells. These mechanisms include type III and type IV secretion systems, which have evolved in pathogenic bacteria as a means of delivering toxins into host cells. When oligomers of NODs recognize their peptide ligands, including bacterial toxins, a conformational change occurs that allows the CARD effector domains of the NOD proteins to recruit multiple copies of the kinase RIP2, forming a signaling complex that has been called the NOD signalosome. The RIP2 kinases in these complexes activate NF-κB, which promotes inflammatory gene expression, similar to TLRs that signal through MyD88, discussed earlier. Both NOD1 and NOD2 appear to be important in innate immune responses to bacterial pathogens in the gastrointestinal tract, such as *Helicobacter pylori* and *Listeria monocytogenes*.

There is great interest in the finding that certain *NOD2* gene polymorphisms increase the risk for an inflammatory disease of the bowel called Crohn's disease. A possible explanation for this association is that the disease-associated NOD2 variants are defective in their ability to sense microbial products, resulting in defective innate responses against commensal and pathogenic organisms in the intestine. If these organisms gain access to the intestinal wall, they may trigger chronic inflammation. Also, gain-of-function mutations of NOD2 that cause increased NOD signaling lead to a systemic inflammatory disease called Blau's syndrome.

The NLRP subfamily of NOD-like receptors respond to cytosolic PAMPs and DAMPs by forming signaling complexes called inflammasomes, which generate active forms of the inflammatory cytokines IL-1 and IL-18 (Fig. 4-4). There are 14 NLRPs (NLR family, pyrin-domain-containing proteins), most of which share a Pyrin effector domain, named after the Greek root *pyro,* meaning "heat," because it was first identified in a mutated gene that is associated with an inherited febrile illness. Inflammasomes containing three of these

NLRPs—IPAF/NLRC4, NLRP3 (also called cryopyrin), and NLRP1—have been well studied. When these NLRPs are activated by the presence of microbial products or changes in the amount of endogenous molecules or ions in the cytosol, they bind other proteins through homotypic interactions between shared structural domains, thereby forming the inflammasome complex. For example, after binding of a ligand, multiple identical NLRP3 proteins interact to form an oligomer, and each NLRP3 protein in the oligomer binds an adaptor protein called ASC. The adaptors then bind an inactive precursor form of the enzyme caspase-1 through interactions of caspase-recruitment domains on both proteins. Caspases are proteases with cysteine residues in their active site that cleave substrate proteins at aspartate residues. Caspase-1 becomes active only after recruitment to the inflammasome complex. Although several other caspases participate in a form of cell death called apoptosis (see Chapter 15), the main

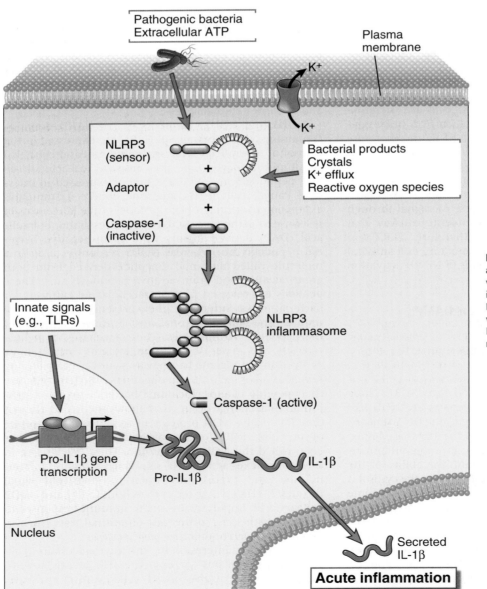

FIGURE 4-4 The inflammasome. The activation of the NLRP3 inflammasome, which processes pro–IL-1 to active IL-1, is shown. Inflammasomes with other NLRP proteins function in a similar way. Various PAMPs or DAMPs induce Pro–IL-1β expression through pattern recognition receptor signaling.

function of caspase-1 is to cleave the inactive cytoplasmic precursor forms of two homologous cytokines called IL-1β and IL-18. Caspase-1 cleavage generates active forms of these cytokines, which then leave the cell and perform various proinflammatory functions. We will describe the action of these cytokines and the inflammatory response in detail later in this chapter. Suffice it to say here that the inflammation induced by IL-1 serves a protective function against the microbes that incite the formation of the inflammasome.

NLRP-inflammasome responses are induced by a wide variety of cytoplasmic stimuli that are often associated with infections and cell stress, including microbial products, environmentally or endogenously derived crystals, and reduction in cytosolic potassium ion (K^+) concentrations (see Fig. 4-4). Microbial products that activate NLRP-inflammasomes include bacterial molecules, such as flagellin, muramyl dipeptide, LPS, and pore-forming toxins, as well as bacterial and viral RNA. Crystalline substances are also potent activators of inflammasomes, and these crystals can be derived from the environment, such as asbestos and silica, or they can be endogenously derived, such as monosodium urate, calcium pyrophosphate dehydrate, and cholesterol. Another endogenous stimulus of inflammasome activation is extracellular ATP, perhaps released from dead cells and transported into the cytoplasm of the responding cell.

The structural diversity of the agents that activate the inflammasome suggests that they do not directly bind to NLRP proteins but may act by inducing a shared set of changes in endogenous cytoplasmic conditions that activate the NLRPs. Reduced cytoplasm potassium ion concentrations may be one such common mechanism because reductions in cellular K^+ induced by some bacterial pore-forming toxins can activate inflammasomes, and many of the other known inflammasome activators cause increased K^+ efflux from cells. Another common mechanism implicated in inflammasome activation is the generation of reactive oxygen species, which are toxic free radicals of oxygen that are often produced during cell injury.

Inflammasome activation of caspase-1 may also cause a form of programmed cell death called **pyroptosis**, characterized by swelling of cells, loss of plasma membrane integrity, and release of inflammatory mediators. Pyroptosis results in the death of certain microbes that gain access to the cytosol and enhances the release of inflammasome-generated IL-1β, which lacks a hydrophobic leader sequence that is required for conventional secretion of proteins from cells. In addition to caspase-1–dependent pyroptosis, a caspase-11–dependent pathway of pyroptosis is required for protection against certain bacteria that readily gain access to the cytosol of host cells, but the innate stimuli that activate this pathway are not yet known.

The discovery that some crystalline substances are potent inflammasome activators has changed our understanding of certain inflammatory diseases. Gout is a painful inflammatory condition of the joints that has long been known to be caused by deposition of monosodium urate crystals in joints. Based on the understanding that urate crystals activate the inflammasome, IL-1 antagonists have been used to effectively treat cases of severe gout that are resistant to conventional anti-inflammatory drugs. Similarly, pseudogout is caused by deposition of calcium pyrophosphate crystals and inflammasome activation. Occupational inhalation of silica and asbestos can cause chronic inflammatory and fibrotic disease of the lung, and there is also interest in the potential of blocking the inflammasome or IL-1 to treat these diseases.

Dysregulated activation of the inflammasome due to autosomal gain-of-function mutations in one or another of its component proteins leads to inappropriately triggered and excess IL-1 production. The result is recurrent attacks of fever and localized inflammation, most commonly in joints and intestines. These disorders are called Cryopyrin Associated Periodic Syndromes (CAPS) and are a subset of a larger group of periodic fever syndromes with similar symptoms caused by excessive production of or responses to inflammatory cytokines. These disorders are also called **autoinflammatory syndromes**, because they are characterized by spontaneous inflammation without an overt inciting trigger. Such diseases are distinct from *autoimmune disorders*, which are disorders of adaptive immunity caused by antibodies and/or T cells reactive with self antigens. Patients with CAPS can be successfully treated with IL-1 antagonists.

A great deal of interest in the inflammasome has recently been generated by findings that it may be activated by excessive amounts of endogenous substances deposited in tissues. These substances include cholesterol crystals in atherosclerosis, free fatty acids and lipids in obesity-associated metabolic syndrome, and β-amyloid in Alzheimer's disease. In all these situations, activation of the inflammasome leads to production of IL-1 and inflammation, which may contribute to the pathogenesis of the diseases. Such findings have spurred clinical trials to alleviate some of these diseases (atherosclerotic heart disease, obesity-associated type 2 diabetes) with IL-1 antagonists.

RIG-Like Receptors

RIG-like receptors (RLRs) are cytosolic sensors of viral RNA that respond to viral nucleic acids by inducing the production of the antiviral type I interferons. RLRs can recognize double-stranded RNA and RNA-DNA heteroduplexes, which include the genomes of RNA viruses and RNA transcripts of RNA and DNA viruses. The two best characterized RLRs are RIG-I (retinoic acid–inducible gene I) and MDA5 (melanoma differentiation-associated gene 5). Both of these proteins contain two N-terminal caspase recruitment domains that interact with other signaling proteins, an RNA-helicase domain, and a C-terminal domain, the latter two being involved in RNA recognition. RIG-I and MDA5 recognize different sets of viral RNAs that are characteristic of distinct viruses, partly based on the length of the RNA ligands. RLRs also can discriminate viral single-stranded RNA from normal cellular single-stranded RNA transcripts. For example, RIG-I will only recognize RNA with a 5′ triphosphate moiety, which is not present in mammalian host cell cytosolic RNA because of addition of a 7-methylguanosine cap or removal of the 5′ triphosphate. RLRs are expressed in a wide variety of cell types, including bone marrow-derived leukocytes and various tissue cells. Therefore, these receptors enable the many cell types susceptible to infection by RNA viruses to participate in innate immune responses to these viruses.

On binding viral RNA, the RLRs initiate signaling events that lead to phosphorylation and activation of IRF3 and IRF7, as well as NF-κB, and these transcription factors induce production of type I interferons.

Cytosolic DNA Sensors and the STING Pathway

Cytosolic DNA sensors (CDSs) are molecules that detect cytosolic DNA and activate signaling pathways that initiate anti-microbial responses, including type 1 interferon production and autophagy. DNA may be released into the cytosol from various intracellular microbes by different mechanisms. Several different cytosolic DNA sensing molecules and pathways have been characterized, including the following:

- *The STING (Stimulator of IFN Genes) pathway, is a major mechanism of DNA-induced activation of type 1 interferon responses.* STING is an endoplasmic reticulum–localized transmembrane protein, which is indirectly activated by microbial DNA in the cytosol. Cytosolic DNA binds to an enzyme called cyclic GMP-AMP synthase (cGAS) that synthesizes a cyclic dinucleotide called cyclic GMP-AMP (cGAMP) after it encounters DNA. cGAMP then interacts with and stimulates STING translocation to Golgi-derived membranes, where it serves as a scaffolding molecule that promotes phosphorylation of IRF3. Phosphorylated IRF3 translocates to the nucleus and induces type 1 interferon gene expression. STING also stimulates autophagy, a mechanism by which cells degrade their own organelles, such as mitochondria, by sequestering them within membrane-bound vesicles and fusing the vesicles with lysosomes. In innate immunity, autophagy is a mechanism to deliver cytosolic microbes to the lysosome, where they are killed by proteolytic enzymes.
- DNA-dependent activator of IFN-regulatory factors (DAI) binds DNA from several microbial sources and activates IRF3, leading to a type I IFN response. DAI also activates the NF-κB pathway.
- RNA polymerase 3 binds microbial DNA, transcribes it into RNA, and the RNA activates the RIG pathway leading to type I interferon expression, as described earlier.
- AIM2 (absent in melanoma-2) is another CDS that recognizes cytosolic dsDNA. It forms a caspase-1–containing inflammasome that processes pro-IL-1β and pro-IL-18.

Other Cell-Associated Pattern Recognition Receptors

Several other types of plasma membrane and cytoplasmic receptors transmit activating signals similar to TLRs that promote inflammatory responses and enhance killing of microbes, or mainly participate in the uptake of microbes into phagocytes (see Table 4-3).

Receptors for Carbohydrates

Receptors that recognize carbohydrates on the surface of microbes facilitate the phagocytosis of the microbes and the secretion of cytokines that promote subsequent adaptive immune responses. These receptors belong to the C-type lectin family, so called because they bind carbohydrates (hence, lectins) in a Ca++-dependent manner (hence, C-type), and have been called CLRs (C-type lectin receptors) to parallel the nomenclature of TLRs and other receptors. Some of the lectins are soluble proteins found in the blood and extracellular fluids (discussed later); others are integral membrane proteins found on the surfaces of macrophages, dendritic cells, and some tissue cells. All of these molecules contain a conserved carbohydrate recognition domain. There are several types of plasma membrane C-type lectins with specificities for different carbohydrates, including mannose, glucose, N-acetylglucosamine, and β-glucans. In general, these cell surface lectins recognize carbohydrate structures found on the cell walls of microorganisms but not mammalian cells. Some of these C-type lectin receptors function in the phagocytosis of microbes, and others have signaling functions that induce protective responses of host cells to microbes.

- *Mannose receptors.* One of the most studied membrane C-type lectins is the **mannose receptor** (CD206), which is involved in phagocytosis of microbes. This receptor recognizes certain terminal sugars on microbial surface carbohydrates, including D-mannose, L-fucose, and *N*-acetyl-D-glucosamine. These terminal sugars are often present on the surface of microorganisms, whereas eukaryotic cell carbohydrates are most often terminated by galactose and sialic acid. Thus, the terminal sugars on microbes can be considered PAMPs. Mannose receptors do not have any known intrinsic signaling functions and are thought to bind microbes as the first step in their ingestion by macrophages and dendritic cells. However, the overall importance of mannose receptor–mediated phagocytic clearance of microbes remains unknown.
- *Dectins.* Dectin-1 (dendritic cell–associated C-type lectin 1) and dectin-2 are dendritic cell receptors that serve as pattern recognition receptors for two life-cycle stages of fungal organisms. Dectin-1 binds β-glucan, which is a major cell wall component of the yeast form of *Candida albicans,* a ubiquitous but potentially pathogenic fungus. Dectin-2 recognizes high-mannose oligosaccharides on the hyphal form of *Candida.* The carbohydrate ligands of dectins are also expressed on some bacteria and other microbes. In response to binding of their ligands, both dectins induce signaling events in dendritic cells that stimulate the production of cytokines and other proteins that promote inflammation and enhance adaptive immune responses. Dectin stimulation of dendritic cells induces the production of some cytokines that promote the differentiation of naive CD4+ T cells to a type of effector T cell called T_H17, which is particularly effective in defense against fungal and some bacterial infections.
- Other dendritic cell carbohydrate receptors include langerin (CD207), mainly expressed by epidermal

Langerhans cells, and DC-SIGN (CD209), expressed on the majority of dendritic cells. DC-SIGN may play a pathogenic role in promoting HIV-1 infection of T cells. The HIV-1 gp120 envelope glycoprotein binds to DC-SIGN on dendritic cells in mucosal tissues, the dendritic cells carry the virus through lymphatics to draining lymph nodes, and the virus is then transferred to and infects CD4+ T cells.

Scavenger Receptors

Scavenger receptors comprise a structurally and functionally diverse collection of cell surface proteins that were originally grouped on the basis of the common characteristic of mediating the uptake of oxidized lipoproteins into cells. Some of these scavenger receptors, including SR-A and CD36, are expressed on macrophages and mediate the phagocytosis of microorganisms. In addition, CD36 functions as a coreceptor in TLR2/6 recognition and response to bacterially derived lipoteichoic acid and diacylated lipopeptides. There is a wide range of molecular structures that bind to each scavenger receptor, including LPS, lipoteichoic acid, nucleic acids, β-glucan, and proteins. The significance of scavenger receptors in innate immunity is highlighted by increased susceptibility to infection in gene knockout mice lacking these receptors and by the observation that several microbial pathogens express virulence factors that block scavenger receptor–mediated recognition and phagocytosis.

Formyl-Peptide Receptors

The **formyl peptide receptor-1** (FPR1), expressed on leukocytes, recognizes bacterial peptides containing *N*-formylmethionyl residues and stimulates directed movement of the cells. Because all bacterial proteins and few mammalian proteins (only those synthesized within mitochondria) are initiated by *N*-formylmethionine, FPR1 enables phagocytes to detect and respond preferentially to bacterial proteins. The bacterial peptide ligands that bind this receptor are some of the most potent chemoattractants for leukocytes. Chemoattractants include several types of diffusible molecules, often produced at sites of infection, that bind to specific receptors on cells and direct their movement toward the source of the chemoattractant. Other chemoattractants, such as the chemokines discussed in Chapter 3, are made by host cells. FPR1 and all other chemoattractant receptors belong to the seven-transmembrane, guanosine triphosphate (GTP)–binding (G) protein–coupled receptor (GPCR) superfamily. These receptors initiate intracellular responses through associated trimeric G proteins (see Chapter 7). The G proteins stimulate many types of cellular responses, including cytoskeletal changes that are responsible for the increased cell motility.

CELLULAR COMPONENTS OF THE INNATE IMMUNE SYSTEM

The cells of the innate immune system serve as sentinels to detect microbes and damaged cells in tissues and perform several functions that are essential for defense against microorganisms. Some cells form physical barriers that impede infections. Several cell types express the various pattern recognition receptors we have just discussed, and after recognizing PAMPs and DAMPs, the cells respond by producing inflammatory cytokines and antiviral proteins and by killing microbes or infected cells. In addition, some of the cells of innate immunity are critical for stimulating subsequent adaptive immune responses.

Epithelial Barriers

Intact epithelial surfaces form physical barriers between microbes in the external environment and host tissue, and epithelial cells produce antimicrobial chemicals that further impede the entry of microbes (Fig. 4-5). The main interfaces between the environment and the mammalian host are the skin and the mucosal surfaces of the gastrointestinal, respiratory, and genitourinary tracts. These interfaces are lined by continuous layers of specialized epithelial cells that serve many physiologic functions, including preventing the entry of microbes. Loss of the integrity of these epithelial layers by trauma or other reasons predisposes an individual to infections.

The protective function of barrier epithelia is in large part physical. The epithelial cells form tight junctions with one another, blocking passage of microbes between the cells. The outer layer of keratin, which accumulates as keratinocytes on the skin surface die, serves to block microbial penetration into deeper layers of the epidermis. Mucus, a viscous secretion containing glycoproteins called mucins, is produced by respiratory, gastrointestinal, and urogenital epithelial cells and physically impairs microbial invasion. The function of these barriers is enhanced by ciliary action in the bronchial tree and peristalsis in the gut, which facilitate elimination of microbes. Although these physical properties alone are very important in

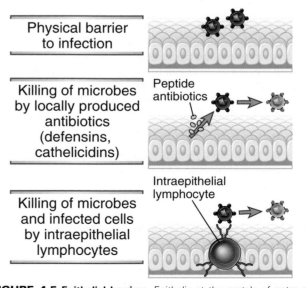

FIGURE 4-5 Epithelial barriers. Epithelia at the portals of entry of microbes provide physical barriers, produce antimicrobial substances, and harbor intraepithelial lymphocytes that are believed to kill microbes and infected cells.

host defense, other epithelial defense mechanisms have evolved to complement the mechanical barrier.

Epithelial cells as well as some leukocytes produce peptides that have antimicrobial properties. Two structurally distinct families of antimicrobial peptides are the defensins and the cathelicidins.

- **Defensins** are small cationic peptides, 29 to 34 amino acids long, that contain both cationic and hydrophobic regions and three intrachain disulfide bonds. Two families of human defensins, named α and β, are distinguished by the location of these bonds. Defensins are produced by epithelial cells of mucosal surfaces and by granule-containing leukocytes, including neutrophils, natural killer cells, and cytotoxic T lymphocytes. The set of defensin molecules produced differs between different cell types. Paneth cells within the crypts of the small bowel are a major producer of α defensins. Paneth cell defensins are sometimes called crypticidins; their function is to limit the amount of microbes in the lumen. Defensins are also produced elsewhere in the bowel, in respiratory mucosal cells, and in the skin. Some defensins are constitutively produced by some cell types, but their secretion may be enhanced by cytokines or microbial products. In other cells, defensins are produced only in response to cytokines and microbial products. The protective actions of the defensins include both direct toxicity to microbes, including bacteria, fungi and enveloped viruses, and the activation of cells involved in the inflammatory response to microbes. Defensins kill microbes by a variety of mechanisms, many of which depend on their ability to insert into and disrupt functions of the microbial membranes.
- **Cathelicidin** is produced by neutrophils and barrier epithelial cells in the skin, gastrointestinal tract, and respiratory tract. Cathelicidin is synthesized as an 18-kD two-domain precursor protein and is proteolytically cleaved into two peptides, each with protective functions. Both precursor synthesis and proteolytic cleavage may be stimulated by inflammatory cytokines and microbial products. The active cathelicidins protect against infections by multiple mechanisms, including direct toxicity to a broad range of microorganisms and the activation of various responses in leukocytes and other cell types that promote eradication of microbes. The C-terminal fragment, called LL-37, can bind and neutralize LPS, a toxic component of the outer wall of gram-negative bacteria that was mentioned earlier. LL-37 also plays an anti-inflammatory role by binding to DNA and blocking AIM2 inflammasome activation.

Barrier epithelia contain certain types of lymphocytes, including intraepithelial T lymphocytes, which recognize and respond to commonly encountered microbes. Intraepithelial T lymphocytes are present in the epidermis of the skin and in mucosal epithelia. Various subsets of intraepithelial lymphocytes are present in different proportions, depending on species and tissue location. These subsets are distinguished mainly by the type of T cell antigen receptors (TCRs) they express. Some intraepithelial T lymphocytes express the conventional αβ form of TCR, which is present on most T cells in lymphoid tissues and

the circulation. Other T cells in epithelia express a form of antigen receptor called the γδ TCR that may recognize peptide and nonpeptide antigens. A common characteristic of these T cells is the limited diversity of their antigen receptors compared with most T cells in the adaptive immune system. The intraepithelial T lymphocytes are believed to recognize a small number of commonly encountered microbial structures. Intraepithelial lymphocytes may function in host defense by secreting cytokines, activating phagocytes, and killing infected cells.

Phagocytes

Cells that have specialized phagocytic functions, primarily macrophages and neutrophils, are the first line of defense against microbes that breach epithelial barriers. We introduced these cell types in Chapter 2, and we will discuss many other details of their functions in the context of the inflammatory response later in this chapter. The essential role that phagocytes play in innate immune defense against microbes is demonstrated by the high rate of lethal bacterial and fungal infections in patients with low blood neutrophil counts caused by bone marrow cancers or cancer therapy and in patients with inherited deficiencies in the functions of phagocytes.

Dendritic Cells

Dendritic cells perform essential recognition and effector roles in innate immunity. Dendritic cells were also introduced in Chapter 2, and we will discuss their role in antigen presentation to T cells in Chapter 6. Recall that dendritic cells, a heterogeneous family of cells with long dendrite-like cytoplasmic processes, are constitutively present in epithelia and most tissues of the body. Because of their placement and morphology, these cells are poised to detect invading microbes. Furthermore, dendritic cells express more different types of TLRs and cytoplasmic pattern recognition receptors than any other cell type, making them the most versatile sensors of PAMPs and DAMPs among all cell types in the body. One particular subset of dendritic cells, called plasmacytoid dendritic cells because their morphology is similar to antibody-producing plasma cells, is a major source of the antiviral cytokines, type I interferons, produced in response to viral infections. This feature of plasmacytoid dendritic cells is due in part to the fact that these cells express abundant amounts of the endosomal TLRs (TLRs 3, 7, 8, 9), which recognize nucleic acids of viruses that have been internalized into the cell. We will discuss the antiviral actions of type I interferons in more detail later in the chapter.

Dendritic cells are uniquely capable of triggering and directing adaptive T cell–mediated immune responses, and this is dependent on their innate immune responses to microbes. This capability reflects the ability of dendritic cells to take up microbial protein antigens, to transport them to lymph nodes where naive T cells home, and to display the protein antigens in a form that the T cells can recognize (see Chapter 6). Importantly, the innate response of dendritic cells to PAMPs, particularly TLR signaling, enhances the ability of dendritic cells to process and present foreign antigens. Furthermore, TLR signaling induces dendritic cell expression of molecules, including costimulators and cytokines, that are needed, in addition to antigen, for the activation of naive T cells and their differentiation into effector T cells. Depending on the nature of the microbe that induces the innate response, a dendritic cell will direct naive T cell differentiation into distinct types of effector cells, such as IFN-γ–producing T_H1 cells or IL-17–producing T_H17 cells. We will discuss the influence of dendritic cells on T cell activation and differentiation in Chapter 9.

Natural Killer Cells and Other Innate Lymphoid Cells

Innate lymphoid cells (ILCs), which were introduced in Chapter 2, are bone marrow–derived cells with lymphocyte morphology that serve diverse antimicrobial functions. These cells arise from a common bone marrow precursor identifiable by expression of the Id2 transcription factor, they depend on IL-7 or, in one case, IL-15 for development, and, unlike lymphocytes of the adaptive immune system, they emerge fully capable of performing effector functions without the need for clonal expansion and differentiation. ILCs use effector mechanisms shared by T cells, particularly the ability to produce various cytokines, but they do not rearrange antigen receptor genes and do not express TCRs. There are three major subsets of innate lymphoid cells, distinguished by the cytokines they produce (Fig. 4-6). Each type can be further divided into additional subsets based on cell surface molecules

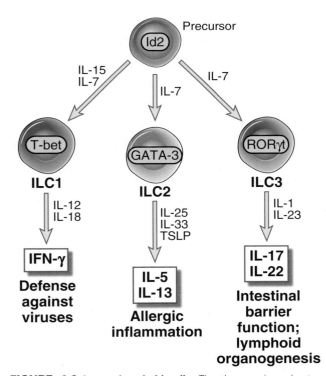

FIGURE 4-6 Innate lymphoid cells. The three major subsets of innate lymphoid cells (ILCs) all develop from a common bone marrow precursor identified by the Id2 transcription factor. Each differentiated subset is distinguished by expression of distinct transcription factors and by cytokines produced when activated, as indicated. The cytokines that drive differentiation into ILC1, 2, or 3 subsets, as well as the cytokines that activate ILCs to produce their own subset-specific cytokines, are shown. The major known functions of the ILCs are also indicated.

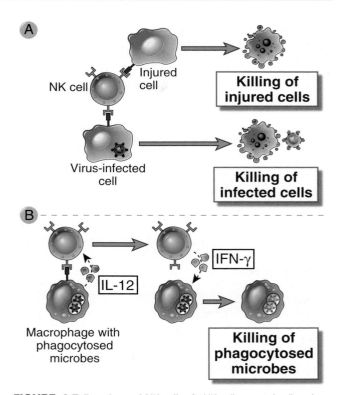

FIGURE 4-7 Functions of NK cells. A, NK cells recognize ligands on infected cells or cells undergoing other types of stress and kill the host cells. In this way, NK cells eliminate reservoirs of infection as well as dysfunctional cells. **B,** NK cells respond to IL-12 produced by macrophages and secrete IFN-γ, which activates the macrophages to kill phagocytosed microbes.

and the effector mechanisms they use to perform their protective functions (discussed shortly).

Natural Killer Cells

Natural killer (NK) cells, the first and best described innate lymphoid cells, are a subtype of type 1 ILCs, which play important roles in innate immune responses mainly against intracellular viruses and bacteria. The term *natural killer* derives from the fact that their major function is killing infected cells, similar to the adaptive immune system's killer cells, the cytotoxic T lymphocytes (CTLs), and they are ready to do so once they develop, without further differentiation (hence *natural*). NK cells constitute 5% to 15% of the mononuclear cells in the blood and spleen. They are rare in other lymphoid organs but are more abundant in certain organs such as the liver and gravid uterus. NK cells in the blood appear as large lymphocytes with numerous cytoplasmic granules. As with all ILCs, NK cells do not express diverse, clonally distributed antigen receptors typical of B and T cells. Rather, they use germline DNA-encoded receptors (discussed later) to distinguish pathogen-infected cells from healthy cells. They can be identified in the blood by expression of CD56 and the absence of the T cell marker CD3. Most human blood NK cells also express CD16, which is involved in recognition of antibody-coated cells.

Functions of NK Cells

The effector functions of NK cells are to kill infected cells and to produce IFN-γ, which activates macrophages to destroy phagocytosed microbes (Fig. 4-7). The mechanism of NK cell–mediated cytotoxicity is essentially the same as that of CD8+ CTLs, which we will describe in detail in Chapter 11. NK cells, like CTLs, have granules containing proteins that mediate killing of target cells. When NK cells are activated, granule exocytosis releases these proteins adjacent to the target cells. One NK cell granule protein, called **perforin**, facilitates the entry of other granule proteins, called **granzymes**, into the cytosol of target cells. The granzymes are enzymes that initiate a sequence of signaling events that cause death of the target cells by apoptosis. By killing cells infected by viruses and intracellular bacteria, NK cells eliminate reservoirs of infection. Early in the course of a viral infection, NK cells are expanded and activated by IL-12 and IL-15, and they kill infected cells before antigen-specific CTLs can become fully active. NK cells may also be important later in the course of viral infection by killing infected cells that have escaped CTL-mediated immune attack by reducing expression of class I MHC molecules. Some tumors, especially those of hematopoietic origin, are targets of NK cells, perhaps because the tumor cells do not express normal levels or types of class I MHC molecules.

NK cell–derived IFN-γ increases the capacity of macrophages to kill phagocytosed bacteria, similar to IFN-γ produced by T cells (see Chapter 10). This IFN-γ–dependent NK cell–macrophage interaction can control an infection with intracellular bacteria such as *Listeria monocytogenes* for several days or weeks and thus allow time for T cell–mediated immunity to develop and eradicate the infection. IFN-γ produced by NK cells in lymph nodes can also direct the differentiation of naive T cells into T_H1 cells (see Chapter 10). Some human NK cells do not express CD16 nor are they cytotoxic, but they do produce abundant IFN-γ. Predictably, depletion of NK cells leads to increased susceptibility to infection by some viruses and intracellular bacteria. In mice lacking T cells, the NK cell response may be adequate to keep infection with such microbes in check for some time, but the animals eventually succumb in the absence of T cell–mediated immunity.

Activating and Inhibitory Receptors of NK Cells

NK cells distinguish infected and stressed cells from healthy cells, and NK cell function is regulated by a balance between signals that are generated from activating receptors and inhibitory receptors. These receptors recognize molecules on the surface of other cells and generate activating or inhibitory signals that promote or inhibit NK responses. The activating receptors stimulate protein kinases that phosphorylate downstream signaling substrates, while inhibitory receptors stimulate phosphatases that counteract the kinases. We will discuss the details of NK receptor signaling later in the chapter. In general, the activating receptors recognize ligands on infected and injured cells, which need to be eliminated, and the inhibitory receptors recognize healthy normal cells, which need to be preserved (Fig. 4-8). When an NK cell interacts with another cell, the outcome is determined by the integration of signals generated from the array of inhibitory and activating receptors that are expressed by the NK cell and that

interact with ligands on the other cell. Engagement of activating receptors stimulates the killing activity of the NK cells resulting in destruction of stressed or infected cells. In contrast, engagement of inhibitory receptors shuts off NK function and prevents destruction of healthy cells. Because of the stochastic nature of their expression, there is significant diversity in the array of activating and inhibitory receptors that different NK cells express in any one individual. The result of this is that individual NK cells even in the same person may respond to different types of microbes or infected cells. Furthermore, the genes encoding many of these receptors are polymorphic, meaning that there are several variants of the genes in the population, so that one person will express a slightly different form of the receptors than another person.

Activating receptors on NK cells recognize a heterogeneous group of ligands, some of which may be expressed on normal cells and others of which are expressed mainly on cells that have undergone stress, are infected with microbes, or are transformed (Fig. 4-9). Many of the NK cell–activating receptors are called **killer cell immunoglobulin (Ig)-like receptors (KIRs)** because they contain a structural domain called an Ig fold, first identified in antibody (also known as Ig) molecules, discussed in Chapter 5. All proteins with Ig folds are members of the Ig superfamily. A second important group of activating NK receptors belong to the family of C-type lectins, which are proteins with carbohydrate-binding properties. Some of the activating receptors appear to bind class I MHC molecules which is an important property of inhibitory receptors, as we will discuss later. The significance of class I MHC recognition by activating receptors is not known. Other activating receptors recognize ligands other than classical MHC molecules. One well-studied NK cell–activating receptor in the C-type lectin family is NKG2D, which binds class I MHC–like proteins, including MIC-A and MIC-B, which are found on virally infected cells and tumor cells but not normal cells. The NKG2D receptor associates with a signaling subunit named DAP10, which has signaling functions that enhance NK cell cytotoxicity against target cells.

Another important activating receptor on NK cells is CD16 (FcγRIIIA), which is a low-affinity receptor for IgG antibodies. Antibody molecules have highly variable antigen-binding ends, and on the opposite end, they have an invariant portion, called the Fc region, that interacts with various other molecules in the immune system. We will describe the structure of antibodies in detail in Chapter 5 but, for now, it is sufficient to know that CD16 binds to the Fc regions of certain types of antibodies called IgG1 and IgG3. CD16 associates with one of three different signaling proteins (e.g., FcεRIγ, ζ, and DAP12 proteins). During an infection, the adaptive immune system produces IgG1 and IgG3 antibodies that bind to microbial antigens expressed on the surface of infected cells, and CD16 on NK cells can bind to the Fc regions of these antibodies. As a result, CD16 generates activating signals, through its associated signaling partners, and the NK cells may kill the infected cells that have been coated with antibody molecules. This process is called **antibody-dependent cell-mediated**

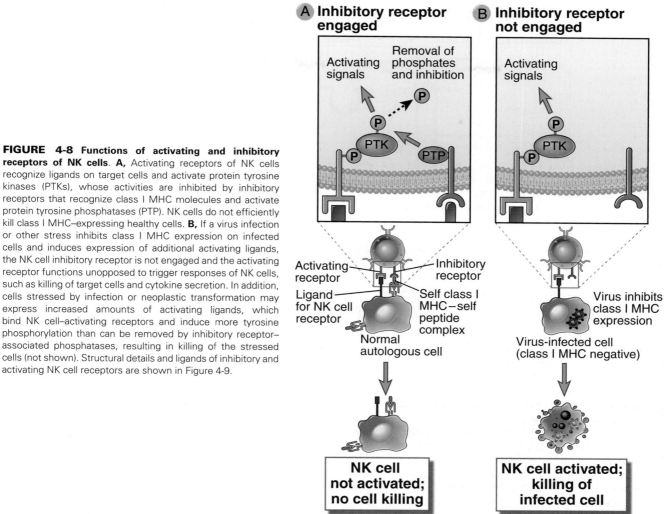

FIGURE 4-8 Functions of activating and inhibitory receptors of NK cells. **A,** Activating receptors of NK cells recognize ligands on target cells and activate protein tyrosine kinases (PTKs), whose activities are inhibited by inhibitory receptors that recognize class I MHC molecules and activate protein tyrosine phosphatases (PTP). NK cells do not efficiently kill class I MHC–expressing healthy cells. **B,** If a virus infection or other stress inhibits class I MHC expression on infected cells and induces expression of additional activating ligands, the NK cell inhibitory receptor is not engaged and the activating receptor functions unopposed to trigger responses of NK cells, such as killing of target cells and cytokine secretion. In addition, cells stressed by infection or neoplastic transformation may express increased amounts of activating ligands, which bind NK cell–activating receptors and induce more tyrosine phosphorylation than can be removed by inhibitory receptor–associated phosphatases, resulting in killing of the stressed cells (not shown). Structural details and ligands of inhibitory and activating NK cell receptors are shown in Figure 4-9.

cytotoxicity; it is an effector function of adaptive immunity, which we will discuss in Chapter 13 when we consider humoral immunity.

Most NK cells express inhibitory receptors that recognize class I major histocompatibility complex (MHC) molecules, which are cell surface proteins normally expressed on all healthy nucleated cells in the body (see Fig. 4-9). A major function of class I MHC molecules, distinct from their role in regulating NK cell activation, is to display peptides derived from cytoplasmic proteins, including microbial proteins, on the cell surface for recognition by CD8+ T lymphocytes. We will describe the structure and function of MHC molecules in relation to T cell antigen recognition in Chapter 6. For now, it is important to understand that NK cells use fundamentally different types of receptors than do T cells to recognize class I MHC molecules. Unlike T cells, many of the NK receptors for class I MHC respond by inhibiting NK activation. This is useful because normal cells express class I MHC molecules, and many viruses and other causes of cell stress lead to a loss of cell surface expression of class I MHC. Thus, NK cells interpret the presence of class I MHC molecules

as markers of normal, healthy self, and their absence is an indication of infection or damage. Thus, NK cells will be inhibited by healthy cells but will not receive inhibitory signals from infected or stressed cells. At the same time, the NK cells are likely to receive activating signals from the same infected cells through activating receptors. The net result will be activation of the NK cell to secrete cytokines and to kill the infected or stressed cell. This ability of NK cells to become activated by host cells that lack class I MHC has been called recognition of missing self.

The largest group of NK inhibitory receptors are the KIRs, which bind a variety of class I MHC molecules. Other inhibitory receptors are lectins, such as the CD94/NKG2A heterodimer, which recognizes a class I MHC molecule called HLA-E. Interestingly, HLA-E displays peptides derived from other class I MHC molecules; so in essence, CD94/NKG2A is a surveillance receptor for several different class I MHC molecules. A third family of NK inhibitory receptors, called the leukocyte Ig-like receptors (LIRs), are also Ig superfamily members that bind class I MHC molecules, albeit with lower affinity than the KIRs, and are more highly expressed on B cells than on NK cells.

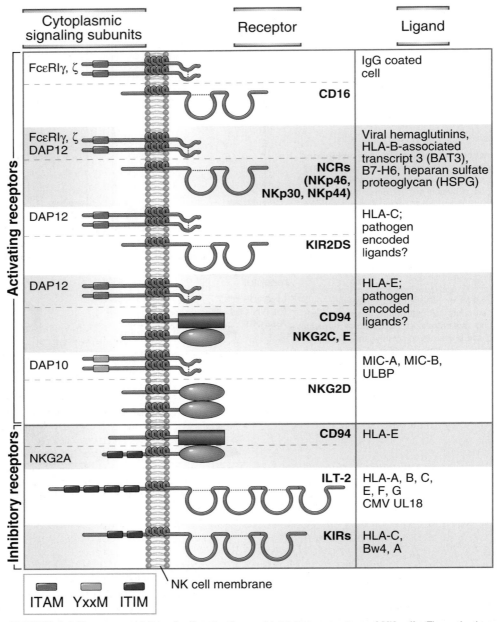

FIGURE 4-9 **Structure and ligands of activating and inhibitory receptors of NK cells**. The activating and inhibitory receptors are indicated in bold. CD16 and the natural cytotoxic receptors (NCRs) associate with ζ chain homodimers, FcεRIγ homodimers, or ζ-FcεRIγ heterodimers. There are multiple different KIRs, with different ligand specificities.

Activating and inhibitory NK receptors contain structural motifs in their cytoplasmic tails, which engage the signaling pathways that respectively promote or inhibit target cell killing and cytokine secretion (see Figs. 4-8 and 4-9). Activating receptors have **immunoreceptor tyrosine-based activation motifs (ITAMs),** which contain tyrosine residues that become phosphorylated by cytoplasmic kinases after ligand binding to the receptors. Other protein kinases are recruited to the modified ITAMs and become activated, and these kinases contribute to further signaling by phosphorylating additional proteins, eventually leading to cytotoxic activity and cytokine secretion. ITAMs also are found in

cytoplasmic tails of other multichain signaling receptors in the immune system, including the antigen receptors on T and B cells, and we will discuss their structure and signaling functions in more detail in Chapter 7. In some activating receptors, a single polypeptide chain contains the ITAM as well as the extracellular ligand-binding portion. In other receptors, the ITAMs are in separate polypeptide chains, such as FcεRIγ, ζ, and DAP12, which do not bind ligand but are noncovalently associated with the ligand-binding chain.

Inhibitory receptors of NK cells have **immunoreceptor tyrosine-based inhibition motifs (ITIMs),** which engage molecules that block the signaling pathways of activating receptors (see Figs. 4-8 and 4-9). ITIMs contain tyrosine residues that are phosphorylated on ligand binding to the inhibitory receptor. This leads to the recruitment and activation of phosphatases, which remove phosphates from several signaling proteins or lipids generated by the signaling pathways downstream of NK activating receptors. The end result is blocking of the signaling functions of activating receptors. ITIMs also are found in cytoplasmic tails of other receptors besides NK inhibitory receptors, and we will discuss their structure and signaling functions in more detail in Chapter 7.

KIR genes are polymorphic, meaning that there are several allelic variants in the human population, and groups of KIR alleles are often inherited together from a single parent. These groups of linked genes are called *KIR* haplotypes. There are two major *KIR* haplotypes and some rarer ones. Haplotypes differ in the number of receptors encoded, and some have more or fewer activating receptors than others. Some haplotypes are associated with increased susceptibility to some diseases, including spontaneous abortion and uveitis.

Cytokines can enhance the functional responses of NK cells. The major cytokines of the innate immune system that stimulate NK function are IL-12, IL-15, IL-18, and type I interferons (discussed later). Each of these cytokines enhances the cytotoxic activity of NK cells, and they can stimulate IFN-γ secretion by the NK cell independent of activating receptors. In addition, IL-12 and IL-15 are important growth factors for NK cells.

Other Innate Lymphoid Cells

The three subsets of innate lymphoid cells, Group 1 (which includes NK cells), Group 2 and Group 3, produce different sets of cytokines, participate in host defense against distinct pathogens, and may be involved in different inflammatory disorders. These subsets are analogous to the T_H1, T_H2 and T_H17 subsets of CD4+ T lymphocytes that secrete some of the same cytokines (see Fig. 4-6). Group 1 ILCs produce IFN-γ and include the cytotoxic and non-cytotoxic NK cells described earlier. Group 2 ILCs, like the T_H2 subset of CD4+ helper T cells, secrete IL-5, IL-9 and IL-13, and express the GATA2 transcription factor. These cells protect mice from parasitic helminthic infections and also contribute to allergic disease. Group 3 ILCs produce IL-22 and/or IL-17 and express the transcription factor RORγt, which are features shared by the T_H17 subset of CD4+ helper T cells. Group 3 ILCs are found at mucosal sites and participate in defense against extracellular bacteria as well as in maintaining the integrity of epithelial barriers. Lymphoid tissue–inducer (LTi) cells are Group 3 ILCs, which, in addition to secreting IL-17 and IL-22, also express membrane lymphotoxin-α and secrete TNF, cytokines that are required for the normal development of lymphoid organs (see Chapter 2).

T and B Lymphocytes with Limited Antigen Receptor Diversity

As we will discuss in greater detail in later chapters, most T and B lymphocytes are components of the adaptive immune system and are characterized by a highly diverse repertoire of specificities for different antigens. However, certain small populations of lymphocytes express antigen receptors that are structurally the same as those of T and B cells, but these receptors have very little diversity. These T and B cell subsets may recognize structures expressed by many different or commonly encountered microbial species. T cells with limited antigen receptor diversity include invariant natural killer T cells (iNKT), γδ T cells, and intraepithelial T cells with αβ TCRs (mentioned earlier). B cell subsets that produce antibodies with a limited set of specificities include B-1 cells and marginal-zone B cells. Although these T and B cells perform similar functions as do their more clonally diverse counterparts, the nature of their specificities places them in a special category of lymphocytes that is akin more to cells of innate immunity than to cells of adaptive immunity. These special T and B cell subsets are described in Chapters 10 and 12, respectively.

Mast Cells

Mast cells are present in the skin and mucosal epithelium and rapidly secrete proinflammatory cytokines and lipid mediators in response to infections and other stimuli. We introduced mast cells in Chapter 2. Recall that these cells contain abundant cytoplasmic granules filled with various inflammatory mediators that are released when the cells are activated, either by microbial products or by a special antibody-dependent mechanism. The granule contents include vasoactive amines (such as histamine) that cause vasodilation and increased capillary permeability, and proteolytic enzymes that can kill bacteria or inactivate microbial toxins. Mast cells also synthesize and secrete lipid mediators (such as prostaglandins) and cytokines (such as TNF). Because mast cells are usually located adjacent to blood vessels (see Fig. 2-1, *B*), their released granule contents rapidly induce changes in the blood vessels that promote acute inflammation. Mast cells express TLRs, and TLR ligands can induce mast cell degranulation. Mast cell–deficient mice are impaired in controlling bacterial infections, probably because of defective innate immune responses. Mast cell products also provide defense against helminths and are responsible for symptoms of allergic diseases. We will return to a detailed discussion of mast cells in relation to allergic diseases in Chapter 20.

SOLUBLE RECOGNITION AND EFFECTOR MOLECULES OF INNATE IMMUNITY

Several different kinds of molecules that recognize microbes and promote innate responses exist in soluble form in the blood and extracellular fluids. These molecules provide early defense against pathogens that are present outside host cells at some stage of their life cycle. The soluble effector molecules function in two major ways.

- By binding to microbes, they act as **opsonins** and enhance the ability of macrophages, neutrophils, and

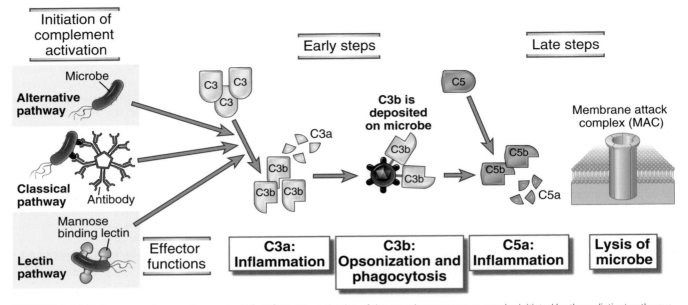

FIGURE 4-10 Pathways of complement activation. The activation of the complement system may be initiated by three distinct pathways, all of which lead to the production of C3b (the early steps). C3b initiates the late steps of complement activation, culminating in the production of peptides that stimulate inflammation (C5a) and polymerized C9, which forms the membrane attack complex, so called because it creates holes in plasma membranes. The principal functions of major proteins produced at different steps are shown. The activation, functions, and regulation of the complement system are discussed in much more detail in Chapter 12.

dendritic cells to phagocytose the microbes. This is because the phagocytic cells express membrane receptors specific for the opsonins, and these receptors can efficiently mediate the internalization of the complex of opsonin and bound microbe.

- After binding to microbes, soluble mediators of innate immunity promote inflammatory responses that bring more phagocytes to sites of infections, and they may also directly kill microbes.

The soluble effector molecules are sometimes called the humoral branch of innate immunity, analogous to the humoral branch of adaptive immunity mediated by antibodies. The major components of the humoral innate immune system are the complement system, collectins, pentraxins, and ficolins, which are described next.

The Complement System

The complement system consists of several plasma proteins that work together to opsonize microbes, to promote the recruitment of phagocytes to the site of infection, and, in some cases, to directly kill the microbes (Fig. 4-10). Complement activation involves proteolytic cascades in which an inactive precursor enzyme, called a zymogen, is altered to become an active protease that cleaves and thereby induces the proteolytic activity of the next complement protein in the cascade. Enzymatic cascades result in tremendous amplification of the amount of proteolytic products that are generated. These products perform the effector functions of the complement system. Besides the complement system, other medically important proteolytic cascades include the blood coagulation pathways

and the kinin-kallikrein system that regulates vascular permeability.

The first step in activation of the complement system is recognition of molecules on microbial surfaces but not host cells, and this occurs in three ways, each referred to as a distinct pathway of complement activation.

- The **classical pathway**, so called because it was discovered first, uses a plasma protein called C1q to detect antibodies bound to the surface of a microbe or other structure (Fig. 4-11). Once C1q binds to the Fc portion of the antibodies, two associated serine proteases, called C1r and C1s, become active and initiate a proteolytic cascade involving other complement proteins. The classical pathway is one of the major effector mechanisms of the humoral arm of adaptive immune responses (see Chapter 13). Innate immune system soluble proteins called pentraxins, which are discussed later, can also bind C1q and initiate the classical pathway.
- The **alternative pathway**, which was discovered later but is phylogenetically older than the classical pathway, is triggered when a complement protein called C3 directly recognizes certain microbial surface structures, such as bacterial LPS. C3 is also constitutively activated in solution at a low level and binds to cell surfaces, but it is then inhibited by regulatory molecules present on mammalian cells. Because microbes lack these regulatory proteins, the spontaneous activation can be amplified on microbial surfaces. Thus, this pathway can distinguish normal self from foreign microbes on the basis of the presence or absence of the regulatory proteins.
- The **lectin pathway** is triggered by a plasma protein called mannose-binding lectin (MBL), which

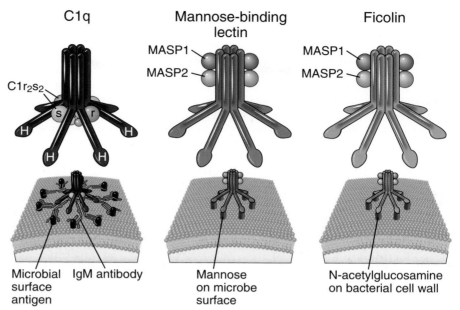

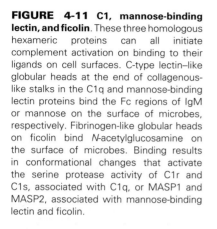

FIGURE 4-11 C1, mannose-binding lectin, and ficolin. These three homologous hexameric proteins can all initiate complement activation on binding to their ligands on cell surfaces. C-type lectin–like globular heads at the end of collagenous-like stalks in the C1q and mannose-binding lectin proteins bind the Fc regions of IgM or mannose on the surface of microbes, respectively. Fibrinogen-like globular heads on ficolin bind *N*-acetylglucosamine on the surface of microbes. Binding results in conformational changes that activate the serine protease activity of C1r and C1s, associated with C1q, or MASP1 and MASP2, associated with mannose-binding lectin and ficolin.

recognizes terminal mannose residues on microbial glycoproteins and glycolipids, similar to the mannose receptor on phagocyte membranes described earlier (see Fig. 4-11). MBL is a member of the collectin family (discussed later) with a hexameric structure similar to the C1q component of the complement system. After MBL binds to microbes, two zymogens called MASP1 (mannose-associated serine protease 1, or mannan-binding lectin-associated serine protease) and MASP2, with similar functions to C1r and C1s, associate with MBL and initiate downstream proteolytic steps identical to the classical pathway.

Recognition of microbes by any of the three complement pathways results in sequential recruitment and assembly of additional complement proteins into protease complexes (see Fig. 4-10). One of these complexes, called **C3 convertase,** cleaves the central protein of the complement system, **C3,** producing C3a and C3b. The larger C3b fragment becomes covalently attached to the microbial surface where the complement pathway was activated. C3b serves as an opsonin to promote phagocytosis of the microbes. The smaller fragment, C3a, is released and stimulates inflammation by acting as a chemoattractant for neutrophils. C3b binds other complement proteins to form a protease called **C5 convertase** that cleaves C5, generating a released peptide (C5a) and a larger fragment (C5b) that remains attached to the microbial cell membranes. C5a is also a chemoattractant; in addition, it induces changes in blood vessels that make them leak plasma proteins and fluid into sites of infections. C5b initiates the formation of a complex of the complement proteins C6, C7, C8, and C9, which are assembled into a membrane pore called the **membrane attack complex** (MAC) that causes lysis of the cells where complement is activated.

The complement system is an essential component of innate immunity, and patients with deficiencies in C3 are highly susceptible to recurrent, often lethal, bacterial infections. Genetic deficiencies in MAC formation (the terminal product of the classical pathway) increase susceptibility to only a limited number of microbes, notably *Neisseria* bacteria, which have thin cell walls that make them especially susceptible to the lytic action of the MAC. We will discuss the complement system in more detail in Chapter 13.

Pentraxins

Several plasma proteins that recognize microbial structures and participate in innate immunity belong to the pentraxin family, which is a phylogenetically old group of structurally homologous pentameric proteins. Prominent members of this family include the short pentraxins C-reactive protein (CRP) and serum amyloid P (SAP) and the long pentraxin PTX3. Both CRP and SAP bind to several different species of bacteria and fungi. The molecular ligands recognized by CRP and SAP include phosphorylcholine and phosphatidylethanolamine, respectively, which are found on bacterial membranes and become exposed on apoptotic cells. CRP, SAP, and PTX3 all activate complement by binding C1q and initiating the classical pathway.

Plasma concentrations of CRP are very low in healthy individuals but can increase up to 1000-fold during infections and in response to other inflammatory stimuli. The increased levels of CRP are a result of increased synthesis by the liver induced by the cytokines IL-6 and IL-1, which are produced by phagocytes as part of the innate immune response. Liver synthesis and plasma levels of several other proteins, including SAP and others unrelated to the pentraxins, also increase in response to IL-1 and IL-6. These plasma proteins are called **acute-phase**

reactants because they are elevated in the blood during acute inflammatory reactions.

PTX3 is produced by several cell types, including dendritic cells, macrophages, and endothelial cells, in response to TLR ligands and inflammatory cytokines, such as TNF, but it is not an acute-phase reactant. PTX3 is also stored in neutrophil granules and released as neutrophils die. PTX3 recognizes various molecules on fungi and selected gram-positive and gram-negative bacteria, and viruses, as well as apoptotic cells. Studies with knockout mice reveal that PTX3 provides protection against these microbes, including the fungus *Aspergillus fumigatus*. PTX3 also contributes to protection against the influenza virus.

Collectins and Ficolins

The **collectins** are a family of trimeric or hexameric proteins, each subunit of which contains a collagen-like tail connected by a neck region to a calcium-dependent (C-type) lectin head. Three members of this family serve as soluble effector molecules in the innate immune system; these are mannose-binding lectin (MBL) and pulmonary surfactant proteins SP-A and SP-D.

Mannose-binding lectin (MBL), which is a soluble pattern recognition receptor that binds carbohydrates with terminal mannose and fucose, was discussed earlier in relation to the lectin pathway of complement activation (see Fig. 4-11). MBL can also function as an opsonin by binding to and enhancing phagocytosis of microbes. Recall that opsonins simultaneously bind microbes and a surface receptor on phagocyte membranes, and in the case of MBL, the surface receptor is called the C1q receptor because it also binds C1q. This receptor mediates the internalization of microbes that are opsonized by MBL. The gene encoding MBL is polymorphic, and certain alleles are associated with impaired hexamer formation and reduced blood levels. Low MBL levels are associated with increased susceptibility to a variety of infections, especially in combination with other immunodeficiency states.

Surfactant protein A (SP-A) and surfactant protein D (SP-D) are collectins with lipophilic properties shared by other surfactants. They are found in the alveoli of the lungs, and their major functions are to maintain the ability of lungs to expand and as mediators of innate immune responses in the lung. They bind to various microorganisms and act as opsonins, facilitating ingestion by alveolar macrophages. SP-A and SP-D can also directly inhibit bacterial growth, and they may activate macrophages. SP-A– and SP-D–deficient mice have impaired abilities to resist a variety of pulmonary infections.

Ficolins are plasma proteins that are structurally similar to collectins. They possess a collagen-like domain, but instead of a C-type lectin domain, they have a fibrinogen-type carbohydrate recognition domain (see Fig. 4-11). Ficolins have been shown to bind several species of bacteria, opsonizing them and activating complement in a manner similar to that of MBL. The molecular ligands of the ficolins include *N*-acetylglucosamine and the lipoteichoic acid component of the cell walls of gram-positive bacteria.

Now that we have discussed the general properties and various components of the innate immune system, including the cells, cellular pathogen recognition receptors, and soluble recognition and effector molecules, we can consider how these various components work to protect against pathogens. The three major ways in which the innate immune system protects against infections is by inducing inflammation, inducing antiviral defense, and stimulating adaptive immunity.

THE INFLAMMATORY RESPONSE

A major way by which the innate immune system deals with infections and tissue injury is to stimulate acute inflammation, which is the accumulation of leukocytes, plasma proteins, and fluid derived from the blood at an extravascular tissue site of infection or injury. The leukocytes and plasma proteins normally circulate in the blood and are recruited to sites of infection and injury, where they perform various effector functions that serve to kill microbes and begin to repair tissue damage. Typically, the most abundant leukocyte that is recruited from the blood into acute inflammatory sites is the neutrophil, but blood monocytes, which become macrophages in the tissue, are increasingly prominent over time and may be the dominant population in some reactions. Among the important plasma proteins that enter inflammatory sites are complement proteins, antibodies, and acute-phase reactants. The delivery of these blood-derived components to the inflammatory site is dependent on reversible changes in blood vessels in the infected or damaged tissue. These changes include increased blood flow into the tissue due to arteriolar dilation, increased adhesiveness of circulating leukocytes to the endothelial lining of venules, and increased permeability of the capillaries and venules to plasma proteins and fluid. All of these changes are induced by cytokines and small-molecule mediators initially derived from resident cells in the tissue, such as mast cells, macrophages, and endothelial cells, in response to PAMP or DAMP stimulation. As the inflammatory process develops, the mediators may be derived from newly arrived and activated leukocytes and complement proteins.

Acute inflammation can develop in minutes to hours and last for days. Chronic inflammation is a process that takes over from acute inflammation if the infection is not eliminated or the tissue injury is prolonged. It usually involves recruitment and activation of monocytes and lymphocytes. Chronic inflammatory sites also often undergo tissue remodeling, with angiogenesis and fibrosis. Although innate immune stimuli may contribute to chronic inflammation, the adaptive immune system may also be involved because cytokines produced by T cells are powerful inducers of inflammation (see Chapter 10). Detailed descriptions of the various mediators and pathologic manifestations of acute and chronic inflammation can be found in pathology textbooks. We will focus our discussion on particular aspects of the acute inflammatory process that have broad relevance to both innate and adaptive immunity and immune-mediated inflammatory diseases.

TABLE 4-4   Cytokines of Innate Immunity

Cytokine	Size	Principal Cell Source	Principal Cellular Targets and Biologic Effects
Tumor necrosis factor (TNF)	17 kD; 51-kD homotrimer	Macrophages, T cells	Endothelial cells: activation (inflammation, coagulation) Neutrophils: activation Hypothalamus: fever Muscle, fat: catabolism (cachexia) Many cell types: apoptosis
Interleukin-1 (IL-1)	17-kD mature form; 33-kD precursors	Macrophages, endothelial cells, some epithelial cells	Endothelial cells: activation (inflammation, coagulation) Hypothalamus: fever Liver: synthesis of acute-phase proteins T cells: T_H17 differentiation
Chemokines (see Table 3-2)	8-12 kD	Macrophages, endothelial cells, T cells, fibroblasts, platelets	Leukocytes: chemotaxis, activation; migration into tissues
Interleukin-12 (IL-12)	Heterodimer of 35-kD and 40-kD subunits	Macrophages, dendritic cells	T cells: T_H1 differentiation NK cells and T cells: IFN-γ synthesis, increased cytotoxic activity
Type I interferons (IFN-α, IFN-β)	IFN-α: 15-21 kD IFN-β: 20-25 kD	IFN-α: macrophages, plasmacytoid dendritic cells IFN-β: fibroblasts	All cells: antiviral state, increased class I MHC expression NK cells: activation
Interleukin-10 (IL-10)	Homodimer of 34-40-kD and 18-kD subunits	Macrophages, T cells (mainly regulatory T cells)	Macrophages, dendritic cells: inhibition of IL-12 production and expression of costimulators and class II MHC molecules
Interleukin-6 (IL-6)	19-26 kD	Macrophages, endothelial cells, T cells	Liver: synthesis of acute-phase proteins B cells: proliferation of antibody-producing cells T cells: T_H17 differentiation
Interleukin-15 (IL-15)	13 kD	Macrophages, others	NK cells: proliferation T cells: proliferation (memory $CD8^+$ cells)
Interleukin-18 (IL-18)	17 kD	Macrophages	NK cells and T cells: IFN-γ synthesis
Interleukin-23 (IL-23)	Heterodimer of unique 19-kD subunit and 40-kD subunit of IL-12	Macrophages and dendritic cells	T cells: maintenance of IL-17–producing T cells
Interleukin-27 (IL-27)	Heterodimer of 28-kD and 13-kD subunits	Macrophages and dendritic cells	T cells: T_H1 differentiation; inhibition of T_H17 cells NK cells: IFN-γ synthesis

The Major Proinflammatory Cytokines TNF, IL-1, and IL-6

One of the earliest responses of the innate immune system to infection and tissue damage is the secretion of cytokines by tissue cells, which is critical for the acute inflammatory response. The cytokines of innate immunity have some important general properties and functions (Table 4-4).

- They are produced mainly by tissue macrophages and dendritic cells, although other cell types, including endothelial and some epithelial cells, can also produce them.
- Most of these cytokines act on cells close to their cell of origin (paracrine action). In some severe infections, enough of the cytokines may be produced that they enter the circulation and act at a distance (endocrine action).
- Different cytokines have similar or overlapping actions, or are functionally unique. One cytokine may stimulate the production of others, thus setting up cascades that amplify the reaction or induce new reactions.

- The cytokines of innate immunity serve several roles: inducing inflammation, inhibiting viral replication, promoting T cell responses, and limiting innate immune responses. These functions are described next and later in the chapter.

Three of the most important proinflammatory cytokines of the innate immune system are TNF, IL-1 (which we have mentioned several times), and IL-6. We will discuss the major features of these cytokines, focusing mainly on TNF and IL-1, before describing their role in acute inflammation.

Tumor Necrosis Factor

Tumor necrosis factor (TNF) is a mediator of the acute inflammatory response to bacteria and other infectious microbes. The name of this cytokine derives from its original identification as a serum substance (factor) that caused necrosis of tumors, now known to be the result of inflammation and thrombosis of tumor blood vessels. TNF is also called TNF-α to distinguish it from the closely related TNF-β, also called lymphotoxin. TNF is produced by macrophages, dendritic cells, and other cell types. In macrophages, it is synthesized as a nonglycosylated type II membrane protein and is expressed as a homotrimer, which is able to bind to one form of TNF receptor. The membrane form of TNF is cleaved by a membrane-associated metalloproteinase, releasing a polypeptide fragment, and three of these polypeptide chains polymerize to form a triangular pyramid-shaped circulating TNF protein (Fig. 4-12). The receptor-binding sites are at the base of the pyramid, allowing simultaneous binding of the cytokine to three receptor molecules.

There are two distinct TNF receptors called type I (TNF-RI) and type II (TNF-RII). The affinities of TNF for its receptors are unusually low for a cytokine, the K_d being only $\sim 1 \times 10^{-9}$ M for binding to TNF-RI and approximately 5×10^{-10} M for binding to TNF-RII. Both TNF receptors are present on most cell types. The TNF receptors are members of a large family of proteins called the TNF receptor superfamily, many of which are involved in immune and inflammatory responses. These receptors exist as trimers in the plasma membrane. Ligand binding to some TNF receptor family members, such as TNF-RI, TNF-RII, and CD40, leads to the recruitment of proteins called TNF receptor–associated factors (TRAFs) to the cytoplasmic domains of the receptors. The TRAFs activate transcription factors, notably NF-κB and AP-1. Cytokine binding to some family members, such as TNF-RI, leads to recruitment of an adaptor protein that activates caspases and triggers apoptosis. Thus, different members of the TNF receptor family can induce gene expression or cell death, and some can do both.

TNF production by macrophages is stimulated by PAMPs and DAMPs. TLRs, NLRs, and RLRs can all induce TNF gene expression, in part by activation of the NF-κB transcription factor. Many different microbial products can therefore induce TNF production. Large amounts of this cytokine may be produced during infections with gram-negative and gram-positive bacteria, which express the TLR ligands LPS and lipoteichoic acid, respectively, and may release these molecules from their cell walls. Septic shock, a life-threatening condition caused when bacteria enter the blood stream, is mediated in large part by TNF. We will discuss septic shock later in this chapter.

Interleukin-1

Interleukin-1 (IL-1) is also a mediator of the acute inflammatory response and has many similar actions as TNF. The major cellular source of IL-1, like that of TNF, is activated mononuclear phagocytes. Unlike TNF, IL-1 is also produced by many cell types other than macrophages, such as neutrophils, epithelial cells (e.g., keratinocytes), and endothelial cells. There are two forms of IL-1, called IL-1α and IL-1β, that are less than 30% homologous to each other, but they bind to the same cell surface receptors and have the same biologic activities. The main biologically active secreted form is IL-1β.

IL-1 production usually requires two distinct signals, one that activates new gene transcription and production of a 33-kD precursor pro–IL-1β polypeptide, and a second that activates the inflammasome to proteolytically cleave the precursor to generate the 17-kD mature IL-1β protein (see Fig. 4-4). As discussed earlier in this chapter, IL-1β gene transcription is induced by TLR and NLR signaling pathways that activate NF-κB, whereas pro–IL-1β cleavage is mediated by the NLRP3 inflammasome. IL-1 is secreted by a nonclassical pathway because, unlike most secreted proteins, neither IL-1α nor IL-1β has hydrophobic signal sequences to target the nascent polypeptide to the endoplasmic reticulum membrane. One possibility is that mature IL-1 is released mainly when infected cells or activated macrophages die. Some pathogenic bacteria induce both inflammasome-mediated processing of IL-1β and IL-18 in macrophages and caspase-1–dependent or caspase-11–dependent cell death (pyroptosis), discussed earlier. TNF can also stimulate phagocytes and other cell types to produce IL-1. This is an example of a cascade of cytokines that have similar biologic activities.

IL-1 mediates its biologic effects through a membrane receptor called the type I IL-1 receptor, which is expressed on many cell types, including endothelial cells, epithelial cells, and leukocytes. This receptor is an integral membrane protein that contains an extracellular ligand-binding Ig domain and a Toll/IL-1 receptor (TIR) signaling domain in the cytoplasmic region, which we described earlier in reference to TLRs. The signaling events that occur when IL-1 binds to the type I IL-1 receptor are similar to those triggered by TLRs and result in the activation of NF-κB and AP-1 transcription factors (see Chapter 7).

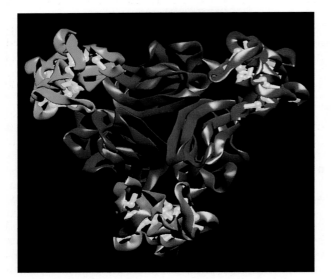

FIGURE 4-12 Structure of the TNF receptor with bound lymphotoxin. The ribbon structure depicts a top view of a complex of three TNF receptors (TNF-RI) and one molecule of the bound cytokine, revealed by x-ray crystallography. Lymphotoxin is a homotrimer in which the three subunits are colored dark blue. The lymphotoxin homotrimer forms an inverted three-sided pyramid with its base at the top and its apex at the bottom. Three TNF-RI molecules, colored magenta, cyan, and red, bind one homotrimer of lymphotoxin, with each receptor molecule interacting with two different lymphotoxin monomers in the homotrimer complex. Disulfide bonds in the receptor are colored yellow. TNF is homologous to lymphotoxin and presumably binds to its receptors in the same way. *(From Banner DW, D'Arcy A, Janes W, Gentz R, Schoenfeld HJ, Broger C, Loetscher H, Lesslauer W: Cell: crystal structure of the soluble human 55 kd TNF receptor–human TNFβ complex: implications for TNF receptor activation, Cell 73:431–445, 1993.)*

The type II IL-1 receptor appears incapable of activating downstream signals.

Interleukin-6

IL-6 is another important cytokine in acute inflammatory responses that has both local and systemic effects. It induces the synthesis of a variety of other inflammatory mediators in the liver, stimulates neutrophil production in the bone marrow, and promotes the differentiation of IL-17–producing helper T cells. IL-6 is synthesized by mononuclear phagocytes, vascular endothelial cells, fibroblasts, and other cells in response to PAMPs and in response to IL-1 and TNF. IL-6 is a homodimer that belongs to the type I cytokine family (see Chapter 7). The receptor for IL-6 consists of a cytokine-binding polypeptide chain and a signal-transducing subunit (called gp130) that is also the signaling component of receptors for other cytokines. The IL-6 receptor engages a signaling pathway that activates the transcription factor STAT3 (see Chapter 7).

Other Cytokines Produced During Innate Immune Responses

In addition to TNF, IL-1, and IL-6, dendritic cells and macrophages activated by PAMPs and DAMPs produce other cytokines that have important roles in innate immune responses (see Table 4-4). We will discuss the main features of some of these cytokines and their roles in innate immunity in this section; interferons and inhibitory cytokines are discussed later in the chapter.

IL-12 is secreted by dendritic cells and macrophages and stimulates IFN-γ production by NK cells and T cells, enhances NK cell and CTL-mediated cytotoxicity, and promotes differentiation of T_H1 cells. IL-12 exists as a disulfide-linked heterodimer of 35-kD (p35) and 40-kD (p40) subunits. The p35 subunit is a member of the type I cytokine family, and the p40 subunit is also a component of the cytokine IL-23, which is involved in the differentiation of T_H17 cells. Therefore, antibodies specific for p40 block both IL-12 and IL-23 and thus inhibit the IL-12–dependent development of T_H1 cells and the IL-23–dependent development of T_H17 cells. These antibodies are approved for the treatment of inflammatory diseases such as inflammatory bowel disease and psoriasis, which are caused by T_H1 and/or T_H17 cytokines.

The principal sources of IL-12 are activated dendritic cells and macrophages. Many cells appear to synthesize the p35 subunit, but macrophages and dendritic cells are the main cell types that produce the p40 component and therefore the biologically active cytokine. During innate immune reactions to microbes, IL-12 is produced in response to TLR and other pattern recognition receptor signaling induced by many microbial stimuli, including bacterial LPS or lipoteichoic acid and virus infections. IFN-γ produced by NK cells or T cells also stimulates IL-12 production, contributing to a positive feedback loop.

The receptor for IL-12 (IL-12R) is a heterodimer composed of β1 and β2 subunits, both of which are members of the type I cytokine receptor family. Both chains are required for high-affinity binding of IL-12 and for signaling, which activates the transcription factor STAT4. Expression of the β2 chain of the IL-12 receptor is itself enhanced by IFN-γ, whose production is stimulated by IL-12. This is another example of a positive amplification loop in immune responses. Studies with gene knockout mice and the phenotype of rare patients with mutations in the IL-12 receptor support the conclusion that IL-12 is important for IFN-γ production by NK cells and T cells and for host resistance to intracellular bacteria and some viruses. For example, patients with mutations in the IL-12 receptor β1 subunit have been described, and they are highly susceptible to infections with intracellular bacteria, notably *Salmonella* and atypical mycobacteria. IL-12 secreted by dendritic cells during antigen presentation to naive CD4+ T cells promotes their differentiation into the T_H1 subset of helper T cells, which are important for defense against intracellular infections (see Chapter 10). This is a key way in which innate immunity shapes adaptive immune responses.

IL-18 enhances the functions of NK cells, similar to IL-12. Recall that the production of IL-18, like that of IL-1, is dependent on the inflammasome. Also like IL-1, IL-18 binds to a receptor that signals through a TIR domain.

IL-15 serves important growth-stimulating and survival functions for both NK cells and T cells. IL-15 is structurally homologous to the T cell growth factor IL-2, and the heterotrimeric IL-15 receptor shares two subunits with the IL-2 receptor. An interesting feature of IL-15 is that it can be expressed on the cell surface bound to the α chain of its receptor and in this form can be presented to and stimulate nearby cells that express a receptor composed of the other two chains (β and γ). IL-15 presented this way by dendritic cells to NK cells in lymph nodes activates signaling pathways that promote NK cell IFN-γ production. IL-15 also serves as a survival factor for NK and memory CD8+ T cells.

IL-25 and IL-33 are structurally unrelated cytokines which stimulate group 2 ILCs, T_H2 cells, and mast cells to produce IL-4, IL-5 and IL-13. The latter cytokines are important for defense against helminthes, but also contribute to allergic disease.

Recruitment of Leukocytes to Sites of Infection

Recruitment of large numbers of neutrophils, followed by monocytes, from blood into tissues typically occurs as part of the acute inflammatory response to infections and tissue injury. The cytokines TNF, IL-1, and IL-6 and chemokines, all of which are secreted at the sites of infection or tissue injury, have multiple effects on vascular endothelial cells, leukocytes, and bone marrow, which together increase the local delivery of cells that can fight infections and repair tissues (see Fig. 3-3). Leukocyte recruitment was described in Chapter 3 and will be only briefly considered here.

Both TNF and IL-1 induce postcapillary venule endothelial cells to express E-selectin and to increase their expression of ICAM-1 and VCAM-1, the ligands for leukocyte integrins. These changes in endothelial adhesion molecule expression are the result of TNF and IL-1 activation of transcription factors, including NF-κB, leading to new adhesion molecule gene transcription. P-selectin expression is also induced on venular endothelial cells at sites of infection and tissue injury, but this is due in large part to the effects of histamine and thrombin, which stimulate the rapid mobilization of P-selectin stored in granules in the endothelial cell to the cell surface.

TNF and IL-1 also stimulate various cells to secrete chemokines, such as CXCL1 and CCL2, that bind to receptors on neutrophils and monocytes, respectively, increase the affinity of leukocyte integrins for their ligands, and stimulate directional movement of leukocytes. The result of increased selectin, integrin, and chemokine expression is an increase in neutrophil and monocyte adhesion to endothelial cells and transmigration through the vessel wall. The leukocytes accumulate in the tissues, forming an inflammatory infiltrate. The actions of TNF on endothelium and leukocytes are critical for local inflammatory responses to microbes. If inadequate quantities of TNF are present (e.g., in patients treated with drugs that block TNF or in TNF gene knockout mice), a consequence may be failure to contain infections.

In addition, TNF, IL-1, and IL-6 produced at inflammatory sites may enter the blood and be delivered to the bone marrow, where they enhance the production of neutrophils from bone marrow progenitors, usually acting in concert with colony-stimulating factors. In this way, these cytokines increase the supply of cells that can be recruited to the sites of infection.

Ingestion and Killing of Microbes by Activated Phagocytes

Neutrophils and macrophages that are recruited into sites of infections ingest microbes into vesicles by the process of phagocytosis and destroy these microbes (Fig. 4-13). Phagocytosis is an active, energy-dependent process of engulfment of large particles (>0.5 μm in diameter) into vesicles. Phagocytic vesicles fuse with lysosomes, where the ingested particles are destroyed. In this way, the mechanisms of killing, which could potentially injure the phagocyte, are isolated from the rest of the cell.

Neutrophils and macrophages express receptors that specifically recognize microbes, and binding of microbes to these receptors is the first step in phagocytosis. Some of these receptors are pattern recognition receptors, including C-type lectins and scavenger receptors, which we discussed earlier. Pattern recognition receptors can contribute to phagocytosis only of organisms that express particular molecular patterns, such as mannose for the

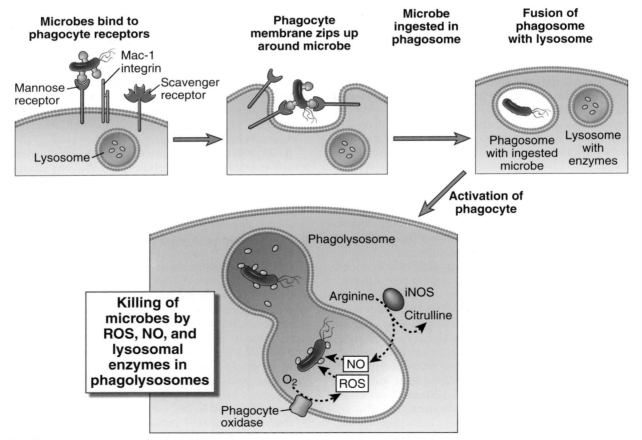

FIGURE 4-13 Phagocytosis and intracellular destruction of microbes. Microbes may be ingested by different membrane receptors of phagocytes; some directly bind microbes, and others bind opsonized microbes. (Note that the Mac-1 integrin binds microbes opsonized with complement proteins, not shown.) The microbes are internalized into phagosomes, which fuse with lysosomes to form phagolysosomes, where the microbes are killed by reactive oxygen and nitrogen species and proteolytic enzymes. *iNOS*, inducible nitric oxide synthase; *NO*, nitric oxide; *ROS*, reactive oxygen species.

mannose receptor. Phagocytes also have high-affinity receptors for certain opsonins, including antibody molecules, complement proteins, and plasma lectins; these receptors are critical for phagocytosis of many different microbes that are coated with the opsonins. One of the most efficient systems for opsonizing microbes is coating them with antibodies. Phagocytes express high-affinity Fc receptors called FcγRI specific for one type of antibody called IgG (see Chapter 13). Thus, if an individual responds to an infection by making IgG antibodies against microbial antigens, the IgG molecules bind to these antigens, the Fc ends of the bound antibodies can interact with FcγRI on phagocytes, and the end result is efficient phagocytosis of the microbes. Antibody-dependent phagocytosis illustrates a link between innate and adaptive immunity—antibodies are a product of the adaptive immune system (B lymphocytes) that engage innate immune system effector cells (phagocytes) to perform their protective functions.

Once a microbe or particle binds to receptors on a phagocyte, the plasma membrane in the region of the receptors begins to redistribute and extends a cup-shaped projection around the microbe. When the protruding membrane cup extends beyond the diameter of the particle, the top of the cup closes over and pinches off the interior of the cup to form an inside-out intracellular vesicle (see Fig. 4-13). This vesicle, called a phagosome, contains the ingested foreign particle, and it breaks away from the plasma membrane. The cell surface receptors also deliver activating signals that stimulate the microbicidal activities of phagocytes. Phagocytosed microbes are destroyed, as described next; at the same time, peptides are generated from microbial proteins and presented to T lymphocytes to initiate adaptive immune responses (see Chapter 6).

Activated neutrophils and macrophages kill phago-cytosed microbes by the action of microbicidal molecules in phagolysosomes (see Fig. 4-13). Signals from various receptors, including pattern recognition receptors (such as TLRs), opsonin receptors (such as Fc and C3 receptors), and receptors for cytokines (mainly IFN-γ) function cooperatively to activate phagocytes to kill ingested microbes. Fusion of phagocytic vacuoles (phagosomes) with lysosomes results in the formation of phagolysosomes, where most of the microbicidal mechanisms are concentrated. Three classes of microbicidal molecules are known to be the most important.

- *Reactive oxygen species.* Activated macrophages and neutrophils convert molecular oxygen into reactive oxygen species (ROS), which are highly reactive oxidizing agents that destroy microbes (and other cells). The primary free radical–generating system is the phagocyte oxidase system. Phagocyte oxidase is a multisubunit enzyme that is assembled in activated phagocytes mainly in the phagolysosomal membrane. Phagocyte oxidase is activated by many stimuli, including IFN-γ and signals from TLRs. The function of this enzyme is to reduce molecular oxygen into ROS such as superoxide radicals, with the reduced form of nicotinamide adenine dinucleotide phosphate (NADPH) acting as a cofactor. Superoxide is enzymatically

dismutated into hydrogen peroxide, which is used by the enzyme myeloperoxidase to convert normally unreactive halide ions into reactive hypohalous acids that are toxic for bacteria. The process by which ROS are produced is called the **respiratory burst** because it occurs during oxygen consumption (cellular respiration). Although the generation of toxic ROS is commonly viewed as the major function of phagocyte oxidase, another function of the enzyme is to produce conditions within phagocytic vacuoles that are necessary for the activity of the proteolytic enzymes discussed earlier. The oxidase acts as an electron pump, generating an electrochemical gradient across the vacuole membrane, which is compensated for by movement of ions into the vacuole. The result is an increase in pH and osmolarity inside the vacuole, which is necessary for elastase and cathepsin G activity. A disease called **chronic granulomatous disease** is caused by an inherited deficiency of one of the components of phagocyte oxidase; this deficiency compromises the capacity of neutrophils to kill certain species of gram-positive bacteria (see Chapter 21).

- *Nitric oxide.* In addition to ROS, macrophages produce reactive nitrogen species, mainly nitric oxide (NO), by the action of an enzyme called inducible nitric oxide synthase (iNOS). iNOS is a cytosolic enzyme that is absent in resting macrophages but can be induced in response to microbial products that activate TLRs, especially in combination with IFN-γ. iNOS catalyzes the conversion of arginine to citrulline, and freely diffusible nitric oxide gas is released. Within phagolysosomes, nitric oxide may combine with hydrogen peroxide or superoxide, generated by phagocyte oxidase, to produce highly reactive peroxynitrite radicals that can kill microbes. The cooperative and redundant function of ROS and nitric oxide is demonstrated by the finding that knockout mice lacking both iNOS and phagocyte oxidase are more susceptible to bacterial infections than single phagocyte oxidase or iNOS knockout animals are.

- *Proteolytic enzymes.* Activated neutrophils and macrophages produce several proteolytic enzymes in the phagolysosomes that function to destroy microbes. One of the important enzymes in neutrophils is elastase, a broad-spectrum serine protease known to be required for killing many types of bacteria. Another important enzyme is cathepsin G. Mouse gene knockout studies have confirmed the essential requirement for these enzymes in phagocyte killing of bacteria.

Neutrophils also kill microbes by extruding their DNA and granule contents, which form extracellular threads on which bacteria and fungi are trapped and killed. The extruded contents, which are called **neutrophil extracellular traps** (NETs), are composed of strands of DNA and histones to which are bound high concentrations of antimicrobial granule contents, including lysozyme, elastase, and defensins. NETs are formed when neutrophils are bound to tissue matrix by the Mac-1 integrin, and they are activated by microbial products.

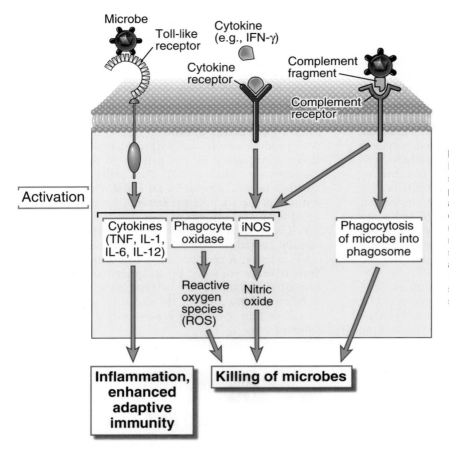

FIGURE 4-14 Functions of macrophages. Macrophages are activated by microbial products such as LPS and by NK cell–derived IFN-γ. The process of macrophage activation leads to the activation of transcription factors, the transcription of various genes, and the synthesis of proteins that mediate the functions of these cells. In adaptive cell-mediated immunity, macrophages are activated by stimuli from T lymphocytes (CD40 ligand and IFN-γ) and respond in essentially the same way (see Fig. 10-7). Macrophages also may be activated by other signals to promote tissue repair and fibrosis (not shown).

The extrusion of nuclear contents during NET formation leads to neutrophil cell death.

Other Functions of Activated Macrophages

In addition to killing phagocytosed microbes, macrophages serve many other functions in defense against infections (Fig. 4-14). Several of these functions are mediated by the cytokines the macrophages produce. We have already described how TNF, IL-1, and chemokines made by phagocytes enhance the inflammatory reactions to microbes and bring in more leukocytes and plasma proteins. Some activated macrophages also produce growth factors for fibroblasts and endothelial cells that participate in the remodeling of tissues after infections and injury. The role of macrophages in cell-mediated immunity is described in Chapter 10.

Macrophages may be activated in different ways, which favor microbicidal and proinflammatory functions, or in contrast, reparative and anti-inflammatory functions. These different types of macrophage activation, called classical and alternative respectively, are discussed in more detail in Chapter 10.

Systemic and Pathologic Consequences of Inflammation

TNF, IL-1, and IL-6 produced during the innate immune response to infection or tissue damage have systemic effects that contribute to host defense and are responsible for many of the clinical manifestations of infection and inflammatory disease (Fig. 4-15).

- *TNF and IL-1 act on the hypothalamus to induce an increase in body temperature (fever).* These cytokines are therefore called endogenous pyrogens (i.e., host-derived fever-causing agents, to distinguish them from LPS, which was considered an exogenous [microbe-derived] pyrogen). This distinction is mainly of historical significance because we now know that even LPS induces fever by the production of the cytokines TNF and IL-1. TNF and IL-1 induce fever by increasing synthesis of prostaglandins in hypothalamic cells. Prostaglandin synthesis inhibitors, such as aspirin, reduce fever by blocking this action of the cytokines. The role of fever in host defense is not well understood but may relate to enhanced metabolic functions of immune cells, impaired metabolic functions of microbes, and changes in the behavior of the febrile host that reduce risk of worsening infections and injury.

- *IL-1 and IL-6 induce hepatocytes to produce acute-phase reactants, including CRP, SAP, and fibrinogen, which are secreted into the blood.* Elevated levels of acute-phase reactants are commonly used clinically as signs of infection or other inflammatory processes. The pentraxins CRP and SAP play protective roles in infections, as we discussed earlier in the chapter, and fibrinogen, the precursor of fibrin, contributes to hemostasis and tissue repair.

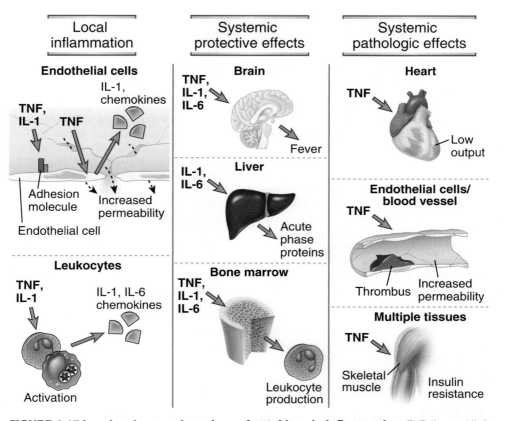

FIGURE 4-15 Local and systemic actions of cytokines in inflammation. TNF, IL-1, and IL-6 have multiple local and systemic inflammatory effects. TNF and IL-1 act on leukocytes and endothelium to induce acute inflammation, and both cytokines induce the expression of IL-6 from leukocytes and other cell types. TNF, IL-1, and IL-6 mediate protective systemic effects of inflammation, including induction of fever, acute-phase protein synthesis by the liver, and increased production of leukocytes by the bone marrow. Systemic TNF can cause the pathologic abnormalities that lead to septic shock, including decreased cardiac function, thrombosis, capillary leak, and metabolic abnormalities due to insulin resistance.

In severe infections, TNF may be produced in large amounts and causes systemic clinical and pathologic abnormalities. If the stimulus for cytokine production is sufficiently strong, the quantity of TNF may be so large that it enters the blood stream and acts at distant sites (see Fig. 4-15). The principal systemic actions of TNF are as follows:

- TNF inhibits myocardial contractility and vascular smooth muscle tone, resulting in a marked decrease in blood pressure, or shock.
- TNF causes intravascular thrombosis, mainly as a result of impairment of the normal anticoagulant properties of the endothelium. TNF stimulates endothelial cell expression of tissue factor, a potent activator of coagulation, and inhibits expression of thrombomodulin, an inhibitor of coagulation. The endothelial alterations are exacerbated by activation of neutrophils, leading to vascular plugging by these cells. The ability of this cytokine to cause necrosis of tumors, which is the basis of its name, is mainly a result of thrombosis of tumor blood vessels.
- Prolonged production of TNF causes wasting of muscle and fat cells, called cachexia. This wasting results from TNF-induced appetite suppression and reduced synthesis of lipoprotein lipase, an enzyme needed to

release fatty acids from circulating lipoproteins so that they can be used by the tissues.

A complication of severe bacterial sepsis is a syndrome called **septic shock**, which may be caused by LPS released from gram-negative bacteria (in which case it is called endotoxin shock) or lipoteichoic acid released from gram-positive bacteria. Septic shock is characterized by vascular collapse, disseminated intravascular coagulation, and metabolic disturbances. This syndrome is due to TLR signaling induced by LPS or lipoteichoic acid, leading to the production of TNF and other cytokines, including IL-12, IFN-γ, and IL-1. The concentration of serum TNF may be predictive of the outcome of severe bacterial infections. Septic shock can be reproduced in experimental animals by administration of LPS, lipoteichoic acid, or TNF. Antagonists of TNF can prevent mortality in the experimental models, but clinical trials with anti-TNF antibodies or with soluble TNF receptors have not shown benefit in patients with sepsis. The cause of this therapeutic failure is not known, but it may be because other cytokines elicit the same responses as TNF.

A syndrome similar to septic shock may occur as a complication of non-infectious disorders, such as severe burns, trauma, pancreatitis, and other serious conditions. This has been called the systemic inflammatory response syndrome (SIRS).

Acute inflammation may cause tissue injury because the effector mechanisms that phagocytes use to kill microbes are also toxic to host tissues. The proteolytic enzymes and reactive oxygen species produced by phagocytes that accumulate at a site of infection can injure host cells and degrade extracellular matrix if they are generated in large quantities, especially if the microbes resist being killed and continue to stimulate the innate immune responses. In fact, at least part of the pathology associated with infections is due to the inflammatory responses and not the direct toxic effects of the microbes. Acute inflammation also causes tissue damage in the setting of autoimmune diseases, in which case neutrophils and macrophages accumulate and become activated secondarily to stimulation of the adaptive immune system by self antigens (see Chapter 15). As in inflammation induced by infections, TNF, IL-1, IL-6, and IL-12 are the key inducers of inflammation in autoimmune diseases. Antagonists against all of these cytokines or their receptors are in clinical use or in trials to reduce inflammation in patients with inflammatory diseases such as rheumatoid arthritis, inflammatory bowel disease, and psoriasis.

THE ANTIVIRAL RESPONSE

The major way by which the innate immune system deals with viral infections is to induce the expression of type I interferons, whose most important action is to inhibit viral replication. Earlier in the chapter, we discussed how several pattern recognition receptors, including some TLRs, NLRs, RLRs, and STING, generate signals that stimulate IFN-α and IFN-β gene expression in many different cell types. The type I interferons are secreted from these cells and act on other cells to prevent the spread of viral infection. In this section, we will describe the major properties of type I interferons and the antiviral effects of these cytokines.

Type I interferons are a large family of structurally related cytokines that mediate the early innate immune response to viral infections. The term *interferon* derives from the ability of these cytokines to interfere with viral infection. There are many type I interferons, which are structurally homologous and are encoded by genes in a single cluster on chromosome 9. The most important type I interferons in viral defense are IFN-α (which actually includes 13 different closely related proteins) and IFN-β, which is a single protein. Plasmacytoid dendritic cells are the major sources of IFN-α, but it also may be produced by mononuclear phagocytes. IFN-β is produced by many cell types. The most potent stimuli for type I interferon synthesis are viral nucleic acids. Recall that RIG-like receptors and DNA sensors in the cytosol and TLRs 3, 7, 8, and 9 in endosomal vesicles recognize viral nucleic acids and initiate signaling pathways that activate the IRF family of transcription factors, which induce type I interferon gene expression (Fig. 4-16).

The receptor for type I interferons, which binds both IFN-α and IFN-β, is a heterodimer of two structurally related polypeptides, IFNAR1 and IFNAR2, which are expressed on all nucleated cells. This receptor signals to activate STAT1, STAT2, and IRF9 transcription factors, which induce expression of several different genes whose protein products contribute to antiviral defense in various ways:

- ***Type I interferons, signaling through the type I interferon receptor, activate transcription of several genes that confer on the cells a resistance to viral infection called an antiviral state*** (Fig. 4-17). Type I interferon–induced genes include double-stranded RNA–activated serine/threonine protein kinase (PKR), which blocks viral transcriptional and translational events, and 2′,5′ oligoadenylate synthetase and RNase L, which promote viral RNA degradation. The antiviral action of type I interferon is primarily a paracrine action in that a virally infected cell secretes interferon to act on and protect neighboring cells that are not yet infected. The effects of type 1 interferons are not specific to viral gene expression, and part of the ability of these cytokines to block the spread of infection is due to their toxicity to host cells that are near infected cells. Interferon secreted by an infected cell may also act in an autocrine fashion to inhibit viral replication in that cell.

- ***Type I interferons cause sequestration of lymphocytes in lymph nodes, thus maximizing the opportunity for encounter with microbial antigens.*** The mechanism for this effect of type I interferons is the induction of a molecule on the lymphocytes, called CD69, which forms a complex with and reduces surface expression of the sphingosine 1-phosphate (S1P) receptor S1PR1. Recall from Chapter 3 that lymphocyte egress from lymphoid tissues depends on S1P binding to S1PR1. Therefore, reduced S1PR1 inhibits this egress and keeps lymphocytes in lymphoid organs.

- ***Type I interferons increase the cytotoxicity of NK cells and CD8+ CTLs and promote the differentiation of naive T cells to the T_H1 subset of helper T cells.*** These effects of type I interferons enhance both innate and adaptive immunity against intracellular infections, including viruses and some bacteria.

- ***Type I interferons upregulate expression of class I MHC molecules and thereby increase the probability that virally infected cells will be recognized and killed by CD8+ CTLs.*** Virus-specific CD8+ CTLs recognize peptides derived from viral proteins bound to class I MHC molecules on the surface of infected cells. (We will discuss the details of T cell recognition of peptide-MHC and CTL killing of cells in Chapters 6 and 11.) Therefore, by increasing the amount of class I MHC synthesized by a virally infected cell, type I interferons will increase the number of viral peptide–class I MHC complexes on the cell surface that the CTLs can see and respond to. The end result is the killing of cells that support viral replication, which is needed to eradicate viral infections.

Thus, the principal activities of type I interferon work in concert to combat viral infections. Knockout mice

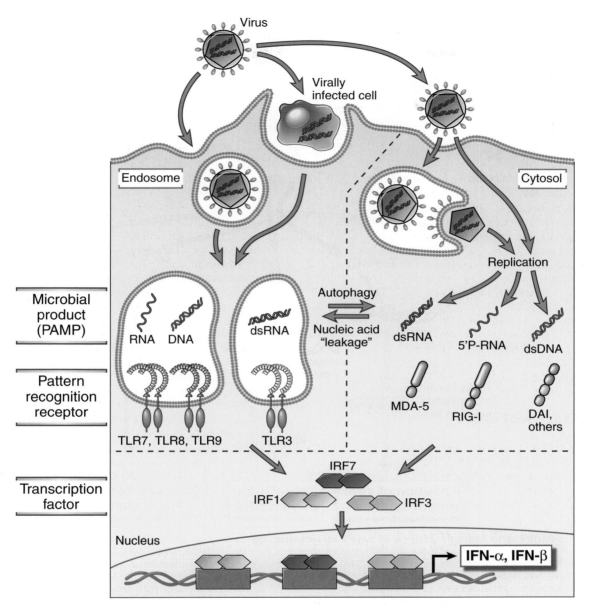

FIGURE 4-16 Mechanisms of induction of type I interferons by viruses. Viral nucleic acids and proteins are recognized by several cellular receptor families (TLRs, the family of cytosolic RIG-like receptors, or RLRs, which include MDA-5, RIG-I, DAI and others, and cytosolic DNA sensors), which activate transcription factors (the IRF proteins) that stimulate the production of type I interferons IFN-α and IFN-β.

lacking the receptor for type I interferons are susceptible to viral infections. IFN-α is in clinical use as an antiviral agent in certain forms of viral hepatitis. IFN-α is also used for the treatment of some tumors, perhaps because it boosts CTL activity or inhibits cell proliferation. IFN-β is used as a therapy for multiple sclerosis, but the mechanism of its beneficial effect in this disease is not known.

Protection against viruses is due, in part, to the activation of intrinsic apoptotic death pathways in infected cells and enhanced sensitivity to extrinsic inducers of apoptosis. Viral proteins synthesized in infected cells may be misfolded, and their accumulation triggers an unfolded protein response that may culminate in apoptosis of the infected cells if the misfolded protein accumulation cannot be corrected. In addition, virally infected cells are hypersensitive to TNF-induced apoptosis. Abundant TNF is made by plasmacytoid dendritic cells and macrophages in response to viral infections, in addition to type I interferons. The type I TNF receptor engages both proinflammatory and proapoptosis death pathways. The dominant pathway that is activated upon TNF binding depends on the state of protein synthesis in the responding cells, and viral infection can shift this balance toward apoptosis.

STIMULATION OF ADAPTIVE IMMUNITY

The innate immune response provides signals that function in concert with antigen to stimulate the proliferation and differentiation of antigen-specific T and B

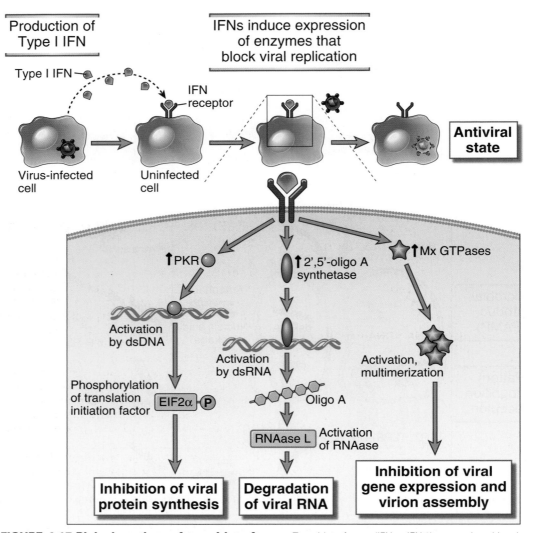

FIGURE 4-17 Biologic actions of type I interferons. Type I interferons (IFN-α, IFN-β) are produced by virus-infected cells in response to intracellular TLR signaling and other sensors of viral RNA. Type I interferons bind to receptors on neighboring uninfected cells and activate JAK-STAT signaling pathways, which induce expression of genes whose products interfere with viral replication. Type I interferons also bind to receptors on infected cells and induce expression of genes whose products enhance the cell's susceptibility to CTL-mediated killing. *PKR*, double stranded RNA-activated protein kinase.

lymphocytes. As the innate immune response is providing the initial defense against microbes, it also sets in motion the adaptive immune response. The activation of lymphocytes requires two distinct signals, the first being antigen and the second being molecules that are produced during innate immune responses to microbes or injured cells (Fig. 4-18). This idea is called the **two-signal hypothesis** for lymphocyte activation. The requirement for antigen (so-called signal 1) ensures that the ensuing immune response is specific. The requirement for additional stimuli triggered by innate immune reactions to microbes (signal 2) ensures that adaptive immune responses are induced when there is a dangerous infection and not when lymphocytes recognize harmless antigens, including self antigens. The molecules produced during innate immune reactions that function as second signals for lymphocyte activation include costimulators (for T cells), cytokines (for both T and B cells), and complement breakdown products (for B cells). We will return

to the nature of second signals for lymphocyte activation in Chapters 9 and 12.

The second signals generated during innate immune responses to different microbes not only enhance the magnitude of the subsequent adaptive immune response but also influence the nature of the adaptive response. A major function of T cell–mediated immunity is to activate macrophages to kill intracellular microbes and to induce robust inflammatory responses, so that a sufficiently large army of phagocytes is called into a site of infection. When phagocytes encounter microbes, TLRs and other pattern recognition receptors stimulate cytokine secretion and T cell–mediated immune responses, which in turn activate and recruit phagocytes to kill microbes. These processes are mediated by cytokines. Thus, the innate immune response to microbes in macrophages stimulates the adaptive T cell response that is effective against such microbes.

By contrast, many extracellular microbes that enter the blood activate the alternative complement pathway,

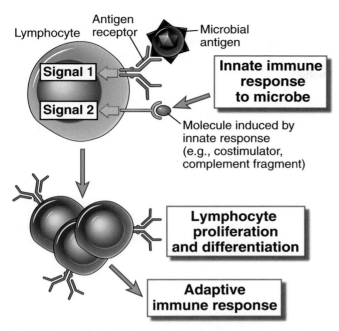

FIGURE 4-18 Stimulation of adaptive immunity by innate immune responses. Antigen recognition by lymphocytes provides signal 1 for the activation of the lymphocytes, and molecules induced on host cells during innate immune responses to microbes provide signal 2. In this illustration, the lymphocytes are B cells, but the same principles apply to T lymphocytes. The nature of second signals differs for B and T cells and is described in later chapters.

which enhances the production of antibodies by B lymphocytes. These antibodies opsonize the microbes and thereby promote their phagocytosis by neutrophils and macrophages, or kill the microbes by complement-dependent mechanisms. Thus, blood-borne microbes induce an innate response (complement activation) that triggers the adaptive response that is designed to eliminate these extracellular pathogens.

Cytokines produced by cells during innate immune responses to microbes stimulate the proliferation and differentiation of lymphocytes in adaptive immune responses. Examples of cytokines secreted by PAMP-stimulated cells acting on B cells, CD4$^+$ T cells, and CD8$^+$ T cells are given here. We have mentioned these cytokines previously, and will discuss the details of their roles in lymphocyte responses in later chapters.

- IL-12 stimulates the differentiation of naive CD4$^+$ T cells to the T$_H$1 subset of effector cells (see Chapter 10).
- IL-1, IL-6, and IL-23 stimulate the differentiation of naive CD4$^+$ T cells to the T$_H$17 subset of effector cells (see Chapter 10).
- IL-15 promotes the survival of memory CD8$^+$ T cells.
- IL-6 promotes the production of antibodies by activated B cells (see Chapter 12).

Adjuvants, which are substances that need to be administered together with purified protein antigens to elicit maximal T cell–dependent immune responses (see Chapter 6), work by stimulating innate immune responses at the site of antigen exposure. Adjuvants are useful in experimental immunology and in clinical vaccines. Many adjuvants in experimental use are microbial products that engage TLRs, such as killed mycobacteria and LPS. The only routinely used adjuvant in human vaccines is alum, which is composed of either aluminum hydroxide or aluminum phosphate, and is a stimulus for inflammasome activation. Among their important effects, adjuvants activate dendritic cells to express more major histocompatibility molecules that are part of the antigen (signal 1) that T cells recognize, increase the expression of costimulators (signal 2) and cytokines needed for T cell activation, and stimulate migration of the dendritic cells to lymph nodes where T cells are located.

MECHANISMS THAT LIMIT INNATE IMMUNE RESPONSES

The magnitude and duration of innate immune responses are regulated by a variety of inhibitory mechanisms that limit potential damage to tissues. Whereas the inflammatory response is critically important for protection against microbes, it has the potential to cause tissue injury and disease. Several mechanisms have evolved to provide a brake on inflammation, and these mechanisms come into play at the same time as or shortly after the initiation of inflammation. Furthermore, the stimuli for the initiation of many of these control mechanisms include the same PAMPs and DAMPs that induce inflammation. We will describe a selected group of these regulatory mechanisms.

IL-10 is a cytokine that is produced by and inhibits activation of macrophages and dendritic cells. IL-10 inhibits the production of various inflammatory cytokines by activated macrophages and dendritic cells, including IL-1, TNF, and IL-12. Because it is both produced by macrophages and inhibits macrophage functions, IL-10 is an excellent example of a negative feedback regulator. Alternatively activated macrophages make more IL-10 than classically activated macrophages. IL-10 is produced by some nonlymphoid cell types (e.g., keratinocytes). IL-10 is also produced by regulatory T cells, and we will discuss the details of IL-10 in this context in Chapter 15.

Mononuclear phagocytes produce a natural antagonist of IL-1 that is structurally homologous to the cytokine and binds to the same receptors but is biologically inactive, so that it functions as a competitive inhibitor of IL-1. It is therefore called **IL-1 receptor antagonist (IL-1RA).** Synthesis of IL-1RA is induced by many of the same stimuli that induce IL-1 production, and some studies in IL-1RA–deficient mice suggest that this inhibitory cytokine is required to prevent inflammatory diseases of joints and other tissues. Recombinant IL-1RA has been developed as a drug for the treatment of rheumatoid arthritis and familial fever syndromes in which IL-1 production is dysregulated. Regulation of IL-1–mediated inflammation may also occur by expression of the type II receptor, which binds IL-1 but does not transduce an activating signal. The major function of this receptor may be to act as a "decoy" that competitively inhibits IL-1 binding to the type I signaling receptor.

Secretion of inflammatory cytokines from a variety of cell types appears to be regulated by the products of autophagy genes. Targeted mutations in different autophagy genes result in enhanced secretion of IL-1 and IL-18 by various cell types and the development of inflammatory bowel disease. The mechanisms by which atophagy proteins impair cytokine synthesis are not well understood; they may regulate inflammasome activation or production of reactive oxygen species. The linkage of polymorphisms in a human autophagy gene with inflammatory bowel disease may be because these proteins affect inflammation or epithelial integrity.

There are numerous negative regulatory signaling pathways that block the activating signals generated by pattern recognition receptors and inflammatory cytokines. Suppressors of cytokine signaling (SOCS) proteins are inhibitors of JAK-STAT signaling pathways linked to cytokine receptors. TLR signaling in macrophages and dendritic cells induces the expression of SOCS proteins, which limit responses of these cells to exogenous cytokines such as type I interferons. Proinflammatory responses of cells to TLR signaling are negatively regulated by SHP-1, an intracellular protein phosphatase that negatively regulates numerous tyrosine kinase–dependent signaling pathways in lymphocytes. There are many other examples of kinases and phosphatases that inhibit TLR, NLR, and RLR signaling.

SUMMARY

* The innate immune system provides the first line of host defense against microbes. The mechanisms of innate immunity exist before exposure to microbes. The cellular components of the innate immune system include epithelial barriers, leukocytes (neutrophils, macrophages, NK cells, lymphocytes with invariant antigen receptors, and mast cells).

* The innate immune system uses cell-associated pattern recognition receptors, present on plasma and endosomal membranes and in the cytosol, to recognize structures called pathogen-associated molecular patterns (PAMPs), which are shared by microbes, are not present on mammalian cells, and are often essential for survival of the microbes, thus limiting the capacity of microbes to evade detection by mutating or losing expression of these molecules. In addition, these receptors recognize molecules made by the host but whose expression or location indicates cellular damage; these are called damage-associated molecular patterns (DAMPs).

* TLRs, present on the cell surface and in endosomes, are the most important family of pattern recognition receptors, recognizing a wide variety of ligands, including bacterial cell wall components and microbial nucleic acids. Cytosolic pattern recognition receptors exist that recognize microbial molecules. These receptors include the RIG-like receptors (RLRs), which recognize viral RNA, cytosolic DNA sensors (CDSs), and NOD-like receptors (NLRs), which recognize bacterial cell wall constituents and also sense intracellular crystals, reactive oxygen species, and various other indicators of infection or cell injury.

* Pattern recognition receptors, including TLRs and RLRs, signal to activate the transcription factors NF-κB and AP-1, which promote inflammatory gene expression, and the IRF transcription factors, which stimulate expression of the antiviral type I interferon genes. The inflammasome, a specialized NLR-containing complex that forms in response to PAMPs and DAMPs, is composed of a NOD-like receptor, an adaptor, and the enzyme caspase-1, the main function of which is to produce active forms of the inflammatory cytokines IL-1 and IL-18.

* Soluble pattern recognition and effector molecules are found in the plasma, including pentraxins (e.g., CRP), collectins (e.g., MBL), and ficolins. These molecules bind microbial ligands and enhance clearance by complement-dependent and complement-independent mechanisms.

* NK cells are one of several kinds of innate lymphoid cells that have effector functions shared by T lymphocytes, but do not express T cell receptors for antigen. NK cells defend against intracellular microbes by killing infected cells and providing a source of the macrophage-activating cytokine IFN-γ. NK cell recognition of infected cells is regulated by a combination of activating and inhibitory receptors. Inhibitory receptors recognize class I MHC molecules, because of which NK cells do not kill normal host cells but do kill cells in which class I MHC expression is reduced, such as virus-infected cells.

* The complement system includes several plasma proteins that become activated in sequence by proteolytic cleavage to generate fragments of the C3 and C5 proteins, which promote inflammation, or opsonize and promote phagocytosis of microbes. Complement activation also generates membrane pores that kill some types of bacteria. The complement system is activated on microbial surfaces and not on normal host cells because microbes lack regulatory proteins that inhibit complement. In innate immune responses, complement is activated mainly spontaneously on microbial cell surfaces and by mannose-binding lectin to initiate the alternative and lectin pathways, respectively.

* The two major effector functions of innate immunity are to induce inflammation, which involves the delivery of microbe-killing leukocytes and soluble effector molecules from blood into tissues, and to block viral infection of cells by the antiviral actions of type 1 interferons. Both types of effector mechanism are induced by the PAMPs and DAMPs, which initiate signaling pathways in tissue cells and leukocytes that activate transcription factors and lead to the expression of cytokines and other inflammatory mediators.

* Several cytokines produced mainly by activated macrophages mediate inflammation. TNF and IL-1 activate endothelial cells, stimulate chemokine production, and increase neutrophil production by the bone marrow. IL-1 and TNF both induce IL-6 production, and all three cytokines mediate systemic effects, including fever and acute-phase protein synthesis by the liver. IL-12 and IL-18 stimulate production of the macrophage-activating cytokine IFN-γ by NK cells and T cells. These cytokines function in innate immune responses to different classes of microbes, and some (IL-1, IL-6, IL-12, IL-18) modify adaptive immune responses that follow the innate immune response.

* Neutrophils and monocytes (the precursors of tissue macrophages) migrate from blood into inflammatory sites during innate immune responses because of the effects of cytokines and chemokines produced by PAMP- and DAMP-stimulated tissue cells.

* Neutrophils and macrophages phagocytose microbes and kill them by producing ROS, nitric oxide, and enzymes in phagolysosomes. Macrophages also produce cytokines that stimulate inflammation and promote tissue remodeling at sites of infection. Phagocytes recognize and respond to microbial products by several different types of receptors, including TLRs, C-type lectins, scavenger receptors, and N-formyl met-leu-phe receptors.

* Molecules produced during innate immune responses stimulate adaptive immunity and influence the nature of adaptive immune responses. Dendritic cells activated by microbes produce cytokines and costimulators that enhance T cell activation and differentiation into effector T cells. Complement fragments generated by the alternative pathway provide second signals for B cell activation and antibody production.

* Innate immune responses are regulated by negative feedback mechanisms that limit potential damage to tissues. IL-10 is a cytokine that is produced by and inhibits activation of macrophages and dendritic cells. Inflammatory cytokine secretion is regulated by autophagy gene products. Negative signaling pathways block the activating signals generated by pattern recognition receptors and inflammatory cytokines.

SUGGESTED READINGS

Pattern Recognition Receptors

Blasius AL, Beutler B: Intracellular Toll-like receptors, *Immunity* 32:305–315, 2010.
Canton J, Neculai D, Grinstein S: Scavenger receptors in homeostasis and immunity, *Nature Reviews Immunology* 13:621–634, 2013.
Chen G, Shaw MH, Kim YG, Nuñez G: Nod-like receptors: role in innate immunity and inflammatory disease, *Annual Review of Pathology* 4:365–398, 2009.
Dixit E, Kagan J: Intracellular pathogen detection by RIG-I-like receptors, *Advances in Immunology* 117:99–125, 2013.
Elinav E, Strowig T, Henao-Mejia J, Flavell RA: Regulation of the antimicrobial response by NLR proteins, *Immunity* 34:665–679, 2011.
Goubau D, Deddouche S, Reis C, Sousa E: Cytosolic sensing of viruses, *Immunity* 38:855–869, 2013.
Hornung V, Latz E: Intracellular DNA recognition, *Nature Reviews Immunology* 10:123–130, 2010.
Janeway CA, Medzhitov R: Innate immune recognition, *Annual Review of Immunology* 20:197–216, 2002.
Kawai T, Akira S: The role of pattern-recognition receptors in innate immunity: update on Toll-like receptors, *Nature Immunology* 11:373–384, 2010.
Latz E, Xiao TS, Stutz A: Activation and regulation of the inflammasome, *Nature Reviews Immunology* 13:397–411, 2013.
Martonez-Pomares L: The mannose receptor, *Journal of Leukocyte Biology* 92:1177–1186, 2012.
Osorio F, Reis e Sousa C: Myeloid C-type lectin receptors in pathogen recognition and host defense, *Immunity* 34:651–664, 2011.
Takeuchi O, Akira S: Pattern recognition receptors and inflammation, *Cell* 140:805–820, 2010.
Wu J, Chen ZJ: Innate immune sensing and signaling of cytosolic nucleic acids, *Annual Review of Immunology* 32:461–488, 2014.

Cells of the Innate Immune System

Amulic B, Cazalet C, Hayes GL, Metzler KD, Zychlinsky A: Neutrophil function: from mechanisms to disease, *Annual Review of Immunology* 30:459–489, 2012.
Dale DC, Boxer L, Liles WC: The phagocytes: neutrophils and monocytes, *Blood* 112:935–945, 2008.
Davies LC, Jenkins SJ, Allen JE, Taylor PR: Tissue-resident macrophages, *Nature Immunology* 14:986–995, 2013.
Flannagan RS, Jaumouille V, Grinstein S: The cell biology of phagocytosis. *Annual Review of Pathology: Mechanisms of Disease* 7:61–98, 2012.
Lanier LL: NK cell recognition, *Annual Review of Immunology* 23:225–274, 2005.
Mócsai A: Diverse novel functions of neutrophils in immunity, inflammation, and beyond, *The Journal of Experimental Medicine* 10:1283–1299, 2013.
Molawi JK, Sieweke MH: Transcriptional control of macrophage identity, self-renewal, and function, *Advances in Immunology* 120:269–300, 2013.
Murray PJ, Wynn TA: Protective and pathogenic functions of macrophage subsets, *Nature Reviews Immunology* 11:723–737, 2011.
Schenten D, Medzhitov R: The control of adaptive immune responses by the innate immune system, *Advances in Immunology* 109:87–124, 2011.
Serbina NV, Jia T, Hohl TM, Pamer EG: Monocyte-mediated defense against microbial pathogens, *Annual Review of Immunology* 26:421–452, 2008.
Sun JC, Lanier LL: NK cell development, homeostasis and function: parallels with CD8+ T cells, *Nature Reviews Immunology* 11:645–5, 2011.
Walker JA, Barlow JL, McKenzie AN: Innate lymphoid cells–how did we miss them? *Nature Reviews Immunology* 13:75–87, 2013.
Vivier E, Tomasello E, Baratin M, Walzer T, Ugolini S: Functions of natural killer cells, *Nature Immunology* 9:503–510, 2008.

Effector Molecules of Innate Immunity

Bottazzi B, Doni A, Garlanda C, Mantovani A: An integrated view of humoral innate immunity: pentraxins as a paradigm, *Annual Review of Immunology* 28:157–183, 2010.
Ivashkiv LB, Donlin LT: Regulation of type I interferon responses, *Nature Reviews Immunology* 14:36–50, 2014.

Lamkanfi M, Dixit VM: Inflammasomes and their roles in health and disease, *Annual Review of Cell and Developmental Biology* 28:137–161, 2012.

Linden SK, Sutton P, Karlsson NG, Korolik V, McGuckin MA: Mucins in the mucosal barrier to infection, *Mucosal Immunology* 1:183–197, 2008.

Rock KL, Latz E, Ontiveros F, Kono H: The sterile inflammatory response, *Annual Review of Immunology* 28:321–342, 2010.

Schroder K, Tschopp J: The inflammasomes, *Cell* 140:821–832, 2010.

Selsted ME, Ouellette AJ: Mammalian defensins in the antimicrobial immune response, *Nature Immunology* 6:551–557, 2005.

Sims JE, Smith DE: The IL-1 family: regulators of immunity, *Nature Reviews Immunology* 10:89–102, 2010.

Van de Wetering JK, van Golde LMG, Batenburg JJ: Collectins: players of the innate immune system, *European Journal of Biochemistry* 271:229–249, 2004.

Diseases Caused by Innate Immunity

Angus DC, van der Poll T: Severe sepsis and septic shock, *New England Journal of Medicine* 369:840–851, 2013.

Deutschman CS, Tracey KJ: Sepsis: current dogma and new perspectives, *Immunity* 40:463–475, 2014.

Park H, Bourla AB, Kastner DL, Colbert RA, Siegel RM: Lighting the fires within: the cell biology of autoinflammatory diseases, *Nature Reviews Immunology* 12:570–580, 2012.

Stearns-Kurosawa DJ, Osuchowski MF, Valentine C, Kurosawa S, Remick DG: The pathogenesis of sepsis, *Annual Review of Pathology* 6:19–48, 2011.

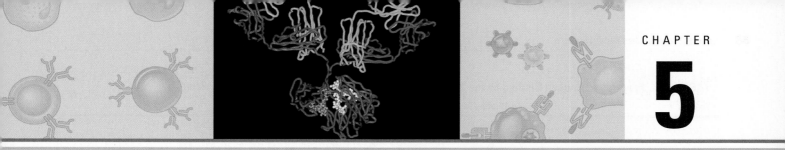

CHAPTER

5

Antibodies and Antigens

Antibodies are circulating proteins that are produced in vertebrates in response to exposure to foreign structures known as antigens. Antibodies are incredibly diverse and specific in their ability to recognize foreign molecular structures and are the mediators of humoral immunity against all classes of microbes. Because these proteins were discovered as serum molecules that provided protection against diphtheria toxin, they were initially called antitoxins. When it was appreciated that similar proteins could be generated against many substances, not just microbial toxins, they were given the general name **antibodies**. The substances that generated or were recognized by antibodies were then called **antigens**. Antibodies, major histocompatibility complex (MHC) molecules (see Chapter 6), and T cell antigen receptors (see Chapter 7) are the three classes of molecules used by the adaptive immune system to bind antigens (Table 5-1). Of these three, antibodies were the first to be discovered, recognize the widest range of antigenic structures, show the greatest ability to discriminate between different

antigens, and bind antigens with the greatest strength. In this chapter we describe the structure and antigen-binding properties of antibodies.

Antibodies are synthesized only by cells of the B lymphocyte lineage and exist in two forms: membrane-bound antibodies on the surface of B lymphocytes function as antigen receptors, and secreted antibodies neutralize toxins, prevent the entry and spread of pathogens, and eliminate microbes. The recognition of antigen by membrane-bound antibodies on naive B cells activates these lymphocytes and initiates a humoral immune response. The activated B cells differentiate into plasma cells that secrete antibodies of the same specificity as the antigen receptor. Secreted forms of antibodies are present in the plasma (the fluid portion of the blood), in mucosal secretions, and in the interstitial fluid of tissues. In the effector phase of humoral immunity, these secreted antibodies bind to antigens and trigger several effector mechanisms that eliminate the antigens.

The elimination of antigen often requires interaction of antibody with other components of the immune system, including molecules such as complement proteins and cells that include phagocytes and eosinophils. Antibody-mediated effector functions include: neutralization of microbes or toxic microbial products; activation of the complement system; opsonization of pathogens for enhanced phagocytosis; antibody-dependent cell-mediated cytotoxicity, by which antibodies target infected cells for lysis by cells of the innate immune system; and antibody-mediated mast cell activation to expel parasitic worms. We will describe these functions of antibodies in detail in Chapter 13.

When blood or plasma forms a clot, antibodies remain in the residual fluid, which is called **serum**. Serum lacks coagulation factors (which are consumed during clot formation) but contains all the other proteins found in plasma. Any serum sample that contains detectable antibody molecules that bind to a particular antigen is commonly called an **antiserum**. The study of antibodies and their reactions with antigens is therefore classically called **serology**. The concentration of antibody molecules in serum specific for a particular antigen is often estimated by determining how many serial dilutions of the serum can be made before binding can no longer be detected;

TABLE 5-1 Features of Antigen Binding by the Antigen-Recognizing Molecules of the Immune System

Feature	Antigen-Binding Molecule		
	Immunoglobulin (Ig)	T cell receptor (TCR)*	MHC molecules*
Antigen-binding site	Made up of three CDRs in V_H and three CDRs in V_L domains	Made up of three CDRs in V_α and three CDRs in V_β domains	Peptide-binding cleft made of α1 and α2 domains (class I MHC) and α1 and β1 domains (class II MHC)
Nature of antigen that may be bound	Macromolecules (proteins, lipids, polysaccharides) and small chemicals	Peptide-MHC complexes	Peptides
Nature of antigenic determinants recognized	Linear and conformational determinants of various macromolecules and chemicals	Linear determinants of peptides; only 2 or 3 amino acid residues of a peptide bound to an MHC molecule	Linear determinants of peptides; only some amino acid residues of a peptide
Affinity of antigen binding	K_d 10^{-7}–10^{-11} M; average affinity of Igs increases during immune response	K_d 10^{-5}–10^{-7} M	K_d 10^{-6}–10^{-9} M; extremely stable binding
On-rate and off-rate	Rapid on-rate, variable off-rate	Slow on-rate, slow off-rate	Slow on-rate, very slow off-rate

CDR, complementarity-determining region; K_d, dissociation constant; MHC, major histocompatibility complex; (only class II molecules depicted); V_H, variable domain of heavy chain Ig; V_L, variable domain of light chain Ig.
*The structures and functions of MHC and TCR molecules are discussed in Chapters 6 and 7, respectively.

sera with a high concentration of antibody molecules specific for a particular antigen are said to have a high titer.

A healthy 70-kg adult human produces about 2 to 3 g of antibodies every day. Almost two thirds of this is an antibody called IgA, which is produced by activated B cells and plasma cells in the walls of the gastrointestinal and respiratory tracts and is actively transported across epithelial cells into the lumens of these tracts. The large amount of IgA produced reflects the large surface areas of these organs.

ANTIBODY STRUCTURE

An understanding of the structure of antibodies has provided important insights into their function. The analysis of antibody structure also laid the foundation for elucidating the mechanisms of antigen receptor diversity, one of the fundamental problems of Immunology that we will consider in depth in Chapter 8.

Early studies of antibody structure relied on antibodies purified from the blood of individuals immunized with various antigens. It was not possible, using this approach, to define antibody structure precisely because serum contains a mixture of different antibodies produced by many clones of B lymphocytes that may each bind to different portions (epitopes) of an antigen (so-called polyclonal antibodies). A major breakthrough in obtaining antibodies whose structures could be elucidated was the discovery that patients with multiple myeloma, a monoclonal tumor of antibody-producing plasma cells, often have large amounts of biochemically identical antibody molecules (produced by the neoplastic clone) in their blood and urine. Immunologists found that these antibodies

could be purified to homogeneity and analyzed. The recognition that myeloma cells make monoclonal immunoglobulins led to the extremely important technology to produce monoclonal antibodies, described later in the chapter. The availability of homogeneous populations of antibodies and monoclonal antibody–producing plasma cells facilitated the detailed structural analysis of antibody molecules and molecular cloning of the genes for individual antibodies. These were major advances in our understanding of the adaptive immune system.

General Features of Antibody Structure

Plasma or serum proteins can be physically separated based on solubility characteristics into albumins and globulins, and may be more precisely separated by migration in an electric field, a process called electrophoresis. Most antibodies are found in the third fastest migrating group of globulins, named **gamma globulins** for the third letter of the Greek alphabet. Another common name for antibody is **immunoglobulin (Ig)**, referring to the immunity-conferring portion of the gamma globulin fraction. The terms *immunoglobulin* and *antibody* are used interchangeably throughout this book.

All antibody molecules share the same basic structural characteristics but display remarkable variability in the regions that bind antigens. This variability of the antigen-binding regions accounts for the capacity of different antibodies to bind a tremendous number of structurally diverse antigens. In every individual, there are millions of different clones of B cells, each producing antibody molecules with the same antigen-binding site and different in this site from the antibodies produced by other clones. The effector functions and common physicochemical properties of antibodies are associated with the non–antigen-binding portions, which exhibit relatively few variations among different antibodies.

An antibody molecule has a symmetric core structure composed of two identical light chains and two identical heavy chains (Fig. 5-1). Both the light chains and heavy chains contain a series of repeating homologous units, each about 110 amino acid residues in length, that fold independently in a globular motif that is called an **Ig domain**, which we introduced in chapters 3 and 4. An Ig domain contains two layers of β-pleated sheet, each layer composed of three to five strands of antiparallel polypeptide chain (Fig. 5-2). The two layers are held together by a disulfide bridge, and adjacent strands of each β sheet are connected by short loops. It is the amino acids in some of these loops that are the most variable and critical for antigen recognition, as discussed later in the chapter.

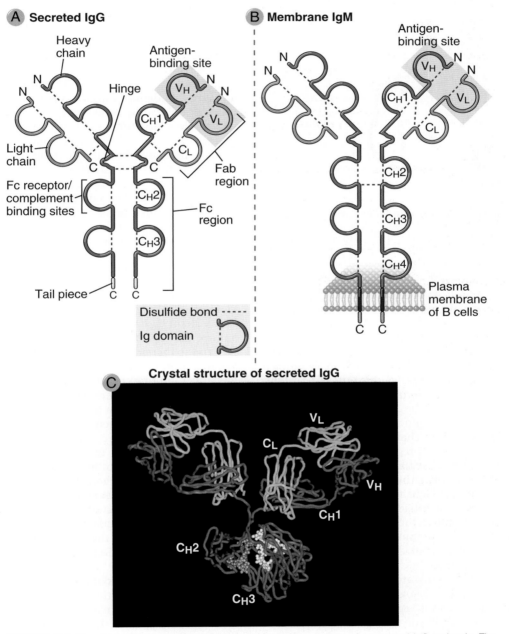

FIGURE 5-1 Structure of an antibody molecule. A, Schematic diagram of a secreted IgG molecule. The antigen-binding sites are formed by the juxtaposition of V_L and V_H domains. The heavy chain C regions end in tail pieces. The locations of complement- and Fc receptor–binding sites within the heavy chain constant regions are approximations. **B,** Schematic diagram of a membrane-bound IgM molecule on the surface of a B lymphocyte. The IgM molecule has one more C_H domain than IgG has, and the membrane form of the antibody has C-terminal transmembrane and cytoplasmic portions that anchor the molecule in the plasma membrane. **C,** Structure of a human IgG molecule as revealed by x-ray crystallography. In this ribbon diagram of a secreted IgG molecule, the heavy chains are colored blue and red, and the light chains are colored green; carbohydrates are shown in gray. *(Courtesy of Dr. Alex McPherson, University of California, Irvine.)*

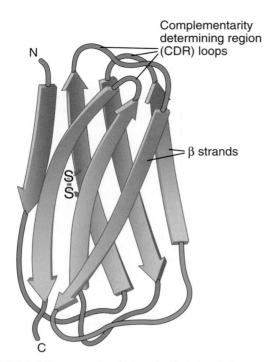

FIGURE 5-2 Structure of an Ig domain. Each domain is composed of two antiparallel arrays of β strands, colored yellow and red, to form two β-pleated sheets held together by a disulfide bond. A constant (C) domain is schematically depicted that contains three and four β strands in the two sheets. Note that the loops connect β strands that are sometimes adjacent in the same β-pleated sheet but that loops sometimes represent connections between the two different sheets that make up an Ig domain. Three loops in each variable domain contribute to antigen binding and are called complementarity determining regions (CDRs).

Both heavy chains and light chains consist of amino-terminal variable (V) regions that participate in antigen recognition and carboxy-terminal constant (C) regions; the C regions of the heavy chains mediate effector functions. In the heavy chains, the V region is composed of one Ig domain, and the C region is composed of three or four Ig domains. Each light chain is composed of one V region Ig domain and one C region Ig domain. Variable regions are so named because their amino acid sequences vary among antibodies made by different B cell clones. The V region of one heavy chain (V_H) and the adjoining V region of one light chain (V_L) form an antigen-binding site (see Fig. 5-1). Because the core structural unit of each antibody molecule contains two heavy chains and two light chains, every antibody molecule has at least two antigen-binding sites.

The C region Ig domains are distant from the antigen-binding site and do not participate in antigen recognition. The heavy chain C regions interact with other effector molecules and cells of the immune system and therefore mediate most of the biologic functions of antibodies. In addition, heavy chains exist in two forms that differ at their carboxy-terminal ends: one form of the heavy chain anchors membrane-bound antibodies in the plasma membranes of B lymphocytes, and the other form is found only in secreted antibodies. The C regions of light chains do not participate in effector functions and are not directly attached to cell membranes.

Heavy and light chains are covalently linked by disulfide bonds formed between cysteine residues in the carboxy terminus of the light chain and the C_H1 domain of the heavy chain. Non-covalent interactions between the V_L and V_H domains and between the C_L and C_H1 domains may also contribute to the association of heavy and light chains. The two heavy chains of each antibody molecule are covalently linked by disulfide bonds. In IgG antibodies, these bonds are formed between cysteine residues in the C_H2 domains, close to the region known as the hinge, described later in the chapter. In other isotypes, the disulfide bonds may be in different locations. Non-covalent interactions (e.g., between the third C_H domains [C_H3]) may also contribute to heavy chain pairing.

The associations between the chains of antibody molecules and the functions of different regions of antibodies were first deduced from experiments in which rabbit IgG was cleaved by proteolytic enzymes into fragments with distinct structural and functional properties. In IgG molecules, the unfolded hinge region between the C_H1 and C_H2 domains of the heavy chain is the segment most susceptible to proteolytic cleavage. If rabbit IgG is treated with the enzyme papain under conditions of limited proteolysis, the enzyme acts on the hinge region and cleaves the IgG into three separate pieces (Fig. 5-3, *A*). Two of the pieces are identical to each other and consist of the complete light chain (V_L and C_L) associated with a V_H-C_H1 fragment of the heavy chain. These fragments retain the ability to bind antigen because each contains paired V_L and V_H domains, and they are called **Fab** (fragment, antigen binding). The third piece is composed of two identical disulfide-linked peptides, each containing the heavy chain C_H2 and C_H3 domains. This piece of IgG has a propensity to self-associate and to crystallize into a lattice and is therefore called **Fc** (fragment, crystallizable). When pepsin (instead of papain) is used to cleave rabbit IgG under limiting conditions, proteolysis occurs distal to the hinge region, generating a F(ab')$_2$ fragment of IgG with the hinge and the interchain disulfide bonds intact and two identical antigen-binding sites (see Fig. 5-3, *B*).

The results of limited papain or pepsin proteolysis of other isotypes besides IgG, or of IgGs of species other than the rabbit, do not always recapitulate the studies with rabbit IgG. However, the basic organization of the antibody molecule deduced from the rabbit IgG proteolysis experiments is common to all Ig molecules of all isotypes and all species. In fact, these experiments provided the first evidence that the antigen recognition functions and the effector functions of Ig molecules are spatially separated.

Many other proteins in the immune system, as well as numerous proteins with no known immunologic function, contain domains with an Ig fold structure—that is, two adjacent β-pleated sheets held together by a disulfide bridge. All molecules that contain this type of domain are said to belong to the **Ig superfamily**, and all gene segments encoding the Ig domains of these molecules are believed to have evolved from one ancestral gene. Ig domains are classified as V-like or C-like on the basis of closest homology to either Ig V or Ig C domains. V domains are formed from a longer polypeptide than are C domains and contain two extra β strands within the

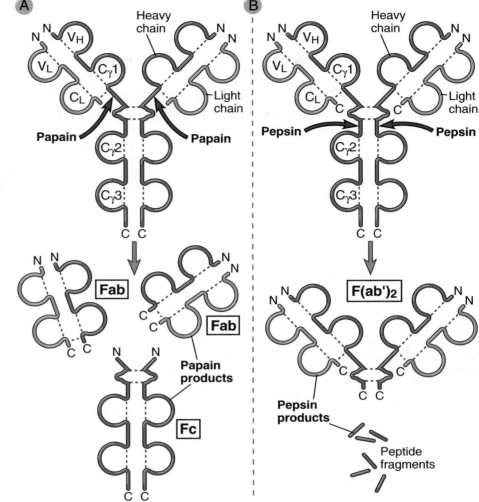

FIGURE 5-3 Proteolytic fragments of an IgG molecule. Rabbit IgG molecules are cleaved by the enzymes papain **(A)** and pepsin **(B)** at the sites indicated by arrows. Papain digestion allows separation of two antigen-binding regions (the Fab fragments) from the portion of the IgG molecule that binds to complement and Fc receptors (the Fc fragment). Pepsin generates a single bivalent antigen-binding fragment, F(ab')$_2$. The structural features deduced by proteolysis of rabbit IgG are common to antibodies of all species.

β sheet sandwich. Some members of the Ig superfamily were described in Chapter 3 (endothelial adhesion molecules ICAM-1 and VCAM-1) and Chapter 4 (NK cell KIR receptors). Examples of Ig superfamily members of relevance in the immune system are depicted in Figure 5-4.

Structural Features of Antibody Variable Regions

Most of the sequence differences and variability among different antibodies are confined to three short stretches in the V region of the heavy chain and to three stretches in the V region of the light chain. These segments of the greatest diversity are known as **hypervariable regions.** They correspond to three protruding loops connecting adjacent strands of the β sheets that make up the V domains of Ig heavy and light chain proteins (Fig. 5-5). The hypervariable regions are each about 10 amino acid residues long, and they are held in place by the more conserved framework sequences that make up the Ig domain of the V region. In an antibody molecule, the three hypervariable regions of a V_L domain and the three hypervariable regions of a V_H domain are brought together to create an antigen-binding surface. The hypervariable loops can

be thought to resemble fingers protruding from each variable domain, with three fingers from the heavy chain and three fingers from the light chain coming together to form the antigen-binding site (Fig. 5-6). Because these sequences form a surface that is complementary to the three-dimensional shape of the bound antigen, the hypervariable regions are also called **complementarity-determining regions (CDRs).** Proceeding from either the V_L or the V_H amino terminus, these regions are called CDR1, CDR2, and CDR3. The CDR3s of both the V_H segment and the V_L segment are the most variable of the CDRs. As we will discuss in Chapter 8, there are special mechanisms for generating more sequence diversity in CDR3 than in CDR1 and CDR2. Sequence differences among the CDRs of different antibody molecules contribute to distinct interaction surfaces and therefore to specificities of individual antibodies. The ability of a V region to fold into an Ig domain is mostly determined by the conserved sequences of the framework regions adjacent to the CDRs. Confinement of the sequence variability to three short stretches allows the basic structure of all antibodies to be maintained despite the variability of specificities among different antibodies.

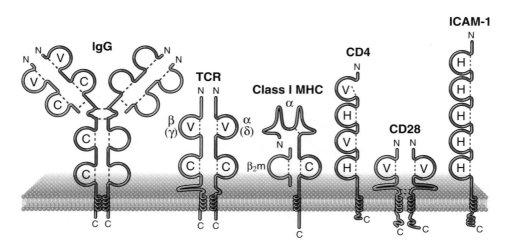

FIGURE 5-4 Examples of Ig superfamily proteins in the immune system. Shown here are a membrane-bound IgG molecule; the T cell receptor; an MHC class I molecule; the CD4 coreceptor of T cells; CD28, a costimulatory receptor on T cells; and the adhesion molecule ICAM-1.

Antigen binding by antibody molecules is primarily a function of the hypervariable regions of V_H and V_L. Crystallographic analyses of antigen-antibody complexes show that the amino acid residues of the hypervariable regions form multiple contacts with bound antigen (see Fig. 5-6). The most extensive contact is with the third hypervariable region (CDR3), which is also the most variable of the three CDRs. However, antigen binding is not solely a function of the CDRs, and framework residues may also contact the antigen. Moreover, in the binding of some antigens, one or more of the CDRs may be outside the region of contact with antigen, thus not participating in antigen binding.

Structural Features of Antibody Constant Regions

Antibody molecules can be divided into distinct classes and subclasses on the basis of differences in the structure

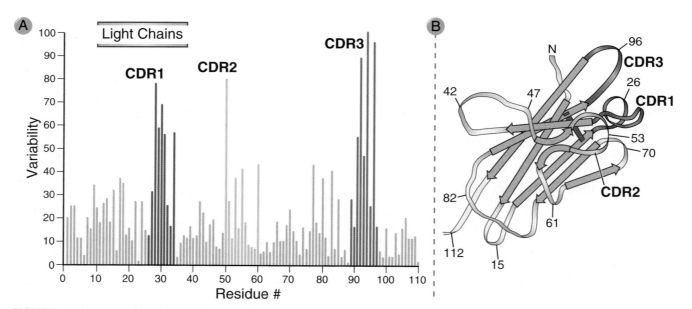

FIGURE 5-5 Hypervariable regions in Ig molecules. A, The vertical lines depict the extent of variability, defined as the number of differences in each amino acid residue among various independently sequenced Ig light chains, plotted against amino acid residue number, measured from the amino terminus. This analysis indicates that the most variable residues are clustered in three "hypervariable" regions, colored in blue, yellow, and red, corresponding to CDR1, CDR2, and CDR3, respectively. Three hypervariable regions are also present in heavy chains (not shown). This way of displaying amino acid variability in Ig molecules is called a Kabat-Wu plot after the two scientists who devised the assay. **B,** Three-dimensional view of the hypervariable CDR loops in a light chain V domain. The V region of a light chain is shown with CDR1, CDR2, and CDR3 loops, colored in blue, yellow, and red, respectively. These loops correspond to the hypervariable regions in the variability plot in **A.** Heavy chain hypervariable regions (not shown) are also located in three loops, and all six loops are juxtaposed in the antibody molecule to form the antigen-binding surface (see Fig. 5-6). *(A, Courtesy of Dr. E. A. Kabat, Department of Microbiology, Columbia University College of Physicians and Surgeons, New York.)*

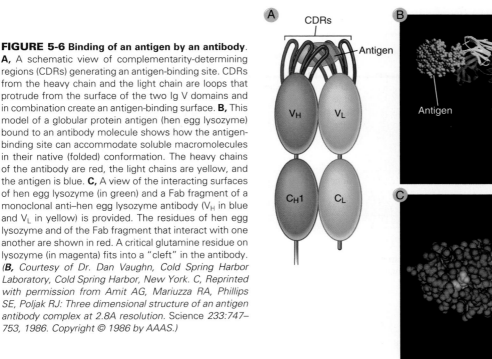

FIGURE 5-6 Binding of an antigen by an antibody.
A, A schematic view of complementarity-determining regions (CDRs) generating an antigen-binding site. CDRs from the heavy chain and the light chain are loops that protrude from the surface of the two Ig V domains and in combination create an antigen-binding surface. **B,** This model of a globular protein antigen (hen egg lysozyme) bound to an antibody molecule shows how the antigen-binding site can accommodate soluble macromolecules in their native (folded) conformation. The heavy chains of the antibody are red, the light chains are yellow, and the antigen is blue. **C,** A view of the interacting surfaces of hen egg lysozyme (in green) and a Fab fragment of a monoclonal anti–hen egg lysozyme antibody (V_H in blue and V_L in yellow) is provided. The residues of hen egg lysozyme and of the Fab fragment that interact with one another are shown in red. A critical glutamine residue on lysozyme (in magenta) fits into a "cleft" in the antibody. (**B,** *Courtesy of Dr. Dan Vaughn, Cold Spring Harbor Laboratory, Cold Spring Harbor, New York. C, Reprinted with permission from Amit AG, Mariuzza RA, Phillips SE, Poljak RJ: Three dimensional structure of an antigen antibody complex at 2.8A resolution.* Science *233:747–753, 1986. Copyright © 1986 by AAAS.*)

of their heavy chain C regions. The classes of antibody molecules are also called **isotypes** and are named IgA, IgD, IgE, IgG, and IgM (Table 5-2). In humans, IgA and IgG isotypes can be further subdivided into closely related subclasses, or subtypes, called IgA1 and IgA2 and IgG1, IgG2, IgG3, and IgG4. (Mice, which are often used in the study of immune responses, differ in that the IgG isotype is divided into the IgG1, IgG2a, IgG2b, and IgG3 subclasses; certain strains of mice, including C57BL/6, lack the gene for IgG2a but synthesize a related isotype called IgG2c). The heavy chain C regions of all antibody molecules of one isotype or subtype have essentially the same amino acid sequence. This sequence is different in antibodies of other isotypes or subtypes. Heavy chains are designated by the letter of the Greek alphabet corresponding to the isotype of the antibody: IgA1 contains α1 heavy chains; IgA2, α2; IgD, δ; IgE, ε; IgG1, γ1; IgG2, γ2; IgG3, γ3; IgG4, γ4; and IgM, μ. In human IgM and IgE antibodies, the C regions contain four tandem Ig domains (see Fig. 5-1). The C regions of IgG, IgA, and IgD contain only three Ig domains. These domains are generically designated $\mathbf{C_H}$ domains and are numbered sequentially from amino terminus to carboxyl terminus (e.g., C_H1, C_H2, and so on). In each isotype, these regions may be designated more specifically (e.g., Cγ1, Cγ2 in IgG).

Different isotypes and subtypes of antibodies perform different effector functions. The reason for this is that most of the effector functions of antibodies are mediated by the binding of heavy chain C regions to Fc receptors (FcRs) on different cells, such as phagocytes, NK cells, and mast cells, and to plasma proteins, such as complement proteins. Antibody isotypes and subtypes differ in their C regions and therefore in what they bind to and what effector functions they perform. The effector functions mediated by each antibody isotype are listed in Table 5-2 and are discussed in more detail later in this chapter and in Chapter 13.

Antibody molecules are flexible, permitting them to bind to different arrays of antigens. Every antibody contains at least two antigen-binding sites, each formed by a pair of V_H and V_L domains. Many Ig molecules can orient these binding sites so that two antigen molecules on a planar (e.g., cell) surface may be engaged at once (Fig. 5-7). This flexibility is conferred, in large part, by a **hinge region** located between C_H1 and C_H2 in certain isotypes. The hinge region varies in length from 10 to more than 60 amino acid residues in different isotypes. Portions of this sequence assume an unfolded and flexible conformation, permitting molecular motion between the C_H1 and C_H2 domains. Some of the greatest differences between the constant regions of the IgG subclasses are concentrated in the hinge. This leads to different overall shapes of the IgG subtypes. In addition, some flexibility of antibody molecules is due to the ability of each V_H domain to rotate with respect to the adjacent C_H1 domain.

There are two classes, or isotypes, of light chains, called κ and λ, that are distinguished by their carboxyl-terminal constant (C) regions. Each antibody molecule has either two identical κ light chains or two identical λ light chains. In humans, about 60% of antibody molecules have κ light chains, and about 40% have λ light chains. Marked changes in this ratio can occur in patients with B cell tumors because the many neoplastic cells, being derived from one B cell clone, produce a single species of antibody molecules, all with the same light chain. In fact, a

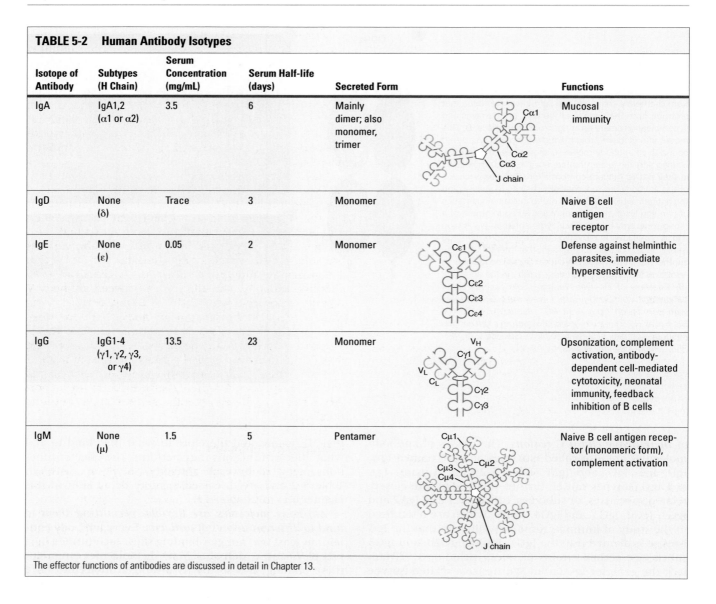

TABLE 5-2   Human Antibody Isotypes

Isotope of Antibody	Subtypes (H Chain)	Serum Concentration (mg/mL)	Serum Half-life (days)	Secreted Form		Functions
IgA	IgA1,2 (α1 or α2)	3.5	6	Mainly dimer; also monomer, trimer		Mucosal immunity
IgD	None (δ)	Trace	3	Monomer		Naive B cell antigen receptor
IgE	None (ε)	0.05	2	Monomer		Defense against helminthic parasites, immediate hypersensitivity
IgG	IgG1-4 (γ1, γ2, γ3, or γ4)	13.5	23	Monomer		Opsonization, complement activation, antibody-dependent cell-mediated cytotoxicity, neonatal immunity, feedback inhibition of B cells
IgM	None (μ)	1.5	5	Pentamer		Naive B cell antigen receptor (monomeric form), complement activation

The effector functions of antibodies are discussed in detail in Chapter 13.

skewed ratio of κ-bearing cells to λ-bearing cells is often used clinically for the diagnosis of B cell lymphomas. In mice, κ-containing antibodies are about 10 times more abundant than λ-containing antibodies. Unlike in heavy chain isotypes, there are no known differences in function between κ-containing antibodies and λ-containing antibodies.

Secreted and membrane-associated antibodies differ in the amino acid sequence of the carboxyl-terminal end of the heavy chain C region. In the secreted form, found in blood and other extracellular fluids, the carboxyl-terminal portion is hydrophilic. The membrane-bound form of antibody contains a carboxyl-terminal stretch that includes two segments: a hydrophobic α-helical transmembrane region, followed by an intracellular juxtamembrane positively charged stretch (Fig. 5-8). The positively charged amino acids bind to negatively charged phospholipid head groups on the inner leaflet of the plasma membrane and help anchor the protein in

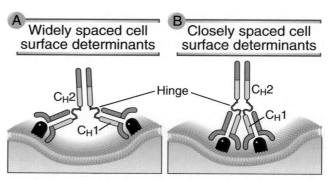

FIGURE 5-7 Flexibility of antibody molecules. The two antigen-binding sites of an Ig monomer can simultaneously bind to two determinants separated by varying distances. In **A,** an Ig molecule is depicted binding to two widely spaced determinants on a cell surface, and in **B,** the same antibody is binding to two determinants that are close together. This flexibility is mainly due to the hinge regions located between the C_H1 and C_H2 domains, which permit independent movement of antigen-binding sites relative to the rest of the molecule.

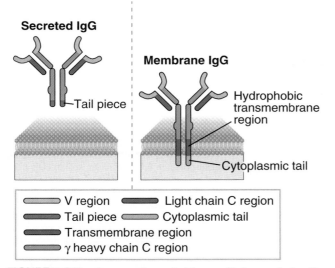

Secreted IgG

Tail piece

Membrane IgG

Hydrophobic transmembrane region

Cytoplasmic tail

V region	Light chain C region
Tail piece	Cytoplasmic tail
Transmembrane region	
γ heavy chain C region	

FIGURE 5-8 Membrane and secreted forms of Ig heavy chains. The membrane forms of the Ig heavy chains, but not the secreted forms, contain transmembrane regions made up of hydrophobic amino acid residues and cytoplasmic domains that differ significantly among the different isotypes. The cytoplasmic portion of the membrane form of the μ chain contains only three residues, whereas the cytoplasmic region of IgG heavy chains (γ heavy chains) contains 20 to 30 residues. The secreted forms of the antibodies end in C-terminal tail pieces, which also differ among isotypes: μ has a long tail piece (21 residues) that is involved in pentamer formation, whereas IgGs have a short tail piece (3 residues).

the membrane. In membrane IgM and IgD molecules, the cytoplasmic portion of the heavy chain is short, only three amino acid residues in length; in membrane IgG and IgE molecules, it is somewhat longer, up to 30 amino acid residues in length.

Secreted IgG and IgE and all membrane Ig molecules, regardless of isotype, are monomeric with respect to the basic antibody structural unit (i.e., they contain two heavy chains and two light chains). In contrast, the secreted forms of IgM and IgA form multimeric complexes in which two or more of the four-chain core antibody structural units are covalently joined. IgM may be secreted as pentamers and hexamers of the core four-chain structure, whereas IgA is often secreted as a dimer. These complexes are formed by interactions between regions called tail pieces that are located at the carboxyl-terminal ends of the secreted forms of μ and α heavy chains (see Table 5-2). Multimeric IgM and IgA molecules also contain an additional 15-kD polypeptide called the joining (J) chain, which is disulfide bonded to the tail pieces and serves to stabilize the multimeric complexes and to transport multimers across epithelial cells from the basolateral to the luminal end. As we will see later, multimeric forms of antibodies bind to antigens more avidly than monomeric forms do, even if both types of antibody contain Fab regions that individually bind the antigen equally well.

Antibodies of different species differ from one another in the C regions and in framework parts of the V regions. Therefore, when Ig molecules from one species are introduced into another (e.g., horse serum antibodies

or mouse monoclonal antibodies injected into humans), the recipient sees them as foreign, mounts an immune response and makes antibodies largely against the C regions of the introduced Ig. The response often creates an illness called serum sickness (see Chapter 19) and thus greatly limits the ability to treat individuals with antibodies produced in other species. Much effort has been devoted to overcoming this problem with mono-clonal antibodies, and we will discuss this issue in more depth later in the chapter.

Smaller sequence differences are present in antibodies from different individuals even of the same species, reflecting inherited polymorphisms in the genes encoding the C regions of Ig heavy and light chains. When a polymorphic variant found in some individuals of a species can be recognized by an antibody, the variants are referred to as **allotypes**, and the antibody that recognizes an allotypic determinant is called an anti-allotypic antibody. The differences between antibody V regions are concentrated in the CDRs and constitute the **idiotypes** of antibodies. An antibody that recognizes some aspect of the CDRs of another antibody is therefore called an anti-idiotypic antibody. There have been interesting theories that individuals produce anti-idiotypic antibodies against their own antibodies that control immune responses, but there is little evidence to support the importance of this potential mechanism of immune regulation.

Monoclonal Antibodies

A tumor of plasma cells (myeloma or plasmacytoma), like most tumors of any cellular origin, is monoclonal and therefore produces antibodies of a single specific-ity. In most cases, the specificity of the tumor-derived antibody is not known, so the myeloma antibody can-not be used to detect or bind to molecules of inter-est. However, the discovery of monoclonal antibodies produced by these tumors led to the idea that it may be possible to produce similar monoclonal antibodies of any desired specificity by immortalizing individual antibody-secreting cells from an animal immunized with a known antigen. A technique to accomplish this was described by Georges Kohler and Cesar Milstein in 1975, and this has proved to be one of the most valu-able advances in all of scientific research and clinical medicine. The method relies on fusing B cells from an immunized animal (typically a mouse) with an immor-tal myeloma cell line and growing the cells under con-ditions in which the unfused normal and tumor cells cannot survive (Fig. 5-9). The resultant fused cells that grow out are called **hybridomas**; each hybridoma makes only one Ig, derived from one B cell from the immunized animal. The antibodies secreted by many hybridoma clones are screened for binding to the anti-gen of interest, and this single clone with the desired specificity is selected and expanded. The products of these individual clones are **monoclonal antibodies**, each specific for a single epitope on the antigen used to immunize the animal and to identify the immortalized antibody-secreting clones.

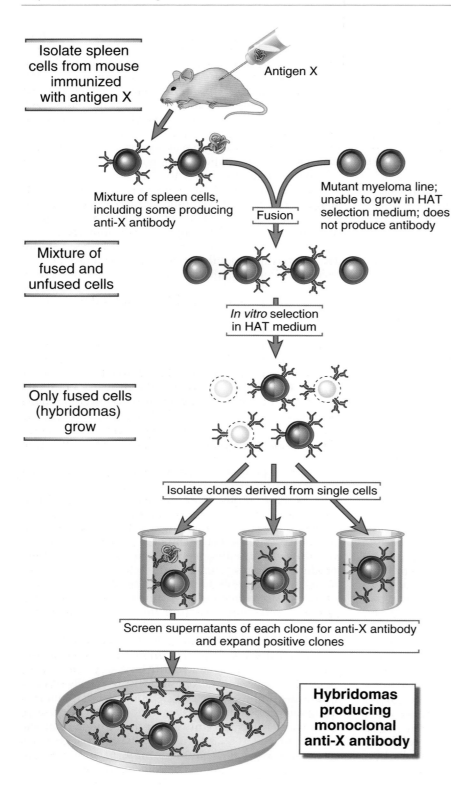

Isolate spleen cells from mouse immunized with antigen X

Antigen X

Mixture of spleen cells, including some producing anti-X antibody

Fusion

Mutant myeloma line; unable to grow in HAT selection medium; does not produce antibody

Mixture of fused and unfused cells

In vitro selection in HAT medium

Only fused cells (hybridomas) grow

Isolate clones derived from single cells

Screen supernatants of each clone for anti-X antibody and expand positive clones

Hybridomas producing monoclonal anti-X antibody

FIGURE 5-9 The generation of monoclonal antibodies. In this procedure, spleen cells from a mouse that has been immunized with a known antigen or mixture of antigens are fused with an enzyme-deficient partner myeloma cell line, with use of chemicals such as polyethylene glycol that can facilitate the fusion of plasma membranes and the formation of hybrid cells that retain many chromosomes from both fusion partners. The myeloma partner used is one that does not secrete its own Ig. These hybrid cells are then placed in a selection medium that permits the survival of only immortalized hybrids; these hybrid cells are then grown as single cell clones and tested for the secretion of the antibody of interest. The selection medium includes hypoxanthine, aminopterin, and thymidine and is therefore called HAT medium. There are two pathways of purine synthesis in most cells, a de novo pathway that needs tetrahydrofolate and a salvage pathway that uses the enzyme hypoxanthine-guanine phosphoribosyltransferase (HGPRT). Myeloma cells that lack HGPRT are used as fusion partners, and they normally survive using de novo purine synthesis. In the presence of aminopterin, tetrahydrofolate is not made, resulting in a defect in de novo purine synthesis and also a specific defect in pyrimidine biosynthesis, namely, in generating TMP from dUMP. Hybrid cells receive HGPRT from the splenocytes and have the capacity for uncontrolled proliferation from the myeloma partner; if they are given hypoxanthine and thymidine, these cells can make DNA in the absence of tetrahydrofolate. As a result, only hybrid cells survive in HAT medium.

Monoclonal antibodies have many practical applications in research and in medical diagnosis and therapy. Some of their common applications include the following:

- *Identification of phenotypic markers unique to particular cell types.* The basis for the modern classification of lymphocytes and other leukocytes is the recognition of individual cell populations by specific monoclonal antibodies. These antibodies have been used to define clusters of differentiation (CD) markers for various cell types (see Chapter 2).
- *Immunodiagnosis.* The diagnosis of many infectious and systemic diseases relies on the detection of particular antigens or antibodies in the blood, urine, or tissues by use of monoclonal antibodies in immunoassays (see Appendix IV).
- *Tumor identification.* Labeled monoclonal antibodies specifc for various cell proteins are used to deteremine the tissue source of tumors by staining histological tumor sections.
- *Therapy.* Advances in medical research have led to the identification of cells and molecules that are involved in the pathogenesis of many diseases. Monoclonal antibodies, because of their exquisite specificity, provide a means of targeting these cells and molecules. A number of monoclonal antibodies are used therapeutically today (Table 5-3). Some examples include antibodies against the cytokine tumor necrosis factor (TNF) used to treat rheumatoid arthritis and other inflammatory diseases, antibodies against CD20 for the treatment of B cell leukemias and for depleting B cells in certain autoimmune disorders, antibodies against epidermal growth factor receptors to target cancer cells, antibodies against vascular endothelial growth factor (a cytokine that promotes angiogenesis) in patients with colon cancer, and so on.
- *Functional analysis of cell surface and secreted molecules.* In biologic research, monoclonal antibodies that bind to cell surface molecules and either stimulate or inhibit particular cellular functions are invaluable tools for defining the functions of surface molecules, including receptors for antigens. Monoclonal antibodies are also widely used to purify selected cell populations from complex mixtures to facilitate the study of the properties and functions of these cells.

One of the limitations of monoclonal antibodies for therapy is that these antibodies are most easily produced by immunizing mice, but patients treated with mouse antibodies may make antibodies against the mouse Ig, called human anti-mouse antibody (HAMA). These anti-Ig antibodies block the function or enhance clearance of the injected monoclonal antibody and can also cause a disorder called serum sickness (see Chapter 19). Genetic engineering techniques have been used to expand the usefulness of monoclonal antibodies. The complementary DNAs (cDNAs) that encode the polypeptide chains of a monoclonal antibody can be isolated from a hybridoma, and these genes can be manipulated in vitro. As discussed earlier, only small portions of the antibody molecule are responsible for binding to antigen; the remainder of the antibody molecule can be thought of as a framework. This structural organization allows the DNA segments encoding the antigen-binding sites from a mouse monoclonal antibody to be inserted into a cDNA encoding a human myeloma protein, creating a hybrid gene. When it is expressed, the resultant hybrid protein, which retains the antigen specificity of the original mouse monoclonal but has the core structure of a human Ig, is referred to as a humanized antibody. Fully human monoclonal antibodies are also in clinical use. These are derived using phage display methods or in mice with B cells expressing human Ig transgenes. Humanized antibodies are far less likely than mouse monoclonals to appear foreign in humans and to induce anti-antibody responses. However, a proportion of subjects receiving fully humanized monoclonal antibodies for therapy develop blocking antibodies, for unknown reasons.

SYNTHESIS, ASSEMBLY, AND EXPRESSION OF Ig MOLECULES

Immunoglobulin heavy and light chains, like most secreted and membrane proteins, are synthesized on membrane-bound ribosomes in the rough endoplasmic reticulum. The protein is translocated into the endoplasmic reticulum, and Ig heavy chains are N-glycosylated during the translocation process. The proper folding of Ig heavy chains and their assembly with light chains are regulated by proteins resident in the endoplasmic reticulum called chaperones. These proteins, which include calnexin and a molecule called BiP (binding protein), bind to newly synthesized Ig polypeptides and ensure that they are retained or targeted for degradation unless they fold properly and assemble into complete Ig molecules. The covalent association of heavy and light chains, stabilized by the formation of disulfide bonds, is part of the assembly process and also occurs in the endoplasmic reticulum. After assembly, the Ig molecules are released from chaperones, transported into the cisternae of the Golgi complex where carbohydrates are modified, and then routed to the plasma membrane in vesicles. Antibodies of the membrane form are anchored in the plasma membrane, and the secreted form is transported out of the cell.

The maturation of B cells from bone marrow progenitors is accompanied by specific changes in Ig gene expression, resulting in the production of Ig molecules in different forms (Fig. 5-10). The earliest cell in the B lymphocyte lineage that produces Ig polypeptides, called the pre-B cell, synthesizes the membrane form of the μ heavy chain. These μ chains associate with proteins called surrogate light chains to form the pre-B cell receptor, and a small proportion of the synthesized pre-B cell receptor is expressed on the cell surface. Immature and mature B cells produce κ or λ light chains, which associate with μ proteins to form IgM molecules. Mature B cells express membrane forms of IgM and IgD (the μ and δ heavy chains associated with κ or λ light chains). These membrane Ig receptors serve as cell surface receptors that recognize antigens and initiate the process of B cell activation. The pre-B cell receptor and the B cell antigen receptor are non-covalently associated with two other

TABLE 5-3   Monoclonal Antibodies in Clinical Use

Target	Effect	Diseases
Inflammatory (Immunological) Diseases		
α4 integrins	Blocking of immune cell egress to intestine and CNS	Crohn's disease, multiple sclerosis
BAFF	Inhibition of B cell survival	Systemic lupus erythematosus
CD3	Depletion of T cells	Transplantation
CD11a	Blocking of inflammatory cell migration	Psoriasis
CD20	Depletion of B cells	B cell lymphomas, rheumatoid arthritis, multiple sclerosis, other autoimmune diseases
CD25 (IL-2Rα)	Inhibition of T cell function	Transplantation
IgE	Blocking of IgE function	Allergy related asthma
IL-6 receptor	Blocking of inflammation	Rheumatoid arthritis
TNF	Blocking of inflammation	Rheumatoid arthritis, Crohn's disease, psoriasis
Cancer		
CD30	Depletion of lymphocytes	Anaplastic large cell lymphoma and Hodgkin lymphoma
CD33	Depletion of myeloid cells; activation of inhibitory signaling in myeloid cells	Acute myelogenous leukemia
CD52	Depletion of lymphocytes	Chronic lymphocytic leukemia
CTLA-4	Activation of T cells	Melanoma
EGFR	Growth inhibition of epithelial tumors	Colorectal, lung, and head and neck cancers
HER2/Neu	Inhibition of EGF signaling; depletion of tumor cells	Breast cancer
PD-1	Activation of effector T cells	Melanoma, renal cell carcinoma, other tumors
PD-L1	Activation of effector T cells	Melanoma, renal cell carcinoma, other tumors
VEGF	Blocking of tumor angiogenesis	Breast cancer, colon cancer, age-related macular degeneration
CD20 (see above)		
Other Diseases		
C5	Blocking of complement-mediated lysis	Paroxysmal nocturnal hemoglobinuria, atypical hemolytic uremic syndrome
Glycoprotein IIb/IIIa	Inhibition of platelet aggregation	Cardiovascular disease
Rank ligand	Blocking of RANK signaling	Post-menopausal osteoporosis, bone metastases of solid tumors
RSV F protein	Blocking of viral entry	Respiratory syncytial virus infection

BAFF, B cell activation factor family; *CTLA-4*, cytotoxic T lymphocyte antigen-4; *EGFR*, epidermal growth factor receptor; *HER2/Neu*, human epidermal growth factor receptor 2/Neu; *PD-1*, program death-1; *PD-L1*, program death ligand-1; *RSV*, respiratory syncytial virus; *TNF*, tumor necrosis factor; *VEGF*, vascular endothelial growth factor.

integral membrane proteins, Igα and Igβ, which serve signaling functions and are essential for surface expression of IgM and IgD. We will discuss the molecular and cellular events in B cell maturation underlying these changes in antibody expression in Chapter 8.

When mature B lymphocytes are activated by antigens and other stimuli, the cells differentiate into antibody-secreting cells. This process is also accompanied by changes in the pattern of Ig production. One such change is the increased production of the secreted form of Ig relative to the membrane form. This alteration occurs at the level of post-transcriptional processing.

The second change is the expression of Ig heavy chain isotypes other than IgM and IgD, called heavy chain isotype (or class) switching. Changes in antibody expression that occur after B cell activation will be discussed in Chapter 12.

Half-Life of Antibodies

The half-life of circulating antibodies is a measure of how long those antibodies remain in blood after secretion from B cells (or after injection in the case of an administered antibody). The half life is the mean time before the

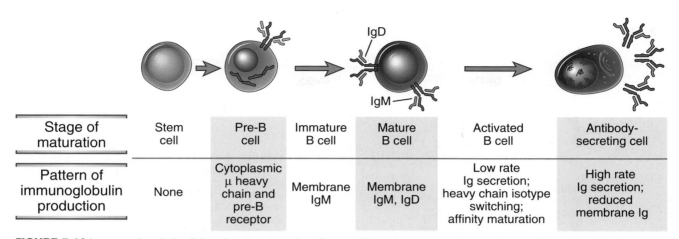

FIGURE 5-10 Ig expression during B lymphocyte maturation. Stages in B lymphocyte maturation are shown with associated changes in the production of Ig heavy and light chains. IgM heavy chains are shown in red, IgD heavy chains in blue, and light chains in green. The molecular events accompanying these changes are discussed in Chapters 8 and 12.

number of antibody molecules is reduced by half. Different antibody isotypes have very different half-lives in circulation. IgE has a very short half-life of about 2 days in the circulation (although cell-bound IgE associated with the high-affinity IgE receptor on mast cells has a very long half-life; see Chapter 20). Circulating IgA has a half-life of about 3 days, and circulating IgM has a half-life of about 4 days. In contrast, circulating IgG molecules have a half-life of about 21 to 28 days.

The long half-life of IgG is attributed to its ability to bind to a specific FcR called the **neonatal Fc receptor** (FcRn), which is also involved in the transport of IgG from the maternal circulation across the placental barrier as well as the transfer of maternal IgG across the intestine in neonates. FcRn structurally resembles MHC class I molecules (described in Chapter 6), and in the placenta and the neonatal intestine, it transports IgG molecules across cells without targeting them to lysosomes. In adult vertebrates, FcRn is found on the surface of endothelial cells, macrophages, and other cell types, and binds to micropinocytosed IgG in acidic endosomes. FcRn does not target bound IgG to lysosomes but recycles to the cell surface and releases it at neutral pH, returning the IgG to the circulation (Fig. 5-11). This intracellular sequestration of IgG away from lysosomes prevents it from being degraded as rapidly as most other serum proteins, including other antibody isotypes, and as a result, IgG has a relatively long half-life. There are differences in the half-lives of the four human IgG isotypes. IgG3 is relatively short-lived because it binds poorly to FcRn. IgG1 and IgG3 are the most long-lived and most efficient in terms of effector functions, as will be discussed in Chapter 13.

The long half-life of IgG has been used to provide a therapeutic advantage for certain injected proteins by producing fusion proteins containing the biologically active part of the protein and the Fc portion of IgG. The Fc portion enables the proteins to bind to the FcRn and thus extends the half-lives of the injected proteins. One therapeutically useful fusion protein is TNFR-Ig, which consists of the extracellular domain of the type II TNF receptor (TNFR) fused to an IgG Fc domain; it is used

to treat certain autoimmune disorders, such as rheumatoid arthritis and psoriasis, in which it blocks the inflammatory actions of TNF. Another therapeutically useful fusion protein is CTLA4-Ig, which contains the extracellular domain of the CTLA-4 receptor, which binds to B7 costimulators (see Fig. 9-7), fused to the Fc portion of human IgG; it has also been used in the treatment of rheumatoid arthritis and may serve more broadly as an immunosuppressive therapeutic.

ANTIBODY BINDING OF ANTIGENS

All of the functions of antibodies are dependent on their ability to specifically bind antigens. We will now consider the nature of antigens and how they are recognized by antibodies.

Features of Biologic Antigens

An antigen is any substance that may be specifically bound by an antibody molecule or T cell receptor. Antibodies can recognize as antigens almost every kind of biologic molecule, including simple intermediary metabolites, sugars, lipids, autacoids, and hormones, as well as macromolecules such as complex carbohydrates, phospholipids, nucleic acids, and proteins. This is in contrast to T cells, which mainly recognize peptides (see Chapter 6).

Although all antigens are recognized by specific lymphocytes or by antibodies, only some antigens are capable of activating lymphocytes. Molecules that stimulate immune responses are called **immunogens**. Macromolecules are effective at stimulating B lymphocytes to initiate humoral immune responses because B cell activation requires the bringing together (cross-linking) of multiple antigen receptors. Small chemicals, such as dinitrophenol, may bind to antibodies and are therefore antigens but they cannot activate B cells on their own (i.e., they are not immunogenic). To generate antibodies specific for such small chemicals, immunologists commonly attach multiple copies of the small molecules to a protein or

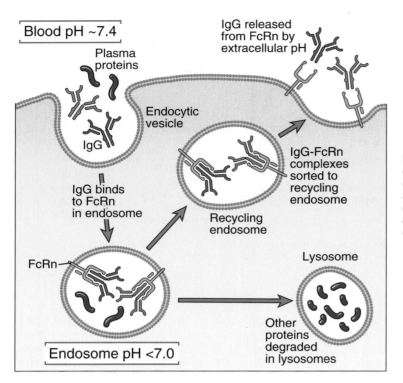

FIGURE 5-11 FcRn contributes to the long half-life of IgG molecules. Micropinocytosed IgG molecules in endothelial cells bind the FcRn, an IgG-binding receptor in the acidic environment of endosomes. In endothelial cells, FcRn directs the IgG molecules away from lysosomal degradation and releases them when vesicles fuse with the cell surface, exposing FcRn-IgG complexes to neutral pH.

polysaccharide before immunization. In these cases, the small chemical is called a **hapten**, and the large molecule to which it is conjugated is called a **carrier**. The hapten-carrier complex, unlike free hapten, can act as an immunogen (see Chapter 12).

Macromolecules, such as proteins, polysaccharides, and nucleic acids, are usually much bigger than the antigen-binding region of an antibody molecule (see Fig. 5-6). Therefore, any antibody binds to only a portion of the macromolecule, which is called a **determinant** or an **epitope**. These two words are synonymous and are used interchangeably throughout this book. Macromolecules typically contain multiple determinants, some of which may be repeated and each of which, by definition, can be bound by an antibody. The presence of multiple identical determinants in an antigen is referred to as **polyvalency** or **multivalency**. Most globular proteins do not contain multiple identical epitopes and are not polyvalent, unless they are in aggregates. In the case of polysaccharides and nucleic acids, many identical epitopes may be regularly spaced, and the molecules are said to be polyvalent. Cell surfaces, including microbes, often display polyvalent arrays of protein or carbohydrate antigenic determinants. Polyvalent antigens can induce clustering of the B cell receptor and thus initiate the process of B cell activation (see Chapter 7).

The spatial arrangement of different epitopes on a single protein molecule may influence the binding of antibodies in several ways. When determinants are well separated, two or more antibody molecules can be bound to the same protein antigen without influencing each other; such determinants are said to be non-overlapping. When two determinants are close to one another, the binding of antibody to the first determinant may cause steric interference with the binding of antibody to the

second; such determinants are said to be overlapping. In rarer cases, binding of one antibody may cause a conformational change in the structure of the antigen, positively or negatively influencing the binding of a second antibody at another site on the protein by means other than steric hindrance. Such interactions are called allosteric effects.

Any available shape or surface on a molecule that may be recognized by an antibody constitutes an antigenic determinant or epitope. Antigenic determinants may be delineated on any type of compound, including but not restricted to carbohydrates, proteins, lipids, and nucleic acids. In the case of proteins, the formation of some determinants depends only on the primary structure, and the formation of other determinants reflects tertiary structure, or conformation (shape) (Fig. 5-12). Epitopes formed by several adjacent amino acid residues are called linear determinants. The antigen-binding site of an antibody can usually accommodate a linear determinant made up of about six amino acids. If linear determinants appear on the external surface or in a region of extended conformation in the native folded protein, they may be accessible to antibodies. In other cases, linear determinants may be inaccessible in the native conformation and appear only when the protein is denatured. In contrast, conformational determinants are formed by amino acid residues that are not in a sequence but become spatially juxtaposed in the folded protein. Antibodies specific for certain linear determinants and antibodies specific for conformational determinants can be used to ascertain whether a protein is denatured or in its native conformation, respectively. Proteins may be subjected to modifications such as glycosylation, phosphorylation, ubiquitination, acetylation, and proteolysis. These modifications, by altering the

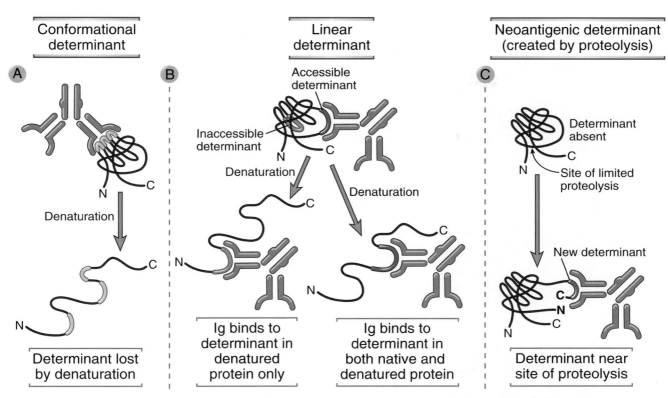

FIGURE 5-12 The nature of antigenic determinants. Antigenic determinants (shown in orange, red, and blue) may depend on protein folding (conformation) as well as on primary structure. Some determinants are accessible in native proteins and are lost on denaturation **(A)**, whereas others are exposed only on protein unfolding **(B)**. Neodeterminants arise from post-synthetic modifications such as peptide bond cleavage **(C)**.

structure of the protein, can produce new epitopes. Such epitopes are called neoantigenic determinants, and they too may be recognized by specific antibodies.

Structural and Chemical Basis of Antigen Binding

The antigen-binding sites of many antibodies are planar surfaces that can accommodate conformational epitopes of macromolecules, allowing the antibodies to bind large macromolecules (see Fig. 5-6). The six CDRs, three from the heavy chain and three from the light chain, can spread out to form a broad surface. In a number of antibodies specific for small molecules, such as monosaccharides and drugs, the antigen is bound in a cleft generated by the close apposition of CDRs from the V_L and V_H domains.

The recognition of antigen by antibody involves noncovalent, reversible binding. Various types of non-covalent interactions may contribute to antibody binding of antigen, including electrostatic forces, hydrogen bonds, van der Waals forces, and hydrophobic interactions. The relative importance of each of these depends on the structures of the binding site of the individual antibody and of the antigenic determinant. The strength of the binding between a single combining site of an antibody and an epitope of an antigen is called the **affinity** of the antibody. The affinity is commonly represented by a dissociation constant (K_d), which indicates how easy it is to separate an antigen-antibody complex into its constituents. A smaller K_d indicates a stronger or higher affinity interaction because a lower concentration of antigen

and of antibody is required for complex formation. The K_d of antibodies produced in typical humoral immune responses usually varies from about 10^{-7} M to 10^{-11} M. Serum from an immunized individual will contain a mixture of antibodies with different affinities for the antigen, depending primarily on the amino acid sequences of the CDRs.

Because the hinge region of antibodies gives them flexibility, a single antibody may attach to a single multivalent antigen by more than one binding site. For IgG or IgE, this attachment can involve, at most, two binding sites, one on each Fab. For pentameric IgM, however, a single antibody may bind at up to 10 different sites (Fig. 5-13). Polyvalent antigens will have more than one copy of a particular determinant. Although the affinity of any one antigen-binding site will be the same for each epitope of a polyvalent antigen, the strength of attachment of the antibody to the antigen must take into account binding of all the sites to all the available epitopes. This overall strength of attachment is called the **avidity** and is much greater than the affinity of any one antigen-binding site. Thus, a low-affinity IgM molecule can still bind tightly to a polyvalent antigen because many low-affinity interactions (up to 10 per IgM molecule) can produce a high-avidity interaction.

Polyvalent antigens are important from the viewpoint of B cell activation, as discussed earlier. Polyvalent interactions between antigen and antibody are also of biologic significance because many effector functions of antibodies are triggered optimally when two or more

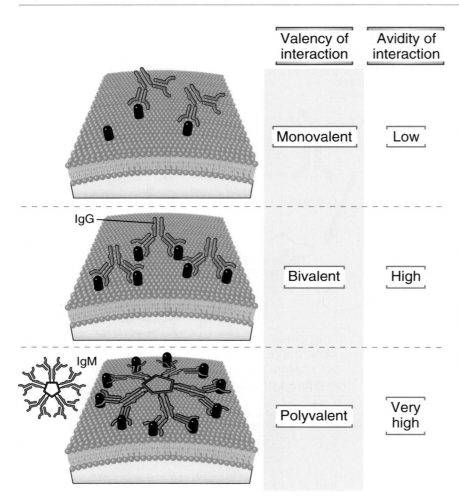

Valency of interaction	Avidity of interaction
Monovalent	Low
Bivalent	High
Polyvalent	Very high

FIGURE 5-13 Valency and avidity of antibody-antigen interactions. Monovalent antigens, or epitopes spaced far apart on cell surfaces, will interact with a single binding site of one antibody molecule. Although the affinity of this interaction may be high, the overall avidity may be relatively low. When repeated determinants on a cell surface are close enough, both the antigen-binding sites of a single IgG molecule can bind, leading to a higher avidity bivalent interaction. The hinge region of the IgG molecule accommodates the shape change needed for simultaneous engagement of both binding sites. IgM molecules have 10 identical antigen-binding sites that can theoretically bind simultaneously with 10 repeating determinants on a cell surface, resulting in a polyvalent, high-avidity interaction.

antibody molecules are brought close together by binding to a polyvalent antigen. If a polyvalent antigen is mixed with a specific antibody in a test tube, the two interact to form **immune complexes** (Fig. 5-14). At the correct concentration, called a zone of equivalence, antibody and antigen form an extensively cross-linked network of attached molecules such that most or all of the antigen and antibody molecules are complexed into large masses. Immune complexes may be dissociated into smaller aggregates either by increasing the concentration of antigen so that free antigen molecules will displace antigen bound to the antibody (zone of antigen excess) or by increasing antibody so that free antibody molecules will displace bound antibody from antigen determinants (zone of antibody excess). If a zone of equivalence is reached in vivo, large immune complexes can form in the circulation. Immune complexes that are trapped or formed in tissues can initiate an inflammatory reaction, resulting in immune complex diseases (see Chapter 19).

STRUCTURE-FUNCTION RELATIONSHIPS IN ANTIBODY MOLECULES

Many structural features of antibodies are critical for their ability to recognize antigens and for their effector functions. In the following section, we will summarize how the structure of antibodies contributes to their functions.

Features Related to Antigen Recognition

Antibodies are able to specifically recognize a wide variety of antigens with varying affinities. All the features of antigen recognition reflect the properties of antibody V regions.

Specificity

Antibodies can be remarkably specific for antigens, distinguishing between small differences in chemical structure. Experiments performed in the early 20th century demonstrated that antibodies made in response to an aminobenzene hapten with a meta-substituted sulfonate group would bind strongly to this hapten but weakly or not at all to ortho- or para-substituted isomers. These antigens are structurally similar and differ only in the location of the sulfonate group on the benzene ring.

The fine specificity of antibodies applies to the recognition of all classes of molecules. For example, antibodies can distinguish between two linear protein determinants differing by only a single conservative amino acid substitution that has little effect on

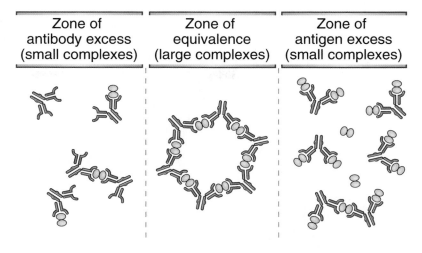

| Zone of antibody excess (small complexes) | Zone of equivalence (large complexes) | Zone of antigen excess (small complexes) |

FIGURE 5-14 Antigen-antibody complexes. The sizes of antigen-antibody (immune) complexes are a function of the relative concentrations of antigen and antibody. Large complexes are formed at concentrations of multivalent antigens and antibodies that are termed the zone of equivalence; the complexes are smaller in relative antigen or antibody excess.

secondary structure. This high degree of specificity is necessary so that antibodies generated in response to the antigens of one microbe usually do not react with structurally similar self molecules or with the antigens of other microbes. However, some antibodies produced against one antigen may bind to a different but structurally related antigen. This is referred to as a **cross-reaction**. Antibodies that are produced in response to a microbial antigen sometimes cross-react with self antigens, and this may be the basis of certain immunologic diseases (see Chapter 19).

Diversity

As we discussed earlier in this chapter, an individual is capable of making a tremendous number of structurally distinct antibodies, perhaps on the order of millions, each with a distinct specificity. The ability of antibodies in any individual to specifically bind a large number of different antigens is a reflection of antibody **diversity**, and the total collection of antibodies with different specificities represents the antibody **repertoire**. The genetic mechanisms that generate such a large antibody repertoire occur exclusively in lymphocytes. This diversity is generated by random recombination of a limited set of inherited germline DNA sequences to form functional genes that encode the V regions of heavy and light chains as well as by the addition of nucleotide sequences during the recombination process. We will discuss these mechanisms in detail in Chapter 8. The millions of resulting variations in structure are concentrated in the antigen-binding hypervariable regions of both heavy and light chains and thereby determine specificity for antigens.

Affinity Maturation

The ability of antibodies to neutralize toxins and infectious microbes is dependent on tight binding of the antibodies. As we have discussed, tight binding is achieved by high-affinity and high-avidity interactions. A mechanism for the generation of high-affinity antibodies involves subtle changes in the structure of the V regions of antibodies during T cell–dependent humoral immune responses to protein antigens. These changes come about by a process of somatic mutation in antigen-stimulated

B lymphocytes that generates new V domain structures, some of which bind the antigen with greater affinity than did the original V domains (Fig. 5-15). Those B cells producing higher affinity antibodies preferentially bind to the antigen and, as a result of selection, become the dominant B cells with each subsequent exposure to the antigen. This process, called **affinity maturation**, results in an increase in the average binding affinity of antibodies for an antigen as a humoral immune response evolves. Thus, an antibody produced during a primary immune response to a protein antigen often has a K_d in the range of 10^{-7} to 10^{-9} M; in secondary responses, the affinity increases, with a K_d of 10^{-11} M or even less. We will discuss the mechanisms of affinity maturation in Chapter 12.

Features Related to Effector Functions

Many of the effector functions of immunoglobulins are mediated by the Fc portions of the molecules, and antibody isotypes that differ in these Fc regions perform distinct functions. We have mentioned previously that the effector functions of antibodies require the binding of heavy chain C regions, which make up the Fc portions, to other cells and plasma proteins. For example, IgG coats microbes and targets them for phagocytosis by neutrophils and macrophages. This occurs because the antigen-complexed IgG molecule is able to bind, through its Fc region, to γ heavy chain–specific FcRs that are expressed on neutrophils and macrophages. In contrast, IgE binds to mast cells and triggers their degranulation because mast cells express IgE-specific FcRs. Another Fc-dependent effector mechanism of humoral immunity is activation of the classical pathway of the complement system. The system generates inflammatory mediators and promotes microbial phagocytosis and lysis. It is initiated by the binding of a complement protein called C1q to the Fc portions of antigen-complexed IgG or IgM. The FcR- and complement-binding sites of antibodies are found within the heavy chain C domains of the different isotypes (see Fig. 5-1). We will discuss the structure and functions of FcRs and complement proteins in Chapter 13.

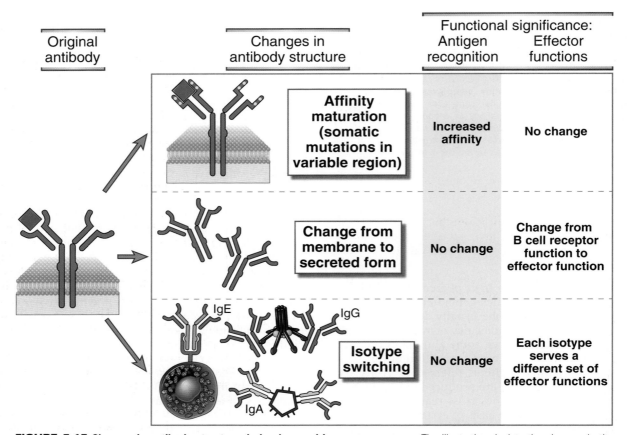

FIGURE 5-15 Changes in antibody structure during humoral immune responses. The illustration depicts the changes in the structure of antibodies that may be produced by the progeny of activated B cells (one clone) and the related changes in function. During affinity maturation, mutations in the V region (indicated by yellow dots) lead to changes in fine specificity without changes in C region–dependent effector functions. Activated B cells may shift production from largely membrane-bound antibodies containing transmembrane and cytoplasmic regions to secreted antibodies. Secreted antibodies may or may not show V gene mutations (i.e., secretion of antibodies occurs before and after affinity maturation). In isotype switching, the C regions change (indicated by color change from purple to green or yellow) without changes in the antigen-binding V region. Isotype switching is seen in membrane-bound and secreted antibodies. We will discuss the molecular basis for these changes in Chapter 12.

The effector functions of antibodies are initiated only by Ig molecules that have bound antigens and not by free Ig. The reason that only antibodies with bound antigens activate effector mechanisms is that two or more adjacent antibody Fc portions are needed to bind to and trigger various effector systems, such as complement proteins and FcRs of phagocytes (see Chapter 13). This requirement for adjacent antibody molecules ensures that the effector functions are targeted specifically toward eliminating antigens that are recognized by the antibody and that circulating free antibodies do not wastefully, and inappropriately, trigger effector responses.

Changes in the isotypes of antibodies during humoral immune responses influence how the responses work to eradicate antigen. After stimulation by an antigen, a single clone of B cells may produce antibodies with different isotypes that nevertheless possess identical V domains and therefore identical antigen specificity. Naive B cells simultaneously produce IgM and IgD that function as membrane receptors for antigens. When these B cells are activated by foreign antigens, typically of microbial origin, they may undergo a process called **isotype** (or **class**) **switching** in which the type of C_H region, and therefore the antibody isotype, produced by the B cell changes, but the V regions and the specificity do not (see Fig. 5-15). As a result of isotype switching, different progeny of the original IgM- and IgD-expressing B cell may produce isotypes and subtypes that are best able to eliminate the antigen. For example, the antibody response to many bacteria and viruses is dominated by IgG antibodies, which promote phagocytosis of the microbes, and the response to helminths consists mainly of IgE, which aids in the destruction of the parasites. Switching to the IgG isotype also prolongs the effectiveness of humoral immune responses because of the long half-life of IgG antibodies. We will discuss the mechanisms and functional significance of isotype switching in Chapter 12.

The heavy chain C regions of antibodies also determine the tissue distribution of antibody molecules. As we mentioned earlier, after B cells are activated, they gradually lose expression of the membrane-bound antibody and express more of it as a secreted protein (see Fig. 5-15). IgA can be secreted efficiently across mucosal epithelia and is the major class of antibody in mucosal secretions and milk (see Chapter 14). Neonates are protected from infections by IgG antibodies they acquire from their mothers through the placenta during gestation and through the intestine early after birth. This transfer of maternal IgG is mediated by the FcRn, which we described earlier as the receptor responsible for the long half-life of IgG antibody.

SUMMARY

* Antibodies, or immunoglobulins, are a family of structurally related glycoproteins produced in membrane-bound or secreted form by B lymphocytes.
* Membrane-bound antibodies serve as receptors that mediate the antigen-triggered activation of B cells.
* Secreted antibodies function as mediators of specific humoral immunity by engaging various effector mechanisms that serve to eliminate the bound antigens.
* The antigen-binding regions of antibody molecules are highly variable, and any one individual has the potential to produce millions of different antibodies, each with distinct antigen specificity.
* All antibodies have a common symmetric core structure of two identical covalently linked heavy chains and two identical light chains, each linked to one of the heavy chains. Each chain consists of two or more independently folded Ig domains of about 110 amino acids containing conserved sequences and intrachain disulfide bonds.
* The *N*-terminal domains of heavy and light chains form the V regions of antibody molecules, which differ among antibodies of different specificities. The V regions of heavy and light chains each contain three separate hypervariable regions of about 10 amino acids that are spatially assembled to form the antigen-combining site of the antibody molecule.
* Antibodies are classified into different isotypes and subtypes on the basis of differences in the heavy chain C regions, which consist of three or four Ig C domains, and these classes and subclasses have different functional properties. The antibody classes are called IgM, IgD, IgG, IgE, and IgA. Both light chains of a single Ig molecule are of the same light chain isotype, either κ or λ, which differ in their single C domains.
* Most of the effector functions of antibodies are mediated by the C regions of the heavy chains, but these functions are triggered by binding of antigens to the combining site in the V region.
* Monoclonal antibodies are produced from a single clone of B cells and recognize a single antigenic determinant. Monoclonal antibodies can be generated in the laboratory and are widely used in research, diagnosis, and therapy.

* Antigens are substances specifically bound by antibodies or T lymphocyte antigen receptors. Antigens that bind to antibodies include a wide variety of biologic molecules, including sugars, lipids, carbohydrates, proteins, and nucleic acids. This is in contrast to most T cell antigen receptors, which recognize only peptide antigens.
* Macromolecular antigens contain multiple epitopes, or determinants, each of which may be recognized by an antibody. Linear epitopes of protein antigens consist of a sequence of adjacent amino acids, and conformational determinants are formed by folding of a polypeptide chain.
* The affinity of the interaction between the combining site of a single antibody molecule and a single epitope is generally represented by the dissociation constant (K_d) calculated from binding data. Polyvalent antigens contain multiple identical epitopes to which identical antibody molecules can bind. Antibodies can bind to two or, in the case of IgM, up to 10 identical epitopes simultaneously, leading to enhanced avidity of the antibody-antigen interaction.
* The relative concentrations of polyvalent antigens and antibodies may favor the formation of immune complexes that may deposit in tissues and cause damage.
* Antibody binding to antigen can be highly specific, distinguishing small differences in chemical structures, but cross-reactions may also occur in which two or more antigens may be bound by the same antibody.
* Several changes in the structure of antibodies made by one clone of B cells may occur in the course of an immune response. B cells initially produce only membrane-bound Ig, but in activated B cells and plasma cells, Ig with the same antigen-binding specificity as the original membrane-bound Ig receptor is secreted. Changes in the use of C region gene segments without changes in V regions are the basis of isotype switching, which leads to changes in effector function without a change in specificity. Point mutations in the V regions of an antibody specific for an antigen lead to increased affinity for that antigen (affinity maturation).

SUGGESTED READINGS

Structure and Function of Antibodies

Corti D, Lanzavecchia A: Broadly neutralizing antiviral antibodies, *Annual Review of Immunology* 31:705–742, 2013.

Danilova N, Amemiya CT: Going adaptive: the saga of antibodies, *Annals of the New York Academy of Sciences* 1168:130–155, 2009.

Fagarasan S: Evolution, development, mechanism and function of IgA in the gut, *Current Opinion in Immunology* 20:170–177, 2008.

Law M, Hengartner L: Antibodies against viruses: passive and active immunization, *Current Opinion in Immunology* 20:486–492, 2008.

Therapeutic Applications of Antibodies

Chan AC, Carter PJ: Therapeutic antibodies for autoimmunity and inflammation, *Nature Reviews Immunology* 10:301–316, 2010.

Kohler G, Milstein C: Continuous culture of fused cells secreting antibody of predetermined specificity, *Nature* 256:495–497, 1975.

Lonberg N: Fully human antibodies from transgenic mouse and phage display platforms, *Current Opinion in Immunology* 20:450–459, 2008.

Weiner LM, Surana R, Wang S: Monoclonal antibodies: versatile platforms for cancer immunotherapy, *Nature Reviews Immunology* 10:317–327, 2010.

Wilson PC, Andrews SF: Tools to therapeutically harness the human antibody response, *Nature Reviews Immunology* 12:709–719, 2012.

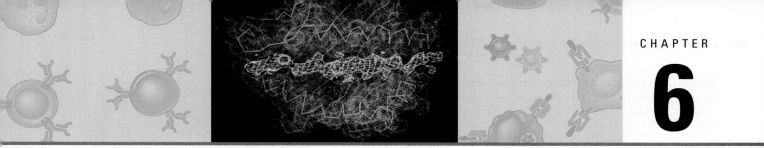

Major Histocompatibility Complex Molecules and Antigen Presentation to T Lymphocytes

The principal functions of T lymphocytes are to eradicate infections by intracellular microbes and to activate other cells, such as macrophages and B lymphocytes. To serve these functions, T cells have to overcome several challenges.

- There are very few naive T cells specific for any one antigen, and this small number has to be able to locate the foreign antigen and eliminate it. Microbes and other antigens may be located at virtually any site in the body. It is impossible for the few T cells specific for any antigen to constantly patrol all the possible tissues where antigens may enter or be produced. Solving this problem requires a specialized system for capturing antigen and bringing it to the lymphoid organs through which T cells circulate and where responses can be initiated. The specialized cells that capture and display antigens and activate T lymphocytes are called **antigen-presenting cells (APCs)**.

- The functions of most T lymphocytes require that they interact with other cells, which may be dendritic cells, macrophages, B lymphocytes, or any infected host cell. To ensure that T cells interact with other cells and not with soluble antigens, T cell antigen receptors are designed to see antigens displayed by cell surface molecules and not antigens on microbes or antigens that are free in the circulation or extracellular fluids. This is in striking contrast to B lymphocytes, whose antigen receptors and secreted products, antibodies, can recognize antigens on microbial surfaces, and soluble antigens as well as cell-associated antigens. The task of displaying host cell–associated antigens for recognition by CD4+ and CD8+ T cells is performed by specialized proteins called **major histocompatibility complex (MHC)** molecules, which are expressed on the surfaces of host cells.

- Different T cells have to be able to respond to microbial antigens in different cellular compartments. For instance, defense against viruses in the circulation has to be mediated by antibodies, and the production of the most effective antibodies requires the participation of CD4+ helper T cells. But if the same virus infects a tissue cell, it becomes inaccessible to the antibody, and its eradication requires that CD8+ cytotoxic T lymphocytes (CTLs) kill the infected cells and eliminate the reservoir of infection. This dichotomy exists because APCs differentially handle antigens derived from extracellular or intracellular locations and present these antigens to the different classes of T cells. MHC molecules play a critical role in segregating antigens from outside versus inside cells and displaying them to different T cell populations.

Thus, antigen capture and display to T cells is a specialized process that is essential for triggering optimal T cell responses. Elucidation of the cell biology and molecular basis of this complex process has been an impressive accomplishment, based on functional experiments, biochemical analyses, and structural biology. In this chapter, we will describe how antigens are captured and displayed to T cells. In Chapter 7, we will describe the antigen receptors of T cells, and in Chapters 9, 10 and 11, we will discuss the activation and effector functions of T lymphocytes.

PROPERTIES OF ANTIGENS RECOGNIZED BY T LYMPHOCYTES

Our current understanding of T cell antigen recognition is the culmination of a vast amount of research that began with studies of the nature of antigens that stimulate cell-mediated immunity. The early experiments showed that the physicochemical forms of antigens that are recognized by T cells are different from those recognized by B lymphocytes and antibodies, and this knowledge led to the discovery of how antigens are seen by T cells. Several features of antigen recognition are unique to T lymphocytes (Table 6-1).

Most T lymphocytes recognize only short peptides, whereas B cells can recognize peptides, proteins, nucleic acids, carbohydrates, lipids, and small chemicals. As a result, T cell–mediated immune responses are usually induced by foreign protein antigens (the natural source of foreign peptides), whereas humoral immune responses are induced by protein and non-protein antigens. Some T cells are specific for small chemical substances such as dinitrophenol, urushiol of poison ivy, β lactams of penicillin antibiotics, and even nickel ions. In these situations, it is likely that the chemicals, called haptens, bind to self proteins, including MHC molecules, and that T cells recognize the hapten-conjugated peptides or altered MHC

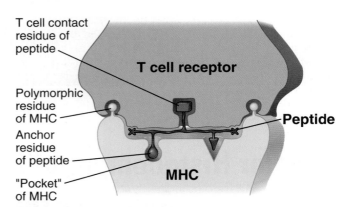

FIGURE 6-1 A model for T cell recognition of a peptide-MHC complex. This schematic illustration shows an MHC molecule binding and displaying a peptide and a T cell receptor recognizing two polymorphic residues of the MHC molecule and one residue of the peptide.

molecules. The peptide specificity of T cells is true for CD4+ and CD8+ cells; as we will discuss at the end of this chapter, there are some small populations of T cells that are capable of recognizing non-protein antigens.

The antigen receptors of CD4+ and CD8+ T cells are specific for peptide antigens that are displayed by MHC molecules (Fig. 6-1). T cell receptors (TCRs) have evolved to be specific for MHC molecules, whose normal function is to display peptides. As we will see in Chapter 8, MHC recognition is also required for the maturation of CD4+ and CD8+ T cells, and this ensures that all mature T cells are restricted to recognizing only MHC molecules with bound antigens. MHC molecules can bind and display peptides and no other chemical structures, and this is why the majority of T cells recognize only peptides. As we will discuss later, MHC molecules are highly polymorphic, and variations in MHC molecules among individuals influence both peptide binding and T cell recognition. A single T cell can recognize a specific peptide displayed by only one of the large number of different MHC molecules that exist. This phenomenon is called **MHC restriction**, and we will describe its molecular basis later in this chapter.

We will start our discussion of antigen presentation by describing how APCs capture antigens and transport them to T cells.

ANTIGEN CAPTURE AND THE FUNCTIONS OF ANTIGEN-PRESENTING CELLS

The realization that various cells other than T cells are needed to present antigens to T lymphocytes came first from studies in which protein antigens that were known to elicit T cell responses were labeled and injected into mice, to ask which cells bound (and, by implication, recognized) these antigens. The result was that the injected antigens were associated mainly with non-lymphoid cells, which was a surprise since it was known that lymphocytes were the cells that responded to foreign antigens. This type of experiment was quickly followed by studies showing that protein antigens that were physically associated with macrophages were much more immunogenic, on a molar basis, than the same antigens injected into mice in

TABLE 6-1 Features of MHC-Dependent Antigen Recognition by T Lymphocytes

Features of Antigens Recognized by T Cells	Explanation
Most T cells recognize peptides and no other molecules.	Only peptides bind to MHC molecules.
T cells recognize linear peptides and not conformational determinants of protein antigens.	Linear peptides bind to clefts of MHC molecules, and protein conformation is lost during the generation of these peptides.
T cells recognize cell-associated and not soluble antigens.	Most T cell receptors recognize only peptide-MHC complexes, and MHC molecules are membrane proteins that display stably bound peptides on cell surfaces.
CD4+ and CD8+ T cells preferentially recognize antigens sampled from the extracellular and cytosolic pools, respectively.	Pathways of assembly of MHC molecules ensure that class II molecules display peptides that are derived from extracellular proteins and taken up into vesicles in APCs and that class I molecules present peptides from cytosolic proteins; CD4 and CD8 bind to nonpolymorphic regions of class II and class I MHC molecules, respectively.

soluble form. In these early experiments, the macrophage populations studied may have contained dendritic cells, since, as we will discuss in the following section, naive T cells are best activated by dendritic cells. Subsequent cell culture experiments showed that purified CD4+ T cells could not respond to protein antigens, but they responded very well if non-T cells such as dendritic cells or macrophages were added to the cultures. These results led to the concept that a critical step in the induction of a T cell response is the presentation of the antigen to T lymphocytes by other cells, which were named *antigen-presenting cells*. The first APCs identified were macrophages, and the responding T cells were CD4+ helper cells. It soon became clear that several cell populations can function as APCs in different situations. By convention, *APC* is still the term used to refer to specialized cells that display antigens to CD4+ T lymphocytes; as we will see later in this chapter, all nucleated cells can display protein antigens to CD8+ T lymphocytes, but they are not all called APCs.

We begin with a discussion of some of the general properties of APCs for CD4+ T lymphocytes.

- *Different cell types function as APCs to activate naive T cells or previously differentiated effector T cells* (Fig. 6-2 and Table 6-2). Dendritic cells are the most effective APCs for activating naive T cells and therefore for initiating T cell responses. Macrophages and B lymphocytes also function as APCs, but mostly for previously activated CD4+ helper T cells rather than for naive T cells. Their roles as APCs are described later in this chapter and in more detail in Chapters 10 and 12. Dendritic

cells, macrophages, and B lymphocytes express class II MHC molecules and other molecules involved in stimulating T cells and are therefore capable of activating CD4+ T lymphocytes. For this reason, these three cell types have been called professional APCs; however, this term is sometimes used to refer only to dendritic cells because this is the only cell type whose major function is to capture and present antigens and the only APC capable of initiating primary T cell responses.

- *APCs display peptide-MHC complexes for recognition by T cells and also provide additional stimuli that are required for the full responses of the T cells.* Since antigen is the first signal, these additional stimuli are sometimes called *second signals*. They are more important for activation of naive T cells than for restimulation of previously activated effector and memory cells. The membrane-bound molecules of APCs that serve to activate T cells are called **costimulators** because they function together with antigen to stimulate T cells. APCs also secrete cytokines that play critical roles in T cell differentiation into effector cells. These costimulators and cytokines are described in Chapters 9 and 10.

- *The antigen-presenting function of APCs is enhanced by exposure to microbial products.* This is one reason that the immune system responds better to microbes than to harmless, non-microbial substances. Dendritic cells and macrophages express Toll-like receptors and other microbial sensors (see Chapter 4) that respond to microbes by increasing the expression of MHC molecules and costimulators, by improving the efficiency

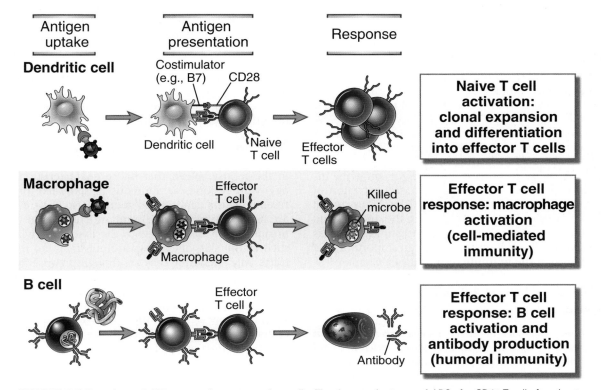

FIGURE 6-2 Functions of different antigen-presenting cells. The three major types of APCs for CD4+ T cells function to display antigens at different stages and in different types of immune responses. Note that effector T cells activate macrophages and B lymphocytes by production of cytokines and by expressing surface molecules; these will be described in later chapters.

TABLE 6-2   Properties and Functions of Antigen-Presenting Cells

| Cell Type | Expression of | | Principal Function |
	Class II MHC	Costimulators	
Dendritic cells	Constitutive; increases with maturation; increased by IFN-γ	Constitutive; expression is increased with TLR signals, IFN-γ, CD40-CD40L interactions	Initiation of T cell responses to protein antigens (priming)
Macrophages	Low or negative; increased by IFN-γ	Expression is increased by TLR signals, IFN-γ, CD40-CD40L interactions	Effector phase of cell-mediated immune responses (T cell–enhanced killing of phagocytosed microbes)
B lymphocytes	Constitutive; increased by IL-4	Expression is increased by T cells (CD40-CD40L interactions), antigen receptor cross-linking	Antigen presentation to CD4+ helper T cells in humoral immune responses (helper T cell–B cell interactions)
Vascular endothelial cells	Inducible by IFN-γ; constitutive in humans	Low; may be inducible	May promote activation of antigen-specific T cells at site of antigen exposure
Various epithelial and mesenchymal cells	Inducible by IFN-γ	Probably none	No known physiologic function; possible role in inflammatory diseases

IFN-γ, interferon-γ; *IL-4*, interleukin-4; *LPS*, lipopolysaccharide.

of antigen presentation, and by activating the APCs to produce cytokines, all of which stimulate T cell responses. In addition, dendritic cells that are activated by microbes express chemokine receptors that stimulate their migration to sites where T cells are present. The induction of optimal T cell responses to purified protein antigens requires that the antigens be administered with substances called **adjuvants.** Adjuvants either are products of microbes, such as killed mycobacteria (used experimentally), or they mimic microbes and enhance the expression of costimulators and cytokines as well as the antigen-presenting functions of APCs.

- *APCs that present antigens to T cells also receive signals from these lymphocytes that enhance their antigen-presenting function.* In particular, CD4+ T cells that are activated by antigen recognition and costimulation express surface molecules, notably one called CD40 ligand (CD154), that binds to CD40 on dendritic cells and macrophages, and the T cells secrete cytokines, such as interferon-γ (IFN-γ), that bind to their receptors on these APCs. The combination of CD40 signals and cytokines activates the APCs, resulting in increased ability to process and present antigens, increased expression of costimulators, and secretion of cytokines that activate the T cells. This bidirectional interaction between APCs displaying the antigen and T lymphocytes that recognize the antigen functions as a positive feedback loop that plays an important role in maximizing the immune response (see Chapter 9).

Role of Dendritic Cells in Antigen Capture and Display

The primary responses of naive T cells are initiated in the peripheral lymphoid organs, to which microbes and protein antigens are transported after being collected from their portal of entry (Fig. 6-3). The common routes through which foreign antigens, such as microbes, enter a host are the skin and the epithelia of the gastrointestinal and respiratory systems. In addition, microbial

antigens may be produced in any tissue that has been colonized or infected by a microbe. The skin, mucosal epithelia, and parenchymal organs contain numerous lymphatic capillaries that drain lymph from these sites and into the regional lymph nodes. Some antigens are transported in the lymph by APCs (primarily dendritic cells) that capture the antigen and enter lymphatic vessels, and other antigens enter the lymphatics in cell-free form. Thus, the lymph contains a sampling of all the soluble and cell-associated antigens present in tissues. The antigens become concentrated in lymph nodes, which are interposed along lymphatic vessels and act as filters that sample the lymph before it reaches the blood (see Chapter 2). Antigens that enter the blood stream may be similarly sampled by the spleen.

The cells that are best able to capture, transport, and present antigens to T cells are the dendritic cells. We next describe their major characteristics and their functions in initiating T cell responses.

Morphology and Populations of Dendritic Cells

Dendritic cells were discovered as a population of cells in the mouse spleen that had a characteristic morphology, with striking membranous or spine-like projections resembling the dendrites of neurons (Fig. 6-4). These cells are present in most tissues and are enriched in lymphoid organs and in interfaces with the external environment, such as the skin and the gastrointestinal and respiratory tracts. Most dendritic cells are thought to arise from adult bone marrow precursors, with the exception of *Langerhans cells* in the skin, which develop from embryonic precursors that take up residence in the skin prior to birth (see Fig. 2-4). It is now clear that there are two major populations of dendritic cells that differ in their phenotypic properties and major functions (Table 6-3).

- **Classical DCs** (also called conventional DCs) were first identified by their morphology and ability to stimulate strong T cell responses, and are the most numerous dendritic cell subset in lymphoid organs. Most induce effective immune responses. The function of these dendritic cells may be to present self antigens to self-reactive T cells and thereby cause inactivation or death of the T cells or generate regulatory T cells. These mechanisms are important for maintaining self-tolerance and preventing autoimmunity (see Chapter 15). On encounter with microbes or cytokines, the dendritic cells become activated: they upregulate costimulatory molecules, produce inflammatory cytokines, and migrate from peripheral tissues into draining lymph nodes, where they initiate T cell responses (discussed later).

Classical dendritic cells may be divided into two major subsets. One, identified by high expression of BDCA-1/CD1c in humans or the CD11b integrin in mice, is most potent at driving CD4+ T cell responses. The other subset, identified by expression of BDCA-3 in humans or, in mice, CD8 in lymphoid tissues or the CD103 integrin in peripheral tissues, is particularly efficient in the process of cross-presentation (described later in this chapter). Some dendritic cells may be derived from monocytes, especially in situations of inflammation.

- **Plasmacytoid DCs** resemble plasma cells morphologically and acquire the morphology and functional properties of dendritic cells only after activation. They develop in the bone marrow from a precursor that also gives rise to classical dendritic cells, and are found in the blood and in small numbers in lymphoid organs. In contrast to classical dendritic cells, plasmacytoid dendritic cells are poorly phagocytic and do not sample environmental antigens. The major function of plasmacytoid dendritic cells is the secretion of large amounts of type I interferons in response to viral infections (see Chapter 4). In viral infections, plasmacytoid dendritic cells also differentiate into cells that resemble classical dendritic cells and play a role in presenting antigens to virus-specific T cells.

Antigen Capture and Transport by Dendritic Cells

Dendritic cells that are resident in epithelia and tissues capture protein antigens and transport the antigens to draining lymph nodes (Fig. 6-5). Resting tissue-resident dendritic cells (sometimes referred to as immature dendritic cells) express membrane receptors, such as C-type lectins, that bind microbes. Dendritic cells use these receptors to capture and endocytose microbes or microbial products and then process the ingested proteins into peptides capable of binding to MHC molecules. Apart from receptor-mediated endocytosis and phagocytosis, dendritic cells can ingest antigens by micropinocytosis and macropinocytosis, processes that do not involve specific recognition receptors but capture whatever might be in the fluid phase in the vicinity of the dendritic cells.

At the time that microbial antigens are being captured, microbial products are recognized by Toll-like receptors and other innate pattern recognition receptors in the dendritic cells and other cells, generating innate immune responses (see Chapter 4). The dendritic cells are activated by these signals and by cytokines, such as tumor necrosis factor (TNF), produced in response to the microbes. The activated dendritic cells (also called mature dendritic cells) lose their adhesiveness for epithelia or tissues and migrate into lymph nodes. The dendritic cells also begin to express

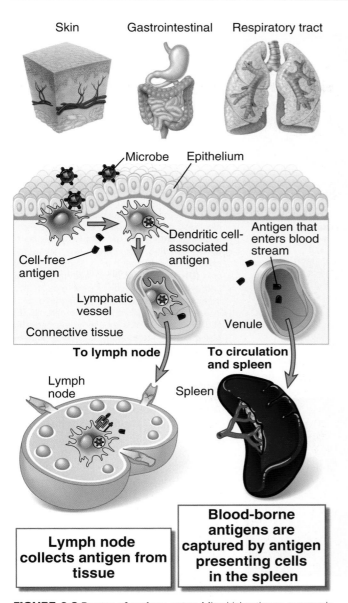

FIGURE 6-3 Routes of antigen entry. Microbial antigens commonly enter through the skin and gastrointestinal and respiratory tracts, where they are captured by dendritic cells and transported to regional lymph nodes. Antigens that enter the blood stream are captured by APCs in the spleen.

of them are derived from myeloid precursors, which migrate from the bone marrow to differentiate locally into resident dendritic cells in lymphoid and non-lymphoid tissues. Similar to tissue macrophages, they constantly sample the environment in which they reside. In the intestine, for example, dendritic cells appear to send out processes that traverse the epithelial cells and project into the lumen, where they may function to capture luminal antigens. Langerhans cells are the dendritic cells that populate the epidermis; they serve the same role for antigens encountered in the skin.

In the absence of infection or inflammation, classical dendritic cells capture tissue antigens and migrate to the draining lymph nodes but do not produce cytokines and membrane molecules that are required to

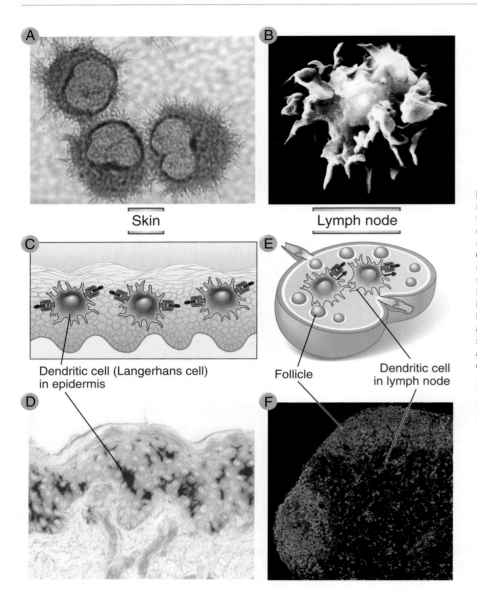

FIGURE 6-4 Dendritic cells. A, Light micrograph of cultured dendritic cells derived from bone marrow precursors. **B,** A scanning electron micrograph of a dendritic cell showing extensive membrane projections. **C, D,** Dendritic cells in the skin, illustrated schematically **(C)** and in a section of the skin **(D)** stained with an antibody specific for Langerhans cells (which appear blue in this immunoenzyme stain). **E, F,** Dendritic cells in a lymph node, illustrated schematically **(E)** and in a section of a mouse lymph node **(F)** stained with fluorescently labeled antibodies against B cells in follicles (green) and dendritic cells in the T cell zone (red). (**A, B,** and **D,** Courtesy of Dr. Y-J Liu, MD, Anderson Cancer Center, Houston, Texas. **F,** Courtesy of Drs. Kathryn Pape and Jennifer Walter, University of Minnesota School of Medicine, Minneapolis.)

TABLE 6-3 The Major Subpopulations of Dendritic Cells

Feature	Classical (Conventional) DCs		Plasmacytoid DCs
	Major	**Cross-Presenting**	
Surface markers	BDCA-1⁺CD1c⁺ (human) CD11c⁺ CD11b⁺ (mice)	BDCA-3/CD141⁺, CLEC9A⁺ (human) CD11c⁺, CD8⁺ in thymus, CD103⁺ in peripheral tissues (mice)	BDCA-2/CD303+ (human) CD11c and CD11b low or negative B220⁺ (mice)
TLRs expressed	High levels of TLR 2, 3, 4, 5, 8, 9	TLR3, 11	High levels of TLR7, 9
Major cytokines produced	IL-12, IL-23, TNF, IL-6	IL-12, IL-23, TNF, IL-6	Type I IFN
Major postulated functions	Innate immunity: source of inflammatory cytokines Adaptive immunity: capture and presentation of antigens mostly to CD4⁺ T cells	Adaptive immunity: capture and cross-presentation of antigens to CD8⁺ T cells	Anti-viral immunity: early innate response; priming of anti-viral T cells

Other subsets of dendritic cells have been described on the basis of the expression of various surface markers or migration from tissue sites (Langerhans-type dendritic cells from epithelia and interstitial dendritic cells from tissues). Note that all DCs express class II MHC molecules. Monocyte-derived dendritic cells, which can be generated from blood monocytes cultured with various cytokines, express CD14 and DC-SIGN, are distinct from the subsets described above, and may develop in vivo during inflammatory reactions. Unactivated dendritic cells of all types may display self antigens and serve to maintain self-tolerance; this postulated function is not listed in the table.

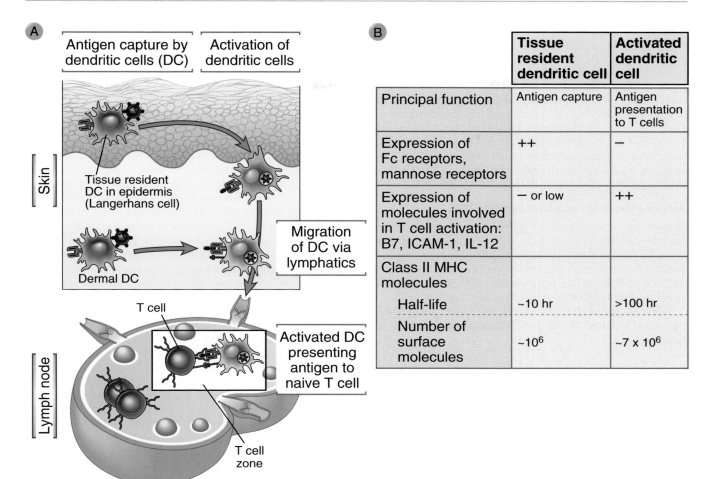

FIGURE 6-5 Role of dendritic cells in antigen capture and presentation. A, Immature dendritic cells (DCs) in the skin (Langerhans cells) or dermis (dermal DCs) capture antigens that enter through the epidermis and transport the antigens to regional lymph nodes. During this migration, the dendritic cells mature and become efficient APCs. **B,** The table summarizes some of the changes during dendritic cell maturation that are important in the functions of these cells.

a chemokine receptor called CCR7 that is specific for two chemokines, CCL19 and CCL21, which are produced in lymphatic vessels and in the T cell zones of lymph nodes. These chemokines attract the dendritic cells bearing microbial antigens into draining lymphatics and ultimately into the T cell zones of the regional lymph nodes. Naive T cells also express CCR7, and this is why naive T cells migrate to the same regions of lymph nodes where antigen-bearing dendritic cells are concentrated (see Chapter 3). The colocalization of antigen-bearing activated dendritic cells and naive T cells maximizes the chance of T cells with receptors for the antigen finding that antigen.

Activation also converts the dendritic cells from cells whose primary function is to capture antigen into cells that are able to present antigens to naive T cells and to activate the lymphocytes. Activated dendritic cells express high levels of MHC molecules with bound peptides as well as costimulators required for T cell activation. Thus, by the time these cells arrive in the lymph nodes, they have developed into potent APCs with the ability to activate T lymphocytes. Naive T cells that recirculate through lymph nodes encounter these APCs, and the T cells that are specific for the displayed peptide-MHC complexes are

activated. This is the initial step in the induction of T cell responses to protein antigens.

Antigens may also be transported to lymphoid organs in soluble form. Resident dendritic cells in the lymph nodes and spleen may capture lymph- and blood-borne antigens, respectively, and also may be driven to mature by microbial products. When lymph enters a lymph node through an afferent lymphatic vessel, it drains into the subcapsular sinus, and some of the lymph enters fibroblast reticular cell (FRC) conduits that originate from the sinus and traverse the cortex (see Chapter 2). Once in the conduits, low–molecular-weight antigens can be extracted by dendritic cells whose processes interdigitate between the FRCs. Other antigens in the subcapsular sinus are taken up by macrophages and dendritic cells, which carry the antigens into the cortex. B cells in the node may also recognize and internalize soluble antigens. Dendritic cells, macrophages, and B cells that have taken up protein antigens can then process and present these antigens to naive T cells and to effector T cells that have been generated by previous antigen stimulation.

The collection and concentration of foreign antigens in lymph nodes are supplemented by other anatomic adaptations that serve similar functions. The mucosal surfaces of the gastrointestinal and respiratory systems, in addition to being drained by lymphatic capillaries, contain specialized collections of secondary lymphoid tissue that can directly sample the luminal contents of these organs for the presence of antigenic material. The best characterized of these mucosal lymphoid organs are Peyer's patches of the ileum and the pharyngeal tonsils (see Chapter 14). APCs in the spleen monitor the blood stream for any antigens that reach the circulation. Such antigens may reach the blood either directly from the tissues or by way of the lymph from the thoracic duct.

Antigen-Presenting Function of Dendritic Cells

Many studies done in vitro and in vivo have established that the induction of primary T cell–dependent immune responses to protein antigens requires the presence of dendritic cells to capture and to present the antigens to the T cells. This was first shown for CD4+ T cell responses but is now known to be true for CD8+ T cells as well.

Several properties of dendritic cells make them the most efficient APCs for initiating primary T cell responses.

- Dendritic cells are strategically located at the common sites of entry of microbes and foreign antigens (in epithelia) and in tissues that may be colonized by microbes.
- Dendritic cells express receptors that enable them to capture and respond to microbes.
- Dendritic cells migrate from epithelia and tissues via lymphatics preferentially into the T cell zones of lymph nodes, and naive T lymphocytes also migrate from the circulation into the same regions of the lymph nodes.
- Mature dendritic cells express high levels of peptide-MHC complexes, costimulators, and cytokines, all of which are needed to activate naive T lymphocytes.

Dendritic cells can ingest infected cells and present antigens from these cells to CD8+ T lymphocytes. Dendritic cells are the best APCs to induce the primary responses of CD8+ T cells, but this poses a special problem because the peptide antigens these lymphocytes recognize must be derived from proteins in the cytosol of the dendritic cells. However, the viral proteins may be produced in any cell type infected by a virus, not necessarily in dendritic cells. Some specialized dendritic cells have the ability to ingest virus-infected cells or cellular fragments, and deliver viral proteins into their cytosol, allowing them to be presented to CD8+ T lymphocytes. This process is called cross-presentation, or cross-priming, and is described later in this chapter.

Functions of Other Antigen-Presenting Cells

Although dendritic cells have a critical role in initiating primary T cell responses, other cell types are also important APCs in different situations (see Fig. 6-2 and Table 6-2).

- *In cell-mediated immune responses, macrophages present the antigens of phagocytosed microbes to effector T cells, which respond by activating the macrophages to kill the microbes.* This process is central to cell-mediated immunity and delayed-type hypersensitivity (see Chapter 10). Circulating monocytes are able to migrate to any site of infection and inflammation, where they differentiate into macrophages and phagocytose and destroy microbes. CD4+ T cells recognize microbial antigens being presented by the macrophages and provide signals that enhance the microbicidal activities of these macrophages.
- *In humoral immune responses, B lymphocytes internalize protein antigens and present peptides derived from these proteins to helper T cells.* This antigen-presenting function of B cells is essential for helper T cell–dependent antibody production (see Chapter 12).
- *All nucleated cells can present peptides, derived from cytosolic protein antigens, to CD8+ CTLs.* All nucleated cells are susceptible to viral infections and cancer-causing mutations. Therefore, it is important that the immune system be able to recognize cytosolic antigens, such as viral antigens and mutated proteins, in any cell type. CD8+ CTLs are the cell population that recognizes these antigens and eliminates the cells in which the antigens are produced. CD8+ CTLs may also recognize phagocytosed microbes if these microbes or their antigens escape from phagocytic vesicles into the cytosol.
- *Other cell types that express class II MHC molecules and may present antigens to T cells include endothelial and some epithelial cells.* Vascular endothelial cells may present antigens to blood T cells that adhere to vessel walls, and this process may contribute to the recruitment and activation of effector T cells in cell-mediated immune reactions. Endothelial cells in grafts are also targets of T cells reacting against graft antigens (see Chapter 17). Various epithelial and mesenchymal cells may express class II MHC molecules in response to the cytokine IFN-γ. The physiologic significance of antigen presentation by these cell populations is unclear. Because most of them do not express costimulators and are not efficient at processing proteins into MHC-binding peptides, it is unlikely that they contribute significantly to the majority of T cell responses. Thymic epithelial cells constitutively express MHC molecules and play a critical role in presenting peptide-MHC complexes to maturing T cells in the thymus as part of the selection processes that shape the repertoire of T cell specificities (see Chapter 8).

THE MAJOR HISTOCOMPATIBILITY COMPLEX (MHC)

The discovery of the fundamental role of the MHC in antigen recognition by CD4+ and CD8+ T cells has revolutionized the field of immunology and paved the way for our current understanding of the activation and functions of lymphocytes.

Discovery of the MHC

The Mouse MHC (H-2 Complex)

The MHC was discovered from studies of tissue transplantation, and it was many years later that the structure and function of MHC molecules were elucidated. It was known from the early days of transplantation that tissues, such as skin, exchanged between non-identical individuals are rejected, whereas the same grafts between identical twins are accepted. This result showed that inherited genes must be involved in the process of tissue rejection. In the 1940s, to analyze the genetic basis of graft rejection, investigators produced inbred mouse strains by repetitive mating of siblings. Inbred mice are homozygous at every genetic locus (i.e., they have two copies of the same allele of every gene, one from each parent), and every mouse of an inbred strain is genetically identical (syngeneic) to every other mouse of the same strain (i.e., they all express the same alleles). Different strains may express different alleles and are said to be allogeneic to one another. By breeding congenic strains of mice that rejected grafts from other strains but were identical for all other genes, these investigators showed that a single genetic region is primarily responsible for rapid rejection of tissue grafts, and this region was called the major histocompatibility locus (*histo,* tissue). The particular locus that was identified in mice was linked to a gene on chromosome 17 encoding a blood group antigen called antigen II, and therefore this region was named histocompatibility-2, or simply H-2. Initially, this locus was thought to contain a single gene that controlled tissue compatibility. However, occasional recombination events occurred within the H-2 locus during interbreeding of different strains, indicating that it actually contained several different but closely linked genes, many of which were involved in graft rejection. The genetic region that controlled graft rejection and contained several linked genes was named the **major histocompatibility complex**. Although not known at the time of the initial experiments, transplant rejection is in large part a T cell–mediated process (see Chapter 17), and therefore it is not surprising that there is a relationship between graft rejection and MHC genes, which encode the peptide-binding MHC molecules that T cells recognize.

The Human MHC (HLA)

The human MHC was discovered by searching for cell surface molecules in one individual that would be recognized as foreign by another individual. This task became feasible when it was discovered that individuals who had received multiple blood transfusions and patients who had received kidney transplants contained antibodies that recognized cells from the blood or kidney donors and that multiparous women had circulating antibodies that recognized paternal cells. The proteins recognized by these antibodies were called **human leukocyte antigens (HLA)** (*leukocyte* because the antibodies were tested by binding to the leukocytes of other individuals, and *antigens* because the molecules were recognized by antibodies). Subsequent analyses showed that as in mice, the inheritance of particular HLA alleles is a major determinant of graft acceptance or rejection (see Chapter 17). Biochemical studies gave the satisfying result that the mouse H-2 proteins and the HLA proteins had similar basic structures. From these results came the conclusion that genes that determine the fate of grafted tissues are present in all mammalian species and are homologous to the H-2 genes first identified in mice; these are called

MHC genes. Other polymorphic genes that contribute to graft rejection to a lesser degree are called minor histocompatibility genes; we will return to these in Chapter 17, when we discuss transplantation immunology.

Immune Response Genes

For almost 20 years after the MHC was discovered, its only documented role was in graft rejection. This was a puzzle to immunologists because transplantation is not a natural phenomenon, and there was no reason that a set of genes should be preserved through evolution if the only function of the genes was to control the rejection of foreign tissue grafts. In the 1960s and 1970s, it was discovered that MHC genes are of fundamental importance for all immune responses to protein antigens. Immunologists found that inbred strains of a single species (guinea pigs or mice) differed in their ability to make antibodies against some simple synthetic polypeptides, and responsiveness was inherited as a dominant Mendelian trait. The relevant genes were called *immune response (Ir) genes,* and they were all found to map to the MHC. We now know that Ir genes are, in fact, MHC genes that encode MHC molecules that differ in their ability to bind and display peptides derived from various protein antigens. Responder strains, which can mount immune responses to a particular polypeptide antigen, inherit MHC alleles whose products can bind peptides derived from these antigens, forming peptide-MHC complexes that can be recognized by helper T cells. These T cells then help B cells to produce antibodies. Non-responder strains express MHC molecules that are not capable of binding peptides derived from the polypeptide antigen, and therefore these strains cannot generate helper T cells or antibodies specific for the antigen. It was also later found that many autoimmune diseases were associated with the inheritance of particular MHC alleles, firmly placing these genes at the center of the mechanisms that control immune responses. Such studies provided the impetus for more detailed analyses of MHC genes and proteins.

The Phenomenon of MHC Restriction

The formal proof that the MHC is involved in antigen recognition by T cells came from the experimental demonstration of MHC restriction by Rolf Zinkernagel and Peter Doherty. In their classic study, reported in 1974, these investigators examined the recognition of virus-infected cells by virus-specific CTLs in inbred mice. If a mouse is infected with a virus, CD8+ CTLs specific for the virus develop in the animal. These CTLs recognize and kill virus-infected cells only if the infected cells express alleles of MHC molecules that are expressed in the animal in which the CTLs were generated (Fig. 6-6). By use of MHC congenic strains of mice whose derivation was described earlier (mice that are identical at every genetic locus except the MHC), it was shown that the CTLs and the infected target cell must be derived from mice that share a class I MHC allele. Thus, the recognition of antigens by CD8+ CTLs is restricted by self class I MHC alleles. Subsequent experiments demonstrated that responses of CD4+ helper T lymphocytes to antigens are restricted by self class II MHC alleles.

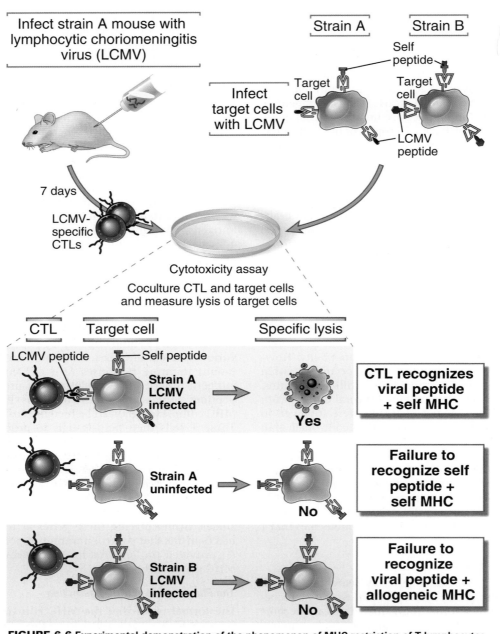

FIGURE 6-6 Experimental demonstration of the phenomenon of MHC restriction of T lymphocytes. Virus-specific cytotoxic T lymphocytes (CTLs) generated from virus-infected strain A mice kill only syngeneic (strain A) target cells infected with that virus. The CTLs do not kill uninfected strain A targets (which express self peptides but not viral peptides) or infected strain B targets (which express different MHC alleles than does strain A). By use of congenic mouse strains that differ only at class I MHC loci, it has been proved that recognition of antigen by CD8+ CTLs is self class I MHC restricted.

We will continue our discussion of the MHC by describing the properties of the genes and then the proteins, and we will conclude by describing how these proteins bind and display foreign antigens.

MHC Genes

The MHC locus contains two types of polymorphic MHC genes, the class I and class II MHC genes, which encode two groups of structurally distinct but homologous proteins, and other non-polymorphic genes whose products are involved in antigen presentation (Fig. 6-7). Class I MHC molecules display peptides to and are recognized by CD8+ T cells, and class II MHC molecules display peptides to CD4+ T cells; these T cell types serve different functions in protection against microbes.

Class I and class II MHC genes are the most polymorphic genes present in any mammalian genome. The studies of the mouse MHC were accomplished with a limited number of strains. Although it was appreciated that mouse MHC genes are polymorphic, only about 20 alleles of each MHC gene were identified in the available

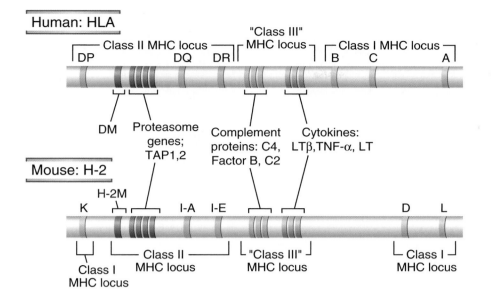

FIGURE 6-7 Schematic maps of human and mouse MHC loci. The basic organization of the genes in the MHC locus is similar in humans and mice. Sizes of genes and intervening DNA segments are not shown to scale. Class II loci are shown as single blocks, but each locus consists of several genes. "Class III" MHC locus refers to genes that encode molecules other than peptide-display molecules; this term is not used commonly.

inbred strains of mice. The human serologic studies were conducted on outbred human populations. A remarkable feature to emerge from the studies of the human MHC genes is the unexpected extent of variation among individuals, called **polymorphism**. In the population, the total number of HLA alleles with different amino acid sequences is estimated to be over 5000, with more than 2500 alleles for the HLA-B locus alone. The variations in MHC molecules (accounting for the polymorphism) result from inheritance of distinct DNA sequences and are not induced by gene recombination (as they are in antigen receptors; see Chapter 8). As we will discuss later in this chapter, the polymorphic residues of MHC molecules determine the specificity of peptide binding and T cell antigen recognition, which has led to the question of why MHC genes are polymorphic. MHC polymorphism may have evolved because it ensures that individuals will be able to deal with the diversity of microbes, and populations will be protected from devastating loss of life from emerging infections. But the selective pressures that have preserved such a vast number of alleles in the population are not understood.

MHC genes are codominantly expressed in each individual. In other words, for a given MHC gene, each individual expresses the alleles that are inherited from each of the two parents. For the individual, this maximizes the number of MHC molecules available to bind peptides for presentation to T cells.

Human and Mouse MHC Loci

In humans, the MHC is located on the short arm of chromosome 6 and occupies a large segment of DNA, extending about 3500 kilobases (kb). (For comparison, a large human gene may extend up to 50 to 100 kb, and the size of the entire genome of the bacterium *Escherichia coli* is approximately 4500 kb.) In classical genetic terms, the MHC locus extends about 4 centimorgans, meaning that crossovers within the MHC occur in about 4% of meioses. A molecular map of the human MHC is shown in Figure 6-8.

The human class I HLA genes were first defined by serologic approaches (antibody binding). There are three class I MHC genes called *HLA-A, HLA-B,* and *HLA-C,* which encode three types of class I MHC molecules with the same names. Class II MHC genes were first identified by use of assays in which T cells from one individual would be activated by cells of another individual (called the mixed lymphocyte reaction; see Chapter 17). There are three class II HLA gene loci called *HLA-DP, HLA-DQ,* and *HLA-DR.* Each class II MHC molecule is composed of a heterodimer of α and β polypeptides, and the *DP, DQ,* and *DR* loci each contains separate genes designated *A* or *B,* encoding α and β chains, respectively, on each copy of chromosome 6. Every individual has two *HLA-DP* genes (called *DPA1* and *DPB1,* encoding α and β chains), two *HLA-DQα* genes (*DQA1, 2*), one *HLA-DQβ* gene (*DQB1*), one *HLA-DRα* gene (*DRA1*), and one or two *HLA-DRβ* genes (*DRB1* and *DRB3, 4* or *5*). The nomenclature of the HLA locus takes into account the enormous polymorphism identified by serologic and molecular methods. Thus, based on modern molecular typing, individual alleles may be called *HLA-A*0201,* referring to the 01 subtype of *HLA-A2,* or *HLA-DRB1*0401,* referring to the 01 subtype of the *DR4B1* gene, and so on.

The mouse MHC, located on chromosome 17, occupies about 2000 kb of DNA, and the genes are organized in an order slightly different from the human MHC gene. One of the mouse class I genes *(H-2K)* is centromeric to the class II region, but the other class I genes are telomeric to the class II region. There are three mouse class I MHC genes called *H-2K, H-2D,* and *H-2L,* encoding three different class I MHC proteins, K, D, and L. These genes are homologous to the human *HLA-A, -B,* and *-C* genes. The MHC alleles of particular inbred strains of mice are designated by lowercase letters (e.g., *a, b*), named for the whole set of MHC genes of the mouse strain in which they were first identified. In the parlance of mouse geneticists, the allele of the *H-2K* gene in a strain with the k-type MHC is called K^k (pronounced K of k), whereas the allele of the *H-2K* gene in a strain with d-type MHC is called K^d (K of d). Similar

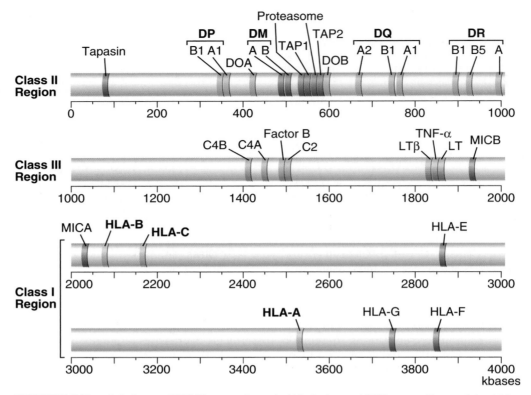

FIGURE 6-8 Map of the human MHC. The genes located within the human MHC locus are illustrated. In addition to the class I and class II *MHC* genes, *HLA-E, HLA-F,* and *HLA-G and the MIC* genes encode class I–like molecules, many of which are recognized by NK cells; *C4, C2,* and *Factor B* genes encode complement proteins; tapasin, DM, DO, TAP, and proteasome encode proteins involved in antigen processing; LTα, LTβ, and TNF encode cytokines. Many pseudogenes and genes whose roles in immune responses are not established are located in the HLA complex but are not shown to simplify the map.

terminology is used for *H-2D* and *H-2L* alleles. Mice have two class II MHC loci called *I-A* and *I-E,* which encode the I-A and I-E molecules, respectively. These are located in the A and E subregions of the Ir region of the MHC and were discovered to be the Ir genes discussed earlier. The mouse class II genes are homologous to human *HLA-DP, DQ,* and *DR* genes. The *I-A* allele found in the inbred mouse strain with the K^k and D^k alleles is called $I-A^k$ (pronounced I A of k). Similar terminology is used for the *I-E* allele. As in humans, there are actually two different genes, designated *A* and *B,* in the *I-A* and *I-E* loci that encode the α and β chains of each class II MHC molecule.

The set of MHC alleles present on each chromosome is called an MHC **haplotype.** For instance, an HLA haplotype of an individual could be HLA-A2, B5, DR3, and so on. All heterozygous individuals, of course, have two HLA haplotypes. Inbred mice, being homozygous, have a single haplotype. Thus, the haplotype of an H-2^d mouse is H-2K^d I-A^d I-E^d D^d L^d.

Expression of MHC Molecules

Because MHC molecules are required to present antigens to T lymphocytes, the expression of these proteins in a cell determines whether foreign (e.g., microbial) antigens in that cell will be recognized by T cells. There are several important features of the expression of MHC molecules that contribute to their role in protecting individuals from diverse microbial infections.

Class I molecules are expressed on virtually all nucleated cells, whereas class II molecules are expressed only on dendritic cells, B lymphocytes, macrophages, and a few other cell types. This pattern of MHC expression is linked to the functions of class I–restricted and class II–restricted T cells. As discussed earlier, class I–restricted CD8$^+$ CTLs kill cells infected with intracellular microbes, such as viruses, as well as tumors that express tumor antigens, and any nucleated cell can harbor a virus or develop into a cancer. Thus, the expression of class I MHC molecules on nucleated cells provides an essential display system for viral and tumor antigens. In contrast, class II–restricted CD4$^+$ helper T lymphocytes have a set of functions that require recognizing antigen presented by a more limited number of cell types. In particular, naive CD4$^+$ T cells need to recognize antigens that are captured and presented by dendritic cells in lymphoid organs. Differentiated CD4$^+$ helper T lymphocytes function mainly to activate (or help) macrophages to eliminate extracellular microbes that have been phagocytosed and to help B lymphocytes to make antibodies that also eliminate extracellular microbes. Class II molecules are expressed mainly on these cell types and provide a system for display of peptides derived from extracellular microbes and proteins.

The expression of MHC molecules is increased by cytokines produced during both innate and adaptive immune responses. Although class I molecules are constitutively expressed on nucleated cells, their expression is increased by the interferons IFN-α, IFN-β, and IFN-γ. The interferons are cytokines produced during the early innate immune response to many viruses (see Chapter 4). Thus, innate immune responses to viruses increase the expression of the MHC molecules that display viral antigens to virus-specific T cells. This is one of the mechanisms by which innate immunity stimulates adaptive immune responses.

The expression of class II molecules is also regulated by cytokines and other signals in different cells. IFN-γ is the principal cytokine involved in stimulating expression of class II molecules in APCs such as dendritic cells and macrophages (Fig. 6-9). IFN-γ may be produced by NK cells during innate immune reactions and by antigen-activated T cells during adaptive immune reactions. The ability of IFN-γ to increase class II MHC expression on APCs is an amplification mechanism in adaptive immunity. As mentioned earlier, the expression of class II molecules also increases in response to signals from Toll-like receptors responding to microbial components, thus promoting the display of microbial antigens. B lymphocytes constitutively express class II molecules and can increase expression in response to antigen recognition and cytokines produced by helper T cells, thus enhancing antigen presentation to helper cells (see Chapter 12). IFN-γ can also increase the expression of MHC molecules on vascular endothelial cells and other non-immune cell types; the role of these cells in antigen presentation to T lymphocytes is unclear, as mentioned earlier. Some cells, such as neurons, never appear to express class II molecules. Following activation, human but not mouse T cells express class II molecules; however, no cytokine has been identified in this response, and its functional significance is unknown.

The rate of transcription is the major determinant of the level of MHC molecule synthesis and expression on the cell surface. Cytokines enhance MHC expression by stimulating the transcription of class I and class II genes in a wide variety of cell types. These effects are mediated by the binding of cytokine-activated transcription factors to DNA sequences in the promoter regions of MHC genes. Several transcription factors may be assembled and bind a protein called the class II transcription activator (CIITA), and the entire complex binds to the class II promoter and promotes efficient transcription. By keeping the complex of transcription factors together, CIITA functions as a master regulator of class II gene expression. Mutations in several of these transcription factors have been identified as the cause of human immunodeficiency diseases associated with defective expression of MHC molecules. The best studied of these disorders is **bare lymphocyte syndrome** (see Chapter 21). Knockout mice lacking CIITA also show reduced or absent class II expression on dendritic cells and B lymphocytes and an inability of IFN-γ to induce class II on all cell types.

The expression of many of the proteins involved in antigen processing and presentation is coordinately regulated. For instance, IFN-γ increases the transcription not only of class I and class II genes but also of several genes whose products are required for class I MHC assembly and peptide display, such as genes encoding the TAP transporter and some of the subunits of proteasomes, discussed later in this chapter.

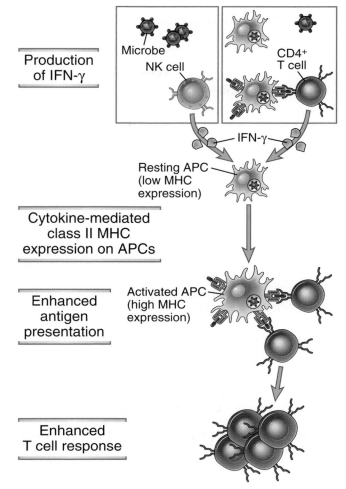

FIGURE 6-9 Enhancement of class II MHC expression by IFN-γ. IFN-γ, produced by NK cells and other cell types during innate immune reactions to microbes or by T cells during adaptive immune reactions, stimulates class II MHC expression on APCs and thus enhances the activation of CD4+ T cells. IFN-γ and type I interferons have a similar effect on the expression of class I MHC molecules and the activation of CD8+ T cells.

MHC Molecules

Biochemical studies of MHC molecules culminated in the solution of the crystal structures for the extracellular portions of human class I and class II molecules. Subsequently, many MHC molecules with bound peptides have been crystallized and analyzed in detail. This knowledge has been enormously informative and, because of it, we now understand how MHC molecules bind and display peptides. In this section, we first summarize the functionally important biochemical features that are common to class I and class II MHC molecules. We then describe the structures of class I and class II proteins, pointing out their significant similarities and differences (Table 6-4).

General Properties of MHC Molecules

All MHC molecules share certain structural characteristics that are critical for their role in peptide display and antigen recognition by T lymphocytes.

- ***Each MHC molecule consists of an extracellular peptide-binding cleft, followed by immunoglobulin (Ig)–like***

TABLE 6-4   Features of Class I and Class II MHC Molecules

Feature	Class I MHC	Class II MHC
Polypeptide chains	α β_2-microglobulin	α and β
Locations of polymorphic residues	$\alpha 1$ and $\alpha 2$ domains	$\alpha 1$ and $\beta 1$ domains
Binding site for T cell coreceptor	CD8 binds mainly to the $\alpha 3$ domain	CD4 binds to a pocket created by parts of $\alpha 2$ and $\beta 2$ domains
Size of peptide-binding cleft	Accommodates peptides of 8-11 residues	Accommodates peptides of 10-30 residues or more
Nomenclature		
Human	HLA-A, HLA-B, HLA-C	HLA-DR, HLA-DQ, HLA-DP
Mouse	H-2K, H-2D, H-2L	I-A, I-E

domains and transmembrane and cytoplasmic domains. Class I molecules are composed of one polypeptide chain encoded in the MHC and a second, non–MHC-encoded chain, whereas class II molecules are made up of two MHC-encoded polypeptide chains. Despite this difference, the overall three-dimensional structures of class I and class II molecules are similar.

- *The polymorphic amino acid residues of MHC molecules are located in and adjacent to the peptide-binding cleft.* This cleft (also called groove) is formed by the folding of the amino termini of the MHC-encoded proteins and is composed of paired α helices forming the two walls of the cleft, resting on a floor made up of an eight-stranded β-pleated sheet. The polymorphic residues, which are the amino acids that vary among different MHC alleles, are located in the floor and walls of this cleft. This portion of the MHC molecule binds peptides for display to T cells, and the antigen receptors of T cells interact with the displayed peptide and also with the α helices of the MHC molecules (see Fig. 6-1). Because of amino acid variability in this region, different MHC molecules bind and display different peptides and are recognized specifically by the antigen receptors of different T cells.

- *The non-polymorphic Ig-like domains of MHC molecules contain binding sites for the T cell molecules CD4 and CD8.* CD4 and CD8 are expressed on distinct subpopulations of mature T lymphocytes and participate, together with antigen receptors, in the recognition of antigen; that is, CD4 and CD8 are T cell coreceptors (see Chapter 7). CD4 binds selectively to class II MHC molecules, and CD8 binds to class I molecules. This is why *CD4$^+$ helper T cells recognize class II MHC molecules displaying peptides, whereas CD8$^+$ T cells recognize class I MHC molecules with bound peptides.* Stated differently, CD4$^+$ T cells are class II MHC restricted, and CD8$^+$ T cells are class I MHC restricted, because binding sites for CD4 and CD8 are on class II and class I MHC molecules, respectively.

Class I MHC Molecules

Class I molecules consist of two non-covalently linked polypeptide chains, an MHC-encoded 44- to 47-kD α chain (or heavy chain) and a non–MHC-encoded 12-kD subunit called β_2-microglobulin (Fig. 6-10). Each α chain is oriented so that about three quarters of the polypeptide

is extracellular, a short hydrophobic segment spans the plasma membrane, and the carboxy-terminal residues are located in the cytoplasm. The amino-terminal $\alpha 1$ and $\alpha 2$ segments of the α chain, each approximately 90 residues long, interact to form a platform of an eight-stranded, antiparallel β-pleated sheet supporting two parallel strands of α helix. This forms the peptide-binding cleft of class I molecules. Its size is large enough (~ 25 Å $\times 10$ Å $\times 11$ Å) to bind peptides of 8 to 11 amino acids in a flexible, extended conformation. The ends of the class I peptide-binding cleft are closed so that larger peptides cannot be accommodated. Therefore, native globular proteins have to be converted into fragments that are small enough and in an extended linear shape so they can bind

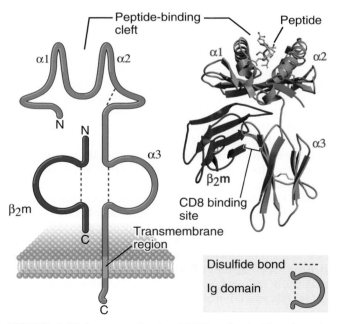

FIGURE 6-10 Structure of a class I MHC molecule. The schematic diagram *(left)* illustrates the different regions of the MHC molecule (not drawn to scale). Class I molecules are composed of a polymorphic α chain non-covalently attached to the non-polymorphic β_2-microglobulin (β_2m). The α chain is glycosylated; carbohydrate residues are not shown. The ribbon diagram *(right)* shows the structure of the extracellular portion of the HLA-B27 molecule with a bound peptide, resolved by x-ray crystallography. *(Courtesy of Dr. P. Bjorkman, California Institute of Technology, Pasadena.)*

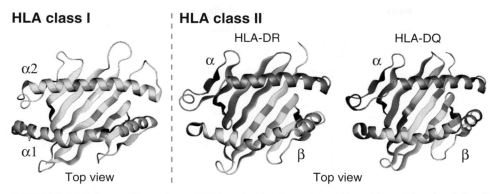

HLA class I

α2

α1

Top view

HLA class II

HLA-DR

α

β

Top view

HLA-DQ

α

β

FIGURE 6-11 Polymorphic residues of MHC molecules. The polymorphic residues of class I and class II MHC molecules are located in the peptide-binding clefts and the α helices around the clefts. The regions of greatest variability among different HLA alleles are indicated in red, of intermediate variability in green, and of the lowest variability in blue. *(Reproduced with permission from Margulies DH, Natarajan K, Rossjohn J, McCluskey J: Major histocompatibility complex [MHC] molecules: structure, function, and genetics. In Paul WE [ed]: Fundamental immunology, 6th ed, Philadelphia, 2008, Lippincott Williams & Wilkins.)*

to MHC molecules and be recognized by T cells (described later). The polymorphic residues of class I molecules are confined to the α1 and α2 domains, where they contribute to variations among different class I alleles in peptide binding and T cell recognition (Fig. 6-11). The α3 segment of the α chain folds into an Ig domain whose amino acid sequence is conserved among all class I molecules. This segment contains most of the binding site for CD8, but β2m and a small part of the lower portion of the α2 domain also contribute. At the carboxy-terminal end of the α3 segment is a stretch of approximately 25 hydrophobic amino acids that traverses the lipid bilayer of the plasma membrane. Immediately following this are approximately 30 residues located in the cytoplasm, which include a cluster of basic amino acids that interact with phospholipid head groups of the inner leaflet of the lipid bilayer and anchor the MHC molecule in the plasma membrane.

β_2-microglobulin, the light chain of class I molecules, is encoded by a gene outside the MHC and is named for its electrophoretic mobility (β_2), size (micro), and solubility (globulin). β_2-microglobulin interacts non-covalently with the α3 domain of the α chain. Like the α3 segment, β_2-microglobulin is structurally homologous to an Ig domain and is invariant among all class I molecules.

The fully assembled class I molecule is a trimer consisting of an α chain, β_2-microglobulin, and a bound peptide, and stable expression of class I molecules on cell surfaces requires the presence of all three components of the trimeric complex. The reason for this is that the interaction of the α chain with β_2-microglobulin is stabilized by binding of peptide antigens to the cleft formed by the α1 and α_2 segments, and conversely, the binding of peptide is strengthened by the interaction of β_2-microglobulin with the α chain. Because peptides are needed to stabilize the MHC molecules and unstable complexes are degraded, only potentially useful peptide-loaded MHC molecules are expressed on cell surfaces.

Most individuals are heterozygous for MHC genes and therefore express six different class I molecules on every cell, containing α chains encoded by the two inherited alleles of *HLA-A, B*, and *C* genes.

Class II MHC Molecules

Class II MHC molecules are composed of two non-covalently associated polypeptide chains, a 32- to 34-kD α chain and a 29- to 32-kD β chain (Fig. 6-12). Unlike class I molecules, the genes encoding both chains of class II molecules are polymorphic and present in the MHC locus.

The amino-terminal α1 and β1 segments of the class II chains interact to form the peptide-binding cleft, which is structurally similar to the cleft of class I molecules. Four strands of the floor of the cleft and one of the α-helical

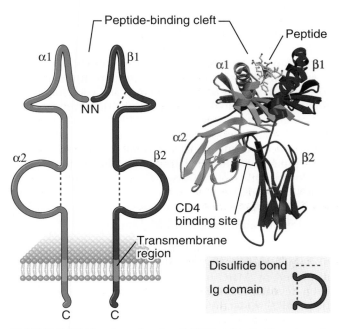

FIGURE 6-12 Structure of a class II MHC molecule. The schematic diagram *(left)* illustrates the different regions of the MHC molecule (not drawn to scale). Class II molecules are composed of a polymorphic α chain non-covalently attached to a polymorphic β chain. Both chains are glycosylated; carbohydrate residues are not shown. The ribbon diagram *(right)* shows the structure of the extracellular portion of the HLA-DR1 molecule with a bound peptide, resolved by x-ray crystallography. *(Courtesy of Dr. P. Bjorkman, California Institute of Technology, Pasadena.)*

walls are formed by the α1 segment, and the other four strands of the floor and the second wall are formed by the β1 segment. The polymorphic residues are located in the α1 and β1 segments, in and around the peptide-binding cleft, as in class I molecules (see Fig. 6-11). In human class II molecules, most of the polymorphism is in the β chain. In class II molecules, the ends of the peptide-binding cleft are open, so that peptides of 30 residues or more can fit.

The α2 and β2 segments of class II molecules, like class I α3 and β2-microglobulin, are folded into Ig domains and are non-polymorphic, that is, they do not vary among alleles of a particular class II gene. Both the α2 and β2 domains of class II molecules contribute to a concavity which accommodates a protrusion from the CD4 protein, thus allowing binding to occur. The carboxy-terminal ends of the α2 and β2 segments continue into short connecting regions followed by approximately 25–amino acid stretches of hydrophobic transmembrane residues. In both chains, the transmembrane regions end with clusters of basic amino acid residues, followed by short hydrophilic cytoplasmic tails. *The fully assembled class II molecule is a trimer consisting of one α chain, one β chain, and a bound antigenic peptide, and stable expression of class II molecules on cell surfaces requires the presence of all three components of the trimer.* As in class I molecules, this ensures that the MHC molecules that end up on the cell surface are the molecules that are serving their normal function of peptide display.

Humans inherit, from each parent, one *DPA* and one *DPB* gene encoding, respectively, the α and β chains of an HLA-DP molecule; one functional *DQA* and one *DQB* gene; one *DRA* and one or two functional *DRB* genes. Thus, each heterozygous individual inherits six to eight class II MHC alleles, three or four from each parent (one set each of *DP* and *DQ,* and one or two of *DR*). Typically, there is not much pairing of MHC proteins from different loci (i.e., DRα with DQβ, and so on), and each haplotype tends to be inherited as a single unit. However, because some haplotypes contain extra DRB loci that produce β chains that assemble with DRα, and some DQα molecules encoded on one chromosome can associate with DQβ molecules produced from the other chromosome, the total number of expressed class II molecules may be more than eight.

Binding of Peptides to MHC Molecules

Following the realization that the immunogenicity of proteins depends on the ability of their peptides to be displayed by MHC molecules, considerable effort has been devoted to elucidating the molecular basis of peptide-MHC interactions and the characteristics of peptides that allow them to bind to MHC molecules. These studies initially relied on functional assays of helper T cells and CTLs responding to APCs that were incubated with different peptides. Direct binding of MHC molecules and peptides has been studied with purified MHC molecules and radioactively or fluorescently labeled peptides in solution, using methods such as equilibrium dialysis and gel filtration. X-ray crystallographic analysis of peptide-MHC complexes has provided definitive information about how peptides sit in the clefts of MHC molecules and about the residues of each that participate in this binding. In the section that follows, we summarize the key features of the interactions between peptides and class I or class II MHC molecules.

Characteristics of Peptide-MHC Interactions

MHC molecules show a broad specificity for peptide binding, in contrast to the fine specificity of antigen recognition by the antigen receptors of lymphocytes. In other words, a single MHC allele, e.g., HLA-A2, can present any one of many different peptides to T cells, but a single T cell will recognize only one of these many possible HLA-A2/peptide complexes. There are several important features of the interactions of MHC molecules and antigenic peptides.

- *Each class I or class II MHC molecule has a single peptide-binding cleft that binds one peptide at a time, but each MHC molecule can bind many different peptides.* One of the earliest lines of evidence supporting this conclusion was the experimental result that different peptides that bind to the same MHC molecule can competitively inhibit one another's presentation, implying that there is only a single peptide-binding cleft in every MHC molecule. The solution of the crystal structures of class I and class II MHC molecules confirmed the presence of a single peptide-binding cleft in these molecules (see Figs. 6-10 and 6-12). It is not surprising that a single MHC molecule can bind multiple peptides because each individual contains only a few different MHC molecules (6 class I and about 8 to 10 class II molecules in a heterozygous individual), and these must be able to present peptides from the enormous number of protein antigens that one is likely to encounter.

- *The peptides that bind to MHC molecules share structural features that promote this interaction.* One of these features is the size of the peptide—class I molecules can accommodate peptides that are 8 to 11 residues long, and class II molecules bind peptides that may be 10 to 30 residues long or longer, the optimal length being 12 to 16 residues. In addition, peptides that bind to a particular allelic form of an MHC molecule contain amino acid residues that allow complementary interactions between the peptide and that allelic MHC molecule. Some of the amino acid residues that promote binding to MHC molecules are described later, when we discuss the structural basis of peptide-MHC interactions. The residues of a peptide that bind to MHC molecules are distinct from those that are recognized by T cells.

- *MHC molecules acquire their peptide cargo during their biosynthesis and assembly inside cells.* Therefore, MHC molecules display peptides derived from microbes that are inside host cells, and this is why MHC-restricted T cells recognize cell-associated microbes and are the mediators of immunity to intracellular microbes. Importantly, class I MHC molecules acquire peptides mainly from cytosolic proteins and class II molecules from proteins in intracellular vesicles. The mechanisms and significance of these processes are discussed later in this chapter.

- *The association of peptides and MHC molecules is a saturable interaction with a very slow off-rate.* In a cell, several chaperones and enzymes facilitate the binding of peptides to MHC molecules (described later). Once formed, most peptide-MHC complexes are stable, and kinetic dissociation constants are indicative of long half-lives that range from hours to many days. This extraordinarily slow off-rate of peptide dissociation from MHC molecules ensures that after an MHC molecule has acquired a peptide, it will display the peptide long enough to maximize the chance that a particular T cell will find the peptide it can recognize and initiate a response.

- *Very small numbers of peptide-MHC complexes are capable of activating specific T lymphocytes.* Because APCs continuously present peptides derived from all the proteins they encounter, only a very small fraction of cell surface peptide-MHC complexes will contain the same peptide. It has been estimated that as few as 100 complexes of a particular peptide with a class II MHC molecule on the surface of an APC can initiate a specific T cell response. This represents less than 0.1% of the total number of class II molecules likely to be present on the surface of the APC.

- *The MHC molecules of an individual do not discriminate between foreign peptides (e.g., those derived from microbial proteins) and peptides derived from the proteins of that individual (self antigens).* Thus, MHC molecules display both self peptides and foreign peptides, and T cells survey these displayed peptides for the presence of foreign antigens. In fact, if the peptides being displayed normally by APCs are purified, most of them turn out to be derived from self proteins. The inability of MHC molecules to discriminate between self and foreign peptides raises two questions. First, how can a T cell recognize and be activated by any foreign antigen if normally all APCs are displaying mainly self peptide–MHC complexes? The answer, as mentioned earlier, is that T cells are remarkably sensitive and need to specifically recognize very few peptide-MHC complexes to be activated. Thus, a newly introduced antigen may be processed into peptides that load enough MHC molecules of APCs to activate T cells specific for that antigen, even though most of the MHC molecules are occupied with self peptides. Also, microbes (the natural source of most foreign antigens) increase the efficiency of antigen presentation and induce the expression of second signals. Second, if individuals process their own proteins and present them in association with their own MHC molecules, why do we normally not develop immune responses against self proteins? The answer to this question is that self peptide–MHC complexes are formed but do not induce autoimmunity because T cells specific for such complexes are killed or inactivated. Therefore, T cells cannot normally respond to self antigens (see Chapter 15).

Structural Basis of Peptide Binding to MHC Molecules

The binding of peptides to MHC molecules is a non-covalent interaction mediated by residues both in the peptides and in the clefts of the MHC molecules. As we will see later, protein antigens are proteolytically cleaved in APCs to generate the peptides that will be bound and displayed by MHC molecules. These peptides bind to the clefts of MHC molecules in an extended conformation. Once bound, the peptides and their associated water molecules fill the clefts, making extensive contacts with the amino acid residues that form the β strands of the floor and the α helices of the walls of the cleft (Fig. 6-13). In the case of class I MHC molecules, association of a peptide with the MHC cleft depends on the binding of the positively charged amino (N) terminus and the negatively charged carboxyl (C) terminus of the peptide to the MHC molecule by electrostatic interactions. In most MHC molecules, the β strands in the floor of the cleft contain pockets where residues of peptides bind. Many class I molecules have a hydrophobic pocket that recognizes one of the following hydrophobic amino acids—valine, isoleucine, leucine, or methionine—at the C-terminal end of the peptide. Some class I molecules have a predilection for a basic residue (lysine or arginine) at the C terminus. In addition, other amino acid residues of a peptide may contain side chains that fit into specific pockets and bind to complementary

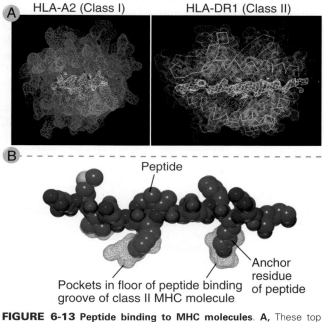

FIGURE 6-13 Peptide binding to MHC molecules. A, These top views of the crystal structures of MHC molecules show how peptides lie in the peptide-binding clefts. The class I molecule shown is HLA-A2, and the class II molecule is HLA-DR1. The cleft of the class I molecule is closed, whereas that of the class II molecule is open. As a result, class II molecules accommodate longer peptides than do class I molecules. **B,** The side view of a cutout of a peptide bound to a class II MHC molecule shows how anchor residues of the peptide hold it in the pockets in the cleft of the MHC molecule. (**A,** *Reprinted with permission of Macmillan Publishers Ltd. from Bjorkman PJ, Saper MA, Samraoui B, Bennett WS, Strominger JL, Wiley DC: Structure of the human class I histocompatibility antigen HLA-A2. Nature 329:506–512, 1987; and Brown J, Jardetzky TS, Gorga JC, Stern LJ, Urban RG, Strominger JL, Wiley DC: Three-dimensional structure of the human class II histocompatibility antigen HLA-DR1. Nature 364:33-39, 1993. **B,** From Scott CA, Peterson PA, Teyton L, Wilson IA: Crystal structures of two I-A^d–peptide complexes reveal that high affinity can be achieved without large anchor residues. Immunity 8:319–329, 1998. Copyright © 1998, with permission from Elsevier Science.*)

amino acids in the MHC molecule through electrostatic interactions (charge-based salt bridges), hydrogen bonding, or van der Waals interactions. Such residues of the peptide are called anchor residues because they contribute most of the favorable interactions of the binding (i.e., anchor the peptide in the cleft of the MHC molecule). Each MHC-binding peptide usually contains only one or two anchor residues, and this presumably allows greater variability in the other residues of the peptide, which are the residues that are recognized by specific T cells. In the case of some peptides binding to MHC molecules, especially class II molecules, specific interactions of peptides with the α-helical sides of the MHC cleft also contribute to peptide binding by forming hydrogen bonds or charge interactions. Class II MHC molecules accommodate larger peptides than class I MHC molecules. These longer peptides extend at either end beyond the floor of the cleft.

Because many of the residues in and around the peptide-binding cleft of MHC molecules are polymorphic (i.e., they differ among various MHC alleles), different alleles favor the binding of different peptides. This is the structural basis for the function of MHC genes as immune response genes; only individuals that express MHC alleles that can bind a particular peptide and display it to T cells can respond to that peptide.

The antigen receptors of T cells recognize both the antigenic peptide and the MHC molecules, with the peptide being responsible for the fine specificity of antigen recognition and the MHC residues accounting for the MHC restriction of the T cells. A portion of the bound peptide is exposed from the open top of the cleft of the MHC molecule, and the amino acid side chains of this portion of the peptide are recognized by the antigen receptors of specific T cells. The same T cell receptor also interacts with polymorphic residues of the α helices of the MHC molecule itself (see Fig. 6-1). Predictably, variations in either the peptide antigen or the peptide-binding cleft of the MHC molecule will alter presentation of that peptide or its recognition by T cells. In fact, one can enhance the immunogenicity of a peptide by incorporating into it a residue that strengthens its binding to commonly inherited MHC molecules in a population.

Because MHC molecules can bind only peptides but most antigens are large proteins, there must be ways by which these proteins are converted into peptides. The conversion is called **antigen processing** and is the focus of the remainder of the chapter.

PROCESSING OF PROTEIN ANTIGENS

The pathways of antigen processing convert protein antigens present in the cytosol or internalized from the extracellular environment into peptides and load these peptides onto MHC molecules for display to T lymphocytes (Fig. 6-14). The mechanisms of antigen processing are designed to generate peptides that have the structural characteristics required for associating with MHC molecules, and to place these peptides in the same cellular location as newly formed MHC molecules with available

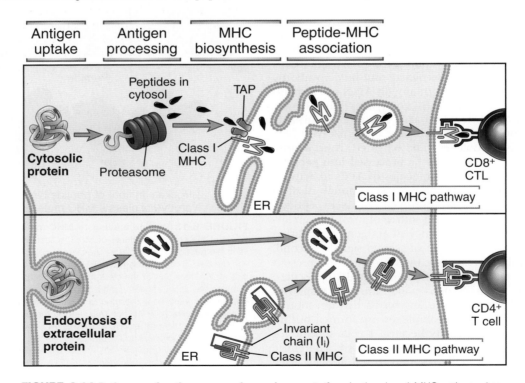

FIGURE 6-14 Pathways of antigen processing and presentation. In the class I MHC pathway *(top panel)*, protein antigens in the cytosol are processed by proteasomes, and peptides are transported into the endoplasmic reticulum (ER), where they bind to class I MHC molecules. In the class II MHC pathway *(bottom panel)*, extracellular protein antigens are endocytosed into vesicles, where the antigens are processed and the peptides bind to class II MHC molecules. Details of these processing pathways are shown in Figures 6-16 and 6-17.

peptide-binding clefts. Peptide binding to MHC molecules occurs before cell surface expression and is an integral component of the biosynthesis and assembly of MHC molecules. In fact, as mentioned earlier, peptide association is required for the stable assembly and surface expression of class I and class II MHC molecules.

Protein antigens that are present in the cytosol (usually synthesized in the cell) generate class I–associated peptides that are recognized by CD8+ T cells, whereas antigens internalized from the extracellular environment into the vesicles of APCs usually generate peptides that are displayed by class II MHC molecules and recognized by CD4+ T cells. The different fates of cytosolic and vesicular antigens are due to the segregated pathways of biosynthesis and assembly of class I and class II MHC molecules (see Fig. 6-14 and Table 6-5). The fundamental difference between the class I MHC and class II MHC pathways resides mainly in the site of peptide degradation. Proteins degraded in proteasomes, many of which are from the cytosol, primarily provide peptides for class I MHC molecules. Only proteins that are degraded in endo-lysosomes provide peptides for class II MHC molecules. The difference between cytosolic and vesicular antigens has been demonstrated experimentally by analyzing the presentation of the same antigen introduced into APCs in different ways (Fig. 6-15). If a protein antigen is produced in the cytoplasm of APCs as the product of a transfected gene (modified so its protein product cannot enter the secretory pathway) or introduced directly into the cytoplasm of the APCs by osmotic shock, peptides derived from the protein are presented by class I MHC molecules and are recognized by CD8+ T cells. In contrast, if the same protein is added in soluble form to APCs and endocytosed into the vesicles of the APCs, peptides (which may be different from the ones presented by class I) are subsequently presented by class II molecules and are recognized by antigen-specific CD4+ T cells.

We first describe these two pathways of antigen processing and then their functional significance.

The Class I MHC Pathway for Processing and Presentation of Cytosolic Proteins

Class I MHC–associated peptides are produced by the proteolytic degradation of mainly cytosolic proteins in proteasomes, and the generated peptides are transported into the endoplasmic reticulum (ER), where they bind to newly synthesized class I molecules. This sequence of events is illustrated in Figure 6-16, and the individual steps are described next.

Sources of Cytosolic Protein Antigens

Most cytosolic protein antigens are synthesized within cells, some are injected into the cytosol via bacterial secretory mechansims, and others are phagocytosed and transported from vesicles into the cytosol. Foreign antigens in the cytosol may be the products of viruses, bacteria, or other intracellular microbes that infect such cells. In tumor cells, various mutated or overexpressed genes may produce protein antigens that are recognized by class I–restricted CTLs (see Chapter 18). Peptides that are presented in association with class I molecules may also be derived from microbes and other particulate antigens that are internalized into phagosomes but escape into the cytosol. Some microbes are able to damage phagosome membranes and create pores through which the microbes and their antigens enter the cytosol. For instance, pathogenic strains of *Listeria monocytogenes* produce a protein called listeriolysin that

TABLE 6-5 Comparative Features of Class I and Class II MHC Pathways of Antigen Processing and Presentation

Feature	Class I MHC Pathway	Class II MHC Pathway
Composition of stable peptide-MHC complex	Polymorphic α chain, β_2-microglobulin, peptide	Polymorphic α and β chains, peptide
Types of APCs	All nucleated cells	Dendritic cells, mononuclear phagocytes, B lymphocytes; endothelial cells, thymic epithelium
Responsive T cells	CD8+ T cells	CD4+ T cells
Source of protein antigens	Mainly cytosolic proteins (usually synthesized in the cell; may enter cytosol from phagosomes); also nuclear and membrane proteins	Endosomal and lysosomal proteins (mostly internalized from extracellular environment)
Enzymes responsible for peptide loading of MHC	Proteasomes	Endosomal and lysosomal proteases (e.g., cathepsins)
Site of peptide loading of MHC	Endoplasmic reticulum	Specialized vesicular compartment
Molecules involved in transport of peptides and loading of MHC molecules	Chaperones, TAP in ER	Chaperones in ER; invariant chain in ER, Golgi and MIIC/CIIV; DM

APC, antigen-presenting cell; *CIIV,* class II vesicle; *ER,* endoplasmic reticulum; *MHC,* major histocompatibility complex; *MIIC,* MHC class II compartment; *TAP,* transporter associated with antigen processing.

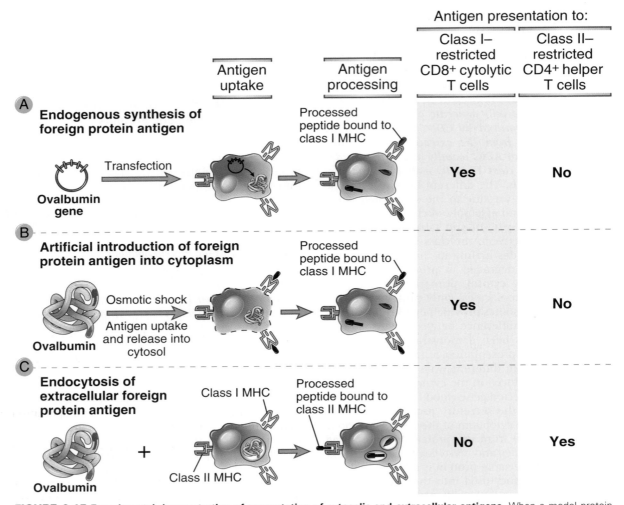

FIGURE 6-15 Experimental demonstration of presentation of cytosolic and extracellular antigens. When a model protein antigen, ovalbumin, is synthesized intracellularly as a result of transfection of its gene modified to lack the *N*-terminal signal sequences **(A)** or when it is introduced into the cytoplasm through membranes made leaky by osmotic shock **(B)**, ovalbumin-derived peptides are presented in association with class I MHC molecules. When ovalbumin is added as an extracellular antigen to an APC that expresses both class I and class II MHC molecules, ovalbumin-derived peptides are presented only in association with class II molecules **(C)**. The measured response of class I–restricted CTLs is killing of the APCs, and the measured response of class II–restricted helper T cells is cytokine secretion.

enables bacteria to escape from vesicles into the cytosol. (This escape is a mechanism that the bacteria may have evolved to resist killing by the microbicidal mechanisms of phagocytes, most of which are concentrated in phagolysosomes.) Once the antigens of the phagocytosed microbes are in the cytosol, they are processed like other cytosolic antigens. In dendritic cells, some antigens that are ingested into vesicles enter the cytosolic class I pathway, in the process called cross-presentation that is described later.

Although microbial proteins that are presented on class I MHC molecules are typically cytosolic, proteins from other cellular compartments may also enter the class I MHC antigen processing pathway. The signal sequences of membrane and secreted proteins are usually cleaved by signal peptidase and degraded proteolytically soon after synthesis and translocation into the ER. This ER processing generates class I–binding

peptides without a need for proteolysis in the cytosol. In addition, nuclear proteins may be processed by proteasomes in the nucleus and presented on class I MHC molecules.

Digestion of Proteins in Proteasomes

The major mechanism for the generation of peptides from cytosolic and nuclear protein antigens is proteolysis by the proteasome. Proteasomes are large multiprotein enzyme complexes with a broad range of proteolytic activity that are found in the cytoplasm and nuclei of most cells. The proteasome appears as a cylinder composed of a stacked array of two inner β rings and two outer α rings, each ring being composed of seven subunits, with a cap-like structure at either end of the cylinder. The proteins in the outer α rings are structural and lack proteolytic activity; in the inner β rings, three of the seven subunits (β1, β2, and β5) are the catalytic sites for proteolysis.

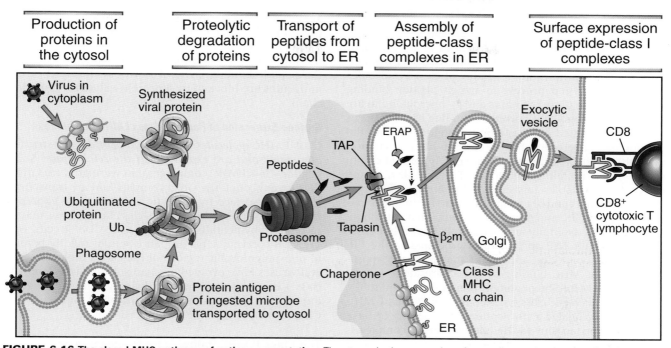

FIGURE 6-16 The class I MHC pathway of antigen presentation. The stages in the processing of cytosolic proteins are described in the text. *ERAP*, endoplasmic reticulum associated peptidase; *ER*, endoplasmic reticulum; *β₂m*, β₂-microglobulin; *TAP*, transporter associated with antigen processing; *Ub*, ubiquitin.

The proteasome performs a basic housekeeping function in cells by degrading many damaged or improperly folded proteins. Protein synthesis normally occurs at a rapid rate, about six to eight amino acid residues being incorporated into elongating chains every second. The process is error prone, and it is estimated that approximately 20% of newly synthesized proteins are misfolded. These newly translated but defective polypeptides, as well as proteins that are damaged by cellular stresses, are targeted for proteasomal degradation by covalent linkage of several copies of a small polypeptide called ubiquitin. Ubiquitinated proteins, with chains of four or more ubiquitins, are recognized by the proteasomal cap and then are unfolded, the ubiquitin is removed, and the proteins are threaded through proteasomes, where they are degraded into peptides. The proteasome has broad substrate specificity and can generate a wide variety of peptides from cytosolic proteins (but usually does not degrade them completely into single amino acids). Interestingly, in cells treated with the cytokine IFN-γ, there is increased transcription and synthesis of three novel catalytic subunits of the proteasome known as β1i, β2i, and β5i, which replace the three catalytic subunits of the β ring of the proteasome. This results in a change in the substrate specificity of the proteasome such that the peptides produced usually contain carboxy-terminal hydrophobic amino acids such as leucine, valine, isoleucine, and methionine or basic residues such as lysine or arginine. These kinds of C termini are typical of peptides that are transported into the class I pathway and bind to class I molecules. This is one mechanism by which IFN-γ enhances antigen presentation, another mechanism being increased expression of MHC molecules (see Fig. 6-9). Thus, proteasomes are organelles whose basic cellular function has been adapted for a specialized role in antigen presentation.

Transport of Peptides from the Cytosol to the Endoplasmic Reticulum

Peptides generated in proteasomes are translocated by a specialized transporter into the ER, where newly synthesized class I MHC molecules are available to bind the peptides. Because antigenic peptides for the class I pathway are generated by proteases the cytosol or the nucleus but class I MHC molecules are synthesized in the ER, a mechanism is needed to deliver cytosolic peptides into the ER. This delivery is mediated by a dimeric protein called **transporter associated with antigen processing (TAP)**, which is a member of the ABC transporter family of proteins, many of which mediate ATP-dependent transport of low–molecular-weight compounds across cellular membranes. The TAP protein is located in the ER membrane, where it mediates the active, ATP-dependent transport of peptides from the cytosol into the ER lumen. Although the TAP heterodimer has a broad range of specificities, it optimally transports peptides ranging from 8 to 16 amino acids in length and containing carboxyl termini that are basic (in humans) or hydrophobic (in humans and mice). As mentioned earlier, these are the characteristics of the peptides that are generated in the proteasome and are able to bind to class I MHC molecules.

On the luminal side of the ER membrane, the TAP protein associates with a protein called tapasin, which also has an affinity for newly synthesized empty class I MHC molecules. Tapasin thus brings the TAP transporter into a complex with the class I MHC molecules that are awaiting the arrival of peptides.

Assembly of Peptide–Class I MHC Complexes in the Endoplasmic Reticulum

Peptides translocated into the ER bind to class I MHC molecules that are associated with the TAP dimer through tapasin. The synthesis and assembly of class I molecules involve a multistep process in which peptide binding plays a key role. Class I α chains and β$_2$-microglobulin are synthesized in the ER. Appropriate folding of the nascent α chains is assisted by chaperone proteins, such as the membrane chaperone calnexin and the luminal chaperone calreticulin. Within the ER, the newly formed empty class I dimers remain linked to the TAP complex. Empty class I MHC molecules, tapasin, and TAP are part of a larger peptide-loading complex in the ER that also includes calnexin, calreticulin, and other components that contribute to class I MHC assembly and loading. Peptides that enter the ER through TAP and peptides produced in the ER, such as signal peptides, are often trimmed to the appropriate size for MHC binding by the ER-resident aminopeptidase (ERAP). The peptide is then able to bind to the cleft of the adjacent class I molecule. Once class I MHC molecules are loaded with peptide, they no longer have an affinity for tapasin, so the peptide–class I complex is released, and it is able to exit the ER and be transported to the cell surface. In the absence of bound peptide, many of the newly formed α chain–β$_2$-microglobulin dimers are unstable and cannot be transported efficiently from the ER to the Golgi complex. These misfolded empty class I MHC complexes are transported into the cytosol and degraded in the proteasomes.

Peptides transported into the ER preferentially bind to class I but not class II MHC molecules for two reasons. First, newly synthesized class I molecules are attached to the luminal aspect of the TAP complex, and they capture peptides rapidly as the peptides are transported into the ER by the TAP. Second, as discussed later, in the ER the peptide-binding clefts of newly synthesized class II molecules are blocked by a protein called the invariant chain.

Surface Expression of Peptide–Class I MHC Complexes

Class I MHC molecules with bound peptides are structurally stable and are expressed on the cell surface. Stable peptide–class I MHC complexes that were produced in the ER move through the Golgi complex and are transported to the cell surface by exocytic vesicles. Once expressed on the cell surface, the peptide–class I complexes may be recognized by peptide antigen–specific CD8+ T cells, with the CD8 coreceptor playing an essential role by binding to non-polymorphic regions of the class I molecule. Several viruses have evolved mechanisms that interfere with class I assembly and peptide loading, emphasizing the importance of this pathway for anti-viral immunity (see Chapter 16).

The Class II MHC Pathway for Processing and Presentation of Vesicular Proteins

The generation of class II MHC–associated peptides from endocytosed antigens involves the proteolytic degradation of internalized proteins in endocytic vesicles and the binding of peptides to class II MHC molecules in vesicles. This sequence of events is illustrated in Figure 6-17, and the individual steps are described next.

Uptake of extracellular proteins into vesicular compartments of APC	Processing of internalized proteins in endosomal/ lysosomal vesicles	Biosynthesis and transport of class II MHC molecules to endosomes	Association of processed peptides with class II MHC molecules in vesicles	Expression of peptide-MHC complexes on cell surface

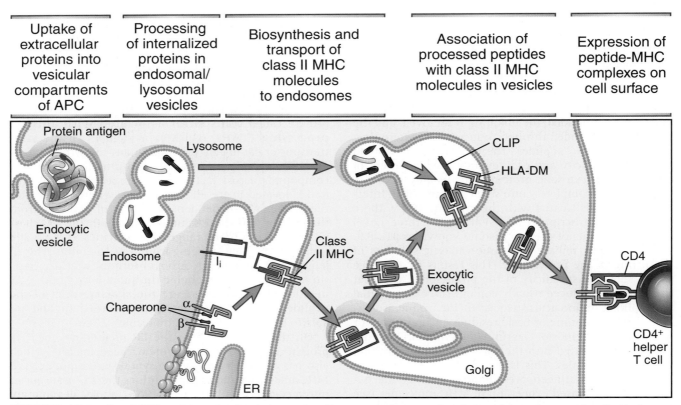

FIGURE 6-17 The class II MHC pathway of antigen presentation. The stages in the processing of extracellular antigens are described in the text. *CLIP*, class II–associated invariant chain peptide; *ER*, endoplasmic reticulum; *I$_i$*, invariant chain.

Generation of Vesicular Proteins

Most class II MHC–associated peptides are derived from protein antigens that are captured from the extracellular environment and internalized into endosomes by specialized APCs. The initial steps in the presentation of an extracellular protein antigen are the binding of the native antigen to an APC and the internalization of the antigen. Different APCs can bind protein antigens in several ways and with varying efficiencies and specificities. Dendritic cells and macrophages express a variety of surface receptors that recognize structures shared by many microbes (see Chapter 4). These APCs use the receptors to bind and internalize microbes efficiently. Macrophages also express receptors for the Fc portions of antibodies and receptors for the complement protein C3b, which bind antigens with attached antibodies or complement proteins and enhance their internalization. Another example of specific receptors on APCs is the surface immunoglobulin on B cells, which, because of its high affinity for antigens, can effectively mediate the internalization of proteins present at very low concentrations in the extracellular fluid (see Chapter 12).

After their internalization, protein antigens become localized in intracellular membrane-bound vesicles called endosomes. The endosomal pathway of intracellular protein traffic communicates with lysosomes, which are denser membrane-bound enzyme-containing vesicles. A subset of class II MHC–rich late endosomes plays a special role in antigen processing and presentation by the class II pathway; this is described later. Particulate microbes are internalized into vesicles called phagosomes, which may fuse with lysosomes, producing vesicles called phagolysosomes or secondary lysosomes. Some microbes, such as mycobacteria and *Leishmania*, may survive and even replicate within phagosomes or endosomes, providing a persistent source of antigens in vesicular compartments.

Proteins other than those ingested from the extracellular milieu can also enter the class II MHC pathway. Some protein molecules destined for secretion may end up in the same vesicles as class II MHC molecules and may be processed instead of being secreted. Less often, cytoplasmic and membrane proteins may be processed and displayed by class II molecules. In some cases, this may result from the enzymatic digestion of cytoplasmic contents, referred to as **autophagy**. In this pathway, cytosolic proteins are trapped within membrane-bound vesicles called autophagosomes; these vesicles fuse with lysosomes, and the cytoplasmic proteins are proteolytically degraded. The peptides generated by this route may be delivered to the same class II–bearing vesicular compartment as are peptides derived from ingested antigens. Autophagy is primarily a mechanism for degrading cellular proteins and recycling their products as sources of nutrients during times of stress. It also participates in the destruction of intracellular microbes, which are enclosed in vesicles and delivered to lysosomes. It is therefore predictable that peptides generated by autophagy will be displayed for T cell recognition. Some peptides that associate with class II molecules are derived from membrane proteins, which may be recycled into the same endocytic pathway as are extracellular proteins. Thus, even viruses, which replicate in the cytoplasm of infected cells, may produce proteins that are degraded into peptides that enter the class II MHC pathway of antigen presentation. This may be a mechanism for the activation of viral antigen–specific CD4+ helper T cells.

Proteolytic Digestion of Proteins in Vesicles

Internalized proteins are degraded enzymatically in late endosomes and lysosomes to generate peptides that are able to bind to the peptide-binding clefts of class II MHC molecules. The degradation of protein antigens in vesicles is an active process mediated by proteases that have acidic pH optima. The most abundant proteases of late endosomes are cathepsins, which are thiol and aspartyl proteases with broad substrate specificities. Several cathepsins contribute to the generation of peptides for the class II pathway. Partially degraded or cleaved proteins bind to the open-ended clefts of class II MHC molecules and are then trimmed enzymatically to their final size. Immunoelectron microscopy and subcellular fractionation studies have defined a class II MHC–rich subset of late endosomes that plays an important role in antigen presentation (Fig. 6-18). In macrophages and human B cells, it is called the MHC class II compartment, or MIIC. (In some mouse B cells, a similar organelle containing

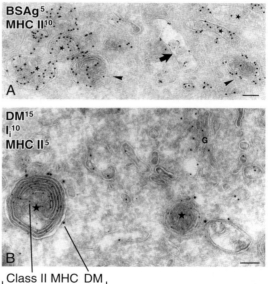

FIGURE 6-18 Morphology of class II MHC–rich endosomal vesicles. **A,** Immunoelectron micrograph of a B lymphocyte that has internalized bovine serum albumin into early endosomes (labeled with 5-nm gold particles, *arrow*) and contains class II MHC molecules (labeled with 10-nm gold particles, *arrowheads*) in MIICs. The internalized albumin will reach the MIICs ultimately. **B,** Immunoelectron micrograph of a B cell showing location of class II MHC molecules and DM in MIICs *(stars)* and invariant chain concentrated in the Golgi (G) complex. In this example, there is virtually no invariant chain detected in the MIIC, presumably because it has been cleaved to generate CLIP. *(**A,** From Kleijmeer MJ, Morkowski S, Griffith JM, Rudensky AY, Geuze HJ: Major histocompatibility complex class II compartments in human and mouse B lymphoblasts represent conventional endocytic compartments. Reproduced from* The Journal of Cell Biology *139:639–649, 1997, by copyright permission of The Rockefeller University Press. **B,** Courtesy of Drs. H. J. Geuze and M. Kleijmeer, Department of Cell Biology, Utrecht University, The Netherlands.)*

class II MHC molecules has been identified and named the class II vesicle.) The MIIC has a characteristic multila-mellar appearance by electron microscopy. Importantly, it contains all of the components required for peptide–class II MHC association, including the enzymes that degrade protein antigens, class II MHC molecules, and two mol-ecules involved in peptide loading of class II MHC mole-cules, the invariant chain and HLA-DM, whose functions are described later.

Biosynthesis and Transport of Class II MHC Molecules to Endosomes

Class II MHC molecules are synthesized in the ER and transported to endosomes with an associated protein, the invariant chain, which occupies the peptide-binding clefts of the newly synthesized class II MHC molecules (Fig. 6-19). The α and β chains of class II MHC molecules are coordinately synthesized and associate with each other in the ER. Nascent class II MHC dimers are structurally unstable, and their folding and assembly are aided by ER-resident chaperones, such as calnexin. The invariant chain (I_i) promotes folding and assembly of class II MHC mol-ecules and directs newly formed class II MHC molecules to the late endosomes and lysosomes where internalized proteins have been proteolytically degraded into peptides. The invariant chain is a trimer composed of three 30-kD subunits, each of which binds one newly synthesized class II MHC αβ heterodimer in a way that blocks the peptide-binding cleft and prevents it from accepting peptides. As a result, class II MHC molecules cannot bind and present peptides they encounter in the ER, leaving such peptides to associate with class I molecules (described earlier). The class II MHC molecules are transported in exocytic vesicles toward the cell surface. During this passage, the vesicles taking class II MHC molecules out of the ER meet and fuse with the endocytic vesicles containing internal-ized and processed antigens. Thus, class II MHC molecules encounter antigenic peptides that have been generated by proteolysis of endocytosed proteins, and the peptide-MHC association occurs in the vesicles.

Association of Processed Peptides with Class II MHC Molecules in Vesicles

Within the endosomal vesicles, the invariant chain dis-sociates from class II MHC molecules by the combined action of proteolytic enzymes and the HLA-DM molecule, and antigenic peptides are then able to bind to the avail-able peptide-binding clefts of the class II molecules (see Fig. 6-19). Because the invariant chain blocks access to the peptide-binding cleft of class II MHC molecules, it must be removed before complexes of peptide and class II MHC molecules can form. The same proteolytic enzymes that generate peptides from internalized proteins, such as cathepsins, also act on the invariant chain, degrading it and leaving only a 24–amino acid remnant called class II–associated invariant chain peptide (CLIP), which sits in the peptide-binding cleft in the same way that other peptides bind to class II MHC molecules. Next, CLIP must be removed so that the cleft becomes accessible to anti-genic peptides produced from extracellular proteins. This removal is accomplished by the action of a molecule called **HLA-DM** (or H-2M in the mouse), which is encoded within the MHC, has a structure similar to that of class II MHC molecules, and colocalizes with class II MHC mol-ecules in the MIIC endosomal compartment. Unlike class II MHC molecules, HLA-DM molecules are not polymor-phic, and they are not expressed on the cell surface. HLA-DM acts as a peptide exchanger, facilitating the removal of CLIP and the addition of other peptides to class II MHC molecules.

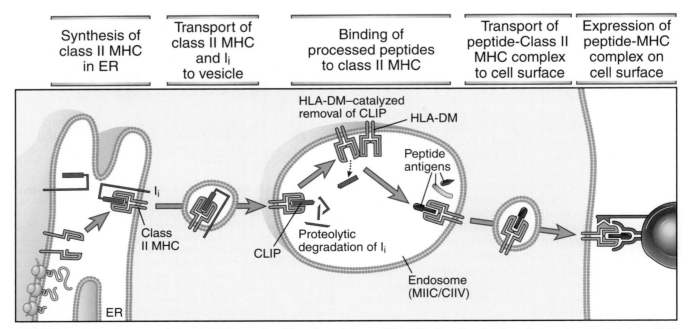

| Synthesis of class II MHC in ER | Transport of class II MHC and I_i to vesicle | Binding of processed peptides to class II MHC | Transport of peptide-Class II MHC complex to cell surface | Expression of peptide-MHC complex on cell surface |

FIGURE 6-19 The functions of class II MHC–associated invariant chain and HLA-DM. Class II molecules with bound invariant chain, or CLIP, are transported into vesicles, where the I_i is degraded and the remaining CLIP is removed by the action of DM. Antigenic peptides generated in the vesicles are then able to bind to the class II molecules. Another class II–like protein, called HLA-DO, may regulate the DM-catalyzed removal of CLIP (*not shown*). *CIIV*, class II vesicle.

If peptides with a higher affinity for the class II MHC cleft than CLIP are available in endosomes they will be able to displace CLIP because of the HLA-DM mediated exchange mechanism. If higher affinity peptides are not available CLIP will remain in the class II MHC cleft and these molecules will not undergo the presumed conformational change and stabilization required to efficiently travel to the cell surface. Because the ends of the class II MHC peptide-binding cleft are open, large peptides may bind and are then trimmed by proteolytic enzymes to the appropriate size for T cell recognition. As a result, the peptides that are actually presented attached to cell surface class II MHC molecules are usually 10 to 30 amino acids long and typically have been generated by this trimming step.

Expression of Peptide–Class II MHC Complexes on the Cell Surface

Class II MHC molecules are stabilized by the bound peptides, and the stable peptide–class II complexes are delivered to the surface of the APC, where they are displayed for recognition by CD4+ T cells. The transport of class II MHC–peptide complexes to the cell surface is believed to occur by fusion of vesiculotubular extensions from the lysosome with the plasma membrane, resulting in delivery of the loaded class II MHC complexes to the cell surface. Once expressed on the APC surface, the peptide–class II complexes are recognized by peptide antigen–specific CD4+ T cells, with the CD4 coreceptor playing an essential role by binding to non-polymorphic regions of the class II molecule. Interestingly, whereas peptide-loaded class II molecules traffic from the late endosomes and lysosomes to the cell surface, other molecules involved in antigen presentation, such as DM, stay in the vesicles and are not expressed in the plasma membrane. The mechanism of this selective traffic is unknown.

Cross-Presentation

Some dendritic cells have the ability to capture and to ingest virus-infected cells or tumor cells and present the viral or tumor antigens to naive CD8+ T lymphocytes (Fig. 6-20). In this pathway, the ingested antigens are transported from vesicles to the cytosol, from where peptides enter the class I pathway. As we discussed earlier, most ingested proteins do not enter the cytosolic class I pathway of antigen presentation. This permissiveness for protein traffic from endosomal vesicles to the cytosol is unique to dendritic cells. (At the same time, the dendritic cells can present class II MHC–associated peptides generated in the vesicles to CD4+ helper T cells, which are often required to induce full responses of CD8+ cells [see Chapter 11].) This process is called **cross-presentation,** or **cross-priming,** to indicate that one cell type (the dendritic cell) can present antigens from another cell (the virus-infected or tumor cell) and prime, or activate, T cells specific for these antigens. Although on face value it may seem that the process of cross-presentation violates the rule that ingested antigens are presented bound to class II MHC molecules, in this situation the ingested antigens are degraded in proteasomes and enter the class I pathway.

Cross-presentation involves the fusion of phagosomes containing the ingested antigens with the ER. Ingested proteins are then translocated from the ER to the cytosol by poorly defined pathways that are likely involved in presentation of proteins degraded in the ER. The proteins that were initially internalized in the phagosome are therefore delivered to the compartment (the cytosol) where proteolysis for the class I pathway normally occurs. These phagocytosed proteins thus undergo proteasomal degradation, and peptides derived from them are transported by TAP back into the ER, where they are assembled with newly synthesized class I MHC molecules as described for the conventional class I pathway.

Physiologic Significance of MHC-Associated Antigen Presentation

So far, we have discussed the specificity of CD4+ and CD8+ T lymphocytes for MHC-associated foreign protein antigens and the mechanisms by which complexes of peptides and MHC molecules are produced. In this section, we will consider how the central role of the MHC

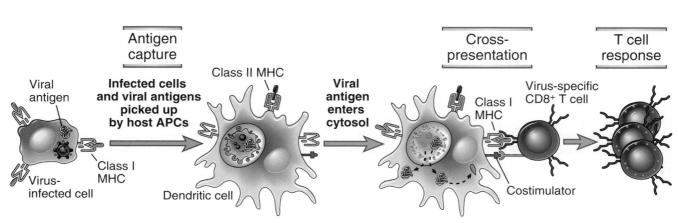

FIGURE 6-20 Cross-presentation of antigens to CD8+ T cells. Cells infected with intracellular microbes, such as viruses, are ingested by dendritic cells, and the antigens of the infectious microbes are transported into the cytosol and processed and presented in association with class I MHC molecules to CD8+ T cells (see also Fig. 6-16). Thus, dendritic cells are able to present endocytosed vesicular antigens by the class I pathway. Note that the same cross-presenting APCs may display class II MHC–associated antigens from the microbe for recognition by CD4+ helper T cells.

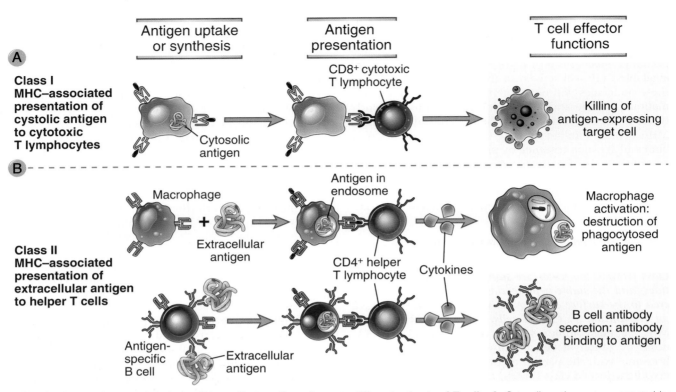

FIGURE 6-21 Presentation of extracellular and cytosolic antigens to different subsets of T cells. A, Cytosolic antigens are presented by nucleated cells to CD8+ CTLs, which kill (lyse) the antigen-expressing cells. **B,** Extracellular antigens are presented by macrophages or B lymphocytes to CD4+ helper T lymphocytes, which activate the macrophages or B cells and eliminate the extracellular antigens.

in antigen presentation influences the nature of T cell responses to different antigens and the types of antigens that T cells recognize.

Nature of T Cell Responses

The presentation of cytosolic versus vesicular proteins by the class I or class II MHC pathways, respectively, determines which subsets of T cells will respond to antigens found in these two pools of proteins and is intimately linked to the functions of these T cells (Fig. 6-21). Endogenously synthesized antigens, such as viral and tumor proteins, are located in the cytosol and are recognized by class I MHC–restricted CD8+ CTLs, which kill the cells producing the intracellular antigens. Conversely, extracellular antigens usually end up in endosomal vesicles and activate class II MHC–restricted CD4+ T cells because vesicular proteins are processed into class II–binding peptides. CD4+ T cells function as helpers to stimulate B cells to produce antibodies and activate macrophages to enhance their phagocytic functions, both mechanisms that serve to eliminate extracellular antigens. Thus, antigens from microbes that reside in different cellular locations selectively stimulate the T cell responses that are most effective at eliminating that type of microbe. This is especially important because the antigen receptors of CTLs and helper T cells cannot distinguish between extracellular and intracellular microbes. By segregating peptides derived from these types of microbes, the MHC molecules guide CD4+ and CD8+ subsets of T cells to respond to the microbes that each subset can best combat.

Immunogenicity of Protein Antigens

MHC molecules determine the immunogenicity of protein antigens in two related ways.

- *The epitopes of complex proteins that elicit the strongest T cell responses are the peptides that are generated by proteolysis in APCs and bind most avidly to MHC molecules.* If an individual is immunized with a protein antigen, in many instances the majority of the responding T cells are specific for only one or a few linear amino acid sequences of the antigen. These are called the **immunodominant** epitopes or determinants. The proteases involved in antigen processing produce a variety of peptides from natural proteins, and only some of these peptides possess the characteristics that enable them to bind to the MHC molecules present in each individual (Fig. 6-22). It is important to define the structural basis of immunodominance because this may permit the efficient manipulation of the immune system with synthetic peptides. An application of such knowledge is the design of vaccines. For example, a viral protein could be analyzed for the presence of amino acid sequences that would form typical immunodominant epitopes capable of binding to MHC molecules with high affinity. Synthetic peptides containing these epitopes may be effective vaccines for eliciting T cell responses against the viral peptide expressed on an infected cell.

- *The expression of particular class II MHC alleles in an individual determines the ability of that individual to respond to particular antigens.* As discussed

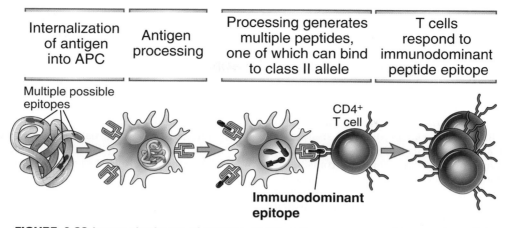

FIGURE 6-22 Immunodominance of peptides. Protein antigens are processed to generate multiple peptides; immunodominant peptides are the ones that bind best to the available class I and class II MHC molecules. The illustration shows an extracellular antigen generating a class II–binding peptide, but this also applies to peptides of cytosolic antigens that are presented by class I MHC molecules.

earlier, the immune response (Ir) genes that control antibody responses are the class II MHC genes. They influence immune responsiveness because various allelic class II MHC molecules differ in their ability to bind different antigenic peptides and therefore to stimulate specific helper T cells. The consequences of inheriting a given MHC allele depend on the nature of the peptide antigens that can bind the MHC molecule encoded by that allele. For example, if the antigen is a peptide from ragweed pollen, the individual who expresses class II molecules capable of binding the peptide would be genetically prone to allergic reactions against pollen. Conversely, some individuals do not respond to vaccines (such as hepatitis B virus surface antigen vaccine), presumably because their HLA molecules cannot bind and display the major peptides of the antigen.

PRESENTATION OF NON-PROTEIN ANTIGENS TO SUBSETS OF T CELLS

Several small populations of T cells are able to recognize non-protein antigens without the involvement of class I or class II MHC molecules. Thus, these populations are exceptions to the rule that T cells can see only MHC-associated peptides. The best defined of these populations are NKT cells and γδ T cells.

NKT cells express markers that are characteristic of both natural killer (NK) cells and T lymphocytes and express αβ T cell receptors with very limited diversity (see Chapter 10). NKT cells recognize lipids and glycolipids displayed by the class I–like non-classical MHC molecule called **CD1.** There are several CD1 proteins expressed in humans and mice. Although their intracellular traffic pathways differ in subtle ways, all CD1 molecules bind and display lipids by a unique mechanism. Newly synthesized CD1 molecules pick up cellular lipids and carry these to the cell surface. From here, the CD1-lipid complexes are endocytosed into endosomes or lysosomes, where lipids that have been ingested from the external environment are captured and

the new CD1-lipid complexes are returned to the cell surface. Thus, CD1 molecules acquire endocytosed lipid antigens during recycling and present these antigens without apparent processing. The NKT cells that recognize the lipid antigens may play a role in defense against microbes, especially mycobacteria (which are rich in lipid components).

γδ T cells are a small population of T cells that express antigen receptor proteins that are similar but not identical to those of CD4$^+$ and CD8$^+$ T cells (see Chapter 10). γδ T cells recognize many different types of antigens, including some proteins and lipids, as well as small phosphorylated molecules and alkyl amines. These antigens are not displayed by MHC molecules, and γδ cells are not MHC restricted. It is not known if a particular cell type or antigen display system is required for presenting antigens to these cells.

SUMMARY

* Most T cells recognize antigens only in the form of peptides displayed by the products of self MHC genes on the surface of APCs. CD4$^+$ helper T lymphocytes recognize antigens in association with class II MHC gene products (class II MHC–restricted recognition), and CD8$^+$ CTLs recognize antigens in association with class I MHC gene products (class I MHC–restricted recognition).

* Specialized APCs, such as dendritic cells, macrophages, and B lymphocytes, capture extracellular protein antigens, internalize and process them, and display class II–associated peptides to CD4$^+$ T cells. Dendritic cells are the most efficient APCs for initiating primary responses by activating naive T cells, and macrophages and B lymphocytes present antigens to differentiated helper T cells in the effector phase of cell-mediated immunity and in humoral immune responses, respectively. All nucleated cells can present class I–associated peptides, derived from cytosolic proteins such as viral and tumor antigens, to CD8$^+$ T cells.

* The MHC is a large genetic region coding for highly polymorphic, codominantly expressed class I and class II MHC molecules.

* Class I MHC molecules are composed of an α (or heavy) chain in a non-covalent complex with a non-polymorphic polypeptide called β_2-microglobulin. Class II MHC molecules contain two MHC-encoded polymorphic chains, an α chain and a β chain. Both classes of MHC molecules consist of an extracellular peptide-binding cleft, a non-polymorphic Ig-like region, a transmembrane region, and a cytoplasmic region. The peptide-binding cleft of MHC molecules has α-helical sides and an eight-stranded antiparallel β-pleated sheet floor. The Ig-like domains of class I and class II MHC molecules contain the binding sites for the T cell coreceptors CD8 and CD4, respectively. The polymorphic residues of MHC molecules are localized to the peptide-binding domain.

* The function of class I and class II MHC molecules is to bind peptide antigens and display them for recognition by antigen-specific T lymphocytes. Peptide antigens associated with class I MHC molecules are recognized by CD8+ T cells, whereas class II MHC–associated peptide antigens are recognized by CD4+ T cells. MHC molecules bind only one peptide at a time, and all of the peptides that bind to a particular MHC molecule share common structural motifs. Every MHC molecule has a broad specificity for peptides and can bind multiple peptides that have common structural features, such as anchor residues.

* The peptide-binding cleft of class I MHC molecules can accommodate peptides that are 6 to 16 amino acid residues in length, whereas the cleft of class II MHC molecules allows larger peptides (up to 30 amino acid residues in length or more) to bind. Some polymorphic MHC residues determine the binding specificities for peptides by forming structures called pockets that interact with complementary residues of the bound peptide, called anchor residues. Other polymorphic MHC residues and some residues of the peptide are not involved in binding to MHC molecules but instead form the structure recognized by T cells.

* Class I MHC molecules are expressed on all nucleated cells, whereas class II MHC molecules are expressed mainly on specialized APCs, such as dendritic cells, macrophages, and B lymphocytes, and a few other cell types, including endothelial cells and thymic epithelial cells. The expression of MHC gene products is enhanced by inflammatory and immune stimuli, particularly cytokines like IFN-γ, which stimulate the transcription of MHC genes.

* Antigen processing is the conversion of native proteins into MHC-associated peptides. This process consists of the introduction of exogenous protein antigens into vesicles of APCs or the synthesis of antigens in the cytosol, the proteolytic degradation of these proteins into peptides, the binding of peptides to MHC molecules, and the display of the peptide-MHC complexes on the APC surface for recognition by T cells. Thus, both extracellular and intracellular proteins are sampled by these antigen-processing pathways, and peptides derived from both normal self proteins and foreign proteins are displayed by MHC molecules for surveillance by T lymphocytes.

* For the class I MHC pathway, cytosolic proteins are proteolytically degraded in the proteasome, generating peptides that bind to class I MHC molecules. These peptides are delivered from the cytosol to the ER by an ATP-dependent transporter called TAP. Newly synthesized class I MHC–β_2-microglobulin dimers in the ER are associated with the TAP complex and receive peptides transported into the ER. Stable complexes of class I MHC molecules with bound peptides move out of the ER, through the Golgi complex, to the cell surface.

* For the class II MHC pathway, extracellular proteins are internalized into endosomes, where these proteins are proteolytically cleaved by enzymes that function at acidic pH. Newly synthesized class II MHC molecules associated with the I_i are transported from the ER to the endosomal vesicles. Here the I_i is proteolytically cleaved, and a small peptide remnant of the I_i, called CLIP, is removed from the peptide-binding cleft of the MHC molecule by the DM molecules. The peptides that were generated from extracellular proteins then bind to the available cleft of the class II MHC molecule, and the trimeric complex (class II MHC α and β chains and peptide) moves to and is displayed on the surface of the cell.

* These pathways of MHC-restricted antigen presentation ensure that most of the body's cells are screened for the possible presence of foreign antigens. The pathways also ensure that proteins from extracellular microbes preferentially generate peptides bound to class II MHC molecules for recognition by CD4+ helper T cells, which activate effector mechanisms that eliminate extracellular antigens. Conversely, proteins synthesized by intracellular (cytosolic) microbes generate peptides bound to class I MHC molecules for recognition by CD8+ CTLs, which function to eliminate cells harboring intracellular infections. The immunogenicity of foreign protein antigens depends on the ability of antigen-processing pathways to generate peptides from these proteins that bind to self MHC molecules.

SUGGESTED READINGS

The Role of Dendritic Cells in Antigen Capture and Presentation

Bousso P: T-cell activation by dendritic cells in the lymph node: lessons from the movies, *Nature Reviews Immunology* 8:675–684, 2008.

Collin M, McGovern N, Haniffa M: Human dendritic cell subsets, *Immunology* 140:22–30, 2013.

Heath WR, Carbone FR: Dendritic cell subsets in primary and secondary T cell responses at body surfaces, *Nature Immunology* 10:1237–1244, 2009.

Merad M, Sathe P, Helft J, Miller J, Mortha A: The dendritic cell lineage: ontogeny and function of dendritic cells and their subsets in the steady state and inflamed setting, *Annual Review of Immunology* 31:563–604, 2013.

Mildner A, Jung S: Development and function of dendritic cell subsets, *Immunity* 40:642–656, 2014.

Satpathy AT, Wu X, Albring JC, Murphy KM: Re(de)fining the dendritic cell lineage, *Nature Immunology* 13:1145–1154, 2012.

Shortman K, Sathe P, Vremec D, Naik S, O'Keeffe M: Plasmacytoid dendritic cell development, *Advances in Immunology* 120:105–126, 2013.

Teijeira A, Russo E, Halin C: Taking the lymphatic route: dendritic cell migration to draining lymph nodes, *Seminars in Immunopathology* 36:261–274, 2014.

Structure of MHC Genes, MHC Molecules, and Peptide-MHC Complexes

Bjorkman PJ, Saper MA, Samraoui B, Bennett WS, Strominger JL, Wiley DC: Structure of the human class I histocompatibility antigen HLA-A2, *Nature* 329:506–512, 1987.

Horton R, Wilming L, Rand V, et al.: Gene map of the extended human MHC, *Nature Reviews Genetics* 5:889–899, 2004.

Marrack P, Scott-Browne JP, Dai S, Gapin L, Kappler JW: Evolutionarily conserved amino acids that control TCR-MHC interaction, *Annual Review of Immunology* 26:171–203, 2008.

Martinez-Borra J, Lopez-Larrea C: The emergence of the major histocompatibility complex, *Advances in Experimental Medicine and Biology* 738:277–289, 2012.

Mazza C, Malissen B: What guides MHC-restricted TCR recognition? *Seminars in Immunology* 19:225–235, 2007.

Reith W, Leibundgut-Landmann S, Waldburger JM: Regulation of MHC class II gene expression by the class II transactivator, *Nature Reviews Immunology* 5:793–806, 2005.

Protein Antigen Processing and MHC-Associated Presentation of Peptide Antigens

Akram A, Inman RD: Immunodominance: a pivotal principle in host response to viral infections, *Clinical Immunology* 143:99–115, 2012.

Basler M, Kirk CJ, Groettrup M: The immunoproteasome in antigen processing and other immunological functions, *Current Opinion in Immunology* 25:74–80, 2013.

Blum JS, Wearsch PA, Cresswell P: Pathways of antigen processing, *Annual Review of Immunology* 31:443–473, 2013.

Chapman HA: Endosomal proteases in antigen presentation, *Current Opinion in Immunology* 18:78–84, 2006.

Hansen TH, Bouvier M: MHC class I antigen presentation: learning from viral evasion strategies, *Nature Reviews Immunology* 9:503–513, 2009.

Neefjes J, Jongsma ML, Paul P, Bakke O: Towards a systems understanding of MHC class I and MHC class II antigen presentation, *Nature Reviews Immunology* 11:823–836, 2011.

Purcell AW, Elliott T: Molecular machinations of the MHC-I peptide loading complex, *Current Opinion in Immunology* 20:75–81, 2008.

Schulze MS, Wucherpfennig KW: The mechanism of HLA-DM induced peptide exchange in the MHC class II antigen presentation pathway, *Current Opinion in Immunology* 24:105–111, 2012.

Stern LJ, Potolicchio I, Santambrogio L: MHC class II compartment subtypes: structure and function, *Current Opinion in Immunology* 18:64–69, 2006.

Trombetta ES, Mellman I: Cell biology of antigen processing in vitro and in vivo, *Annual Review of Immunology* 23:975–1028, 2005.

Vyas JM, Van der Veen AG, Ploegh HL: The known unknowns of antigen processing and presentation, *Nature Reviews Immunology* 8:607–618, 2008.

Watts C: The endosome-lysosome pathway and information generation in the immune system, *Biochim Biophys Acta* 14-21:2012, 1824.

Cross-Presentation

Joffre OP, Segura E, Savina A, Amigorena S: Cross-presentation by dendritic cells, *Nature Reviews Immunology* 12:557–569, 2012.

Kurts C, Robinson BW, Knolle PA: Cross-priming in health and disease, *Nature Reviews Immunology* 10:403–414, 2010.

Lin ML, Zhan Y, Villadangos JA, Lew AM: The cell biology of cross-presentation and the role of dendritic cell subsets, *Immunology and Cell Biology* 86:353–362, 2008.

"Non-Classical" Antigen Presentation

Adams EJ, Luoma AM: The adaptable major histocompatibility complex (MHC) fold: structure and function of nonclassical and MHC class I-like molecules, *Annual Review of Immunology* 31:529–561, 2013.

Cohen NR, Garg S, Brenner MB: Antigen presentation by CD1: lipids, T cells, and NKT cells in microbial immunity, *Advances in Immunology* 102:1–94, 2009.

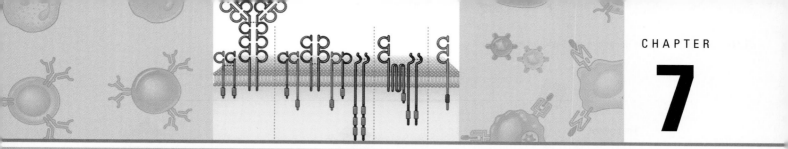

CHAPTER

7

Immune Receptors and Signal Transduction

The idea that cells have specific surface receptors that can be triggered by external ligands came from one of the founders of modern immunology. Paul Ehrlich, in his "side chain theory," published in 1897, conceived of antibodies on the surface of immune cells that recognize antigens and instruct the immune cell to release more of the same antibody. Cell surface receptors for hormones were discovered many decades later, in the second half of the twentieth century, but well before the identification of antigen receptors on lymphocytes in the early 1980s.

Cell surface receptors serve two major functions—the induction of intracellular signaling and the adhesion of one cell to another or to the extracellular matrix. Signal transduction broadly refers to the intracellular biochemical pathways that are activated in cells after the binding of ligands to specific receptors. Most but not all signaling receptors are located in the plasma membrane. Signaling initiated by these receptors typically involves an initial cytosolic phase when the cytoplasmic portion of the receptor or of proteins that interact with the receptor may be post-translationally modified. This often leads to the activation or nuclear translocation of transcription factors that are silent in resting cells, followed by a nuclear phase when transcription factors orchestrate changes in gene expression (Fig. 7-1). Some signal transduction pathways stimulate cell motility or activate granule exocytosis from the cytoplasm without a change in gene expression. Signal transduction can result in a number of different consequences for a cell, including acquisition of new functions, induction of differentiation, commitment to a specific lineage, protection from cell death, initiation of proliferative and growth responses, and induction of cell cycle arrest or of death by apoptosis.

Antigen receptors on B and T lymphocytes are among the most sophisticated signaling machines known, and they will form a large part of the focus of this chapter. We will initially provide a broad overview of signal transduction, followed by a discussion of signaling mediated by clonally distributed antigen receptors in lymphocytes and by structurally related immune receptors found mainly in cells of the innate immune system. When discussing antigen receptors in T and B cells, we will examine the role of other receptors called coreceptors and costimulatory receptors that enhance lymphocyte activation by the antigen receptor, and we will discuss the role of inhibitory

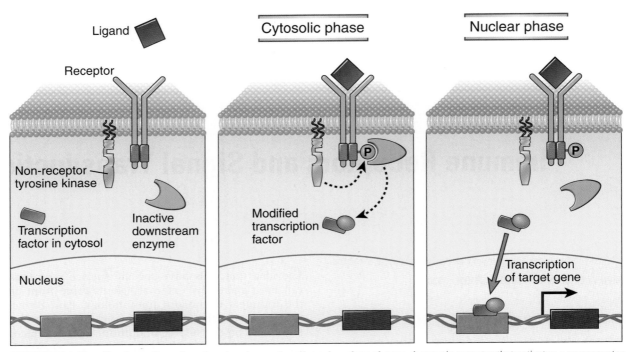

FIGURE 7-1 Signaling from the cell surface involves cytosolic and nuclear phases. A generic receptor that activates a non-receptor tyrosine kinase after it binds ligand is shown. In the cytosolic signaling phase, the non-receptor kinase phosphorylates a key tyrosine residue on the cytoplasmic tail of the receptor, as a result of which the phosphotyrosine-containing receptor tail is able to recruit a downstream enzyme that is activated once it is recruited. In the cytosolic phase, this activated downstream enzyme post-translationally modifies a specific transcription factor that is located in the cytoplasm. In this simplified example, the cytosolic phase has only a single enzymatic event, but many actual signal transduction pathways involve multiple steps. In the nuclear phase, this modified transcription factor enters the nucleus and induces the expression of target genes that have a binding site in the promoter or in some other regulatory region that can bind to this modified transcription factor and facilitate transcription.

receptors in T, B, and NK cells. We will also consider different categories of cytokine receptors and signal transduction mechanisms initiated by these receptors. Finally, to illustrate the steps in the activation of a prototypic transcription factor, we will examine the major pathway that leads to the activation of NF-κB, a transcription factor of relevance to both innate and adaptive immunity.

OVERVIEW OF SIGNAL TRANSDUCTION

Receptors that initiate signaling responses are generally integral membrane proteins present on the plasma membrane, where their extracellular domains recognize soluble secreted ligands or structures that are attached to the plasma membrane of a neighboring cell or cells. Another category of receptors, nuclear receptors, are intracellular transcription factors that are activated by lipid-soluble ligands that can cross the plasma membrane.

The initiation of signaling from a cell surface receptor may require ligand-induced clustering of receptor proteins, called cross-linking, or may involve a conformational alteration of the receptor induced by its association with ligand. Both mechanisms of signal initiation typically result in the creation of a novel geometric shape in the cytosolic portion of the receptor that promotes interactions with other signaling molecules.

A common early event in signal transduction is the enzymatic addition of a phosphate residue on a tyrosine, *serine, or threonine side chain in the cytosolic portion of a receptor or in an adaptor protein.* The enzymes that add phosphate groups onto amino acid side chains are called **protein kinases**. Many of the initiating events in lymphocyte signaling depend on protein kinases that phosphorylate specific tyrosine residues, and these enzymes are therefore called **protein tyrosine kinases**. Other protein kinases that are involved in distinct signaling pathways are serine/threonine kinases, which phosphorylate serine or threonine residues. Some enzymes activated downstream of signaling receptors phosphorylate lipid substrates; they are therefore known as **lipid kinases**. For every type of phosphorylation event, there is also a specific phosphatase, an enzyme that can remove the phosphate residue and thus modulate signaling. These phosphatases play important, usually inhibitory, roles in signal transduction.

Phosphorylation of proteins is not the only post-translational modification that drives signal transduction. Many other modifications can facilitate signaling events. A type of modification that we will describe later in this chapter is the covalent addition of ubiquitin molecules that either target proteins for degradation or drive signal transduction in many cells, including lymphocytes. Many important protein signaling molecules are modified by the addition of lipids that may help localize these proteins to a specialized region of the plasma membrane in order for them to efficiently interact with other signaling molecules that are also targeted to this membrane

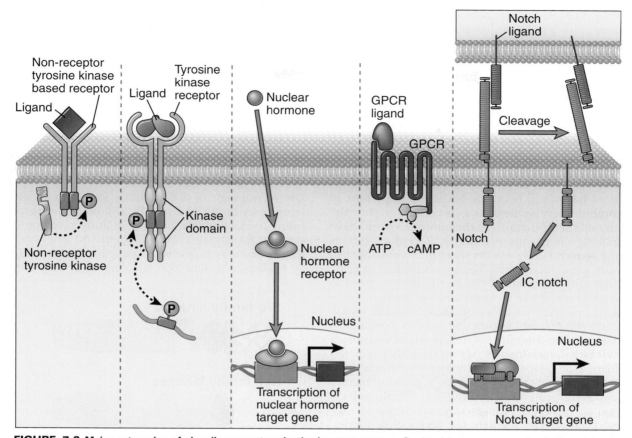

FIGURE 7-2 Major categories of signaling receptors in the immune system. Depicted here are a receptor that uses a non-receptor tyrosine kinase, a receptor tyrosine kinase, a nuclear receptor that binds its ligand and can then influence transcription, a seven-transmembrane G protein–coupled receptor (GPCR), and Notch, which recognizes a ligand on a distinct cell and is cleaved, yielding an intracellular fragment (IC Notch) that can enter the nucleus and influence transcription of specific target genes.

micro-domain. Some transcription factors are functionally modified by acetylation, and the *N*-terminal tails of histones can be acetylated and methylated in order to modulate gene expression, DNA replication, and DNA recombination events.

Cellular receptors are grouped into several categories based on the signaling mechanisms they use and the intracellular biochemical pathways they activate (Fig. 7-2):

- Receptors that use **non-receptor tyrosine kinases.** In this category of membrane receptors, the cytoplasmic tails of the ligand-binding polypeptides have no intrinsic catalytic activity, but a separate intracellular tyrosine kinase, known as a non-receptor tyrosine kinase, participates in receptor activation by phosphorylating specific motifs on the receptor or on other proteins associated with the receptor (see Fig. 7-1). A family of receptors called immune receptors, some of which recognize antigens while others recognize the Fc portions of antibodies, all use non-receptor tyrosine kinases to initiate signaling. Apart from the immune receptor family, some cytokine receptors, discussed later in this chapter, use non-receptor tyrosine kinases. Integrins, key adhesion receptors in the immune system, also signal by activating non-receptor tyrosine kinases.

- **Receptor tyrosine kinases (RTKs)** are integral membrane proteins that activate an intrinsic tyrosine kinase domain (or domains) located in the cytoplasmic tails of the receptors when they are cross-linked by multivalent extracellular ligands. An example of an RTK relevant to blood cell formation is the c-Kit protein. Other examples of RTKs include the insulin receptor, the epidermal growth factor receptor, and the platelet-derived growth factor receptor.

- **Nuclear receptors.** These receptors are typically located in or migrate into the nucleus, where they function as transcription factors. The binding of a lipid-soluble ligand to its nuclear receptor results in the ability of the latter either to induce transcription or to repress gene expression. Nuclear hormone receptors, such as the vitamin D receptor and the glucocorticoid receptor, can influence events that range from development of the immune system to modulation of cytokine gene expression.

- **G protein–coupled receptors (GPCRs)** are receptors that function by activating associated GTP-binding proteins (G proteins). They are polypeptides that traverse the plasma membrane seven times, because of which they are sometimes called serpentine receptors. A conformational change induced by the binding of ligand to this type of receptor permits the activation of an associated heterotrimeric G protein by the exchange of bound GDP with GTP. The activated G protein initiates downstream signaling events.

Examples of this category of receptors that are relevant to immunity and inflammation include receptors for leukotrienes, prostaglandins, histamine, complement fragments C3a and C5a, bacterial formyl peptides, and all chemokines (see Chapter 3). Different types of G proteins linked to distinct GPCRs may activate or inhibit different downstream effectors. Two major enzymes that GPCRs activate are adenylate cyclase, which converts ATP to the effector molecule cAMP, capable of activating numerous cellular responses, and phospholipase C, which also triggers multiple signals as discussed later.

- **Other classes of receptors.** Other categories of receptors have long been known to be important in embryonic development and in certain mature tissues, and their functions in the immune system have begun to emerge more recently. Receptor proteins of the **Notch** family are involved in development in a wide range of species. The association of specific ligands with receptors of this family leads to proteolytic cleavage of the receptor and the nuclear translocation of the cleaved cytoplasmic domain (intracellular Notch), which functions as a component of a transcription complex. Notch proteins contribute to cell fate determination during lymphocyte development (see Chapter 8) and may also influence the activation of mature lymphocytes. A group of ligands called **Wnt** proteins can influence lymphopoiesis. Signaling through transmembrane receptors for these proteins can regulate the levels of β-catenin, which facilitates the transcriptional activity of proteins that contribute to B and T cell development, as discussed in Chapter 8. Numerous other signaling receptors and pathways first discovered in non–immune cell populations are now beginning to be studied in the context of lymphocyte biology. We will not attempt to comprehensively consider all of these pathways in this chapter.

Modular Signaling Proteins and Adaptors

Signaling molecules are often composed of distinct modules, each with a specific binding or catalytic function. The discovery of tyrosine phosphorylation represented a major breakthrough in the study of cellular signaling pathways. It was subsequently discovered that the sequence of amino acids surrounding specific phosphorylated tyrosine residues contributes to the interaction of tyrosine-phosphorylated proteins with other signaling molecules. The study of non-receptor tyrosine kinases has shown us that signaling molecules contain distinct modules, or domains, each of which has different functions. The cellular homologue of the transforming protein of the Rous sarcoma virus, called c-Src, is the prototype for an immunologically important family of non-receptor tyrosine kinases known as **Src family kinases**. c-Src contains unique domains, including **Src homology 2** (SH2) and **Src homology 3** (SH3) domains. It also contains a catalytic tyrosine kinase domain and an N-terminal lipid addition domain that facilitates the covalent addition of a myristic acid molecule to the protein. The myristate helps target Src family kinases to the plasma membrane. The

modular structures of three families of tyrosine kinases that are important in the immune system are depicted in Figure 7-3.

SH2 domains are composed of about 100 amino acids folded into a particular conformation, and they bind to phosphotyrosine-containing peptides in certain proteins. In antigen receptor signaling, Src family kinases phosphorylate tyrosine residues present in particular motifs in the cytoplasmic tails of proteins that are part of the receptor complex (described later). These phosphotyrosine motifs in the antigen receptor complex then serve as binding sites for SH2 domains present in tyrosine kinases of the Syk family, such as Syk and ZAP-70 (see Fig. 7-3). The recruitment of a Syk family kinase to an antigen receptor by means of a specific SH2 domain–phosphotyrosine interaction is a key step in antigen receptor activation. SH3 domains are also about 100 amino acids in length, and they help mediate protein-protein interactions by binding to proline-rich stretches in certain proteins.

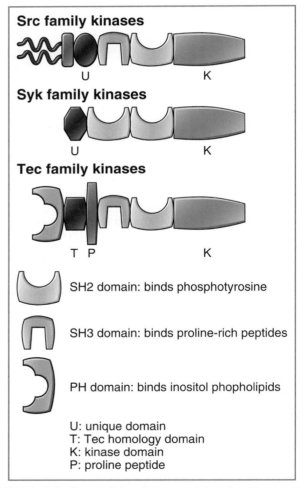

Src family kinases

U   K

Syk family kinases

U   K

Tec family kinases

T P   K

SH2 domain: binds phosphotyrosine

SH3 domain: binds proline-rich peptides

PH domain: binds inositol phopholipids

U: unique domain
T: Tec homology domain
K: kinase domain
P: proline peptide

FIGURE 7-3 The modular structure of tyrosine kinases that influence lymphocyte activation. Modules include SH2 domains that bind specific phosphotyrosine-containing polypeptides, SH3 domains that recognize proline-rich stretches in polypeptides, PH domains that recognize PIP3 or other phosphatidylinositol-derived lipids, and Tec homology domains found in tyrosine kinases of the Tec family. Tyrosine kinase families depicted are the Src family kinases, which include c-Src, Lyn, Fyn, and Lck; the Syk family kinases, which include Syk and ZAP-70; and the Tec family kinases, which include Tec, Btk, and Itk.

Another type of modular domain, called the pleckstrin homology (PH) domain, can recognize specific phospholipids. The PH domains in a number of signaling molecules, including the TEC family tyrosine kinase Btk, recognize phosphatidylinositol trisphosphate (PIP3), a lipid moiety on the inner leaflet of the plasma membrane.

Adaptor proteins function as molecular hubs that physically link different enzymes and promote the assembly of complexes of signaling molecules. Adaptors may be integral membrane proteins such as LAT (linker for the activation of T cells) (Fig. 7-4), or they may be cytosolic proteins such as BLNK (B cell linker), SLP-76 (SH2 domain–containing linker protein of 76 kD), and GADS (Grb-2–related adaptor protein downstream of Shc). A typical adaptor may contain a few specific domains that mediate protein-protein interactions, such as SH2 and SH3 domains, among others (there are many more types of modular domains not mentioned here). Adaptors often contain some proline-rich stretches that can bind other proteins that contain SH3 domains, and they also often contain tyrosine residues that may be phosphorylated by tyrosine kinases and serve as docking sites for other signaling molecules. The amino acid residues that are close to a tyrosine moiety that is phosphorylated determine which specific SH2 domains may bind that site. For instance, an upstream or initiating tyrosine kinase may phosphorylate a YxxM motif (where Y represents tyrosine, M represents methionine, and x refers to any amino acid) in an adaptor protein, and this may permit binding of an SH2 domain in the lipid kinase phosphatidylinositol 3-kinase (PI3-kinase). A proline-rich stretch in the same adaptor protein may bind a specific SH3 domain in a distinct downstream tyrosine kinase. Thus, tyrosine phosphorylation of the adaptor can result in a downstream tyrosine kinase and PI3-kinase being perched next to each other, resulting in the phosphorylation and activation of PI3-kinase. Signal transduction can therefore be visualized as a kind of social networking phenomenon. An initial signal (tyrosine phosphorylation, for instance) results in proteins being brought close to one another at designated hubs (adaptors), resulting in the activation of specific enzymes that eventually influence the nuclear localization or activity of specific downstream transcription factors or induce other cellular events, such as actin polymerization.

THE IMMUNE RECEPTOR FAMILY

Immune receptors are a unique family of receptor complexes typically made up of integral membrane proteins of the immunoglobulin (Ig) superfamily that are involved in ligand recognition, associated with other transmembrane signaling proteins that have unique tyrosine-containing motifs in their cytoplasmic tails. Whereas the signaling components are generally separate proteins from those involved in ligand recognition, in a few members of the family, the receptor consists of a single chain in which the extracellular domain is involved in ligand recognition and the cytoplasmic tail contains tyrosine residues that contribute to signaling. The signaling proteins of the immune receptor family are often positioned close to non-receptor tyrosine kinases of the Src family, which possess *N*-terminal lipid anchors that tether them to the inner leaflet of the plasma membrane.

The cytoplasmic tyrosine-containing motifs on the signaling proteins of the immune receptor family are generally one of two different types. **ITAMs** (**immunoreceptor tyrosine-based activating motifs**) are found on receptors involved in cell activation and have the sequence $YxxL/I(x)_{6-8}YxxL/I$, where *Y* represents a tyrosine residue, *L* represents leucine, *I* represents isoleucine, and *x* refers to any amino acid. Both tyrosine residues in ITAM motifs can be phosphorylated by Src family kinases when immune receptors are activated. Tyrosine-phosphorylated ITAMs recruit a distinct tyrosine kinase of the Syk/ZAP-70 family, which contains tandem SH2 domains that each bind to one of the two phosphorylated YxxL/I motifs of the ITAM. Binding of the Syk (or ZAP-70) kinase to an ITAM causes a conformational change that activates the kinase, leading to additional signaling events that drive immune cell activation. Some immune receptors inhibit cellular responses, and signaling chains in these receptors may contain a slightly different tyrosine-containing motif that is called an **ITIM** (**immunoreceptor tyrosine-based inhibitory motif**),

FIGURE 7-4 Selected adaptors that participate in lymphocyte activation. On the left, LAT, an integral membrane protein that functions as an adaptor, and two cytosolic adaptors, GADS and SLP-76, are shown in a non-activated T cell. On the right, after T cell activation, LAT is tyrosine phosphorylated and is shown to have recruited PLCγ (which simultaneously binds to the membrane phospholipid PIP3) and the GADS adaptor, both of which contain SH2 domains. A proline-rich amino acid stretch in SLP-76 associates with an SH3 domain of GADS, and tyrosine-phosphorylated SLP-76 recruits Vav.

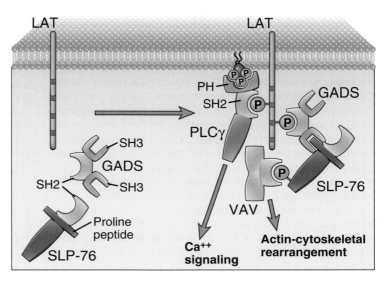

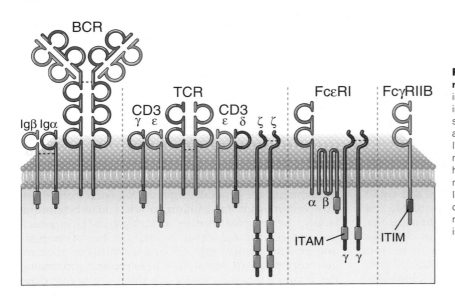

FIGURE 7-5 Selected members of the immune receptor family. Four selected members of the immune receptor family are depicted. Typically, immune receptors that activate immune cells have separate polypeptide chains for recognition and associated polypeptide chains that contain cytosolic ITAMs. Examples shown here include the B cell receptor (BCR), the T cell receptor (TCR), and the high-affinity receptor for IgE (FcεRI). Inhibitory receptors in the immune system typically have ITIM motifs on the cytosolic portion of the same chain that uses its extracellular domain for ligand recognition. The inhibitory receptor shown, FcγRIIB, is found on B cells and myeloid cells.

which has the consensus sequence V/L/IxYxxL, where V refers to valine. Phosphorylated ITIMs recruit tyrosine or inositol lipid phosphatases, enzymes that remove phosphate residues from phosphotyrosine moieties or from certain lipid phosphates and thus counteract ITAM-based immune receptor activation.

Members of the immune receptor family include antigen receptors on B cells and T cells, the IgE-specific Fc receptor on mast cells, and IgG-specific activating and inhibitory Fc receptors on innate immune cells and B lymphocytes (Fig. 7-5). These immune receptors form complexes with ITAM-containing proteins that are involved in signal transduction, including the ζ chain and CD3 proteins of the T cell receptor (TCR) complex, Igα and Igβ proteins associated with membrane Ig molecules, the antigen receptors of B cells, and components of several Fc receptors and of the NKG2D activating receptor on natural killer (NK) cells (see Chapter 4). The inhibitory receptors, including CD22, FcγRIIB, and several inhibitory NK cell receptors, contain ITIMs in their cytoplasmic domains or in associated proteins.

General Features of Antigen Receptor Signaling

Signaling downstream of T and B cell antigen receptors is characterized by a similar sequence of events, consisting of the following.

- Receptor ligation typically involves the clustering of receptors by multivalent ligands and results in activation of an associated Src family kinase. Receptor ligation may also induce the unfolding of the cytoplasmic tail of a polypeptide chain that is part of the receptor. The unfolding event (or conformational change) may allow previously hidden tyrosine residues of a cytosolic ITAM motif to become available for phosphorylation by a Src family kinase.
- The activated Src family kinase phosphorylates available tyrosines in the ITAMs of signaling proteins that are part of the receptor complex.
- The two phosphorylated tyrosines in a single ITAM are recognized by a Syk family tyrosine kinase that has tandem SH2 domains that each bind to an ITAM phosphotyrosine.

- Recruitment of the Syk family kinase to the phosphorylated ITAM results in the activation of this tyrosine kinase and the subsequent tyrosine phosphorylation of adaptor proteins and enzymes that activate distinct signaling pathways downstream of the immune receptor.

This sequence of events is described in more detail in the context of T cell and B cell receptor signaling later in this chapter.

Alterations in the strength of TCR and B cell receptor (BCR) signaling influence the responses of lymphocytes during their development and activation. In other words, the presence of different numbers of activated signaling molecules induced by antigen-ligated receptors is interpreted differently by lymphocytes. For instance, during maturation of T cells in the thymus, weak antigen receptor signals are required for positive selection, the process that preserves useful cells by matching coreceptors to the appropriate MHC molecules, and gradations of signal strength may determine positive selection of developing T cells into the CD4 or CD8 lineage (see Chapter 8). In contrast, strong antigen receptor signals during maturation may contribute to lymphocyte death by apoptosis. The strength of TCR and BCR signaling may also differentially influence the type of immune response that is generated by a given antigen.

Antigen receptor signaling is fine-tuned and modulated by three mechanisms that are unique to this class of receptors.

- *Progressive ITAM use.* One of the ways in which different quantities of signal output might be generated by antigen receptors is the phosphorylation of different numbers of ITAM tyrosines after receptor engagement. The TCR complex has six signaling chains and ten ITAMs, and increasing numbers of ITAMs may be phosphorylated with stronger or prolonged binding of antigen to the TCR. The number of ITAMs phosphorylated may therefore provide a cytosolic interpretation of the affinity of the antigen that binds to the TCR, and antigen affinity can thus influence the nature of the cellular response at different stages of differentiation and activation. The BCR has only two ITAMs, but because this number increases when multiple receptor proteins are cross-linked by multivalent antigens, the degree of cross-linking by antigens may determine the number of ITAMs that might be used and thus generate different responses to antigens of differing affinity and valency.

- *Increased cellular activation by coreceptors.* A **coreceptor** is a transmembrane signaling protein on a lymphocyte that can facilitate antigen receptor activation by simultaneously binding to the same antigen complex that is recognized by the antigen receptor. The coreceptor brings with it signaling enzymes linked to its cytoplasmic tail and can thereby facilitate ITAM phosphorylation and activation of the antigen receptor when antigen draws it into the vicinity of the antigen receptor. Coreceptors on T cells are the CD4 and CD8 proteins that demarcate two functionally distinct subsets. Complement receptor type 2 (CR2/CD21) is the coreceptor on B cells (see Chapter 12).
- *Modulation of signaling by inhibitory receptors.* Key **inhibitory receptors** in T cells include CTLA-4 and PD-1, whereas important inhibitory signals in B cells are delivered through receptors such as CD22 and FcγRIIB, among others. The roles of these inhibitors are discussed later in this chapter.

In addition, antigen receptor signals may, in some circumstances, cooperate with signals from proteins called **costimulatory receptors** that add yet another level of control to the process of lymphocyte activation. Costimulatory receptors provide so-called *second signals* for lymphocytes (antigen recognition provides the first signal) and ensure that immune responses are optimally triggered by infectious pathogens and substances that mimic microbes, which are the agents that induce or activate costimulators (see Figs. 4-18 and 9-3). Unlike coreceptors, costimulatory receptors do not recognize components of the same ligands as do antigen receptors; signal outputs downstream of costimulatory receptors are integrated with the signals derived from the antigen receptor, and these signals cooperate to fully activate lymphocytes. The prototypic costimulatory receptor is CD28 on T cells, which is activated by the costimulatory molecules B7-1 (CD80) and B7-2 (CD86), ligands induced on antigen-presenting cells (APCs) as a result of their exposure to microbes (see Chapter 9).

THE T CELL RECEPTOR COMPLEX AND T CELL SIGNALING

The TCR was discovered in the early 1980s, at around the same time that the structure of major histocompatibility complex (MHC) molecules associated with peptides, the ligands for T cells, was being defined (see Chapter 6). This was years after the B cell antigen receptor and Ig genes were characterized. The methods used to search for the proteins of the TCR and the genes encoding them relied on the assumption that they would be similar to Ig proteins and genes. We now know that TCRs are similar to

antibodies, but there are important differences between these two types of antigen receptors (Table 7-1).

The Structure of the T Cell Receptor for Antigen

The antigen receptor of MHC-restricted CD4+ helper T cells and CD8+ cytotoxic T lymphocytes (CTLs) is a heterodimer consisting of two transmembrane polypeptide chains, designated TCR α and β, covalently linked to each other by a disulfide bridge between extracellular cysteine residues (Fig. 7-6). These T cells are called αβ T cells. A less common type of TCR is composed of TCR γ and δ chains, and the cells on which it is expressed are called γδ T cells. Each TCR α and β chain consists of one Ig-like N-terminal variable (V) domain, one Ig-like constant (C) domain, a hydrophobic transmembrane region, and a short cytoplasmic region. Thus, the extracellular portion of the TCR αβ heterodimer is structurally similar to the antigen-binding fragment (Fab) of an Ig molecule, which is made up of the V and C regions of a light chain and the V region and one C region of a heavy chain (see Chapter 5).

The V regions of the TCR α and β chains contain short stretches of amino acids where the variability between different TCRs is concentrated, and these form the hypervariable or complementarity-determining regions (CDRs). Three CDRs in the α chain and three similar regions in the β chain together form the part of the TCR that specifically recognizes peptide-MHC complexes (Fig. 7-7). The β chain V domain contains a fourth hypervariable region that does not appear to participate in antigen recognition but is the binding site for microbial products called superantigens (see Chapter 15). Each

TABLE 7-1 Properties of Lymphocyte Antigen Receptors: T Cell Receptor and Immunoglobulins

	T Cell Receptor (TCR)	Immunoglobulin (Ig)
Components	α and β chains	Heavy and light chains
Number of Ig domains	One V domain and one C domain in each chain	Heavy chain: one V domain, three or four C domains Light chain: one V domain and one C domain
Number of CDRs involved in antigen binding	Six (three in each chain)	Six (three in each chain)
Associated signaling molecules	CD3 and ζ	Igα and Igβ
Affinity for antigen (K_d)	10^{-5}–10^{-7} M	10^{-7}–10^{-11} M (secreted Ig)
Changes After Cellular Activation		
Production of secreted form	No	Yes
Isotope switching	No	Yes
Somatic mutations	No	Yes

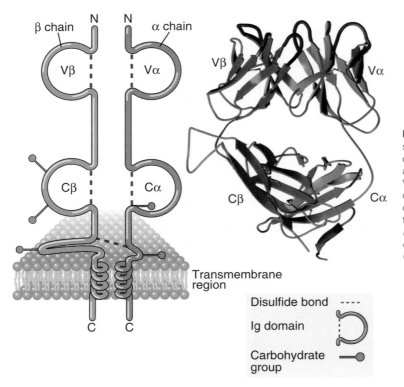

FIGURE 7-6 Structure of the T cell receptor. The schematic diagram of the αβ TCR *(left)* shows the domains of a typical TCR specific for a peptide-MHC complex. The antigen-binding portion of the TCR is formed by the V_β and V_α domains. The ribbon diagram *(right)* shows the structure of the extracellular portion of a TCR as revealed by x-ray crystallography. The hypervariable segment loops that form the peptide-MHC binding site are at the top. *(Modified from Bjorkman PJ: MHC restriction in three dimensions: a view of T cell receptor/ligand interactions, Cell 89:167–170, 1997. Copyright © Cell Press.)*

TCR chain, like Ig heavy and light chains, is encoded by multiple gene segments that are joined together during the maturation of T lymphocytes (see Chapter 8).

The C regions of both α and β chains continue into short hinge regions, which contain cysteine residues that contribute to a disulfide bond linking the two chains. Each hinge is followed by a hydrophobic transmembrane portion, an unusual feature of which is the presence of positively charged amino acid residues, including a lysine residue (in the α chain) or a lysine and an arginine residue (in the β chain). These residues interact with negatively charged residues present in the transmembrane portions of other polypeptides (those of the CD3 complex and ζ) that are part of the TCR complex. Both TCR

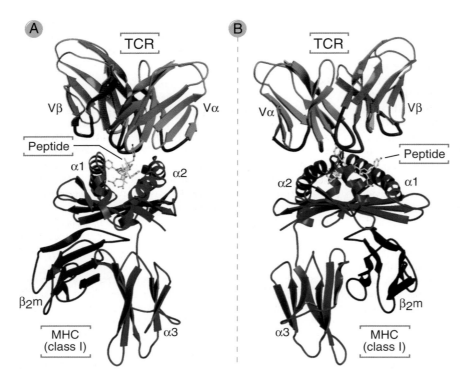

FIGURE 7-7 Binding of a TCR to a peptide-MHC complex. The V domains of a TCR are shown interacting with a human class I MHC molecule, HLA-A2, presenting a viral peptide *(in yellow)*. **A** is a front view and **B** is a side view of the x-ray crystal structure of the trimolecular MHC-peptide-TCR complex. *(From Bjorkman PJ: MHC restriction in three dimensions: a view of T cell receptor/ligand interactions, Cell 89:167–170, 1997. Copyright © Cell Press.)*

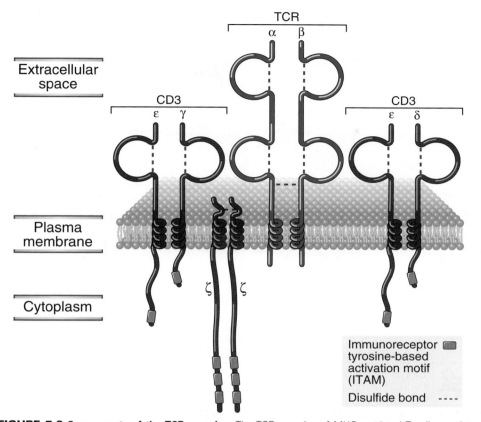

FIGURE 7-8 Components of the TCR complex. The TCR complex of MHC-restricted T cells consists of the αβ TCR non-covalently linked to the CD3 and ζ proteins. The association of these proteins with one another is mediated by charged residues in their transmembrane regions *(not shown)*.

α and β chains have carboxyl-terminal cytoplasmic tails that are 5 to 12 amino acids long. Like membrane Ig on B cells (see later), these cytoplasmic regions are too small to transduce signals, and molecules physically associated with the TCR serve the signal-transducing functions of this antigen receptor complex.

The CD3 and ζ proteins are non-covalently associated with the TCR αβ heterodimer to form the TCR complex, and when the TCR recognizes antigen, these associated proteins transduce the signals that lead to T cell activation. The components of the TCR complex are illustrated in Figures 7-8 and 7-9. The CD3 proteins and the ζ chain are identical in all T cells regardless of specificity, which is consistent with their role in signaling and not in antigen recognition. The CD3 proteins are also required for surface expression of the complete receptor complex on T cells.

The CD3 γ, δ, and ε proteins are homologous to each other. The *N*-terminal extracellular regions of the γ, δ, and ε chains of CD3 each contains a single Ig-like domain, and therefore these three proteins are members of the Ig superfamily. The transmembrane segments of all three CD3 chains contain a negatively charged aspartic acid residue that binds to positively charged residues in the transmembrane domains of the TCR α and β chains. Each TCR complex contains one TCR αβ heterodimer associated with one CD3 γε heterodimer, one CD3 δε heterodimer, and one disulfide-linked ζ homodimer.

The cytoplasmic domains of the CD3 γ, δ, and ε proteins range from 44 to 81 amino acid residues in length,

and each of these domains contains one ITAM. The ζ chain has a short extracellular region of nine amino acids, a transmembrane region containing a negatively charged aspartic acid residue (similar to the CD3 chains), and a long cytoplasmic region (113 amino acids) that contains three ITAMs. It is normally expressed as a homodimer. The ζ chain is also associated with signaling receptors on lymphocytes other than T cells, such as the Fcγ receptor (FcγRIII) of NK cells.

Signal Initiation by the T Cell Receptor

Ligation of the TCR by MHC-peptide ligands results in the clustering of coreceptors with the antigen receptor and phosphorylation of ITAM tyrosine residues. Phosphorylation of ITAM tyrosines initiates signal transduction and the activation of downstream tyrosine kinases, which in turn phosphorylate tyrosine residues on other adaptor proteins. The subsequent steps in signal transduction are generated by the specific recruitment of key enzymes that each initiate distinct downstream signaling pathways.

It is thought that the TCR, like other immune receptors, is activated when multiple receptor molecules are brought together by binding to adjacent antigenic epitopes. However, cross-linking of the TCR poses a challenge because the induction of receptor clustering would require a high density of identical MHC-peptide complexes on APCs, and APCs generally express very few MHC molecules containing

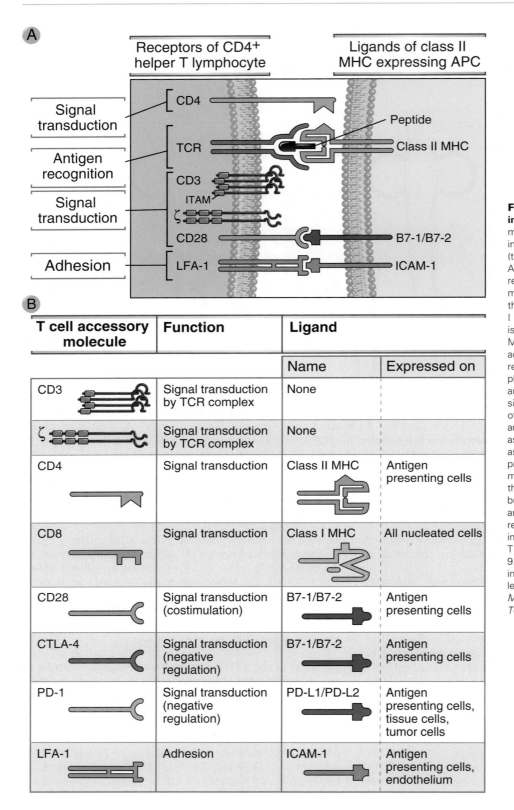

B

T cell accessory molecule	Function	Ligand	
		Name	Expressed on
CD3	Signal transduction by TCR complex	None	
ζ	Signal transduction by TCR complex	None	
CD4	Signal transduction	Class II MHC	Antigen presenting cells
CD8	Signal transduction	Class I MHC	All nucleated cells
CD28	Signal transduction (costimulation)	B7-1/B7-2	Antigen presenting cells
CTLA-4	Signal transduction (negative regulation)	B7-1/B7-2	Antigen presenting cells
PD-1	Signal transduction (negative regulation)	PD-L1/PD-L2	Antigen presenting cells, tissue cells, tumor cells
LFA-1	Adhesion	ICAM-1	Antigen presenting cells, endothelium

FIGURE 7-9 Ligand-receptor pairs involved in T cell activation. A, The major surface molecules of CD4+ T cells involved in the activation of these cells (the receptors) and the molecules on APCs (the ligands) recognized by the receptors are shown. CD8+ T cells use most of the same molecules, except that the TCR recognizes peptide–class I MHC complexes, and the coreceptor is CD8, which recognizes class I MHC. Immunoreceptor tyrosine-based activation motifs (ITAMs) are the regions of signaling proteins that are phosphorylated on tyrosine residues and become docking sites for other signaling molecules. CD3 is composed of three polypeptide chains, named γ, δ, and ε, arranged in two pairs (γε and δε) as shown in Figure 7-8; we show CD3 as three protein chains. **B,** The important properties of the major accessory molecules of T cells, so called because they participate in responses to antigens but are not the receptors for antigen, are summarized. CTLA-4 (CD152) is a receptor for B7 molecules that delivers inhibitory signals; its role in shutting off T cell responses is described in Chapter 9. *APC,* antigen-presenting cell; *ICAM-1,* intercellular adhesion molecule 1; *LFA-1,* leukocyte function-associated antigen 1; *MHC,* major histocompatibility complex; *TCR,* T cell receptor.

the same peptide, perhaps as few as 100 per cell, that may be recognized by a given TCR (see Chapter 6). How, then, is the signal from the TCR initiated? Recognition of MHC-peptide complexes may induce a conformational change in the TCR, making the ITAMs associated with the linked CD3 or ζ chains available for tyrosine phosphorylation by Src family kinases. The CD4 and CD8 coreceptors (described next) greatly facilitate the activation process by bringing Lck (which is loosely associated with the tail of the coreceptor proteins) close to the CD3 and ζ ITAMs. The actual mechanism of signal initiation remains to be conclusively determined. Eventually, a stable interface is formed between the

T cell and the APC, known as the immunologic synapse (discussed later).

The Role of the CD4 and CD8 Coreceptors in T Cell Activation

CD4 and CD8 are T cell coreceptors that bind to non-polymorphic regions of MHC molecules and facilitate signaling by the TCR complex during T cell activation (see Fig. 7-9). These proteins are called *coreceptors* because they bind to MHC molecules and thus recognize a part of the same ligand (peptide-MHC complexes) that interacts with the TCR. Mature αβ T cells express either CD4 or CD8, but not both. CD8 and CD4 interact with class I and class II MHC molecules, respectively, and are responsible for the class I or class II MHC restriction of these subsets of T cells (see Fig. 7-9 and Chapter 6).

CD4 and CD8 are transmembrane glycoprotein members of the Ig superfamily (Fig. 7-10). CD4 is expressed as a monomer on the surface of peripheral T cells and thymocytes and is also present at lower levels on mononuclear phagocytes and some dendritic cells. The human immunodeficiency virus (HIV) uses CD4 as a receptor to gain entry into T lymphocytes and other immune cells that express the molecule. CD4 has four extracellular Ig-like domains, a hydrophobic transmembrane region, and a highly basic cytoplasmic tail 38 amino acids long. The two *N*-terminal Ig-like domains of the CD4 protein bind to the non-polymorphic α2 and β2 domains of the class II MHC molecule.

Most CD8 molecules exist as disulfide-linked heterodimers composed of two related chains called CD8α and CD8β (see Fig. 7-10). Both the α chain and the β chain have a single extracellular Ig domain, a hydrophobic transmembrane region, and a highly basic cytoplasmic tail that is about 25 amino acids long. The Ig domain of CD8 binds mainly to the non-polymorphic α3 domain of class I MHC molecules, and also interacts with portions

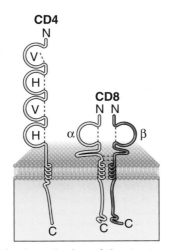

FIGURE 7-10 A schematic view of the structure of the CD4 and CD8 coreceptors. The CD4 protein is an integral membrane monomer consisting of four extracellular Ig domains, a transmembrane domain, and a cytoplasmic tail. The CD8 protein is either a disulfide-linked αβ integral membrane heterodimer or a disulfide linked αα homodimer *(not shown)*. Each chain has a single extracellular Ig domain. The cytoplasmic portions of both CD4 and CD8 can associate with Lck *(not shown)*.

of the α2 domain and with β2 microglobulin. Some activated and memory T cells express CD8 αα homodimers, and this different form may have inhibitory rather than activating functions, presumably because it is excluded from signaling microdomains called lipid rafts. These homodimers are also present on a subset of murine dendritic cells (see Chapter 6).

The cytoplasmic tails of both CD4 and CD8 bind the Src family kinase Lck. The ability of the extracellular domains of these coreceptors to bind to MHC molecules helps these proteins to be drawn adjacent to the TCR that contacts the same MHC-peptide complex on the APC. As a result, on the cytosolic face of the membrane, Lck is brought in close proximity to the ITAMs in CD3 and ζ proteins and phosphorylates the tyrosine residues in these ITAMs, thus facilitating the subsequent recruitment and activation of the ZAP-70 tyrosine kinase.

Activation of Tyrosine Kinases and a Lipid Kinase During T Cell Activation

Phosphorylation of proteins and lipids plays a central role in the transduction of signals from the TCR complex and coreceptors. Even before TCR activation there is some basal tyrosine phosphorylation of ITAM tyrosines and some recruitment of ZAP-70, described below, to these phosphorylated ITAMs. Within seconds of TCR ligation, Lck is brought close to the tyrosine residues within the ITAMs of the CD3 and ζ chains, which are thus more extensively phosphorylated (Fig. 7-11). In addition to coreceptor-associated Lck, another Src family kinase that is found in physical association with the TCR complex is CD3-associated Fyn, and it may contribute to basal ITAM tyrosine phosphorylation. Knockout mice lacking Lck exhibit some defects in TCR signaling and T cell development, and double knockout mice lacking both Lck and Fyn have even more severe defects.

The tyrosine-phosphorylated ITAMs in the ζ chain are docking sites for the Syk family tyrosine kinase called **ZAP-70** (ζ-associated protein of 70 kD). ZAP-70 contains two SH2 domains that can bind to ITAM phosphotyrosines. As discussed earlier, each ITAM has two tyrosine residues, and both of these must be phosphorylated to provide a docking site for one ZAP-70 molecule. The bound ZAP-70 becomes a substrate for the adjacent Lck after TCR recognition of antigen, and Lck phosphorylates specific tyrosine residues of ZAP-70. As a result, ZAP-70 acquires its own tyrosine kinase activity and is then able to phosphorylate a number of other cytoplasmic signaling molecules. A critical threshold of ZAP-70 activity may be needed before downstream signaling events will proceed, and this threshold is achieved by the recruitment of multiple ZAP-70 molecules to the phosphorylated ITAMs on the ζ chains and on CD3 tails.

Another signaling pathway in T cells involves the activation of **PI3-kinase**, which phosphorylates a specific membrane-associated inositol lipid (Fig. 7-12). This enzyme is recruited to the TCR complex and associated adaptor proteins and generates phosphatidylinositol trisphosphate (PIP3) from phosphatidylinositol bisphosphate (PIP2), which is located on the inner leaflet of the plasma membrane. Certain signaling proteins in the

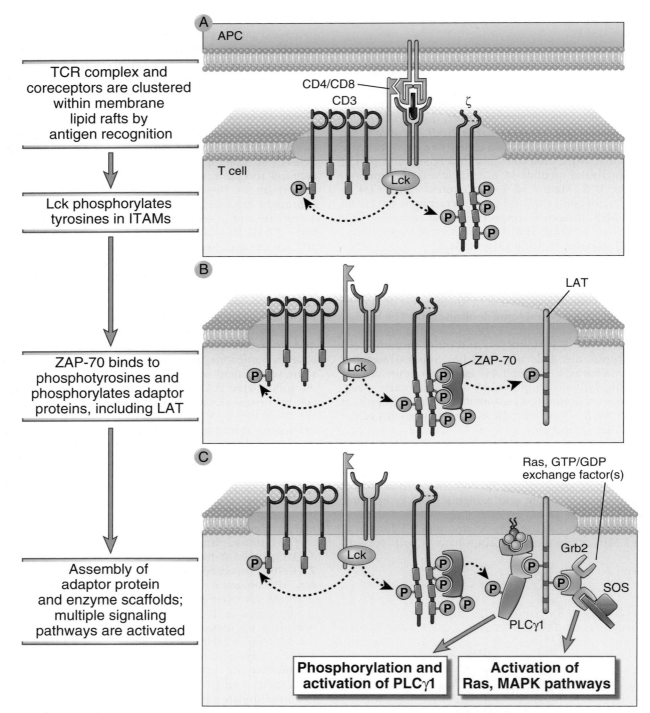

FIGURE 7-11 Early tyrosine phosphorylation events in T cell activation. On antigen recognition, there is clustering of TCR complexes with coreceptors (CD4, in this case). CD4-associated Lck becomes active and phosphorylates tyrosines in the ITAMs of CD3 and ζ chains **(A)**. ZAP-70 binds to the phosphotyrosines of the ζ chains and is itself phosphorylated and activated. (The illustration shows one ZAP-70 molecule binding to two phosphotyrosines of one ITAM in the ζ chain, but it is likely that initiation of a T cell response requires the assembly of multiple ZAP-70 molecules on each ζ chain.) Active ZAP-70 then phosphorylates tyrosines on various adaptor molecules, such as LAT **(B)**. The adaptors become docking sites for cellular enzymes such as PLCγ1 and exchange factors that activate Ras and other small G proteins upstream of MAP kinases **(C)**, and these enzymes activate various cellular responses.

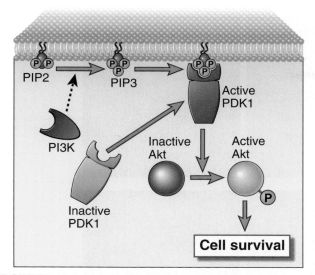

FIGURE 7-12 Role of PI3-kinase in T cell responses. Membrane PIP3, generated by PI3-kinase (PI3K), activates PDK1, which phosphorylates and activates the Akt kinase, which in turn phosphorylates downstream targets that are involved in cell survival.

cytosol have specialized PH domains that have an affinity for PIP3, and, as a result, PH domain–containing proteins can bind to the inside of the cell membrane only when PIP3 is generated. Examples of PH domain–containing proteins include tyrosine kinases such as Itk in T cells and Btk in B cells. Another important PIP3-dependent kinase is PDK1, which is required for the phosphorylation and activation of an important downstream kinase called Akt. Activated Akt phosphorylates crucial targets and contributes to cell survival in a number of ways, including the inactivation of pro-apoptotic members of the Bcl-2 family.

Recruitment and Modification of Adaptor Proteins

Activated ZAP-70 phosphorylates several adaptor proteins that are able to bind signaling molecules (see Fig. 7-11). A key early event in T cell activation is the ZAP-70–mediated tyrosine phosphorylation of adaptor proteins such as SLP-76 and LAT. Phosphorylated LAT directly binds PLCγ1, a key enzyme in T cell activation (discussed later), and coordinates the recruitment of several other adaptor proteins, including SLP-76, GADS, and Grb-2, to the cluster of TCR and TCR-associated proteins, sometimes referred to as the signalosome. Thus, LAT serves to bring a variety of downstream components of TCR signaling pathways close to their upstream activators. Because the function of many of these adaptors depends on their tyrosine phosphorylation by active ZAP-70, only antigen recognition (the physiologic stimulus for ZAP-70 activation) triggers the signal transduction pathways that lead to functional T cell responses.

Formation of the Immunologic Synapse

When the TCR complex recognizes MHC-associated peptides on an APC, several T cell surface proteins and intracellular signaling molecules are rapidly mobilized to the site of T cell–APC contact (Fig. 7-13). This region of physical contact between the T cell and the APC forms a bull's-eye–like structure that is called an **immunologic synapse** or a supramolecular activation cluster (SMAC). The T cell molecules that are rapidly mobilized to the center of the synapse include the TCR complex (the TCR, CD3, and ζ chains), CD4 or CD8 coreceptors, receptors for costimulators (such as CD28), enzymes such as PKC-θ, and adaptor proteins that associate with the cytoplasmic tails of the transmembrane receptors. At this region of the synapse, called the c-SMAC (for central supramolecular activation cluster), the distance between the T cell plasma membrane and that of the APC is about 15 nm. Integrins remain at the periphery of the synapse, where they function to stabilize the binding of the T cell to the APC, forming the peripheral portion of the SMAC called the p-SMAC. In this outer part of the synapse, the two membranes are about 40 nm apart. Many signaling molecules found in synapses are initially localized to regions of the plasma membrane that have a lipid content different from the rest of the cell membrane and are called lipid rafts or glycolipid-enriched microdomains. TCR and costimulatory receptor signaling is initiated in these rafts, and signaling initiates cytoskeletal rearrangements that allow rafts to coalesce and form the immunologic synapse.

Immunologic synapses may serve a number of functions during and after T cell activation.

- The synapse forms a stable contact between an antigen-specific T cell and an APC displaying that antigen and becomes the site for assembly of the signaling machinery of the T cell, including the TCR complex, coreceptors, costimulatory receptors, and adaptors. Although TCR signal transduction is clearly initiated before the formation of the synapse and is required for synapse formation, the immunologic synapse itself may provide a unique interface for TCR triggering. T cell activation needs to overcome the problems of a generally low affinity of TCRs for peptide-MHC ligands and the presence of few MHC molecules displaying any one peptide on an APC. The synapse represents a site at which repeated engagement of TCRs may be sustained by this small number of peptide-MHC complexes on the APC, thus facilitating prolonged and effective T cell signaling.

- The synapse may ensure the specific delivery of secretory granule contents and cytokines from a T cell to APCs or targets that are in contact with the T cell. Vectorial delivery of secretory granules containing perforin and granzymes from CTLs to target cells has been shown to occur at the synapse (see Chapter 11). Similarly, CD40L-CD40 interactions are facilitated by the accumulation of these molecules on the T cell and APC interfaces of the immunologic synapse. Some cytokines are also secreted in a directed manner into the synaptic cleft, from where they are preferentially delivered to the cell that is displaying antigen to the T lymphocyte.

- The synapse may also be an important site for the turnover of signaling molecules, primarily by monoubiquitination and delivery to late endosomes and lysosomes. This degradation of signaling proteins may contribute to the termination of T cell activation and is discussed later.

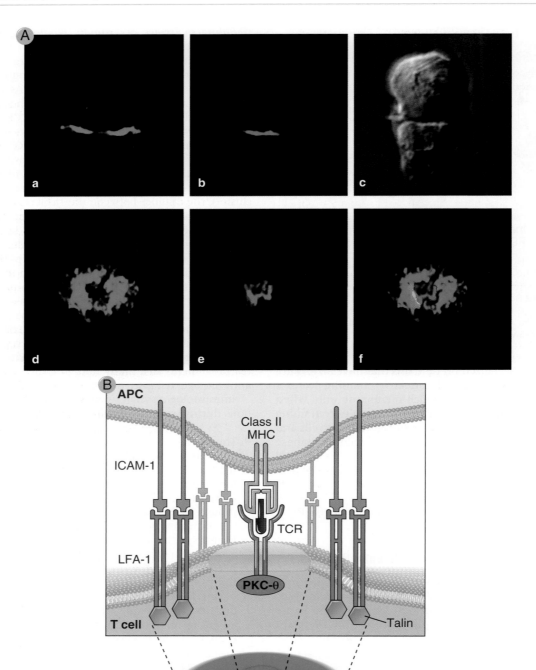

FIGURE 7-13 The immunologic synapse. A, This figure shows two views of the immunologic synapse in a T cell–APC conjugate (shown as a Nomarski image in panel c). Talin, a protein that associates with the cytoplasmic tail of the LFA-1 integrin, was revealed by an antibody labeled with a green fluorescent dye, and PKC-θ, which associates with the TCR complex, was visualized by antibodies conjugated to a red fluorescent dye. In panels a and b, a two-dimensional optical section of the cell contact site along the x-y axis is shown, revealing the central location of PKC-θ and the peripheral location of talin, both in the T cell. In panels d to f, a three-dimensional view of the entire region of cell-cell contact along the x-z axis is provided. Note, again, the central location of PKC-θ and the peripheral accumulation of talin. **B,** A schematic view of the synapse, showing talin and LFA-1 in the p-SMAC (green) and PKC-θ and the TCR in the c-SMAC (red). *(**A,** Reprinted with permission of Macmillan Publishers Ltd. from Monks CRF, Freiburg BA, Kupfer H, Sciaky N, Kupfer A: Three dimensional segregation of supramolecular activation clusters in T cells, Nature 395:82–86. Copyright © 1998.)*

MAP Kinase Signaling Pathways in T Lymphocytes

Small guanine nucleotide–binding proteins (G proteins) activated by antigen recognition stimulate at least three different mitogen-activated protein (MAP) kinases, which in turn activate distinct transcription factors. G proteins are involved in diverse activation responses in different cell types. Two major members of this family activated downstream of the TCR are Ras and Rac. Each activates a different component or set of transcription factors, and together they mediate many cellular responses of T cells.

- The **Ras** pathway is triggered in T cells after TCR ligation, leading to the activation of the extracellular receptor–activated kinase (ERK), a prominent member of the MAP kinase family, and eventually to the activation of downstream transcription factors. Ras is loosely attached to the plasma membrane through covalently attached lipids. In its inactive form, the guanine nucleotide–binding site of Ras is occupied by guanosine diphosphate (GDP). When the bound GDP is replaced by guanosine triphosphate (GTP), Ras undergoes a conformational change and can then recruit or activate various cellular enzymes, the most important of which is c-Raf. Activation of Ras by GDP/GTP exchange is seen in response to the engagement of many types of receptors in many cell populations, including the TCR complex in T cells. Mutated Ras proteins that are constitutively active (i.e., they constantly assume the GTP-bound conformation) are associated with neoplastic transformation of many cell types. Non-mutated Ras proteins are active GTPases that convert the GTP bound to Ras into GDP, thus returning Ras to its normal, inactive state.

The mechanism of Ras activation in T cells involves the adaptor proteins LAT and Grb-2 (Fig. 7-14). When LAT is phosphorylated by ZAP-70 at the site of TCR clustering, it serves as the docking site for the SH2 domain of Grb-2. Once attached to LAT, Grb-2 recruits the Ras GTP/GDP exchange factor called SOS (so named because it is the mammalian homologue of a *Drosophila* protein called son of sevenless) to the plasma membrane. SOS catalyzes GTP for GDP exchange on Ras. This generates the GTP-bound form of Ras (written as Ras·GTP), which then activates a MAP kinase cascade of three kinases. Ras·GTP directly activates a kinase called Raf, the first kinase in this cascade. Raf then phosphorylates and activates a dual-specificity kinase called MEK-1, which in turn phosphorylates the third kinase in the cascade, called ERK, on closely spaced threonine and tyrosine residues. ERK is a MAP kinase and MEK-1 is called a MAP kinase-kinase (a kinase that activates a MAP kinase). The activated ERK translocates to the nucleus and phosphorylates a protein called Elk, and phosphorylated Elk stimulates transcription of c-Fos, a component of the activation protein 1 (AP-1) transcription factor.

- In parallel with the activation of Ras through recruitment of Grb-2 and SOS, the adaptors phosphorylated by TCR-associated kinases also recruit and activate a GTP/GDP exchange protein called **Vav** that acts on another

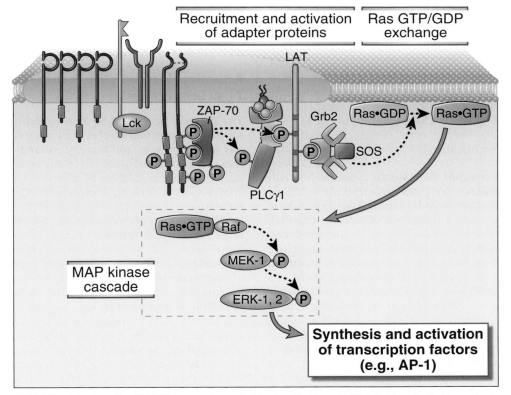

FIGURE 7-14 The Ras-MAP kinase pathway in T cell activation. ZAP-70 that is activated by antigen recognition phosphorylates membrane-associated adaptor proteins (such as LAT), which then bind another adaptor, Grb-2, which provides a docking site for the GTP/GDP exchange factor SOS. SOS converts Ras·GDP to Ras·GTP. Ras·GTP activates a cascade of enzymes, which culminates in the activation of the MAP kinase ERK. A parallel Rac-dependent pathway generates another active MAP kinase, JNK *(not shown)*.

small guanine nucleotide–binding protein called **Rac** (see Fig. 7-14). The Rac·GTP that is generated initiates a parallel MAP kinase cascade, resulting in the activation of a distinct MAP kinase called c-Jun *N*-terminal kinase (JNK). JNK is sometimes called stress-activated protein (SAP) kinase because in many cells it is activated by various forms of noxious stimuli. Activated JNK then phosphorylates c-Jun, the second component of the AP-1 transcription factor. A third member of the MAP kinase family, in addition to ERK and JNK, is p38, and it too is activated by Rac·GTP and in turn activates various transcription factors. Rac·GTP also induces cytoskeletal reorganization and may play a role in the clustering of TCR complexes, coreceptors, and other signaling molecules into the synapse.

The activities of ERK and JNK are eventually shut off by the action of dual-specificity protein tyrosine/threonine phosphatases. These phosphatases are induced or activated by ERK and JNK themselves, providing a negative feedback mechanism to terminate T cell activation.

Calcium- and PKC-Mediated Signaling Pathways in T Lymphocytes

TCR signaling leads to the activation of the γ1 isoform of the enzyme phospholipase C (PLCγ1), and the products of PLCγ1-mediated hydrolysis of membrane lipids activate enzymes that induce specific transcription factors in T cells (Fig. 7-15). PLCγ1, a cytosolic enzyme specific for inositol phospholipids, is recruited to the plasma membrane by tyrosine-phosphorylated LAT within minutes of ligand binding to the TCR. Here, the enzyme is phosphorylated by ZAP-70 and by other kinases, such as the Tec family kinase called Itk. Phosphorylated PLCγ1 catalyzes the hydrolysis of the plasma membrane phospholipid phosphatidylinositol 4,5-bisphosphate (PIP2), generating two breakdown products, the soluble sugar triphosphate, inositol 1,4,5-trisphosphate (IP3), and membrane-bound diacylglycerol (DAG). IP3 and DAG then activate two distinct downstream signaling pathways in T cells.

IP3 produces a rapid increase in cytosolic free calcium within minutes after T cell activation. IP3 diffuses through the cytosol to the endoplasmic reticulum, where it binds to its receptor, a ligand-gated calcium channel, and stimulates release of membrane-sequestered calcium stores. The released calcium causes a rapid rise (during a few minutes) in the cytosolic free calcium ion concentration, from a resting level of about 100 nM to a peak of 600 to 1000 nM. The depletion of endoplasmic reticulum calcium is sensed by an endoplasmic reticulum membrane protein called STIM1, which activates a plasma membrane ion channel called a CRAC (calcium release–activated calcium) channel. The result is an influx of extracellular calcium that sustains cytosolic levels at about 300 to 400 nM for more than 1 hour. A key component of the CRAC channel is a protein called Orai; mutations in the gene encoding this protein are the cause of a rare human immunodeficiency disease. Cytosolic free calcium acts as a signaling molecule by binding to a ubiquitous calcium-dependent regulatory

protein called calmodulin. Calcium-calmodulin complexes activate several enzymes, including a protein serine/threonine phosphatase called calcineurin that is important for transcription factor activation, as discussed later.

Diacylglycerol (DAG), the second breakdown product of PIP2, is a membrane-bound lipid that activates the enzyme protein kinase C (PKC). There are several isoforms of PKC that participate in the generation of active transcription factors, discussed later. The combination of elevated free cytosolic calcium and DAG activates certain isoforms of membrane-associated PKC by inducing a conformational change that makes the catalytic site of the kinase accessible to its substrates. Numerous downstream proteins are phosphorylated by PKC. The PKC-θ isoform localizes to the immunologic synapse and is involved in the activation and nuclear translocation of the nuclear factor κB (NF-κB) transcription factor. Pathways of NF-κB activation are discussed later in this chapter.

So far, we have described several signal transduction pathways initiated by ligand binding to the TCR that result in the activation of different types of enzymes: small G protein–MAP kinase pathways leading to activation of kinases such as ERK and JNK; a PLCγ1-calcium–dependent pathway leading to activation of the phosphatase calcineurin; and a DAG-dependent pathway leading to activation of PKC. Each of these pathways contributes to the expression of genes encoding proteins needed for T cell clonal expansion, differentiation, and effector functions. In the following section, we will describe the mechanisms by which these different signaling pathways stimulate the transcription of various genes in T cells.

Activation of Transcription Factors That Regulate T Cell Gene Expression

The enzymes generated by TCR signaling activate transcription factors that bind to regulatory regions of numerous genes in T cells and thereby enhance transcription of these genes (Fig. 7-16). Much of our understanding of the transcriptional regulation of genes in T cells is based on analyses of cytokine gene expression. The transcriptional regulation of most cytokine genes in T cells is controlled by the binding of transcription factors to nucleotide sequences in the promoter and enhancer regions of these genes. For instance, the promoter located 5′ of the coding exons of the *IL2* gene contains a segment of approximately 300 base pairs in which are located binding sites for several different transcription factors. All of these sites must be occupied by transcription factors for maximal transcription of the *IL2* gene. Different transcription factors are activated by different cytoplasmic signal transduction pathways, and the requirement for multiple transcription factors accounts for the need to activate many signaling pathways after antigen recognition. The same principles are true for the induced expression of many genes in T cells, including those encoding cytokine receptors and effector molecules, although different genes may be responsive to different combinations of transcription factors.

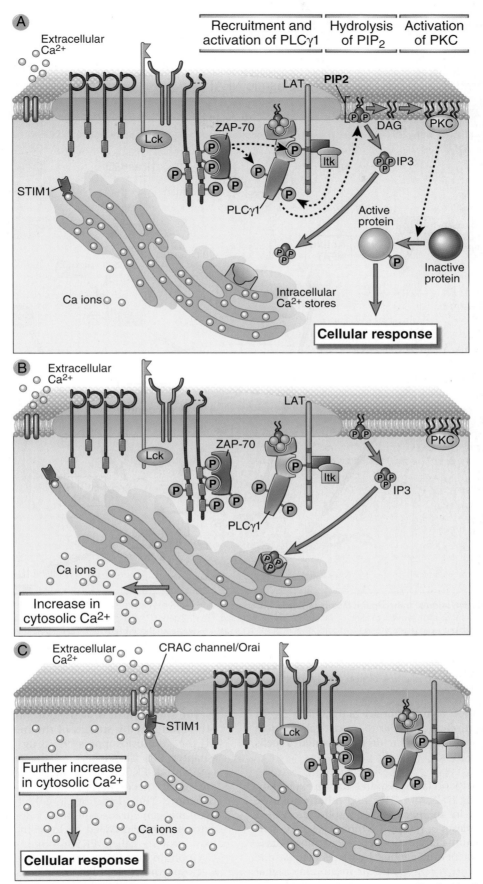

FIGURE 7-15 T cell signaling downstream of PLCγ1. A, The LAT adaptor protein that is phosphorylated on T cell activation binds the cytosolic enzyme PLCγ1, which is phosphorylated by ZAP-70 and other kinases, such as Itk, and activated. Active PLCγ1 hydrolyzes membrane PIP2 to generate IP3, which stimulates an increase in cytosolic calcium, and DAG, which activates the enzyme PKC. **B,** IP3 causes depletion of endoplasmic reticulum calcium, which is sensed by STIM1. PKC induces numerous cellular responses. **C,** STIM1 induces the opening of the CRAC channel that facilitates entry of extracellular calcium into the cytosol. Orai is a component of the CRAC channel. Increased cytosolic calcium together with PKC activate various transcription factors, leading to cellular responses.

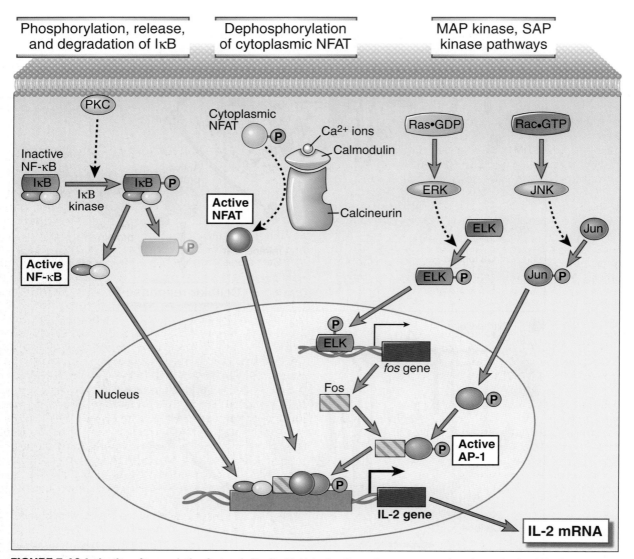

FIGURE 7-16 Activation of transcription factors in T cells. Multiple signaling pathways converge in antigen-stimulated T cells to generate transcription factors that stimulate expression of various genes (in this case, the *IL-2* gene). The calcium-calmodulin pathway activates NFAT, and the Ras and Rac pathways generate the two components of AP-1. Less is known about the link between TCR signals and NF-κB activation. (NF-κB is shown as a complex of two subunits, which in T cells are typically the p50 and p65 proteins, named for their molecular sizes in kilodaltons.) PKC is important in T cell activation, and the PKC-θ isoform is particularly important in activating NF-κB. These transcription factors function coordinately to regulate gene expression. Note also that the various signaling pathways are shown as activating unique transcription factors, but there may be considerable overlap, and each pathway may play a role in the activation of multiple transcription factors.

Three transcription factors that are activated in T cells by antigen recognition and appear to be critical for most T cell responses are nuclear factor of activated T cells (NFAT), AP-1, and NF-κB.

- **NFAT** is a transcription factor required for the expression of genes encoding IL-2, IL-4, TNF, and other cytokines. NFAT is present in an inactive, serine-phosphorylated form in the cytoplasm of resting T lymphocytes. It is activated by the calcium-calmodulin–dependent phosphatase **calcineurin**. Calcineurin dephosphorylates cytoplasmic NFAT, thereby uncovering a nuclear localization signal that permits NFAT to translocate into the nucleus. Once it is in the nucleus, NFAT binds to the regulatory regions of *IL2, IL4,* and other cytokine genes, usually in association with other transcription factors, such as AP-1.

The mechanism of activation of NFAT was discovered indirectly by studies of the mechanism of action of the immunosuppressive drug cyclosporine (see Chapter 17). This drug and the functionally similar compound, FK506, are natural products of fungi and are widely used therapeutic agents to treat allograft rejection. They function largely by blocking T cell cytokine gene transcription. Cyclosporine binds to a cytosolic protein called cyclophilin, and FK506 binds to a protein called FK506-binding protein (FKBP). Cyclophilin and FKBP are also called immunophilins. Cyclosporine-cyclophilin complexes and FK506-FKBP complexes bind to and inhibit calcineurin and thereby block translocation of NFAT into the nucleus.

- **AP-1** is a transcription factor found in many cell types; it is specifically activated in T lymphocytes by

TCR-mediated signals. AP-1 is actually the name for a family of DNA-binding factors composed of dimers of two proteins that bind to one another through a shared structural motif called a leucine zipper. The best characterized AP-1 factor is composed of the proteins Fos and Jun. TCR-induced signals lead to the appearance of active AP-1 in the nucleus of T cells. As discussed previously, the formation of active AP-1 typically involves synthesis of the Fos protein and phosphorylation of preexisting Jun protein, both stimulated by MAP kinases. AP-1 appears to physically associate with other transcription factors in the nucleus, and it works best in combination with NFAT. Thus, AP-1 activation represents a convergence point of several TCR-initiated signaling pathways.

- **NF-κB** is a transcription factor that is activated in response to TCR signals and is essential for cytokine synthesis. NF-κB proteins are homodimers or heterodimers of proteins that are homologous to the product of a cellular proto-oncogene called c-*rel* and are important in the transcription of many genes in diverse cell types, particularly in innate immune cells (see Chapter 4). The NF-κB pathway is also important for responses to Toll-like receptor and cytokine signaling, and is discussed in depth at the end of this chapter.

The links between different signaling proteins, activation of transcription factors, and functional responses of T cells are often difficult to establish because there are complex and incompletely understood interactions between signaling pathways. Also, for the sake of simplicity, we often discuss signaling as a set of linear pathways, but it is likely that this does not reflect the more complex and interconnected reality. Finally, we have focused on selected pathways to illustrate how antigen recognition may lead to biochemical alterations, but it is clear that many other signaling molecules are also involved in antigen-induced lymphocyte activation.

An additional mechanism by which T cell activation is regulated involves **microRNAs (miRNAs)**. miRNAs are small non-coding RNAs that are transcribed from DNA but are not translated into proteins. The function of miRNAs is to inhibit expression of specific genes. miRNAs are initially generated in the nucleus as longer primary transcripts that are processed by an endoribonuclease called Drosha into shorter pre-miRNAs that have a stem loop structure and can be exported into the cytosol. In the cytosol, the pre-miRNA is processed by another endoribonuclease called Dicer into a short double-stranded miRNA 21 to 22 base pairs in length, one strand of which can be used to pair with a complementary sequence in a number of cellular messenger RNAs (mRNAs). These mRNAs associate with miRNAs and proteins called Argonaute proteins to form complexes known as RISC (RNA-induced silencing complex). If the 6-8–base pair miRNA seed sequence is not perfectly complementary to the mRNA, the mRNA is prevented from being translated efficiently. mRNAs may be targeted for degradation when complementarity is perfect. In either case, the result is a reduction in the abundance of proteins encoded by genes targeted by miRNAs. In activated T cells, the expression of the majority of miRNAs is globally reduced. In addition, the Argonaute protein is ubiquitinated and degraded, further compromising miRNA function and enhancing the expression of a large number of proteins required for cell cycle progression downstream of T cell activation. Specific miRNAs modulate gene expression in different types of T cells, as we will discuss in Chapter 8.

Modulation of T Cell Signaling by Protein Tyrosine Phosphatases

Tyrosine phosphatases remove phosphate moieties from tyrosine residues on proteins and generally inhibit TCR signaling. Two tyrosine phosphatases that serve an important inhibitory role in lymphocytes and other hematopoietic cells are called SHP-1 and SHP-2 (for SH2 domain–containing phosphatases 1 and 2). Inhibitory phosphatases are typically recruited to ITIMs in the cytoplasmic tails of inhibitory receptors that are themselves phosphorylated by tyrosine kinases induced during lymphocyte activation. These phosphatases inhibit signal transduction by removing phosphate moieties from tyrosine residues in key signaling molecules and thus functionally antagonize tyrosine kinases. Another inhibitory phosphatase that does not act on phosphoproteins but rather is specific for an inositol phospholipid is called SHIP (SH2 domain–containing inositol phosphatase). Like SHP-1 and SHP-2, SHIP binds to phosphorylated ITIM sequences on specific inhibitory receptors. SHIP removes a phosphate group from phosphatidylinositol (3,4,5)-triphosphate (PIP3), a phospholipid in the inner leaflet of the plasma membrane, and thus antagonizes PI3-kinase signaling in lymphocytes.

Although most phosphatases attenuate lymphocyte signaling, one tyrosine phosphatase, CD45, facilitates lymphocyte activation. The CD45 protein is a receptor tyrosine phosphatase expressed in all hematopoietic cells. It is an integral membrane protein whose cytoplasmic tail contains tandem protein tyrosine phosphatase domains. CD45 dephosphorylates inhibitory tyrosine residues in Src family kinases in general (including Lck and Fyn in T cells) and thus contributes to the generation of active kinases.

Costimulatory Receptor Signaling in T Cells

Costimulatory signals are delivered by receptors that recognize ligands that are induced on APCs by microbes and cooperate with TCR signals to promote activation of the T cells. The two-signal hypothesis for T cell activation was introduced in Chapters 1 and 4. In immunologic jargon, the response by the TCR to MHC and peptide on an APC is referred to as signal 1. T cells are fully activated only when a foreign peptide is recognized in the context of the activation of the innate immune system by a pathogen or some other cause of inflammation. Costimulatory ligands represent the danger signals (or signal 2) induced on antigen-presenting cells by microbes. Foreignness must combine with a sense of danger for optimal T cell activation to occur.

The CD28 Family of Costimulatory Receptors

The best defined costimulators for T lymphocytes are a pair of related proteins, called B7-1 (CD80) and B7-2 (CD86), which are expressed on activated dendritic cells, macrophages, and B lymphocytes. The **CD28** molecule on T cells, which recognizes the B7 proteins, is the principal costimulatory receptor for delivery of second signals for T cell activation. The biologic roles of the B7 and CD28 protein families are discussed in Chapter 9.

Another activating member of the CD28 family is a receptor called ICOS (inducible costimulator), which plays an important role in T follicular helper cell development and will be discussed in Chapters 9 and 12.

The CD2/SLAM Family of Costimulatory Receptors

Proteins other than CD28 family members also contribute to T cell activation and differentiation. One family of proteins that plays a role in the activation of T cells and NK cells is structurally related to a receptor called CD2. CD2 is a glycoprotein present on more than 90% of mature T cells, on 50% to 70% of thymocytes, and on NK cells. The molecule contains two extracellular Ig domains, a hydrophobic transmembrane region, and a long (116 amino acid residues) cytoplasmic tail. The principal ligand for CD2 in humans is a molecule called leukocyte function-associated antigen 3 (LFA-3, or CD58), also a member of the CD2 family. LFA-3 is expressed on a wide variety of hematopoietic and non-hematopoietic cells, either as an integral membrane protein or as a phosphatidylinositol-anchored membrane molecule. In mice, the principal ligand for CD2 is CD48, which is also a member of the CD2 family and is distinct from but structurally similar to LFA-3.

CD2 functions both as an intercellular adhesion molecule and as a signal transducer. Although mice lacking only CD28 have significant immune defects, while mice lacking only CD2 do not, mice lacking both CD28 and CD2 have more profound defects. This indicates that CD28 may compensate for the loss of CD2, an example of the redundancy of costimulatory receptors of T cells.

A distinct subgroup of the CD2 family of proteins is known as the **SLAM** (signaling lymphocytic activation molecule) family. SLAM, like all members of the CD2 family, is an integral membrane protein that contains two extracellular Ig domains and a long cytoplasmic tail. The cytoplasmic tail of SLAM, but not of CD2, contains a specific tyrosine-based motif, TxYxxV/I (where T is a threonine residue, Y is a tyrosine residue, V is a valine, I is an isoleucine, and x is any amino acid) known as an immunoreceptor tyrosine-based switch motif (ITSM) that is distinct from the ITAM and ITIM motifs found in other activating and inhibitory receptors. It is called a switch motif because in some receptors, this motif can orchestrate a switch from the binding of a tyrosine phosphatase SHP-2 to binding a tyrosine kinase, such as Fyn, depending on the absence or presence, respectively, of an adaptor called SAP (SLAM-associated protein). Thus, the ITSM can mediate a change from an inhibitory to an activating function.

The extracellular Ig domains of SLAM are involved in homophilic interactions. SLAM on a T cell can interact with SLAM on a dendritic cell and, as a result, the cytoplasmic tail of SLAM may deliver signals to T cells. The ITSM motif binds to SAP, and the latter forms a bridge between SLAM and Fyn (a Src family kinase that is also physically linked to CD3 proteins in T cells). SLAM and other members of the SLAM family function as costimulatory receptors in T cells, NK cells, and some B cells. As we will discuss in Chapter 21, mutations in the *SH2D1A* gene encoding SAP are the cause of a disease called X-linked lymphoproliferative syndrome (XLP).

An important member of the SLAM family in NK cells, CD8⁺ T cells, and γδ T cells is called **2B4**. Like SLAM, the cytoplasmic tail of 2B4 contains ITSM motifs, binds to the SAP adaptor protein, and signals by recruiting Fyn. Defective 2B4 signaling may contribute in a major way to the immune deficit in patients with X-linked lymphoproliferative syndrome.

Metabolic Changes During T Cell Activation

When lymphocytes are activated, they need to increase their metabolic activity to cope with the increased demands of the cellular response. This phenomenon has been best studied in T cells. Upon activation by antigen and costimulators, T cells increase the transport of glucose and change their energy production from mitochondrial oxidative phosphorylation to glycolysis, even in the presence of abundant oxygen, a phenomenon known as aerobic glycolysis (Fig. 7-17). This phenomenon, also known as the Warburg effect, was first described in tumor cells but is now recognized as an important mechanism used by many proliferating cells. Although glycolysis generates less ATP, the energy store, than does oxidative phosphorylation, glycolysis does not use substrates other than glucose, such as amino acids and lipids, and thus preserves these to provide the building blocks needed to support the responses of the activated lymphocytes. This altered mechanism of energy production in lymphocytes may be important not just for cellular proliferation but also for the differentiation of T cells into effector cells, and for the production of effector cytokines.

THE B LYMPHOCYTE ANTIGEN RECEPTOR COMPLEX

The B lymphocyte antigen receptor is a transmembrane form of an antibody molecule associated with two signaling chains. We described the structure of antibodies in detail in Chapter 5. Here we will focus on some salient features of the membrane forms of Ig and their associated proteins and discuss how they deliver signals to B cells. Because the signaling pathways are much like those in T cells, we will summarize these without great detail. However, there are both similarities and significant differences between B and T cell antigen receptors (see Table 7-1).

Structure of the B Cell Receptor for Antigen

Membrane IgM and IgD, the antigen receptors of naive B cells, have short cytoplasmic tails consisting of only three amino acids (lysine, valine, and lysine). These tails are too small to transduce signals generated after the recognition of antigen. Ig-mediated signals are transduced by two

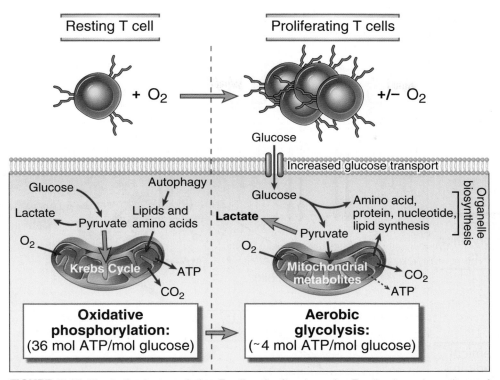

FIGURE 7-17 Metabolic changes during T cell activation. In resting T cells, the major pathway of energy generation is mitochondrial oxidative phosphorylation. Upon activation, there is a switch to aerobic glycolysis, which generates less energy but preserves and produces the building blocks for cellular organelle biosynthesis, which is required for cell proliferation and functional responses.

other molecules called Igα and Igβ that are disulfide linked to one another and are expressed in B cells non-covalently associated with membrane Ig (Fig. 7-18). These proteins each contain an ITAM motif in their cytoplasmic tails, are required for the transport of membrane Ig molecules to the cell surface, and together with membrane Ig form the **B cell receptor (BCR) complex**. B cell receptor complexes in class-switched B cells, including memory B cells, contain membrane immunoglobulins that may be of the IgG, IgA, or IgE classes (see Chapter 12).

Signal Initiation by the B Cell Receptor

Signal initiation by antigens occurs by cross-linking of the BCR and is facilitated by the coreceptor for the BCR. It is thought that cross-linking of membrane Ig by multivalent antigens brings Src family kinases together and, by promoting their physical interaction, fully activates these enzymes, enabling them to phosphorylate the tyrosine residues on the ITAMs of Igα and Igβ. It is also possible that as in T cells, antigen binding facilitates a conformational change in BCR-associated ITAMs, making them accessible to already active Src family kinases that modify ITAM tyrosines. The phosphorylation of ITAM tyrosine residues triggers all subsequent signaling events downstream of the BCR (Fig. 7-19). Cross-linked Ig receptors enter lipid rafts, where many adaptor proteins and signaling molecules are concentrated. Igα and Igβ are loosely connected to Src family tyrosine kinases such as Lyn, Fyn, and Blk, and these enzymes are also linked by lipid anchors to the inside of the plasma membrane. The phosphorylated tyrosine residues in the ITAMs of Igα and

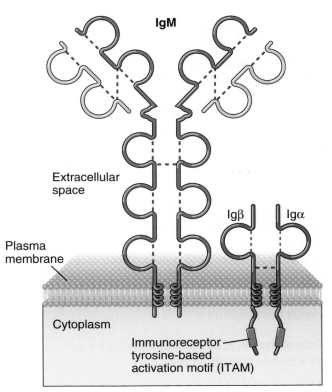

FIGURE 7-18 B cell antigen receptor complex. Membrane IgM (and IgD) on the surface of mature B cells is associated with the invariant Igβ and Igα molecules, which contain ITAMs in their cytoplasmic tails that mediate signaling functions. Note the similarity to the TCR complex.

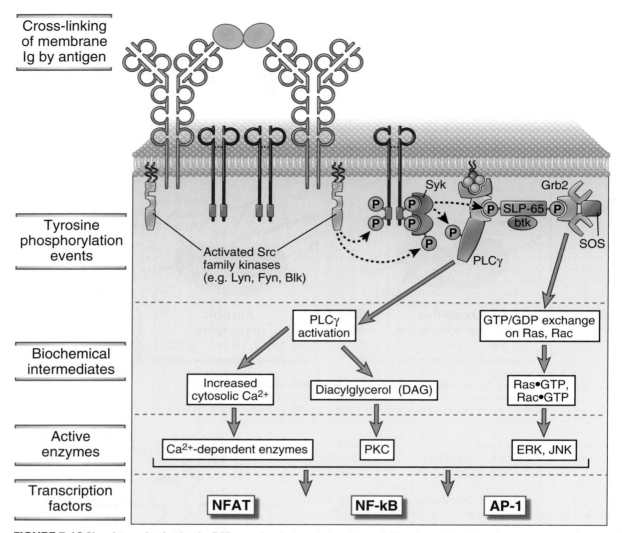

FIGURE 7-19 Signal transduction by the BCR complex. Antigen-induced cross-linking of membrane Ig on B cells leads to clustering and activation of Src family tyrosine kinases and tyrosine phosphorylation of the ITAMs in the cytoplasmic tails of the Igα and Igβ molecules. This leads to docking of Syk and subsequent tyrosine phosphorylation events as depicted. Several signaling cascades follow these events, as shown, leading to the activation of several transcription factors. These signal transduction pathways are similar to those described in T cells.

Igβ provide a docking site for the tandem SH2 domains of the Syk tyrosine kinase. Syk is activated when it associates with phosphorylated tyrosines of ITAMs and may itself be phosphorylated on specific tyrosine residues by BCR-associated Src family kinases, leading to further activation. If the antigen is monovalent and incapable of cross-linking multiple Ig molecules, some signaling may nevertheless occur, but additional activation by helper T cells may be necessary to fully activate B cells, as discussed in Chapter 12.

Role of the CR2/CD21 Complement Receptor as a Coreceptor for B Cells

The activation of B cells is enhanced by signals that are provided by complement proteins and the CD21 coreceptor complex, which link innate immunity to the adaptive humoral immune response (Fig. 7-20). The complement system consists of a collection of plasma proteins that are activated either by binding to antigen-complexed

antibody molecules (the classical pathway) or by binding directly to some microbial surfaces and polysaccharides in the absence of antibodies (the alternative and lectin pathways) (see Chapters 4 and 13). Thus, polysaccharides and other microbial components may activate the complement system directly, during innate immune responses. Proteins and other antigens that do not activate complement directly may be bound by preexisting antibodies or by antibodies produced early in the response, and these antigen-antibody complexes activate complement by the classical pathway. Recall that complement activation results in the proteolytic cleavage of complement proteins. The key component of the system is a protein called C3, and its cleavage results in the production of a molecule called C3b that binds covalently to the microbe or antigen-antibody complex. C3b is further degraded into a fragment called C3d, which remains bound to the microbial surface or on the antigen-antibody complex. B lymphocytes express a receptor for C3d that is called the type 2 complement receptor (CR2, or CD21). The

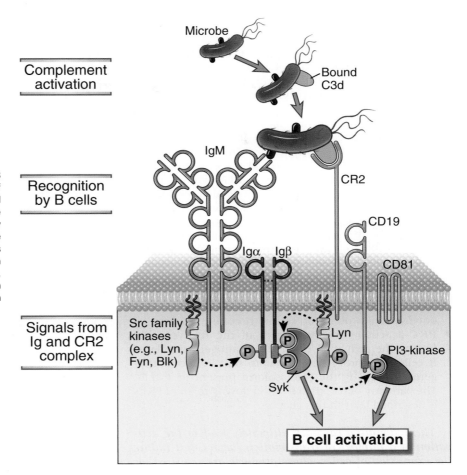

FIGURE 7-20 Role of complement in B cell activation. B cells express a complex of the CR2 complement receptor, CD19, and CD81. Microbial antigens that have bound the complement fragment C3d can simultaneously engage both the CR2 molecule and the membrane Ig on the surface of a B cell. This leads to the initiation of signaling cascades from both the BCR complex and the CR2 complex, because of which the response to C3d-antigen complexes is greatly enhanced compared with the response to antigen alone.

complex of C3d and antigen or C3d and antigen-antibody complex binds to B cells, with the membrane Ig recognizing antigen and CR2 recognizing the bound C3d (see Fig. 7-19).

CR2 is expressed on mature B cells as a complex with two other membrane proteins, CD19 and CD81 (also called TAPA-1). The CR2-CD19-CD81 complex is often called the B cell coreceptor complex because CR2 binds to antigens through attached C3d at the same time that membrane Ig binds directly to the antigen. Binding of C3d to the B cell complement receptor brings CD19 in proximity to BCR-associated kinases, and the cytoplasmic tail of CD19 rapidly becomes tyrosine phosphorylated. Phosphorylation of the tail of CD19 results in the efficient recruitment of Lyn, a Src family kinase that can amplify BCR signaling by greatly enhancing the phosphorylation of ITAM tyrosines in Igα and Igβ. Phosphorylated CD19 also activates other signaling pathways, notably one dependent on the enzyme PI3-kinase, which in turn further augment signaling initiated by antigen binding to membrane Ig. PI3-kinase is required for the activation of Btk and PLCγ2 because these enzymes must bind to PIP3 on the inner leaflet of the plasma membrane to be fully activated, in a manner analogous to that shown for PDK1 activation in T cells in Figure 7-12. The net result of coreceptor activation is that the response of the antigen-stimulated B cell is greatly enhanced.

Signaling Pathways Downstream of the B Cell Receptor

After antigen binding to the BCR, Syk and other tyrosine kinases activate numerous downstream signaling pathways that are regulated by adaptor proteins (see Fig. 7-19). The cross-linking of the BCR or the activation of the BCR by a coreceptor-dependent mechanism results in ITAM phosphorylation and recruitment of Syk to the ITAM, followed by the activation of this dual SH2 domain–containing kinase. Activated Syk phosphorylates critical tyrosine residues on adaptor proteins such as SLP-65 (SH2-binding leukocyte phosphoprotein of 65 kD, also called BLNK, or B cell linker protein). This facilitates the recruitment to these adaptor proteins of other SH2 domain– and phosphotyrosine-binding (PTB) domain–containing enzymes, including guanine nucleotide exchange proteins that can separately activate Ras and Rac, PLCγ2, and the Btk tyrosine kinase, among others. Recruitment facilitates the activation of these downstream effectors, each generally contributing to the activation of a distinct signaling pathway.

- The **Ras-MAP kinase pathway** is activated in antigen-stimulated B cells. The GTP/GDP exchange factor SOS is recruited to BLNK through the binding of the Grb-2 adaptor protein; Ras is then converted by this exchange factor from an inactive GDP-bound form to an active

GTP-bound form. Activated Ras contributes to the activation of the ERK MAP kinase pathway discussed earlier in the context of T cell signaling. In a parallel fashion, the activation of the small G protein Rac may contribute to the activation of the JNK MAP kinase pathway.

- A specific **phosphatidylinositol-specific phospholipase C (PLC)** is activated in response to BCR signaling, and this in turn facilitates the activation of downstream signaling pathways. In B cells, the dominant isoform of PLC is the γ2 isoform, whereas T cells express the related γ1 isoform of the enzyme. PLCγ2 becomes active when it binds to BLNK and is phosphorylated by Syk and Btk. As described in the context of TCR signaling, active PLC breaks down membrane PIP2 to yield soluble IP3 and leaves DAG in the plasma membrane. IP3 mobilizes calcium from intracellular stores, leading to a rapid elevation of cytoplasmic calcium, which is subsequently augmented by an influx of calcium from the extracellular milieu. In the presence of calcium, DAG activates some isoforms of protein kinase C (mainly PKC-β in B cells), which phosphorylate downstream proteins on serine/threonine residues.

- **PKC-β** activation downstream of the BCR contributes to the activation of NF-κB in antigen-stimulated B cells. This process is similar to that in T cells triggered by PKC-θ, the PKC isoform present in T cells. The pathway of NF-κB activation downstream of PKCs is described later in this chapter.

These signaling cascades ultimately lead to the activation of a number of transcription factors that induce the expression of genes whose products are required for functional responses of B cells. Some of the transcription factors that are activated by antigen receptor–mediated signal transduction in B cells are Fos (downstream of Ras and ERK activation), JunB (downstream of Rac and JNK activation), and NF-κB (downstream of Btk, PLCγ2, and PKC-β activation). We described these earlier when we discussed T cell signaling pathways. These and other transcription factors, many not mentioned here, are involved in stimulating proliferation and differentiation of B cells (see Chapter 12).

As in T cells, our knowledge of antigen-induced signaling pathways in B cells and their links with subsequent functional responses is incomplete. We have described some of these pathways to illustrate the main features, but others may play important roles in B cell activation. The same signaling pathways are used by membrane IgM and IgD on naive B cells and by IgG, IgA, and IgE on B cells that have undergone isotype switching because all of these membrane isotypes associate with Igα and Igβ.

THE ATTENUATION OF IMMUNE RECEPTOR SIGNALING

Activation of lymphocytes has to be tightly controlled to limit immune responses against microbes in order to avoid collateral damage to host tissues. In addition, the immune system needs mechanisms that will prevent reactions against self antigens. We will describe the

biology of these control mechanisms in later chapters, notably Chapter 15. Attenuation of signaling is essential to prevent uncontrolled inflammation and lymphoproliferation. Here we discuss the biochemical mechanisms that serve to limit and terminate lymphocyte activation.

Inhibitory signaling in lymphocytes is mediated primarily by inhibitory receptors and also by enzymes known as E3 ubiquitin ligases that mark certain signaling molecules for degradation. Inhibitory receptors typically recruit and activate phosphatases that counter signaling events induced by antigen receptors (Fig. 7-21). The functional responses of all cells are regulated by a balance between stimulatory and inhibitory signals, and we will first describe, from a broad mechanistic standpoint, how inhibitory receptors may function in NK cells, T cells, and B cells. We will then describe how ubiquitin E3 ligases may attenuate signaling in lymphocytes. The biologic relevance of signal attenuation through inhibitory receptors in NK cells, T cells, and B cells is addressed in Chapters 4, 9, and 12, respectively.

Inhibitory Receptors of NK Cells, B Cells, and T Cells

Most but not all inhibitory receptors in the immune system contain ITIM motifs in their cytoplasmic tails that can recruit SH2 domain–containing phosphatases and thus attenuate signaling in a broadly similar manner (see Fig 7-21). Inhibitory receptors play key roles in NK

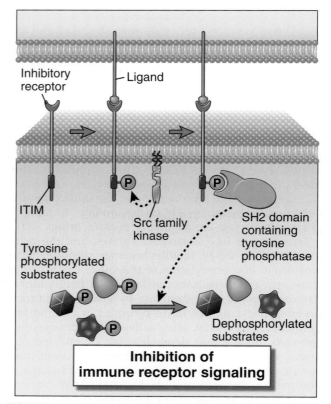

FIGURE 7-21 Inhibitory signaling in lymphocytes. A schematic depiction is provided of an inhibitory receptor with an extracellular ligand-binding domain and a cytosolic ITIM motif. Ligand binding results in phosphorylation of the ITIM tyrosine by a Src family kinase, followed by recruitment of an SH2 domain–containing tyrosine phosphatase that can attenuate immune receptor signaling.

cells, T cells, and B cells as well as in other cells of innate immunity.

In NK cells, inhibitory receptors called KIRs (see Chapter 4) contain extracellular Ig domains that can recognize class I HLA molecules, and a subset of these receptors contains cytosolic ITIM motifs. The CD94/NKG2A inhibitory receptor binds to an atypical class I MHC molecule called HLA-E, and the NKG2A chain of this dimer contains cytosolic ITIM motifs.

Tyrosine residues on the ITIMs of these and other inhibitory receptors can be phosphorylated by Src family kinases linked to lymphocyte activation and, as described earlier, recruit SH2 domain–containing tyrosine phosphatases such as SHP-1 and SHP-2 and an SH2 domain–containing inositol phosphatase called SHIP. SHP-1 and SHP-2 attenuate tyrosine kinase–initiated signaling from activating receptors in NK cells as well as from the BCR and TCR in B and T cells, respectively. SHIP removes phosphate moieties from PIP3 and thus inhibits PI3-kinase activity in lymphocytes, NK cells, and innate immune cells.

The prototypical inhibitory receptor of the CD28 family, **CTLA-4** (also called CD152), has the ability to inhibit T cell responses induced on activated T cells and has a higher affinity than CD28 for B7 proteins. CTLA-4 is involved in the maintenance of unresponsiveness (tolerance) to self antigens and is discussed in this context in Chapter 15. Another inhibitory receptor of the same family is called **PD-1** (programmed death 1), and this is also discussed in Chapter 15. CTLA-4 contains a tyrosine-containing motif in its tail that may be inhibitory; PD-1 contains cytosolic ITIM and ITSM motifs, and its cytosolic tail is critical for the initiation of inhibitory signals. The key inhibitory receptors in B cells include FcγRIIB and CD22/Siglec-2 (see Chapter 12). FcγRIIB, an important attenuator of signaling in activated B cells as well as in dendritic cells and macrophages, can bind IgG-containing immune complexes through extracellular Ig domains. It primarily recruits SHIP and antagonizes PI3-kinase signaling. This receptor dampens B cell activation in the latter part of a humoral immune response and will be discussed in more detail in Chapter 12.

E3 Ubiquitin Ligases and the Degradation of Signaling Proteins

One of the major ways of degrading cytosolic and nuclear proteins involves the covalent attachment of ubiquitin residues to these proteins. Although ubiquitination of proteins is frequently linked to the degradation of these proteins in proteasomes, proteins can be ubiquitinated in a number of ways, each form of ubiquitination serving a very different function. In the context of signal transduction, two different types of ubiquitination mediate signal attenuation on the one hand and signal generation on the other.

Ubiquitination was briefly discussed in Chapter 6 in the context of class I MHC–based antigen processing and presentation. Ubiquitin is a 76–amino acid protein that is activated in an ATP-dependent fashion by an E1 enzyme, then carried by an E2 enzyme, and then transferred to lysine residues on specific substrates that are recognized by specific E3 ubiquitin ligases. In many cases, after the C terminus of a ubiquitin moiety is covalently linked to a lysine residue on a target protein, the C-terminal ends of subsequent ubiquitin moieties may be covalently attached to lysine residues on the preceding ubiquitin to generate a polyubiquitin chain. The shape of the polyubiquitin chain is very different depending on which specific lysine residue on the preceding ubiquitin molecule in the chain is the site for covalent binding of the next ubiquitin molecule, and the shape of the ubiquitin chain has important functional consequences. If lysine in position 48 of the first ubiquitin moiety forms an isopeptide bond with the C terminus of the next ubiquitin and so on, a lysine-48 type of ubiquitin chain will be generated that can be recognized by the proteasomal cap, and the protein will be targeted for degradation in the proteasome. Some E3 ligases generate a different type of polyubiquitin chain called a lysine-63 type of chain, which does not target proteins for degradation but instead generates a structure for latching the marked proteins onto other specific proteins; this is important in NF-κB signaling, as discussed later. For some functions, in particular targeting membrane proteins to lysosomes rather than to proteasomes, only a single ubiquitin moiety may need to be attached to a protein target.

Several E3 ligases are found in T cells; some of them are involved in signal activation and others in signal attenuation. The prototype of E3 ligases involved in terminating T cell responses is Cbl-b, but several others serve similar functions. Recruitment of Cbl-b to the TCR complex and associated adaptor proteins leads to the monoubiquitination, endocytosis, and lysosomal degradation of the TCR complex, and this may be a mechanism for the attenuation of TCR signaling (Fig. 7-22). CD28 signals block the inhibitory activity of Cbl-b, and this is one mechanism by which costimulation augments TCR signals. In knockout mice lacking Cbl-b, the T cells respond to antigen even without CD28-mediated costimulation and produce abnormally high amounts of IL-2. These mice develop autoimmunity as a result of the enhanced activation of their T cells.

CYTOKINE RECEPTORS AND SIGNALING

Cytokines, the secreted messenger molecules of the immune system, have been mentioned in previous chapters and will be throughout the book. Here we will describe receptors for cytokines and their mechanisms of signaling.

All cytokine receptors consist of one or more transmembrane proteins whose extracellular portions are responsible for cytokine binding and whose cytoplasmic portions are responsible for initiation of intracellular signaling pathways. For most cytokine receptors, these signaling pathways are activated by ligand-induced receptor clustering, bringing together the cytoplasmic portions of two or more receptor molecules, and thus inducing the activity of unique non-receptor tyrosine kinases. In the case of the TNF receptor family of cytokine receptors, preformed receptor trimers apparently undergo a conformational change after contacting their cognate trimeric ligands.

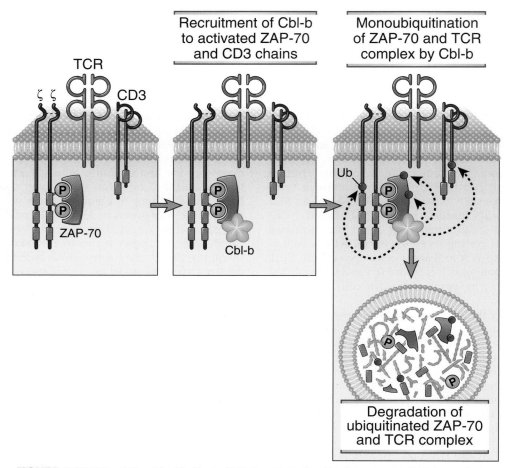

FIGURE 7-22 Role of the ubiquitin ligase Cbl-b in terminating T cell responses. Cbl-b is recruited to the TCR complex, where it facilitates the monoubiquitination of CD3, ZAP-70, and other proteins of the TCR complex. These proteins are targeted for proteolytic degradation in lysosomes and other organelles *(not shown)*.

Classes of Cytokine Receptors

The most widely used classification of cytokine receptors is based on structural homologies of the extracellular cytokine-binding domains and shared intracellular signaling mechanisms (Fig. 7-23). Signaling mechanisms utilized by individual families are considered in the section that follows.

Type I Cytokine Receptors (Hematopoietin Receptor Family)

Type I cytokine receptors are dimers or trimers that typically consist of unique ligand-binding chains and one or more signal-transducing chains, which are often shared by receptors for different cytokines. These chains contain one or two domains with a conserved pair of cysteine residues and a membrane proximal peptide stretch containing a tryptophan-serine-X-tryptophan-serine (WSXWS) motif, where X is any amino acid (Fig. 7-23, *A*). The conserved sequences of the receptors form structures that bind cytokines that have four α-helical bundles and are referred to as type I cytokines, but the specificity for individual cytokines is determined by amino acid residues that vary from one receptor to another. This receptor family can be divided into subgroups based on structural homologies or the use of shared signaling polypeptides (Fig. 7-23, *B*). One group

contains a signaling component called the common γ chain (CD132); in this group are the receptors for IL-2, IL-4, IL-7, IL-9, IL-15, and IL-21. A distinct subgroup of type I receptors includes receptors that share a common β chain (CD131) subunit. This subgroup includes the receptors for IL-3, IL-5, and GM-CSF. Another subgroup of receptors uses the gp130 signaling component, and this includes the receptors for IL-6, IL-11, and IL-27. All of the type I cytokine receptors engage JAK-STAT signaling pathways.

Type II Cytokine Receptors (Interferon Receptor Family)

The type II receptors are similar to type I receptors by virtue of possessing two extracellular domains with conserved cysteines, but type II receptors do not contain the WSXWS motif. These receptors consist of one ligand-binding polypeptide chain and one signal-transducing chain. All of the type II cytokine receptors, like the type I receptors, engage JAK-STAT signaling pathways. This family includes receptors for type I and type II interferons and for IL-10, IL-20, and IL-22.

TNF Receptor Family

These receptors are part of a large family of preformed trimers (some of which recognize membrane-associated ligands and are not considered cytokine receptors) with

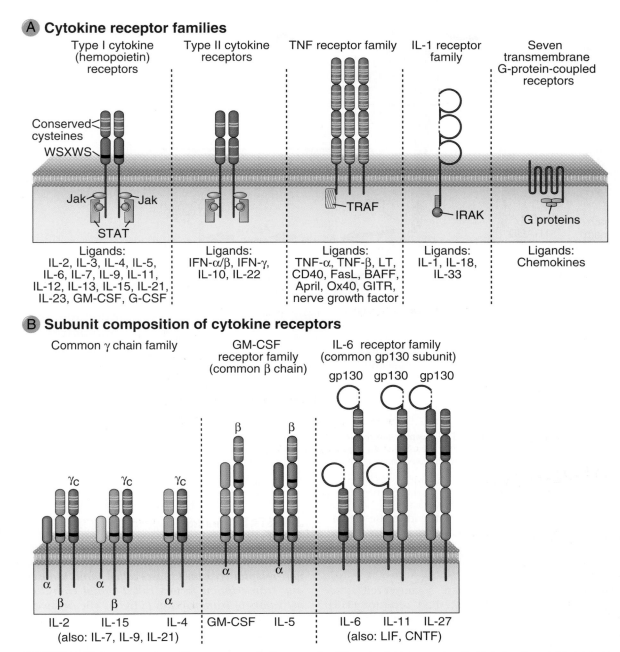

A Cytokine receptor families

Type I cytokine (hemopoietin) receptors	Type II cytokine receptors	TNF receptor family	IL-1 receptor family	Seven transmembrane G-protein-coupled receptors

Conserved cysteines
WSXWS
Jak   Jak
STAT
TRAF
IRAK
G proteins

Ligands:
IL-2, IL-3, IL-4, IL-5, IL-6, IL-7, IL-9, IL-11, IL-12, IL-13, IL-15, IL-21, IL-23, GM-CSF, G-CSF

Ligands:
IFN-α/β, IFN-γ, IL-10, IL-22

Ligands:
TNF-α, TNF-β, LT, CD40, FasL, BAFF, April, Ox40, GITR, nerve growth factor

Ligands:
IL-1, IL-18, IL-33

Ligands:
Chemokines

B Subunit composition of cytokine receptors

Common γ chain family

GM-CSF receptor family (common β chain)

IL-6 receptor family (common gp130 subunit)

gp130   gp130   gp130

γc   γc   γc

β   β

α   α   α

α   α

β   β   α

IL-2   IL-15   IL-4
(also: IL-7, IL-9, IL-21)

GM-CSF   IL-5

IL-6   IL-11   IL-27
(also: LIF, CNTF)

FIGURE 7-23 Structure of cytokine receptors. A, Receptors for different cytokines are classified into families on the basis of conserved extracellular domain structures and signaling mechanisms. Representative cytokines or other ligands that bind to each receptor family are listed below the schematic drawings. *WSXWS,* tryptophan-serine-X-tryptophan-serine. **B,** Groups of cytokine receptors share identical or highly homologous subunit chains. Selected examples of cytokine receptors in each group are shown.

conserved cysteine-rich extracellular domains and shared intracellular signaling mechanisms that typically stimulate gene expression but in some cases induce apoptosis. Some important receptors of this family, most of which will be discussed in other chapters in their biologic contexts, include the TNF receptors TNFRI and TNFRII, the CD40 protein, Fas, the lymphotoxin receptor, and the BAFF receptor family. The ligands for these receptors also form trimers. Some of these ligands are membrane bound, whereas others are soluble.

Binding of the ligands to the preformed trimeric receptors typically induces a conformational change

and recruits adaptor proteins to the receptor complex. These adaptors in turn recruit enzymes that include both E3 ubiquitin ligases, which mediate non-degradatory polyubiquitination, and protein kinases, which initiate downstream signaling. In the case of the TNF receptor illustrated in Figure 7-24, the receptor recruits the adaptor protein TRADD (TNF receptor–associated death domain), and TRADD in turn can recruit proteins called TRAFs (TNF receptor associated factors), which possess a unique type of E3 ligase activity that will be discussed in the section on NF-κB signaling. The type I TNF receptor (there are two different receptors for TNF) and Fas

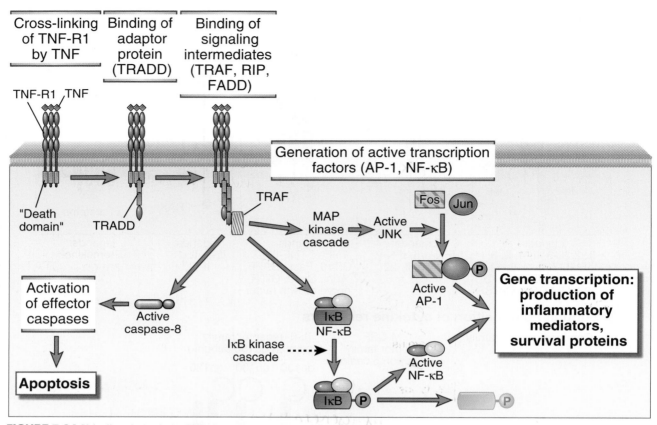

FIGURE 7-24 Signaling through the TNF receptor can result in NF-κB and MAP kinase activation or in the induction of apoptotic death. Ligation of the type I TNF receptor results in the recruitment of an adaptor protein called TRADD, which in turn can activate TRAF molecules (E3 ubiquitin ligases) and the RIP1 kinase. Downstream consequences include the activation of the NF-κB pathway and the JNK MAP kinase pathway or the induction of apoptotic death.

(CD95) can also recruit adaptors that lead to the activation of caspase-8, and these receptors can thereby induce apoptosis in certain cells.

IL-1 Family

The receptors of this family share a conserved cytosolic sequence, called the Toll-like/IL-1 receptor (TIR) domain, and engage similar signal transduction pathways that induce new gene transcription. We discussed Toll-like receptor (TLR) signaling in Chapter 4. Briefly, engagement of the IL-1R or of TLRs results in receptor dimerization and the recruitment of one or more of four known TIR domain–containing adaptors to the TIR domain of the cytoplasmic tail of the receptor. The adaptors link TLRs to different members of the IRAK (IL-1R–associated kinase) family. IRAKs can in turn link adaptors to TRAF6, an E3 ubiquitin ligase required for NF-κB activation. Other events downstream of TLR signaling include MAP kinase activation and the phosphorylation of IRF3 and IRF7, inducers of type I interferon transcription. The latter aspect of TLR signaling has been considered in the context of the antiviral state in Chapter 4. Different adaptors link TLRs to NF-κB signaling and to MAP kinase activation, or to delayed activation of NF-κB and the activation of IRF3. The mechanisms connecting IL-1R/TLR signaling and NF-κB activation are discussed later.

JAK-STAT Signaling

Cytokine receptors of the type I and type II receptor families engage signal transduction pathways that involve non-receptor tyrosine kinases called Janus kinases (JAKs) and transcription factors called signal transducers and activators of transcription (STATs). The discovery of the JAK-STAT pathways came from biochemical and genetic analyses of interferon signaling. There are four known Janus kinases (JAKs1 to 3 and TYK2) and seven STATs (STATs1 to 4, 5a, 5b, and 6).

The sequence of events in the JAK-STAT signaling pathways is now well defined (Fig. 7-25). Inactive JAK enzymes are non-covalently attached to the cytoplasmic domains of type I and type II cytokine receptors. When two receptor molecules are brought together by binding of a cytokine molecule, the receptor-associated JAKs are activated and phosphorylate tyrosine residues in the cytoplasmic portions of the clustered receptors. Some of these phosphotyrosine moieties of the receptors are then recognized and bind to Src homology 2 (SH2) domains of monomeric cytosolic STAT proteins. The STAT proteins are thus brought close to JAKs and are phosphorylated by these receptor-associated kinases. The SH2 domain of one STAT monomer is able to bind to a phosphotyrosine residue on an adjacent STAT protein. The STAT dimers that are generated migrate to the

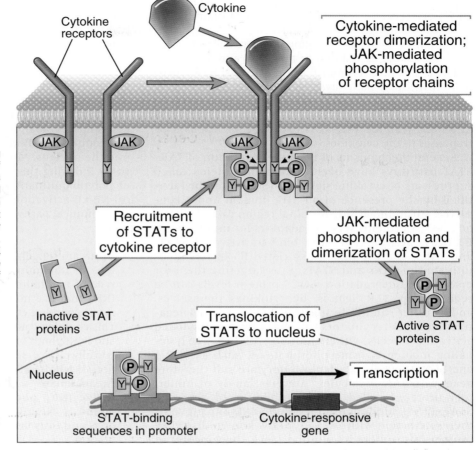

FIGURE 7-25 JAK-STAT signaling induced by cytokines. Ligation of receptors for type I and type II cytokines results in the activation of an associated JAK tyrosine kinase, the phosphorylation of the receptor tail, and the recruitment of an SH2 domain–containing activator of transcription (STAT) to the receptor. The recruited STAT is activated by JAK phosphorylation, dimerizes, enters the nucleus, and turns on the expression of cytokine target genes.

nucleus, where they bind to specific DNA sequences in the promoter regions of cytokine-responsive genes and activate gene transcription.

An intriguing question is how the specificity of responses to many different cytokines is achieved, given the limited numbers of JAKs and STATs used by the various cytokine receptors. The likely answer is that unique amino acid sequences in the different cytokine receptors provide the scaffolding for specifically binding, and thereby activating, different combinations of JAKs and STATs. The SH2 domains of different STAT proteins selectively bind to phosphotyrosines and flanking residues of different cytokine receptors. This is largely responsible for the activation of particular STATs by various cytokine receptors and therefore for the specificity of cytokine signaling. Several type I and type II cytokine receptors are heterodimers of two different polypeptide chains, each of which binds a different JAK. Furthermore, two different STATs may heterodimerize on phosphorylation. Therefore, there is a significant amount of combinatorial diversity in the signaling that can be generated from a limited number of JAK and STAT proteins.

Several JAKs and STATs are relevant to human disease and are targets of therapeutic agents. The subset of type I cytokine receptor family members that use the common γ chain (CD132; see Figure 7-23, B) all use

the JAK3 kinase for signaling. JAK3 is the only JAK kinase that is not expressed ubiquitously; its expression is largely restricted to immune cells and it is only activated by common γ chain–containing cytokine receptors. As discussed in Chapter 21, the common γ chain is encoded by an X-linked gene and mutations in this gene are the cause of X-linked severe combined immunodeficiency disease (X-SCID). Autosomal recessive mutations in the gene encoding JAK3 contribute to a similar phenotype. Type I cytokine receptors of the IL-6 family (see Figure 7-23, B) use JAK2 to activate STAT3. A number of other cytokines also activate STAT3. As discussed in Chapters 4 and 10, IL-6 signaling contributes to inflammation both in the context of innate immunity and the generation of T_H17 responses. Heterozygous dominant negative mutations in STAT3 are one of the causes of the hyper IgE syndrome, also called Job's syndrome, an immunodeficiency associated with defects in T_H17 responses (see Chapter 21). Activating mutations in STAT3 are characteristic features of large granular lymphocytic leukemias that involve expansions of NK cells or CD8+ T cells. In general, loss-of-function germline mutations in certain JAKs and STATs contribute to primary immunodeficiency syndromes, and activating somatic mutations in STATs are associated with a host of malignancies. JAK antagonists have been developed for the treatment of some leukemias that have mutations in this pathway, and more recently for the treatment of inflammatory diseases including rheumatoid arthritis.

Cytokines activate signaling pathways and transcription factors in addition to the JAKs and STATs. For instance, the IL-2 receptor β chain activates Ras-dependent MAP kinase pathways that may be involved in gene transcription and growth stimulation. Other cytokine receptors may similarly activate other signaling pathways in concert with the JAK-STAT pathways to elicit biologic responses to the cytokines.

Several mechanisms of negative regulation of JAK-STAT pathways have been identified. Proteins called suppressors of cytokine signaling (SOCS) can be identified by the presence of an SH2 domain and a conserved 40–amino acid C-terminal region called a SOCS box. SOCS proteins serve as adaptors for multisubunit E3 ligase activity. They can bind to activated STATs and JAKs, and the tightly associated E3 ligases ubiquitinate the JAKs and STATs, thus targeting them for proteasomal degradation. SOCS protein levels can be regulated by TLR ligands, by cytokines themselves, and by other stimuli. In this way, SOCS serve as negative feedback regulators of the cytokine-mediated activation of cells. Other inhibitors of JAK-STAT signaling include tyrosine phosphatases, such as SHP-1 and SHP-2, which can dephosphorylate and therefore deactivate JAK molecules. Another family of inhibitory proteins, called protein inhibitors of activated STAT (PIAS), binds phosphorylated STATs and prevents their interaction with DNA. It is now known that PIAS proteins also interact with and block the function of other transcription factors associated with cytokine signaling, including NF-κB and SMADs (transcription factors downstream of members of the TGF-β receptor family).

Pathways of NF-κB Activation

NF-κB is a transcription factor that plays a central role in inflammation, lymphocyte activation, cell survival, and the formation of secondary lymphoid organs. It is also an important player in lymphocyte development and in the pathogenesis of many cancers, including malignant neoplasms derived from activated lymphocytes. NF-κB is activated by many cytokine and TLR stimuli and by antigen recognition and is discussed here as the prototype of a transcription factor with fundamental roles in innate and adaptive immunity.

There are five NF-κB proteins. The domain that is common to all NF-κB proteins is a DNA-binding domain called a Rel homology domain. For a transcription factor to be active, it must both bind DNA and contain an activation domain that can facilitate transcriptional initiation. Three NF-κB proteins have both Rel homology domains and activation domains. These are p65/RelA, RelB, and c-Rel. NF-κB1/p50 and NF-κB2/p52 proteins contain a DNA-binding Rel homology domain but lack activation domains. NF-κB1 typically forms active heterodimers with p65/RelA or with c-Rel, and these heterodimers are typically considered canonical NF-κB heterodimers (Fig. 7-26). Canonical NF-κB heterodimers

reside in the cytosol bound to an inhibitor of NF-κB called **IκBα**. Canonical NF-κB heterodimers are activated by a number of signaling receptors that drive inflammation or lymphocyte activation.

As we have noted earlier in this chapter, TLRs, the BCR, the TCR, and many cytokine receptors of the TNF and IL-1R family activate NF-κB, and we will examine the common pathway involved in activating canonical NF-κB signaling. This NF-κB pathway induces the tagging and degradation of IκBα, allowing the unfettered heterodimeric NF-κB transcription factor to migrate into the nucleus. Most receptors that activate NF-κB do so by inducing this pathway. Two very different types of polyubiquitination events are required for canonical NF-κB activation. There are a few common steps in the canonical pathway that apply to all upstream signal inputs.

- Upstream signaling leads to the activation of a unique type of ubiquitin E3 ligase that can add a lysine-63 type of ubiquitin chain to a protein called NEMO or IKKγ that is a non-catalytic subunit of a trimeric enzyme complex called the IκB kinase (IKK) complex. This complex contains two other subunits called IKKα and IKKβ, both of which have the potential to be catalytically active serine/threonine kinases. Ubiquitination of NEMO allows IKKβ to be activated by an upstream kinase.
- Active IKKβ phosphorylates the inhibitory protein bound to NF-κB, IκBα, on two specific serine residues and thus tags this protein for lysine-48 ubiquitination.
- Polyubiquitinated IκBα is targeted for degradation in the proteasome, and the canonical NF-κB heterodimer is then free to enter the nucleus (see Fig. 7-26).

We discussed earlier how TCR and BCR signaling contributes to the activation of PKC-θ and PKC-β, respectively. These PKCs can phosphorylate a protein called CARMA1 that forms a complex with two proteins called Bcl-10 and MALT1. The CARMA1/MALT1/Bcl-10 complex can contribute to the activation of a lysine-63 type of ubiquitin E3 ligase called TRAF6. Active TRAF6 can activate TAK1 and also add a lysine-63 ubiquitin chain to NEMO, thus facilitating the activation of IKKβ. TLRs and the IL-1R also activate TRAF6 to initiate IKK activation. Many members of the TNF receptor family, including the TNF receptor and CD40, can activate canonical NF-κB signaling through the activation of other TRAF proteins such as TRAF2, TRAF3, and TRAF5.

Heterodimers of NF-κB2 and RelB make up a non-canonical form of NF-κB, and these heterodimers are activated by a separate signaling pathway that is particularly important for lymphoid organ biogenesis and the survival of naive B lymphocytes. The two key receptors that induce the non-canonical or alternative NF-κB pathway, the LTβR (lymphotoxin β receptor) and the BAFFR (BAFF receptor), activate an IKK-like complex that contains IKKα homodimers. This leads to ubiquitination and degradation of a part of the NF-κB2–RelB dimer and release of the active protein.

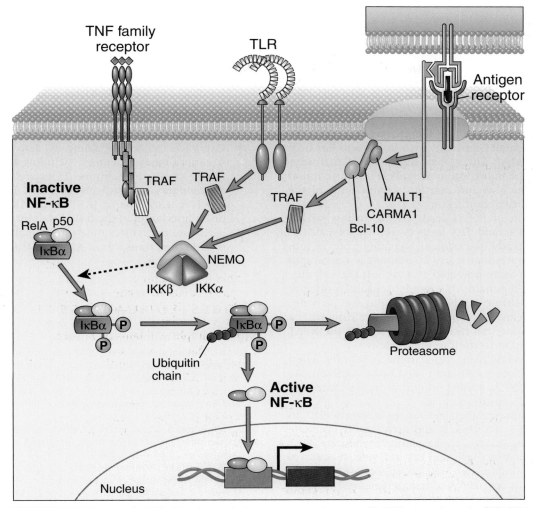

FIGURE 7-26 The canonical NF-κB pathway. Antigen receptors activate specific PKCs that activate the CARMA1/ Bcl-10/MALT1 complex, which in turn contributes to the induction of a TRAF E3 ligase that can polyubiquitinate NEMO/IKKγ, a component of the IκB kinase (IKK) complex, forming lysine-63–linked ubiquitin chains. This leads to the phosphorylation and activation of IKKβ by an upstream kinase. IKKβ phosphorylates the inhibitor of NF-κB (IκBα) and targets it for lysine-48 polyubiquitination and proteasomal degradation. Degradation of IκBα leads to the entry of active NF-κB into the nucleus. TLRs, members of the IL-1R family, and many members of the TNF receptor family activate TRAF family members that can activate this pathway.

SUMMARY

* Signaling receptors, typically located on the cell surface, generally initiate signaling in the cytosol, followed by a nuclear phase during which gene expression is altered.

* Many different types of signaling receptors contribute to innate and adaptive immunity, the most prominent category being immune receptors that belong to a receptor family in which non-receptor tyrosine kinases phosphorylate tyrosine-containing ITAM motifs on the cytoplasmic tails of proteins in the receptor complex.

* Some of the other types of receptors of interest in immunology include those of the receptor tyrosine kinase family, nuclear receptors, heterotrimeric G protein–coupled serpentine receptors, and receptors of the Notch family.

* Antigen receptors on T and B cells, as well as Ig Fc receptors, are members of the immune receptor family.

* Antigen receptors can produce widely varying outputs, depending on the affinity and valency of the antigen that can recruit different numbers of ITAMs.

* Coreceptors, such as CD4 or CD8 on T cells and CD21 (CR2) on B cells, enhance signaling from antigen receptors. Coreceptors bind to the same antigen complex that is being recognized by the antigen receptor.

* Signaling from antigen receptors can be attenuated by inhibitory receptors.

* The TCR complex is made up of the TCR α and β chains that contribute to antigen recognition and the ITAM-containing signaling chains CD3 γ, δ, and ε as well as the ζ homodimer. The CD3 chains each contain one ITAM, whereas each ζ chain contains three ITAMs.

* TCR ligation results in tyrosine phosphorylation of CD3 and ζ ITAMs by Src family kinases and the recruitment of ZAP-70 to the phospho-ITAMs, each SH2 domain of ZAP-70 binding to one phosphorylated tyrosine of the ITAM.
* Activated ZAP-70 phosphorylates tyrosine residues on adaptors, and downstream enzymes are recruited to the signalosome.
* Enzymes that mediate the exchange of GTP for GDP on small G proteins such as Ras and Rac help initiate MAP kinase pathways. These pathways lead to the induction or activation of transcription factors such as Jun and Fos, components of the AP-1 transcription factor.
* Activation of PLCγ1 leads to the release of IP3 from PIP2, and IP3 induces release of calcium from intracellular stores. Depletion of calcium from intracellular stores facilitates the opening of CRAC, a store-operated channel on the cell surface that maintains the raised intracellular calcium levels. Calcium binds to calmodulin and activates downstream proteins including calcineurin, a phosphatase that facilitates the entry of the NFAT transcription factor into the nucleus.
* Diacylglycerol is generated in the membrane when PLCγ1 releases IP3 from PIP2. DAG can activate PKC-θ, which, among other things, can contribute to NF-κB activation.
* A lipid kinase called PI3-kinase converts PIP2 to PIP3. PIP3 can recruit and activate PH domain–containing proteins to the plasma membrane. PIP3 activates Itk in T cells and Btk in B cells. It activates PDK1, a kinase that can phosphorylate a downstream kinase called Akt that mediates cell survival.
* Costimulatory receptors initiate signaling separately from antigen receptors, but signaling outputs from antigen receptors and costimulatory receptors synergize in the nucleus. The major costimulatory receptor in T cells is CD28.
* T cell signaling can be inhibited by phosphatases that may be recruited by inhibitory receptors such as CTLA-4 and PD-1.
* T cell signaling is also attenuated by ubiquitin E3 ligases that can contribute to the monoubiquitination and lysosomal degradation of activated signaling proteins.
* The B cell receptor is made up of membrane-bound immunoglobulin and an associated disulfide-linked Igα and Igβ heterodimer. Both Igα and Igβ contain ITAM motifs in their cytoplasmic tails. Signaling pathways linked to the BCR are broadly similar to signaling pathways downstream of the TCR
* Attenuation of immune receptor signaling in B cells, T cells, and NK cells, among others, is mediated by inhibitory receptors that frequently contain inhibitory tyrosine–containing motifs or ITIMs in their cytoplasmic tails.
* Another important mechanism of signal attenuation involves the ubiquitination of signaling proteins by E3 ubiquitin ligases.

* Cytokine receptors can be divided into a few broad categories based on structural considerations and mechanisms of signaling.
* Many cytokine receptors use non-receptor tyrosine kinases called JAKs to phosphorylate transcription factors called STATs.
* Some cytokine receptors such as those of the TNF receptor family activate either canonical or non-canonical NF-κB signaling.
* Canonical NF-κB signaling is activated downstream of many receptors, including TNF receptor family cytokine receptors, TLRs and IL-1R family members, and antigen receptors. The pathway involves activation of IKKβ in the IKK complex, phosphorylation of the IκBα inhibitor by activated IKKβ, ubiquitination and proteasomal degradation of IκBα, and transport of NF-κB to the nucleus.

SUGGESTED READINGS

Signaling by Immune Receptors

Call ME, Wucherpfennig KW: Common themes in the assembly and architecture of activating immune receptors, *Nature Reviews Immunology* 7:841–850, 2007.

Cannons JL, Tangye SG, Schwartzberg PL: SLAM family receptors and SAP adaptors in immunity, *Annual Review of Immunology* 29:665–705, 2011.

Vallabhapurapu S, Karin M: Regulation and function of NF-κB transcription factors in the immune system, *Annual Review of Immunology* 27:693–733, 2009.

Yuan JS, Kousis PC, Suliman S, Visan I, Guidos CJ: Functions of notch signaling in the immune system: consensus and controversies, *Annual Review of Immunology* 28:343–365, 2010.

T Cell Receptor Structure and Signaling

Brownlie RJ, Zamoyska R: T cell receptor signaling networks: branched, diversified, and bonded, *Nature Reviews Immunology* 13:257–269, 2013.

Burkhardt JK, Carrizosa E, Shaffer MH: The actin cytoskeleton in T cell activation, *Annual Review of Immunology* 26:233–259, 2008.

Fooksman DR, Vardhana S, Vasiliver-Shamis G, Liese J, Blair DA, Waite J, Sacristan C, Victora GD, Zanin-Zhorov A, Dustin ML: Functional anatomy of T cell activation and synapse formation, *Annual Review of Immunology* 28:79–105, 2010.

Gallo EM, Cante-Barrett K, Crabtree GR: Lymphocyte calcium signaling from membrane to nucleus, *Nature Immunology* 7:25–32, 2006.

Hogan PG, Lewis RS, Rao A: Molecular basis of calcium signaling in lymphocytes: STIM and ORAI, *Annual Review of Immunology* 28:491–533, 2010.

Kuhns MS, Davis MM, Garcia KC: Deconstructing the form and function of the TCR/CD3 complex, *Immunity* 24:133–139, 2006.

MacIver NJ, Michalek RD, Rathmell JC: Metabolic regulation of T lymphocytes, *Annual Review of immunology* 31:259–283, 2013.

Okkenhaug K: Signaling by the phosphoinositide 3-kinase family in immune cells, *Annual Review of immunology* 31:675–704, 2013.

Pearce EL, Poffenberger MC, Chang CH, Jones RG: Fueling immunity: insights into metabolism and lymphocyte function, *Science* 342:1242454, 2013.

Rudolph MG, Stanfield RL, Wilson IA: How TCRs bind MHCs, peptides, and coreceptors, *Annual Review of Immunology* 24:419–466, 2006.

Smith-Garvin JE, Koretzky GA, Jordan MS: T cell activation, *Annual Review of Immunology* 27:591–619, 2009.

van der Merwe P, Dushek O: Mechanisms for T cell receptor triggering, *Nature Reviews Immunology* 11:47–55, 2011.

Waickman AT, Powell JD: Mammalian target of rapamycin integrates diverse inputs to guide the outcome of antigen recognition in T cells, *Journal of Immunology* 188:4721–4729, 2012.

B Cell Receptor Structure and Signaling

Harwood NE, Batista FD: Early events in B cell activation, *Annual Review of Immunology* 28:185–210, 2010.

Kurosaki T, Shinohara H, Baba Y: B cell signaling and fate decision, *Annual Review of Immunology* 28:21–55, 2010.

Signal Attenuation in Lymphocytes

Acuto O, Bartolo VD, Michel F: Tailoring T-cell receptor signals by proximal negative feedback mechanisms, *Nature Reviews Immunology* 8:699–712, 2008.

Pao LI, Badour K, Siminovitch KA, Neel BG: Nonreceptor protein-tyrosine phosphatases in immune cell signaling, *Annual Review of Immunology* 25:473–523, 2007.

Smith KG, Clatworthy MR: FcγRIIB in autoimmunity and infection: evolutionary and therapeutic implications, *Nature Reviews Immunology* 10:328–343, 2010.

Sun SC: Deubiquitylation and regulation of the immune response, *Nature Reviews Immunology* 8:501–511, 2008.

Cytokine Receptors

O'Shea JJ, Holland SM, Staudt LM: JAKs and STATs in immunity, immunodeficiency, and cancer, *New England Journal of Medicine* 368:161–170, 2013.

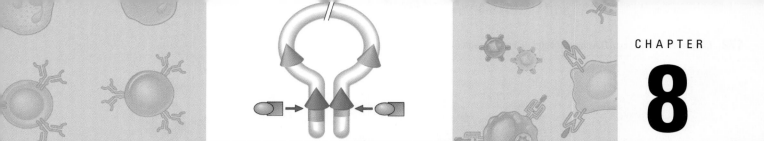

Lymphocyte Development and Antigen Receptor Gene Rearrangement

Lymphocytes express highly diverse antigen receptors that are capable of recognizing a wide variety of foreign substances. This diversity is generated during the development of mature B and T lymphocytes from precursor cells that do not express antigen receptors and cannot recognize and respond to antigens. The process by which lymphocyte progenitors in the thymus and bone marrow differentiate into mature lymphocytes that populate peripheral lymphoid tissues is called lymphocyte development or lymphocyte maturation. (The terms development and maturation are used interchangeably in this context.) The large collection of distinct antigen receptors—and therefore specificities—expressed by B and T lymphocytes are produced during the maturation of these cells. Maturation is initiated by signals from cell surface receptors that have two main roles: They promote the proliferation of progenitors, and they initiate the rearrangement of specific antigen receptor genes. The rearrangement of antigen receptor genes is a key event in the commitment of a progenitor cell to the B or T lymphocyte lineage.

We begin this chapter by considering the process of commitment to the B and T lymphocyte lineages and discussing some common principles and mechanisms of B and T cell development. This is followed by a description of the processes that are unique to the development of B cells and then of those unique to T cells.

OVERVIEW OF LYMPHOCYTE DEVELOPMENT

The maturation of B and T lymphocytes involves a series of events that occur in the generative lymphoid organs (Fig. 8-1). These events include the following:

- The *commitment of progenitor cells* to the B lymphoid or T lymphoid lineage.
- *Proliferation* of progenitors and immature committed cells at specific early stages of development, providing a large pool of cells that can generate useful lymphocytes.
- The *sequential and ordered rearrangement of antigen receptor genes* and the expression of antigen receptor proteins. (The terms rearrangement and recombination are used interchangeably.)
- *Selection events* that preserve cells that have produced functional antigen receptor proteins and eliminate potentially dangerous cells that strongly recognize self antigens. These checkpoints during development ensure that lymphocytes that express functional receptors with useful specificities will mature and enter the peripheral immune system.

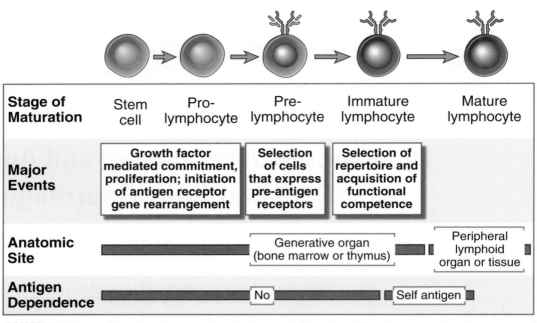

FIGURE 8-1 Stages of lymphocyte maturation. Development of both B and T lymphocytes involves the sequence of maturational stages shown. B cell maturation is illustrated, but the basic stages of T cell maturation are similar.

● *Differentiation of B and T cells into functionally and phenotypically distinct subpopulations.* B cells develop into follicular, marginal zone, and B-1 cells, and T cells develop into CD4+ and CD8+ αβ T lymphocytes, NKT cells and γδ T cells. The specialized functions of these different lymphocyte populations are discussed in later chapters.

Commitment to the B and T Cell Lineages and Proliferation of Progenitors

Pluripotent stem cells in the fetal liver and bone marrow, known as hematopoietic stem cells (HSCs), give rise to all lineages of blood cells, including lymphocytes. HSCs mature into common lymphoid progenitors that can give rise to B cells, T cells, innate lymphoid cells, and some dendritic cells (Fig. 8-2). The maturation of B cells from progenitors committed to this lineage occurs mostly in the bone marrow and before birth in the fetal liver. Fetal liver–derived stem cells give rise mainly to a type of B cell called a B-1 cell, whereas bone marrow–derived HSCs give rise to the majority of circulating B cells (follicular B cells) as well as a subset of B cells called marginal zone B cells. Precursors of T lymphocytes leave the fetal liver before birth and the bone marrow later in life and circulate to the thymus, where they complete their maturation. The majority of T cells, which are αβ T cells, develop from bone marrow–derived HSCs, whereas most γδ T cells arise from fetal liver HSCs. In general, the B and T cells that are generated early in fetal life have less diverse antigen receptors. Despite their different anatomic locations, the early maturation events of both B and T lymphocytes are fundamentally similar.

Commitment to the B or T lineage depends on instructions received from several cell surface receptors, which induce specific transcriptional regulators that drive a common lymphoid progenitor to specifically assume a B cell or a T cell fate. The cell surface receptors and transcription factors that contribute to commitment induce expression of the proteins involved in antigen receptor gene rearrangements, described later in the chapter, and make particular antigen receptor gene loci accessible to these proteins. In the case of developing B cells, the immunoglobulin (Ig) heavy chain locus, originally in an inaccessible chromatin configuration, is opened up so that it becomes accessible to the proteins that will mediate Ig gene rearrangement and expression. In developing αβ T cells, the T cell receptor (TCR) β gene locus is made available first. In addition to genes involved in the process of antigen receptor gene rearrangement, genes that drive the further differentiation of T and B cells are expressed at this stage.

Different sets of transcription factors drive the development of the B and T cell lineages from uncommitted precursors (see Fig. 8-2). The Notch-1 and GATA-3 transcription factors commit developing lymphocytes to the T cell lineage. The Notch family of proteins are cell surface molecules that are proteolytically cleaved when they interact with specific ligands on neighboring cells. The cleaved intracellular portions of Notch proteins migrate to the nucleus and modulate the expression of specific target genes. Notch-1 is activated in lymphoid progenitor cells and together with GATA3 it induces expression of a number of genes that are required for the further development of αβ T cells. Some of these genes encode components of the pre-TCR and proteins required for V(D)J recombination, described later. The EBF, E2A, and Pax-5 transcription factors induce the expression of genes required for B cell development. These include genes encoding the Rag-1 and Rag-2 proteins, surrogate light chains, and the Igα and Igβ proteins that contribute to signaling through the pre–B cell

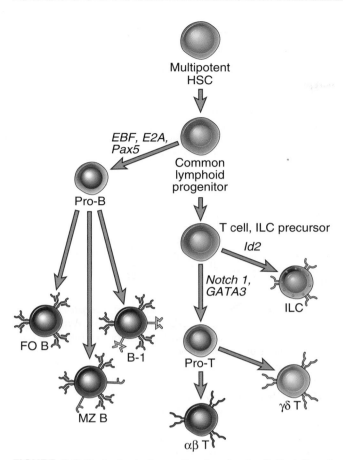

FIGURE 8-2 Pluripotent stem cells give rise to distinct B and T lineages. Hematopoietic stem cells (HSCs) give rise to distinct progenitors for various types of blood cells. One of these progenitor populations *(shown here)* is called a common lymphoid progenitor (CLP). CLPs give rise mainly to B and T cells but may also contribute to NK cells and some dendritic cells *(not depicted here).* Pro-B cells can eventually differentiate into follicular (FO) B cells, marginal zone (MZ) B cells, and B-1 cells. Pro-T cells may commit to either the αβ or γδ T cell lineages. Commitment to different lineages is driven by various transcription factors, indicated in italics. *ILC*, innate lymphoid cells.

and, as a result, profound deficiencies in mature T and B cells. Mutations in the common γ chain, a protein that is shared by the receptors for several cytokines including IL-2, IL-7, and IL-15 among others, give rise to an immunodeficiency disorder in humans called **X-linked severe combined immunodeficiency disease (X-SCID)** (see Chapter 21). This disease is characterized by a block in T cell and NK cell development, but normal B cell development, reflecting the requirement for IL-7 in T cell development in humans and of IL-15 for NK cells.

The greatest proliferative expansion of lymphocyte precursors occurs after successful rearrangement of the genes encoding one of the two chains of the T or B cell antigen receptor, producing a pre-antigen receptor (described later). Signals generated by pre-antigen receptors are responsible for far more expansion of developing lymphocytes than are cytokines such as IL-7.

Epigenetics, MicroRNAs, and Lymphocyte Development

Many nuclear events in lymphocyte development are regulated by epigenetic mechanisms. Epigenetics refers to mechanisms that control gene expression (as well as gene rearrangement in developing lymphocytes) that go beyond the actual sequence of DNA in individual genes. DNA exists in chromosomes tightly bound to histones and non-histone proteins, forming what is known as chromatin. DNA in chromatin is wound around a protein core of histone octamers, forming structures called nucleosomes, which may be either well separated from other nucleosomes or densely packed. Chromatin may therefore exist as relatively loosely packed structures, called euchromatin, wherein genes are available and are transcribed, or as very tightly packed structures called heterochromatin in which genes are maintained in a silenced state. The structural organization of portions of chromosomes therefore varies in different cells, making certain genes available for transcription factors to bind to while these very same genes may be unavailable to transcription factors in other cells.

The mechanisms that make genes available or unavailable in chromatin are considered to be epigenetic mechanisms. These include the methylation of DNA on certain cytosine residues that generally silences genes, post-translational modifications of the histone tails of nucleosomes (e.g., acetylation, methylation, and ubiquitination) that may render genes either active or inactive depending on the histone modified and the nature of the modification, active remodeling of chromatin by protein machines called remodeling complexes that can also either enhance or suppress gene expression, and the silencing of gene expression by non-coding RNAs.

Several critical components of lymphocyte development are regulated by epigenetic mechanisms.

● Histone modifications in antigen receptor gene loci are required for recruitment of proteins that mediate gene recombination to form functional antigen receptor genes.

receptor and the B cell receptor. The role of these receptors in B cell development will be considered later in this chapter.

During B and T cell development, committed progenitor cells proliferate first in response to cytokines and later in response to signals generated by a pre-antigen receptor that select cells that have successfully rearranged the first set of antigen receptor genes. Proliferation ensures that a large enough pool of progenitor cells will be generated to eventually provide a highly diverse repertoire of mature, antigen-specific lymphocytes. In rodents, the cytokine interleukin-7 (IL-7) drives proliferation of both early T and B cell progenitors; in humans, IL-7 is required for the proliferation of T cell progenitors but not of progenitors in the B lineage. IL-7 is produced by stromal cells in the bone marrow and by epithelial and other cells in the thymus. Mice with targeted mutations in either the IL-7 gene or the IL-7 receptor gene show defective maturation of lymphocyte precursors beyond the earliest stages

- CD4 vs. CD8 lineage commitment during T cell development depends on epigenetic mechanisms that silence the expression of the CD4 gene in CD8$^+$ T cells. Silencing involves chromatin modifications that place the CD4 gene into an inaccessible heterochromatin state.

- In Chapter 7, we discussed microRNAs (miRNAs) in the context of T cell activation. They contribute in significant ways to modulating gene and protein expression during development as well. As mentioned in Chapter 7, Dicer is a key enzyme in miRNA generation. Deletion of Dicer in the T lineage results in a preferential loss of regulatory T cells and the consequent development of an autoimmune phenotype similar to that seen in the absence of FoxP3 (discussed in Chapters 15 and 21). The loss of Dicer in the B lineage results in a block at the pro-B to pre-B cell transition (discussed in more detail in the section that follows), primarily by being permissive for the apoptosis of pre-B cells. Members of a specific miRNA family, the miR17-92 family, play a key role in preventing the death by apoptosis of pre-B cells by directly inhibiting the expression of Bim, a pro-apoptotic Bcl-2 family protein, and by also inhibiting the expression of PTEN, an inositol phosphatase that contributes positively to the induction of Bim expression. Gene ablation studies have revealed that other specific miRNAs are also involved in other steps in both B and T cell development.

Antigen Receptor Gene Rearrangement and Expression

The rearrangement of antigen receptor genes is the key event in lymphocyte development that is responsible for the generation of a diverse repertoire. As we discussed in Chapter 7, each clone of B or T lymphocytes produces an antigen receptor with a unique antigen-binding structure. In any individual, there may be 10^7 or more different B and T lymphocyte clones, each with a unique receptor. The ability of each individual to generate these enormously diverse lymphocyte repertoires has evolved in a way that does not require an equally large number of distinct antigen receptor genes; otherwise, a large proportion of the genome would be devoted to encoding the vast number of Ig and TCR molecules. Functional antigen receptor genes are produced in immature B cells in the bone marrow and in immature T cells in the thymus by a process of gene rearrangement, which is able to generate a large number of variable region–encoding exons using a relatively small fraction of the genome. In any given developing lymphocyte, one of many variable region gene segments is randomly selected and joined to a downstream DNA segment. The DNA rearrangement events that lead to the production of antigen receptors are not dependent on or influenced by the presence of antigens. In other words, as the clonal selection hypothesis had proposed, diverse antigen receptors are generated and expressed before encounter with antigens (see Fig. 1-7). We will discuss the molecular details of antigen receptor gene rearrangement later in this chapter.

Selection Processes That Shape the B and T Lymphocyte Repertoires

The process of lymphocyte development contains numerous intrinsic steps, called checkpoints, at which the developing cells are tested and continue to mature only if a preceding step in the process has been successfully completed. One of these checkpoints is based on the successful production of one of the polypeptide chains of the two-chain antigen receptor protein, and a second checkpoint requires the assembly of a complete receptor. The requirement for traversing these checkpoints ensures that only lymphocytes that have successfully completed antigen receptor gene rearrangement processes, and are therefore likely to be functional, are selected to mature. Additional selection processes operate after antigen receptors are expressed and serve to eliminate potentially harmful, self-reactive lymphocytes and to commit developing cells to particular lineages. We will next summarize the general principles of these selection events.

Pre-antigen receptors and antigen receptors deliver signals to developing lymphocytes that are required for the survival of these cells and for their proliferation and continued maturation (Fig. 8-3). Pre-antigen receptors, called pre-BCRs in B cells and pre-TCRs in T cells, are signaling structures expressed during B and T cell development, which contain only one of the two polypeptide chains present in a mature antigen receptor. Pre-BCRs contain the Ig μ heavy chain, and pre-TCRs contain the TCR β chain. In order to express Ig μ or TCR β proteins, B or T cells must undergo antigen receptor gene rearrangements. This involves the opening of a particular receptor gene locus (such as a TCR gene locus in T cells and an Ig gene locus in B cells) and the joining of DNA segments in this locus to generate a functional antigen receptor gene. During this process, bases are randomly added or removed between the gene segments being joined together, thus maximizing variability among receptors. In developing B cells, the first antigen receptor gene to be completely rearranged is the Ig heavy chain (IgH) gene. (Although the usual convention is to use italics for gene names, in this chapter we refer to genes, gene loci, gene segments and exons, and these are not italicized, for simplicity.) In αβ T cells, the β chain of the TCR is rearranged first. Cells of the B lymphocyte lineage that successfully rearrange their Ig heavy chain genes express the μ heavy chain protein and assemble a pre-antigen receptor known as the pre-BCR. In an analogous fashion, developing T cells that make a productive TCR β chain gene rearrangement synthesize the TCR β chain protein and assemble a pre-antigen receptor known as the pre-TCR. Only about one in three developing B and T cells that rearranges an antigen receptor gene makes an in-frame rearrangement and is therefore capable of generating a proper full-length protein. If cells make out-of-frame rearrangements at the Ig μ or TCR β chain loci, the pre-antigen receptors are not expressed, the cells do not receive necessary survival signals, and they undergo programmed cell death. The assembled pre-BCR and pre-TCR complexes provide signals for survival, for proliferation, for the phenomenon of allelic exclusion (discussed later), and for the further development of early B and

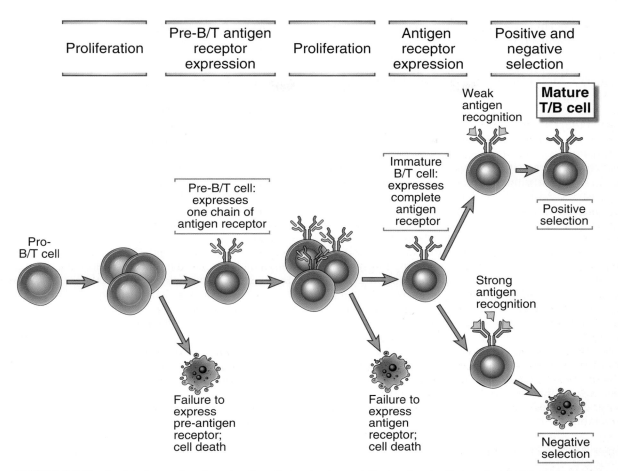

FIGURE 8-3 Checkpoints in lymphocyte maturation. During development, the lymphocytes that express receptors required for continued proliferation and maturation are selected to survive, and cells that do not express functional receptors die by apoptosis. Positive selection and negative selection further preserve cells with useful specificities. The presence of multiple checkpoints ensures that only cells with useful receptors complete their maturation.

T lineage cells. Thus, expression of the pre-antigen receptor is the first checkpoint during lymphocyte development.

Developing B and T cells next express complete antigen receptors and are selected for survival based on what those receptors can or cannot recognize. Lymphocytes that have successfully navigated the pre-antigen receptor checkpoint go on to rearrange and express genes encoding the second chain of the BCR or TCR, and express the complete antigen receptor while they are still immature. At this immature stage, potentially harmful cells that strongly recognize self structures may be eliminated or induced to alter their antigen receptors, and cells that express useful antigen receptors may be preserved (see Fig. 8-3). A process called **positive selection** facilitates the survival of potentially useful lymphocytes, and this developmental event is linked to lineage commitment, the process by which lymphocyte subsets are generated. In the T cell lineage, positive selection ensures the maturation of T cells whose receptors recognize self MHC molecules. Also, the expression of the appropriate coreceptor on a T cell (CD8 or CD4) is matched to the recognition of the appropriate type of MHC molecule (class I MHC or class II MHC, respectively). Mature T cells whose precursors were positively selected by self MHC molecules in the thymus are

able to recognize foreign peptide antigens displayed by the same self MHC molecules on antigen-presenting cells in peripheral tissues. In the B cell lineage, positive selection preserves receptor-expressing cells and is coupled to the generation of different subsets, discussed later.

Negative selection is the process that eliminates or alters developing lymphocytes whose antigen receptors bind strongly to self antigens present in the generative lymphoid organs. Both developing B and T cells are susceptible to negative selection during a short period after antigen receptors are first expressed. Developing T cells with a high affinity for self antigens are eliminated by apoptosis, a phenomenon known as **clonal deletion**. Strongly self-reactive immature B cells may be induced to make further Ig gene rearrangements and thus evade self-reactivity. This phenomenon is called **receptor editing**. If editing fails, the self-reactive B cells die, also called clonal deletion. Negative selection of immature lymphocytes is an important mechanism for maintaining tolerance to many self antigens; this is also called **central tolerance** because it develops in the central (generative) lymphoid organs (see Chapter 15).

With this introduction, we will proceed to a more detailed discussion of lymphocyte maturation, starting with the key event in the process, the rearrangement and expression of antigen receptor genes.

REARRANGEMENT OF ANTIGEN RECEPTOR GENES IN B AND T LYMPHOCYTES

The genes that encode diverse antigen receptors of B and T lymphocytes are generated by the rearrangement in individual lymphocytes of different variable (V) region gene segments with diversity (D) and joining (J) gene segments. A novel rearranged exon for each antigen receptor gene is generated by fusing a specific distant upstream V gene segment to a downstream segment on the same chromosome. This specialized process of site-specific gene rearrangement is called **V(D)J recombination.** Elucidation of the mechanisms of antigen receptor gene rearrangement, and therefore of the underlying basis for the generation of immune diversity, represents one of the landmark achievements of modern immunology.

The first insights into how millions of different antigen receptors could be generated from a limited amount of coding DNA in the genome came from analyses of the amino acid sequences of Ig molecules. These analyses showed that the polypeptide chains of many different antibodies of the same isotype shared identical sequences at their C-terminal ends (corresponding to the constant domains of antibody heavy and light chains) but differed considerably in the sequences at their N-terminal ends that correspond to the variable domains of immunoglobulins (see Chapter 5). Contrary to one of the central tenets of molecular genetics, enunciated as the one gene–one polypeptide hypothesis, it was postulated in 1965 that each antibody chain is actually encoded by at least two genes, one variable and the other constant, and that the two are physically combined at the level of DNA or of messenger RNA (mRNA) to eventually give rise to functional Ig proteins. Formal proof of this hypothesis came more than a decade later when Susumu Tonegawa demonstrated that the structure of Ig genes in the cells of an antibody-producing tumor, called a myeloma or plasmacytoma, is different from that in embryonic tissues or in nonlymphoid tissues not committed to Ig production. These differences arise because DNA segments that are separated within the inherited loci encoding Ig heavy and light chains are brought together and joined only in developing B cells but not in other tissues or cell types. Similar rearrangements were found to occur during T cell development in the loci encoding the polypeptide chains of TCRs. Antigen receptor gene rearrangement is best understood by first describing the unrearranged, or germline, organization of Ig and TCR genes and then describing their rearrangement during lymphocyte maturation.

Germline Organization of Ig and TCR Genes

The germline organizations of Ig and TCR genetic loci are fundamentally similar and are characterized by spatial segregation of many different sequences that encode variable domains and relatively few sequences that encode constant domains of receptor proteins; distinct variable region sequences are joined to constant region sequences

in different lymphocytes. We will first describe the Ig loci and then the TCR loci.

Organization of Ig Gene Loci

Three separate loci encode, respectively, all of the Ig heavy chains, the Ig κ light chain, and the Ig λ light chain. Each locus is on a different chromosome. The organization of human Ig genes is illustrated in Figure 8-4, and the relationship of gene segments after rearrangement to the domains of the Ig heavy and light chain proteins is shown in Figure 8-5, *A*. Ig genes are organized in essentially the same way in all mammals, although their chromosomal locations and the number and sequence of different gene segments in each locus may vary.

At the 5′ end of each Ig locus, there is a cluster of V (variable) genes, with each V gene in the cluster being about 300 base pairs long. The numbers of V genes vary considerably among the different Ig loci and among different species. For example, in humans there are about 35 V genes in the human κ light chain locus, about 30 in the λ locus and about 45 functional V genes in the heavy chain locus, whereas in mice, the κ locus has about 30 V genes, the λ light chain locus has only two V genes and the heavy chain locus has more than 1000 V genes, of which about 250 are functional. The V gene segments for each locus are spaced over large stretches of DNA, up to 2000 kilobases long. Located 5′ of each V segment is a leader exon that encodes the 20 to 30 N-terminal residues of the translated protein. These residues are moderately hydrophobic and make up the leader (or signal) peptide. Signal sequences are found in all newly synthesized secreted and transmembrane proteins and are involved in guiding nascent polypeptides being translated on membrane-bound ribosomes into the lumen of the endoplasmic reticulum. Here, the signal sequences are rapidly cleaved, and they are not present in the mature proteins. Upstream of each leader exon is a V gene promoter at which transcription can be initiated, but, as discussed later, this occurs most efficiently after rearrangement.

At varying distances 3′ of the V genes are several J (joining) segments that are closely linked to downstream constant region exons. J segments are typically 30 to 50 base pairs long and are separated by non-coding sequences. Between the V and J segments in the IgH locus, there are additional segments known as D (diversity) segments. D segments are not found in Ig light chain loci. As for V genes, the numbers of D and J genes vary in different Ig loci and different species.

Each Ig locus has a distinct arrangement and number of C region genes. In humans, the Ig κ light chain locus has a single C gene (C_κ), and the λ light chain locus has four functional C genes (C_λ). The Ig heavy chain locus has nine C genes (C_H), arranged in a tandem array, that encode the C regions of the nine different Ig isotypes and subtypes (see Chapter 5). The C_κ and C_λ genes are each composed of a single exon that encodes the entire C domain of the light chains. In contrast, each C_H gene is composed of five or six exons. Three or four exons (each similar in size to a V gene segment) each encode a C_H domain of the Ig heavy chain, and two smaller exons code for the carboxyl-terminal ends of the membrane form of each Ig heavy chain, including the transmembrane and cytoplasmic domains of the heavy chains (see Fig. 8-5, *A*).

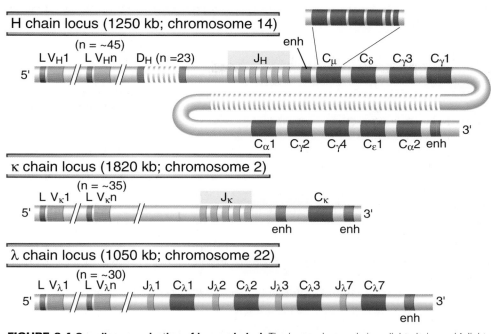

FIGURE 8-4 Germline organization of human Ig loci. The human heavy chain, κ light chain, and λ light chain loci are shown. Only functional genes are shown; pseudogenes have been omitted for simplicity. Exons and introns are not drawn to scale. Each C_H gene is shown as a single box but is composed of several exons, as illustrated for C_μ. Gene segments are indicated as follows: *L,* leader (often called signal sequence); *V,* variable; *D,* diversity; *J,* joining; *C,* constant; *enh,* enhancer. In this and in subsequent figures the tubular structures depict double stranded segments of chromosomes with the 5′ and 3′ ends referring to the coding strands.

In an Ig light chain protein (κ or λ), the V domain is encoded by the V and J gene segments; in the Ig heavy chain protein, the V domain is encoded by the V, D, and J gene segments (see Fig. 8-5, *A*). In the case of the Ig H and TCR β V domains, the junctional residues between the rearranged V and D segments and the D and J segments as well as the sequences of the D and J segments themselves make up the third hypervariable region, also known as complementarity-determining region 3 or CDR3. The junctional sequences between the rearranged V and J segments as well as the J segment itself make up the third hypervariable region of Ig light chains. CDR1 and CDR2 are encoded in each germline V gene segment itself. The V and C domains of Ig molecules share structural features, including a tertiary structure called the Ig fold. As we discussed in Chapter 5, proteins that include this structure are members of the Ig superfamily.

Noncoding sequences in the Ig loci play important roles in recombination and gene expression. As we will see later, sequences that dictate recombination of different gene segments are found adjacent to each coding segment in Ig genes. Also present are V gene promoters and other *cis*-acting regulatory elements, such as locus control regions, enhancers, and silencers, which regulate gene expression at the level of transcription.

Organization of TCR Gene Loci

Each germline TCR locus is arranged in a very similar way to the Ig loci described earlier, with a 5′ cluster of several V gene segments, followed by D segments (in the β and δ loci only), followed by cluster of J segments, all upstream of C region genes (Fig. 8-6). In the human β locus there about 50 V, 2D and 12 J gene segments, and in the α locus there are 45 V and 50 J segments. The γ and δ loci overall have fewer gene segments than the α and β loci, with a total of only 7 V genes. Upstream of each TCR V gene is an exon that encodes a leader peptide, and upstream of each leader exon is a promoter for each V gene. In the TCR β and δ proteins, the V domain is encoded by the V, D, and J gene segments, and in the TCR α or γ proteins, the V domain is encoded by the V and J gene segments. There are two C genes in each of the human TCR β and TCR γ loci, each of which has its own associated 5′ cluster of J segments, and only one C gene in each of the α and γ loci. Each TCR C region gene is composed of four exons encoding the extracellular C region Ig domain, a short hinge region, the transmembrane segment, and the cytoplasmic tail.

The relationship of the TCR gene segments and the corresponding portions of TCR proteins that they encode is shown in Figure 8-5, *B*. As in Ig molecules, the TCR V and C domains assume an Ig fold tertiary structure, and thus the TCR is a member of the Ig superfamily of proteins.

V(D)J Recombination

The germline organization of Ig and TCR loci described in the preceding section exists in all cell types in the body. The germline genes cannot be transcribed into mRNAs that encode functional antigen receptor proteins. Functional antigen receptor genes are created only in developing B and T lymphocytes after DNA rearrangement

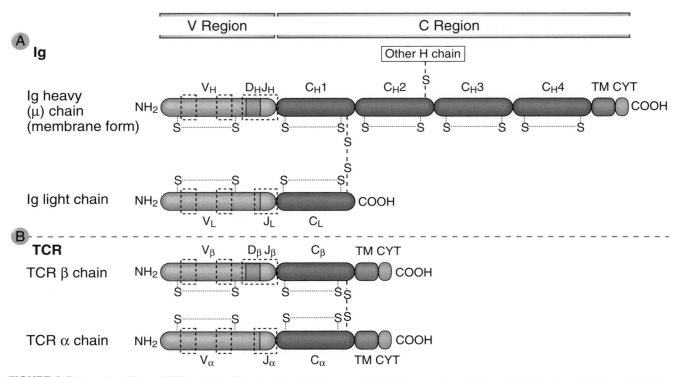

FIGURE 8-5 Domains of Ig and TCR proteins. The domains of Ig heavy and light chains are shown in **A,** and the domains of TCR α and β chains are shown in **B.** The relationships between the Ig and TCR gene segments and the domain structure of the antigen receptor polypeptide chains are indicated. The V and C regions of each polypeptide are encoded by different gene segments. The locations of intrachain and interchain disulfide bonds (S-S) are approximate. Areas in the dashed boxes are the hypervariable (complementarity-determining) regions. In the Ig μ chain and the TCR α and β chains, transmembrane (TM) and cytoplasmic (CYT) domains are encoded by separate exons.

events that bring randomly chosen V, (D), and J gene segments into contiguity.

The process of V(D)J recombination at any Ig or TCR locus involves selection of one V gene, one D segment (when present), and one J segment in each lymphocyte and rearrangement of these segments to form a single V(D)J exon that will code for the variable region of an antigen receptor protein (Fig. 8-7). In the Ig light chain and TCR α and γ loci, which lack D segments, a single rearrangement event joins a randomly selected V gene to an equally randomly selected J segment. The Ig H and TCR β and δ loci contain D segments, and at these loci two distinct rearrangement events must be separately initiated, first joining a D to a J and then a V segment to the fused DJ segment. Each rearrangement event involves a number of sequential steps. First, the chromatin must be opened in specific regions of the chromosome to make antigen receptor gene segments accessible to the enzymes that mediate recombination. Next, two selected gene segments must be brought next to one another across a considerable chromosomal distance. Double-stranded breaks are then introduced at the coding ends of these two segments, nucleotides are added or removed at the broken ends, and finally the processed ends are ligated to produce clonally unique but diverse antigen receptor genes that can be efficiently transcribed. The C regions lie downstream of the rearranged V(D)J exon separated by the germline J-C intron. This rearranged gene is transcribed to form a primary (nuclear) RNA transcript. Subsequent RNA splicing brings together

the leader exon, the V(D)J exon, and the C region exons, forming an mRNA that can be translated on membrane-bound ribosomes to produce one of the chains of the antigen receptor. The use of different combinations of V, D, and J gene segments and the addition and removal of nucleotides at the junctions contribute to the tremendous diversity of antigen receptors, as we will discuss in more detail later.

Recognition Signals That Drive V(D)J Recombination

Lymphocyte-specific proteins that mediate V(D)J recombination recognize certain DNA sequences called recombination signal sequences (RSSs), located 3′ of each V gene segment, 5′ of each J segment, and flanking each side of every D segment (Fig. 8-8, *A*). The RSSs consist of a highly conserved stretch of 7 nucleotides, called the heptamer, usually CACAGTG, located adjacent to the coding sequence, followed by a spacer of exactly 12 or 23 nonconserved nucleotides, followed by a highly conserved AT-rich stretch of 9 nucleotides, called the nonamer. The 12- and 23-nucleotide spacers roughly correspond to one or two turns of a DNA helix, respectively, and they presumably bring two distinct heptamers into positions that are simultaneously accessible to the enzymes that catalyze the recombination process.

During V(D)J recombination, double-stranded breaks are generated between the heptamer of the RSS and the adjacent V, D, or J coding sequence. In Ig light chain V-to-J recombination, for example, breaks will be made 3′ of a V segment and 5′ of a J segment. The intervening

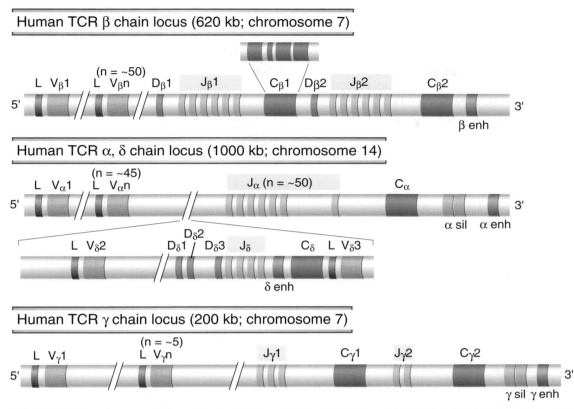

FIGURE 8-6 Germline organization of human TCR loci. The human TCR β, α, γ, and δ chain loci are shown, as indicated. Exons and introns are not drawn to scale, and nonfunctional pseudogenes are not shown. Each C gene is shown as a single box but is composed of several exons, as illustrated for $C_\beta 1$. Gene segments are indicated as follows: *L*, leader (usually called signal sequence); *V*, variable; *D*, diversity; *J*, joining; *C*, constant; *enh*, enhancer; *sil*, silencer (sequences that regulate *TCR* gene transcription).

double-stranded DNA, containing signal ends (the ends that contain the heptamer and the rest of the RSS), is removed in the form of a circle, and the V and J coding ends are joined (Fig. 8-8, B). In some V genes, especially in the Ig κ locus, the RSSs are 3′ of a Vκ and 3′ of Jκ, and therefore do not face each other. In these cases, the

intervening DNA is inverted and the V and J segments are properly aligned; the fused RSSs are not deleted but retained in the chromosome (Fig. 8-8, C). Most Ig and TCR gene rearrangements occur by deletion; inversion is the basis of up to 50% of rearrangements in the Ig κ locus. Recombination occurs between two segments only if one

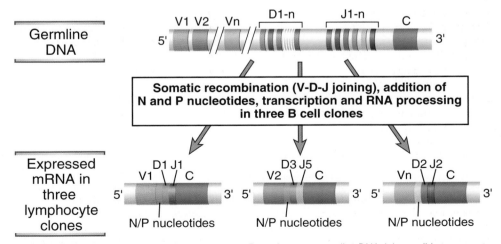

FIGURE 8-7 Diversity of antigen receptor genes. From the same germline DNA, it is possible to generate recombined DNA sequences and mRNAs that differ in their V-D-J junctions. In the example shown, three distinct antigen receptor mRNAs are produced from the same germline DNA by the use of different gene segments and the addition of nucleotides to the junctions.

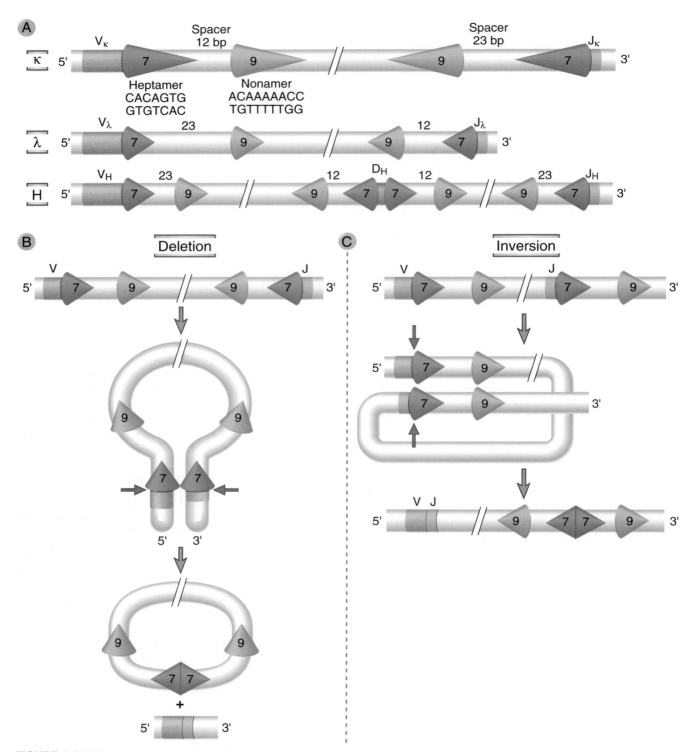

FIGURE 8-8 V(D)J recombination. The DNA sequences and mechanisms involved in recombination in the Ig gene loci are depicted. The same sequences and mechanisms apply to recombinations in the TCR loci. **A,** Conserved heptamer (7 bp) and nonamer (9 bp) sequences, separated by 12- or 23-bp spacers, are located adjacent to V and J segments (for κ and λ loci) or to V, D, and J segments (in the H chain locus). The V(D)J recombinase recognizes these recombination signal sequences and brings the exons together. **B, C,** Recombination of V and J exons may occur by deletion of intervening DNA and ligation of the V and J segments **(B)** or, if the RSS is 3′ of a J segment, by inversion of the DNA followed by ligation of adjacent gene segments **(C)**. Red arrows indicate the sites where germline sequences are cleaved before their ligation to other Ig or TCR gene segments.

of the segments is flanked by a 12-nucleotide spacer and the other is flanked by a 23-nucleotide spacer; this is called the 12/23 rule. A coding segment with an RSS with a spacer spanning a single turn of the DNA helix therefore always recombines with a coding segment with an RSS with a spacer that covers two turns of the helix. The type of the flanking RSSs (one turn or two turns) ensures that the appropriate gene segments will recombine. For example, in the Ig heavy chain locus, the RSSs flanking both V and J segments have 23-nucleotide spacers (two turns) and therefore cannot join directly; D-to-J recombination occurs first, followed by V-to-DJ recombination, and this is possible because the D segments are flanked on both sides by 12-nucleotide spacers, allowing D-J and then V-DJ joining. The RSSs described here are unique to Ig and TCR genes. Therefore, V(D)J recombination can occur in antigen receptor genes but not in other genes.

One of the consequences of V(D)J recombination is that the process brings promoters located immediately 5′ of V genes close to downstream enhancers that are located in the J-C introns and also 3′ of the C region genes (Fig. 8-9). These enhancers maximize the transcriptional activity of the V gene promoters and are thus important for high-level transcription of rearranged V genes in lymphocytes. Because Ig and TCR genes are sites for multiple DNA recombination events in B and T cells, and because these sites become transcriptionally active after recombination, genes from other loci can be abnormally translocated to these loci and, as a result, may be aberrantly transcribed. In tumors of B and T lymphocytes, oncogenes are often translocated to Ig or TCR gene loci. Such chromosomal translocations are frequently accompanied by enhanced transcription of the oncogenes and are one of the factors promoting the development of lymphoid tumors.

The Mechanism of V(D)J Recombination

Rearrangement of Ig and TCR genes represents a special kind of non-homologous DNA recombination event, mediated by the coordinated activities of several enzymes, some of which are found only in developing lymphocytes, whereas others are ubiquitous DNA double-stranded break repair (DSBR) enzymes. Although the mechanism of V(D)J recombination is fairly well understood and will be described here, how exactly specific loci are made accessible to the machinery involved in recombination remains to be determined. It is likely that the accessibility of the Ig and TCR loci to the enzymes that mediate recombination is regulated in developing B and T cells by several mechanisms, including epigenetic alterations in chromatin structure and DNA as discussed earlier, and basal transcriptional activity in the gene loci.

The process of V(D)J recombination can be divided into four distinct events that flow sequentially from one to the next (Fig. 8-10):

1. *Synapsis:* Portions of the chromosome on which the antigen receptor gene is located are made accessible to the recombination machinery. Two selected coding segments and their adjacent RSSs are brought

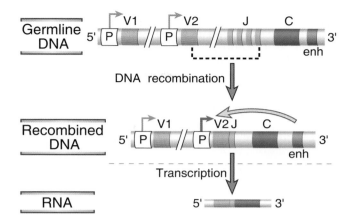

FIGURE 8-9 Transcriptional regulation of Ig genes. V-D-J recombination brings promoter sequences (shown as P) close to the enhancer (enh). The enhancer promotes transcription of the rearranged V gene (V2, whose active promoter is indicated by a bold green arrow). Many receptor genes have an enhancer in the J-C intron and another 3′ of the C region. Only the 3′ enhancer is depicted here.

together by a chromosomal looping event and held in position for subsequent cleavage, processing, and joining.

2. *Cleavage:* Double-stranded breaks are enzymatically generated at RSS-coding sequence junctions by machinery that is lymphoid specific. Two proteins encoded by lymphoid-specific genes, called **recombination-activating gene 1** and **recombination-activating gene 2** (*RAG1* and *RAG2*), form a complex, containing two molecules of each protein, that plays an essential role in V(D)J recombination. The Rag-1/Rag-2 complex is also known as the **V(D)J recombinase.** The Rag-1 protein, in a manner similar to a restriction endonuclease, recognizes the DNA sequence at the junction between a heptamer and a coding segment and cleaves it, but it is enzymatically active only when complexed with the Rag-2 protein. The Rag-2 protein may help link the Rag-1/Rag-2 tetramer to other proteins, including accessibility factors that bring these proteins to specific open receptor gene loci at specific times and at defined stages of lymphocyte development. Rag-1 and Rag-2 contribute to holding together gene segments during the process of chromosomal folding or synapsis. Rag-1 then makes a nick (on one DNA strand) between the coding end and the heptamer. The released 3′ OH of the coding end then attacks a phosphodiester bond on the other DNA strand, forming a covalent hairpin. The signal end (including the heptamer and the rest of the RSS) does not form a hairpin and is generated as a blunt double-stranded DNA terminus that undergoes no further processing. This double-stranded break results in a closed hairpin of one coding segment being held in apposition to the closed hairpin of the other coding end and two blunt recombination signal ends being placed next to each other. Rag-1 and Rag-2, apart from generating the double-stranded breaks, also hold the hairpin ends and the blunt ends together before the modification of the coding ends and the process of ligation.

RAG genes are lymphoid specific and are expressed only in developing B and T cells. Rag proteins are expressed mainly in the G_0 and G_1 stages of the cell cycle and are inactivated in proliferating cells. It is thought that limiting DNA cleavage and recombination

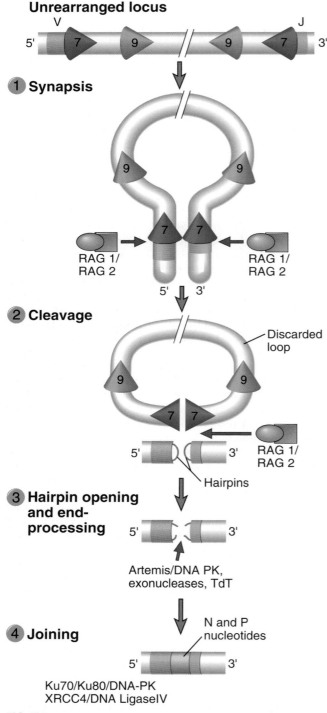

Unrearranged locus

① **Synapsis**

② **Cleavage**

③ **Hairpin opening and end-processing**

Artemis/DNA PK, exonucleases, TdT

④ **Joining**

N and P nucleotides

Ku70/Ku80/DNA-PK
XRCC4/DNA LigaseIV

FIGURE 8-10 Sequential events during V(D)J recombination. Synapsis and cleavage of DNA at the heptamer/coding segment boundary are mediated by Rag-1 and Rag-2. The coding end hairpin is opened by the Artemis endonuclease, and broken ends are repaired by the non-homologous end joining machinery present in all cells. Note that the two strands of DNA are shown in the hairpins but not in other schematic illustrations of genes.

to the G_0 and G_1 stages minimizes the risk of generating inappropriate DNA breaks during DNA replication or during mitosis. Mice without functional *Rag1* or *Rag2* genes (*Rag* knockout mice) fail to develop B or T lymphocytes, and Rag-1 or Rag-2 deficiency is also a rare cause of SCID, in which patients also lack all lymphocytes.

3. *Hairpin opening and end-processing:* The broken coding ends are modified by the addition or removal of bases, and thus greater diversity is generated. After the formation of double-stranded breaks, hairpins must be resolved (opened up) at the coding junctions, and bases may be added to or removed from the coding ends to ensure even greater diversification. **Artemis** is an endonuclease that opens up the hairpins at the coding ends. In the absence of Artemis, hairpins cannot be opened, and mature T and B cells cannot be generated. Mutations in ARTEMIS are a rare cause of SCID, similar to patients with *RAG1* or *RAG2* mutations. (see Chapter 21). A lymphoid-specific enzyme, called terminal deoxynucleotidyl transferase (TdT), adds bases to broken DNA ends and will be discussed later in the chapter in the context of junctional diversity.

4. *Joining:* The broken coding ends as well as the signal ends are brought together and ligated by a double-stranded break repair process found in all cells that is called nonhomologous end joining. A number of ubiquitous factors participate in nonhomologous end joining. Ku70 and Ku80 are DNA end-binding proteins that bind to the breaks and recruit the catalytic subunit of DNA-dependent protein kinase (DNA-PK), a double-stranded DNA repair enzyme. This enzyme is defective in mice carrying the severe combined immunodeficiency *(scid)* mutation, and mutations in the gene encoding this enzyme have also been discovered in human SCID patients (see Chapter 21). Like *Rag*-deficient mice, *scid* mice fail to produce mature lymphocytes. DNA-PK also phosphorylates and activates Artemis, which, as mentioned before, is involved in end processing. Ligation of the processed broken ends is mediated by DNA ligase IV and XRCC4, the latter being a non-catalytic but essential subunit of the ligase.

Generation of Diversity in B and T Cells

The diversity of the B and T cell repertoires is created by random combinations of germline gene segments being brought together and by random addition or deletion of sequences at the junctions between the segments before they are united. Several genetic mechanisms contribute to this diversity, and the relative importance of each mechanism varies among the different antigen receptor loci (Table 8-1).

● *Combinatorial diversity. V(D)J rearrangement brings together multiple germline gene segments that may combine randomly, and different combinations produce different antigen receptors.* The maximum possible number of combinations of these gene segments is the product of the numbers of V, J, and (if present) D gene

TABLE 8-1 Contributions of Different Mechanisms to the Generation of Diversity in Ig and TCR Genes

Mechanism	Ig			TCR αβ		TCR γδ	
	Heavy Chain	κ	λ	α	β	γ	δ
Variable (V) segments	45	35	30	45	50	5	2
Diversity (D) segments	23	0	0	0	2	0	3
D segments read in all three reading frames	Rare	—		—	Often	—	Often
N region diversification	V-D, D-J	None		V-J	V-D, D-J	V-J	V-D1, D1-D2, D1-J
Joining (J) segments	6	5	4	55	12	5	4
Total potential repertoire with junctional diversity	~10^{11}			~10^{16}		~10^{18}	

The potential number of antigen receptors with junctional diversity is much greater than the number that can be generated only by combinations of V, D, and J gene segments. Note that although the upper limit on the numbers of Ig and TCR proteins that may be expressed is very large, it is estimated that each individual contains on the order of 10^7 clones of B and T cells with distinct specificities and receptors; in other words, only a fraction of the potential repertoire may actually be expressed.

segments at each antigen receptor locus. Therefore, the amount of combinatorial diversity that can be generated at each locus reflects the number of germline V, J, and D gene segments at that locus. After synthesis of antigen receptor proteins, combinatorial diversity is further enhanced by the juxtaposition of two different, randomly generated V regions (i.e., V_H and V_L in Ig molecules and V_α and V_β in TCR molecules). Therefore, the total combinatorial diversity is theoretically the product of the combinatorial diversity of each of the two associating chains. The actual degree of combinatorial diversity in the expressed Ig and TCR repertoires in any individual is likely to be considerably less than the theoretical maximum. This is because not all recombinations of gene segments are equally likely to occur, and not all pairings of Ig heavy and light chains or TCR α and β chains may form functional antigen receptors. Importantly, because the numbers of V, D, and J segments in each locus are limited (see Table 8-1), the maximum possible numbers of combinations are on the order of thousands. This is, of course, much less than the actual diversity of antigen receptors in mature lymphocytes.

- *Junctional diversity. The largest contribution to the diversity of antigen receptors is made by the removal or addition of nucleotides at the junctions of the V and D, D and J, or V and J segments at the time these segments are joined.* One way in which this can occur is if endonucleases remove nucleotides from the germline sequences at the ends of the recombining gene segments. In addition, new nucleotide sequences, not present in the germline, may be added at junctions (Fig. 8-11). As described earlier, coding segments (e.g., V and J gene segments) that are cleaved by Rag-1 form hairpin loops whose ends are often cleaved asymmetrically by the enzyme Artemis so that one DNA strand is longer than the other. The shorter strand has to be extended with nucleotides complementary to the longer strand before the ligation of the two segments. The longer strand serves as a template for the addition of short lengths of nucleotides called P nucleotides, and this process introduces new sequences at

the V-D-J junctions. Another mechanism of junctional diversity is the random addition of up to 20 non–template-encoded nucleotides called N nucleotides (see Fig. 8-11). N region diversification is more common in Ig heavy chains and in TCR β and γ chains than in Ig κ or λ chains. This addition of new nucleotides is mediated by the enzyme **terminal deoxynucleotidyl transferase (TdT).** In mice rendered deficient in TdT by gene knockout, the diversity of B and T cell repertoires is substantially less than in normal mice. The addition of P nucleotides and N nucleotides at the recombination sites may introduce frameshifts, theoretically generating termination codons in two of every three joining events (if the total number of added bases is not a multiple of three). These genes cannot produce functional proteins, but such inefficiency is the price that is paid for generating diversity.

Because of junctional diversity, antibody and TCR molecules show the greatest variability at the junctions of V and C regions, which form the third hypervariable region, or CDR3 (see Fig. 8-5). In fact, because of junctional diversity, the numbers of different amino acid sequences that are present in the CDR3 regions of Ig and TCR molecules are much greater than the numbers that can be encoded by germline gene segments. The CDR3 regions of Ig and TCR molecules are also the most important portions of these molecules for determining the specificity of antigen binding (see Chapters 5 and 7). Thus, the greatest diversity in antigen receptors is concentrated in the regions of the receptors that are the most important for antigen binding.

Although the theoretical limit to the number of Ig and TCR proteins that can be produced is enormous (see Table 8-1), the actual number of antigen receptors on B or T cells expressed in each individual is probably on the order of only 10^7. This may reflect the fact that most receptors, which are generated by random DNA recombination, do not pass the selection processes needed for maturation.

A clinical application of our knowledge of junctional diversity is the determination of the clonality of lymphoid tumors that have arisen from B or T cells. This laboratory

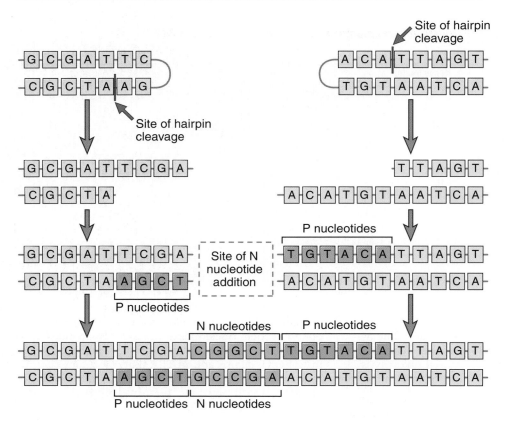

FIGURE 8-11 Junctional diversity. During the joining of different gene segments, addition or removal of nucleotides may lead to the generation of novel nucleotide and amino acid sequences at the junction. Nucleotides (P sequences) may be added to asymmetrically cleaved hairpins in a templated manner. Other nucleotides (N regions) may be added to the sites of V-D, V-J, or D-J junctions in a non-templated manner by the action of the enzyme TdT. These additions generate new sequences that are not present in the germline.

test is commonly used to identify monoclonal tumors of lymphocytes and to distinguish tumors from polyclonal proliferations. Because every lymphocyte clone expresses a unique antigen receptor CDR3 region, the sequence of nucleotides at the V(D)J recombination site serves as a specific marker for each clone. Thus, by measuring the length or determining the sequence of the junctional regions of Ig or TCR genes in different B or T cell proliferations, using polymerase chain reaction assays, one can establish whether these lesions arose from a single clone (indicating a tumor) or independently from different clones (implying non-neoplastic proliferation of lymphocytes). The same method may be used to identify small numbers of tumor cells in the blood or tissues.

With this background, we proceed to a discussion of B lymphocyte development and then the maturation of T cells.

B LYMPHOCYTE DEVELOPMENT

The principal events during the maturation of B lymphocytes are the rearrangement and expression of Ig genes in a precise order, selection and proliferation of developing B cells at the pre-antigen receptor checkpoint, and selection of the mature B cell repertoire. Before birth, B lymphocytes develop from committed precursors in the fetal liver, and after birth, B cells are generated in the bone marrow. The majority of B lymphocytes arise from adult bone marrow progenitors that initially do not express Ig. These precursors develop into immature B cells that express

membrane-bound IgM molecules, and then leave the bone marrow to mature further, primarily in the spleen. Cells that mature into follicular B cells in the spleen express IgM and IgD on the cell surface and acquire the ability to recirculate and populate all peripheral lymphoid organs. These follicular B cells home to lymphoid follicles and are able to recognize and respond to foreign antigens. The development of a mature B cell from a lymphoid progenitor is estimated to take 2 to 3 days in humans.

Stages of B Lymphocyte Development

During their maturation, cells of the B lymphocyte lineage go through distinguishable stages, each characterized by distinct cell surface markers and a specific pattern of Ig gene expression (Fig. 8-12). The major stages and the events in each are described next.

The Pro-B and Pre-B Stages of B Cell Development

The earliest bone marrow cell committed to the B cell lineage is called a pro-B cell. Pro-B cells do not produce Ig, but they can be distinguished from other immature cells by the expression of B lineage–restricted surface molecules such as CD19 and CD10. Rag-1 and Rag-2 proteins are first expressed at this stage, and the first recombination of Ig genes occurs at the heavy chain locus. This recombination brings together one D and one J gene segment, with deletion of the intervening DNA (Fig. 8-13, *A*). The D segments that are 5′ of the rearranged D segment and the J segments that are 3′ of the rearranged J segment are deleted by this recombination (e.g., D1 and J2 to J6 in Fig. 8-13, *A*). After the D-J recombination event, one of the

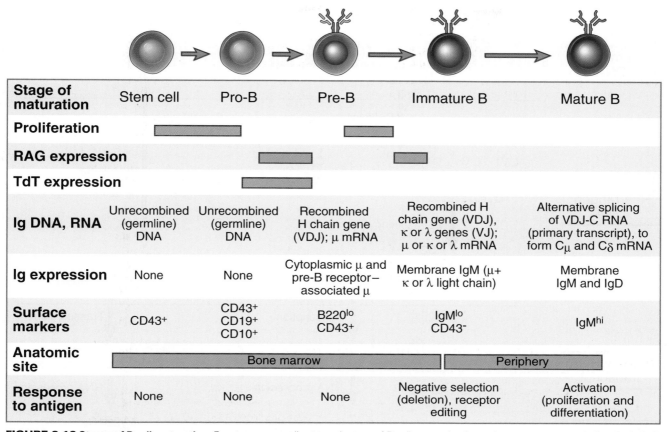

FIGURE 8-12 Stages of B cell maturation. Events corresponding to each stage of B cell maturation from a bone marrow stem cell to a mature B lymphocyte are illustrated. Several surface markers in addition to those shown have been used to define distinct stages of B cell maturation.

Stage of maturation	Stem cell	Pro-B	Pre-B	Immature B	Mature B
Proliferation					
RAG expression					
TdT expression					
Ig DNA, RNA	Unrecombined (germline) DNA	Unrecombined (germline) DNA	Recombined H chain gene (VDJ); μ mRNA	Recombined H chain gene (VDJ), κ or λ genes (VJ); μ or κ or λ mRNA	Alternative splicing of VDJ-C RNA (primary transcript), to form C_μ and C_δ mRNA
Ig expression	None	None	Cytoplasmic μ and pre-B receptor–associated μ	Membrane IgM (μ+ κ or λ light chain)	Membrane IgM and IgD
Surface markers	CD43+	CD43+ CD19+ CD10+	B220lo CD43+	IgMlo CD43-	IgMhi
Anatomic site	Bone marrow			Periphery	
Response to antigen	None	None	None	Negative selection (deletion), receptor editing	Activation (proliferation and differentiation)

many 5′ V genes is joined to the DJ unit, giving rise to a rearranged VDJ exon. At this stage, all V and D segments between the rearranged V and D genes are also deleted. V-to-DJ recombination at the Ig H chain locus occurs only in committed B lymphocyte precursors and is a critical event in Ig expression because only the rearranged V gene is subsequently transcribed. The TdT enzyme, which catalyzes the non-templated addition of junctional N nucleotides, is expressed most abundantly during the pro-B stage when VDJ recombination occurs at the Ig H locus and levels of TdT decrease before light chain gene V-J recombination is complete. Therefore, junctional diversity attributed to addition of N nucleotides is more prominent in rearranged heavy chain genes than in light chain genes.

The heavy chain C region exons remain separated from the VDJ complex by DNA containing the distal J segments and the J-C intron. The rearranged Ig heavy chain gene is transcribed to produce a primary transcript that includes the rearranged VDJ complex and the C_μ exons. The C_μ nuclear RNA is cleaved downstream of one of two consensus polyadenylation sites, and multiple adenine nucleotides, called poly-A tails, are added to the 3′ end. This nuclear RNA undergoes splicing, an RNA processing event in which the introns are removed and exons joined together. In the case of the μ RNA, introns between the leader exon and the VDJ exon, between the VDJ exon and the first exon of the C_μ locus, and between each of the subsequent constant region exons of C_μ are removed, thus giving rise to a spliced mRNA for the μ

heavy chain. If the mRNA is derived from an Ig locus at which rearrangement was productive, translation of the rearranged μ heavy chain mRNA leads to synthesis of the μ protein. For a rearrangement to be productive (in the correct reading frame), bases must be added or removed at junctions in multiples of three. This ensures that the rearranged Ig gene will be able to correctly encode an Ig protein. Approximately half of all pro-B cells make productive rearrangements at the Ig H locus on at least one chromosome and can thus go on to synthesize the μ heavy chain protein. Only cells that make productive rearrangements survive and differentiate further.

Once a productive Ig μ rearrangement is made, a cell ceases to be called a pro-B cell and has differentiated into the pre-B stage. **Pre-B cells** are developing B lineage cells that express the Ig μ protein but have yet to rearrange their light chain loci. The pre-B cell expresses the μ heavy chain on the cell surface, in association with other proteins, in a complex called the pre-B cell receptor, which has several important roles in B cell maturation.

The Pre-B Cell Receptor

Complexes of μ heavy chain, surrogate light chains, and signal-transducing proteins called Igα and Igβ form the pre-antigen receptor of the B lineage, known as the pre-B cell receptor (pre-BCR). The μ heavy chain associates with the λ5 and V pre-B proteins, also called surrogate light chains because they are structurally homologous to κ and λ light chains but are invariant (i.e., they are identical

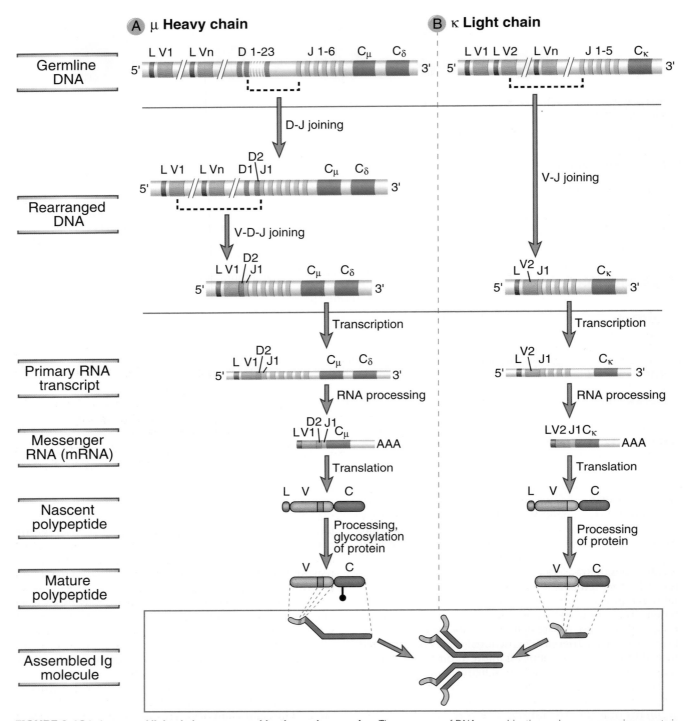

FIGURE 8-13 Ig heavy and light chain gene recombination and expression. The sequence of DNA recombination and gene expression events is shown for the Ig μ heavy chain **(A)** and the Ig κ light chain **(B)**. In the example shown in **A,** the V region of the μ heavy chain is encoded by the exons V1, D2, and J1. In the example shown in **B,** the V region of the κ chain is encoded by the exons V2 and J1.

in all pre-B cells) and are synthesized only in pro-B and pre-B cells (Fig. 8-14, *A*). Igα and Igβ also form part of the B cell receptor in mature B cells (see Chapter 7). Signals from the pre-BCR are responsible for the largest proliferative expansion of B lineage cells in the bone marrow. It is not known what the pre-BCR recognizes; the consensus view at present is that this receptor functions in a ligand-independent manner and that it is activated by the process

of assembly. The importance of pre-BCRs is illustrated by studies of knockout mice and rare cases of human deficiencies of these receptors. For instance, in mice, knockout of the gene encoding the μ chain or one of the surrogate light chains results in markedly reduced numbers of mature B cells because development is blocked at the pro-B stage.

The expression of the pre-BCR is the first checkpoint in B cell maturation. Numerous signaling molecules linked

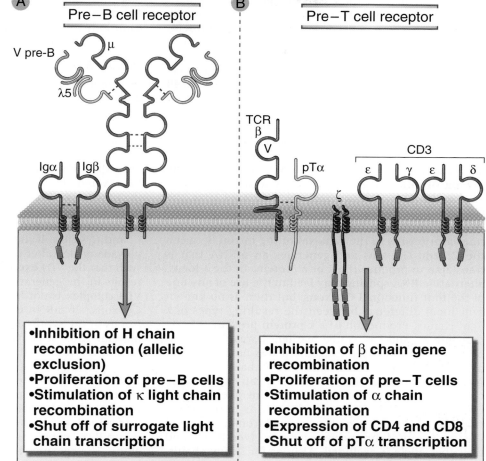

FIGURE 8-14 Pre–B cell and pre–T cell receptors. The pre–B cell receptor **(A)** and the pre–T cell receptor **(B)** are expressed during the pre–B cell and pre–T cell stages of maturation, respectively, and both receptors share similar structures and functions. The pre-B cell receptor is composed of the μ heavy chain and an invariant surrogate light chain. The surrogate light chain is composed of two proteins, the V pre-B protein, which is homologous to a light chain V domain, and a λ5 protein that is covalently attached to the μ heavy chain by a disulfide bond. The pre-T cell receptor is composed of the TCR β chain and the invariant pre-T α (pTα) chain. The pre–B cell receptor is associated with the Igα and Igβ signaling molecules that are part of the BCR complex in mature B cells (see Chapter 9), and the pre–T cell receptor associates with the CD3 and ζ proteins that are part of the TCR complex in mature T cells (see Chapter 7).

to both the pre-BCR and the BCR are required for cells to successfully negotiate the pre-BCR–mediated checkpoint at the pro-B to pre-B cell transition. A kinase called Bruton's tyrosine kinase (Btk) is activated downstream of the pre-BCR and is required for delivery of signals from this receptor that mediate survival, proliferation, and maturation at and beyond the pre-B cell stage. In humans, mutations in the *BTK* gene result in the disease called **X-linked agammaglobulinemia (XLA)**, which is characterized by a failure of B cell maturation (see Chapter 21). In a mouse strain called Xid (for X-linked immunodeficiency), mutations in *btk* result in a less severe B cell defect because murine pre-B cells express a second Btk-like kinase called Tec that partially compensates for the defective Btk.

The pre-BCR regulates further rearrangement of Ig genes in two ways. First, if a μ protein is produced from the recombined heavy chain locus on one chromosome and forms a pre-BCR, this receptor signals to irreversibly inhibit rearrangement of the Ig heavy chain locus on the other chromosome. If the first rearrangement is nonproductive, the heavy chain allele on the other chromosome can complete VDJ rearrangement at the Ig H locus. Thus, in any B cell clone, one heavy chain allele is productively rearranged and expressed, and the other is either retained in the germline configuration or nonproductively rearranged. As a result, an individual B cell can

express an Ig heavy chain protein encoded by only one of the two inherited alleles. This phenomenon is called **allelic exclusion**, and it ensures that every B cell will express a single receptor, thus maintaining clonal specificity. If both alleles undergo nonproductive Ig H gene rearrangements, the developing cell cannot produce Ig heavy chains, cannot generate a pre-BCR–dependent survival signal, and thus undergoes programmed cell death. Ig heavy chain allelic exclusion involves changes in chromatin structure in the heavy chain locus that limit accessibility to the V(D)J recombinase.

The second way in which the pre-BCR regulates the production of the antigen receptor is by stimulating κ light chain gene rearrangement. However, μ chain expression is not absolutely required for light chain gene recombination, as shown by the finding that knockout mice lacking the μ gene do initiate light chain gene rearrangements in some developing B cells (which, of course, cannot express functional antigen receptors and proceed to maturity). The pre-BCR also contributes to the inactivation of surrogate light chain gene expression as pre-B cells mature.

Immature B Cells

Following the pre-B cell stage, each developing B cell initially rearranges a κ light chain gene. If the rearrangement is in-frame, it will produce a κ light chain protein, which associates with the previously synthesized μ chain to produce a complete IgM protein. If the κ locus is not productively rearranged, the cell can rearrange the λ locus and again produce a complete IgM molecule. (Induction of λ light chain gene rearrangement occurs mainly when Ig κ-expressing B cell receptors are self-reactive, as we will discuss later.) The IgM-expressing B cell is called an **immature B cell**. DNA recombination in the κ light chain locus occurs in a similar manner as in the Ig heavy chain locus (see Fig. 8-13, *B*). There are no D segments in the light chain loci, and therefore recombination involves only the joining of one V segment to one J segment, forming a VJ exon. This VJ exon remains separated from the C region by an intron, and this separation is retained in the primary RNA transcript. Splicing of the primary transcript results in the removal of the intron between the VJ and C exons and generates an mRNA that is translated to produce the κ or λ protein. In the λ locus, alternative RNA splicing may lead to the use of any one of the four functional C_λ exons, but there is no known functional difference between the resulting types of λ light chains. Production of a κ protein prevents λ rearrangement, and, as stated earlier, λ rearrangement occurs only if the κ rearrangement was nonproductive or if a self-reactive rearranged κ light chain is deleted. As a result, an individual B cell clone can express only one of the two types of light chains; this phenomenon is called light chain isotype exclusion. As in the heavy chain locus, a κ or λ gene is expressed from only one of the two parental chromosomes in any given B cell, and the other allele is excluded. Also, as for heavy chains, if both alleles of both κ and λ chains are nonfunctionally rearranged in a developing B cell, that cell fails to receive survival signals that are normally generated by the BCR and dies.

The assembled IgM molecules are expressed on the cell surface in association with Igα and Igβ, where they function as specific receptors for antigens. In cells that are not strongly self-reactive, the BCR provides ligand-independent tonic signals that keep the B cell alive and also mediate the shutoff of *RAG* gene expression, thus preventing further Ig gene rearrangement. Immature B cells do not proliferate and differentiate in response to antigens. In fact, if they recognize antigens in the bone marrow with high avidity, which may occur if the B cells express receptors for multivalent self antigens that are present in the bone marrow, the B cells may undergo receptor editing or cell death, as described later. These processes are important for the negative selection of strongly self-reactive B cells. Immature B cells that are not strongly self-reactive leave the bone marrow and complete their maturation in the spleen before migrating to other peripheral lymphoid organs.

Subsets of Mature B Cells

Distinct subsets of B cells develop from different progenitors (Fig. 8-15). Fetal liver–derived HSCs are the precursors of B-1 cells. Bone marrow–derived HSCs give rise to the majority of B cells. These cells rapidly pass through two transitional stages and can commit to development either into **marginal zone B cells** or into **follicular B cells**. The affinity of the B cell receptor for self antigens may contribute to whether a maturing B cell will differentiate into a follicular or a marginal zone B cell.

Follicular B Cells

Most mature B cells belong to the follicular B cell subset and produce IgD in addition to IgM. Each of these B cells coexpresses μ and δ heavy chains using the same VDJ exon to generate the V domain and in association with the same κ or λ light chain to produce two membrane receptors with the same antigen specificity. Simultaneous expression in a single B cell of the same rearranged VDJ exon on two transcripts, one including C_μ exons and the other C_δ exons, is achieved by alternative RNA splicing (Fig. 8-16). A long primary RNA transcript is produced containing the rearranged VDJ unit as well as the C_μ and C_δ genes. If the primary transcript is cleaved and polyadenylated after the μ exons, introns are spliced out such that the VDJ exon is contiguous with C_μ exons; this results in the generation of a μ mRNA. If, however, the VDJ complex is not linked to C_μ exons but is spliced to C_δ exons, a δ mRNA is produced. Subsequent translation results in the synthesis of a complete μ or δ heavy chain protein. Thus, selective polyadenylation and alternative splicing allow a B cell to simultaneously produce mature mRNAs and proteins of two different heavy chain isotypes. The precise mechanisms that regulate the choice of polyadenylation or splice acceptor sites by which the rearranged VDJ is joined to either C_μ or C_δ are poorly understood, as are the signals that determine when and why a B cell expresses both IgM and IgD rather than IgM alone. The coexpression of IgM and IgD is accompanied by the ability to recirculate and the acquisition of functional competence, and this is why IgM+IgD+ B cells are also called **mature B cells**. This correlation between expression of IgD and acquisition of functional competence has led to the suggestion that IgD is the essential activating receptor of mature B cells. However, there is no evidence for a functional difference between membrane IgM and membrane IgD. Moreover, knockout of the Ig δ gene in mice does not have a significant impact on the maturation or antigen-induced responses of B cells. Follicular B cells are also often called recirculating B cells because they migrate from one lymphoid organ to the next, residing in specialized niches known as B cell follicles (see Chapter 2). In these niches, the B cells are maintained, in part, by survival signals delivered by a cytokine of the tumor necrosis factor (TNF) family called BAFF or BLyS (see Chapter 12).

Mature, naive B cells are responsive to antigens, and unless the cells encounter antigens that they recognize with high affinity and respond to, they die in a few months. In Chapter 12, we will discuss how these cells respond to antigens and how the pattern of Ig gene expression changes during antigen-induced B cell differentiation.

B-1 and Marginal Zone B Cells

A subset of B lymphocytes, called B-1 cells, expresses limited antigen receptor diversity and may serve unique functions. These cells develop from fetal liver–derived

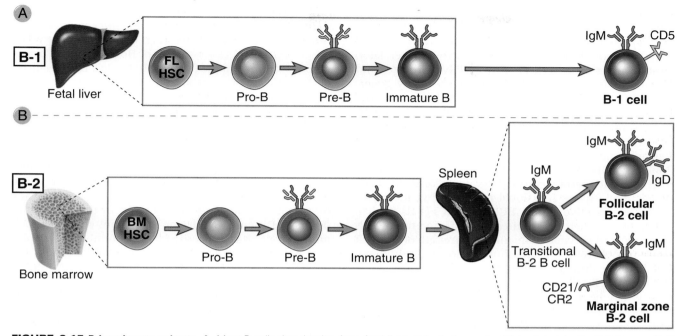

FIGURE 8-15 B lymphocyte subsets. A, Most B cells that develop from fetal liver–derived stem cells differentiate into the B-1 lineage. **B,** B lymphocytes that arise from bone marrow precursors after birth give rise to the B-2 lineage. Two major subsets of B lymphocytes are derived from B-2 B cell precursors. Follicular B cells are recirculating lymphocytes; marginal zone B cells are abundant in the spleen in rodents but can also be found in lymph nodes in humans.

HSCs and are best defined in rodents. Most murine B-1 cells express the CD5 molecule. In adults, large numbers of B-1 cells are found as a self-renewing population in the peritoneum and mucosal sites. B-1 cells develop earlier during ontogeny than follicular and marginal zone B cells do, express a relatively limited repertoire of V genes, and exhibit far less junctional diversity than conventional B cells (because TdT is not expressed in the fetal liver). B-1 cells spontaneously secrete IgM antibodies that often react with microbial polysaccharides and lipids as well as oxidized lipids produced by

lipid peroxidation. These antibodies are sometimes called natural antibodies because they are present in individuals without overt immunization, although it is possible that microbial flora in the gut are the source of antigens that stimulate their production. B-1 cells contribute to rapid antibody production against microbes in particular tissues, such as the peritoneum. At mucosal sites, as many as half the IgA-secreting cells in the lamina propria may be derived from B-1 cells. B-1 cells are analogous to γδ T cells in that they both have antigen receptor repertoires of limited diversity, and they are both presumed to respond to antigens that are commonly encountered in epithelial interfaces with the external environment.

In humans, B-1–like cells have been described, but CD5 is not a defining marker for these cells because it is also found on transitional B cells and some activated B cell populations.

Marginal zone B cells are located primarily in the vicinity of the marginal sinus in the spleen and are similar to B-1 cells in terms of their limited diversity and their ability to respond to polysaccharide antigens and to generate natural antibodies. Marginal zone B cells exist in both mice and humans and express IgM and the CD21 coreceptor. In mice, marginal zone B cells exist only in the spleen, whereas in humans, they can be found in the spleen as well as in lymph nodes. Marginal zone B cells respond very rapidly to blood-borne microbes and differentiate into short-lived IgM-secreting plasma cells. Although they generally mediate T cell–independent humoral immune responses to circulating pathogens, marginal zone B cells also appear capable of mediating some T cell–dependent immune responses.

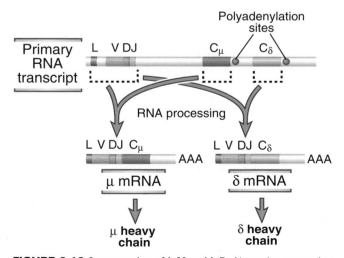

FIGURE 8-16 Coexpression of IgM and IgD. Alternative processing of a primary RNA transcript results in the formation of a μ or δ mRNA. Dashed lines indicate the H chain segments that are joined by RNA splicing.

Selection of the Mature B Cell Repertoire

The repertoire of mature B cells is positively selected from the pool of immature B cells. As we will see later, positive selection is well defined in T lymphocytes and is responsible for matching the TCRs on newly generated CD8+ and CD4+ T cells with their ability to recognize self class I and class II MHC molecules, respectively. There is no comparable restriction for B cell antigen recognition. Nevertheless, positive selection appears to be a general phenomenon primarily geared to identification of lymphocytes that have completed their antigen receptor gene rearrangement program successfully. Only B cells that express functional membrane Ig molecules receive constitutive (tonic) BCR-derived signals, which, as described earlier, are required to keep immature B cells alive. Self antigens may influence the strength of the BCR signal and thereby the subsequent choice of peripheral B cell lineage during B cell maturation.

Immature B cells that recognize self antigens with high avidity may be induced to change their specificities by a process called **receptor editing**. Self antigen recognition by immature B cells induces reactivation of *RAG* genes and the rearrangement and production of a new Ig light chain, allowing the cell to express a different (edited) B cell receptor that is not self-reactive. The original VJκ exon encoding the variable domain of an autoreactive light chain gene is typically deleted and replaced by a new rearrangement involving an upstream Vκ and a downstream Jκ gene segment. If the editing process fails to generate an in-frame productive κ light chain rearrangement on either chromosome, the activated immature B cell may then go on to rearrange the λ light chain locus that is located on a different chromosome. Almost all B cells bearing λ light chains are therefore cells that were once self-reactive and have undergone receptor editing.

If receptor editing fails, the immature B cells that express high-affinity receptors for self antigens and encounter these antigens in the bone marrow or the spleen may die by apoptosis. This process is also called **negative selection**. The antigens mediating negative selection—usually abundant or polyvalent self antigens such as nucleic acids, membrane bound lipids, and membrane proteins—deliver strong signals to IgM-expressing immature B lymphocytes that happen to express receptors specific for these self antigens. Both receptor editing and deletion are responsible for maintaining B cell tolerance to self antigens that are present in the bone marrow (see Chapter 15).

Once the transition is made to the IgM+ IgD+ mature B cell stage, antigen recognition leads to proliferation and differentiation, not to receptor editing or apoptosis. As a result, mature B cells that recognize antigens with high affinity in peripheral lymphoid tissues are activated, and this process leads to humoral immune responses. Follicular B cells make most of the helper T cell–dependent antibody responses to protein antigens (see Chapter 12).

T LYMPHOCYTE DEVELOPMENT

The development of mature T lymphocytes from committed progenitors involves the sequential rearrangement and expression of TCR genes, cell proliferation, antigen-induced selection, and commitment to phenotypically and functionally distinct subsets* (Fig. 8-17). In many ways, this is similar to B cell maturation. However, T cell maturation has some unique features that reflect the specificity of the majority of T lymphocytes for self MHC–associated peptide antigens and the need for a special microenvironment for selecting cells with this specificity.

Role of the Thymus in T Cell Maturation

The thymus is the major site of maturation of T cells. This function of the thymus was first suspected because of immunologic deficiencies associated with the lack of a thymus. The congenital absence of the thymus, as occurs in DiGeorge syndrome in humans or in the nude mouse strain, is characterized by low numbers of mature T cells in the circulation and peripheral lymphoid tissues and severe deficiencies in T cell–mediated immunity (see Chapter 21). If the thymus is removed from a neonatal mouse, this animal fails to develop mature T cells. The thymic anlage develops from the endoderm of the third pharyngeal pouch and the underlying neural crest–derived mesenchyme and is subsequently populated by bone marrow–derived precursors. The thymus involutes with age and is virtually undetectable in post-pubertal humans, resulting in a somewhat reduced output of mature T cells. However, maturation of T cells continues throughout adult life, as indicated by the successful reconstitution of the immune system in adult recipients of bone marrow transplants. It may be that the remnant of the involuted thymus is adequate for some T cell maturation. Because memory T cells have a long life span (perhaps longer than 20 years in humans) and accumulate with age, the need to generate new T cells decreases as individuals age.

T lymphocytes originate from precursors that arise in the fetal liver and adult bone marrow and seed the thymus. These precursors are multipotent progenitors that enter the thymus from the blood stream, crossing the endothelium of a post-capillary venule in the corticomedullary junction region of the thymus. In mice, immature lymphocytes are first detected in the thymus on the eleventh day of the normal 21-day gestation. This corresponds to about week 7 or 8 of gestation in humans. Developing T cells in the thymus are called **thymocytes**. The most immature thymocytes are found in the subcapsular sinus and outer cortical region of the thymus. From here, the thymocytes migrate into and through the cortex, where most of the subsequent maturation events occur. It is in the cortex that the thymocytes first express γδ and αβ TCRs. The αβ T cells mature into CD4+ class II MHC–restricted or CD8+ class I MHC–restricted T cells as they leave the cortex and enter the medulla. From the medulla, CD4+ and CD8+ single-positive thymocytes exit the thymus through the circulation. We will discuss the maturation of αβ T cells in the following sections and γδ T cells later in the chapter.

The thymic environment provides stimuli that are required for the proliferation and maturation of thymocytes. Many of these stimuli come from thymic cells other than the maturing T cells. Within the cortex,

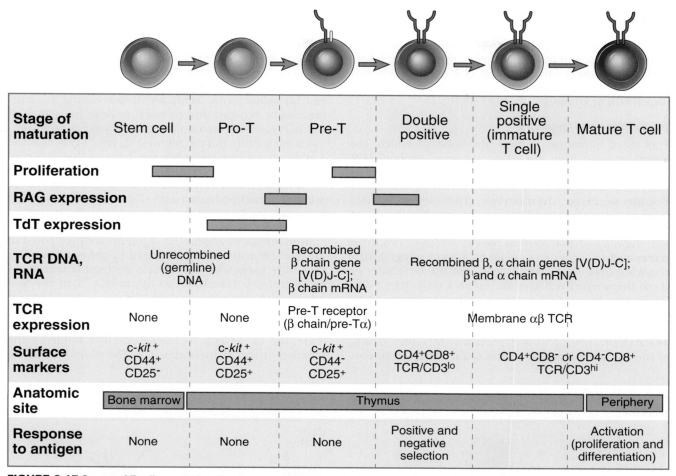

Stage of maturation	Stem cell	Pro-T	Pre-T	Double positive	Single positive (immature T cell)	Mature T cell
Proliferation						
RAG expression						
TdT expression						
TCR DNA, RNA	Unrecombined (germline) DNA		Recombined β chain gene [V(D)J-C]; β chain mRNA	Recombined β, α chain genes [V(D)J-C]; β and α chain mRNA		
TCR expression	None	None	Pre-T receptor (β chain/pre-Tα)	Membrane αβ TCR		
Surface markers	c-*kit*⁺ CD44⁺ CD25⁻	c-*kit*⁺ CD44⁺ CD25⁺	c-*kit*⁺ CD44⁻ CD25⁺	CD4⁺CD8⁺ TCR/CD3^{lo}	CD4⁺CD8⁻ or CD4⁻CD8⁺ TCR/CD3^{hi}	
Anatomic site	Bone marrow	Thymus				Periphery
Response to antigen	None	None	None	Positive and negative selection		Activation (proliferation and differentiation)

FIGURE 8-17 Stages of T cell maturation. Events corresponding to each stage of T cell maturation from a bone marrow stem cell to a mature T lymphocyte are illustrated. Several surface markers in addition to those shown have been used to define distinct stages of T cell maturation.

thymic cortical epithelial cells form a meshwork of long cytoplasmic processes, around which thymocytes must pass to reach the medulla. Epithelial cells of a distinct type known as medullary thymic epithelial cells are also present in the medulla, and may serve a unique role in presenting self antigens for the negative selection of developing T cells (see Chapter 15). Bone marrow–derived dendritic cells are present at the corticomedullary junction and within the medulla, and macrophages are present primarily within the medulla. The migration of thymocytes through this anatomic arrangement allows physical interactions between the thymocytes and these other cells that are necessary for the maturation and selection of the T lymphocytes. Epithelial and dendritic cells in the thymus express class I and class II MHC molecules. The interactions of maturing thymocytes with these MHC molecules are essential for the selection of the mature T cell repertoire, as we will discuss later.

The movement of cells into and through the thymus is driven by chemokines. The progenitors of thymocytes express the chemokine receptor CCR9, which binds to the chemokine CCL25, which is produced in the thymic cortex. Entry of precursors into the thymus is dependent on CCL25 and CCR9. Chemokines such as CCL21 and

CCL19, which are recognized by the CCR7 chemokine receptor on thymocytes, mediate the guided movement of developing T cells from the cortex to the medulla. Eventually, newly formed T lymphocytes, which express the sphingosine 1-phosphate receptor (see Chapter 3), exit the thymic medulla following a gradient of sphingosine-1 phosphate into the blood stream.

Thymic stromal cells, including epithelial cells, secrete IL-7, which was mentioned earlier as a critical lymphopoietic growth factor. The rates of cell proliferation and apoptotic death are extremely high in cortical thymocytes. A single precursor gives rise to many progeny, and 95% of these cells die by apoptosis before reaching the medulla. The cell death is due to a combination of factors including failure to productively rearrange the TCR β chain gene and thus to fail the pre-TCR/β selection checkpoint (described later), failure to be positively selected by self MHC molecules in the thymus, and self antigen–induced negative selection (see Fig. 8-3).

Stages of T Cell Maturation

During T cell maturation, there is a precise order in which TCR genes are rearranged and in which the TCR and CD4

and CD8 coreceptors are expressed (Fig. 8-18; see also Fig. 8-17). In the mouse, surface expression of the γδ TCR occurs first, 3 to 4 days after precursor cells first arrive in the thymus, and the αβ TCR is expressed 2 or 3 days later. In human fetal thymuses, γδ TCR expression begins at about 9 weeks of gestation, followed by expression of the αβ TCR at 10 weeks.

Double-Negative Thymocytes

The most immature cortical thymocytes, which are recent arrivals from the bone marrow, contain TCR genes in their germline configuration and do not express TCR, CD3, ζ chains, CD4, or CD8; these cells are called **double-negative thymocytes**. Thymocytes at this stage are also considered to be at the pro-T cell stage of maturation. The majority (>90%) of the double-negative thymocytes that survive thymic selection processes will ultimately give rise to αβ TCR–expressing, MHC-restricted CD4+ and CD8+ T cells, and the remainder of these thymocytes will give rise to γδ T cells. Rag-1 and Rag-2 proteins are first expressed at the double-negative stage of T cell development and are required for the rearrangement of TCR genes. D_β-to-J_β rearrangements at the TCR β chain locus occur first; these involve either joining of the $D_\beta 1$ gene segment to one of the six $J_\beta 1$ segments

or joining of the $D_\beta 2$ segment to one of the six $J_\beta 2$ segments (Fig. 8-19, *A*). V_β-to-DJ_β rearrangements occur at the transition between the pro-T stage and the subsequent pre-T stage during αβ T cell development. The DNA sequences between the segments undergoing rearrangement, including D, J, and possibly $C_\beta 1$ genes (if $D_\beta 2$ and $J_\beta 2$ segments are used), are deleted during this rearrangement process. The primary nuclear transcripts of the TCR β genes contain the intron between the recombined VDJ_β exon and the relevant C_β gene (as well as the 3 additional introns between the 4 exons that make up each C_β gene, displayed in the figure as a single exon for convenience). Poly-A tails are added after cleavage of the primary transcript downstream of consensus polyadenylation sites located 3′ of the C_β region, and the sequences between the VDJ exon and C_β are spliced out to form a mature mRNA in which VDJ segments are juxtaposed to the first exon of either of the two C_β genes (depending on which J segment was selected during the rearrangement process). Translation of this mRNA gives rise to a full-length TCR β chain protein. The two C_β genes appear to be functionally interchangeable, and an individual T cell never switches from one C gene to another. Furthermore, the use of either C_β gene does not influence the function or specificity of the TCR. The promoters in the

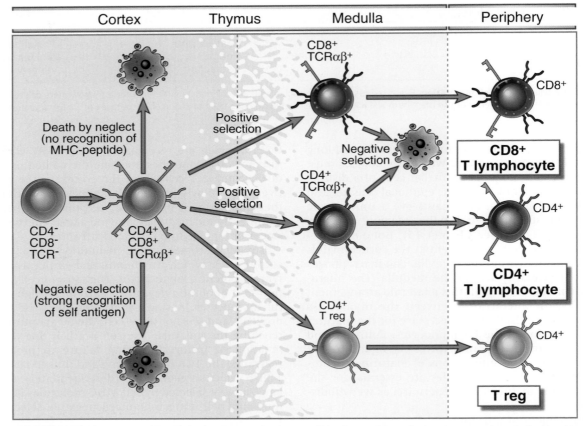

FIGURE 8-18 Maturation of T cells in the thymus. Precursors of T cells travel from the bone marrow through the blood to the thymus. In the thymic cortex, progenitors of αβ T cells express TCRs and CD4 and CD8 coreceptors. Selection processes eliminate self-reactive T cells in the cortex at the double-positive (DP) stage and also single-positive (SP) medullary thymocytes. They promote survival of thymocytes whose TCRs bind self MHC molecules with low affinity. Functional and phenotypic differentiation into CD4+CD8− or CD8+CD4− T cells occurs in the medulla, and mature T cells are released into the circulation. Some double-positive cells differentiate into regulatory T cells (see Chapter 15). The development of γδ T cells is not shown.

5′ flanking regions of V_β genes function together with a powerful enhancer that is located 3′ of the $C_\beta 2$ gene once V genes are brought close to the C gene by VDJ recombination. This proximity of the promoter to the enhancer is responsible for high-level T cell–specific transcription of the rearranged TCR β chain gene.

Pre-T Cell Receptor

If a productive (i.e., in-frame) rearrangement of the TCR β chain gene occurs in a given double-negative T cell, the

TCR β chain protein is expressed on the cell surface in association with an invariant protein called pre-Tα and with CD3 and ζ proteins to form the pre-T cell receptor (pre-TCR) complex (see Fig. 8-14, *B*). The pre-TCR mediates the selection of the developing pre-T cells that productively rearrange the β chain of the TCR. After the addition and removal of bases during gene rearrangement, roughly half of all developing pre-T cells contain new bases in the TCR β chain gene that are a multiple of three (on at least one TCR β chromosome), and therefore only approximately

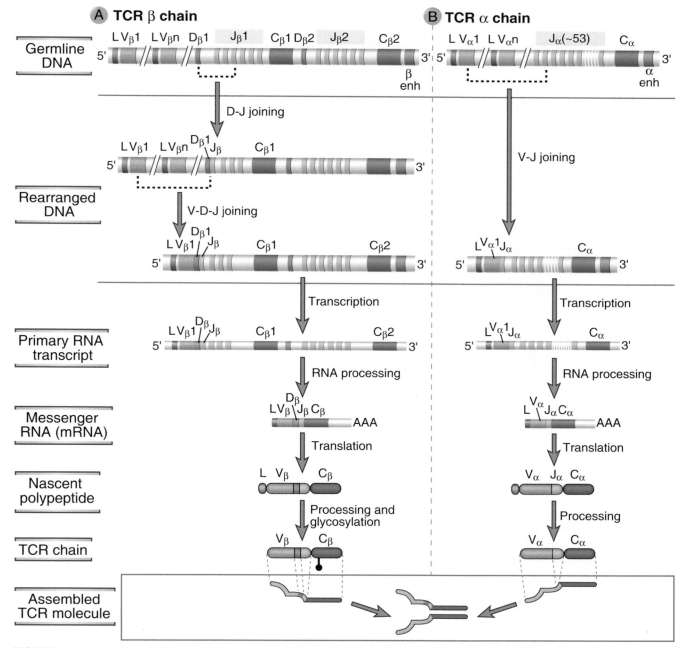

FIGURE 8-19 TCR α and β chain gene recombination and expression. The sequence of recombination and gene expression events is shown for the TCR β chain **(A)** and the TCR α chain **(B)**. In the example shown in A, the variable (V) region of the rearranged TCR β chain includes the $V_\beta 1$ and $D_\beta 1$ gene segments and the third J segment in the $J_\beta 1$ cluster. The constant (C) region in this example is encoded by the exons of the $C_\beta 1$ gene, depicted for convenience as a single exon. Note that at the TCR β chain locus, rearrangement begins with D-to-J joining followed by V-to-DJ joining. In humans, 14 J_β segments have been identified, and not all are shown in the figure. In the example shown in **B,** the V region of the TCR α chain includes the $V_\alpha 1$ gene and the second J segment in the J_α cluster (this cluster is made up of at least 61 J_α segments in humans; not all are shown here).

half of all developing pre-T cells successfully express a TCR β protein. The function of the pre-TCR complex in T cell development is similar to that of the surrogate light chain–containing pre-BCR complex in B cell development. Signals from the pre-TCR mediate the survival of pre-T cells that have productively rearranged the TCR β chain gene and contribute to the largest proliferative expansion during T cell development. Pre-TCR signals also initiate recombination at the TCR α chain locus and drive the transition from the double-negative to the double-positive stage of thymocyte development (discussed later). These signals also inhibit further rearrangement of the TCR β chain locus largely by limiting accessibility of the other allele to the recombination machinery. This results in β chain allelic exclusion (i.e., mature T cells express only one of the two inherited β chain alleles). As in pre-B cells, it is not known what, if any, ligand the pre-TCR recognizes. Pre-TCR signaling, like pre-BCR signaling, is generally believed to be initiated in a ligand-independent manner, dependent on the successful assembly of the pre-TCR complex. Pre-TCR signaling is mediated by a number of cytosolic kinases and adaptor proteins that are also linked to TCR signaling (see Chapter 7). The essential function of the pre-TCR complex in T cell maturation has been demonstrated by numerous studies with genetically mutated mice, in which lack of any component of the pre-TCR complex (i.e., the TCR β chain, pre-Tα, CD3, ζ, or Lck) results in a block in the maturation of T cells at the double-negative stage.

Double-Positive Thymocytes

At the next stage of T cell maturation, thymocytes express both CD4 and CD8 and are called double-positive thymocytes. The expression of CD4 and CD8 is essential for subsequent selection events, discussed later. The rearrangement of the TCR α chain genes and the expression of TCR αβ heterodimers occur in the CD4+CD8+ double-positive population soon after cells cross the pre-TCR checkpoint (see Figs. 8-17 and 8-18). A second wave of *RAG* gene expression late in the pre-T stage promotes TCR α gene recombination. Because there are no D segments in the TCR α locus, rearrangement consists of the joining of only V and J segments (see Fig. 8-19, *B*). The large number of J_α segments permits multiple attempts at productive V-J joining on each chromosome, thereby increasing the probability that a functional αβ TCR will be produced. In contrast to the TCR β chain locus, where production of the protein and formation of the pre-TCR suppress further rearrangement, there is little or no allelic exclusion in the α chain locus. Therefore, productive TCR α rearrangements may occur on both chromosomes, and if this happens, the T cell will express two α chains. In fact, up to 30% of mature peripheral T cells do express two different TCRs, with different α chains but the same β chain. It is possible that only one of the two different TCRs participates in self MHC-driven positive selection, described later. Transcriptional regulation of the α chain gene occurs in a similar manner to that of the β chain. There are promoters 5′ of each V_α gene that have low-level activity and are responsible for high-level T cell–specific transcription when brought close to an α chain enhancer located 3′ of the Cα gene. Unsuccessful

rearrangements of the TCR α gene on both chromosomes lead to a failure of positive selection (discussed later). Thymocytes of the αβ T cell lineage that fail to make a productive rearrangement of the TCR α chain gene will die by apoptosis.

TCR α gene expression in the double-positive stage leads to the formation of the complete αβ TCR, which is expressed on the cell surface in association with CD3 and ζ proteins. The coordinate expression of CD3 and ζ proteins and the assembly of intact TCR complexes are required for surface expression. Rearrangement of the TCR α gene results in deletion of the TCR δ locus that lies between V segments (common to both α and δ loci) and J_α segments (see Fig. 8-6). As a result, this T cell is no longer capable of becoming a γδ T cell and is completely committed to the αβ T cell lineage. The expression of *RAG* genes and further TCR gene recombination cease after this stage of maturation.

Double-positive cells that successfully undergo selection processes go on to mature into CD4+ or CD8+ T cells, which are called single-positive thymocytes. Thus, the stages of T cell maturation in the thymus can readily be distinguished by the expression of CD4 and CD8 (Fig. 8-20). This phenotypic maturation is accompanied by commitment to different functional programs upon activation in secondary lymphoid organs. CD4+ cells acquire the ability to produce cytokines in response to subsequent antigen stimulation and to express effector molecules (such as CD40 ligand) that activate B lymphocytes, dendritic cells, and macrophages, whereas CD8+ cells become capable of

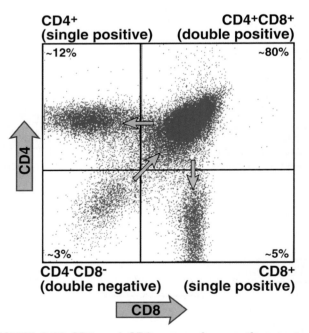

FIGURE 8-20 CD4 and CD8 expression on thymocytes and positive selection of T cells in the thymus. The maturation of thymocytes can be followed by changes in expression of the CD4 and CD8 coreceptors. A two-color flow cytometric analysis of thymocytes using anti-CD4 and anti-CD8 antibodies, each tagged with a different fluorochrome, is illustrated. The percentages of all thymocytes contributed by each major population are shown in the four quadrants. The least mature subset is the CD4−CD8− (double-negative) cells. Arrows indicate the sequence of maturation.

producing molecules that kill other cells. Mature single-positive thymocytes enter the thymic medulla and then leave the thymus to populate peripheral lymphoid tissues.

Selection Processes in the Maturation of MHC-Restricted αβ T Cells

The selection of developing T cells is dependent on recognition of antigen (peptide-MHC complexes) in the thymus and is responsible for preserving useful cells and eliminating potentially harmful ones. The immature, or unselected, repertoire of T lymphocytes consists of cells whose receptors may recognize any peptide antigen (self or foreign) displayed by any MHC molecule (also self or foreign). In addition, receptors may theoretically be expressed that do not recognize any peptide–MHC molecule complex. In every individual, the only useful T cells are the ones specific for foreign peptides presented by that individual's MHC molecules, that is, self MHC molecules. When double-positive thymocytes first express αβ TCRs, these receptors encounter self peptides (the only peptides normally present in the thymus) displayed by self MHC molecules (the only MHC molecules available to display peptides) mainly on thymic epithelial cells in the cortex. The outcome of this recognition is determined primarily by the strength of the encounter between TCRs and self antigen–MHC complexes. **Positive selection** is the process that preserves T cells that recognize self MHC (with self peptides) with low avidity. This recognition preserves cells that can see antigens displayed by that individual's MHC molecules. At the same time, the cells become committed to the CD4 or CD8 lineage based on whether the TCR on an individual cell respectively recognizes MHC class II or MHC class I molecules. Also, in every individual, T cells that recognize self antigens with high avidity are potentially dangerous because such recognition may trigger autoimmunity. **Negative selection** is the process in which thymocytes whose TCRs bind strongly to self peptide antigens in association with self MHC molecules are deleted (see Fig. 8-18). The net result of these selection processes is that the repertoire of mature T cells that leaves the thymus is self MHC–restricted and tolerant to many self antigens, and only the useful cells complete their maturation. In the sections that follow, we will discuss the details of positive and negative selection.

Positive Selection of Thymocytes: Development of the Self MHC–Restricted T Cell Repertoire

Positive selection is the process in which thymocytes whose TCRs bind with low avidity (i.e., weakly) to self peptide–self MHC complexes are stimulated to survive (see Fig. 8-18). Double-positive thymocytes are produced without antigenic stimulation and begin to express αβ TCRs with randomly generated specificities, which are likely biased toward recognition of MHC-like structures. In the thymic cortex, these immature cells encounter epithelial cells that are displaying a variety of self peptides bound to class I and class II MHC molecules. Weak recognition of these self peptide–self MHC complexes promotes the survival of the T cells. Thymocytes whose receptors do not recognize self MHC molecules are permitted to die by a default pathway of apoptosis; this phenomenon is called death

by neglect (see Fig. 8-18). Thus, positive selection ensures that T cells are self MHC–restricted.

During the transition from double-positive to single-positive cells, thymocytes with class I MHC–restricted TCRs become CD8⁺CD4⁻, and cells with class II MHC–restricted TCRs become CD4⁺CD8⁻. Immature, double-positive T cells express TCRs that may recognize either self class I or self class II MHC. Two models have been proposed to explain the process of lineage commitment, as a result of which coreceptors are correctly matched with the TCRs that recognize a specific class of MHC molecules. The stochastic or probabilistic model suggests that the commitment of immature T cells toward either lineage depends on the random probability of a double-positive cell differentiating into a CD4⁺ or a CD8⁺ T cell. In this model, a cell that recognizes self class I MHC may randomly differentiate into a CD8⁺ T cell (with the appropriate coreceptor) and survive or into a CD4⁺ T cell (with the wrong coreceptor) that may fail to receive survival signals. In this process of random differentiation into single-positive cells, the coreceptor would fail to be matched with recognition of the right class of MHC molecules approximately half the time.

A more widely accepted view is that the process of lineage commitment linked to positive selection is not a random process but is driven by specific signals that instruct the T cell to become CD4⁺ or CD8⁺. Instructional models suggest that class I MHC– and class II MHC–restricted TCRs deliver different signals that actively induce expression of the correct coreceptor and shut off expression of the other coreceptor. It is known that double-positive cells go through a stage at which they express high CD4 and low CD8. If the TCR on such a cell is class I MHC–restricted, when it sees the appropriate class I MHC and self peptide, it will receive a weak signal because levels of the CD8 coreceptor are low and, in addition, CD8 associates less well with the Lck tyrosine kinase than CD4 does. These weak signals activate transcription factors such as Runx3 that maintain the CD8⁺ T cell phenotype by regulating the expression of CD8 and downstream transcription factors, and commit the CD8⁺ T cell to become a cytotoxic T lymphocyte after full maturation and antigen activation. Conversely, if the TCR on the cell is class II MHC–restricted, when it sees class II MHC, it will receive a stronger signal because CD4 levels are high and CD4 associates relatively well with Lck. These strong signals activate the transcription factor GATA3, which commits cells toward a CD4 fate, and induces the expression of a repressor called ThPoK, which prevents the expression of defining genes of CD8⁺ T cells.

Peptides bound to MHC molecules on thymic epithelial cells play an essential role in positive selection. In Chapter 6, we described how cell surface class I and class II MHC molecules always contain bound peptides. These MHC-associated peptides on thymic antigen-presenting cells probably serve two roles in positive selection—first, they promote stable cell surface expression of MHC molecules, and second, they may influence the specificities of the T cells that are selected. It is also clear from a variety of experimental studies that some peptides are better than others in supporting positive selection, and different peptides differ in the repertoires of T cells they select. These results suggest that specific antigen recognition, and not just MHC recognition, has some role in positive selection. One consequence of self peptide–induced positive selection is that the T cells that mature have the capacity to recognize self peptides. We mentioned in Chapter 2 that the survival of naive lymphocytes before encounter with foreign antigens requires survival signals that are apparently generated by recognition of self antigens in peripheral lymphoid organs. The same self peptides that mediate positive selection of double-positive thymocytes in the thymus may be involved in keeping naive, mature (single-positive) T cells alive in peripheral organs, such as the lymph nodes and spleen.

The model of positive selection based on weak recognition of self antigens raises a fundamental question: How does positive selection driven by weak recognition of self antigens produce a repertoire of mature T cells specific for foreign antigens? The likely answer is that positive selection allows many different T cell clones to survive and differentiate, and many of these T cells that recognize self peptides with low affinity will, after maturing, fortuitously recognize foreign peptides with a high enough affinity to be activated and to generate useful immune responses.

Negative Selection of Thymocytes: Central Tolerance

Thymocytes whose receptors recognize peptide-MHC complexes in the thymus with high avidity undergo apoptosis (called negative selection) or differentiate into regulatory T cells (see Fig. 8-18). Among the double-positive T cells that are generated in the thymus, some may express TCRs that recognize self antigens with high affinity. The peptides present in the thymus are self peptides derived from widely expressed protein antigens as well as from some proteins believed to be restricted to particular tissues. (Recall that microbes that enter through the common routes, i.e., epithelia, are captured and transported to lymph nodes and tend to not enter the thymus.) In immature T cells, a major consequence of high-avidity antigen recognition is the triggering of apoptosis, leading to death, or deletion, of the cells. Therefore, many of the immature thymocytes that express high-affinity receptors for self antigens in the thymus die, resulting in negative selection of the T cell repertoire. This process eliminates the potentially most harmful self-reactive T cells and is one of the mechanisms ensuring that the immune system does not respond to many self antigens, a phenomenon called self-tolerance. Tolerance induced in immature lymphocytes by recognition of self antigens in the generative (or central) lymphoid organs is also called central tolerance, to be contrasted with peripheral tolerance induced in mature lymphocytes by self antigens in peripheral tissues. We will discuss the mechanisms and physiologic importance of immunologic tolerance in more detail in Chapter 15.

The deletion of immature self-reactive T cells may occur both at the double-positive stage in the cortex and in newly generated single-positive T cells in the medulla. The thymic antigen-presenting cells that mediate negative selection are primarily bone marrow–derived dendritic cells and macrophages, both abundant in the medulla, and medullary thymic epithelial cells, whereas cortical epithelial cells are especially (and perhaps uniquely) effective at inducing positive selection. Double-positive T cells are drawn to the thymic medulla by chemokines. In the medulla, medullary thymic epithelial cells express a nuclear protein called **AIRE (autoimmune regulator)** that induces the expression of a number of tissue-specific genes in the thymus. These genes are normally expressed only in specific peripheral organs. Their AIRE-dependent expression in the thymus makes many tissue-specific peptides available for presentation to developing T cells, facilitating the deletion (negative selection) of these cells. A mutation in the gene that encodes AIRE results in an autoimmune polyendocrine syndrome, underscoring the importance of AIRE in mediating central tolerance to tissue-specific antigens (see Chapter 15).

The mechanism of negative selection in the thymus is the induction of death by apoptosis. Unlike the phenomenon of death by neglect, which occurs in the absence of positive selection, in negative selection, active death-promoting signals are generated when the TCR of immature thymocytes binds with high affinity to antigen. The induction by TCR signaling of a proapoptotic protein called Bim probably plays a crucial role in the induction of mitochondrial leakiness and thymocyte apoptosis during negative selection (see Chapter 15). It is also clear that whereas high-avidity antigen recognition by immature T cells triggers apoptosis, the same recognition by mature lymphocytes, in concert with other signals, initiates T cell responses (see Chapter 9). The biochemical basis of this fundamental difference is not defined.

Recognition of self antigens in the thymus can generate a population of CD4+ regulatory T cells that function to prevent autoimmune reactions (see Chapter 15). It is not clear what factors determine the choice between the two alternative fates of immature T cells that recognize self antigens with high avidity, namely, deletion of immature T cells and the development of regulatory T cells. It is possible that slightly lower avidity interactions than those required for deletion may lead to the development of regulatory T cells, but clear evidence for this kind of fine discrimination is lacking.

γδ T Lymphocytes

TCR αβ- and γδ-expressing thymocytes are separate lineages with a common precursor. In fetal thymuses, the first TCR gene rearrangements involve the γ and δ loci. Recombination of TCR γ and δ loci proceeds in a fashion similar to that of other antigen receptor gene rearrangements, although the order of rearrangement appears to be less rigid than in other loci. In a developing double-negative T cell, rearrangement of TCR β, γ, or δ loci is initially possible. If a cell succeeds in productively rearranging its TCR γ as well as its TCR δ loci before it makes a productive TCR β rearrangement, it is selected into the γδ T cell lineage. This happens in about 10% of developing double-negative T cells. About 90% of the time, a productive TCR β gene rearrangement is made first. In this situation, pre-TCR signaling selects these cells to mature into the αβ T cell lineage, and eventual deletion of TCR δ when TCR α is rearranged (the TCR δ locus is embedded in the TCR α locus) results in irreversible commitment to the αβ lineage.

The diversity of the γδ T cell repertoire is theoretically even greater than that of the αβ T cell repertoire, in part because the heptamer-nonamer recognition sequences adjacent to D segments permit D-to-D joining. Paradoxically, however, the actual diversity of expressed γδ TCRs is limited because only a few of the available V, D, and J segments are used in mature γδ T cells, for unknown reasons. This limited diversity is reminiscent of the limited diversity of the B-1 subset of B lymphocytes and is in keeping with the concept that γδ T cells serve as an early defense against a limited number of commonly encountered microbes at epithelial barriers. The functions of γδ T cells are described in Chapter 10.

Another small population, called NKT cells, also develops in the thymus; these are described in Chapter 10 as well.

SUMMARY

* B and T lymphocytes arise from a common bone marrow–derived precursor that becomes committed to the lymphocyte lineage. B cell maturation proceeds in the bone marrow, whereas early T cell progenitors migrate to and complete their maturation in the thymus. Early maturation is characterized by cell proliferation induced by cytokines, mainly IL-7, leading to an expansion in the numbers of lymphocytes that have just committed to individual lineages.

* Extracellular signals induce the activation of transcription factors that induce the expression of lineage-specific genes and open up specific antigen receptor gene loci at the level of chromatin accessibility.

* B and T cell development involves the somatic rearrangement of antigen receptor gene segments and the initial expression of the Ig heavy chain μ protein in B cell precursors and TCR β molecules in T cell precursors. The initial expression of pre-antigen receptors and the subsequent expression of antigen receptors are essential for the survival, expansion, and maturation of developing lymphocytes and for selection processes that lead to a diverse repertoire of useful antigen specificities.

* The antigen receptors of B and T cells are encoded by receptor genes made up of a limited number of gene segments that are spatially segregated in the germline antigen receptor loci but are somatically recombined in developing B and T cells.

* Separate loci encode the Ig heavy chain, Ig κ light chain, Ig λ light chain, TCR β chain, TCR α and δ chains, and TCR γ chain. These loci contain V, J, and, in the Ig heavy chain and TCR β and δ loci only, D gene segments. The J segments are located immediately 5' of exons encoding constant domains, and V segments are a large distance upstream of the J segments. When present, D segments are between the V and J clusters. Somatic rearrangement of both Ig and TCR loci involves the joining of D and J segments in the loci that contain D segments, followed by the joining of the V segment to the recombined DJ segments in these loci or direct V-to-J joining in the other loci.

* This process of somatic gene recombination is mediated by a recombinase enzyme complex made up of the lymphocyte-specific components Rag-1 and Rag-2.

* The diversity of the antibody and TCR repertoires is generated by the combinatorial associations of multiple germline V, D, and J gene segments and junctional diversity generated by the addition or removal of random nucleotides at the sites of recombination. These mechanisms generate the most diversity at the junctions of the segments that form the third hypervariable regions of both antibody and TCR polypeptides.

* B cell maturation occurs in stages characterized by different patterns of Ig gene rearrangement and expression. In the earliest B cell precursors, called pro-B cells, Ig genes are initially in the germline configuration, and D to J rearrangement occurs at the Ig heavy chain locus.

* At the pro-B to pre-B cell transition, V-D-J recombination is completed at the Ig H chain locus. A primary RNA transcript containing the VDJ exon and Ig C gene exons is produced, and the VDJ exon is spliced to the μ C region exons of the heavy chain RNA to generate a mature mRNA that is translated into the μ heavy chain protein in cells in which an in-frame rearrangement has occurred. The pre-BCR is formed by pairing of the μ chain with surrogate light chains and by association with the signaling molecules Igα and Igβ. This receptor delivers survival and proliferation signals and also signals to inhibit rearrangement on the other heavy chain allele (allelic exclusion).

* As cells differentiate into immature B cells, V-J recombination occurs initially at the Ig κ locus, and light chain proteins are expressed. Heavy and light chains are then assembled into intact IgM molecules and expressed on the cell surface. Immature B cells leave the bone marrow to populate peripheral lymphoid tissues, where they complete their maturation. At the mature B cell stage, synthesis of μ and δ heavy chains occurs in parallel mediated by alternative splicing of primary heavy chain RNA transcripts, and membrane IgM and IgD are expressed.

* During B lymphocyte maturation, immature B cells that express high-affinity antigen receptors specific for self antigens present in the bone marrow are induced to edit their receptor genes, or these cells are eliminated. Receptor editing involves further rearrangement at the Ig κ locus and may also involve Ig λ light chain gene rearrangement. B cells that express λ light chains are frequently cells that have undergone receptor editing.

* T cell maturation in the thymus also progresses in stages distinguished by the pattern of expression of antigen receptor genes, CD4 and CD8 coreceptor molecules, and by the location of developmental events within the thymus. The earliest T lineage immigrants to the thymus do not express TCRs or CD4 or CD8 molecules. The developing T cells within the thymus, called thymocytes, initially populate the outer cortex, where they undergo proliferation, rearrangement of TCR genes, and induce surface expression of CD3, TCR, CD4, and CD8 molecules. As the cells mature, they migrate from the cortex to the medulla.

* The least mature thymocytes, called pro-T cells, are CD4$^-$CD8$^-$ (double-negative), and the *TCR* genes are initially in the germline configuration at this stage. Rearrangement of the TCR β, δ, and γ chain genes occurs at this stage.

* At the pre-T stage, thymocytes remain double-negative, but V-D-J recombination is completed at the TCR β chain locus. Primary β chain transcripts are expressed and processed to bring a VDJ exon adjacent to a C_β segment, and TCR β chain polypeptides are produced. In cells in which rearrangement has been productive, the TCR β chain associates with the invariant pre-Tα protein to form a pre-TCR. The pre-TCR transduces signals that inhibit rearrangement on the other β chain allele (allelic exclusion) and promotes differentiation to the stage of dual CD4 and CD8 expression and further proliferation of immature thymocytes. At the CD4+CD8+ (double-positive) stage of T cell development, V-J recombination occurs at the TCR α locus, α chain polypeptides are produced, and low levels of TCR are expressed on the cell surface.

* Selection processes drive maturation of TCR-expressing, double-positive thymocytes and shape the T cell repertoire toward self MHC restriction and self-tolerance.

* Positive selection of CD4+CD8+ TCR αβ thymocytes requires low-avidity recognition of peptide-MHC complexes on thymic epithelial cells, leading to a rescue of the cells from programmed death. As TCR αβ thymocytes mature, they move into the medulla and become either CD4+CD8$^-$ or CD8+CD4$^-$. Lineage commitment accompanies positive selection. It results in the matching of TCRs that recognize MHC class I with CD8 expression and the silencing of CD4; TCRs that recognize MHC class II molecules are matched with CD4 expression and the loss of CD8 expression.

* Negative selection of CD4+CD8+ TCR αβ double-positive thymocytes occurs when these cells recognize, with high avidity, antigens that are present in the thymus. This process is responsible for tolerance to many self-antigens. Medullary thymocytes continue to be negatively selected, and cells that are not clonally deleted acquire the ability to differentiate into either naive CD4+ or CD8+ T cells and finally emigrate to peripheral lymphoid tissues.

SUGGESTED READINGS

Early B Cell Development and V(D)J Recombination

Clark MR, Mandal M, Ochiai K, Singh H: Orchestrating B cell lymphopoiesis through interplay of IL-7 receptor and pre-B cell receptor signaling, *Nature Reviews Immunology* 14:69–80, 2014.

Cobaleda C, Busslinger M: Developmental plasticity of lymphocytes, *Current Opinion in Immunology* 20:139–148, 2008.

Jenkinson EJ, Jenkinson WE, Rossi SW, Anderson G: The thymus and T-cell commitment: the right choice for Notch? *Nature Reviews Immunology* 6:551–555, 2006.

Johnson K, Reddy KL, Singh H: Molecular pathways and mechanisms regulating the recombination of immunoglobulin genes during B-lymphocyte development, *Advances in Experimental Medicine and Biology* 650:133–147, 2009.

Jung D, Giallourakis C, Mostoslavsky R, Alt FW: Mechanism and control of V(D)J recombination at the immunoglobulin heavy chain locus, *Annual Review of Immunology* 24:541–570, 2006.

Nemazee D: Receptor editing in lymphocyte development and central tolerance, *Nature Reviews Immunology* 6:728–740, 2006.

Schatz DG, Ji Y: Recombination centers and the orchestration of V(D)J recombination, *Nature Reviews Immunology* 11:251–263, 2011.

T Cell Development

Boehm T: Thymus development and function, *Current Opinion in Immunology* 20:178–184, 2008.

Carpenter AC, Bosselut R: Decision checkpoints in the thymus, *Nature Immunology* 11:666–673, 2010.

Godfrey DI, Stankovic S, Baxter AG: Raising the NKT cell family, *Nature Immunology* 11:197–206, 2010.

Kyewski B, Klein L: A central role for central tolerance, *Annual Review of Immunology* 24:571–606, 2006.

Maillard I, Fang T, Pear WS: Regulation of lymphoid development, differentiation, and function by the Notch pathway, *Annual Review of Immunology* 23:945–974, 2005.

Rodewald HR: Thymus organogenesis, *Annual Review of Immunology* 26:355–388, 2008.

Rothenberg EV, Moore JE, Yui MA: Launching the T-cell-lineage developmental programme, *Nature Reviews Immunology* 8:9–21, 2008.

Singer A, Adoro S, Park JH: Lineage fate and intense debate: myths, models and mechanisms of CD4 versus CD8 lineage choice, *Nature Reviews Immunology* 8:788–801, 2008.

Stritesky GL, Jameson SC, Hogquist KA: Selection of self-reactive T cells in the thymus, *Annual Review of Immunology* 30:95–114, 2012.

Taniuchi I, Ellmeier W: Transcriptional and epigenetic regulation of CD4/CD8 lineage choice, *Advances in Immunology* 110:71–110, 2011.

MicroRNAs and Lymphocyte Development

Lodish HF, Zhou B, Liu G, Chen CZ: Micromanagement of the immune system by microRNAs, *Nature Reviews Immunology* 8:120–130, 2008.

O'Connell RM, Rao DS, Baltimore D: microRNA regulation of inflammatory responses, *Annual Review of Immunology* 30:295–312, 2012.

Xiao C, Rajewsky K: MicroRNA control in the immune system: basic principles, *Cell* 136:26–36, 2009.

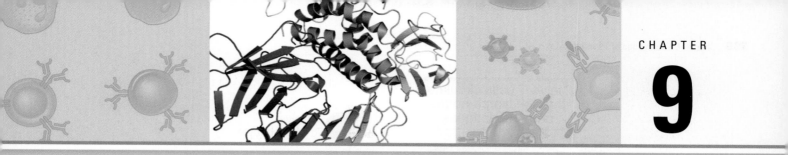

Activation of T Lymphocytes

The process of T cell activation generates, from a small pool of naive lymphocytes specific for an antigen, a large number of effector cells with the same specificity that function to eliminate that antigen and a population of long-lived memory cells that can rapidly react against the antigen in case it is reintroduced. A fundamental characteristic of the T cell response, like all adaptive immune responses, is that it is highly specific for the antigen that elicits the response. Both the initial activation of naive T cells and the effector phases of T cell–mediated adaptive immune responses are triggered by recognition of the antigen by the antigen receptors of T lymphocytes. In Chapter 6, we described the specificity of T cells for peptide fragments, derived from protein antigens, which are bound to and displayed by self major histocompatibility complex (MHC) molecules. In Chapter 7, we described the antigen receptors and other molecules of T cells that are involved in the activation of the cells by antigens, and the biochemical signals initiated by these receptors. In this chapter, we will describe the biology of T cell activation. We begin with a brief overview of T cell activation, discuss the role of costimulators and other signals provided by antigen-presenting cells (APCs) in T cell activation, and describe the sequence of proliferation and differentiation that occurs when CD4+ and CD8+ T cells recognize foreign antigens.

The generation and functions of differentiated CD4+ effector cells are described in Chapter 10 and of CD8+ effector T cells in Chapter 11. Thus, Chapters 9, 10, and 11 together cover the biology of T lymphocyte activation and function in cell-mediated immunity.

OVERVIEW OF T LYMPHOCYTE ACTIVATION

The initial activation of naive T lymphocytes occurs mainly in secondary lymphoid organs, through which these cells normally circulate and where they may encounter antigens presented by mature dendritic cells (Fig. 9-1). Clones of T lymphocytes, each with a different specificity, are generated in the thymus before antigen exposure. Naive T lymphocytes, which have not recognized and responded to antigens, circulate throughout the body in a resting state, and they acquire powerful functional capabilities only after they are activated. This activation of naive T lymphocytes occurs in specialized lymphoid organs, where the naive lymphocytes and APCs are brought together (see Chapters 2 and 6).

Naive T lymphocytes move around within lymphoid organs transiently interacting with many dendritic cells, and stop when they find the antigen for which they express specific receptors. Dendritic cells in lymphoid organs may be presenting many different antigens. T cells are in constant motion, mainly guided by the fibroblast reticular network, a matrix substratum produced by fibroblastic reticular cells in the T cell zone of the lymphoid organs. Antigen recognition results in the generation of biochemical signals that lead to rapid arrest of the T cells. This process stabilizes the contact between the T cells and the relevant antigen-expressing APC, and allows the activation program of the T cell to be initiated.

Antigen recognition together with other activating stimuli induces several responses in T cells: cytokine secretion; proliferation, leading to an increase in the numbers of cells in the antigen-specific clones (called clonal expansion); and differentiation of the naive cells into effector and memory lymphocytes (Fig. 9-2). In addition, the process of T cell activation is associated with changes in the expression of numerous surface molecules, many of which play important roles in inducing and regulating the responses. Cytokines drive the proliferation and differentiation of antigen-activated T cells. Clonal expansion

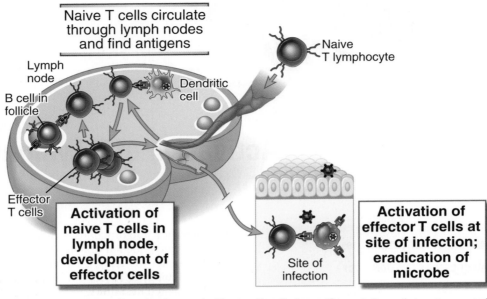

FIGURE 9-1 Activation of naive and effector T cells by antigen. Antigens that are transported by dendritic cells to lymph nodes are recognized by naive T lymphocytes that recirculate through these lymph nodes. The T cells are activated to differentiate into effector cells, which may remain in the lymphoid organs to help B lymphocytes or migrate to sites of infection, where the effector cells are again activated by antigens and perform their various functions, such as macrophage activation.

and differentiation are enhanced by several positive feedback amplification mechanisms. For example, activated T cells deliver signals back to the APCs, further increasing their ability to activate T cells. At the same time, some surface molecules expressed on activated T cells as well as cytokines secreted by these cells have regulatory functions that serve to establish safe limits to the response. The steps in T cell responses and the nature of the positive and negative feedback loops are described later in this chapter.

Antigen-presenting cells not only display antigens but also provide the stimuli that guide the magnitude and nature of the T cell response. These stimuli include surface molecules and secreted cytokines. Different types of APCs may express distinct signals that induce the development of different types of effector cells. We will describe these roles of APCs in instructing T cells how to respond later in this chapter and in Chapter 10.

Effector T cells recognize antigens in lymphoid organs or in peripheral nonlymphoid tissues and are activated to perform functions that are responsible for the elimination of microbes and, in disease states, for tissue damage. Whereas naive cells are activated mainly in lymphoid organs, differentiated effector cells may respond to antigens and carry out their functions in any tissue (see Fig. 9-1). The process of differentiation from naive to effector cells gives the cells the capacity to perform specialized functions and the ability to migrate to any site of infection or inflammation. At these sites, the effector cells again encounter the antigen for which they are specific and respond in ways that serve to eliminate the source of the antigen. Effector T cells of the CD4+ lineage secrete cytokines and express cell surface molecules that can trigger other immune cells; these effector cells are classified into subpopulations on the basis of their cytokine profiles and functions (see Chapter 10). Some of these differentiated

helper cells activate macrophages to kill phagocytosed microbes; others secrete cytokines that recruit leukocytes and thus stimulate inflammation; others enhance mucosal barrier functions; and yet others remain in lymphoid organs and help B cells to differentiate into cells that secrete antibodies. CD8+ cytotoxic T lymphocytes (CTLs), the effector cells of the CD8+ lineage, kill infected cells and tumor cells that display class I MHC–associated antigens and also secrete cytokines that activate macrophages and cause inflammation.

Memory T cells that are generated by T cell activation are long-lived cells with an enhanced ability to react against the antigen. These cells are present in the recirculating lymphocyte pool and are abundant in mucosal tissues and the skin as well as in lymphoid organs. After a T cell response wanes, there are many more memory cells of the responding clone than there were naive T cells before the response. These memory cells respond rapidly to subsequent encounter with the antigen and generate new effector cells that eliminate the antigen.

T cell responses decline after the antigen is eliminated by effector cells. This process of contraction is important for returning the immune system to a state of equilibrium, or homeostasis. It occurs mainly because the majority of antigen-activated effector T cells die by apoptosis. One reason for this is that as the antigen is eliminated, lymphocytes are deprived of survival stimuli that are normally provided by the antigen and by the costimulators and cytokines produced during inflammatory reactions to the antigen. It is estimated that more than 90% of the antigen-specific T cells that arise by clonal expansion die by apoptosis as the antigen is cleared. In addition, inhibitory pathways activated by antigen recognition function to control the magnitude and duration of the response.

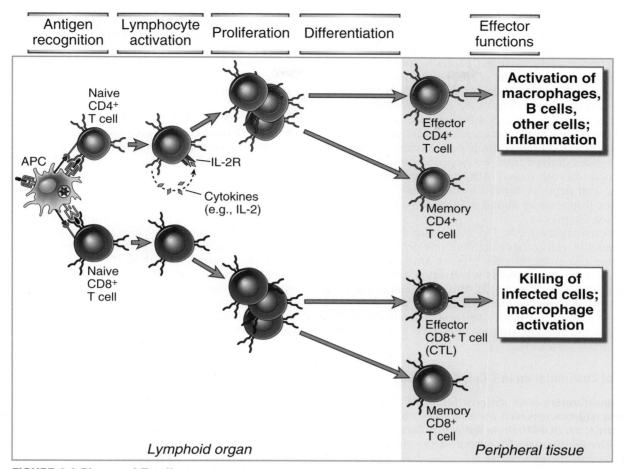

FIGURE 9-2 Phases of T cell responses. Antigen recognition by T cells induces cytokine (e.g., IL-2) secretion, particularly in CD4+ T cells, clonal expansion as a result of cell proliferation, and differentiation of the T cells into effector cells or memory cells. In the effector phase of the response, the effector CD4+ T cells respond to antigen by producing cytokines that have several actions, such as the recruitment and activation of leukocytes and activation of B lymphocytes, while CD8+ CTLs respond by killing other cells.

With this overview, we will proceed to a discussion of the signals required for T cell activation and the steps that are common to CD4+ and CD8+ T cells. We will conclude with a discussion of memory cells and the decline of immune responses.

SIGNALS FOR T LYMPHOCYTE ACTIVATION

The proliferation of T lymphocytes and their differentiation into effector and memory cells require antigen recognition, costimulation, and cytokines. In this section, we will summarize the nature of antigens recognized by T cells and discuss specific costimulators and their receptors that contribute to T cell activation. Cytokines are discussed later in this chapter and in Chapter 10.

Recognition of Antigen

Antigen is always the necessary first signal for the activation of lymphocytes, ensuring that the resultant immune response is specific for the antigen. Because CD4+ and CD8+ T lymphocytes recognize peptide-MHC complexes displayed by APCs, they can respond only to protein

antigens, the natural source of peptides, or to chemicals that modifiy proteins. In addition to the TCR recognizing peptides displayed by MHC molecules, several other T cell surface proteins participate in the process of T cell activation (see Fig. 7-9). These include adhesion molecules, which stabilize the interaction of the T cells with APCs; coreceptors, which deliver biochemical signals that work in concert with signals from the TCR complex; and costimulators, which are described later. The biochemical signals delivered by antigen receptors and coreceptors are discussed in Chapter 7.

Activation of naive T cells requires recognition of antigen presented by dendritic cells. This critical role of dendritic cells in initiating T cell responses is because these APCs are at the appropriate location to interact with naive T cells (see Chapter 6). In addition, the activation of naive T cells is dependent on signals such as costimulators (discussed later) that are highly expressed by dendritic cells. Protein antigens that cross epithelial barriers or are produced in tissues are captured by dendritic cells and transported to lymph nodes. Antigens that enter the circulation may be captured by dendritic cells in the spleen. If these antigens are components of microbes or are administered with adjuvants (as in vaccines), the resulting innate immune response leads to the activation of dendritic cells and the expression of costimulators. Dendritic cells with captured antigens migrate to the T cell zones of draining lymph nodes. As discussed in Chapter 6, both naive T cells and mature dendritic cells are drawn to the T cell zones of secondary lymphoid organs by chemokines produced at these sites that engage the CCR7 chemokine receptor on the cells. By the time the mature dendritic cells reach the T cell areas, they display antigenic peptides on MHC molecules and also express costimulators. Dendritic cells present peptides derived from endocytosed protein antigens in association with class II MHC molecules to naive CD4+ T cells, and peptides derived from cytosolic and nuclear proteins displayed by class I MHC molecules to CD8+ T cells (see Chapter 6).

Differentiated effector T cells can respond to antigens presented by cells other than dendritic cells. In humoral immune responses, B cells present antigens to helper T cells and are the recipients of activating signals from the helper cells (see Chapter 12); in cell-mediated immune responses, macrophages present antigens to and respond to CD4+ T cells (see Chapter 10); and virtually any nucleated cell can present antigen to and be killed by CD8+ CTLs (see Chapter 11).

Role of Costimulation in T Cell Activation

The proliferation and differentiation of naive T cells require signals provided by molecules on APCs, called costimulators, in addition to antigen-induced signals (Fig. 9-3). The requirement for costimulatory signals was first suggested by the experimental finding that T cell antigen receptor signaling alone (e.g., induced by anti-CD3 antibodies that cross-link TCR-CD3 complexes, mimicking antigen) resulted in lower responses than those seen with antigens presented by activated APCs. This result indicated that APCs express molecules that are required, in addition to antigen, for T cell activation. These molecules are called **costimulators**, and the second signal for T cell activation is called **costimulation** because it functions together with antigen (signal 1) to stimulate T cells. In the absence of costimulation, T cells that encounter antigens either fail to respond and die by apoptosis or enter a state of prolonged unresponsiveness (see Chapter 15).

The B7:CD28 Family of Costimulators

The best characterized costimulatory pathway in T cell activation involves the T cell surface receptor CD28, which binds the costimulatory molecules B7-1 (CD80) and B7-2 (CD86) expressed on activated APCs. CD28 was discovered when antibodies against human T cell surface molecules were screened for their ability to enhance T cell responses when added together with an activating anti-CD3 antibody. This was soon followed by the identification of the ligands for CD28, called B7 and later shown to be two homologous proteins, named B7-1 (CD80) and B7-2 (CD86). The essential role of CD28 and B7-1 and B7-2 (often collectively called B7) in T cell activation has been established not only by experiments with cross-linking antibodies but also by the severe T cell immune deficiency caused by knockout of genes encoding these proteins in mice and by the ability of agents that bind to and block B7 molecules to inhibit a variety of T cell responses in experimental animals and in humans. The development of therapeutic agents based on these principles is described later.

B7-1 and B7-2 are structurally similar integral membrane single-chain glycoproteins, each with two extracellular immunoglobulin (Ig)–like domains. CD28 is a disulfide-linked homodimer, each subunit of which has a single extracellular Ig domain. It is expressed on more than 90% of CD4+ T cells and on 50% of CD8+ T cells in humans (and on all naive T cells in mice).

The expression of B7 costimulators is regulated and ensures that T lymphocyte responses are initiated only when needed. The B7 molecules are expressed mainly on APCs, including dendritic cells, macrophages, and B

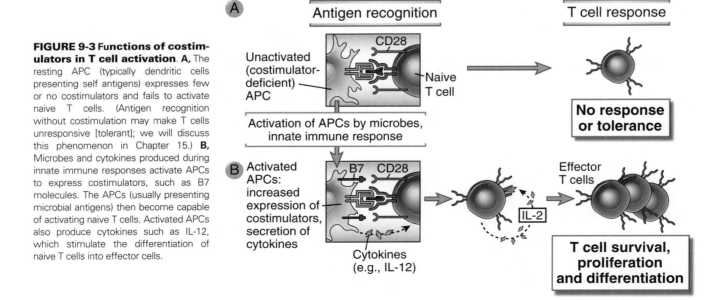

FIGURE 9-3 Functions of costimulators in T cell activation. A, The resting APC (typically dendritic cells presenting self antigens) expresses few or no costimulators and fails to activate naive T cells. (Antigen recognition without costimulation may make T cells unresponsive [tolerant]; we will discuss this phenomenon in Chapter 15.) **B,** Microbes and cytokines produced during innate immune responses activate APCs to express costimulators, such as B7 molecules. The APCs (usually presenting microbial antigens) then become capable of activating naive T cells. Activated APCs also produce cytokines such as IL-12, which stimulate the differentiation of naive T cells into effector cells.

lymphocytes. They are absent or expressed at low levels on resting APCs and are induced by various stimuli, including microbial products that engage Toll-like receptors and cytokines such as interferon-γ (IFN-γ) produced during innate immune reactions to microbes. The induction of costimulators by microbes and by the cytokines of innate immunity promotes T cell responses to microbial antigens. This is an excellent illustration of the role of innate immune responses in enhancing adaptive immunity (see Chapter 4). In addition, activated CD4+ T cells themselves enhance the expression of B7 costimulators on the APCs by a pathway dependent on CD40, described later, providing a feedback loop that serves to amplify T cell responses. Of all potential APCs, mature dendritic cells express the highest levels of costimulators and, as a result, are the most potent stimulators of naive T cells. The temporal patterns of expression of B7-1 and B7-2 differ; B7-2 is expressed constitutively at low levels and induced rapidly after activation of APCs, whereas B7-1 is induced hours or days later.

In Chapter 6, we mentioned the essential role of **adjuvants** in inducing primary T cell responses to protein antigens such as vaccines. Many adjuvants are products of microbes, or mimic microbes, and one of their major functions in T cell activation is to stimulate the expression of costimulators on APCs.

Unactivated, or resting, APCs in normal tissues are capable of presenting self antigens to T cells, but because these tissue APCs express only low levels of costimulators, potentially self-reactive T cells that see the self antigens are not activated and may be rendered permanently unresponsive (see Chapter 15). Regulatory T cells, which are important for tolerance to self antigens (see Chapter 15), are also dependent on B7:CD28-mediated costimulation for their generation and maintenance. It is possible that the low levels of B7 costimulators that are constitutively expressed by resting APCs function together with the self antigens that are displayed by these APCs to maintain regulatory T cells.

CD28 signals work in cooperation with antigen recognition to promote the survival, proliferation, and differentiation of the specific T cells. Costimulatory signaling via CD28 amplifies signaling pathways that are also induced downstream of the T cell receptor (see Chapter 7) and may trigger additional signals that cooperate with TCR-induced signals (Fig. 9-4). PI3-kinase is recruited to the cytoplasmic tail of CD28, and this in turn activates the downstream pro-survival kinase Akt as well as Itk and PLCγ, which can trigger calcium signaling. CD28 can also contribute to the activation of the JNK MAP kinase via the Rac small G protein and can amplify the activation of the NF-κB pathway. The net result of these signaling pathways is the increased expression of anti-apoptotic proteins such as Bcl-2 and Bcl-X$_L$, which promote survival of T cells; increased metabolic activity of T cells; enhanced proliferation of the T cells; production of cytokines such as IL-2; and differentiation of the naive T cells into effector and memory cells. Previously activated effector and memory T cells are less dependent on costimulation by the B7:CD28 pathway than are naive

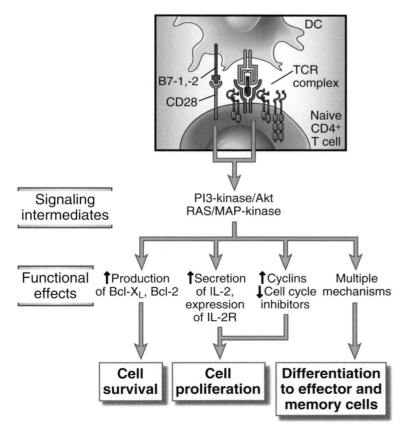

FIGURE 9-4 Mechanisms of T cell costimulation by CD28. CD28 engagement induces signaling pathways that enhance or work together with TCR signals to stimulate the expression of survival proteins, cytokines, and cytokine receptors; to promote cell proliferation; and to induce differentiation toward effector and memory cells by activating various transcription factors (not shown, see Chapters 10 and 11). These differentiation events may be secondary to the increased clonal expansion and may also involve increased production of various transcription factors.

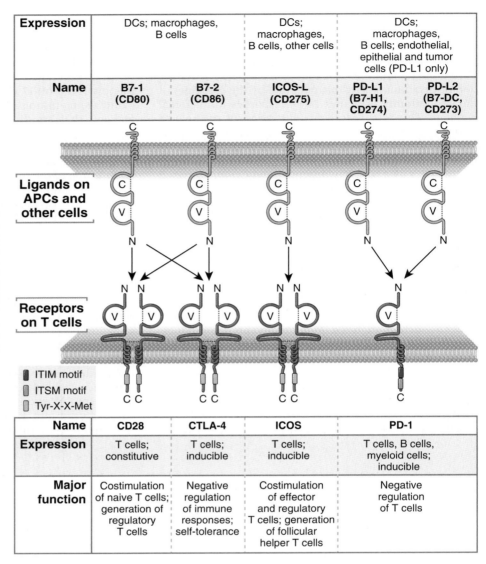

FIGURE 9-5 The major members of the B7 and CD28 families. The known B7 family ligands expressed on APCs and CD28 family receptors expressed on T cells are shown, with their expression patterns and likely major functions. Other widely distributed molecules with limited homology to B7, such as B7-H3 and B7-H4, have been identified, but their physiologic roles are not yet established. Other inhibitory receptors have also been defined, such as BTLA, but these are not homologous to CD28 and are not shown.

Expression	DCs; macrophages, B cells		DCs; macrophages, B cells, other cells	DCs; macrophages, B cells; endothelial, epithelial and tumor cells (PD-L1 only)	
Name	B7-1 (CD80)	B7-2 (CD86)	ICOS-L (CD275)	PD-L1 (B7-H1, CD274)	PD-L2 (B7-DC, CD273)

Ligands on APCs and other cells

Receptors on T cells

- ITIM motif
- ITSM motif
- Tyr-X-X-Met

Name	CD28	CTLA-4	ICOS	PD-1
Expression	T cells; constitutive	T cells; inducible	T cells; inducible	T cells, B cells, myeloid cells; inducible
Major function	Costimulation of naive T cells; generation of regulatory T cells	Negative regulation of immune responses; self-tolerance	Costimulation of effector and regulatory T cells; generation of follicular helper T cells	Negative regulation of T cells

cells. This property of effector and memory cells enables them to respond to antigens presented by various APCs that may reside in nonlymphoid tissues and may express no or low levels of B7. For instance, the differentiation of CD8+ T cells into effector CTLs requires costimulation, but effector CTLs can kill other cells that do not express costimulators.

Numerous receptors homologous to CD28 and their ligands homologous to B7 have been identified, and these proteins regulate T cell responses both positively and negatively (Fig. 9-5). Following the demonstration of the importance of B7 and CD28, several other proteins structurally related to B7-1 and B7-2 or to CD28 were identified. A surprising conclusion has emerged that some of the members of the B7:CD28 families are involved in T cell activation (and are thus costimulators) and others are critical inhibitors of T cells (and are sometimes called coinhibitors). The costimulatory receptor other than CD28 whose function is best understood is **ICOS** (inducible costimulator, CD278). Its ligand, called ICOS-L (CD275), is expressed on dendritic cells, B cells, and other cell populations. ICOS plays an essential role in

T cell–dependent antibody responses, particularly in the germinal center reaction. It is required for the development and activation of follicular helper T cells, which are essential for the formation of germinal centers and for the generation of high-affinity B cells in these structures (see Chapter 12).

The outcome of T cell activation is influenced by a balance between engagement of activating and inhibitory receptors of the CD28 family. The inhibitory receptors of the CD28 family are **CTLA-4** (cytotoxic T lymphocyte antigen 4) and **PD-1** (programmed death 1). (The names of these two proteins do not accurately reflect their distribution or function.) The concept that a balance between activating and inhibitory receptors controls the magnitude of responses in the immune system was discussed in Chapter 4 in the context of natural killer (NK) cells (see Fig. 4-8). A similar idea is applicable to responses of T and B lymphocytes, although the receptors involved are quite different. Because the inhibitory receptors CTLA-4 and PD-1 are involved in the phenomenon of tolerance, and abnormalities in their expression or function cause autoimmune diseases, we will discuss

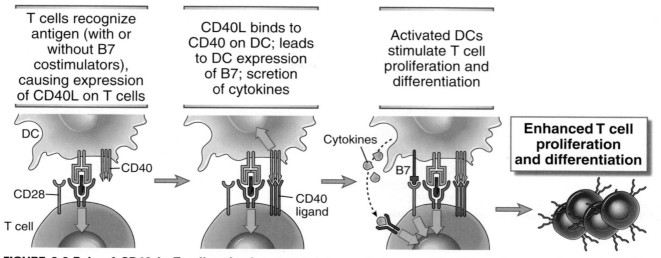

FIGURE 9-6 Role of CD40 in T cell activation. Naive T cells are activated by peptide-MHC complexes on activated APCs. Antigen recognition by T cells together with some costimulation *(not shown)* induces the expression of CD40 ligand (CD40L) on the activated T cells. CD40L engages CD40 on APCs and may stimulate the expression of more B7 molecules and the secretion of cytokines that activate T cells. Thus, CD40L on the T cells makes the APCs better at promoting and amplifying T cell activation.

them in more detail in Chapter 15, when we consider immunological tolerance and autoimmunity. Suffice it to say here that CD28 and CTLA-4 provide an illustrative example of two receptors that recognize the same ligands (the B7 molecules) but have opposite functional effects on T cell activation. CTLA-4 is a high-affinity receptor for B7, and it has been postulated that it is engaged when B7 levels on APCs are low (as on resting APCs displaying self antigens). CD28 has a 20- to 50-fold lower affinity for B7, and it may be engaged when B7 levels are relatively high (e.g., after exposure to microbes). According to this model, the level of B7 expression on APCs—low with self antigens, high with microbes—determines the relative engagement of CTLA-4 or CD28, respectively, and this in turn determines if responses are terminated (because of CTLA-4 engagement) or initiated (because of CD28 signals). Once engaged, CTLA-4 may competitively inhibit access of CD28 to B7 molecules on APCs, remove B7 from the surface of APCs, or deliver inhibitory signals that block activating signals from the TCR and CD28 (see Chapter 15).

Although many of the costimulators and the inhibitory receptors may have overlapping functions, the major physiologic roles of different members of these families may be different. It is believed that the CD28:B7 interaction is most important for initiating T cell responses by activating naïve T cells; ICOS:ICOS-ligand interactions are critical for helper T cell-dependent antibody responses; CTLA-4:B7 interactions inhibit the initial activation of T lymphocytes in secondary lymphoid organs; and PD1:PD-ligand interactions inhibit the activation of effector cells, especially in peripheral tissues.

Other Costimulatory Pathways

Many other T cell surface molecules, including CD2 and integrins, have been shown to deliver costimulatory signals in vitro, but their physiologic role in promoting T cell activation is less clear than that of the CD28 family. We have discussed the functions of CD2 family proteins

in Chapter 7 and of integrins in Chapter 3. Several other receptors that belong to the large tumor necrosis factor (TNF) receptor (TNFR) superfamily, and their ligands, which are homologous to TNF, have been shown to stimulate and to inhibit T cells under various experimental conditions. Many of the receptors are expressed on activated T cells and are believed to be involved in the development, maintenance, and functions of effector cells. Ox40 (CD134) is a TNFR family member expressed on activated CD4+ and CD8+ T cells that functions to maintain cell survival and sustained responses. Its ligand is expressed on activated APCs. Other members of this family that have been implicated in stimulating and suppressing lymphocyte responses include 4-1BB (CD137), which is also expressed on activated T cells. Some TNFR family members, such as CD27, are expressed on memory T cells; their physiologic function is not defined. The roles of these proteins in controlling normal and pathologic immune responses remain areas of active investigation.

The interaction of CD40L on T cells with CD40 on APCs enhances T cell responses by activating the APCs. CD40 ligand (CD40L) is a TNF superfamily membrane protein that is expressed primarily on activated T cells, and CD40 is a member of the TNFR superfamily expressed on B cells, macrophages, and dendritic cells. The functions of CD40 in activating macrophages in cell-mediated immunity and activating B cells in humoral immune responses are described in Chapters 10 and 12, respectively. Activated helper T cells express CD40L, which engages CD40 on the APCs and activates the APCs to make them more potent by enhancing their expression of B7 molecules and secretion of cytokines such as IL-12 that promote T cell differentiation (Fig. 9-6). This phenomenon is sometimes called licensing because activated T cells license APCs to become more powerful stimulators of immune responses. Thus, the CD40 pathway indirectly amplifies T cell responses by inducing costimulators on APCs, but CD40L does not by itself function as a costimulator for T cells.

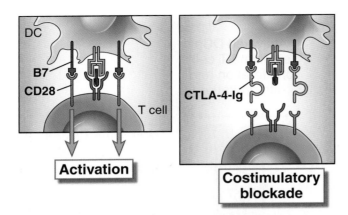

FIGURE 9-7 The mechanism of therapeutic costimulatory blockade. A fusion protein of the extracellular portion of CTLA-4 and the Fc tail of an IgG molecule is used to bind to and block B7 molecules, thus preventing their interaction with the activating receptor CD28 and inhibiting T cell activation.

Therapeutic Costimulatory Blockade

Based on the understanding of these costimulatory pathways, new therapeutic agents have been developed for controlling injurious immune responses (Fig. 9-7). CTLA-4–Ig, a fusion protein consisting of the extracellular domain of CTLA-4 and the Fc portion of human IgG, binds to B7-1 and B7-2 and blocks the B7:CD28 interaction. The reason for the use of the extracellular domain of CTLA-4 rather than of CD28 to block B7 molecules is that CTLA-4 has a higher affinity for B7 than does CD28. Attachment of the Fc portion of IgG increases the in vivo half-life of the protein. CTLA-4-Ig is an approved therapy for rheumatoid arthritis and transplant rejection, and clinical trials are currently assessing its efficacy in the treatment of other inflammatory diseases, such as psoriasis and Crohn's disease. Inhibitors of the CD40L:CD40 pathway are also in clinical trials for transplant rejection and chronic inflammatory diseases.

Antibodies that block the CTLA-4 and PD-1 inhibitory receptors are approved or in clinical trials for the immunotherapy of tumors; they work by removing the brakes on T cell activation and enabling the cancer-bearing individual to mount more effective anti-tumor immune responses (see Chapter 18). As one might predict from the role of CTLA-4 in maintaining self-tolerance, blocking of this inhibitory receptor induces autoimmune reactions in some patients.

FUNCTIONAL RESPONSES OF T LYMPHOCYTES

The earliest responses of antigen-stimulated T cells consist of changes in the expression of various surface molecules, including cytokine receptors, as well as the secretion of cytokines. These are followed by proliferation of the antigen-specific cells, driven in part by the secreted cytokines, and then by differentiation of the activated cells into effector and memory cells. In the remainder of this chapter, we will describe these steps, their underlying mechanisms, and their functional consequences.

Changes in Surface Molecules During T Cell Activation

After the initiation of activation by antigen recognition and costimulator binding, there are characteristic changes in the expression of various surface molecules in T cells, which are best defined in CD4⁺ helper cells (Fig. 9-8). Many of the molecules that are expressed in activated T cells are also involved in the functional responses of the T cells. Some of the functionally important molecules induced after recognition of antigen and costimulators are the following:

- *CD69.* Within a few hours, T cells increase their expression of CD69, a plasma membrane protein. This protein binds to and reduces surface expression of the sphingosine 1-phosphate receptor S1PR1, which we described in Chapter 3 as a receptor that mediates egress of T cells from lymphoid organs. The consequence of decreased S1PR1 expression is that activated T cells are retained in lymphoid organs long enough to receive the signals that initiate their proliferation and differentiation into effector and memory cells. After cell division, CD69 expression decreases, the activated T cells reexpress high levels of S1PR1, and therefore effector and memory cells can exit the lymphoid organs (see Chapter 3).
- *CD25 (IL-2Rα).* The expression of this cytokine receptor enables activated T cells to respond to the growth-promoting cytokine IL-2. This process is described later.
- *CD40 ligand (CD40L, CD154).* Within 24 to 48 hours after antigen recognition, T cells express high levels of the ligand for CD40. The expression of CD40L enables activated T cells to mediate their key effector functions, which are to help macrophages and B cells. In addition, as discussed earlier, CD40L on the T cells activates dendritic cells to become better APCs, thus providing a positive feedback mechanism for amplifying T cell responses.
- *CTLA-4 (CD152).* The expression of CTLA-4 on T cells also increases within 24 to 48 hours after antigen recognition. We mentioned CTLA-4 earlier as a member of the CD28 family that functions as an inhibitor of T cell activation and thus as a regulator of the response. The mechanism of action of CTLA-4 is described in Chapter 15 (see Fig. 15-5).
- *Adhesion molecules and chemokine receptors.* During activation, T cells reduce expression of molecules that bring them to the lymphoid organs (such as L-selectin [CD62L] and the chemokine receptor CCR7) and increase the expression of molecules that are involved in their migration to peripheral sites of infection and tissue injury (such as the integrins LFA-1 and VLA-4, the ligands for E- and P-selectins, and various chemokine receptors). These molecules and their roles in T cell migration were described in Chapter 3. Activation also increases the expression of CD44, a receptor for the extracellular matrix molecule hyaluronan. Binding of CD44 to its ligand helps to retain effector T cells in the tissues at sites of infection and tissue damage (see Chapter 10).

Cytokines in Adaptive Immune Responses

Cytokines play critical roles in adaptive immunity. These cytokines have some general properties.

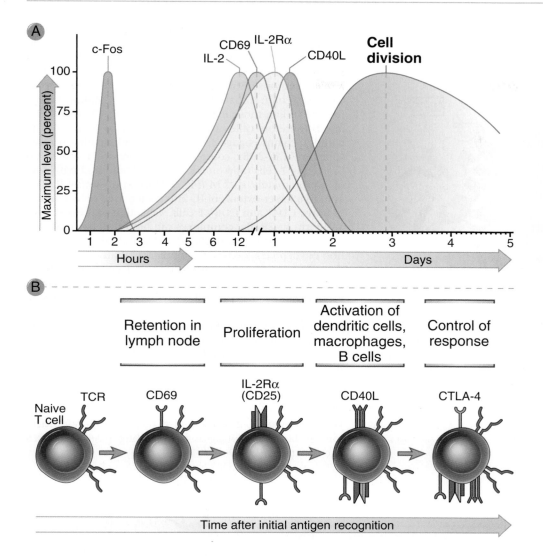

FIGURE 9-8 Changes in surface molecules after T cell activation. **A,** The approximate kinetics of expression of selected molecules during activation of T cells by antigens and costimulators are shown. The illustrative examples include a transcription factor (c-Fos), a cytokine (IL-2), and surface proteins. These proteins are typically expressed at low levels in naive T cells and are induced by activating signals. CTLA-4 is induced 1 to 2 days after initial activation. The kinetics are estimates and will vary with the nature of the antigen, its dose and persistence, and the type of adjuvant. **B,** The major functions of selected surface molecules are shown and described in the text. *CD40L,* CD40 ligand; *IL-2R,* IL-2 receptor

- In adaptive immune responses, CD4⁺ helper T cells make the largest amount and variety of cytokines, but cytokines made by CD8⁺ T cells and B cells also play important roles. Cytokines secreted by dendritic cells and other APCs serve critical functions in the development of T cell responses.

- Cytokines produced during adaptive immune responses are involved in the proliferation and differentiation of antigen-stimulated T and B cells and in the effector functions of T cells.

- Most of these cytokines act on the cells that produce them (autocrine action) or on nearby cells (paracrine action).

The roles of cytokines in the effector functions of T cells are described in Chapters 10 and 11. Here we discuss interleukin-2, the prototype of a T cell–derived cytokine that stimulates T cell responses.

IL-2 Secretion and IL-2 Receptor Expression

Interleukin-2 (IL-2) is a growth, survival, and differentiation factor for T lymphocytes that plays a major role in the induction of T cell responses and in the control of

immune responses. Because of its ability to support proliferation of antigen-stimulated T cells, IL-2 was originally called T cell growth factor (TCGF). It acts on the same cells that produce it or on adjacent cells (i.e., it functions as an autocrine or paracrine cytokine).

IL-2 is produced mainly by CD4⁺ T lymphocytes early after recognition of antigen and costimulators. Activation of T cells stimulates transcription of the *IL 2* gene and synthesis and secretion of the protein. IL-2 production is rapid and transient, starting within 1 to 2 hours after antigen recognition, peaking at about 8 to 12 hours, and declining by 24 hours. CD4⁺ T cells secrete IL-2 into the immunologic synapse formed between the T cell and APC (see Chapter 7). IL-2 receptors on T cells also tend to localize to the synapse, so that the cytokine and its receptor reach sufficiently high local concentrations to initiate cellular responses.

Secreted IL-2 is a 14- to 17-kD globular glycoprotein containing four α helices (Fig. 9-9). It is the prototype of the four–α-helical cytokines that interact with type I cytokine receptors (see Chapter 7).

Functional IL-2 receptors are transiently expressed on activation of naive and effector T cells; regulatory T cells always express high-affinity IL-2 receptors. The IL-2 receptor (IL-2R) consists of three non-covalently associated

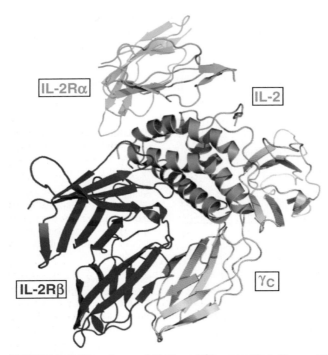

FIGURE 9-9 Structure of IL-2 and its receptor. The crystal structure of IL-2 and its trimeric receptor shows how the cytokine interacts with the three chains of the receptor. *(Reproduced from Wang X, Rickert M, Garcia KC: Structure of the quaternary complex of interleukin-2 with its α, β, and γc receptors, Science 310:1159-1163, 2005, with the permission of the publishers. Courtesy of Drs. Patrick Lupardus and K. Christopher Garcia, Stanford University School of Medicine, Palo Alto, California.)*

proteins, IL-2Rα (CD25), IL-2/15Rβ (CD122), and γ_c (CD132). Of the three chains, only IL-2Rα is unique to the IL-2R. IL-2 binds to the α chain alone with low affinity, and this does not lead to any detectable cytoplasmic signaling or biologic response. The β chain is also part of the IL-15 receptor. The γ chain is shared with a number of cytokine receptors, including those for IL-4, IL-7, IL-9, IL-15, and IL-21, and is therefore called the common γ chain (γ_c). Both the β and γ_c chains engage JAK-STAT signaling pathways (see Chapter 7). IL-2Rβγ_c complexes are expressed at low levels on resting T cells (and on NK cells) and bind IL-2 with a K_d of approximately 10^{-9} M (Fig. 9-10). Expression of IL-2Rα and, to a lesser extent, of IL-2Rβ is increased on activation of naive CD4$^+$ and CD8$^+$ T cells. Cells that express IL-2Rα and form IL-2Rαβγ_c complexes can bind IL-2 more tightly, with a K_d of approximately 10^{-11} M, and growth stimulation of such cells occurs at a similarly low IL-2 concentration. IL-2, produced in response to antigen stimulation, is a stimulus for induction of IL-2Rα, providing a feedback mechanism by which T cell responses amplify themselves. CD4$^+$ regulatory T cells (see Chapter 15) express the complete IL-2R complex and are thus poised to respond to the cytokine. Chronic T cell stimulation leads to shedding of IL-2Rα, and an increased level of shed IL-2Rα in the serum is used clinically as a marker of strong antigenic stimulation (e.g., acute rejection of a transplanted organ).

Functions of IL-2

The biology of IL-2 is fascinating because it plays critical roles in both promoting and controlling T cell responses and functions (Fig. 9-11).

FIGURE 9-10 Regulation of IL-2 receptor expression. Resting (naive) T lymphocytes express the IL-2Rβγ_c complex, which has a moderate affinity for IL-2. Activation of the T cells by antigen, costimulators, and IL-2 itself leads to expression of the IL-2Rα chain and increased levels of the high-affinity IL-2Rαβγ complex.

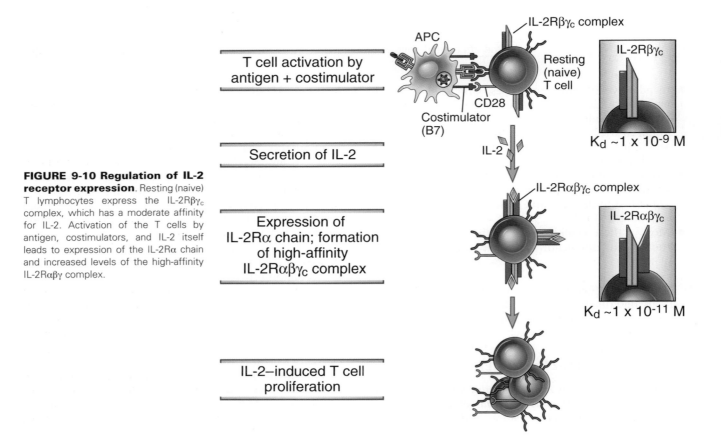

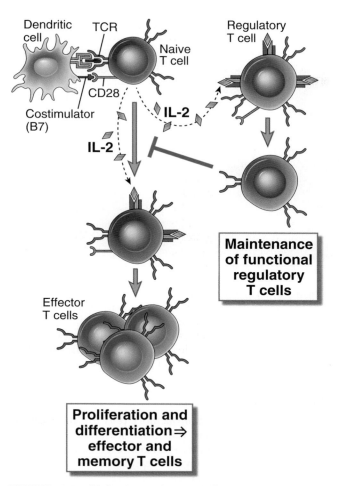

FIGURE 9-11 Biologic actions of IL-2. IL-2 stimulates the survival, proliferation and differentiation of T lymphocytes, acting as an autocrine growth factor. IL-2 also maintains functional regulatory T cells and thus controls immune responses (e.g., against self antigens).

- *IL-2 stimulates the survival, proliferation, and differentiation of antigen-activated T cells.* IL-2 promotes survival of cells by inducing the anti-apoptotic protein Bcl-2. It stimulates cell cycle progression through the synthesis of cyclins and by relieving a block in cell cycle progression through degradation of the cell cycle inhibitor p27. In addition, IL-2 increases production of effector cytokines, such as IFN-γ and IL-4, by T cells.
- *IL-2 is required for the survival and function of regulatory T cells,* which suppress immune responses against self and other antigens. Knockout mice lacking IL-2 or IL-2R α or β chains develop uncontrolled T and B cell proliferation and autoimmune disease because of defects in regulatory T cells. This finding suggests that other growth factors can replace IL-2 for expansion of effector T cells, but no other cytokine can replace IL-2 for the maintenance of functional regulatory T cells. We will discuss this role of IL-2 in more detail in Chapter 15, when we describe the properties and functions of regulatory T cells. An interesting feature of this function of IL-2 is that regulatory T cells do not produce significant amounts of the cytokine, implying that they depend for their survival on IL-2 made by other T cells responding to antigens.

- *IL-2 has also been shown to stimulate the proliferation and differentiation of NK cells and B cells in vitro.* The physiologic importance of these actions is not established.

Clonal Expansion of T Cells

T cell proliferation in response to antigen recognition is mediated by a combination of signals from the antigen receptor, costimulators, and autocrine growth factors, primarily IL-2. The cells that recognize antigen produce IL-2 and also preferentially respond to it, ensuring that the antigen-specific T cells are the ones that proliferate the most. The result of this proliferation is an increase in the size of the antigen-specific clones, known as **clonal expansion,** which generates the large number of cells required to eliminate the antigen from a small pool of naive antigen-specific lymphocytes. Before antigen exposure, the frequency of naive T cells specific for any antigen is 1 in 10^5 to 10^6 lymphocytes. After microbial antigen exposure, the frequency of CD8+ T cells specific for that microbe may increase to as many as 1 in 3 CD8+ T lymphocytes, representing a >50,000-fold expansion of antigen-specific CD8+ T cells, and the number of specific CD4+ cells increases up to 1 in 100 CD4+ lymphocytes (Fig. 9-12). Studies in mice first showed this tremendous expansion of the antigen-specific population in some acute viral infections and, remarkably, it occurred within as little as 1 week after infection. Equally remarkable was the finding that during this massive antigen-specific clonal expansion, bystander T cells not specific for the virus did not proliferate. The expansion of T cells specific for Epstein-Barr virus and human immunodeficiency virus (HIV) in acutely infected humans is also on this order of magnitude.

Differentiation of Activated T Cells into Effector Cells

Many of the progeny of the antigen-stimulated cells differentiate into effector cells. Effector cells of the CD4+ lineage express surface molecules and secrete cytokines that activate other cells (B lymphocytes, macrophages, and dendritic cells). Whereas naive CD4+ T cells produce mostly IL-2 on activation, effector CD4+ T cells are capable of producing a large number and variety of cytokines that have diverse biologic activities. Effector CD8+ cells are cytotoxic and kill infected cells. Because there are important differences in effector cells of the CD4+ and CD8+ lineages, we will describe their development and functions separately in Chapters 10 and 11.

Development of Memory T Cells

T cell–mediated immune responses to an antigen usually result in the generation of memory T cells specific for that antigen, which may persist for years, even a lifetime. Memory cells provide effective defense against pathogens that are prevalent in the environment and may be repeatedly encountered. The success of vaccination is attributed in large part to the ability to generate memory cells on initial antigen exposure. Edward Jenner's classic experiment of successful vaccination of a child against smallpox is a demonstration of a memory response. Despite the

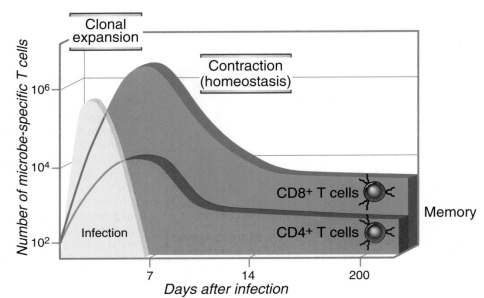

FIGURE 9-12 Clonal expansion of T cells. The numbers of CD4+ and CD8+ T cells specific for microbial antigens and the expansion and decline of the cells during immune responses are illustrated. The numbers are approximations based on studies of model microbial and other antigens in inbred mice.

importance of immunologic memory, many fundamental questions about the generation of memory cells have still not been answered.

Memory cells may develop from effector cells along a linear pathway, or effector and memory populations follow divergent differentiation and are two alternative fates of lymphocytes activated by antigen and other stimuli (Fig. 9-13). The mechanisms that determine whether an individual antigen-stimulated T cell will become a short-lived effector cell or enter the long-lived memory cell pool are not established. The signals that drive the development of memory cells are also not fully understood. One possibility is that the types of transcription factors that are induced during T cell activation influence the choice between the development of effector or memory cells. For instance, expression of the transcription factor T-bet drives differentiation toward effector cells in CD4+ and CD8+ populations, whereas expression of a different transcription factor Blimp-1 promotes the generation of memory cells. Whether induction of these transcription factors is a random (stochastic) process or is influenced by specific external signals is not yet clear.

Properties of Memory T Cells

The defining properties of memory cells are their ability to survive in a quiescent state after antigen is eliminated and to mount larger and enhanced responses to antigens than do naive cells. Several features of memory cells account for these properties.

- ***Memory cells express increased levels of anti-apoptotic proteins, which may be responsible for their prolonged survival.*** Whereas naive T cells live for weeks or months and are replaced by mature cells that develop in the thymus, memory T cells may survive for months or years. Thus, as humans age in an environment in

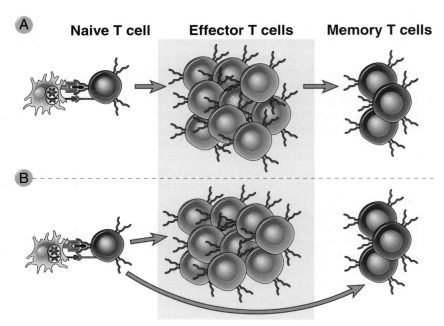

FIGURE 9-13 Development of memory T cells. In response to antigen and costimulation, naive T cells differentiate into effector and memory cells. **A,** According to the linear model of memory T cell differentiation, most effector cells die and some survivors develop into the memory population. **B,** According to the branched differentiation model, effector and memory cells are alternative fates of activated T cells.

which they are constantly exposed and responding to infectious agents, the proportion of memory cells induced by these microbes compared with naive cells progressively increases. In individuals older than 50 years of age or so, half or more of circulating T cells may be memory cells. The anti-apoptotic proteins that promote memory cell survival include Bcl-2 and Bcl-X$_L$, which prevent cytochrome c release from mitochondria and thus block apoptosis induced by a deficiency of survival signals (see Fig. 15-7). The presence of these proteins allows memory cells to survive even after antigen is eliminated and innate immune responses have subsided, when the normal signals for T cell survival and proliferation are no longer present.

- *Memory cells respond more rapidly to antigen stimulation than do naive cells specific for the same antigen.* The rapid response of memory cells to antigen challenge has been documented in many studies done in humans and experimental animals. For example, in studies in mice, naive T cells respond to antigen in vivo in 5 to 7 days, and memory cells respond within 1 to 3 days (see Fig. 1-4). A possible explanation for this enhanced responsiveness is that the gene loci for cytokines and other effector molecules are fixed in an accessible state in memory cells, in part because of changes in methylation and acetylation of histones. As a result, these genes are poised to respond rapidly to antigen challenge.
- *The number of memory T cells specific for any antigen is greater than the number of naive cells specific for the same antigen.* As we discussed earlier, proliferation leads to a large clonal expansion in all immune responses and differentiation of naive lymphocytes into effector cells, most of which die after the antigen is eliminated. The surviving cells of the expanded clone are memory cells, and they are typically 10- to 100-fold more numerous than the pool of naive cells before antigen encounter. The increased clone size is a major reason that antigen challenge in a previously immunized individual induces a more robust response than the first immunization in a naive individual. As expected, the size of the memory pool is proportional to the size of the naive antigen-specific population.
- *Memory cells are able to migrate to peripheral tissues and respond to antigens at these sites.* As we have previously discussed, naive T cells migrate preferentially to secondary lymphoid organs, but memory cells can migrate to virtually any tissue. These differences are related to differences in the expression of adhesion molecules and chemokine receptors. In addition, memory T cells are less dependent on costimulation than are naive cells, allowing memory cells to respond to antigens presented by a wide range of APCs in peripheral tissues; in contrast, as we have discussed earlier in this chapter and in Chapter 6, naive T cells are dependent on antigen presentation by mature dendritic cells in lymphoid organs.
- *Memory cells undergo slow proliferation, and this ability to self-renew may contribute to the long life span of the memory pool.* The cycling of these cells may be driven by cytokines. Because of the capacity for self-renewal, memory cells have been likened to stem cells.
- *The maintenance of memory cells is dependent on cytokines but does not require antigen recognition.* The most important cytokine for the maintenance of memory CD4$^+$ and CD8$^+$ T cells is IL-7, which also plays a key role in early lymphocyte development (see Chapter 8) and in the survival of naive T cells (see Chapter 2). Predictably, high expression of the IL-7 receptor (CD127) is characteristic of memory T cells. Memory CD8$^+$ T cells also depend on the related cytokine IL-15 for their survival. IL-7 and IL-15 induce the expression of anti-apoptotic proteins and stimulate low-level proliferation, both of which maintain populations of memory T cells for long periods. The ability of memory cells to survive without antigen recognition has been best demonstrated by experiments in mice in which antigen receptors are genetically deleted after mature lymphocytes have developed. In these mice, the number of naive lymphocytes drops rapidly but memory cells are maintained.

The most reliable phenotypic markers for memory T cells appear to be the surface expression of the IL-7 receptor and a protein of unknown function called CD27, and the absence of markers of naive and recently activated T cells (see Table 2-3). In humans, most naive T cells express the 200-kD isoform of the surface molecule CD45 called CD45RA (for "restricted A") and most memory T cells express a 180-kD isoform of CD45 called CD45RO (see Chapter 2).

Both CD4$^+$ and CD8$^+$ memory T cells are heterogeneous and can be subdivided into subsets based on their homing properties and functions. **Central memory** T cells express the chemokine receptor CCR7 and L-selectin and home mainly to lymph nodes. They have a limited capacity to perform effector functions when they encounter antigen, but they undergo brisk proliferative responses and generate many effector cells on antigen challenge. **Effector memory** T cells, on the other hand, do not express CCR7 or L-selectin and home to peripheral sites, especially mucosal tissues. On antigenic stimulation, effector memory T cells produce effector cytokines such as IFN-γ or rapidly become cytotoxic, but they do not proliferate much. This effector subset, therefore, is poised for a rapid response to a repeated exposure to a microbe, but complete eradication of the infection may also require large numbers of effectors generated from the pool of central memory T cells. It is unclear if all memory T cells can be classified into central and effector memory cells.

Memory T cells are also heterogeneous in terms of cytokine profiles. For example, some CD4$^+$ memory T cells may be derived from precursors before commitment to the T$_H$1, T$_H$2, or T$_H$17 phenotype (described in Chapter 10), and when activated by reexposure to antigen and cytokines, they can differentiate into any of these subsets. Other memory T cells may be derived from fully differentiated T$_H$1, T$_H$2, or T$_H$17 effectors and retain their respective cytokine profiles on reactivation. Memory CD8$^+$ T cells may also exist that have some of the phenotypic characteristics of differentiated CTLs.

DECLINE OF T CELL RESPONSES

Elimination of antigen leads to contraction of the T cell response, and this decline is responsible for maintaining homeostasis in the immune system. There are several reasons that the response declines. As the antigen is eliminated and the innate immune response associated with antigen exposure abates, the signals that normally keep activated lymphocytes alive and proliferating are no longer active. As mentioned earlier, costimulation and growth factors like IL-2 stimulate expression of the anti-apoptotic proteins Bcl-2 and Bcl-X_L in the activated lymphocytes, and these proteins keep cells viable. As the level of costimulation and the amount of available IL-2 decrease, the levels of anti-apoptotic proteins in the cells drop. At the same time, growth factor deprivation activates sensors of cellular stress (such as the BH3-only protein Bim), which trigger the mitochondrial pathway of apoptosis and are no longer opposed by the anti-apoptotic proteins (see Fig. 15-8). The net result of these changes is that most of the cells that were produced by activation die and the generation of newly activated cells declines, so the pool of antigen-activated lymphocytes contracts.

There has been much interest in the possibility that various regulatory mechanisms contribute to the normal contraction of immune responses. Such mechanisms might include the inhibitory receptors CTLA-4 and PD-1, apoptosis induced by death receptors of the TNF receptor superfamily (such as TNFRI and Fas), and regulatory T cells.

SUMMARY

* T cell responses are initiated by signals that are generated by TCR recognition of peptide-MHC complexes on the surface of an APC and through signals provided at the same time by costimulators expressed on APCs.
* The best-defined costimulators are members of the B7 family, which are recognized by receptors of the CD28 family expressed on T cells. The expression of B7 costimulators on APCs is increased by encounter with microbes, providing a mechanism for generating optimal responses against infectious pathogens. Some members of the CD28 family inhibit T cell responses, and the outcome of T cell antigen recognition is determined by the balance between engagement of activating and inhibitory receptors of this family.
* T cell responses to antigen and costimulators include changes in the expression of surface molecules, synthesis of cytokines and cytokine receptors, cellular proliferation, and differentiation into effector and memory cells.
* The surface molecules whose expression is induced on T cell activation include proteins that are involved in retention of T cells in lymphoid organs, growth factors for cytokines, effector and regulatory molecules, and molecules that influence migration of the T cells.
* Shortly after activation, T cells produce the cytokine IL-2 and express high levels of the functional IL-2 receptor. IL-2 drives the proliferation of the cells, which can result in marked expansion of antigen-specific clones.

* Some activated T cells may differentiate into memory cells, which survive for long periods and respond rapidly to antigen challenge. The maintenance of memory cells is dependent on cytokines such as IL-7, which may promote the expression of anti-apoptotic proteins and stimulate low-level cycling. Memory T cells are heterogeneous and consist of populations that differ in migration properties and functional responses.
* T cell responses decline after elimination of the antigen, thus returning the system to rest. The decline is largely because the signals for continued lymphocyte activation are also eliminated.

SELECTED READINGS

T Cell Activation

Huppa JB, Davis MM: The interdisciplinary science of T-cell recognition, *Advances in Immunology* 119:1–50, 2013.

Jenkins MK, Moon JJ: The role of naïve T cell precursor frequency and recruitment in dictating immune response magnitude, *Journal of Immunology* 188:4135–4140, 2012.

Costimulation: B7, CD28, and More

Chen L, Flies DB: Molecular mechanisms of T cell co-stimulation and co-inhibition, *Nature Reviews Immunology* 13:227–242, 2013.

Croft M: The TNF family in T cell differentiation and function—unanswered questions and future directions, *Seminars in Immunology*, 2014, Mar 5, (epub).

Greenwald RJ, Freeman GJ, Sharpe AH: The B7 family revisited, *Annual Review of Immunology* 23:515–548, 2005.

T Cell Cytokines

Boyman O, Sprent J: The role of interleukin-2 during homeostasis and activation of the immune system, *Nature Reviews Immunology* 12:180–190, 2012.

Huse M, Quann EJ, Davis MM: Shouts, whispers and the kiss of death: directional secretion in T cells, *Nature Immunology* 9:1105–1111, 2008.

Liao W, Lin JX, Leonard WJ: Interleukin-2 at the crossroads of effector responses, tolerance, and immunotherapy, *Immunity* 38:13–25, 2013.

Rochman Y, Spolski R, Leonard WJ: New insights into the regulation of T cells by γ_c family cytokines, *Nature Reviews Immunology* 9:169–173, 2009.

Memory T Cells

Mueller SN, Gebhardt T, Carbone FR, Heath WR: Memory T cell subsets, migration patterns, and tissue residence, *Annual Review of Immunology* 31:137–161, 2013.

Pepper M, Jenkins MK: Origin of CD4+ effector and central memory T cells, *Nature Immunology* 12:467–471, 2011.

Sallusto F, Lanzavecchia A: Heterogeneity of CD4+ memory T cells: functional modules for tailored immunity, *European Journal of Immunology* 39:2076–2082, 2009.

Sprent J, Surh CD: Normal T cell homeostasis: the conversion of naive cells into memory-phenotype cells, *Nature Immunology* 12:478–484, 2011.

Differentiation and Functions of CD4+ Effector T Cells

The functions of CD4+ effector T cells are to recruit and activate phagocytes (macrophages and neutrophils) and other leukocytes that destroy intracellular and some extracellular microbes, and to help B lymphocytes to produce antibodies. CD4+ T lymphocytes are critical for phagocyte-mediated elimination of microbes, whereas CD8+ effector cells are responsible for the eradication of microbes, typically viruses, that infect and replicate inside all cells, including nonphagocytic cells (Fig. 10-1). For historical reasons, **cell-mediated immunity** refers to the process of CD4+ T cell–stimulated phagocyte-mediated killing of microbes. Some CD4+ T cells activate cells other than phagocytes, such as eosinophils, to destroy particular types of microbes. Although these reactions are not included in the original definition of cell-mediated immunity, they are important functions of effector T cells. In this chapter, we will describe the role of CD4+ T cells in eliminating microbes. At the end, we will discuss some less numerous populations of T cells whose major functions are mediated by secreted cytokines. The differentiation and function of CD8+ effector cells are discussed in Chapter 11, and the role of helper T cells in antibody responses is considered in Chapter 12.

OVERVIEW OF CELL-MEDIATED IMMUNITY

Cell-mediated immunity is the type of host defense that is mediated by T lymphocytes, and it serves as a defense mechanism against intracellular and phagocytosed microbes. Historically, immunologists divided adaptive immunity into humoral immunity, which can be adoptively transferred from an immunized donor to a naive host by antibodies in the absence of cells, and cell-mediated immunity, which can be adoptively transferred only by viable T lymphocytes. The effector phase of humoral immunity is triggered by the recognition of antigen by secreted antibodies. Therefore, humoral immunity neutralizes and eliminates extracellular microbes and toxins that are accessible to antibodies, but it is not effective against microbes inside cells. Conversely, in cell-mediated immunity, the effector phase is initiated by the recognition of antigens by T cells. T lymphocytes recognize protein antigens of microbes that are displayed on the surfaces of infected cells as peptides bound to self major histocompatibility complex (MHC) molecules. Therefore, cell-mediated immunity is effective against cell-associated microbes, including phagocytosed and other intracellular microbes. Defects in cell-mediated immunity result in increased susceptibility to infection by viruses and intracellular bacteria as well as some extracellular bacteria and fungi that are normally eliminated by phagocytes. T cell–mediated reactions are also important in allograft rejection

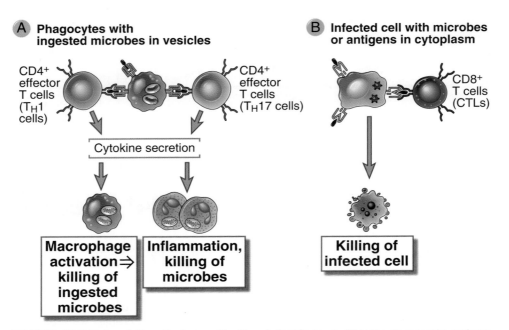

FIGURE 10-1 Role of T cells in eradicating infections. A, CD4+ T cells recognize antigens of phagocytosed and extracellular microbes and produce cytokines that activate the phagocytes to kill the microbes and stimulate inflammation. CD8+ T cells can also secrete cytokines and participate in similar reactions. **B,** CD8+ cytotoxic T lymphocytes (CTLs) recognize antigens of microbes residing in the cytosol of infected cells and kill the cells.

(see Chapter 17), anti-tumor immunity (see Chapter 18), and immune-mediated inflammatory diseases (see Chapter 19).

The sequence of events in the responses of CD4+ T cells involves the initial activation of these cells in lymphoid organs to generate effector and memory cells, migration of effector cells to sites of infection, and elimination of infectious pathogens at these sites (Fig. 10-2). We described the early steps in the activation of T cells in Chapter 9, and we will describe the subsequent steps in the generation and functions of effector CD4+ T cells in this chapter.

Effector CD4+ T cells are generated by antigen recognition in secondary lymphoid organs but most of them leave these organs and migrate to peripheral sites of infection where they function in microbe elimination. This migration of effector (and memory) T cells to sites of infection is dependent on endothelial adhesion molecules and chemokines expressed at these sites (see Chapter 3). Although migration is largely independent of antigen, T cells that recognize antigen in extravascular tissues may be preferentially retained there. Once in the tissues, the T cells encounter microbial antigens presented by macrophages and other antigen-presenting cells (APCs). T cells that specifically recognize antigens receive signals through their antigen receptors that increase the affinity of integrins for their ligands. Two of these integrins, VLA-4 and VLA-5, bind to fibronectin in extracellular matrices, and a third adhesion molecule, CD44, which is also highly expressed on activated T cells, binds to hyaluronan. As a result, antigen-specific effector and memory T cells that encounter the antigen are preferentially retained at the extravascular site.

T cells not specific for the antigen that migrate into a site of inflammation may die in the tissue or return through lymphatic vessels to the circulation.

Some CD4+ T cells that are activated in secondary lymphoid organs do not exit the organs but migrate into lymphoid follicles within the organs, where they help B cells to produce high-affinity antibodies of different isotypes. The best-defined of these helper T cells are called follicular helper T cells; these cells and their functions in humoral immune responses are described in Chapter 12.

In cell-mediated immune responses against phagocytosed microbes, T cells specifically recognize microbial antigens but phagocytes actually destroy the pathogens. Thus, effector T cells of the CD4+ lineage link specific recognition of microbes with the recruitment and activation of other leukocytes that destroy the microbes. This fundamental concept was first appreciated from studies of cell-mediated immunity to the intracellular bacterium *Listeria monocytogenes* (Fig. 10-3). It was shown in the 1950s that mice previously infected with a low dose of *Listeria* were protected from challenge with higher doses that were lethal in previously uninfected animals. Protection could be transferred to naive animals with lymphocytes (later shown to be T lymphocytes) from the infected mice but not with serum, the fluid fraction of clotted blood that contains antibodies. In vitro, the bacteria were killed not by T cells from immune animals but by activated macrophages, emphasizing the central role of macrophages in the execution of effector function.

Ingestion and elimination of microbes by phagocytes is also an important reaction of innate immunity, but T cells greatly enhance this function of phagocytes. As we

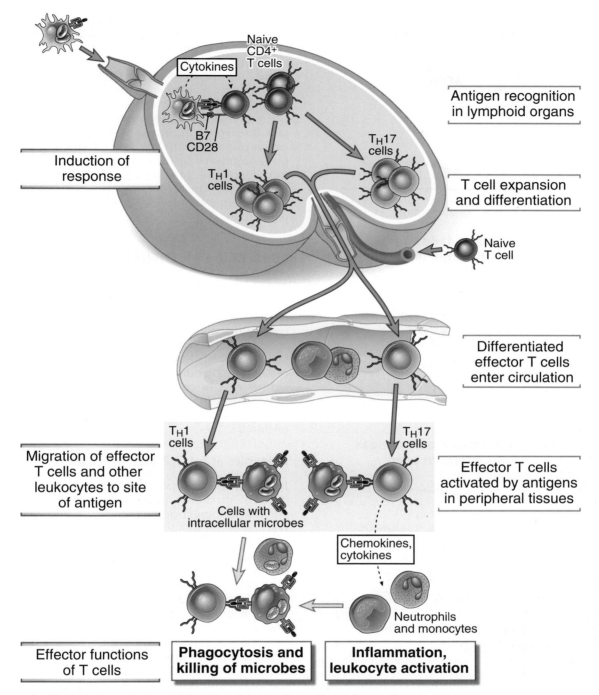

FIGURE 10-2 Reactions of CD4⁺ T cells in cell-mediated immunity. Induction of response: CD4⁺ T cells recognize peptides that are derived from protein antigens and presented by dendritic cells in peripheral lymphoid organs. The T lymphocytes are stimulated to proliferate and differentiate into effector (and memory) cells, which enter the circulation. Migration of effector T cells and other leukocytes to the site of antigen: Effector T cells and other leukocytes migrate through blood vessels in peripheral tissues by binding to endothelial cells that have been activated by cytokines produced in response to infection in these tissues. Effector functions of T cells: Effector T cells recognize the antigen in the tissues and respond by secreting cytokines that recruit more leukocytes and activate phagocytes to eradicate the infection.

discussed in Chapter 4, phagocytes recognize microbes and are activated by microbial ligands, and they are potent at destroying a variety of microbes. However, many infectious pathogens have evolved to resist this mechanism of innate immunity and can survive and even replicate inside macrophages. In these situations, T cells recognize microbial protein antigens and recruit and activate phagocytes, enabling them to eradicate infections that may not be combated by innate immunity alone. CD4⁺ effector T cells activate phagocytes via surface molecules, principally CD40 ligand, and secreted cytokines. We will see how these signals cooperate when

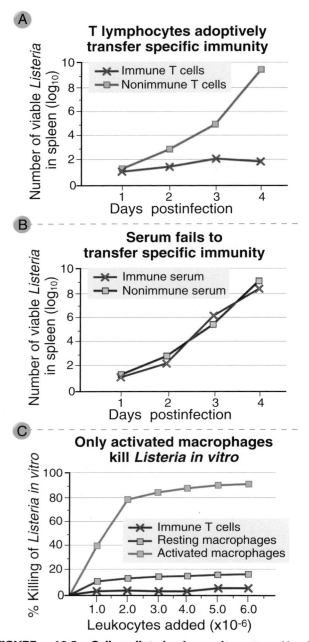

FIGURE 10-3 Cell-mediated immunity to *Listeria monocytogenes.* Immunity to *L. monocytogenes* is measured by inhibition of bacterial growth in the spleens of animals inoculated with a known dose of viable bacteria. Such immunity can be transferred to normal mice by T lymphocytes **(A)** but not by serum **(B)** from syngeneic mice previously immunized with killed or low doses of *L. monocytogenes*. In an in vitro assay of cell-mediated immunity, the bacteria are actually killed by activated macrophages and not by T cells **(C)**.

we discuss the activation of macrophages later in this chapter and of B cells in Chapter 12.

Inflammation, consisting of leukocyte recruitment and activation, accompanies many of the reactions of CD4+ T lymphocytes and may damage normal tissues. This T cell–dependent injurious reaction is called **delayed-type hypersensitivity (DTH)**, the term *hypersensitivity* referring to tissue damage caused by an immune response. DTH frequently occurs together with

protective cell-mediated immunity against microbes and may be the cause of much of the pathology associated with certain types of infection (see Chapters 16 and 19).

Because the functions of CD4+ T cells are mediated in large part by cytokines, there has been great interest in defining these cytokines, which cells produce them, and how they function. One of the most important discoveries in immunology has been the identification of populations of CD4+ effector T cells that can be distinguished by the cytokines they produce and the transcription factors they express. We will begin with a description of the major properties of these subsets, and then describe the development and functions of each population.

SUBSETS OF CD4+ EFFECTOR T CELLS

Three major subsets of CD4+ effector T cells, called T_H1, T_H2, and T_H17, function in host defense against different types of infectious pathogens and are involved in different types of tissue injury in immunologic diseases (Fig. 10-4). A fourth subset, called follicular helper T cells, is important for antibody responses (see Chapter 12). Regulatory T cells are another distinct population of CD4+ T cells. They are not effector cells; rather, their function is to control immune reactions to self and foreign antigens, and they are described in Chapter 15 in the context of immunologic tolerance.

Properties of T_H1, T_H2, and T_H17 Subsets

It was appreciated many years ago that host responses to different infections varied greatly, as did the reactions in different immunologic diseases. For instance, the immune reaction to intracellular bacteria like *Mycobacterium tuberculosis* is dominated by activated macrophages, whereas the reaction to helminthic parasites consists of the production of IgE antibody and the activation of eosinophils. Furthermore, in many chronic autoimmune diseases, tissue damage is caused by inflammation with accumulation of neutrophils and macrophages, whereas in allergic disorders, the lesions contain abundant eosinophils along with other leukocytes. The realization that all of these phenotypically diverse immunologic reactions are dependent on CD4+ T cells raised an obvious question: How can the same CD4+ cells elicit such different responses? The answer, as we now know, is that CD4+ T cells consist of subsets of effector cells that produce distinct sets of cytokines, elicit quite different reactions, and are involved in host defense against different microbes as well as in distinct types of immunologic diseases. The first subsets that were discovered were called types 1 and 2 helper T cells, or T_H1 and T_H2. The T_H17 subset, so named because its characteristic cytokine is IL-17, was discovered many years after T_H1 and T_H2 cells were first described. T_H17 cells were identified as the T cells responsible for some CD4+ T cell-mediated inflammatory diseases that could not be attributed to the T_H1 and T_H2 subsets.

The defining characteristics of differentiated subsets of effector cells are the cytokines they produce, the

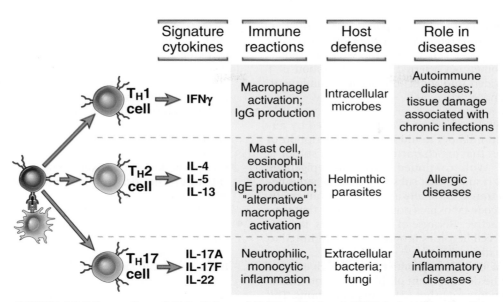

FIGURE 10-4 Properties of T$_H$1, T$_H$2, and T$_H$17 subsets of CD4+ helper T cells. Naive CD4+ T cells may differentiate into distinct subsets of effector cells in response to antigen, costimulators, and cytokines. The columns to the right list the major differences between the best-defined subsets.

transcription factors they express, and epigenetic changes in specific cytokine gene loci. These characteristics of each subset are described below.

The signature cytokines produced by the major CD4+ T cell subsets are IFN-γ for T$_H$1 cells; IL-4, IL-5, and IL-13 for T$_H$2 cells; and IL-17 and IL-22 for T$_H$17 cells (see Fig. 10-4). The cytokines produced by these T cell subsets determine their effector functions and roles in diseases. The cytokines also participate in the development and expansion of the respective subsets (described later).

T$_H$1, T$_H$2, and T$_H$17 cells each have distinct patterns of homing, in large part defined by the chemokine receptors and adhesion molecules they express, which direct them to migrate into different sites of infections. We discussed the control of lymphocyte migration in Chapter 3. T$_H$1, but not T$_H$2, cells express high levels of the chemokine receptors CXCR3 and CCR5, which bind to chemokines elaborated in tissues during innate immune responses. Therefore, T$_H$1 cells tend to be abundant at sites of infection where the infectious agents trigger strong innate immune reactions; these agents include many bacteria and viruses. T$_H$1 cells also express high levels of ligands for E-selectin and P-selectin, which assist in the migration of these cells to sites of strong inflammation (where the selectins are expressed on the endothelium). In contrast, T$_H$2 cells express the chemokine receptors CCR3, CCR4, and CCR8, which recognize chemokines that are highly expressed at sites of helminthic infection or allergic reactions, particularly in mucosal tissues, and so T$_H$2 cells tend to migrate to these tissues. T$_H$17 cells express CCR6, which binds the chemokine CCL20, which is produced by various tissue cells and macrophages in some bacterial and fungal infections.

These differentiated T cell populations are identifiable in immune reactions and have provided many valuable insights into lymphocyte responses. Nevertheless, there are some important caveats with the idea that all effector CD4+ T cells can be classified into clear subsets based on defined criteria.

- Many effector CD4+ T cells produce various combinations of cytokines or only some of the cytokines characteristic of a particular subset and are not readily classifiable into separable populations. For instance, in many inflammatory reactions, there may be T cells that produce both IFN-γ (characteristic of T$_H$1 cells) and IL-17 (typical of T$_H$17 cells). Conversely, some cells may produce cytokines that are not characteristic of any of the three subsets (such as IL-9) or are only some of the cytokines produced by a particular subset. This restricted cytokine profile has led to an expanding nomenclature describing these populations (such as T$_H$9, T$_H$22, and so on). It is not known whether populations with mixed or limited cytokine patterns are intermediates in the development of the classical polarized effector cells or are themselves fixed populations.

- It is also clear that some of these differentiated effector T cells may convert from one cytokine profile to another by changes in activation conditions. The extent and significance of such plasticity are topics of active research.

- Although differentiated CD4+ effector T cells are considered the source of many cytokines in protective and pathologic adaptive immune responses, the same cytokines may be produced by other cell types, such as γδ T cells and innate lymphoid cells. For instance, in some inflammatory reactions dominated by IL-17, CD4+ T$_H$17 cells account for only 30% to 35% of the cytokine-producing cells, the remainder being other cell populations.

Development of T$_H$1, T$_H$2, and T$_H$17 Subsets

Differentiated T$_H$1, T$_H$2, and T$_H$17 cells all develop from naive CD4+ T lymphocytes, mainly in response to cytokines *present early during immune responses, and differentiation involves transcriptional activation and epigenetic modification of cytokine genes.* The process of differentiation, which is sometimes referred to as polarization of T cells, can be divided into induction, stable commitment, and amplification.

- *Induction.* Cytokines act on T cells stimulated by antigen and costimulators to induce the transcription of cytokine genes that are characteristic of each subset.
- *Commitment.* With continued activation, epigenetic modifications result in that subset's cytokine genes being fixed in a transcriptionally active state. Conversely, genes that encode cytokines not produced by that subset remain inactive. Because of these changes, the differentiating T cell becomes progressively committed to one specific pathway.
- *Amplification.* Cytokines produced by any given subset promote the development of this subset and inhibit differentiation toward other CD4+ subpopulations. The net result is the accumulation of cells of one subset.

There are several important general features of T cell subset differentiation.

- *The cytokines that drive the development of CD4+ T cell subsets are produced by APCs (primarily dendritic cells and macrophages) and other immune cells (such as NK cells and basophils or mast cells) present in the lymphoid organ where the immune response is initiated.* Dendritic cells that encounter microbes and display microbial antigens are activated to produce cytokines (as well as costimulators) as part of innate immune responses to the microbes (see Chapter 4). Different microbes may stimulate dendritic cells to produce distinct sets of cytokines, perhaps because the microbes are recognized by different microbial sensors in the cells. Other cells of innate immunity, such as NK cells and mast cells, also produce cytokines that influence the pattern of T cell subset development.
- *Stimuli other than cytokines may also influence the pattern of helper T cell differentiation.* Some studies indicate that different subsets of dendritic cells selectively promote either T_H1 or T_H2 differentiation; the same principle may be true for T_H17 cells. In addition, the genetic makeup of the host is an important determinant of the pattern of T cell differentiation. Some inbred strains of mice develop T_H2 responses to the same microbes that stimulate T_H1 differentiation in most other strains. Strains of mice that develop T_H2-dominant responses are susceptible to infections by intracellular microbes (see Chapter 16).
- *The distinct cytokine profiles of differentiated cell populations are controlled by particular transcription factors that activate cytokine gene expression, and by chromatin modifications affecting accessibility to the promoters and regulatory elements of cytokine genes that these transcription factors bind to.* The transcription factors are themselves activated or induced by signals from antigen receptors, innate immune receptors, costimulators, and other cytokine receptors. Each subset expresses its own characteristic set of transcription

factors. As the subsets become increasingly polarized, the gene loci encoding that subset's signature cytokines undergo histone modifications (such as changes in methylation and acetylation) and other chromatin remodeling events, so that these loci remain accessible to RNA polymerase and transcription factors, whereas the loci for other cytokines (those not produced by that subset) are in an inaccessible chromatin state. These epigenetic changes ensure that each subset can produce only its characteristic collection of cytokines. It is likely that epigenetic changes in cytokine gene loci correlate with stable phenotypes, and before these changes are established, the subsets may be plastic and convertible.

- *Each subset of differentiated effector cells produces cytokines that promote its own development and may suppress the development of the other subsets.* This feature of T cell subset development provides a powerful amplification mechanism. For instance, IFN-γ secreted by T_H1 cells promotes further T_H1 differentiation and inhibits the generation of T_H2 and T_H17 cells. Similarly, IL-4 produced by T_H2 cells promotes T_H2 differentiation, and IL-21 produced by T_H17 cells enhances T_H17 differentiation. Thus, each subset amplifies itself and may inhibit the other subsets. For this reason, once an immune response develops along one effector pathway, it becomes increasingly polarized in that direction, and the most extreme polarization is seen in chronic infections or in chronic exposure to environmental antigens, when the immune stimulation is prolonged.
- *Differentiation of each subset is induced by the types of microbes that the subset is best able to combat.* For instance, the development of T_H1 cells is driven by intracellular microbes, against which the principal defense is T_H1 mediated. By contrast, the immune system responds to helminthic parasites by the development of T_H2 cells, and the cytokines produced by these cells are critical for combating helminths. Similarly, T_H17 responses are induced by some bacteria and fungi and are most effective at defending against these microbes. The generation and effector functions of these differentiated T cells are an excellent illustration of the concept of specialization of adaptive immunity, which refers to the ability of the immune system to respond to different microbes in ways that are optimal for combating those microbes.

With this background, we will proceed to a description of the development and functions of each subset.

THE T_H1 SUBSET

The T_H1 subset is induced by microbes that are ingested by and activate phagocytes, and is the major effector T cell population in phagocyte-mediated host defense, the central reaction of cell-mediated immunity. T_H1 cells have long been considered the key mediators of cellular immunity, although we now realize that other effector T cells also contribute to this form of host defense.

Development of T$_H$1 Cells

T$_H$1 differentiation is driven mainly by the cytokines IL-12 and IFN-γ and occurs in response to microbes that activate dendritic cells, macrophages, and NK cells (Fig. 10-5). The differentiation of antigen-activated CD4$^+$ T cells to T$_H$1 effectors is stimulated by many intracellular bacteria, such as *Listeria* and mycobacteria, and by some parasites, such as *Leishmania*, all of which infect dendritic cells and macrophages. T$_H$1 differentiation is also stimulated by viruses and by protein antigens administered with strong adjuvants. A common feature of these infections and immunization conditions is that they elicit innate immune reactions that are associated with the production of certain cytokines, including IL-12, IL-18, and type I interferons. All of these

cytokines promote T$_H$1 development; of these, IL-12 is probably the most potent. Knockout mice lacking IL-12 are extremely susceptible to infections with intracellular microbes. IL-18 synergizes with IL-12, and type I interferons may be important for T$_H$1 differentiation in response to viral infections, especially in humans. Other microbes stimulate NK cells to produce IFN-γ, which is itself a strong T$_H$1-inducing cytokine and also acts on dendritic cells and macrophages to induce more IL-12 secretion. Once T$_H$1 cells have developed, they secrete IFN-γ, which promotes more T$_H$1 differentiation and thus amplifies the reaction. In addition, IFN-γ inhibits the differentiation of naive CD4$^+$ T cells to the T$_H$2 and T$_H$17 subsets, thus promoting the polarization of the immune response in one direction. T cells may further enhance cytokine production by dendritic cells and macrophages, by virtue of CD40 ligand (CD40L) on activated T cells engaging CD40 on the APCs and stimulating IL-12 secretion.

IFN-γ and IL-12 stimulate T$_H$1 differentiation by activating the transcription factors T-bet, STAT1, and STAT4 (see Fig. 10-5). T-bet, a member of the T-box family of transcription factors, is induced in naive CD4$^+$ T cells in response to antigen and IFN-γ. IFN-γ also activates the transcription factor STAT1, which in turn stimulates expression of T-bet. T-bet then promotes IFN-γ production through a combination of direct transcriptional activation of the *IFN-γ* gene and by inducing chromatin remodeling of the IFN-γ promoter region. The ability of IFN-γ to stimulate T-bet expression and the ability of T-bet to enhance IFN-γ transcription set up a positive amplification loop that drives differentiation of T cells toward the T$_H$1 phenotype. IL-12 contributes to T$_H$1 commitment by binding to receptors on antigen-stimulated CD4$^+$ T cells and activating the transcription factor STAT4, which further enhances IFN-γ production.

Functions of T$_H$1 Cells

The principal function of T$_H$1 cells is to activate macrophages to ingest and destroy microbes (Fig. 10-6). The same reaction of T$_H$1-mediated macrophage activation is involved in injurious delayed-type hypersensitivity, which is a component of many inflammatory diseases, and in granulomatous inflammation, which is typical of tuberculosis and is also seen in some other infectious and inflammatory disorders. These pathologic reactions are described in Chapter 19. T$_H$1 cells, or follicular helper T cells that produce the T$_H$1 cytokine IFN-γ, also stimulate the production of some IgG antibodies, especially in rodents.

Before discussing the activation of macrophages and how they destroy microbes, we will describe the properties of interferon-γ (IFN-γ), the cytokine responsible for most of the specialized functions of T$_H$1 cells.

Interferon-γ

IFN-γ is the principal macrophage-activating cytokine and serves critical functions in immunity against intracellular microbes. IFN-γ is also called immune or type II interferon. Although its name interferon implies antiviral activity, it is not a potent antiviral cytokine, and it

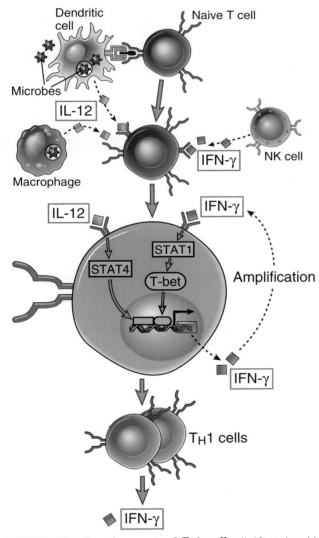

FIGURE 10-5 Development of T$_H$1 cells. IL-12 produced by dendritic cells and macrophages in response to microbes, including intracellular microbes, and IFN-γ produced by NK cells (all part of the early innate immune response to the microbes) activate the transcription factors T-bet, STAT1, and STAT4, which stimulate the differentiation of naive CD4$^+$ T cells to the T$_H$1 subset. IFN-γ produced by the T$_H$1 cells amplifies this response and inhibits the development of T$_H$2 and T$_H$17 cells.

functions mainly as an activator of effector cells of the immune system.

IFN-γ is a homodimeric protein belonging to the type II cytokine family (see Chapter 7). In addition to CD4⁺ T$_H$1 cells, NK cells and CD8⁺ T cells also produce IFNγ. NK cells secrete IFN-γ in response to activating ligands on the surface of infected or stressed host cells (see Chapter 4) or in response to IL-12; in this setting, IFN-γ functions as a mediator of innate immunity. In adaptive immunity, T cells produce IFN-γ in response to antigen recognition, and production is enhanced by IL-12 and IL-18.

The receptor for IFN-γ is composed of two structurally homologous polypeptides belonging to the type II cytokine receptor family, called IFNγR1 and IFNγR2. IFN-γ binds to and induces the dimerization of the two receptor chains. This leads to activation of the associated JAK1 and JAK2 kinases and ultimately to phosphorylation and dimerization of STAT1, which stimulates transcription of several genes (see Chapter 7). IFN-γ–induced genes encode many different molecules that mediate the biologic activities of this cytokine, described next.

The functions of IFN-γ are important in cell-mediated immunity against intracellular microbes (see Fig. 10-6).

- **IFN-γ activates macrophages to kill phagocytosed microbes.** Macrophage activation resulting in increased microbicidal activity is called **classical macrophage activation**, to be contrasted with an alternative activation pathway that is induced by T$_H$2 cytokines; these types of macrophage activation are described in more detail later. In innate immune reactions, IFN-γ is produced by NK cells and acts on macrophages together with Toll-like receptor (TLR) signals delivered by microbes (see Chapter 4) to trigger macrophage activation. In adaptive cell-mediated immunity, IFN-γ produced by T$_H$1 cells works together with CD40 ligand, also expressed by the T cells, to activate macrophages.
- **IFN-γ acts on B cells to promote switching to certain IgG subclasses, notably IgG2a or IgG2c (in mice), and to inhibit switching to IL-4–dependent isotypes, such as IgE.** The IgG subclasses induced by IFN-γ bind to Fcγ receptors on phagocytes and activate complement, and both mechanisms promote the phagocytosis of opsonized microbes (see Chapter 12). Thus, IFN-γ induces antibody responses that also participate in phagocyte-mediated elimination of microbes, in concert with the direct macrophage-activating effects of this cytokine. The mechanism of isotype switching and the role of cytokines in this process are described in Chapter 12. The major source of IFN-γ in antibody responses may be follicular helper T cells that produce this cytokine, and not classical T$_H$1 cells (see Chapter 12). This action of IFN-γ on B cells is better established in mice than in humans.
- **IFN-γ promotes the differentiation of CD4⁺ T cells to the T$_H$1 subset and inhibits the development of T$_H$2 and T$_H$17 cells.** These actions of IFN-γ serve to amplify the T$_H$1 response and were described earlier.
- **IFN-γ stimulates expression of several different proteins that contribute to enhanced MHC-associated antigen**

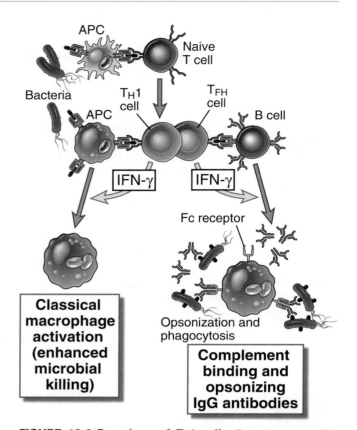

FIGURE 10-6 Functions of T$_H$1 cells. T$_H$1 cells secrete IFN-γ, which acts on macrophages to increase phagocytosis and killing of microbes in phagolysosomes and on B lymphocytes to stimulate production of IgG antibodies that opsonize microbes for phagocytosis. Help for antibody production may be provided not by classical T$_H$1 cells, most of which migrate out of lymphoid organs to sites of infection and inflammation, but by follicular helper T (T$_{FH}$) cells that remain in lymphoid organs and produce IFN-γ. The role of IFN-γ in antibody production is established in mice but not in humans. T$_H$1 cells also produce TNF, which activates neutrophils and promotes inflammation *(not shown)*.

presentation and the initiation and amplification of T cell–dependent immune responses (see Fig. 6-9). These proteins include MHC molecules; many proteins involved in antigen processing, including the transporter associated with antigen processing (TAP) and components of the proteasome; HLA-DM; and B7 costimulators on APCs.

The actions of IFN-γ together result in increased ingestion of microbes and the destruction of the ingested pathogens. Individuals with rare inherited inactivating mutations in the IFN-γ receptor and knockout mice lacking IFN-γ or the IFN-γ receptor or molecules required for T$_H$1 differentiation or IFN-γ signaling (IL-12 or IL-12 receptor, T-bet, STAT1) are susceptible to infections with intracellular microbes, such as mycobacteria, because of defective macrophage-mediated killing of the microbes.

Other T$_H$1 Cytokines

In addition to IFN-γ, T$_H$1 cells produce TNF and various chemokines, which contribute to the recruitment of leukocytes and enhanced inflammation. Somewhat surprisingly, T$_H$1 cells are also important sources of

IL-10, which functions mainly to inhibit dendritic cells and macrophages and thus to suppress T$_H$1 activation. This is an example of a negative feedback loop in T cell responses.

T$_H$1-Mediated Classical Macrophage Activation and Killing of Phagocytosed Microbes

T$_H$1 cells activate macrophages by contact-mediated signals delivered by CD40L-CD40 interactions and by IFN-γ (Fig. 10-7). When the T$_H$1 cells are stimulated by antigen, the cells express CD40L on their surface and secrete IFN-γ. The actions of IFN-γ on macrophages, described earlier, synergize with the actions of CD40 ligand, and together they are potent stimuli for macrophage activation. CD40 signals activate the transcription factors nuclear factor κB (NF-κB) and activation protein 1 (AP-1) and, as discussed earlier, IFN-γ activates the transcription factor STAT1. These transcription factors together stimulate the expression of several enzymes in the phagolysosomes of macrophages,

including phagocyte oxidase, which induces the production of reactive oxygen species (ROS); inducible nitric oxide synthase (iNOS), which stimulates the production of nitric oxide (NO); and lysosomal enzymes. The requirement for interactions between the surface molecules CD40 on the macrophages and CD40L on the T cells ensures that macrophages that are presenting antigens to the T cells (i.e., the macrophages that are harboring intracellular microbes) are also the macrophages that will be in contact with T cells and thus most efficiently activated by the T cells.

Activated macrophages kill phagocytosed microbes mainly by the actions of reactive oxygen species, nitric oxide, and lysosomal enzymes. All of these potent microbicidal agents are produced within the lysosomes of macrophages and kill ingested microbes after phagosomes fuse with lysosomes (see Fig. 4-12). These toxic substances may also be released into adjacent tissues, where they kill extracellular microbes and may cause damage to normal tissues.

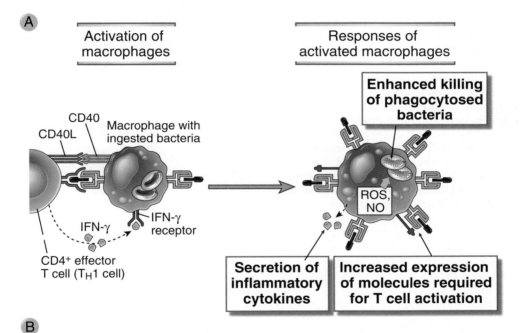

Macrophage response	Role in cell-mediated immunity
Production of reactive oxygen species, nitric oxide, increased lysosomal enzymes	Killing of microbes in phagolysosomes (effector function of macrophages)
Secretion of cytokines (TNF, IL-1, IL-12) and chemokines	TNF, IL-1, chemokines: leukocyte recruitment (inflammation)
	IL-12: T$_H$1 differentiation, IFN-γ production
Increased expression of B7 costimulators, MHC molecules	Increased T cell activation (amplification of T cell response)

FIGURE 10-7 Macrophage activation by T$_H$1 cells. A,** Macrophages are activated by CD40L-CD40 interactions and by IFN-γ expressed by T$_H$1 cells and perform several functions that kill microbes, stimulate inflammation, and enhance the antigen-presenting capacity of the cells. **B, The principal responses of macrophages activated by the classical activation pathway, and their roles in T cell–mediated host defense, are listed. Macrophages are also activated during innate immune reactions and perform similar functions (see Chapter 4).

Inherited immunodeficiencies, as well as gene knockout mice, have established the critical importance of CD40-CD40L interactions, in addition to IFN-γ, in cell-mediated immunity against intracellular pathogens. Humans with inherited mutations in CD40L (**X-linked hyper-IgM syndrome**) and mice in which the gene for CD40 or CD40L is knocked out are highly susceptible to infections with otherwise harmless intracellular microbes, including the intracellular fungus *Pneumocystis jiroveci* (see Chapter 21), which require T cell–dependent macrophage activation in order to be eradicated. As expected, these patients and knockout mice also have defects in helper T cell–dependent antibody production.

Activated macrophages are involved in several other reactions of host defense (see Fig. 10-7). They stimulate inflammation through the secretion of cytokines, mainly TNF, IL-1, and chemokines, and short-lived lipid mediators such as prostaglandins, leukotrienes, and platelet-activating factor. The collective action of these macrophage-derived mediators of inflammation is to recruit more leukocytes, which improves the host's ability to destroy infectious organisms. Activated macrophages amplify cell-mediated immune responses by becoming more efficient APCs because of increased levels of molecules involved in antigen processing and increased surface expression of class II MHC molecules and costimulators, and by producing cytokines (such as IL-12) that stimulate T lymphocyte differentiation into effector cells.

Some tissue injury may normally accompany T$_H$1 cell–mediated immune reactions to microbes because the microbicidal products released by activated macrophages and neutrophils are capable of injuring normal tissue and do not discriminate between microbes and host tissue. However, this tissue injury is usually limited in extent and duration, and it resolves as the infection is cleared. As mentioned earlier, delayed hypersensitivity is an example of a T$_H$1-mediatied reaction that can cause significant tissue injury (see Chapter 19).

THE T$_H$2 SUBSET

The T$_H$2 subset is the mediator of phagocyte-independent defense, in which eosinophils and mast cells play central roles. These reactions are important for the eradication of helminthic infections and perhaps also for elimination of other microbes in mucosal tissues. They are also central to the development of allergic diseases (see Chapter 20).

Development of T$_H$2 Cells

T$_H$2 differentiation is stimulated by the cytokine IL-4 and occurs in response to helminths and allergens (Fig. 10-8). Helminths and allergens cause chronic T cell stimulation, often without the strong innate immune responses that are required for T$_H$1 differentiation. Thus, T$_H$2 cells may develop in response to microbes and antigens that cause persistent or repeated T cell stimulation without much inflammation or the production of pro-inflammatory

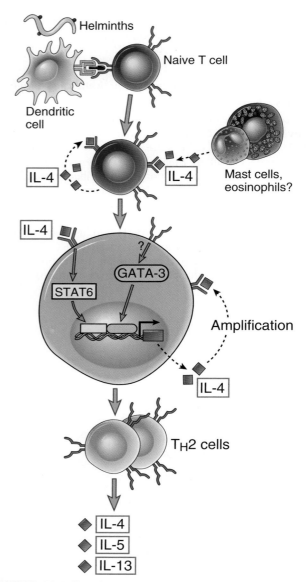

FIGURE 10-8 Development of T$_H$2 cells. IL-4 produced by activated T cells themselves or by mast cells and eosinophils, especially in response to helminths, activates the transcription factors GATA-3 and STAT6, which stimulate the differentiation of naive CD4⁺ T cells to the T$_H$2 subset. IL-4 produced by the T$_H$2 cells amplifies this response and inhibits the development of T$_H$1 and T$_H$17 cells.

cytokines that drive T$_H$1 and T$_H$17 responses. The dependence of T$_H$2 differentiation on IL-4 raises an interesting question: Because differentiated T$_H$2 cells are the major source of IL-4 during immune responses to protein antigens, where does the IL-4 come from before T$_H$2 cells develop? In some situations, such as helminthic infections, IL-4 produced by mast cells and, possibly, other cell populations, such as innate lymphoid cells, may contribute to T$_H$2 development. Another possibility is that antigen-stimulated CD4⁺ T cells secrete small amounts of IL-4 from their initial activation. If the antigen is persistent and present at high concentrations, the local concentration of IL-4 gradually increases. If the antigen also does not trigger inflammation with attendant IL-12

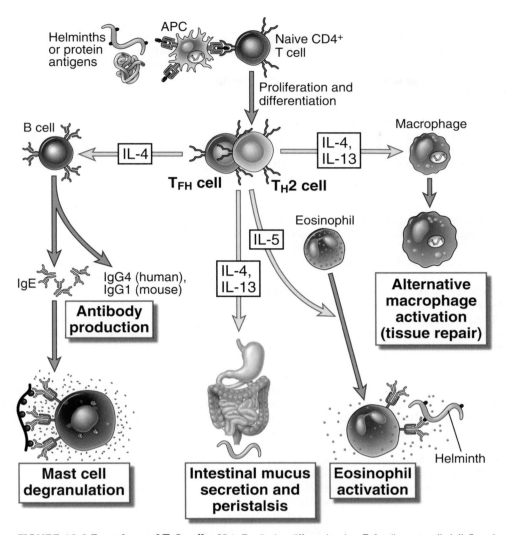

FIGURE 10-9 Functions of T$_H$2 cells. CD4$^+$ T cells that differentiate into T$_H$2 cells secrete IL-4, IL-5, and IL-13. IL-4 (and IL-13) act on B cells to stimulate production of antibodies that bind to mast cells, such as IgE. Help for antibody production may be provided by T$_{FH}$ cells that produce T$_H$2 cytokines and reside in lymphoid organs, and not by classical T$_H$2 cells. IL-4 is also an autocrine growth and differentiation cytokine for T$_H$2 cells. IL-5 activates eosinophils, a response that is important for defense against helminthic infections. IL-4 and IL-13 are involved in immunity at mucosal barriers, induce an alternative pathway of macrophage activation, and inhibit classical T$_H$1-mediated macrophage activation.

production, the result is increasing differentiation of T cells to the T$_H$2 subset. Once T$_H$2 cells have developed, the IL-4 they produce serves to amplify the reaction and inhibits the development of T$_H$1 and T$_H$17 cells.

IL-4 stimulates T$_H$2 development by activating the transcription factor STAT6, which, together with TCR signals, induces expression of GATA-3 (see Fig. 10-8). GATA-3 is a transcription factor that acts as a master regulator of T$_H$2 differentiation, enhancing expression of the T$_H$2 cytokine genes IL-4, IL-5, and IL-13, which are located in the same genetic locus. GATA-3 works by directly interacting with the promoters of these genes and also by causing chromatin remodeling, which opens up the locus for accessibility to other transcription factors. This is similar to the way in which T-bet influences IFN-γ expression. GATA-3 functions to stably commit differentiating cells toward the T$_H$2 phenotype, enhancing its own expression through a positive feedback loop. Furthermore, GATA-3 blocks T$_H$1

differentiation by inhibiting expression of the signaling chain of the IL-12 receptor. Knockout mice lacking IL-4, STAT6, or GATA-3 are deficient in T$_H$2 responses.

Functions of T$_H$2 Cells

T$_H$2 cells stimulate IgE-, mast cell- and eosinophil-mediated reactions that serve to eradicate helminthic infections (Fig. 10-9). Helminths are too large to be phagocytosed by neutrophils and macrophages and may be more resistant to the microbicidal activities of these phagocytes than are most bacteria and viruses. Therefore, special mechanisms are needed for defense against helminthic infections. The functions of T$_H$2 cells are mediated by IL-4, which induces IgE antibody responses; IL-5, which activates eosinophils; and IL-13, which has diverse actions. We will first describe the properties of these cytokines and then their roles in host defense.

Interleukin-4

IL-4 is the signature cytokine of the T_H2 subset and functions as both an inducer and an effector cytokine of these cells. It is a member of the type 1 four–α-helical cytokine family. The principal cellular sources of IL-4 are CD4+ T lymphocytes of the T_H2 subset and activated mast cells, but other tissue cells also produce this cytokine. The IL-4 receptor of lymphoid cells consists of a cytokine-binding α chain that is a member of the type I cytokine receptor family, associated with the $γ_c$ chain shared by other cytokine receptors. This IL-4R$αγ_c$ receptor signals by a JAK-STAT pathway involving JAK1, JAK3, and STAT6, and by a pathway that involves the insulin response substrate (IRS) called IRS-2. The STAT6 protein induces transcription of genes that account for many of the actions of this cytokine. IL-4 also binds to the IL-13 receptor (described later).

IL-4 has important actions on several cell types.

- *IL-4 stimulates B cell Ig heavy chain class switching to the IgE isotype.* The mechanisms of class switching are described in Chapter 12. Knockout mice lacking IL-4 have less than 10% of normal IgE levels. IgE antibodies play a role in eosinophil-mediated defense against helminthic (and some arthropod) infections. IgE is also the principal mediator of immediate hypersensitivity (allergic) reactions, and production of IL-4 is important for the development of allergies (see Chapter 20). IL-4 also enhances switching to IgG4 (in humans, or the homologous IgG1 in mice) and inhibits switching to the IgG2a and IgG2c isotypes in mice, both of which are stimulated by IFN-γ. This is one of several reciprocal antagonistic actions of IL-4 and IFN-γ. IL-13 can also contribute to switching to the IgE isotype. The effector cells that stimulate isotype switching may be T_{FH} cells that produce IL-4, and perhaps IL-13, and not classical T_H2 cells (see Chapter 12).
- *IL-4 stimulates the development of T_H2 effector cells from naive CD4+ T cells, and functions as an autocrine growth factor for differentiated T_H2 cells.* This function of IL-4 was described earlier.
- *IL-4, together with IL-13, contributes to an alternative form of macrophage activation that is distinct from the macrophage response to IFN-γ.* IL-4 and IL-13 suppress IFN-γ–mediated classical macrophage activation and thus inhibit defense against intracellular microbes.
- *IL-4 (and IL-13) stimulate peristalsis in the gastrointestinal tract, and IL-13 increases mucus secretion from airway and gut epithelial cells.* Both actions contribute to elimination of microbes at epithelial surfaces.
- *IL-4 and IL-13 stimulate the recruitment of leukocytes,* notably eosinophils, by promoting the expression of adhesion molecules on endothelium and the secretion of chemokines that bind chemokine receptors expressed on eosinophils.

Interleukin-13

IL-13 is structurally and functionally similar to IL-4 and also plays a key role in defense against helminths (see Chapter 16) and in allergic diseases (see Chapter 20).

IL-13 is a member of the type 1 four–α-helical cytokine family, with limited sequence homology but significant structural similarity to IL-4. IL-13 is produced mainly by the T_H2 subset, but basophils, eosinophils, and NKT cells may also produce the cytokine. The functional IL-13 receptor is a heterodimer of the IL-4Rα chain and the IL-13Rα1 chain. This complex can bind both IL-4 and IL-13 with high affinity and also signals through a JAK1, JAK3, and STAT6 pathway. The receptor is expressed on a wide variety of cells, including B cells, mononuclear phagocytes, dendritic cells, eosinophils, basophils, fibroblasts, endothelial cells, and bronchial epithelial cells. T cells do not express the IL-13 receptor.

IL-13 works together with IL-4 in defense against helminths and in allergic inflammation. Some of the actions of IL-13 overlap those of IL-4, and others are distinct. IL-13 functions with IL-4 to induce alternative macrophage activation, which contributes to tissue repair and fibrosis. IL-13 stimulates mucus production by airway epithelial cells, an important component of allergic reactions such as asthma. As mentioned before, both IL-13 and IL-4 can activate B cells to switch to IgE and some IgG isotypes and recruit leukocytes. Unlike IL-4, IL-13 is not involved in T_H2 differentiation.

Interleukin-5

IL-5 is an activator of eosinophils and serves as the principal link between T cell activation and eosinophilic inflammation. It is a homodimer of a polypeptide containing a four–α-helical domain and is a member of the type I cytokine family. It is produced by T_H2 cells and by activated mast cells. The IL-5 receptor is a heterodimer composed of a unique α chain and a common β chain ($β_c$), which is also part of the IL-3 and granulocyte-macrophage colony-stimulating factor (GM-CSF) receptors (see Fig. 7-23). The major IL-5–induced signaling pathway involves JAK2 and STAT3.

The principal actions of IL-5 are to activate mature eosinophils and to stimulate the growth and differentiation of eosinophils. Activated eosinophils are able to kill helminths. Eosinophils express Fc receptors specific for IgE and some IgG antibodies and are thereby able to bind to microbes, such as helminths, that are opsonized by these antibodies. IL-5 also stimulates the production of IgA antibodies.

Roles of T_H2 Cells in Host Defense

T_H2 cells function in defense against helminthic infections by several mechanisms (see Fig. 10-9).

- *IgE- and eosinophil-mediated reactions.* IL-4 (and IL-13), secreted by T_H2 cells or by T_{FH} cells that make these cytokines, stimulates the production of helminth-specific IgE antibodies, which opsonize the helminths and promote the binding of eosinophils. IL-5 activates the eosinophils, and these cells release their granule contents, including major basic protein and major cationic protein, which are capable of destroying even the tough integuments of helminths (see Chapters 16 and 20).
- *Activation of mast cells.* Mast cells express high-affinity Fcε receptors that are responsible for coating the cells with IgE, and may be activated by antigens that

bind the IgE, resulting in degranulation. The granule contents of mast cells include vasoactive amines, and mast cells secrete cytokines such as TNF and chemokines, and lipid mediators, all of which induce local inflammation that helps to destroy the parasites. Mast cell mediators are also responsible for the vascular abnormalities and inflammation in allergic reactions (see Chapter 20).

- *Host defense at mucosal barriers.* Cytokines produced by T$_H$2 cells are involved in blocking entry and promoting expulsion of microbes from mucosal organs, by increased mucus production and intestinal peristalsis. Thus, T$_H$2 cells play an important role in host defense at the barriers with the external environment, sometimes called **barrier immunity.**
- *Alternative macrophage activation.* IL-4 and IL-13 activate macrophages to express enzymes that promote collagen synthesis and fibrosis. The macrophage response to T$_H$2 cytokines has been called **alternative macrophage activation** (Fig. 10-10) to distinguish it from the activation induced by IFN-γ, which was characterized first (and hence the designation *classical*) and which results in potent microbicidal functions and inflammation (see Fig. 10-7). Alternatively

activated macrophages may serve to initiate repair after diverse types of tissue injury. These macrophages, as well as T$_H$2 cells themselves, induce scarring and fibrosis by secreting growth factors that stimulate fibroblast proliferation (platelet-derived growth factor), collagen synthesis (IL-13, transforming growth factor-β [TGF-β]), and new blood vessel formation or angiogenesis (fibroblast growth factor). T$_H$2 cytokines also suppress classical macrophage activation and interfere with protective T$_H$1-mediated immune responses to intracellular infections (see Chapter 16). Suppression of classical macrophage activation occurs, in part, because IL-4 stimulates production of cytokines such as IL-10 and TGF-β by alternatively activated macrophages that inhibit T$_H$1 development and function.

THE T$_H$17 SUBSET

The T$_H$17 subset is primarily involved in recruiting leukocytes and inducing inflammation. These reactions are critical for destroying extracellular bacteria and fungi, and also contribute significantly to inflammatory diseases.

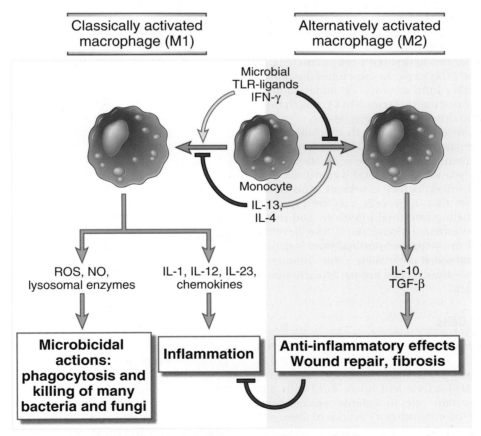

FIGURE 10-10 Classical and alternative macrophage activation. Subsets of activated macrophages are shown. Different stimuli activate monocytes-macrophages to develop into functionally distinct populations. Classically activated macrophages are induced by microbial products and cytokines, particularly IFN-γ, and are microbicidal and involved in potentially harmful inflammation. Alternatively activated macrophages are induced by IL-4 and IL-13 produced by T$_H$2 cells and other leukocytes and function to control inflammation; they may also promote tissue repair and fibrosis.

Development of T_H17 Cells

The development of T_H17 cells is stimulated by pro-inflammatory cytokines produced in response to bacteria and fungi (Fig. 10-11). Various bacteria and fungi act on dendritic cells and stimulate the production of cytokines including IL-6, IL-1, and IL-23, all of which promote differentiation of CD4+ T cells to the T_H17 subset. Engagement of the lectin-like receptor Dectin-1 on dendritic cells by fungal glucans is a signal for the production of these cytokines. The combination of cytokines that drive T_H17 cell development may be produced not only in response to particular microbes, such as fungi, but also when cells infected with various bacteria and fungi undergo apoptosis and are ingested by dendritic cells. Whereas IL-6 and IL-1 stimulate the early steps in T_H17 differentiation, IL-23 may be more important for the proliferation and maintenance of differentiated T_H17 cells. A surprising aspect of T_H17 differentiation is that TGF-β, which is produced by many cell types and is an anti-inflammatory cytokine (see Chapter 15), promotes the development of proinflammatory T_H17 cells when other mediators of inflammation, such as IL-6 or IL-1, are present. T_H17 differentiation is inhibited by IFN-γ and IL-4; therefore, strong T_H1 and T_H2 responses tend to suppress T_H17 development.

The development of T_H17 cells is dependent on the transcription factors RORγt and STAT3 (see Fig. 10-11). TGF-β and the inflammatory cytokines, mainly IL-6 and IL-1, work cooperatively to induce the production of RORγt, a transcription factor that is a member of the retinoic acid receptor family. RORγt is a T cell–restricted protein encoded by the *RORC* gene, so sometimes the protein may be called RORc. Inflammatory cytokines, notably IL-6, activate the transcription factor STAT3, which functions with RORγt to drive the T_H17 response.

T_H17 cells appear to be abundant in mucosal tissues, particularly of the gastrointestinal tract, suggesting that the tissue environment influences the generation of this subset, perhaps by providing high local concentrations of TGF-β and innate inflammatory cytokines. This observation also suggests that T_H17 cells may be especially important in combating intestinal infections and in the development of intestinal inflammation. The development of T_H17 cells in the gastrointestinal tract is dependent on the local microbial population; some commensal bacteria of the *Clostridium* species are particularly potent inducers of T_H17 cells.

Functions of T_H17 Cells

T_H17 cells combat microbes by recruiting leukocytes, mainly neutrophils, to sites of infection (Fig. 10-12). Because neutrophils are a major defense mechanism against extracellular bacteria and fungi, T_H17 cells play an especially important role in defense against these infections. Most of the inflammatory actions of these cells are mediated by IL-17, but other cytokines produced by this subset may also contribute.

Interleukin-17

IL-17 is an unusual cytokine because neither it nor its receptor is homologous to any other known

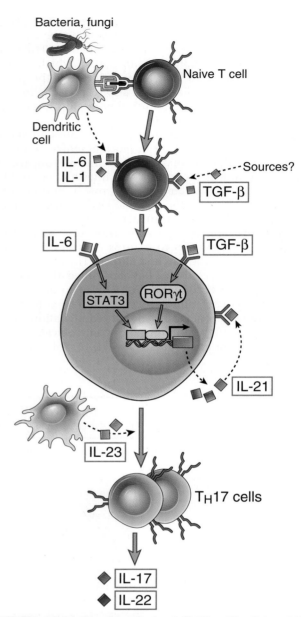

FIGURE 10-11 Development of T_H17 cells. IL-1 and IL-6 produced by APCs and transforming growth factor-β (TGF-β) produced by various cells activate the transcription factors RORγt and STAT3, which stimulate the differentiation of naive CD4+ T cells to the T_H17 subset. IL-23, which is also produced by APCs, especially in response to fungi, stabilizes the T_H17 cells. TGF-β may promote T_H17 responses indirectly by suppressing T_H1 and T_H2 cells, both of which inhibit T_H17 differentiation *(not shown)*. IL-21 produced by the T_H17 cells amplifies this response.

cytokine-receptor pair. The IL-17 family includes six structurally related proteins, of which IL-17A and IL-17F are the most similar, and the immunologic functions of this cytokine family seem to be mediated primarily by IL-17A. IL-17A and IL-17F are produced by T_H17 cells, whereas the other members of the family are produced by diverse cell types. IL-17 receptors are multimeric and expressed on a wide range of cells. Their structure and signaling mechanisms are not well defined.

IL-17 is an important link between T cell–mediated adaptive immunity and the acute inflammatory

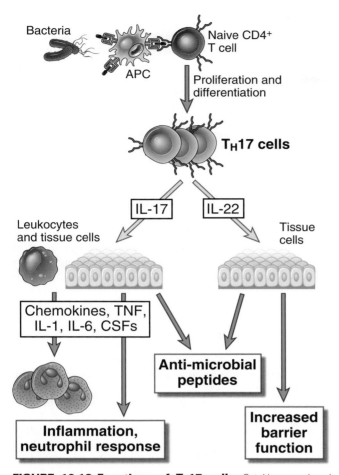

FIGURE 10-12 Functions of T$_H$17 cells. Cytokines produced by T$_H$17 cells stimulate local production of chemokines that recruit neutrophils and other leukocytes, increase production of antimicrobial peptides (defensins), and promote epithelial barrier functions.

response, which we discussed in Chapter 4 as one of the major reactions of innate immunity. The term *immune inflammation* is sometimes used to indicate the strong acute inflammatory reaction that may accompany T cell responses; in many cases, these reactions are more florid than what is seen in innate immunity alone. IL-17 has several important functions in host defense.

- *IL-17 induces neutrophil-rich inflammation.* It stimulates the production of chemokines and other cytokines (such as TNF) that recruit neutrophils and, to a lesser extent, monocytes to the site of T cell activation. It also enhances neutrophil generation by increasing the production of G-CSF and the expression of its receptors. Recruited neutrophils ingest and destroy bacteria and fungi.
- *IL-17 stimulates the production of antimicrobial substances,* including defensins, from numerous cell types (see Chapters 4 and 13).

Other T$_H$17 Cytokines

IL-22 is a member of the type II cytokine family. It is produced by activated T cells, particularly T$_H$17 cells,

and by some NK cells and group 3 innate lymphoid cells. IL-22 is produced in epithelial tissues, especially of the skin and gastrointestinal tract, and serves to maintain epithelial integrity, mainly by promoting the barrier function of epithelia, by stimulating repair reactions, and by inducing production of anti-microbial peptides. IL-22 also contributes to inflammation, in part by stimulating epithelial production of chemokines, and may therefore be involved in tissue injury in inflammatory diseases.

IL-21 is produced by activated CD4$^+$ T cells, including T$_H$17 cells and follicular helper T cells. It has a wide variety of effects on B and T cells and NK cells. The IL-21 receptor belongs to the type I cytokine receptor family, consists of a ligand-binding chain and the γ_c subunit, and activates a JAK-STAT signaling pathway in which STAT3 is especially prominent. An important function of IL-21 is in antibody responses, especially the reactions that occur in germinal centers (see Chapter 12). IL-21 is required for the generation of follicular helper T cells and stimulates B cells in germinal centers. IL-21 has also been shown to promote the differentiation of T$_H$17 cells, especially in humans, providing an autocrine pathway for amplifying T$_H$17 responses. Some of the other reported actions of IL-21 include increasing the proliferation, differentiation, and effector function of CD8$^+$ T cells and NK cells.

Roles of T$_H$17 Cells in Host Defense

The principal effector function of T$_H$17 cells is to destroy extracellular bacteria and fungi, mainly by inducing neutrophilic inflammation (see Fig. 10-12). The recruited neutrophils ingest and kill extracellular microbes. The importance of this role of T$_H$17 cells is illustrated by the inherited disease called **Job's syndrome** (or hyper-IgE syndrome), which is caused by mutations in STAT3 and is characterized by increased susceptibility to cutaneous fungal and bacterial infections. Patients present with multiple bacterial and fungal abscesses of the skin, resembling the biblical accounts of the punishments visited on Job. Defective T$_H$17 responses are also associated with chronic mucocutaneous candidiasis.

T$_H$1 and T$_H$17 cells function cooperatively in phagocyte-mediated elimination of microbes in cell-mediated immunity. Prior to the discovery of the T$_H$17 subset, it was thought that cell-mediated immunity was the purview of T$_H$1 cells, a concept bolstered by classical experimental analyses of this reaction occurring in the spleen. We now know that in many tissue infections, T$_H$17 cells are probably the most important effector T cells for recruiting phagocytes (neutrophils and monocytes) to the site of infection. This process of cell recruitment is driven by chemokines produced by the T cells and by other cells in the tissue responding to T cell cytokines and to the microbes themselves. Once the phagocytes are brought to the site of infection, they may be activated by T$_H$1 cells to ingest and destroy the microbes.

T$_H$17 cells contribute to the pathogenesis of many inflammatory diseases. T$_H$17 responses have been associated with psoriasis, inflammatory bowel disease, rheumatoid arthritis, and multiple sclerosis. Agents that block the development or functions of T$_H$17 cells are in clinical trials for several of these diseases, and have shown impressive efficacy in psoriasis. These antagonists are not effective in inflammatory bowel disease and perhaps in rheumatoid arthritis as well, so the role of T_H17 cells in these diseases is uncertain. T_H1 and T_H17 cells may both be present in the lesions in various inflammatory diseases, and their relative contribution to the development and propagation of the disorders is an area of active research.

FUNCTIONS OF OTHER T CELL SUBSETS

In addition to CD4+ and CD8+ T cells, there are smaller populations of T cells that have distinct features and probably serve specialized functions in host defense. The best defined of these subsets are γδ T cells and NKT cells. Both of these subsets have common characteristics that distinguish them from CD4+ and CD8+ T cells.

- γδ T cells and NKT cells recognize a wide variety of antigens, many of which are not peptides, and these are not displayed by class I and class II MHC molecules on APCs.
- The antigen receptors of many γδ T cells and NKT cells have limited diversity, suggesting that both cell types may have evolved to recognize a small group of microbial antigens. Because of this feature, these T cells are often said to be at the crossroads of innate and adaptive immunity.
- Both cell types are abundant in epithelial tissues, such as the gastrointestinal tract.

Because of these unusual properties, γδ T cells and NKT cells are postulated to serve special roles in host defense, similar to the roles of innate lymphoid cells (see Chapter 4). Their common functions may include the following:

- Early defense against microbes encountered at epithelia, before adaptive immune responses have developed
- Surveillance against stressed cells, such as cells that have undergone DNA damage or are infected, and elimination of these cells
- Production of cytokines that influence later adaptive immune responses.

γδ T Cells

The antigen receptor of MHC-restricted CD4+ and CD8+ T lymphocytes is a heterodimer composed of α and β chains (see Chapter 7). There is a second type of clonally distributed receptor composed of heterodimers of γ and δ chains, which are homologous to the α and β chains of the TCRs found on CD4+ and CD8+ T lymphocytes. T cells expressing the γδ TCR represent a lineage distinct from the more numerous αβ-expressing T cells. The percentages of γδ T cells vary widely in different tissues and species, but overall, less than 5% of all T cells express this form of TCR. The γδ heterodimer associates with the CD3 and ζ proteins in the same way as TCR αβ heterodimers do, and TCR-induced signaling events typical of αβ-expressing T cells are also observed in γδ T cells. Although the theoretical potential diversity of the γδ TCR is even greater

than the diversity of the αβ TCR, in reality, only a limited number of γ and δ V regions are expressed in some subsets of these cells, and there is little or no junctional diversity.

Different populations of γδ T cells may develop at distinct times during ontogeny, contain different V regions in their antigen receptors, reside in different tissues, and have a limited capacity to recirculate among these tissues. In mice, many skin γδ T cells develop in neonatal life and express one particular TCR with essentially no variability in the V region, whereas many of the γδ T cells in the vagina, uterus, and tongue appear later and express another TCR with a different V region. The limited diversity of the γδ TCRs in many tissues suggests that the ligands for these receptors may be invariant and conserved among cell types or microbes commonly encountered in these tissues. One intriguing feature of γδ T cells is their abundance in epithelial tissues of certain species. For example, more than 50% of lymphocytes in the small bowel mucosa of mice and chickens, called intraepithelial lymphocytes, are γδ T cells. In mouse skin, many of the intraepidermal T cells express the γδ receptor. Equivalent cell populations are not as abundant in humans; only about 10% of human intestinal intraepithelial T cells express the γδ TCR. γδ T cells in lymphoid organs express more diverse TCRs than the epithelial γδ cells.

γδ T cells do not recognize MHC-associated peptide antigens and are not MHC restricted. Some γδ T cell clones recognize small phosphorylated molecules, alkyl amines, or lipids that are commonly found in mycobacteria and other microbes and that may be presented by non-classical class I MHC–like molecules. Other γδ T cells recognize protein or non-protein antigens that do not require processing or any particular type of APCs for their presentation. Many γδ T cells are triggered by microbial heat shock proteins. A working hypothesis for the specificity of γδ T cells is that they may recognize antigens that are frequently encountered at epithelial boundaries between the host and the external environment.

A number of biologic activities have been ascribed to γδ T cells, including secretion of cytokines and killing of infected cells, but the function of these cells remains poorly understood. It has been postulated that this subset of T cells may initiate immune responses to microbes at epithelia, before the recruitment and activation of antigen-specific αβ T cells. However, mice lacking γδ T cells, created by targeted disruption of the γ or δ TCR gene, have little or no immunodeficiency and only a modest increase in susceptibility to infections by some intracellular bacteria. Intriguingly, in the inflammatory skin disease psoriasis, IL-17 plays an important pathogenic role, and in a mouse model, the earliest IL-17–producing cells in lesions appear to be γδ T cells. It is not known if this is the case in other inflammatory disorders, or what the γδ cells are recognizing or how much they are contributing to the development of the disease.

NKT Cells

A small population of T cells also expresses markers that are found on NK cells, such as CD56; these are called

NKT cells. The TCR α chains expressed by a subset of NKT cells have limited diversity, and, in humans, these cells are characterized by a V region encoded by a rearranged Vα24-Jα18 gene segment, with little or no junctional diversity, associated with one of three β chains. Because of this limited diversity, these cells are also called invariant NKT (iNKT) cells. Other NKT cells exist that have quite diverse antigen receptors. All NKT cell TCRs recognize lipids that are bound to class I MHC–like molecules called CD1 molecules. NKT cells and other lipid antigen–specific T cells are capable of rapidly producing cytokines such as IL-4 and IFN-γ, after activation, and they may help marginal zone B cells to produce antibodies against lipid antigens. NKT cells may mediate protective innate immune responses against some pathogens, such as mycobacteria (which have lipid-rich cell walls), and invariant NKT cells may even regulate adaptive immune responses primarily by secreting cytokines. However, the roles of these cells in protective immunity or disease in humans are unclear.

Having concluded our discussion of the functions of CD4+ effector T cells and some less common T cell populations, in Chapter 11 we will consider effector cells of the CD8+ lineage, whose major roles are in defense against viral infections.

SUMMARY

* Cell-mediated immunity is the adaptive immune response stimulated by microbes inside host cells. It is mediated by T lymphocytes and can be transferred from immunized to naive individuals by T cells and not by antibodies.

* CD4+ helper T lymphocytes may differentiate into specialized effector T_H1 cells that secrete IFN-γ, which mediate defense against intracellular microbes, or into T_H2 cells that secrete IL-4 and IL-5, which favor IgE- and eosinophil/mast cell–mediated immune reactions against helminths, or into T_H17 cells, which promote inflammation and mediate defense against extracellular fungi and bacteria.

* The differentiation of naive CD4+ T cells into subsets of effector cells is induced by cytokines produced by APCs, by the T cells themselves, and by other cells. The differentiation program is governed by transcription factors that promote cytokine gene expression in the T cells and epigenetic changes in cytokine gene loci, which may be associated with stable commitment to a particular subset. Each subset produces cytokines that increase its own development and inhibit the development of the other subsets, thus leading to increasing polarization of the response.

* CD4+ T_H1 cells recognize antigens of microbes that have been ingested by phagocytes and activate the phagocytes to kill the microbes. The activation of macrophages by T_H1 cells is mediated by IFN-γ and CD40L-CD40 interactions. Activated macrophages kill phagocytosed microbes ingested into phagolysosomes by the actions of reactive oxygen and nitrogen species and enzymes (called classical macrophage activation). Activated macrophages also stimulate inflammation and can damage tissues.

* CD4+ T_H2 cells recognize antigens produced by helminths and other microbes as well as environmental antigens associated with allergies. IL-4, secreted by activated T_H2 cells or T_{FH} cells, promotes B cell isotype switching and production of IgE, which may coat helminths and mediate mast cell degranulation and inflammation. IL-5 secreted by activated T_H2 cells activates eosinophils to release granule contents that destroy helminths but may also damage host tissues. IL-4 and IL-13 together provide protection at epithelial barriers and induce an alternative form of macrophage activation that generates macrophages that control inflammation and mediate tissue repair and fibrosis.

* CD4+ T_H17 cells stimulate neutrophil-rich inflammatory responses that eradicate extracellular bacteria and fungi. T_H17 cells may also be important in mediating tissue damage in autoimmune diseases.

* Both T_H1 and T_H17 cells contribute to cell-mediated immunity, each subset serving different roles in the phagocyte-mediated eradication of infections.

* γδ T cells and NKT cells are T cells that express receptors of limited diversity and recognize various antigens without a requirement for MHC-associated presentation. These cells produce cytokines and likely contribute to host defense and inflammatory diseases.

SELECTED READINGS

Differentiation and Functions of CD4+ T Cell Subsets of Effector Cells: T_H1, T_H2, and T_H17

Annunziato F, Romagnani S: Heterogeneity of human effector CD4+ T cells, *Arthritis Research and Therapy* 11:257–264, 2009.

Baumjohann D, Ansel KM: Micro-RNA-mediated regulation of T helper cell differentiation and plasticity, *Nature Reviews Immunology* 13:666–678, 2013.

Dong C: T_H17 cells in development: an updated view of their molecular identity and genetic programming, *Nature Reviews Immunology* 8:337–348, 2008.

Kanno Y, Golnaz V, Hirahara K, Singleton K, O'Shea JJ: Transcriptional and epigenetic control of T helper cell specification: molecular mechanisms underlying commitment and plasticity, *Annual Review of Immunology* 30:707–731, 2012.

Korn T, Bettelli E, Oukka M, Kuchroo VK: IL-17 and T_H17 cells, *Annual Review of Immunology* 27:485–517, 2009.

Littman DR, Rudensky AY: TH17 and regulatory T cells in mediating and restraining inflammation, *Cell* 140:845–858, 2010.

Locksley RM: Nine lives: plasticity among helper T cell subsets, *Journal of Experimental Medicine* 206:1643–1646, 2009.

McGeachy MJ, Cua DJ: Th17 cell differentiation: the long and winding road, *Immunity* 28:445–453, 2008.

Murphy KM, Stockinger B: Effector T cell plasticity: flexibility in the face of changing circumstances, *Nature Immunology* 11:674–680, 2010.

Paul WE, Zhu J: How are T_H2 responses initiated and amplified? *Nature Reviews Immunology* 10:225–235, 2010.

Pulendran B, Artis D: New paradigms in type 2 immunity, *Science* 337:431–435, 2012.

Steinman L: A brief history of T$_H$17, the first major revision in the T$_H$1/ T$_H$2 hypothesis of T cell–mediated tissue damage, *Nature Medicine* 13:139–145, 2007.

Zhu J, Yamane H, Paul WE: Differentiation of effector CD4 T cell populations, *Annual Review of Immunology* 28:445–489, 2010.

Activation of Macrophages

Billiau A, Matthys P: Interferon-γ: a historical perspective, *Cytokine and Growth Factor Reviews* 20:97–113, 2009.

Gordon S, Martinez FO: Alternative activation of macrophages: mechanisms and functions, *Immunity* 32:593–604, 2010.

Sica A, Mantovani A: Macrophage plasticity and polarization: in vivo veritas, *Journal of Clinical Investigation* 122:787–795, 2012.

Van Dyken SJ, Locksley RM: Interleukin-4- and interleukin-13-mediated alternatively activated macrophages: roles in homeostasis and disease, *Annual Review of Immunology* 31:317–343, 2013.

Other T Cell Populations

Bendelac A, Savage PB, Teyton L: The biology of NKT cells, *Annual Review of Immunology* 25:297–336, 2007.

Chien Y-H, Meyer C, Bonneville M. γδ T cells: first line of defense and beyond, *Annual Review of Immunology* 32:121–155, 2014.

Godfrey DI, Stankovic S, Baxter AG: Raising the NKT cell family, *Nature Immunology* 11:197–206, 2010.

Vantourout D, Hayday A: Six-of-the-best: unique contributions of γδ T cells to immunology, *Nature Reviews Immunology* 13:88–100, 2013.

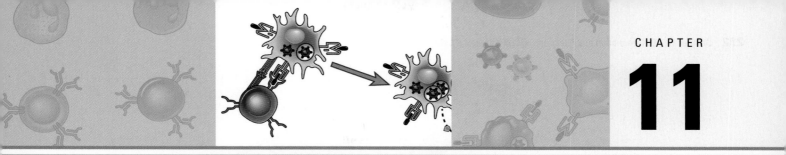

Differentiation and Functions of CD8⁺ Effector T Cells

Viruses have evolved to use various cell surface molecules to gain entry into host cells and to use the host cell's genetic and protein synthetic machinery to replicate and disseminate from one cell to another. Viruses can infect and survive in a wide variety of cells. The viruses cannot be destroyed if the infected cells lack intrinsic microbicidal mechanisms, or if the viruses are in the cytosol where they are inaccessible to these killing mechanisms. In these situations, the only way to eradicate the established infection is to kill the infected cell, releasing the virus from its home and crippling its ability to survive and replicate. This function of killing cells with viruses in the cytosol is mediated by **CD8⁺ cytotoxic T lymphocytes (CTLs)**, the effector cells of the CD8⁺ lineage (see Fig. 10-1, *B*). Cytokines produced by effector CD8⁺ T cells also contribute to the elimination of a variety of intracellular microbes. In addition to their role in defense against microbes, the second important function of CD8⁺ CTLs is the eradication of many tumors. These cells also play critical roles in the acute rejection of organ allografts.

In Chapter 6 we discussed the nature of the peptide-MHC complexes that are recognized by CD8⁺ T cells. We discussed the early steps of activation of T cells in Chapter 9. There we mentioned some of the features of activation of CD8⁺ cells, including their remarkable clonal expansion following activation by antigen and other signals. The differentiation of naive CD8⁺ cells, which lack killing ability, into functional CTLs has several special characteristics that should be considered separately. In this chapter, we will describe how functionally effective CTLs are produced and how they kill other cells, and then discuss the roles of CTLs in host defense.

DIFFERENTIATION OF CD8⁺ T CELLS INTO CYTOTOXIC T LYMPHOCYTES

The activation of naive CD8⁺ T cells requires antigen recognition and second signals, and proceeds in steps much like those for other T cell responses (Fig. 11-1). However, the activation of naive CD8⁺ T cells is dependent on a specific pathway of antigen presentation in a specialized subset of dendritic cells and may also require CD4⁺ T cell help.

Differentiation of CD8⁺ T cells into effector CTLs involves acquisition of the machinery to kill target cells. The infected or tumor cell that is killed by CTLs is commonly called the target cell. Naive CD8⁺ cells recognize antigens but need to proliferate and differentiate to generate a sufficiently large pool of CTLs to destroy the source of the antigen. Within the cytoplasm of differentiated CTLs are numerous modified lysosomes (called granules) that contain proteins, including perforin and granzymes, whose function is to kill other cells (described later). In addition, differentiated CTLs are capable of secreting cytokines, mostly IFN-γ, that function to activate phagocytes.

The molecular events in CTL differentiation involve transcription of genes encoding these effector molecules. Two transcription factors that are required for this program of new gene expression are T-bet (which we discussed in relationship to T_H1 differentiation in Chapter 10) and eomesodermin, which is structurally related to T-bet. T-bet and eosmesodermin contribute to the high level expression of perforin, granzymes, and some cytokines, especially interferon-γ.

Nature of Antigen and Antigen-Presenting Cells for Activation of CD8⁺ T Lymphocytes

The activation of naive CD8⁺ T cells, like that of all naive T cells, is best initiated by antigens presented by dendritic cells.

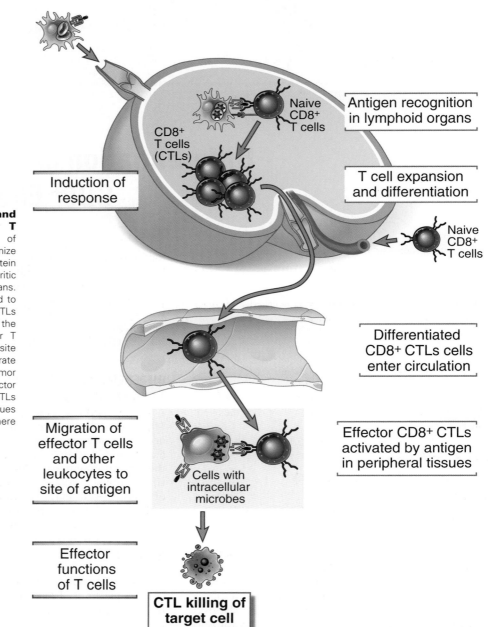

FIGURE 11-1 Induction and effector phases of CD8⁺ T cell responses. Induction of response: CD8⁺ T cells recognize peptides that are derived from protein antigens and presented by dendritic cells in peripheral lymphoid organs. The T lymphocytes are stimulated to proliferate and differentiate into CTLs (and memory cells), which enter the circulation. Migration of effector T cells and other leukocytes to the site of antigen: Effector T cells migrate to tissues at sites of infection, tumor growth, or graft rejection. Effector functions of T cells: CD8⁺ CTLs recognize the antigen in the tissues and respond by killing the cells where the antigen is produced.

This requirement raises the problem that the antigens recognized by CD8⁺ T cells may be viruses that infect many cell types, including cells other than dendritic cells, or they may be antigens of tumors that are also derived from a variety of cell types. The class I MHC pathway of antigen presentation to CD8⁺ T cells requires that protein antigens be present in the cytosol of infected cells so that these proteins can be degraded in proteasomes and can then enter the endoplasmic reticulum via the TAP transporter. Proteins from a virus that infects a specific cell type such as liver cells can access the cytosol and proteasomes in these cells but are unable to do so in most antigen presenting cells (APCs) since these APCs are not infected by the virus and do not endogenously synthesize viral antigen. As we discussed in Chapter 6, the immune system deals with this problem by the process of cross-presentation. In this process, specialized dendritic cells ingest infected cells, tumor cells, or proteins expressed by these cells, transfer the protein antigens into the cytosol, and process the antigens to enter the class I MHC antigen presentation pathway for recognition by CD8⁺ T cells (see Fig. 6-20). Only some subsets of dendritic cells are efficient at cross-presentation and, therefore, these dendritic cell subsets are crucial for naive CD8⁺ T cell activation. Results from experiments in mice suggest that the most efficient cross-presenting APCs are the lymphoid tissue dendritic cells that express CD8 or the peripheral tissue subset that express the CD103 integrin (see Chapter 6). The corresponding specialized cross-presenting dendritic cells in human tissues express high levels of CD141, also known as BDCA-3. In addition, plasmacytoid dendritic cells may also cross-present proteins derived from viruses in the blood to naive CD8⁺ T cells in the spleen.

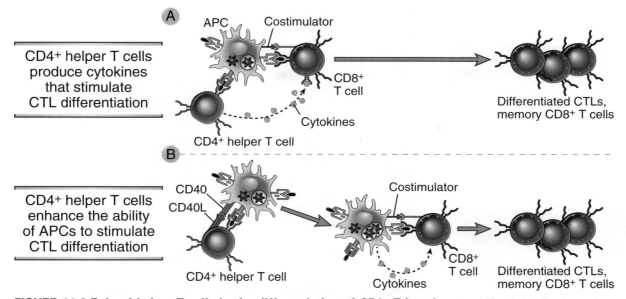

FIGURE 11-2 Role of helper T cells in the differentiation of CD8+ T lymphocytes. CD4+ helper T cells promote the development of CD8+ CTLs and memory cells by secreting cytokines that act directly on the CD8+ cells **(A)** or by activating APCs to become more effective at stimulating the differentiation of the CD8+ T cells **(B)**.

In addition to presenting antigens in the form of peptide-MHC complexes, dendritic cells likely also provide costimulation via B7 or other molecules (see Chapter 9).

Role of Helper T Cells

The full activation of naive CD8+ T cells and their differentiation into functional CTLs and memory cells may require the participation of CD4+ helper cells. In other words, helper T cells can provide second signals for CD8+ T cells. Helper T cells are activated by antigen presented on class II MHC molecules and by B7 costimulators expressed on dendritic cells.

The requirement for helper cells may vary according to the type of antigen exposure. In the setting of a strong innate immune response to a microbe, or if APCs are directly infected by the microbe, CD4+ T cell help may not be critical. CD4+ helper T cells may be required for CD8+ T cell responses to latent viral infections, organ transplants, and tumors, all of which tend to elicit relatively weak innate immune reactions. The varying importance of CD4+ T cells in the development of CTL responses is illustrated by studies with mice that lack helper T cells. In these mice, some viral infections fail to generate effective CTLs or CD8+ memory cells and are not eradicated, whereas other viruses do stimulate effective CTL responses. A lack of CD4+ T cell helper function is the accepted explanation for the defects in CTL generation seen in individuals infected with HIV, which infects and eliminates only CD4+ T cells. There is also evidence that CD4+ helper cells are more important for the generation of CD8+ memory T cells than for the differentiation of naive CD8+ T cells into effector CTLs.

Helper T cells may promote CD8+ T cell activation by several mechanisms (Fig. 11-2).

- Helper T cells may secrete cytokines that stimulate the differentiation of CD8+ T cells. The nature of these cytokines is discussed in the section that follows.
- Activated helper T cells express CD40 ligand (CD40L), which may bind to CD40 on antigen-loaded dendritic cells. This interaction activates the APCs to make them more efficient at stimulating the differentiation of CD8+ T cells, in part by inducing the expression of costimulators. This process has been termed *licensing* of the APCs.

Role of Cytokines

Several cytokines contribute to the differentiation of CD8+ T cells and the maintenance of effector and memory cells of this lineage.

- IL-2 promotes proliferation and differentiation of CD8+ T cells into CTLs and memory cells. CD8+ cells express the β and γ chains of the IL-2 receptor and may express high levels of the α chain after activation (see Chapter 9).
- IL-12 and type I IFNs have both been shown to stimulate the differentiation of naive CD8+ T cells into effector CTLs. These cytokines may be produced by different dendritic cell populations during the innate immune response to viral and some bacterial infections. Recall that the same cytokines are involved in the differentiation of CD4+ T cells into T_H1 cells. This similarity may reflect the fact that development of both effector populations, T_H1 cells and CTLs, is dependent on similar transcription factors, such as T-bet (for both) and the related eomesodermin (for CTLs).
- IL-15 is important for the survival of memory CD8+ IL-15 may be produced by many cell types, including

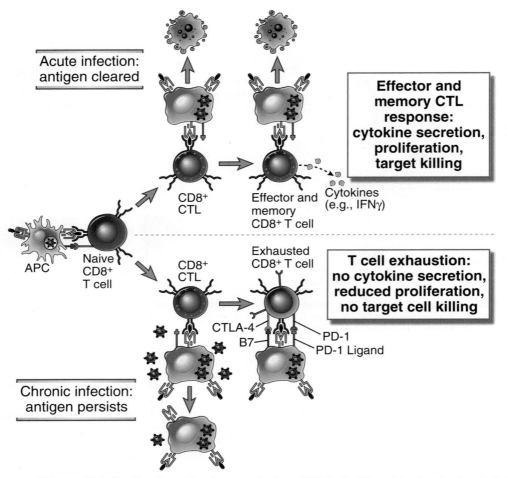

FIGURE 11-3 T cell exhaustion. In acute infections, CD8+ T cells differentiate into CTLs that eliminate the infected cells. In situations of persistent or chronic antigen exposure, the response of CD8+ T cells is suppressed by the expression and engagement of PD-1 and other inhibitory receptors.

dendritic cells. Mice lacking IL-15 show a significant loss of memory CD8+ T cells.

- IL-21 produced by activated CD4+ T cells has been shown to play a role in the induction of CD8+ T cell memory and the prevention of CD8+ T cell exhaustion (discussed in the section that follows).

Inhibition of CD8+ T Cell Responses: The Concept of T Cell Exhaustion

In some chronic viral infections, the responses of CD8+ T cells may be initiated but gradually extinguished, a phenomenon that is called exhaustion (Fig. 11-3). The term *exhaustion* has been used to imply that the effector response does develop but is actively shut down (unlike in *tolerance*, when lymphocytes typically fail to develop into effector cells). This phenomenon of exhaustion was first described in a chronic viral infection in mice, and was implicated in the prolonged persistence of the virus. Exhausted CD8+ T cells show numerous functional and phenotypic changes, including reduced production of IFN-γ and increased expression of multiple

inhibitory receptors, notably PD-1 (see Chapter 9). One documented mechanism of termination of the response is inhibitory signals from PD-1 that block the activation of CTLs. The same phenomenon of PD-1–mediated T cell exhaustion may contribute to the chronicity of some viral infections in humans, such as HIV and hepatitis C virus (HCV), and to the ability of some tumors to evade the immune response (see Chapter 18). Antibodies that block PD-1 are effective in the immunotherapy of tumors and are being tested in chronic viral infections. Exhaustion may have evolved as a means to attenuate the tissue-damaging consequences of chronic viral infection.

EFFECTOR FUNCTIONS OF CD8+ CYTOTOXIC T LYMPHOCYTES

CD8+ CTLs eliminate intracellular microbes mainly by killing infected cells (see Fig. 10-1, *B*). In addition to direct cell killing, CD8+ T cells secrete IFN-γ and thus contribute to classical macrophage activation in host defense and in hypersensitivity reactions. Here we discuss the mechanisms by which differentiated CTLs kill cells harboring microbes.

Mechanisms of CTL-Mediated Cytotoxicity

CTL-mediated killing involves specific recognition of target cells and delivery of proteins that induce cell death. CTLs kill targets that express the same class I MHC–associated antigen that triggered the proliferation and differentiation of naive CD8+ T cells from which they are derived and do not kill adjacent uninfected cells that do not express this antigen. In fact, even the CTLs themselves are not injured during the killing of antigen-expressing targets. This specificity of CTL effector function ensures that normal cells are not injured by CTLs reacting against infected cells. The killing is highly specific because close apposition, known as a **synapse** (see Chapter 7), is formed at the site of contact of the CTL and the antigen-expressing target, and the molecules that actually perform the killing are secreted into the synapse and cannot diffuse to other nearby cells.

The process of CTL-mediated killing of targets consists of antigen recognition, activation of the CTLs, delivery of the **lethal hit** that kills the target cells, and release of the CTLs (Fig. 11-4). Each of these steps is controlled by specific molecular interactions.

Recognition of Antigen and Activation of CTLs

The CTL binds and reacts to the target cell by using its antigen receptor, coreceptor (CD8), and adhesion molecules. To be efficiently recognized by CTLs, target cells must express class I MHC molecules complexed to a peptide (the complex serves as the ligand for the T cell receptor [TCR] and also binds to the CD8 coreceptor) and intercellular adhesion molecule 1 (ICAM-1, the principal ligand for the LFA-1 integrin). The CTLs and their target cells form tight conjugates (Fig. 11-5). This immune synapse (see Chapter 7) formed between the two cells is characterized by a ring of close apposition between the CTL and target cell membranes, mediated by LFA-1 binding to ICAM-1, and an enclosed gap or space inside the ring. Distinct regions of the CTL membrane can be observed by immunofluorescence microscopy within the ring, including a signaling patch, which includes the TCR, protein kinase C-θ, and Lck, and a secretory domain, which appears as a gap to one side of the signaling patch. This interaction results in the initiation of biochemical signals that activate the CTL, which are essentially the same as the signals involved in the activation of helper T cells. Cytokines and costimulators provided by dendritic cells, which are required for the differentiation of naive CD8+ T cells into CTLs, are not necessary for triggering the effector function of CTLs (i.e., target cell killing). Therefore, once CD8+ T cells specific for an antigen have differentiated into fully functional CTLs, they can kill any nucleated cell that displays that antigen.

In addition to the T cell receptor, CD8+ CTLs express receptors that are also expressed by NK cells, which contribute to both regulation and activation of CTLs. Some of these receptors belong to the killer immunoglobulin receptor (KIR) family, discussed in Chapter 4, and recognize class I MHC molecules on target cells but are not specific for a particular peptide-MHC complex. These

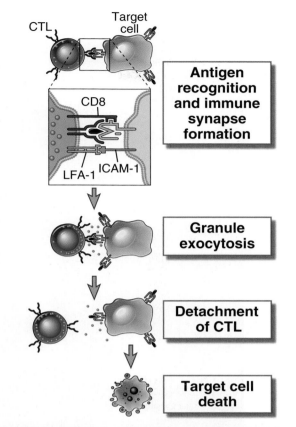

FIGURE 11-4 Steps in CTL-mediated lysis of target cells. A CTL recognizes the antigen-expressing target cell and is activated. Activation results in the release of granule contents from the CTL into the target cell through the area of contact (the immunologic synapse). Granule contents deliver a lethal hit to the target. The CTL may detach and kill other target cells. The formation of conjugates between a CTL and its target and activation of the CTL also require interactions between accessory molecules (LFA-1, CD8) on the CTL and their specific ligands (ICAM-1 and class I MHC, respectively) on the target cell *(not shown)*.

KIRs transduce inhibitory signals that may serve to prevent CTLs from killing normal cells. In addition, CTLs express the NKG2D receptor, described in Chapter 4, that recognizes class I MHC–like molecules MIC-A, MIC-B, and ULBP, expressed on stressed (infected or transformed) cells. NKG2D may serve to deliver signals that act together with TCR recognition of antigen to enhance killing activity.

Killing of Target Cells by CTLs

Within a few minutes after a CTL's antigen receptor recognizes its antigen on a target cell, the CTL delivers granule proteins into the target cell that lead to apoptotic death of the target cell. Target cell death occurs during the 2 to 6 hours following antigen recognition and proceeds even if the CTL detaches. Thus, the CTL is said to deliver a lethal hit to the target cell. The principal mechanism of CTL-mediated target cell killing is the delivery of cytotoxic proteins stored within cytoplasmic granules (also called secretory lysosomes) to the target cell, thereby triggering apoptosis of the target cell (Fig. 11-6). As discussed earlier, CTL recognition of the target cell leads to activation

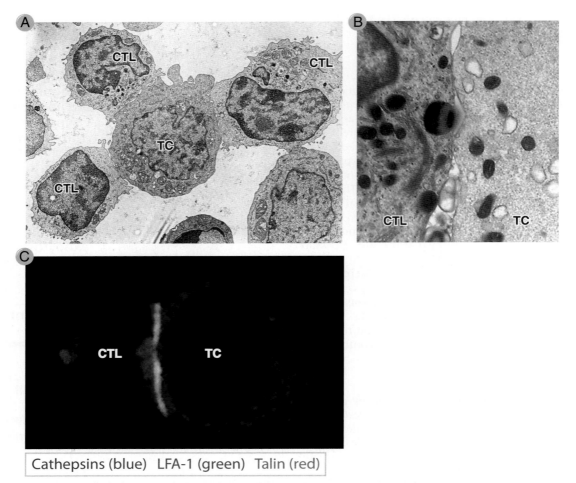

Cathepsins (blue) LFA-1 (green) Talin (red)

FIGURE 11–5 Formation of conjugates between CTLs and a target cell. A, Electron micrograph of three CTLs from a cloned cell line specific for the human MHC molecule HLA-A2 binding to an HLA-A2–expressing target cell (TC) within 1 minute after the CTLs and targets are mixed. Note that in the CTL on the upper left, the granules have been redistributed toward the target cell. **B,** Electron micrograph of the point of membrane contact between a CTL *(left)* and target cell *(right)*. Two CTL granules are near the synapse. Several mitochondria are also visible. **C,** Confocal fluorescence micrograph of an immune synapse between a CTL *(left)* and target cell *(right)* stained with antibodies against cathepsins in a secretory granule *(blue)*, LFA-1 *(green)*, and the cytoskeletal protein talin *(red)*. The image demonstrates the central location of the secretory granule and the peripheral location of the adhesion molecule LFA-1 and associated cytoskeletal protein talin. (**A,** *Courtesy of Dr. P. Peters, Netherlands Cancer Institute, Amsterdam.* **B,** *Reprinted from Stinchcombe JC, Bossi G, Booth S, Griffiths GM: The immunological synapse of CTL contains a secretory domain and membrane bridges,* Immunity *8:751-761, 2001. Copyright © Cell Press, with permission from Elsevier.* **C,** *Reprinted from Stinchcombe JC, Griffiths GM: The role of the secretory immunological synapse in killing by CD8⁺ CTL,* Seminars in Immunology *15:301-205. Copyright © 2003 Elsevier Science Ltd., with permission from Elsevier.)*

of the CTL, one consequence of which is cytoskeleton reorganization. In this process, the microtubule organizing center of the CTL moves to the area of the cytoplasm near the contact with the target cell. The cytoplasmic granules of the CTL are transported along microtubules and become concentrated in the region of the synapse, and the granule membrane fuses with the plasma membrane at the secretory domain. Membrane fusion results in exocytosis of the CTL's granule contents into the confined space within the synaptic ring, between the plasma membranes of the CTL and target cell.

The major cytotoxic proteins in the granules of CTLs (and NK cells) are granzymes and perforin. **Granzymes** A, B, and C are serine proteases that share a His-Asp-Ser sequence in their catalytic domains. Granzyme B cleaves proteins after aspartate residues, and is the only one unequivocally shown to be required for CTL cytotoxicity in vivo. It can activate caspases that induce cell death (the executioner caspases). **Perforin** is a membrane-perturbing molecule that is homologous to the C9 complement protein. The granules also contain a sulfated proteoglycan, **serglycin**, which serves to assemble a complex containing granzymes and perforin.

The main function of perforin is to facilitate delivery of the granzymes into the cytosol of the target cell. How this is accomplished is still not well understood. Perforin can polymerize and form aqueous pores in the target cell membrane, but these pores may not be of sufficient

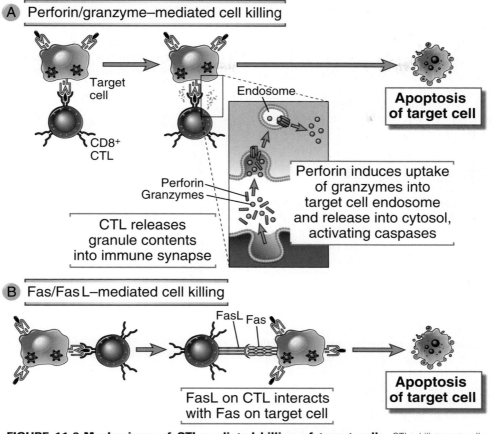

A Perforin/granzyme–mediated cell killing

Target cell

CD8⁺ CTL

Endosome

Apoptosis of target cell

Perforin Granzymes

Perforin induces uptake of granzymes into target cell endosome and release into cytosol, activating caspases

CTL releases granule contents into immune synapse

B Fas/FasL–mediated cell killing

FasL Fas

Apoptosis of target cell

FasL on CTL interacts with Fas on target cell

FIGURE 11-6 Mechanisms of CTL-mediated killing of target cells. CTLs kill target cells by two main mechanisms. **A,** Complexes of perforin and granzymes are released from the CTL by granule exocytosis and enter target cells. The granzymes are delivered into the cytoplasm of the target cells by a perforin-dependent mechanism, and they induce apoptosis. **B,** FasL is expressed on activated CTLs, engages Fas on the surface of target cells, and induces apoptosis.

size to allow granzymes to enter. According to a current model, complexes of granzyme B, perforin, and serglycin are discharged from the CTL onto the target cell, and perforin insertion into the target cell membrane elicits a membrane repair process, which leads to internalization of both the perforin and granzymes into endosomes. Perforin may then act on the endosomal membrane to facilitate the release of the granzymes into the target cell cytosol. Once in the cytosol, the granzymes cleave various substrates, including caspases, and initiate apoptotic death of the cell. For example, granzyme B activates caspase-3 as well as the Bcl-2 family member Bid, which triggers the mitochondrial pathway of apoptosis (see Fig. 15-8). Another protein found in human CTL (and NK cell) granules, called granulysin, can alter the permeability of target cell and microbial membranes, but its importance in cell killing by CTLs is not established.

CTLs also use a granule-independent mechanism of killing that is mediated by interactions of membrane molecules on the CTLs and target cells. On activation, CTLs express a membrane protein called **Fas ligand (FasL)** that binds to the death receptor Fas, which is expressed on many cell types. This interaction also results in activation of caspases and apoptosis of Fas-expressing targets (see Fig. 15-8). Studies with

knockout mice lacking perforin, granzyme B, or FasL indicate that perforin and granzyme B are the principal mediators of killing by CD8⁺ CTLs. Some CD4⁺ T cells, found in the intestine and often induced in viral infections, express perforin and granzymes and are also capable of killing target cells (which, of course, must express class II MHC–associated peptides to be recognized by the CD4⁺ cells).

After delivering the lethal hit, the CTL is released from its target cell, which usually occurs even before the target cell goes on to die. CTLs themselves are not injured during target cell killing, probably because the directed granule exocytosis process during CTL-mediated killing preferentially delivers granule contents into the target cell and away from the CTL. In addition, CTL granules contain a proteolytic enzyme called cathepsin B, which is delivered to the CTL surface on granule exocytosis, where it degrades errant perforin molecules that come into the vicinity of the CTL membrane.

Cytokine Production by CD8⁺ Effector T Cells

CD8⁺ T cells produce the macrophage-activating cytokine IFN-γ. In fact, the secretion of IFN-γ in response to specific peptides is a sensitive assay for the frequency of antigen-specific CD8+ T cells in a population of lymphocytes. The production of this cytokine is another similarity between CD8+ cells and T_H1 cells. It is likely that both of these T cell subsets contribute to IFN-γ–induced phagocytic clearance of ingested microbes. CD8+ cells may also play a role in some cytokine–induced inflammatory reactions, such as contact sensitivity skin reactions induced by environmental chemicals, where IFN-γ–producing CD8+ T cells often arrive earlier than and outnumber CD4+ T cells.

ROLES OF CD8+ CTLs IN HOST DEFENSE

In infections by intracellular microbes, the killing activity of CTLs is important for eradication of the reservoir of infection (see Fig. 10-1, *B*). This is particularly important in two types of situations, when cells cannot destroy microbes that infect them. First, most viruses live and replicate in cells that lack the phagosome/lysosome machinery for destroying microbes (such as hepatitis viruses in liver cells). Second, even in phagocytes, some microbes escape from vesicles and live in the cytosol, where microbicidal mechanisms are ineffective because these mechanisms are largely restricted to vesicles (to protect the cells from damage). Such infections can be eliminated only by destroying the infected cells, and in adaptive immune responses, CD8+ CTLs are the principal mechanism for killing infected cells (see Fig. 16-4). In addition, the caspases that are activated in target cells by granzymes and FasL cleave many substrates and activate enzymes that degrade DNA, but they do not distinguish between host and microbial proteins. Therefore, by activating nucleases in target cells, CTLs can initiate the destruction of microbial DNA as well as the target cell genome, thereby eliminating potentially infectious DNA. The massive expansion of CD8+ T cells that follows infections (see Fig. 9-12) provides a large pool of CTLs to combat these infections. Defects in the development and activity of CTLs result in increased susceptibility to viral and some bacterial infections and reactivation of latent virus infections (such as infection by the Epstein-Barr virus), which are normally kept in check by virus-specific CTLs.

In addition to their role in eliminating virus-infected cells, CTLs have been shown to be crucial for host defense against certain intracellular bacteria, including *Mycobacterium tuberculosis*, and in the clearance of a number of other organisms including the protozoon parasite that causes malaria (see Chapter 16).

Destruction of infected cells by CTLs is a cause of tissue injury in some infectious diseases. For instance, in infection by hepatitis B and C viruses, the infected liver cells are killed by the host CTL (and NK cell) response and not by the viruses. These viruses are not cytopathic, but the host senses and reacts against the infectious microbe and is not able to distinguish microbes that are intrinsically harmful or relatively harmless (see Chapter 19).

CTLs are important mediators of tumor immunity and the rejection of organ transplants. These roles of CTLs are described in later chapters.

SUMMARY

* T cells of the CD8+ subset proliferate and differentiate into cytotoxic T lymphocytes (CTLs), which express cytotoxic granules and can kill infected cells.
* The differentiation of CD8+ T cells into functional CTLs and memory cells requires recognition of antigen presented by dendritic cells, signals from CD4+ helper T cells in some situations, costimulation, and cytokines. Differentiation to CTLs involves the acquisition of the machinery to kill target cells, and is driven by various transcription factors.
* In some situations of chronic antigen exposure (such as tumors and chronic viral infections), CD8+ T cells initiate a response but begin to express inhibitory receptors that suppress the response, a process called exhaustion.
* CD8+ CTLs kill cells that express peptides derived from cytosolic antigens (e.g., viral antigens) that are presented in association with class I MHC molecules. CTL-mediated killing is mediated mainly by granule exocytosis, which releases granzymes and perforin. Perforin facilitates granzyme entry into the cytoplasm of target cells, and granzymes initiate several pathways of apoptosis.
* CD8+ T cells also secrete IFN-γ and thus may participate in defense against phagocytosed microbes and in DTH reactions.

SELECTED READINGS

Activation of CD8+ T Cells

Castellino F, Germain RN: Cooperation between CD4+ and CD8+ T cells: when, where, and how, *Annual Review of Immunology* 24:519–540, 2006.

Kaech SM, Cui W: Transcriptional control of effector and memory CD8+ T cell differentiation, *Nature Reviews Immunology* 12:749–761, 2012.

Masopust D, Vezys V, Wherry EJ, Ahmed R: A brief history of CD8+ T cells, *European Journal of Immunology* 37:S103–S110, 2007.

Wherry EJ. T cell exhaustion. *Nature Immunology* 12:492–499, 2011.

Williams MA, Bevan MJ: Effector and memory CTL differentiation, *Annual Review of Immunology* 25:171–192, 2007.

Zhang N, Bevan MJ: CD8+ T cells: foot soldiers of the immune system, *Immunity* 35:161–168, 2011.

Functions of Cytotoxic T Lymphocytes

Bossi G, Griffiths GM: CTL secretory lysosomes: biogenesis and secretion of a harmful organelle, *Seminars in Immunology* 17:87–94, 2005.

Lieberman J: The ABCs of granule-mediated cytotoxicity: new weapons in the arsenal, *Nature Reviews Immunology* 3:361–370, 2003.

Wong P, Pamer EG: CD8 T cell responses to infectious pathogens, *Annual Review of Immunology* 21:29–70, 2003.

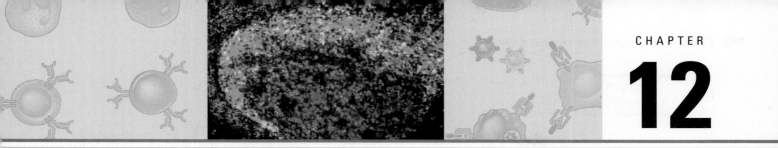

B Cell Activation and Antibody Production

Humoral immunity is mediated by secreted antibodies, which are produced by cells of the B lymphocyte lineage. This chapter describes the molecular and cellular events of the humoral immune response, in particular the stimuli that induce B cell proliferation and differentiation and how these stimuli influence the type of antibody that is produced. The mechanisms by which antibodies eliminate microbes are described in Chapter 13.

OVERVIEW OF HUMORAL IMMUNE RESPONSES

The earliest studies of adaptive immunity were devoted to analyses of serum antibodies produced in response to microbes, toxins, and model antigens. Much of our current understanding of adaptive immune responses and the cellular interactions that take place during such responses has evolved from studies of antibody production. We begin with a summary of some of the key features of B cell activation and antibody production.

- *The activation of B cells results in their proliferation, leading to clonal expansion, followed by differentiation, culminating in the generation of antibody-secreting plasma cells and memory B cells* (Fig. 12-1). As we discussed in Chapter 8, mature antigen-responsive B lymphocytes develop from bone marrow precursors before antigenic stimulation and populate peripheral lymphoid organs, which are the sites where lymphocytes interact with foreign antigens. Humoral immune responses are initiated by the recognition of antigens by specific B lymphocytes. Antigen binds to membrane immunoglobulin M (IgM) and IgD on mature, naive B cells and activates these cells. Activation leads to proliferation of antigen-specific cells and their differentiation, generating antibody-secreting plasma cells and memory B cells. A single B cell may, within a week, give rise to as many as 5000 antibody-secreting cells, which collectively produce more than 10^{12} antibody molecules per day. This tremendous expansion is needed to keep pace with rapidly dividing microbes. Some activated B cells begin to produce antibodies other than IgM and IgD; this process is called **heavy chain isotype (class) switching**. As a humoral immune response

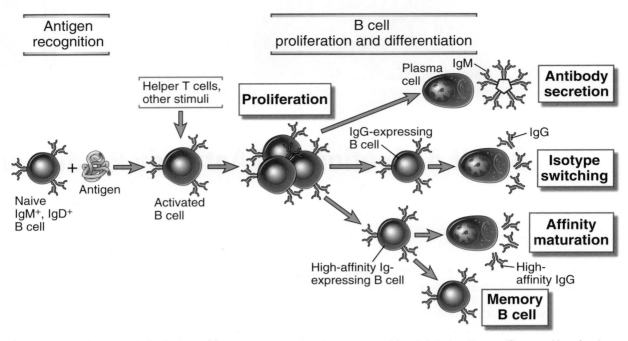

FIGURE 12-1 Phases of the humoral immune response. The activation of B cells is initiated by specific recognition of antigens by the surface Ig receptors of the cells. Antigen and other stimuli, including helper T cells, stimulate the proliferation and differentiation of the specific B cell clone. Progeny of the clone may differentiate into plasma cells that produce IgM or other Ig isotypes (e.g., IgG), may undergo affinity maturation, or may persist as memory cells.

develops, activated B cells that produce antibodies that bind to antigens with increasing affinity progressively dominate the response; this process is called **affinity maturation.**

- *The type and amount of antibodies produced vary according to the type of antigen driving the immune response, the involvement of T cells, a prior history of antigen exposure, and the anatomic site at which activation occurs.* The influence of these factors on the humoral immune response is discussed in detail later in this chapter.

- *Antibody responses to protein antigens require that the antigen be internalized by specific B cells, processed, and peptides presented to CD4+ helper T lymphocytes, which then activate the B cells.* For this reason, proteins are classified as **T-dependent antigens**. The term *helper T lymphocyte* arose from the realization that T cells stimulate, or help, B lymphocytes to produce antibodies. A specialized type of helper T cell, called a **follicular helper T cell**, facilitates the formation of germinal centers, which are structures generated in lymphoid organs where several aspects of T-dependent humoral immune responses occur.

- *Antibody responses to multivalent non-protein antigens with repeating determinants, such as polysaccharides, some lipids, and nucleic acids, do not require antigen-specific helper T lymphocytes.* Multivalent antigens (so called because each antigen molecule contains multiple identical epitopes) are therefore called **T-independent antigens**. These responses are elicited by engagement of the B cell receptor (BCR) and may be enhanced by the signals from other receptors on the B cells.

- *Activated B cells differentiate into antibody-secreting plasma cells.* In T-dependent responses, the plasma cells or their precursors migrate from germinal centers in the peripheral lymphoid organs, where they are produced, to the bone marrow, where they may live for many years. These long-lived plasma cells continuously secrete antibodies that provide immediate protection whenever a microbe recognized by those antibodies infects the individual.

- *Some progeny of B cells activated in a T-dependent manner may differentiate into memory cells.* These memory T cells survive in a resting state without secreting antibodies for many years, but they mount rapid responses on subsequent encounters with the antigen.

- *Isotype switching and affinity maturation are typically seen in helper T cell–dependent humoral immune responses to protein antigens.* Both of these processes result from the stimulation of B cells by helper T cells. The T cell signals that drive isotype switching and affinity maturation, and their molecular mechanisms and functional significance, are discussed later in the chapter.

- *Primary and secondary antibody responses to protein antigens differ qualitatively and quantitatively* (Fig. 12-2). Primary responses result from the activation of previously unstimulated naive B cells, whereas secondary responses are due to the stimulation of expanded clones of memory B cells. Therefore, the secondary response develops more rapidly than does the primary response, and larger amounts of antibodies are produced in the secondary response. Heavy chain isotype switching and affinity maturation also increase with repeated exposure to protein antigens.

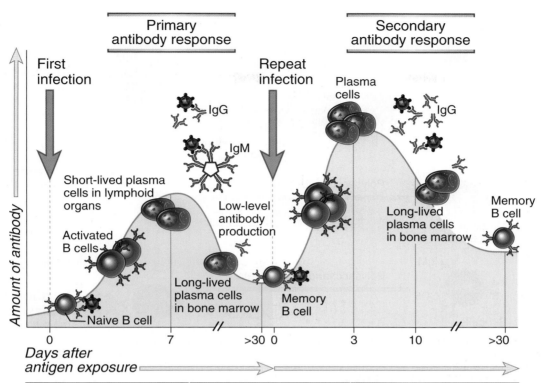

Feature	Primary response	Secondary response
Peak response	Smaller	Larger
Antibody isotype	Usually IgM > IgG	Relative increase in IgG and, under certain situations, in IgA or IgE
Antibody affinity	Lower average affinity, more variable	Higher average affinity (affinity maturation)
Induced by	All immunogens	Mainly protein antigens

FIGURE 12-2 Primary and secondary humoral immune responses. In a primary immune response, naive B cells are stimulated by antigen, become activated, and differentiate into antibody-secreting cells that produce antibodies specific for the eliciting antigen. A secondary immune response is elicited when the same antigen stimulates memory B cells, leading to production of greater quantities of specific antibody than are produced in the primary response. Note that the characteristics of secondary antibody responses summarized in the table are typical of T-dependent antibody responses to protein antigens.

- *Distinct subsets of B cells respond preferentially to different types of antigens* (Fig. 12-3). Follicular B cells in peripheral lymphoid organs primarily make antibody responses to protein antigens that require collaboration with helper T cells. Marginal zone B cells in the spleen and other lymphoid tissues recognize multivalent antigens, such as blood-borne polysaccharides, and mount primarily T-independent antibody responses. B-1 cells in mucosal tissues and the peritoneum also mediate largely T-independent responses.

With this background, we proceed to a discussion of B cell activation, starting with the interaction of antigen with B cells. We will then describe the role of helper T cells in B cell responses to protein antigens and the mechanisms of isotype switching and affinity maturation. We conclude with a discussion of T-independent antibody responses.

ANTIGEN RECOGNITION AND ANTIGEN-INDUCED B CELL ACTIVATION

To initiate antibody responses, antigens have to be captured and transported to the B cell areas of lymphoid organs. The antigens then initiate the process of B cell activation, often working in concert with other signals that are generated during innate immune responses triggered by microbes during infections or by adjuvants in vaccines. We will next describe these early events in B cell activation.

Antigen Capture and Delivery to B Cells

Most mature naive B lymphocytes are follicular B cells (sometimes also called recirculating B cells) that constantly recirculate in the blood and migrate from one secondary lymphoid organ to the next in search of antigen. Follicular

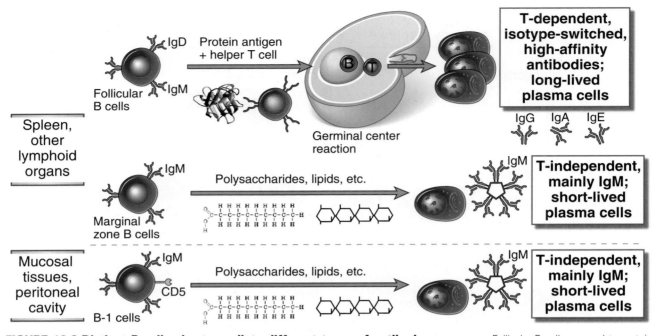

FIGURE 12-3 Distinct B cell subsets mediate different types of antibody responses. Follicular B cells respond to protein antigens and thus initiate T-dependent antibody responses. T-independent responses to multivalent antigens are mediated mainly by marginal zone B cells in the spleen and B-1 cells in mucosal sites. These functional distinctions between subsets are not absolute.

B cells enter secondary lymphoid tissues (spleen, lymph nodes, mucosal lymphoid tissues) through blood vessels located in the T cell zones, and then they migrate into the follicles, the B cell zones of these tissues. The movement into lymphoid follicles is guided by the chemokine CXCL13 secreted by follicular dendritic cells, the major stromal cell type in the follicle, as well as by other stromal cells. CXCL13 binds to the CXCR5 chemokine receptor on the recirculating naive B cells and attracts these cells into the follicles. As we will discuss later, the same chemokine-receptor pair is also important during immune responses because it can attract a subset of activated T cells to the follicle.

Antigen may be delivered to naive B cells in lymphoid organs in different forms and by multiple routes. Antigens that enter by crossing an epithelial barrier as well as antigens in the circulation are collected and brought to the follicles by several mechanisms (Fig. 12-4).

- Most antigens from tissue sites are transported to lymph nodes by afferent lymphatic vessels that drain into the subcapsular sinus of the nodes. Soluble antigens, generally smaller than 70 kD, may reach the B cell zone through conduits that extend between the subcapsular sinus and the follicle and interact directly with specific B cells.
- Subcapsular sinus macrophages capture large microbes and antigen-antibody complexes and deliver these to follicles, which lie under the sinus.
- Many relatively large antigens that enter the node through afferent lymphatic vessels are not captured by subcapsular sinus macrophages and are too large to enter the conduits. These antigens may be captured in the medullary region by resident dendritic

cells and transported into follicles, where they can activate B cells.

- Antigens in immune complexes may bind to complement receptors (in particular the complement receptor type 2 or CR2) on marginal zone B cells, and these cells can transfer the immune complex–containing antigens to follicular B cells.
- Immune complexes may also bind to the complement receptor CR2 on the surface of follicular dendritic cells and the antigens in these complexes are then presented to antigen-specific B cells.
- Blood-borne pathogens may be captured by plasmacytoid dendritic cells in the blood and transported to the spleen, where they may be delivered to marginal zone B cells.
- Polysaccharide antigens can be captured by macrophages in the marginal zone of splenic lymphoid follicles and displayed or transferred to B cells in this area.

In all of these cases, *the antigen that is presented to B cells is generally in its intact, native conformation and is not processed by antigen-presenting cells.* This, of course, is one of the important distinctions between the forms of antigens recognized by B and T lymphocytes (see Chapter 6).

Activation of B Cells by Antigens and Other Signals

Antigen and cytokines play important roles in the survival of naive B cells. Naive follicular B cells survive for limited periods until they encounter antigen (see Chapter 2). Follicular B cell survival depends on signals from the BCR as well as on inputs received from a tumor necrosis factor (TNF) superfamily cytokine called BAFF

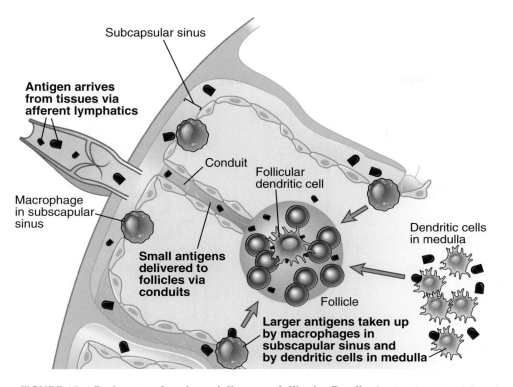

FIGURE 12-4 Pathways of antigen delivery to follicular B cells. Small antigens are delivered to B cells in follicles through afferent lymphatics and via conduits, and larger antigens by subcapsular sinus macrophages or by dendritic cells in the medulla.

(B cell–activating factor of the TNF family, also known as BLyS, for B lymphocyte stimulator), which provides maturation and survival signals through the BAFF receptor. BAFF and a related ligand, APRIL, can activate two other receptors, TACI and BCMA, which participate in later stages of B cell activation and differentiation (and will be discussed later). These cytokines are produced mainly by myeloid cells in lymphoid follicles and in the bone marrow.

The activation of antigen-specific B lymphocytes is initiated by the binding of antigen to membrane Ig molecules, which, in conjunction with the associated Igα and Igβ proteins, make up the antigen receptor complex of mature B cells. The B lymphocyte antigen receptor, described in Chapter 7, serves two key roles in B cell activation. First, binding of antigen to the receptor delivers biochemical signals to the B cells that initiate the process of activation (see Chapter 7). Second, the receptor internalizes the bound antigen into endosomal vesicles, and if the antigen is a protein, it is processed into peptides that may be presented on the B cell surface for recognition by helper T cells. This antigen-presenting function of B cells will be considered later in the context of T-dependent B cell activation.

Although antigen recognition can initiate B cell responses, by itself it is usually inadequate to stimulate significant B cell proliferation and differentiation. For full responses to be induced, other stimuli cooperate with BCR engagement, including complement proteins, pattern recognition receptors, and, in the case of protein antigens, helper T cells (discussed later).

B cell activation is facilitated by the CR2/CD21 coreceptor on B cells, which recognizes complement fragments covalently attached to the antigen or that are part of immune complexes containing the antigen (Fig. 12-5, *A*). Complement activation is typically seen with microbes, which activate this system in the absence of antibodies by the alternative and lectin pathways, and in the presence of antibodies, by the classical pathway (see Chapters 4 and 13). In all of these situations, complement fragments are generated that bind to the microbes. One of these fragments, called C3d, is recognized by the complement receptor CR2 (also called CD21), which enhances the strength of BCR signaling and thus functions as a coreceptor for B cells (see Chapter 7). Some non-microbial polysaccharides also activate complement by the alternative or lectin pathway, and this is one reason that such antigens are able to induce antibody responses without T cell help.

Microbial products engage Toll-like receptors on B cells, which also enhances B cell activation (Fig. 12-5, *B*). Human B cells express several TLRs, including TLR5, which recognizes bacterial flagellin; endosomal TLR7, which recognizes single-stranded RNA; and TLR9, which is specific for unmethylated CpG-rich DNA in endosomes (see Chapter 4). Murine B cells (but not human cells) also express TLR4 on the cell surface, which recognizes LPS. These pattern recognition receptors provide signals that enhance or cooperate with those from the B cell receptor during B cell activation. In addition, the activation of myeloid cells through pattern recognition receptors can promote B cell activation indirectly in two ways. Dendritic cells activated through TLRs contribute significantly

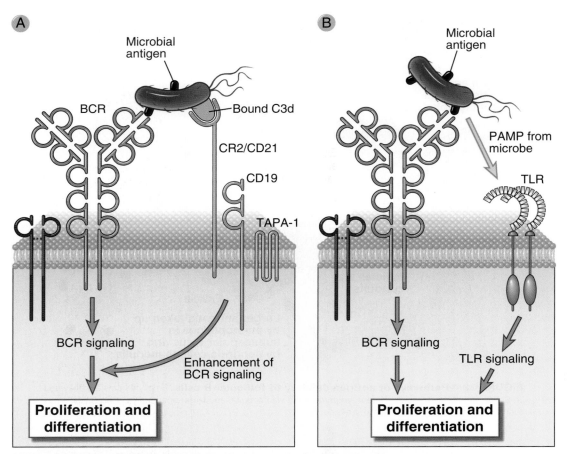

FIGURE 12-5 Role of CR2 and Toll-like receptors in B cell activation. In immune responses to microbes, activation of B cells through the BCR may be enhanced by complement-coated antigen that can ligate both the BCR and complement receptor 2 (CR2) **(A)**, and also by the simultaneous activation of Toll-like receptors (TLRs) on B cells by molecules (pathogen-associated molecular patterns [PAMPs]) derived from the microbe **(B)**.

to helper T cell activation, which stimulate B cells in responses to protein antigens. Myeloid cells activated by TLRs may secrete APRIL and BAFF, cytokines that can induce T-independent B cell responses.

Functional Responses of B Cells to Antigens

Distinct cellular events are induced by antigen-mediated cross-linking of the BCR by different types of antigens: multivalent antigens initiate B cell proliferation and differentiation, and protein antigens prepare B cells for subsequent interactions with helper T cells. Antigen receptor cross-linking by some antigens can stimulate several important changes in B cells (Fig. 12-6). In response to multivalent antigens, the previously resting cells enter into the G₁ stage of the cell cycle, and this is accompanied by increases in cell size, cytoplasmic RNA, and biosynthetic organelles such as ribosomes. Some activated B cells differentiate into short-lived antibody-secreting plasma cells. Survival of the stimulated B cells is enhanced as a result of the production of anti-apoptotic proteins, notably Bcl-2 (see Fig. 15-8). Activation of B cells by antigen results in increased expression of class II major histocompatibility complex (MHC) molecules and B7 costimulators, because of which antigen-stimulated B cells are more efficient activators of helper T lymphocytes than are naive B cells.

The expression of receptors for several T cell–derived cytokines is also increased, which enables antigen-stimulated B lymphocytes to respond to cytokines secreted by helper T cells. The expression of chemokine receptors may change, resulting in movement of the B cells out of the follicles.

The importance of signaling by the BCR complex for the subsequent responses of the cells varies with the nature of the antigen. Most T-independent antigens, such as polysaccharides, contain multiple identical epitopes on each molecule or displayed on a cell surface. Such multivalent antigens can effectively cross-link many B cell antigen receptors and initiate responses even though they are not recognized by helper T lymphocytes. In contrast, many naturally occurring globular protein antigens possess only one copy of each epitope per molecule. Therefore, such protein antigens cannot simultaneously bind to and cross-link multiple Ig molecules, and their ability to activate the BCR is limited, so they do not typically induce signals that can drive B cell proliferation and differentiation. They are, however, sufficient to influence survival, induce changes in chemokine receptor expression, and promote antigen endocytosis. Some protein antigens may be displayed as multivalent arrays on the surfaces of microbes or cells, or they may be multivalent because they are in aggregates.

Protein antigens are also internalized by the BCR, processed, and presented as peptides bound to MHC

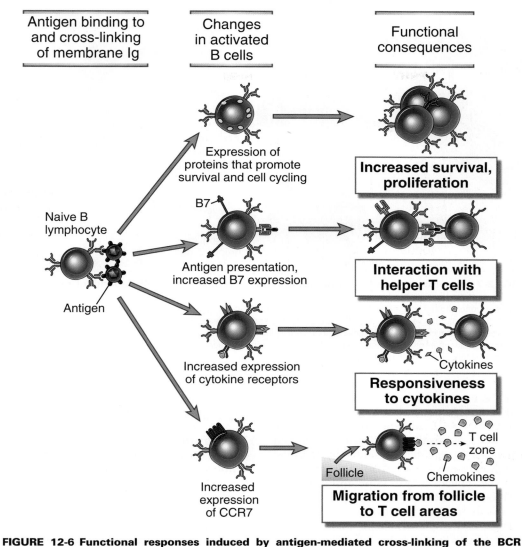

Antigen binding to and cross-linking of membrane Ig	Changes in activated B cells	Functional consequences

FIGURE 12-6 Functional responses induced by antigen-mediated cross-linking of the BCR complex. Antigen-induced cross-linking of the B cell antigen receptor induces several cellular responses including: production of proteins that promote survival and proliferation, expression costimulators and cytokine receptors that promote interactions with and responsiveness to helper T cells, and migration of the cells toward T cells as a result of the expression of CCR7.

molecules to helper T cells, which are potent stimulators of B lymphocyte proliferation and differentiation. In fact, in T-dependent responses, a major function of membrane Ig is not to drive proliferation and differentiation but to facilitate binding and internalization of the antigen for subsequent presentation to helper T cells.

After specific B cells recognize antigens, the subsequent steps in humoral immune responses are very different in T-dependent and T-independent responses. We will next describe the activation of B cells by protein antigens and helper T cells.

HELPER T CELL–DEPENDENT ANTIBODY RESPONSES TO PROTEIN ANTIGENS

The helper function of T lymphocytes was discovered by experiments performed in the late 1960s, which showed that antibody responses required cooperation of two different cell populations that were later determined to be B cells and T cells. These classic experimental studies were among the first formal proof of the importance of interactions between two different cell populations in the immune system. It took many years to establish that most helper T cells are CD4+CD8− lymphocytes that recognize peptide antigens presented by class II MHC molecules. One of the important accomplishments of immunology has been the elucidation of the mechanisms of T-B cell interactions and the actions of helper T cells in antibody responses.

The Sequence of Events During T Cell–Dependent Antibody Responses

Protein antigens are recognized by specific B and T lymphocytes in peripheral lymphoid organs, and the activated cell populations come together in these organs to initiate humoral immune responses (Fig. 12-7). The interaction

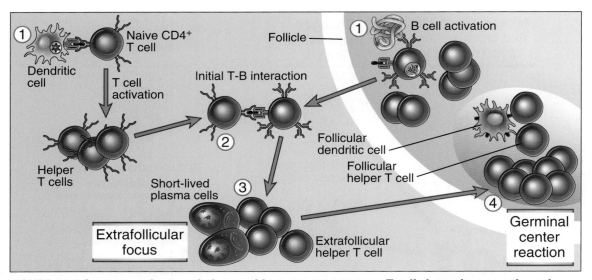

FIGURE 12-7 Sequence of events in humoral immune responses to T cell–dependent protein antigens. (1) Immune responses are initiated by the recognition of antigens by B cells and CD4+ T cells. (2) The activated lymphocytes migrate toward one another and interact, resulting in B cell proliferation and differentiation. (3) Restimulation of B cells by helper T cells in extrafollicular sites leads to early isotype switching and short-lived plasma cell generation, while activation of T cells by B cells results in the induction of follicular helper T cells. (4) The late events occur in germinal centers and include somatic mutation and the selection of high-affinity cells (affinity maturation), additional isotype switching, memory B cell generation, and the generation of long-lived plasma cells.

between helper T cells and B lymphocytes is initiated by the recognition of the same protein antigen by both cell types and follows a precise sequence of events. Naive CD4+ T cells are activated in the T cell zones by antigen (in the form of processed peptides) presented by dendritic cells, and differentaite into helper T cells. Naive B cells are activated in the follicles by the same antigen (in its native conformation) transported there. The helper T cells and activated B cells migrate toward one another and interact at the edges of the follicles, where the initial antibody response develops. Some of the cells migrate back into follicles to form germinal centers, where the more specialized antibody responses are induced. Next we will describe each of these steps in detail.

Initial Activation and Migration of Helper B Cells and T Cells

The activation of specific B and T cells by the same antigen is essential for their functional interaction and brings them into proximity to enhance the likelihood of the antigen-specific B and T cells locating one another (Fig. 12-8). The frequency of naive B cells or T cells specific for a given epitope of an antigen is as low as 1 in 10^5 to 1 in 10^6 lymphocytes, and the specific B and T cells have to find each other and physically interact to generate strong antibody responses. This is accomplished in part by regulated movement of the cells following antigen recognition. Helper T cells downregulate

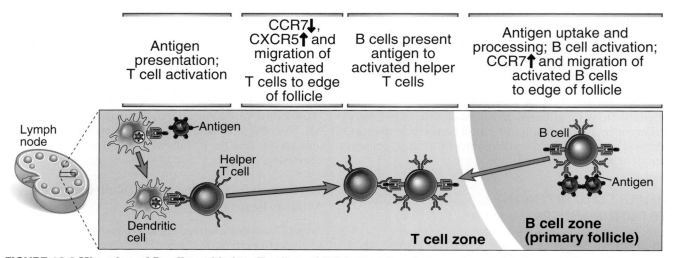

FIGURE 12-8 Migration of B cells and helper T cells and T-B interaction. Antigen-activated helper T cells and B cells move toward one another in response to chemokine signals and make contact adjacent to the edge of primary follicles.

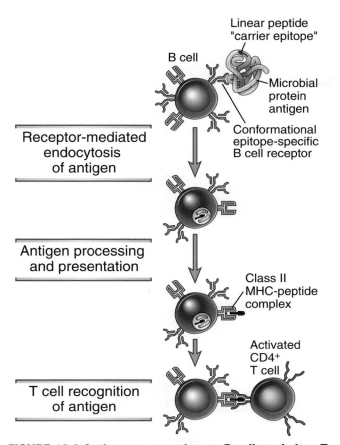

Linear peptide
"carrier epitope"

B cell

Microbial
protein
antigen

Conformational
epitope-specific
B cell receptor

**Receptor-mediated
endocytosis
of antigen**

**Antigen processing
and presentation**

Class II
MHC-peptide
complex

Activated
CD4+
T cell

**T cell recognition
of antigen**

FIGURE 12-9 Antigen presentation on B cells to helper T cells. Protein antigens recognized by membrane Ig are endocytosed and processed, and peptide fragments are presented in association with class II MHC molecules. Helper T cells recognize MHC-peptide complexes on the B cells and then stimulate B cell responses. In responses to hapten-carrier conjugates, the hapten (the B cell epitope) is recognized by a specific B cell, the conjugate is endocytosed, the carrier protein is processed in the B cell, and peptides from the carrier (the T cell epitopes) are presented to the helper T cell.

Antigen Presentation by B Cells and the Hapten-Carrier Effect

Protein antigens that are recognized by specific B cell antigen receptors are endocytosed and processed to generate peptides that bind to class II MHC molecules and are presented to CD4+ T cells (Fig. 12-9). This class II MHC pathway of antigen presentation was described in detail in Chapter 6. The peptides that are presented by the B cell to a helper T cell are the same peptides that initially activated the precursor naive CD4+ T cell when they were presented by dendritic cells in the T cell zone. Because the BCR recognizes an epitope of the native protein with high affinity, specific B cells bind and present the antigen much more efficiently (i.e., at much lower concentrations) than do other B cells not specific for the antigen. This is why B cells specific for an antigen respond preferentially to that antigen, compared with other cells. A protein antigen that elicits a T-dependent B cell response therefore makes use of at least two epitopes when activating specific B cells: A surface epitope on the native protein is recognized with high specificity by a B cell, and an internal linear peptide epitope is subsequently released from the protein, binds to class II MHC molecules, and is recognized by helper T cells. The antibodies that are eventually secreted are usually specific for conformational determinants of the native antigen because membrane Ig on B cells is capable of binding conformational epitopes of proteins, and the same Ig is secreted by plasma cells derived from those B cells. This feature of B cell antigen recognition determines the fine specificity of the antibody response and is independent of the fact that helper T cells recognize only linear epitopes of processed peptides. In fact, a single B lymphocyte specific for a native epitope may bind and endocytose a protein and present multiple different peptides complexed with class II MHC molecules to different helper T cells, but the resultant antibody response remains specific for the native protein.

The principles outlined here for T-B cell collaboration help explain a phenomenon that is known as the **hapten-carrier effect**. Analysis of antibody responses to hapten-carrier conjugates provided among the earliest demonstrations of how antigen presentation by B lymphocytes contributes to the development of humoral immune responses. Haptens, such as dinitrophenol, are small chemicals that can be bound by specific antibodies but are not immunogenic by themselves. If, however, haptens are coupled to proteins, which serve as carriers, the conjugates are able to induce antibody responses against the haptens. There are three important characteristics of anti-hapten antibody responses to hapten-protein conjugates. First, such responses require both hapten-specific B cells and protein (carrier)–specific helper T cells. Second, to stimulate a response, the hapten and carrier portions have to be physically linked and cannot be administered separately. Third, the interaction is class II MHC restricted, that is, the helper T cells cooperate only with B lymphocytes that express class II MHC molecules that are identical to those that were involved in the initial activation of naive T cells by dendritic cells. All of these features of antibody responses to hapten-protein conjugates can be explained by the antigen-presenting functions of B lymphocytes.

the chemokine receptor CCR7 and increase the expression of CXCR5 and, as a result, leave the T cell zone and migrate toward the follicle. As mentioned earlier, CXCL13, the ligand for CXCR5, is secreted by follicular dendritic cells and other follicular stromal cells, and it attracts activated CD4+ T cells toward the follicle. Also as discussed earlier, B cells respond to these antigens by reducing cell surface expression of the chemokine receptor CXCR5 and increasing expression of CCR7. As a result, activated B cells migrate toward the T cell zone drawn by a gradient of CCL19 and CCL21, the ligands for CCR7. B cells activated by protein antigens can also express CD69, which blocks surface expression of sphingosine 1-phosphate receptors, causing retention of activated B cells in lymph nodes (see Chapter 3). The net result of these changes is that antigen-activated T and B lymphocytes are drawn toward each other.

Protein antigens are endocytosed by the B cell and presented in a form that can be recognized by helper T cells, and this represents the next step in the process of T-dependent B cell activation.

Hapten-specific B cells bind the antigen through the hapten determinant, endocytose the hapten-carrier conjugate, and present peptides derived from the carrier protein to carrier-specific helper T lymphocytes (see Fig. 12-9). Thus, the two cooperating lymphocytes recognize different epitopes of the same complex antigen. The hapten is responsible for efficient internalization of the carrier protein into the B cell, which explains why hapten and carrier must be physically linked. The requirement for MHC-associated antigen presentation for T cell activation accounts for the MHC restriction of T cell–B cell interactions.

The characteristics of humoral responses elucidated for hapten-carrier conjugates apply to all protein antigens in which one intrinsic determinant, usually a native conformational determinant, is recognized by B cells (and is therefore analogous to the hapten) and another determinant in the form of a class II MHC–associated linear peptide, is recognized by helper T cells (and is analogous to the carrier that is the source of the peptide). The hapten-carrier effect is the basis for the development of conjugate vaccines, which contain carbohydrate epitopes recognized by B cells attached to proteins recognized by T cells, discussed later in this chapter.

Role of CD40L:CD40 Interaction in T-Dependent B Cell Activation

On activation, helper T cells express CD40 ligand (CD40L), which engages its receptor, CD40, on antigen-stimulated B cells and induces B cell proliferation and differentiation, initially in extrafollicular foci and later in germinal centers (Fig. 12-10). Recall that CD40 is a member of the TNF receptor superfamily (see Chapter 10). Its ligand, CD40L (CD154), is a trimeric membrane protein that is homologous to TNF. CD40 is constitutively expressed on B cells, and CD40L is expressed on the surface of helper T cells after activation by antigen and costimulators. When these activated helper T cells interact physically with antigen-presenting B cells, CD40L recognizes CD40 on the B cell surface. CD40L binding to CD40 results in conformational alteration of preformed CD40 trimers, and this induces the association of cytosolic proteins called TRAFs (TNF receptor–associated factors) with the cytoplasmic domain of CD40. The TRAFs recruited to CD40 initiate enzyme cascades that lead to the activation and nuclear translocation of transcription factors, including NF-κB and AP-1, which collectively stimulate B cell proliferation and increased synthesis and secretion of Ig. Similar signaling pathways are activated by TNF receptors (see Chapter 7). CD40-induced transcription factor induction is also crucial for subsequent germinal center reactions, as we will discuss later. T cell–mediated dendritic cell and macrophage activation also involves the interaction of CD40L on activated helper T cells with CD40 on dendritic cells and macrophages (see Chapters 6 and 10).

Mutations in the *CD40L* gene result in a disease called the **X-linked hyper-IgM syndrome**, which is characterized by defects in antibody production, isotype switching, affinity maturation, and memory B cell generation in response to protein antigens, as well as deficient cell-mediated immunity (see Chapter 21). Similar abnormalities are seen in *CD40* or *CD40L* gene knockout mice.

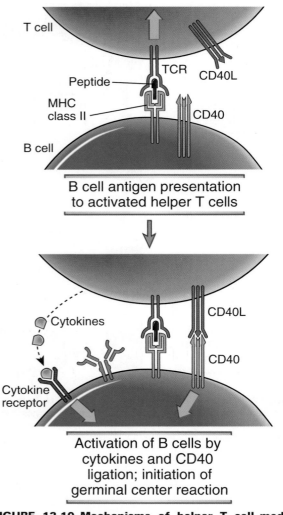

B cell antigen presentation to activated helper T cells

Activation of B cells by cytokines and CD40 ligation; initiation of germinal center reaction

FIGURE 12-10 Mechanisms of helper T cell–mediated B cell activation. Helper T cells that are activated by recognizing antigens presented by B cells express CD40L, which binds to CD40 on B cells and stimulates B cell proliferation and differentiation. Cytokines produced by the helper T cells also contribute to B cell responses.

Interestingly, a DNA virus called the Epstein-Barr virus (EBV) infects human B cells and induces their proliferation. This may lead to immortalization of the cells and the development of lymphomas. The cytoplasmic tail of a transforming protein of EBV called LMP1 (latent membrane protein 1) associates with the same TRAF molecules as does the cytoplasmic domain of CD40, and this apparently triggers B cell proliferation. Thus, EBV LMP1 is functionally homologous to a physiologic B cell signaling molecule, and EBV has apparently co-opted a normal pathway of B lymphocyte activation for its own purpose, which is to promote survival and proliferation of cells that the virus has infected.

In addition to CD40L on helper T cells activating B cells, helper T cells also secrete cytokines that contribute to B cell responses. The best defined roles of T cell–derived cytokines in humoral immune responses are in isotype switching, described later. Several cytokines have

TABLE 12-1   Extrafollicular and Germinal Center B Cell Responses

Feature	Extrafollicular	Follicular/Germinal Center
Localization	Medullary cords of lymph nodes and at junctions between T cell zone and red pulp of spleen	Secondary follicles
CD40 signals	Required	Required
Specialized T cell help	Extrafollicular helper T cells	T_{FH} cells in germinal center
AID expression	Yes	Yes
Class switching	Yes, limited	Yes, extensive
Somatic hypermutation	Low rate	High rate
Antibody affinity	Low	High
Terminally differentiated B cells	Short-lived plasma cells (life span of ~3 days)	Long-lived plasma cells, which migrate to bone marrow or MALT, and memory cells
B cell transcription factors	Blimp-1	Bcl-6

AID, activation-induced cytidine deaminase; *Bcl-6*, B cell lymphoma 6; *Blimp-1*, B lymphocyte–induced maturation protein 1; *MALT*, mucosa-associated lymphoid tissue; *T_{FH}*, follicular helper T cell.
Adapted from Vinuesa CG, Sanz I, Cook MC: Dysregulation of germinal centres in autoimmune disease, *Nature Reviews Immunology* 9:845-857, 2009.

also been implicated in the early steps of B cell proliferation and differentiation, but it is not clear if any are actually essential for these responses.

After the initial interaction of B cells with helper T cells at the interface between the follicle and the T cell zone, subsequent activation of B cells by helper T cells can occur at two different locations, one outside the follicles in an extrafollicular focus, and the other in the germinal centers of follicles. The nature of the B cell response differs in these locations (Table 12-1).

Extrafollicular B Cell Activation

B cell activation in the extrafollicular focus provides an early antibody response to protein antigens and sets up the formation of the more slowly developing but more effective germinal center response. Extrafollicular foci of T-dependent B cell activation produce low-affinity antibodies that can circulate and limit the spread of an infection. The extrafollicular response also helps generate follicular helper T cells (T_{FH} cells) that migrate into the follicle and are required for germinal center formation. Some antigen-activated B cells from the extrafollicular focus also return to the follicle, participate in germinal center formation, and undergo changes that result in a more potent and long-lasting antibody response. Each such focus may produce 100 to 200 antibody-secreting plasma cells. In the spleen, extrafollicular foci develop in the outer portions of the T cell–rich periarteriolar lymphoid sheath (PALS) or between the T cell zone and the red pulp, and these collections of cells are also called PALS foci. Similar T-dependent foci are observed in the medullary cords of lymph nodes.

B cells that are activated by helper T cells through CD40L in the extrafollicular foci undergo limited isotype switching. The antibody-secreting cells that are generated in extrafollicular foci, including circulating plasmablasts and tissue plasma cells, are mostly short-lived, and these cells do not acquire the ability to migrate to distant sites such as the bone marrow. The small amount of antibody produced in these foci may contribute to the formation of immune complexes (containing antigen, antibody, and perhaps complement) that are trapped by follicular dendritic cells in lymphoid follicles. Follicular dendritic cells then release chemokines, perhaps in response to the immune complexes, that draw in a few (perhaps only one or two) activated B cells from the extrafollicular focus into the follicle to initiate the germinal center reaction.

The Germinal Center Reaction

The characteristic events of helper T cell–dependent antibody responses, including affinity maturation, isotype switching, and generation of long-lived plasma cells and memory B cells, occur primarily in organized structures called germinal centers that are created within lymphoid follicles during T-dependent immune responses. The development of germinal centers and the complex process of genetic diversification of activated B cells and survival of the fittest that occurs in these sites is called the germinal center reaction.

Germinal centers develop about 4 to 7 days after the initiation of a T-dependent B cell response. At this time, a few of the B cells that are activated in extrafollicular foci migrate back into the follicle and begin to proliferate rapidly, forming a distinct region of the follicle (Fig. 12-11). This region was named the *germinal center* by morphologists because of the belief that new cells were generated there, long before its functional significance was understood. Each fully formed germinal center contains cells derived from only one or a few antigen-specific B cell clones. Within the germinal center is a dark zone that is densely packed with rapidly proliferating B cells. The doubling time of these proliferating germinal center B cells, also called centroblasts, is estimated to be 6 to 12 hours, so that within 5 days, a single lymphocyte may

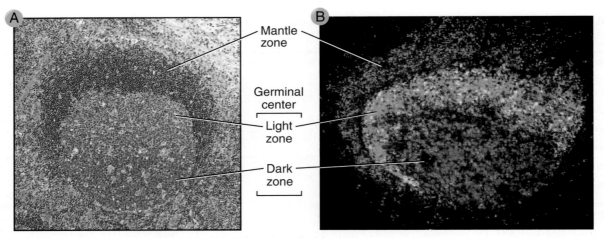

FIGURE 12-11 Germinal centers in secondary lymphoid organs. A, The germinal center is within the follicle and includes a basal dark zone and an adjacent light zone. **B,** The light zone contains follicular dendritic cells, stained with an anti-CD23 antibody (green), and the dark zone contains proliferating B cells, stained with an anti-Ki67 antibody (red), which detects cycling cells. (**A,** Courtesy of Dr. James Gulizia, Department of Pathology, Brigham and Women's Hospital, Boston, Massachusetts. **B,** Modified from Liu YJ, Johnson GD, Gordon J, MacLennan IC: Germinal centres in T-cell–dependent antibody responses, Immunology Today 13:17-21. Copyright © 1992 with permission from Elsevier.)

give rise to as many as 5000 progeny. The progeny of the proliferating B cells in the germinal center are smaller cells, sometimes called centrocytes, which undergo differentiation and selection processes in the light zone, described later. B cells in germinal centers express a transcriptional repressor known as Bcl-6 (B cell lymphoma gene 6), whose role is described later when we consider the transcriptional regulation of B cell fate.

The architecture of lymphoid follicles and the germinal center reaction within follicles depend on the presence of **follicular dendritic cells (FDCs)**. FDCs are found only in lymphoid follicles and express complement receptors (CR1, CR2, and CR3) and Fc receptors. These molecules are involved in displaying antigens for the selection of germinal center B cells, as described later. FDCs do not express class II MHC molecules and are not derived from progenitors in the bone marrow. Thus, in spite of their name, they are distinct from the class II MHC–expressing dendritic cells that capture antigens in tissues and transport them to lymphoid organs where they present peptides to T lymphocytes. The long cytoplasmic processes of FDCs form a meshwork around which germinal centers are formed.

The germinal center reaction consists of sequential steps (Fig. 12-12). Proliferating B cells accumulate in the dark zone of the germinal center, which contains neither FDCs nor T cells. The small non-dividing progeny of the B cells migrate to the adjacent light zone, where they come into close contact with the processes of the abundant FDCs and also form intimate contacts with T_{FH} cells, and this is where subsequent selection events occur. The rim of naive B cells in the follicle, surrounding the germinal center, is called the mantle zone.

Germinal center formation is dependent on CD40L on T_{FH} cells interacting with CD40 on B cells. These interactions are critical for B cell proliferation, which is required for expansion of B cells in germinal centers, and also for isotype switching and affinity maturation. Germinal center formation is defective in humans and in mice with genetic

defects in T cell development or activation or with mutations of either CD40 or its ligand, discussed earlier.

The Induction of Follicular Helper T Cells

Within 4 to 7 days after antigen exposure, activated antigen-specific B cells induce some previously activated T cells to differentiate into T_{FH} cells, which express high levels of the chemokine receptor CXCR5, are drawn into lymphoid follicles by CXCL13, the ligand for CXCR5, and play critical roles in germinal center formation and function. In addition to CXCR5, T_{FH} cells express ICOS (inducible costimulator), PD-1 (programmed death-1), the cytokine IL-21, and the transcription factor Bcl-6. T_{FH} cells have a phenotype that makes them distinct from the T_H1, T_H2, and T_H17 subsets of effector T cells described in Chapter 10.

Differentiation of T_{FH} cells from naive CD4+ T cells requires two steps: initial activation by antigen-presenting dendritic cells and subsequent activation by B cells (Fig. 12-13). The choice between a T_H1, T_H2 or T_H17 fate on the on hand or a T_{FH} fate on the other depends partly on the strength of the initial interaction between peptide–class II MHC complexes on dendritic cells and the T cell receptor on naive CD4+ T cells. Strong TCR activation by dendritic cells induces expression of the Bcl-6 transcriptional repressor and low levels of the α chain of the IL-2 receptor (IL-2R) on CD4+ T cells. This initial expression of moderate levels of Bcl-6 combined with weak IL-2R signaling inhibits the acquisition of a T_H1, T_H2 or T_H17 cell fate. Some of these activated T cells begin to express CXCR5. The differentiation of T_{FH} cells is completed by the activation of the nascent T_{FH} cells by activated B cells. A number of molecules on B cells and helper T cells are known to play key roles in the generation of T_{FH} cells. The costimulator ICOS, which is related to CD28 and is expressed on T_{FH} cells, is essential for the germinal center reaction. The interaction of ICOS with ICOS ligand on activated B cells promotes the

Activation of B cells
and migration
into germinal center

↓

B cell proliferation

↓

Somatic mutation and
affinity maturation;
isotype switching

↓

Exit of high-affinity
antibody-secreting cells,
and memory B cells

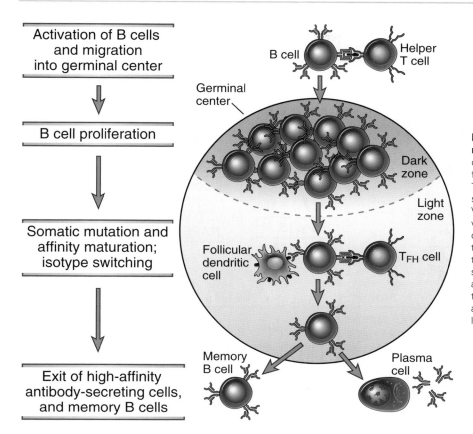

FIGURE 12-12 The germinal center reaction in a lymph node. Activated B cells migrate into the follicle and proliferate, forming the dark zone of the germinal center. These B cells undergo extensive isotype switching and somatic hypermutation of Ig V genes, and migrate into the light zone, where they encounter follicular dendritic cells displaying antigen and T_{FH} cells. B cells with the highest affinity Ig receptors are selected to survive, and they differentiate into antibody-secreting cells and memory B cells. The antibody-secreting cells leave and reside in the bone marrow as long-lived plasma cells, and the memory B cells enter the recirculating lymphocyte pool.

differentiation of T cells into T_{FH} cells. The interactions between activated B cells and helper T cells are mediated by integrins and by members of the SLAM family of costimulators. A signaling molecule that associates with these SLAM family proteins in T_{FH} cells is called SAP, and SAP signaling stabilizes the expression of transcriptional regulators, particularly Bcl-6, that are required for T_{FH} cell development. SAP is mutated in patients with a disease known as X-linked lymphoproliferative syndrome, which is associated with defects in antibody and cytotoxic T cell responses (see Chapter 21).

The defining cytokine of T_{FH} cells is IL-21. This cytokine is required for germinal center development and contributes to the generation of plasma cells in the germinal center reaction. IL-21 secreted by T_{FH} cells also facilitates

germinal center B cell selection events and the differentiation of activated B cells into plasmablasts. In addition to IL-21, T_{FH} cells secrete other cytokines, including IFN-γ or IL-4, and likely low levels of IL-17 as well, and all of these cytokines participate in isotype switching.

T_{FH} cells play several important roles in the activation and differentiation of B cells in the germinal center reaction. These roles depend on several signals, including ICOSL, CD40L, and IL-21, and will be discussed in detail below.

Heavy Chain Isotype (Class) Switching

In T-dependent responses, some of the progeny of activated IgM- and IgD-expressing B cells undergo heavy chain isotype (class) switching and produce antibodies

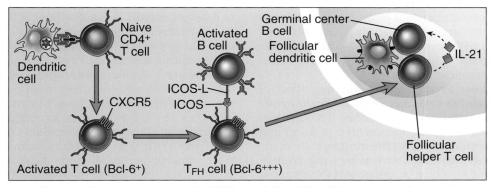

FIGURE 12-13 Molecular events in follicular helper T cell generation. The generation of T_{FH} cells requires sequential activation of T cells, first by dendritic cells and then by activated B cells. The differentiated T_{FH} cells migrate into germinal centers, where they activate B cells.

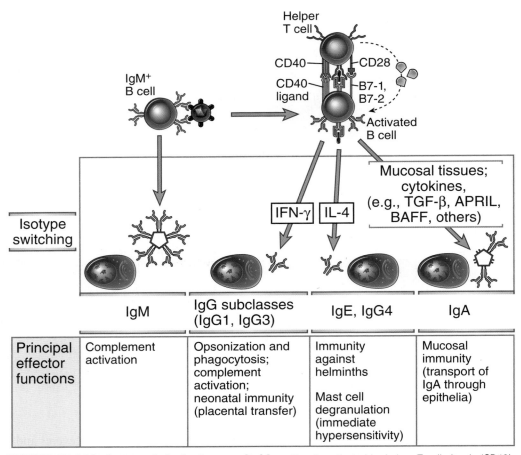

| IgM | IgG subclasses (IgG1, IgG3) | IgE, IgG4 | IgA |

	IgM	IgG subclasses (IgG1, IgG3)	IgE, IgG4	IgA
Principal effector functions	Complement activation	Opsonization and phagocytosis; complement activation; neonatal immunity (placental transfer)	Immunity against helminths Mast cell degranulation (immediate hypersensitivity)	Mucosal immunity (transport of IgA through epithelia)

FIGURE 12-14 Ig heavy chain isotype switching. B cells activated by helper T cell signals (CD40L, cytokines) undergo switching to different Ig isotypes, which mediate distinct effector functions. Selected examples of switched isotypes are shown. The role of IFN-γ in directing specific isotype switching events has been established only in rodents.

with heavy chains of different classes, such as γ, α, and ε (Fig. 12-14). Some isotype switching occurs in B cells in extrafollicular foci, driven by extrafollicular helper T cells, but much more occurs in germinal centers, driven by T$_{FH}$ cells. The capacity of B cells to produce different antibody isotypes provides a remarkable plasticity in humoral immune responses by generating antibodies that perform distinct effector functions and are involved in defense against different types of infectious agents. B cells change the isotypes of the antibodies they produce by changing the constant regions of the heavy chains but the specificity of the antibodies (which is determined by the variable regions) remains unaltered. The molecular mechanisms responsible for the change in heavy chain constant regions are described below.

Isotype switching in response to different types of microbes is regulated by cytokines produced by the helper T cells that are activated by these microbes. IFN-γ induces B cell switching to IgG (best documented in mice) and IL-4 induces switching to IgE. The response to many viruses and intracellular bacteria involves the production of IgG antibodies, which block entry of the microbes into host cells and also promote phagocytosis by macrophages. Viruses and many bacteria activate helper T cells of the T$_H$1 subset, which produce the cytokine IFN-γ and

also likely induce T$_{FH}$ cells to make increased amounts of IFN-γ. The humoral response to many helminthic parasites is mainly driven by IgE antibodies, which participate in eosinophil- and mast cell–mediated elimination of the helminths (see Chapters 13 and 16); IgE antibodies also mediate immediate hypersensitivity (allergic) reactions (see Chapter 20). Helminths likely influence T$_{FH}$ cell differentiation and induce these helper T cells to produce T$_H$2-type cytokines during the germinal center reaction.

In addition, B cells in different anatomic sites switch to different isotypes, in part because of the cytokines produced at these sites. Specifically, B cells in mucosal tissues switch to IgA, which is the antibody class that is most efficiently transported through epithelia into mucosal secretions, where it defends against microbes that try to enter through the epithelia (see Chapter 14). Switching to IgA is stimulated by transforming growth factor-β (TGF-β), which is produced by many cell types, including helper T cells, in mucosal and other tissues. Cytokines of the TNF family, BAFF and APRIL, also stimulate switching to IgA. Because these cytokines are produced by myeloid cells, they can stimulate IgA responses in the absence of T cell help. Some individuals who inherit mutant versions of the *TACI* gene, which encodes a receptor for these cytokines, have a selective deficiency of IgA production (see Chapter 21).

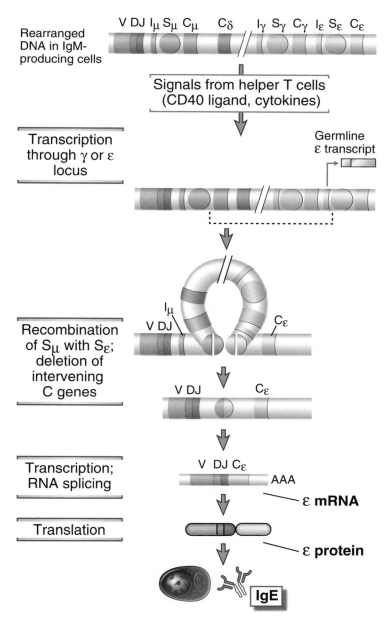

Rearranged DNA in IgM-producing cells

V DJ I_μ S_μ C_μ C_δ I_γ S_γ C_γ I_ε S_ε C_ε

Signals from helper T cells (CD40 ligand, cytokines)

Transcription through γ or ε locus

Germline ε transcript

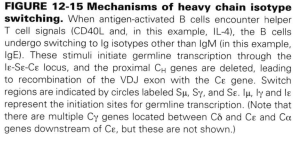

Recombination of S_μ with S_ε; deletion of intervening C genes

I_μ
V DJ
C_ε

V DJ C_ε

Transcription; RNA splicing

V DJ C_ε AAA

ε mRNA

Translation

ε protein

IgE

FIGURE 12-15 Mechanisms of heavy chain isotype switching. When antigen-activated B cells encounter helper T cell signals (CD40L and, in this example, IL-4), the B cells undergo switching to Ig isotypes other than IgM (in this example, IgE). These stimuli initiate germline transcription through the I_ε-S_ε-C_ε locus, and the proximal C_H genes are deleted, leading to recombination of the VDJ exon with the C_ε gene. Switch regions are indicated by circles labeled S_μ, S_γ, and S_ε. I_μ, I_γ and I_ε represent the initiation sites for germline transcription. (Note that there are multiple C_γ genes located between C_δ and C_ε and C_α genes downstream of C_ε, but these are not shown.)

CD40 signals work together with cytokines to induce isotype switching. CD40 engagement induces the enzyme activation-induced deaminase (AID), which, as we will see later, is crucial for both isotype switching and affinity maturation. The requirement for CD40 signaling and AID to promote isotype switching in B cells is well documented by analysis of mice and humans lacking CD40, CD40-ligand, or AID. In all these cases, the antibody response to protein antigens is dominated by IgM antibodies, and there is limited switching to other isotypes.

The molecular mechanism of isotype switching is a process called switch recombination, in which the Ig heavy chain DNA in B cells is cut and recombined such that a previously formed VDJ exon that encodes the V domain is placed adjacent to a downstream C region, and the intervening DNA is deleted (Fig. 12-15). These DNA recombination events involve nucleotide sequences called switch regions, which are located in the introns

between the J and C segments at the 5' ends of each C_H locus, other than the δ gene. Switch regions are 1 to 10 kilobases long, contain numerous tandem repeats of GC-rich DNA sequences, and are found upstream of every heavy chain gene. Upstream of each switch region is a small exon called the I exon (for initiator of transcription) preceded by an I region promoter. Signals from cytokines and CD40 induce transcription from a particular I region promoter reading through the I exon, switch region, and adjacent C_H exons. These transcripts are known as germline transcripts. They are not translated into proteins but are required for isotype switching to proceed. Germline transcripts are found at both the μ locus and the downstream heavy chain locus to which an activated B cell is being induced to switch. At each participating switch region, the germline transcript facilitates the generation of DNA double-stranded breaks, as described later. The DNA break in the upstream (μ) switch region is joined to the break in the downstream selected switch region. As a result, the rearranged VDJ exon just upstream of the μ switch region in the IgM-producing B cell recombines with the Ig heavy chain gene located immediately after the transcriptionally active downstream switch region. Cytokines determine which C_H region will undergo germline transcription. For instance, IL-4 induces germline transcription through the I_ε-S_ε-C_ε locus (see Fig. 12-15). This leads first to the production of germline ε transcripts in an IgM-expressing B cell and then to recombination of the S_μ switch region with the S_ε switch region. The intervening DNA is lost, and the VDJ exon is thus brought adjacent to C_ε. The end result is the production of IgE with the same V domain as that of the original IgM produced by that B cell.

The key enzyme required for isotype switching (and affinity maturation, described later) is **activation-induced deaminase (AID)**. As we mentioned earlier, AID expression is activated mainly by CD40 signals from T_{FH} cells. The enzyme deaminates cytosines in single-stranded DNA templates, converting cytosine (C) residues to uracil (U) residues (Fig. 12-16). Switch regions are rich in G and C bases, and switch region transcripts tend to form stable DNA-RNA hybrids involving the coding (top) strand of DNA, thus freeing up the bottom or non-template strand, which forms an open single-stranded DNA loop called an R-loop. The R-loop is where a large number of C residues in the switch DNA sequence are converted to U residues by AID. An enzyme called uracil N-glycosylase removes the U residues, leaving abasic sites. The ApeI endonuclease and probably other endonucleases cleave these abasic sites, generating a nick at each position. Some nicks are generated on the upper strand as well in an AID-dependent manner, but it is less clear how that happens. Nicks on both strands contribute to double-stranded breaks both in the S_μ region and in the downstream switch region that is involved in a particular isotype switch event. The double-stranded breaks in the two switch regions are joined together (repaired) by use of the machinery involved in double-stranded break repair by non-homologous end joining. In this process, the DNA between the two switch regions is deleted, and the net result is that the original rearranged V region becomes adjacent to a new constant region.

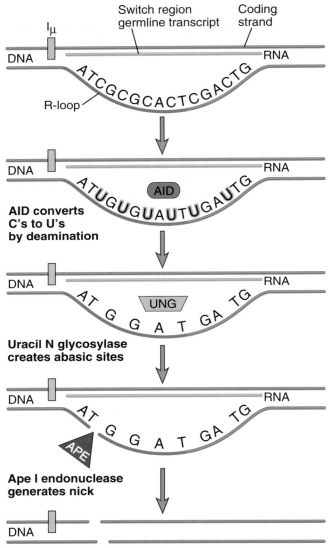

AID converts C's to U's by deamination

Uracil N glycosylase creates abasic sites

Ape I endonuclease generates nick

Eventual double-strand breaks in switch region

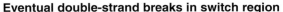

FIGURE 12-16 Mechanism by which AID and germline transcription collaborate to generate double-stranded breaks at switch regions. Germline transcripts form DNA-RNA hybrids in the switch region and AID deaminates C residues to generate U residues in single-stranded DNA. Uracil N-glycosylase (UNG) removes U residues to generate abasic sites where the ApeI endonuclease creates nicks that lead to a double-stranded break.

Affinity Maturation: Somatic Mutation of Ig Genes and Selection of High-Affinity B Cells

Affinity maturation is the process that leads to increased affinity of antibodies for a particular antigen as a T-dependent humoral response progresses, and it is the result of somatic mutation of Ig genes followed by selective survival of the B cells producing the antibodies with the highest affinities. The process of affinity maturation generates antibodies with an increased ability to bind antigens and thus to more efficiently neutralize and eliminate microbes (Fig. 12-17). Helper T cells and CD40:CD40L interactions are required for somatic mutation to be initiated, and, as a result, affinity maturation is observed only in antibody responses to T-dependent protein antigens.

In proliferating germinal center B cells in the dark zone, Ig V genes undergo point mutations at an extremely high rate. This rate is estimated to be 1 in 10^3 V gene base pairs per cell division, which is about a thousand times higher than the spontaneous rate of mutation in other mammalian genes. For this reason, mutation in Ig V genes is also called **somatic hypermutation**. The V genes of expressed heavy and light chains in each B cell contain a total of about 700 nucleotides; this implies that mutations will accumulate in expressed V regions at an average rate of almost one per cell division. Ig V gene mutations continue to occur in the progeny of individual B cells. As a result, any B cell clone can accumulate more and more mutations during its life in the germinal center. It is estimated that as a consequence of somatic mutations, the nucleotide sequences of IgG antibodies derived from one clone of B cells can diverge as much as 5% from the original germline sequence. This usually translates to up to 10 amino acid substitutions. Several features of these mutations are noteworthy. First, the

mutations are clustered in the V regions, mostly in the antigen-binding complementarity-determining regions (Fig. 12-18). Second, there are far more mutations in IgG than in IgM antibodies. Third, the presence of mutations correlates with increasing affinities of the antibodies for the antigen that induced the response.

The mechanisms underlying somatic mutation in Ig genes are partially understood. It is clear that the rearranged Ig VDJ exon becomes highly susceptible to mutation, suggesting enhanced susceptibility of this region to DNA-binding factors that identify rearranged V regions for mutation. The enzyme AID, discussed earlier in the context of isotype switching, plays an essential role in affinity maturation. Its DNA deaminase activity converts C residues to U residues at hotspots for mutation. The U's may be changed to T's when DNA replication occurs, thus generating a common type of C to T mutation, or the U may be excised by uracil N-glycosylase, and the abasic site thus generated is repaired by an error-prone repair process, eventually generating substitutions with any of the four DNA nucleotides at each site of AID-induced cytidine deamination. These error-prone repair processes extend mutations to residues beyond the C residues that are targeted by AID.

Repeated stimulation by T cell–dependent protein antigens leads to increasing numbers of mutations in the Ig genes of antigen-specific germinal center B cells. Some of these mutations are likely to be useful because they will generate high-affinity antibodies. However, many of the mutations may result in a decline or even in a loss of antigen binding. Therefore, the next and crucial step

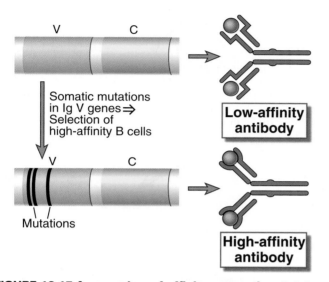

FIGURE 12-17 An overview of affinity maturation. Early in the immune response, low-affinity antibodies are produced. During the germinal center reaction, somatic mutation of Ig V genes and selection of B cells with high-affinity antigen receptors result in the production of antibodies with high affinity for antigen.

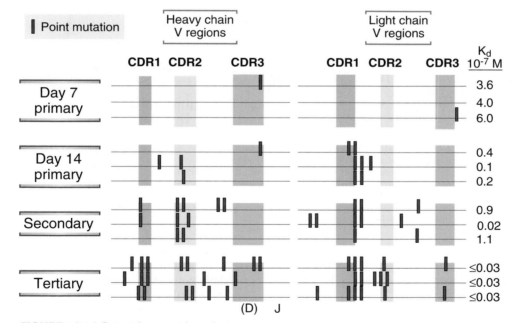

FIGURE 12-18 Somatic mutations in *Ig V* genes. Hybridomas were produced from spleen cells of mice immunized 7 or 14 days previously with a hapten, oxazolone, coupled to a protein and from spleen cells obtained after secondary and tertiary immunizations with the same antigen. Hybridomas producing oxazolone-specific monoclonal antibodies were produced, and the nucleotide sequences of the V genes encoding the Ig heavy and light chains were determined. Mutations in V genes increase with time after immunization and with repeated immunizations and are clustered in the complementarity-determining regions (CDRs). The location of CDR3 in the heavy chains is approximate. The affinities of the antibodies produced also tend to increase with more mutations, as indicated by the lower dissociation constants (Kd) for hapten binding. *(Modified from Berek C, Milstein C: Mutation drift and repertoire shift in maturation of the immune response,* Immunological Reviews *96:23-41, 1987, Blackwell Publishing.)*

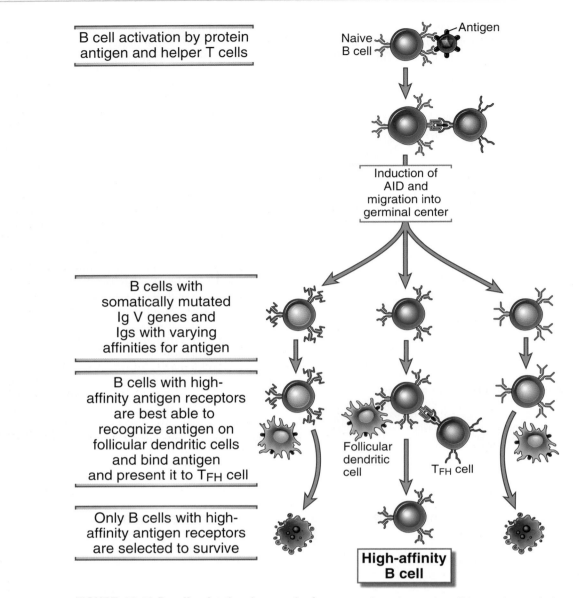

B cell activation by protein antigen and helper T cells

Naive B cell

Antigen

Induction of AID and migration into germinal center

B cells with somatically mutated Ig V genes and Igs with varying affinities for antigen

B cells with high-affinity antigen receptors are best able to recognize antigen on follicular dendritic cells and bind antigen and present it to T_{FH} cell

Only B cells with high-affinity antigen receptors are selected to survive

Follicular dendritic cell

T_{FH} cell

High-affinity B cell

FIGURE 12-19 B cell selection in germinal centers. Somatic mutation of V genes in germinal center B cells generates antibodies with different affinities for antigen. Binding of the B cells to antigen displayed on follicular dendritic cells is necessary to rescue the B cells from programmed cell death. B cells may also present antigen to germinal center T_{FH} cells, which promote B cell survival. The B cells with the highest affinity for antigen thus have a selective advantage for survival as the amount of available antigen decreases during an immune response. This leads to an average increase in the affinity of antibodies for antigen as the humoral immune response progresses.

in the process of affinity maturation is the selection of the most useful, high-affinity B cells, a type of Darwinian natural selection that ensures survival of the best B cells (fittest in terms of antigen binding).

B cells that bind antigens in germinal centers with high affinity are selected to survive (Fig. 12-19). The early response to antigen results in the production of antibodies, some of which form complexes with residual antigen and may activate complement. Follicular dendritic cells express receptors for the Fc portions of antibodies and for products of complement activation, including C3b and C3d. These receptors bind and display antigens that are complexed with antibodies and complement products. Antigen may also be displayed in free form in the

germinal center. Meanwhile, germinal center B cells that have undergone somatic mutation migrate into the FDC-rich light zone of the germinal center. These B cells die by apoptosis unless they are rescued by recognition of antigen. B cells with high-affinity receptors for the antigen are best able to bind the antigen when it is present at low concentrations, and these B cells survive preferentially because of several mechanisms. First, antigen recognition by itself induces expression of anti-apoptotic proteins of the Bcl-2 family. Second, high-affinity B cells will preferentially endocytose and present the antigen and interact with the limiting numbers of T_{FH} cells in the germinal center. These helper T cells may signal via CD40L to promote the survival of the B cells with which they interact. Third, some T_{FH} cells express Fas ligand, which can recognize the death receptor Fas on germinal center B cells and deliver an apoptotic signal. High-affinity B cells, which are best able to recognize and respond to antigen, may activate endogenous inhibitors of Fas when their BCRs recognize antigen and thus be protected from death, while low-affinity B cells are killed.

As more antibody is produced, more of the antigen is eliminated and less is available in the germinal centers. Therefore, the B cells that will be able to specifically bind this antigen and to be rescued from death need to express antigen receptors with higher and higher affinity for the antigen. As a result, as the antibody response to an antigen progresses, the B cells that are selected to survive in germinal centers produce Ig of increasing affinity for the antigen. This selection process results in affinity maturation of the antibody response. Because somatic mutation also generates many B cells that do not express high-affinity receptors for antigen and cannot therefore be selected to survive, the germinal centers are sites of tremendous apoptosis.

Somatic mutation occurs in the basal dark zone of germinal centers in B cells called centroblasts, which contain nuclear AID, and these mutated cells may repeatedly cycle between the basal dark zone and the apical light zone, where they differentiate into morphologically distinct cells called centrocytes. Eventually, high-affinity centrocytes may be selected in the light zone by antigen, with help from T_{FH} cells, and may undergo additional isotype switching. The selected cells then either differentiate into memory B cells or into high-affinity antibody-secreting precursors of plasma cells that exit the germinal center.

The DNA breaks associated with somatic hypermutation and isotype switching set the stage for chromosomal translocations of various oncogenes into Ig gene loci, producing tumors of B cells (lymphomas). This explains why many lymphomas develop from germinal center B cells. Germinal centers may also contribute to the pathogenesis of autoimmunity if somatic mutation drives a B cell clone in the germinal center to become strongly self-reactive.

B Cell Differentiation into Antibody-Secreting Plasma Cells

Plasma cells are morphologically distinct, terminally differentiated B cells committed to abundant antibody production (see Chapter 2). They are generated after the activation of B cells through signals from the BCR, CD40, TLRs, and other receptors including cytokine receptors.

There are two types of plasma cells.

- Short-lived plasma cells are generated during T-independent responses and early during T cell–dependent responses in extrafollicular B cell foci, described earlier. These cells are generally found in secondary lymphoid organs and in peripheral non-lymphoid tissues.
- Long-lived plasma cells are generated in T-dependent germinal center responses to protein antigens. Signals from the B cell antigen receptor and IL-21 cooperate in the generation of plasma cells and their precursors, called **plasmablasts**. Plasmablasts are found mainly in

the circulation, where they can be identified as antibody-secreting cells that do not express CD20, a marker of mature B cells. Plasmablasts generated in germinal centers enter the circulation and home to the bone marrow where they differentiate into long-lived plasma cells. These plasma cells are maintained by cytokines of the BAFF family that bind to a plasma cell membrane receptor called BCMA, thus allowing the cells to survive for long periods, often as long as the life span of the host. Typically 2 to 3 weeks after immunization with a T cell–dependent antigen, the bone marrow becomes a major site of antibody production. Plasma cells in the bone marrow may continue to secrete antibodies for months or even years after the antigen is no longer present. These antibodies can provide immediate protection if the antigen is encountered later. It is estimated that almost half the antibody in the blood of a healthy adult is produced by long-lived plasma cells and is specific for antigens that were encountered in the past. Secreted antibodies enter the circulation and mucosal secretions, but mature plasma cells do not recirculate.

The differentiation of B cells into antibody-secreting plasma cells involves major structural alterations in components of the endoplasmic reticulum and secretory pathway, and increased Ig production as well as a change in Ig heavy chains from the membrane to the secreted form. The cell enlarges dramatically, and the ratio of the area of the cytoplasm to the nucleus observed under a microscope (see Fig. 2-8) also undergoes a striking increase. The endoplasmic reticulum becomes prominent, and the cell is transformed into a secretory cell that bears little or no resemblance to a B lymphocyte. Many of these alterations are most striking in the transition from plasmablast to mature plasma cell.

The change in Ig production from the membrane form (characteristic of B cells) to the secreted form (in plasma cells) is the result of changes in the carboxyl terminal of the Ig heavy chain (Fig. 12-20). For instance, in membrane μ, $C_{\mu}4$ is followed by a short spacer, 26 hydrophobic residues, and a cytoplasmic tail of three amino acids (lysine, valine, and lysine). In secreted IgM, on the other hand, the $C_{\mu}4$ domain is followed by a tail piece containing polar amino acids. This transition from membrane to secreted Ig is caused by alternative RNA processing of the heavy chain messenger RNA (mRNA). The primary RNA transcript in all IgM-producing B cells contains the rearranged VDJ cassette, the four C_{μ} exons coding for the constant (C) region domains, and the two exons encoding the transmembrane and cytoplasmic domains. Alternative processing of this transcript, which is regulated by RNA cleavage and the choice of polyadenylation sites, determines whether or not the transmembrane and cytoplasmic exons are included in the mature mRNA. If they are included, the μ chain produced contains the amino acids that make up the transmembrane and cytoplasmic segments and is therefore anchored in the lipid bilayer of the plasma membrane. If, on the other hand, the transmembrane segment is excluded from the μ chain, the carboxyl terminus consists of about 20 amino acids constituting the tail piece. Because this protein does not have a stretch of hydrophobic amino acids or a positively

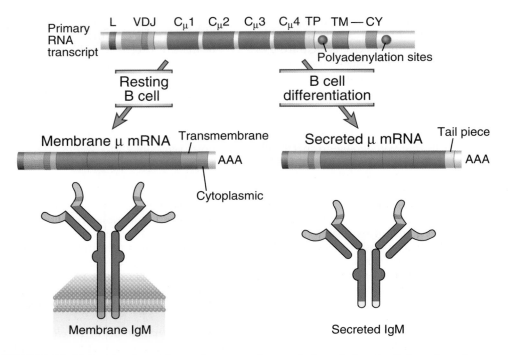

FIGURE 12-20 Production of membrane and secreted μ chains in B lymphocytes. Alternative processing of a primary RNA transcript results in the formation of mRNA for the membrane or secreted form of the μ heavy chain. B cell differentiation results in an increasing fraction of the μ protein produced as the secreted form. TP, TM, and CY refer to tail piece, transmembrane, and cytoplasmic segments, respectively. Cμ1, Cμ2, Cμ3, and Cμ4 are four exons of the Cμ gene.

charged cytoplasmic tail, it cannot remain anchored in the endoplasmic reticulum membrane, and is secreted. Thus, each B cell can synthesize both membrane and secreted Ig. Most of the Ig heavy chain mRNA in a plasma cell is cleaved at the upstream polyadenylation site, so most of this mRNA is of the secretory form. All C_H genes contain similar membrane exons, and all heavy chains can be potentially expressed in membrane-bound and secreted forms. The secretory form of the δ heavy chain is rarely made, however, so that IgD is usually present only as a membrane protein.

Generation of Memory B Cells

Memory B cells are generated during the germinal center reaction and are capable of making rapid responses to subsequent introduction of antigen. Because memory cells are generated mainly in germinal centers, they are seen in T-dependent immune responses and usually emerge in parallel with memory helper T cells. Some of the B cells that are activated in the germinal centers acquire the ability to survive for long periods, apparently without continuing antigenic stimulation. These memory B cells express high levels of the anti-apoptotic protein Bcl-2, which contributes to their long life span. Some memory B cells may remain in the lymphoid organ where they were generated, whereas others exit germinal centers and recirculate between the blood and lymphoid organs. Memory cells typically express high-affinity (mutated) antigen receptors and Ig molecules of switched isotypes more commonly than do naive B lymphocytes. The production of large quantities of isotype-switched,

high-affinity antibodies is greatly accelerated after secondary exposure to antigens, and this can be attributed to the activation of memory cells in germinal centers. Many of the features of secondary antibody responses to protein antigens, and their differences from primary responses (see Fig. 12-2), reflect the differences between responses of memory cells and naive B cells, respectively.

Effective vaccines against microbes and microbial toxins must induce both affinity maturation and memory B cell formation, and these events will occur only if the vaccines are able to activate helper T cells. This concept has been applied to the design of vaccines for some bacterial infections in which the target antigen is a capsular polysaccharide, which is incapable of stimulating T cells. In these cases, the polysaccharide is covalently linked to a foreign protein to form the equivalent of a hapten-carrier conjugate, which does activate helper T cells. Such vaccines, which are called **conjugate vaccines**, more readily induce high-affinity antibodies and memory cells than do polysaccharide vaccines without linked proteins. Conjugate vaccines have proved particularly effective at inducing protective immunity in infants and young children, who are less able to make strong T-independent responses to polysaccharides than are adults.

Role of Transcriptional Regulators in Determining the Fate of Activated B Cells

The outcome of B cell differentiation is regulated by the induction and activation of different transcription factors. It is clear from the discussion so far that activated B cells can follow several fates. They can develop into short-lived or long-lived plasma cells, which secrete large amounts of antibodies, or into long-lived memory cells, which do not secrete antibodies but survive for prolonged periods and respond rapidly to antigen challenge. In Chapter 10, we discussed the concept that T cell fates are determined in large part by the expression of various transcriptional activators and repressors. The same general principle applies to the fates of activated B cells. The major transcription factors involved in determining the fate of germinal center B cells are the following:

- **Bcl-6.** In germinal center B cells, signals delivered through CD40 and the IL-21 receptor induce the expression of Bcl-6, which functions as a transcriptional repressor to maintain the germinal center reaction, particularly the massive proliferation of germinal center B cells. Bcl-6 represses the expression of cyclin-dependent kinase inhibitors and thus cooperates with transcriptional activators such as c-Myb to orchestrate rapid cell cycle entry of germinal center B cells. Bcl-6 also represses p53, a transcription factor that mediates cell cycle arrest and apoptotic cell death after DNA damage. As a result, centroblasts can tolerate the DNA damage that accompanies somatic hypermutation and isotype switching and do not undergo apoptosis. Bcl-6 antagonizes another transcriptional repressor called Blimp-1, which is required for plasma cell development (see below), and thus prevents cells in the germinal center from differentiating into plasma cells during the massive proliferation that is characteristic of the germinal center reaction.
- **Blimp-1 and IRF4.** Blimp-1, a transcriptional repressor, and IRF4, a transcriptional activator, are induced in some of the activated B cells and commit these cells to a plasma cell fate. In addition to suppressing Bcl-6, to maintain the germinal center B cell reaction, Blimp-1 suppresses a second transcription factor, Pax5, which is required for the maintenance of mature B cells. Thus, Blimp-1 is permissive for plasma cell development. IRF4 contributes to the expression of XBP-1, a transcription factor that plays a critical role in the unfolded protein response. XBP-1 protects developing plasma cells from the injurious consequences of unfolded proteins (which are produced as a side effect of the massive increase in protein synthesis) and contributes to the maturation of plasma cells and the enhanced synthesis of Ig seen in these cells.
- The transcription factors that delineate memory B cell development remain to be identified. It appears that some of the progeny of an antigen-stimulated B cell clone express low levels of IRF4, and these become functionally quiescent, self-renewing, long-lived memory cells. Whereas high levels of IRF4 lead to plasma cell differentiation, lower levels of IRF4 are insufficient to drive an activated B cell toward plasma cell differentiation and thus may be permissive for memory B cell generation.

ANTIBODY RESPONSES TO T-INDEPENDENT ANTIGENS

Many non-protein antigens, such as polysaccharides and lipids, stimulate antibody production in the absence of

TABLE 12-2   Properties of Thymus-Dependent and Thymus-Independent Antigens

	Thymus-Dependent Antigen	Thymus-Independent Antigen
Chemical nature	Proteins	Polymeric antigens, especially polysaccharides; also glycolipids, nucleic acids
Features of Antibody Response		
Isotype switching	Yes; IgG, IgE, and IgA	Little or no; may be some IgG and IgA
Affinity maturation	Yes	No
Secondary response (memory B cells)	Yes	Only seen with some antigens (e.g., polysaccharides)

helper T cells, and these antigens and the responses they elicit are termed thymus independent or T independent (TI). These antibody responses differ in several respects from responses to T cell–dependent protein antigens (Table 12-2). The antibodies that are produced in the absence of T cell help are generally of low affinity and consist mainly of IgM, with limited isotype switching to some IgG subtypes and also to IgA.

Subsets of B Cells That Respond to T-Independent Antigens

The marginal zone and B-1 subsets of B cells are especially important for antibody responses to TI antigens. Whereas responses to T-dependent protein antigens are largely mediated by follicular B cells, other B cell subsets may be the primary responders to TI antigens (see Fig. 12-3). Marginal zone B cells are a distinct population of B cells that mainly respond to polysaccharides. After activation, these cells differentiate into short-lived plasma cells that produce mainly IgM. B-1 cells represent another lineage of B cells that responds readily to TI antigens mainly in the peritoneum and in mucosal sites.

T-independent antibody responses may be initiated in the spleen, bone marrow, peritoneal cavity, and mucosal sites. Macrophages located in the marginal zones surrounding lymphoid follicles in the spleen are particularly efficient at trapping polysaccharides when these antigens are injected intravenously. TI antigens may persist for prolonged periods on the surfaces of marginal zone macrophages, where they are recognized by specific B cells.

Mechanisms of T-Independent Antibody Responses

T-independent antigens are capable of stimulating B cell proliferation and differentiation in the absence of T cell help. The most important TI antigens are polysaccharides, glycolipids, and nucleic acids, all of which induce specific antibody production in T cell–deficient animals. These antigens cannot be processed and presented in association with MHC molecules, and therefore they cannot be recognized by CD4+ helper T cells. Most TI antigens are multivalent, being composed of repeated identical antigenic epitopes. Such multivalent antigens may induce maximal cross-linking of the BCR complex on specific B cells, leading to activation without a requirement for cognate T cell help. In addition, many polysaccharides activate the complement system by the alternative pathway, generating C3d, which binds to the antigen and is recognized by CR2, thus augmenting B cell activation (see Fig. 12-5). Membrane proteins at a high density on a microbial surface may be functionally multivalent and may function in a T-independent as well as T-dependent manner. As mentioned earlier, TI responses may also be facilitated by additional signals derived from microbial products that activate TLRs on B cells.

Although TI responses typically show little isotype switching, some T-independent non-protein antigens do induce Ig isotypes other than IgM. In humans, the dominant antibody class induced by pneumococcal capsular polysaccharide is IgG2. In mice engineered to lack CD40, IgE and many IgG subclasses are barely detectable in the serum, but levels of IgG3 (which resembles human IgG2) and IgA in the serum are reduced to only about half their normal levels. Cytokines produced by non–T cells may stimulate isotype switching in TI responses. As described earlier, in the absence of T cells, BAFF and APRIL produced by cells of myeloid origin, such as dendritic cells and macrophages, can induce the synthesis of AID in antigen-activated B cells through a receptor of the BAFF receptor family called TACI. This may be further facilitated by the activation of TLRs on these B cells. In addition, cytokines such as TGF-β that help mediate the IgA switch are secreted by many non-lymphoid cells at mucosal sites and may contribute to the generation of IgA antibodies directed against non-protein antigens (see Chapter 14).

Protection Mediated by T-Independent Antibodies

The practical significance of TI antigens is that many bacterial cell wall polysaccharides belong to this category, and humoral immunity is the major mechanism of host defense against infections by such encapsulated bacteria. For this reason, individuals with congenital or acquired deficiencies of humoral immunity are especially susceptible to life-threatening infections with encapsulated bacteria, such as pneumococcus, meningococcus, and *Haemophilus*.

TI antigens also contribute to the generation of **natural antibodies**, which are present in the circulation of normal individuals and are apparently produced without overt exposure to pathogens. Most natural antibodies are low-affinity anti-carbohydrate antibodies, postulated to be produced by peritoneal B-1 cells stimulated by bacteria that colonize the gastrointestinal tract and by marginal zone B cells in the spleen. A remarkably large proportion of the natural antibodies in humans and mice are specific for oxidized lipids, including phospholipid head groups such as lysophosphatidylcholine and phosphorylcholine, which are found on bacterial membranes and on apoptotic cells but are not exposed on the surface of healthy host cells. Some experimental evidence indicates that the natural antibodies specific for

these phospholipids provide protection against bacterial infections and facilitate the phagocytosis of apoptotic cells. The anti-ABO blood group antibodies, another example of natural antibodies, recognize certain glycolipids (blood group antigens) expressed on the surface of many cell types, including blood cells. Blood group antigens and antibodies are important for blood transfusions and transplantation but not for host defense and are discussed in Chapter 17.

Despite their inability to specifically activate helper T cells, many polysaccharide vaccines, such as the pneumococcal vaccine, induce quite long-lived protective immunity. Rapid and large secondary responses typical of memory (but without much isotype switching or affinity maturation) may also occur on secondary exposure to these carbohydrate antigens.

ANTIBODY FEEDBACK: REGULATION OF HUMORAL IMMUNE RESPONSES BY Fc RECEPTORS

Secreted antibodies inhibit continuing B cell activation by forming antigen-antibody complexes that simultaneously bind to antigen receptors and inhibitory Fcγ receptors on antigen-specific B cells (Fig. 12-21). This is the explanation for a phenomenon called **antibody feedback**, which refers to the downregulation of antibody production by secreted IgG antibodies. IgG antibodies inhibit B cell activation by forming complexes with the antigen, and these complexes bind to a B cell receptor for the Fc portions of the IgG, called the Fcγ receptor II (FcγRIIB, or CD32). (We will discuss Fc receptors in Chapter 13.) The cytoplasmic tail of FcγRIIB contains an immunoreceptor tyrosine-based inhibition motif (ITIM) (see Chapter 7). When the Fcγ receptor of B cells is engaged, the ITIM on the cytosolic tail of the receptor is phosphorylated on tyrosine residues, and it forms a docking site for the inositol 5-phosphatase SHIP (SH2 domain–containing inositol phosphatase). The recruited SHIP hydrolyses a phosphate on the signaling lipid intermediate phosphatidylinositol trisphosphate (PIP_3) and inactivates this molecule. By this mechanism, engagement of FcγRII terminates the B cell response to antigen. The antigen-antibody complexes simultaneously interact with the antigen receptor (through the antigen) and with FcγRIIB (through the antibody), and this brings the inhibitory phosphatases close to the antigen receptors whose signaling is blocked.

Fc receptor–mediated antibody feedback is a physiologic control mechanism in humoral immune responses because it is triggered by secreted antibody and blocks further antibody production. We stated earlier in this chapter that antibodies can also amplify antibody production by activating complement and generating C3d. It is not clear under which circumstances secreted antibodies provide complement-mediated amplification or Fc receptor–mediated inhibition. A likely scenario is that early in humoral immune responses, IgM antibodies (which activate complement but do not bind to the Fcγ receptor) are involved in amplification, whereas increasing production of IgG leads to feedback inhibition.

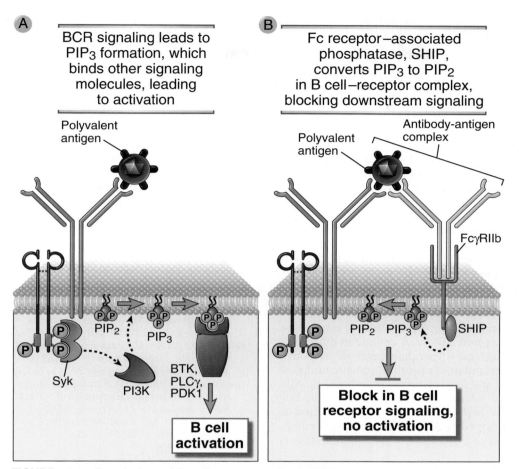

FIGURE 12-21 Regulation of B cell activation by FcγRIIB. A, Antigen-antibody complexes can simultaneously bind to membrane Ig (through antigen) and the FcγRIIB receptor through the Fc portion of the antibody. **B,** As a consequence of this simultaneous ligation of receptors, phosphatases associated with the cytoplasmic tail of the FcγRIIB inhibit signaling by the BCR complex and block B cell activation.

The importance of FcγRIIB-mediated inhibition is demonstrated by the uncontrolled antibody production seen in mice in which the gene encoding this receptor has been knocked out. A polymorphism in the *FcγRIIB* gene has been linked to susceptibility to the autoimmune disease systemic lupus erythematosus in humans.

B cells express another inhibitory receptor called CD22, which is a sialic acid–binding lectin; its natural ligand is not known, nor is it known exactly how CD22 is engaged during physiologic B cell responses. However, knockout mice lacking CD22 show greatly enhanced B cell activation. The cytoplasmic tail of this molecule contains ITIM tyrosine residues, which, when phosphorylated by the Src family kinase Lyn, bind the SH2 domain of the tyrosine phosphatase SHP-1. SHP-1 removes phosphates from the tyrosine residues of several enzymes and adaptor proteins involved in BCR signaling and thus abrogates B cell activation. A mouse strain called *motheaten*, which develops severe autoimmunity with uncontrolled B cell activation and autoantibody production, has a naturally occurring mutation in SHP-1. Conditional deletion of SHP-1 as well as the engineered loss of Lyn in B cells leads to a breakdown of peripheral B cell tolerance and the development of autoimmunity.

SUMMARY

* In humoral immune responses, B lymphocytes are activated by antigen and secrete antibodies that act to eliminate the antigen. Both protein and non-protein antigens can stimulate antibody responses. B cell responses to protein antigens require the contribution of CD4+ helper T cells specific for the antigen.

* Helper T cell–dependent B cell responses to protein antigens require initial activation of naive T cells in the T cell zones and of B cells in lymphoid follicles in lymphoid organs. The activated lymphocytes migrate toward one another and interact at the edges of follicles, where the B cells present the antigen to helper T cells.

* Activated helper T cells express CD40L, which engages CD40 on the B cells, and the T cells secrete cytokines that bind to cytokine receptors on the B cells. The combination of CD40 and cytokine signals stimulates B cell proliferation and differentiation.

* Stimulation of activated B cells at extrafollicular sites by helper T cells leads to the formation of

extrafollicular foci where some isotype switching occurs and short-lived plasma cells are generated.

* Some activated helper T cells differentiate into specialized T$_{FH}$ cells that express high levels of ICOS and CXCR5 and secrete IL-21. T$_{FH}$ cells and activated B cells migrate into the follicle, and T$_{FH}$ cells activate these specific B cells to initiate the formation of germinal centers. The late events in T cell–dependent antibody responses, including extensive isotype switching, somatic mutation, affinity maturation, generation of memory B cells, and induction of long-lived plasma cells, take place within germinal centers.

* Helper T cell–derived signals, including CD40L and cytokines, induce isotype switching in B cells by a process of switch recombination, leading to the production of various Ig isotypes. Isotype switching requires the induction of AID, a cytidine deaminase that converts cytosine to uracil in single-stranded DNA, and different cytokines allow AID to access distinct downstream heavy chain loci.

* Affinity maturation occurs in germinal centers and leads to increased affinity of antibodies during the course of a T cell–dependent humoral response. Affinity maturation is a result of somatic mutation of Ig heavy and light chain genes induced by AID, followed by selective survival of the B cells that produce the high-affinity antibodies and bind to antigen displayed by FDCs in the germinal centers. T$_{FH}$ cells also participate in selection of high-affinity B cells.

* Some of the progeny of germinal center B cells differentiate into antibody-secreting plasma cells that migrate to the bone marrow. Other progeny become memory B cells that live for long periods, recirculate between lymph nodes and spleen, and respond rapidly to subsequent exposures to antigen by differentiating into high-affinity antibody secretors. The expression of various transcription factors controls the differentiation of activated B cells into plasma cells or memory cells.

* T-independent (TI) antigens are generally non-protein antigens that induce humoral immune responses without the involvement of helper T cells. Many TI antigens, including polysaccharides, membrane glycolipids, and nucleic acids, are multivalent, can cross-link multiple membrane Ig molecules on a B cell, and activate complement, thereby activating the B cells without T cell help. TLR activation on B cells by microbial products facilitates T-independent B cell activation. TI antigens stimulate antibody responses in which there is limited heavy chain class switching, affinity maturation, or memory B cell generation because these features are largely dependent on helper T cells, which are not activated by non-protein antigens. However, some T-independent isotype switching can be induced by TLR stimulation by microbes, which may lead to the production of cytokines of the TNF family that activate B cells to induce AID.

* Antibody feedback is a mechanism by which humoral immune responses are downregulated when enough antibody has been produced and soluble antibody-antigen complexes are present. B cell membrane Ig and the receptor on B cells for the Fc portions of IgG, called FcγRIIB, are clustered together by antibody-antigen complexes. This activates an inhibitory signaling cascade through the cytoplasmic tail of FcγRIIB that terminates the activation of the B cell.

SELECTED READINGS

B Cell Subsets and B Cell Activation

Cerutti A, Cols M, Puga I: Marginal zone B cells: virtues of innate-like antibody-producing lymphocytes, *Nature Reviews Immunology* 13:118–132, 2013.

Gonzalez SF, Degn SE, Pitcher LA, Woodruff M, Heesters BA, Carroll MC: Trafficking of B cell antigen in lymph nodes, *Annual Review of Immunology* 29:215–233, 2011.

Goodnow CC, Vinuesa CG, Randall KL, Mackay F, Brink R: Control systems and decision making for antibody production, *Nature Immunology* 11:681–688, 2010.

Martin F, Chan AC: B cell immunobiology in disease: evolving concept from the clinic, *Annual Review of Immunology* 24:467–496, 2006.

Mauri C, Bosma A: Immune regulatory function of B cells, *Annual Review of immunology* 30:221–241, 2012.

Rickert RC: New insights into pre-BCR and BCR signalling with relevance to B cell malignancies, *Nature Reviews Immunology* 13:578–591, 2013.

Yuseff MI, Pierobon P, Reversat A, Lennon-Dumenil AM: How B cells capture, process and present antigens: a crucial role for cell polarity, *Nature Reviews Immunology* 13:475–486, 2013.

T Follicular Helper Cells and the Germinal Center Reaction

Crotty S: Follicular helper CD4 T cells, *Annual Review of Immunology* 29:621–663, 2011.

Crotty S, Johnston RJ, Schoenberger SP: Effectors and memories: Bcl-6 and Blimp-1 in T and B lymphocyte differentiation, *Nature Immunology* 11:114–120, 2010.

McHeyzer-Williams M, Okitsu S, Wang N, McHeyzer-Williams L: Molecular programming of B cell memory, *Nature Reviews Immunology* 12:24–34, 2012.

Tangye SG, Ma CS, Brink R, Deenick EK: The good, the bad and the ugly - T$_{FH}$ cells in human health and disease, *Nature Reviews Immunology* 13:412–426, 2013.

Victora GD, Nussenzweig MC: Germinal centers, *Annual Review of Immunology* 30:429–457, 2012.

Vinuesa CG, Sanz I, Cook MC: Dysregulation of germinal centres in autoimmune disease, *Nature Reviews Immunology* 9:845–857, 2009.

AID, Class Switching, and Somatic Mutation

Cerutti A: The regulation of IgA class switching, *Nature Reviews Immunology* 8:421–434, 2008.

Delker RK, Fugmann S, Papavasiliou FN: A coming-of-age story: activation-induced cytidine deaminase turns 10, *Nature Immunology* 10:1147–1153, 2009.

Kato L, Stanlie A, Begum NA, Kobayashi M, Aida M, Honjo T: An evolutionary view of the mechanism for immune and genome diversityn, *Journal of Immunology* 188:3559–3566, 2012.

Liu M, Schatz DG: Balancing AID and DNA repair during somatic hypermutation, *Trends in Immunology* 30:173–181, 2009.

Neuberger MS: Antibody diversification by somatic mutation: from Burnet onwards, *Immunology and Cell Biology* 86:124–132, 2008.

Peled JU, Kuang FL, Iglesias-Ussel MD, Roa S, Kalis SL, Goodman MF, Scharff MD: The biochemistry of somatic hypermutation, *Annual Review of Immunology* 26:481–511, 2008.

Stavnezer J, Guikema JE, Schrader CE: Mechanism and regulation of class switch recombination, *Annual Review of Immunology* 26:261–292, 2008.

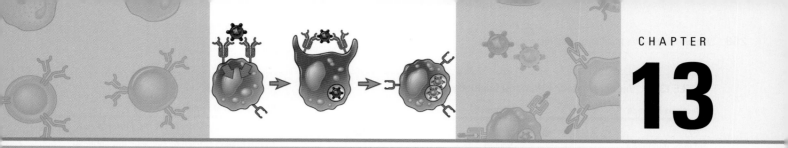

Effector Mechanisms of Humoral Immunity

Humoral immunity is mediated by secreted antibodies, and its physiologic function is defense against extracellular microbes and microbial toxins. This type of immunity contrasts with cell-mediated immunity, the other effector arm of the adaptive immune system, which is mediated by T lymphocytes and functions to eradicate microbes that infect and live within host cells (see Chapters 10 and 11). Humoral immunity is the form of immunity that can be transferred from immunized to naive individuals with serum. The types of microorganisms that are combated by humoral immunity are extracellular bacteria, fungi, and even obligate intracellular microbes such as viruses, which are targets of antibodies before they infect cells or when they are released from infected cells. Defects in antibody production result in increased susceptibility to infection with many microbes, including bacteria, fungi, and viruses. Currently used vaccines induce protection primarily by stimulating the production of antibodies

(Table 13-1). Apart from their crucial protective roles, antibodies can be harmful and mediate tissue injury in allergic individuals and in certain autoimmune diseases. In this chapter, we will discuss the effector mechanisms that are used by antibodies to eliminate antigens. The structure of antibodies is described in Chapter 5 and the process of antibody production in Chapter 12.

OVERVIEW OF HUMORAL IMMUNITY

Before we discuss the principal mechanisms by which antibodies provide protection against microbes, we will summarize some of the salient features of antibody-mediated host defense.

- ***The main functions of antibodies are to neutralize and eliminate infectious microbes and microbial toxins*** (Fig. 13-1). As we will see later, antibody-mediated elimination of antigens involves a number of effector mechanisms and requires the participation of various cellular and humoral components of the immune system, including phagocytes and complement proteins.
- ***Antibodies are produced by plasma cells in secondary lymphoid organs and bone marrow, and antibodies perform their effector functions at sites distant from their production.*** Antibodies produced in the lymph nodes, spleen, and bone marrow may enter the blood and then circulate throughout the body. Antibodies produced in mucosa-associated lymphoid tissues are transported across epithelial barriers into the lumens of mucosal organs, such as the intestine and the airways, where these secreted antibodies block the entry of ingested and inhaled microbes (see Chapter 14). Antibodies are also actively transported across the placenta into the circulation of the developing fetus. Occasionally, antibodies may be produced in peripheral non-lymphoid tissues, at sites of infection or chronic inflammation. In cell-mediated immunity, activated T lymphocytes are able to migrate to peripheral sites of infection and inflammation, but they are not transported into mucosal secretions or across the placenta.
- ***The antibodies that mediate protective immunity may be derived from short-lived or long-lived antibody-producing***

TABLE 13-1   Vaccine-Induced Humoral Immunity

Infectious Disease	Vaccine*	Mechanism of Protective Immunity
Polio	Oral attenuated poliovirus	Neutralization of virus by mucosal IgA antibody
Tetanus, diphtheria	Toxoids	Neutralization of toxin by systemic IgG antibody
Hepatitis A or B	Recombinant viral envelope proteins	Neutralization of virus by mucosal IgA or systemic IgG antibody
Pneumococcal pneumonia, Haemophilus	Conjugate vaccines composed of bacterial capsular polysaccharide attached to a carrier protein	Opsonization and phagocytosis mediated by IgM and IgG antibodies, directly or secondary to complement activation

*Selected examples of vaccines that work by stimulating protective humoral immunity are listed.

plasma cells. The first exposure to an antigen, either by infection or by vaccination, leads to the activation of naive B lymphocytes and their differentiation into antibody-secreting plasma cells and memory cells (see Chapter 12). Subsequent exposure to the same antigens leads to the activation of memory B cells and a larger and more rapid antibody response. Plasma cells generated early in an immune response or from marginal zone B cells or B-1 cells in T-independent immune responses tend to be short-lived. In contrast, class-switched, high-affinity antibody-secreting plasma cells, which are produced in germinal centers during T-dependent responses to protein antigens, migrate to the bone marrow and persist at this site, where they continue to produce antibodies for years after the antigen is eliminated. Much of the immunoglobulin G (IgG) found in the serum of normal individuals is derived from these long-lived plasma cells that were induced by the responses of naive and memory B cells to various antigens throughout the life of the individual. If an immune individual is exposed to a previously encountered microbe, the level of circulating antibody produced by the long-lived plasma cells provides immediate protection against the infection. At the same time, activation of memory B cells generates a larger burst of antibody that provides a second and more effective wave of protection.

- *Many of the effector functions of antibodies are mediated by the heavy chain constant regions of Ig molecules, and different Ig heavy chain isotypes serve distinct*

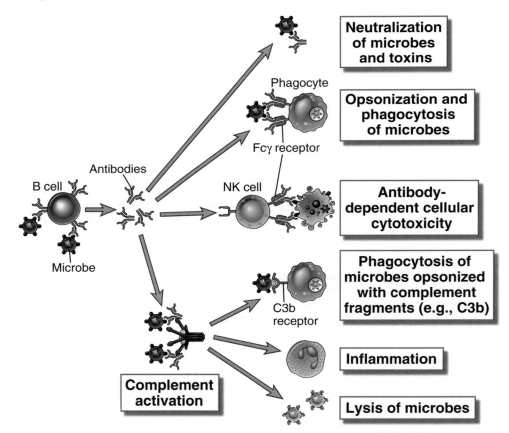

FIGURE 13-1 Effector functions of antibodies. Antibodies against microbes (and their toxins, not shown) neutralize these agents, opsonize them for phagocytosis, sensitize them for antibody-dependent cellular cytotoxicity, and activate the complement system. These various effector functions may be mediated by different antibody isotypes.

TABLE 13-2 Functions of Antibody Isotypes

Antibody Isotype	Isotype-Specific Effector Functions
IgG	Opsonization of antigens for phagocytosis by macrophages and neutrophils
	Activation of the classical pathway of complement
	Antibody-dependent cell-mediated cytotoxicity mediated by natural killer cells
	Neonatal immunity: transfer of maternal antibody across the placenta and gut
	Feedback inhibition of B cell activation
IgM	Activation of the classical pathway of complement
	Antigen receptor of naive B lymphocytes*
IgA	Mucosal immunity: secretion of IgA into the lumens of the gastrointestinal and respiratory tracts
IgE	Mast cell degranulation (immediate hypersensitivity reactions)
IgD	Antigen receptor of naive B lymphocytes*

*These functions are mediated by membrane-bound and not secreted antibodies.

effector functions (Table 13-2). For instance, some IgG subclasses (IgG1 and IgG3) bind to phagocyte Fc receptors and promote the phagocytosis of antibody-coated particles; IgM and some subclasses of IgG (IgG1, IgG2, and IgG3 but not IgG4) activate the complement system; and IgE binds to the Fc receptors of mast cells and triggers their activation. Each of these effector mechanisms will be discussed later in this chapter. The humoral immune system is specialized in such a way that different microbes or antigen exposures stimulate B cell switching to the Ig isotypes that are best for combating these microbes. The major stimuli for isotype switching during the process of B cell activation are cytokines together with CD40 ligand expressed by activated follicular helper T cells (see Chapter 12). Neutralization is the only function of antibodies that is mediated entirely by binding of antigen and does not require participation of the Ig constant regions.

- *Although many effector functions of antibodies are mediated by the Ig heavy chain constant regions, all these functions are triggered by the binding of antigens to the variable regions.* The binding of antibodies to a multivalent antigen, such as a polysaccharide or a repeated epitope on a microbial surface, brings the Fc regions of antibodies close together, and this clustering of antibody molecules leads to complement activation and allows the antibodies to bind to and activate Fc receptors on phagocytes. The requirement for antigen binding ensures that antibodies activate various effector mechanisms only when they are needed, that is, when the antibodies encounter and specifically bind antigens, not when the antibodies are circulating in an antigen-free form.

With this introduction to humoral immunity, we proceed to a discussion of the various functions of antibodies in host defense.

NEUTRALIZATION OF MICROBES AND MICROBIAL TOXINS

Antibodies against microbes and microbial toxins block the binding of these microbes and toxins to cellular receptors (Fig. 13-2). In this way, antibodies inhibit, or neutralize, the infectivity of microbes as well as the potential injurious effects of microbial toxins. Many microbes enter host cells by the binding of particular microbial surface molecules to membrane proteins or lipids on the surface of host cells. For example, influenza viruses use their envelope hemagglutinin to infect respiratory epithelial cells, and Gram-negative bacteria use pili to attach to and infect a variety of host cells. Antibodies that bind to these microbial structures interfere with the ability of the microbes to interact with cellular receptors by means of steric hindrance and may thus prevent infection. In some cases, antibodies may bind to a microbe and induce conformational changes in surface molecules that prevent the microbe from interacting with cellular receptors; such interactions are examples of the allosteric effects of antibodies. Many microbial toxins mediate their pathologic effects also by binding to specific cellular receptors. For instance, tetanus toxin binds to receptors in the motor end plate of neuromuscular junctions and inhibits neuromuscular transmission, which leads to paralysis, and diphtheria toxin binds to cellular receptors and enters various cells, where it inhibits protein synthesis. Antibodies against such toxins sterically hinder the interactions of toxins with host cells and thus prevent the toxins from causing tissue injury and disease.

Antibody-mediated neutralization of microbes and toxins requires only the antigen-binding regions of the antibodies. Therefore, such neutralization may be mediated by antibodies of any isotype in the circulation and in mucosal secretions and can experimentally also be mediated by Fab or F(ab')$_2$ fragments of specific antibodies, which lack the Fc regions of the heavy chains. Most neutralizing antibodies in the blood are of the IgG isotype; in mucosal organs, they are largely of the IgA isotype. The most effective neutralizing antibodies are those with high affinities for their antigens. High-affinity antibodies are produced by the process of affinity maturation (see Chapter 12). Many prophylactic vaccines work by stimulating the production of high-affinity neutralizing antibodies (see Table 13-1). A mechanism that microbes have developed to evade host immunity is to mutate the genes encoding surface antigens that are the targets of neutralizing antibodies (see Chapter 16).

ANTIBODY-MEDIATED OPSONIZATION AND PHAGOCYTOSIS

Antibodies of the IgG isotype coat (opsonize) microbes and promote their phagocytosis by binding to Fc receptors on phagocytes. Mononuclear phagocytes and neutrophils

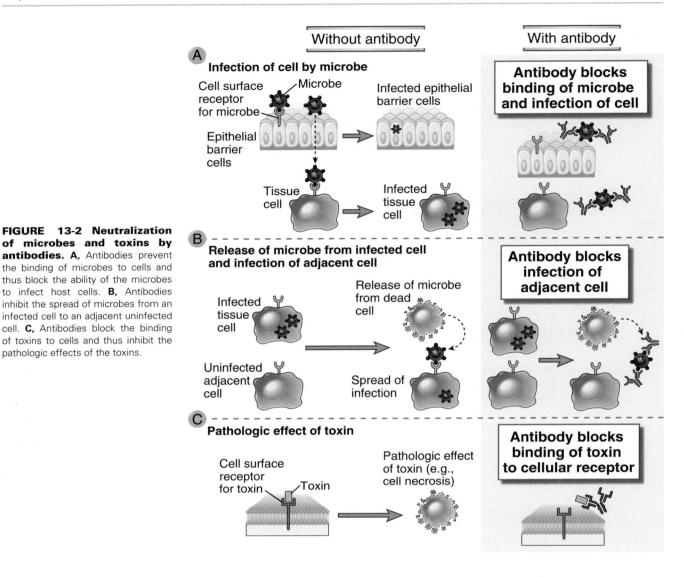

FIGURE 13-2 Neutralization of microbes and toxins by antibodies. A, Antibodies prevent the binding of microbes to cells and thus block the ability of the microbes to infect host cells. **B,** Antibodies inhibit the spread of microbes from an infected cell to an adjacent uninfected cell. **C,** Antibodies block the binding of toxins to cells and thus inhibit the pathologic effects of the toxins.

ingest microbes as a prelude to intracellular killing and degradation. These phagocytes express a variety of surface receptors that directly bind microbes and ingest them, even without antibodies, providing one mechanism of innate immunity (see Chapter 4). The efficiency of this process is markedly enhanced if the phagocyte can bind the particle with high affinity. Mononuclear phagocytes and neutrophils express receptors for the Fc portions of IgG antibodies that specifically bind antibody-coated particles. Microbes may also be coated by a product of complement activation called C3b and are phagocytosed by binding to a leukocyte receptor for C3b (described later in this chapter). The process of coating particles to promote phagocytosis is called **opsonization**, and substances that perform this function, including antibodies and complement proteins, are called **opsonins**.

Leukocyte Fc Receptors

Leukocytes express Fc receptors that bind to the constant regions of antibodies, and thereby promote the phagocytosis of Ig-coated particles and deliver signals that regulate the activities of the leukocytes; other Fc receptors mediate the transport of antibodies to various sites. Fc receptors for different Ig heavy chain isotypes are expressed on many leukocyte populations and serve diverse functions in immunity. Of these Fc receptors, the ones that are most important for phagocytosis of opsonized particles are receptors for the heavy chains of IgG antibodies, called Fcγ receptors, and these are the receptors that will be primarily considered in this chapter. In Chapter 20, we will discuss the Fc receptors that bind to IgE. In Chapter 5, we described the neonatal Fc receptor (FcRn), which is expressed in the placenta, and on vascular endothelium and other cell types. In Chapter 14, we will discuss the poly-Ig receptor, which is involved in the transcytosis of IgA and IgM.

Fcγ receptors have been classified into three groups, I, II and III, based on their affinities for heavy chains of different IgG subclasses. Different Fc receptors are also expressed on different cell types (Table 13-3). In general, IgG1- and IgG3-containing immune complexes bind efficiently to activating Fc receptors and IgG2-containing complexes do not bind well. IgG4 has a very

TABLE 13-3   Fc Receptors

FcR	Affinity for Immunoglobulin	Cell Distribution	Function
FcγRI (CD64)	High ($K_d < 10^{-9}$ M); binds IgG1 and IgG3, can bind monomeric IgG	Macrophages, neutrophils; also eosinophils	Phagocytosis; activation of phagocytes
FcγRIIA (CD32)	Low ($K_d > 10^{-7}$ M)	Macrophages, neutrophils; eosinophils, platelets	Phagocytosis; cell activation
FcγRIIB (CD32)	Low ($K_d > 10^{-7}$ M)	B lymphocytes, macrophages, dendritic cells, other cells	Feedback inhibition of various cellular responses
FcγRIIC (CD32)	Low ($K_d > 10^{-7}$ M)	Macrophages, neutrophils, NK cells	Phagocytosis, cell activation
FcγRIIIA (CD16)	Low ($K_d > 10^{-6}$ M)	NK cells	Antibody-dependent cell-mediated cytotoxicity
FcγRIIIB (CD16)	Low ($K_d > 10^{-6}$ M); GPI-linked protein	Neutrophils	Phagocytosis (inefficient)
FcεRI	High ($K_d > 10^{-10}$ M); binds monomeric IgE	Mast cells, basophils, eosinophils	Cell activation (degranulation)
FcεRII (CD23)	Low ($K_d > 10^{-7}$ M)	B lymphocytes, eosinophils, Langerhans cells	Unknown
FcαR (CD89)	Low ($K_d > 10^{-6}$ M)	Neutrophils, eosinophils, monocytes	Cell activation?

GPI, glycophosphatidylinositol; *NK,* natural killer.

low affinity for activating Fc receptors and the biological function of this antibody isotype is poorly understood. The engagement of most Fc receptors results in cellular activation, except for FcγRIIB, which is an inhibitory receptor. All Fcγ receptors contain a ligand-binding chain, called the α chain, that recognizes IgG heavy chains. Differences in specificities or affinities of each FcγR for the various IgG isotypes are based on differences in the structure of these α chains. All Fc receptors are optimally activated by antibodies bound to their antigens and not by free, circulating antibodies. In all of the FcRs except FcγRII, the α chain is associated with one or more additional polypeptide chains involved in signal transduction (Fig. 13-3). Signaling functions of FcγRII are mediated by the cytoplasmic tail of this single chain receptor.

The three major groups of IgG-specific Fc receptors have multiple isoforms that may differ in structure and function (see Table 13-3); these are described below. The FcRn has a unique function and was discussed in Chapter 5.

- **FcγRI** (CD64) is the major phagocyte Fcγ receptor. It is expressed on macrophages and neutrophils and binds IgG1 and IgG3 with high affinity (K_d of 10^{-8} to 10^{-9} M). (In mice, FcγRI preferentially binds IgG2a and IgG2b/2c antibodies.) The large extracellular amino-terminal region of the Fc-binding α chain folds into three tandem Ig-like domains. The α chain of FcγRI is associated with a disulfide-linked homodimer of a signaling protein called the FcR γ chain. This γ chain is also found in the signaling complexes associated with FcγRIII, FcαR, and FcεRI. The γ chain has only a short extracellular amino terminus but a large cytoplasmic carboxyl terminus, which is structurally homologous to the ζ chain of the T cell receptor (TCR) complex. Like the TCR ζ chain, the FcR γ chain contains an immunoreceptor tyrosine-based activation motif (ITAM) that couples receptor clustering to activation of protein tyrosine kinases. FcγRI, like

the high-affinity receptor for IgE (see Chapter 20), is constantly saturated with its Ig ligands. Triggering of Fc receptors requires that receptors be clustered in the plane of the membrane, and clustering and consequent activation by FcγRI are mediated by the cross-linking of receptor-bound IgG molecules by multivalent antigens.

Transcription of the *FcγRI* gene and expression of FcγRI on macrophages are stimulated by interferon-γ (IFN-γ). The antibody isotypes that bind best to Fcγ receptors (such as IgG2a in mice) are also produced in part as a result of IFN-γ–mediated isotype switching of B cells. In addition, IFN-γ directly stimulates the microbicidal activities of phagocytes (see Chapter 11).

- **FcγRII** (CD32) binds human IgG subtypes (IgG1 and IgG3) with a low affinity (K_d 10^{-6} M). In humans, gene duplication and diversification have resulted in the generation of three forms, called FcγRII A, B, and C. These isoforms have similar extracellular domains and ligand specificities but differ in cytoplasmic tail structure, cell distribution, and functions. FcγRIIA is expressed by neutrophils and mononuclear phagocytes and participates in the phagocytosis of opsonized particles, while FcγRIIC is expressed in mononuclear phagocytes, neutrophils, and NK cells. The cytoplasmic tails of FcγRIIA and FcγRIIC contain ITAMs and, on clustering by IgG1- or IgG3-coated particles or cells, can deliver an activation signal to phagocytes. FcγRIIB is an inhibitory receptor expressed on myeloid cells and B cells and is the only Fc receptor on B cells. Its function is described later.

- **FcγRIII** (CD16) is also a low-affinity receptor for IgG. The extracellular ligand-binding portion of FcγRIII is similar to FcγRII in structure, affinity, and specificity for IgG. This receptor exists in two forms, encoded by separate genes. The FcγRIIIA isoform is a transmembrane protein expressed mainly on NK cells. FcγRIIIA associates with homodimers of the FcR γ chain, homodimers of the TCR ζ chain, or heterodimers

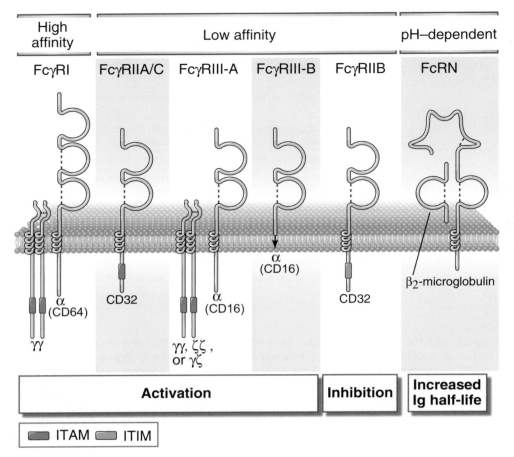

FIGURE 13-3 Subunit composition of Fcγ receptors. Schematic models of the different human Fc receptors illustrate the Fc-binding α chains and the signaling subunits. FcγRIII-B is a glycophosphatidylinositol anchored membrane protein with no known signaling functions. FcγRIIA and IIC are structurally similar low-affinity activating receptors with slightly different patterns of expression. Note that although FcγRIIA/C and FcγRIIB are both designated CD32, they are different proteins with distinct functions (see text). The neonatal FcR (FcRn) resembles class I MHC molecules structurally but does not have a peptide-binding cleft.

composed of the FcR γ chain and the ζ chain. This association is necessary for the cell surface expression and function of these FcRs because intracellular activating signals are delivered through the ITAMs in these signaling chains. The FcγRIIIB isoform is a glycophosphatidylinositol (GPI)–linked protein expressed on neutrophils; it does not mediate phagocytosis or trigger neutrophil activation, and its function is poorly understood.

In addition to these Fcγ receptors, there are receptors for the heavy chains of IgE and IgA (see Table 13-3). We will describe FcεRI in Chapter 20, in the context of mast cell activation. The function of FcαR is not well established.

Role of Fcγ Receptors in Phagocytosis and Activation of Phagocytes

Binding of Fc receptors on phagocytes to multivalent antibody-coated particles leads to engulfment of the particles and the activation of phagocytes (Fig. 13-4). The IgG subtypes that bind best to these receptors (IgG1 and IgG3) are the most efficient opsonins for promoting phagocytosis. As discussed earlier, FcγRI (CD64) is the high-affinity Fcγ receptor on phagocytic cells, and it is the most important receptor for phagocytosis of opsonized particles.

Opsonized particles are internalized into vesicles known as phagosomes, which fuse with lysosomes, and the phagocytosed particles are destroyed in these phagolysosomes. Activation requires cross-linking of the FcRs by several adjacent Ig molecules (e.g., on antibody-coated microbes or in immune complexes). Cross-linking of the ligand-binding α chains of an FcR results in signal transduction events that are similar to those that occur after antigen receptor cross-linking in lymphocytes (see Chapter 7). These include Src kinase–mediated tyrosine phosphorylation of the ITAMs in the signaling chains of the FcRs; SH2 domain–mediated recruitment of Syk family kinases to the ITAMs; activation of phosphatidylinositol 3-kinase; recruitment of adaptor molecules, including SLP-76 and BLNK; and recruitment of enzymes such as phospholipase Cγ and Tec family kinases. These events lead to generation of inositol trisphosphate and diacylglycerol and sustained calcium mobilization.

These signaling pathways induce a number of responses in leukocytes, including transcription of genes encoding cytokines, inflammatory mediators and microbicidal enzymes, and mobilization of the cytoskeleton leading to phagocytosis, granule exocytosis, and cell migration. The major microbiocidal substances produced in the activated phagocytes are reactive oxygen species, nitric oxide, and hydrolytic enzymes. These are the same substances produced by phagocytes activated in innate immune responses, discussed in Chapter 4. The same microbicidal substances may damage tissues; this mechanism of antibody-mediated tissue injury is important

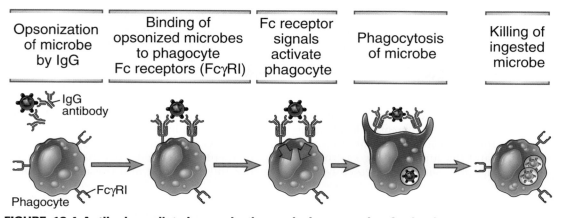

FIGURE 13-4 Antibody-mediated opsonization and phagocytosis of microbes. Antibodies of certain IgG subclasses bind to microbes and are then recognized by Fc receptors on phagocytes. Signals from the Fc receptors promote the phagocytosis of the opsonized microbes and activate the phagocytes to destroy these microbes. The microbicidal mechanisms of phagocytes are described in Chapters 4 (see Fig. 4-13) and 10 (see Fig. 10-7).

in hypersensitivity diseases (see Chapter 19). Knockout mice lacking the ligand-binding α chain of FcγRI or the signal-transducing FcR γ chain are defective in antibody-mediated defense against microbes and do not develop some forms of IgG antibody-mediated tissue injury, thus demonstrating the essential role of Fc receptors in these processes.

Inhibitory Signaling by the FcγRIIB Receptor

The FcγRIIB receptor is an inhibitory Fc receptor that was described earlier in the context of inhibitory signaling in B cells and the phenomenon of antibody feedback (see Chapter 12). FcγRIIB is also expressed on dendritic cells, neutrophils, macrophages, and mast cells and may play a role in regulating the responses of these cells to activating Fc receptors and other stimuli. A somewhat empirical but often useful treatment of many auto immune diseases is the intravenous administration of pooled human IgG, called intravenous immunoglobulin (IVIG). IVIG may both increase the expression of FcγRIIB and bind to the receptor and deliver inhibitory signals to B lymphocytes and other cells, thus reducing antibody production and dampening inflammation. Another mechanism by which IVIG may ameliorate disease is by competing with circulating autoantibodies for the neonatal Fc receptor, which results in enhanced clearance of the autoantibodies (see Chapter 5).

Antibody-Dependent Cell-Mediated Cytotoxicity

Natural killer (NK) cells and other leukocytes bind to antibody-coated cells by Fc receptors and destroy these cells. This process is called antibody-dependent cell-mediated cytotoxicity (ADCC) (Fig. 13-5). It was first described as a function of NK cells, which use their Fc receptor, FcγRIIIA, to bind to antibody-coated cells. FcγRIIIA (CD16) is a low-affinity receptor that binds clustered IgG molecules displayed on cell surfaces but does not bind circulating monomeric IgG. Therefore, ADCC occurs only when the target cell is coated with antibody molecules, and free IgG in plasma neither activates NK cells nor competes effectively with

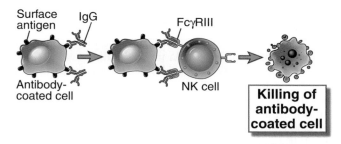

FIGURE 13-5 Antibody-dependent cell-mediated cytotoxicity. Antibodies of certain IgG subclasses bind to cells (e.g., infected cells), and the Fc regions of the bound antibodies are recognized by an Fcγ receptor on NK cells. The NK cells are activated and kill the antibody-coated cells.

cell-bound IgG for binding to FcγRIII. Engagement of FcγRIII by antibody-coated target cells activates the NK cells to synthesize and secrete cytokines such as IFN-γ as well as to discharge the contents of their granules, which mediate the killing functions of this cell type (see Chapter 4). ADCC can be readily demonstrated in vitro, but its role in host defense against microbes is not definitively established. It is likely an important mechanism for the elimination of cells that are coated by certain therapeutic monoclonal antibodies, such as B cells and B cell–derived tumor cells that are targeted by anti-CD20 antibody.

Antibody-Mediated Clearance of Helminths

Antibodies, eosinophils, and mast cells function together to mediate the killing and expulsion of some helminthic parasites. Helminths (worms) are too large to be engulfed by phagocytes, and their integuments are relatively resistant to the microbicidal products of neutrophils and macrophages. They can, however, be killed by a toxic cationic protein, known as the major basic protein, present in the granules of eosinophils. IgE antibodies and, to a lesser extent, IgG and IgA antibodies that coat helminths can bind to Fc receptors on eosinophils and cause the degranulation of these cells, releasing the basic protein and other eosinophil granule contents that kill the parasites. The high-affinity Fcε receptor of eosinophils (FcεRI) lacks the signaling β chain and can signal only through the associated γ chain. In addition to activating eosinophils, IgE antibodies that recognize antigens on the surface of the helminths may initiate local mast cell degranulation through the high-affinity IgE receptor (see Chapter 20). Mast cell mediators may induce bronchoconstriction and increased local motility, contributing to the expulsion of worms from sites such as the airways and the lumen of the gastrointestinal tract. Chemokines and cytokines released by activated mast cells may attract eosinophils and cause their degranulation as well.

THE COMPLEMENT SYSTEM

The complement system is one of the major effector mechanisms of humoral immunity and is also an important effector mechanism of innate immunity. We briefly discussed the role of complement in innate immunity in Chapter 4. Here we will describe the activation and regulation of complement in more detail.

The name *complement* is derived from experiments performed by Jules Bordet shortly after the discovery of antibodies. He demonstrated that if fresh serum containing an antibacterial antibody is added to the bacteria at physiologic temperature (37°C), the bacteria are lysed. If, however, the serum is heated to 56°C or more, it loses its lytic capacity. This loss of lytic capacity is not due to decay of antibody activity because antibodies are relatively heat stable, and even heated serum is capable of agglutinating the bacteria. Bordet concluded that the serum must contain another heat-labile component that assists, or complements, the lytic function of antibodies, and this component was later given the name **complement**.

The complement system consists of serum and cell surface proteins that interact with one another and with other molecules of the immune system in a highly regulated manner to generate products that function to eliminate microbes. Complement proteins are plasma proteins that are normally inactive; they are activated only under particular conditions to generate products that mediate various effector functions of complement. Several features of complement activation are essential for its normal function.

- *The complement system is activated by microbes and by antibodies that are attached to microbes and other antigens.* The mechanisms of initial activation are described later.
- *Activation of complement involves the sequential proteolysis of proteins to generate enzyme complexes with proteolytic activity.* Proteins that acquire proteolytic enzymatic activity by the action of other proteases are called zymogens. The process of sequential zymogen activation, a defining feature of a proteolytic enzyme cascade, is also characteristic of the coagulation and kinin systems. Proteolytic cascades allow tremendous amplification because each enzyme molecule activated at one step can generate multiple activated enzyme molecules at the next step.

- *The products of complement activation become covalently attached to microbial cell surfaces, to antibodies bound to microbes and to other antigens, and to apoptotic bodies.* In the fluid phase, complement proteins are inactive or only transiently active (for seconds), and they become stably activated after they are attached to microbes, antibodies, or dying cells. Many of the biologically active cleavage products of complement proteins also bind covalently to microbes, antibodies, and tissues in which the complement is activated. This characteristic ensures that the full activation and therefore the biologic functions of the complement system are limited to microbial cell surfaces or to sites of antibodies bound to antigens and do not occur in the blood.
- *Complement activation is inhibited by regulatory proteins that are present on normal host cells and absent from microbes.* The regulatory proteins are an adaptation of normal cells that minimize complement-mediated damage to host cells. Microbes lack these regulatory proteins, which allows complement activation to occur on microbial surfaces. Apoptotic bodies lack membrane-bound complement inhibitors but can recruit inhibitory proteins from the blood, thus reducing complement activation and the degree of inflammation.

Pathways of Complement Activation

There are three major pathways of complement activation: the classical pathway, which is activated by certain isotypes of antibodies bound to antigens; the alternative pathway, which is activated on microbial cell surfaces in the absence of antibody; and the lectin pathway, which is activated by a plasma lectin that binds to mannose residues on microbes (Fig. 13-6). The names *classical* and *alternative* arose because the classical pathway was discovered and characterized first, but the alternative pathway is phylogenetically older. Although the pathways of complement activation differ in how they are initiated, all of them result in the generation of enzyme complexes that are able to cleave the most abundant complement protein, C3. The alternative and lectin pathways are effector mechanisms of innate immunity, whereas the classical pathway is a major mechanism of adaptive humoral immunity.

The central event in complement activation is proteolysis of the complement protein C3 to generate biologically active products and the subsequent covalent attachment of a product of C3, called C3b, to microbial cell surfaces or to antibody bound to antigen (see Fig. 13-6). Complement activation depends on the generation of two proteolytic complexes: the **C3 convertase,** which cleaves C3 into two proteolytic fragments called C3a and C3b; and the **C5 convertase**, which cleaves C5 into C5a and C5b. By convention, the proteolytic products of each complement protein are identified by lowercase letter suffixes, *a* referring to the smaller product and *b* to the larger one. C3b becomes covalently attached to the microbial cell surface or to the antibody molecules at the site of complement activation. All of the biologic functions of complement are dependent on

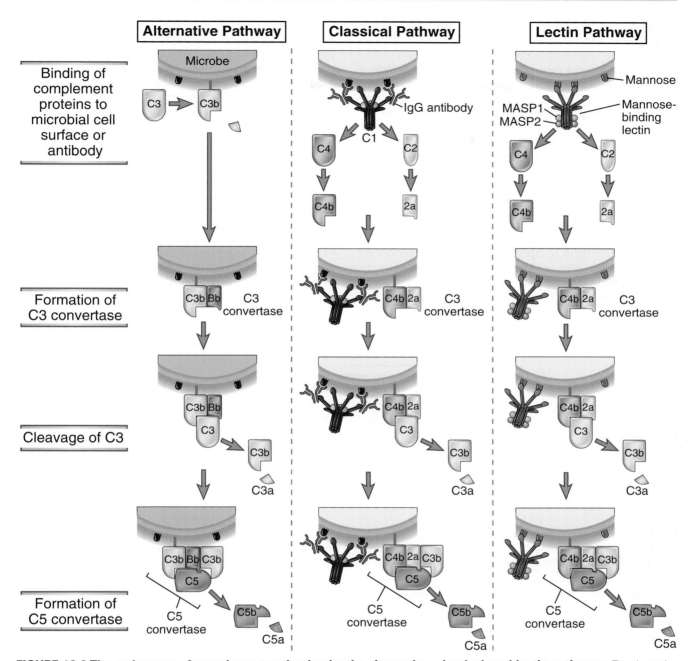

FIGURE 13-6 The early steps of complement activation by the alternative, classical, and lectin pathways. The alternative pathway is activated by C3b binding to various activating surfaces, such as microbial cell walls; the classical pathway is initiated by C1 binding to antigen-antibody complexes; and the lectin pathway is activated by binding of a plasma lectin to microbes. The C3b that is generated by the action of the C3 convertase binds to the microbial cell surface or the antibody and becomes a component of the enzyme that cleaves C5 (C5 convertase) and initiates the late steps of complement activation. The late steps of all three pathways are the same *(not shown)*, and complement activated by all three pathways serves the same functions.

the proteolytic cleavage of C3. For example, complement activation promotes phagocytosis because C3b becomes covalently linked to microbes, and phagocytes (neutrophils and macrophages) express receptors for C3b. Peptides produced by proteolysis of C3 (and other complement proteins) stimulate inflammation. The C5 convertase assembles after the prior generation of C3b, and this convertase contributes both to inflammation (by generation of the C5a fragment) and to the formation of pores in the membranes of microbial targets. The

pathways of complement activation differ in how C3b is produced but follow a common sequence of reactions after the cleavage of C5.

With this background, we proceed to more detailed descriptions of the alternative, classical, and lectin pathways.

The Alternative Pathway

The alternative pathway of complement activation results in the proteolysis of C3 and the stable attachment of its breakdown product C3b to microbial surfaces, without a role for antibody (Fig. 13-7 and Table 13-4). Normally, C3 in plasma is being continuously cleaved at a low rate to generate C3b in a process that is called C3 tickover. The C3 protein contains a reactive thioester bond that is buried in a region of the protein known as the thioester domain. When C3 is cleaved, the C3b molecule undergoes a dramatic conformational change and the thioester domain flips out (a massive shift of about 85 Å), exposing the previously hidden reactive thioester bond. A small amount of the C3b may become covalently attached to the surfaces of cells, including microbes, through the thioester domain, which reacts with the amino or hydroxyl groups of cell surface proteins or polysaccharides to form amide or ester bonds (Fig. 13-8). If these bonds are not formed, the C3b remains in the fluid phase, and the exposed and reactive thioester bond is quickly hydrolyzed, rendering the protein inactive. As a result, further complement activation cannot proceed.

When C3b undergoes its post-cleavage conformational change, a binding site for a plasma protein called Factor B is also exposed. Factor B then binds to the C3b protein that is now covalently tethered to the surface of a microbial or host cell. Bound factor B is in turn cleaved by a plasma serine protease called Factor D, releasing a small fragment called Ba and generating a larger fragment called Bb that remains attached to C3b. The C3bBb complex is the alternative pathway C3 convertase, and it functions to cleave more C3 molecules, thus setting up an amplification sequence. Even when C3b is generated by the classical or lectin pathways, it can form a complex with Bb, and this complex is able to cleave more C3. Thus, the alternative pathway C3 convertase functions to amplify complement activation when it is initiated by the alternative, classical, or lectin pathways. When C3 is broken down, C3b remains attached to cells and C3a is released. This soluble fragment has several biologic activities that are discussed later.

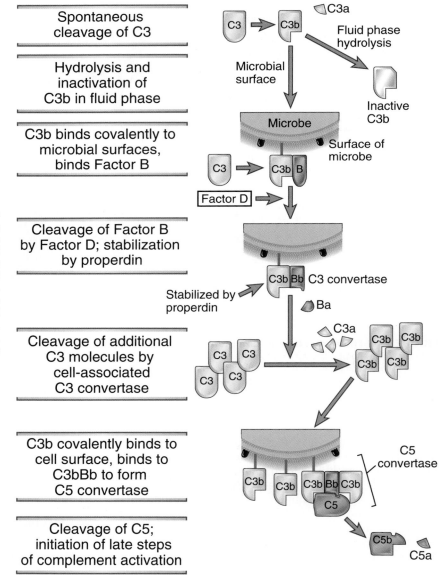

FIGURE 13-7 The alternative pathway of complement activation. Spontaneous hydrolysis of plasma C3 leads to the formation of a fluid-phase C3 convertase (not shown) and the generation of C3b. If the C3b is deposited on the surfaces of microbes, it binds Factor B and forms the alternative pathway C3 convertase. This convertase cleaves C3 to produce more C3b, which binds to the microbial surface and participates in the formation of a C5 convertase. The C5 convertase cleaves C5 to generate C5b, the initiating event in the late steps of complement activation.

TABLE 13-4 Proteins of the Alternative Pathway of Complement

Protein	Structure	Serum Concentration (μg/mL)	Function
C3	185 kD (α subunit, 110 kD; β subunit, 75 kD)	1000-1200	C3b binds to the surface of the microbe, where it functions as an opsonin and as a component of C3 and C5 convertases. C3a stimulates inflammation (anaphylatoxin).
Factor B	93-kD monomer	200	Bb is a serine protease and the active enzyme of the C3 and C5 convertases.
Factor D	25-kD monomer	1-2	Plasma serine protease cleaves factor B when it is bound to C3b.
Properdin	Composed of up to four 56-kD subunits	25	Properdin stabilizes C3 convertases (C3bBb) on microbial surfaces.

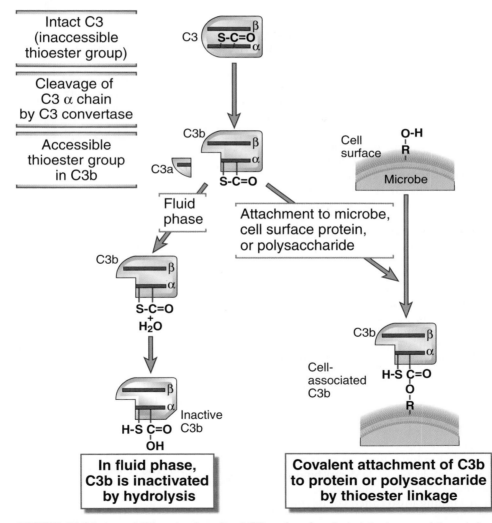

FIGURE 13-8 Internal thioester bonds of C3 molecules. Proteolytic cleavage of the α chain of C3 converts it into a metastable form in which the internal thioester bonds are exposed and susceptible to nucleophilic attack by oxygen atoms (as shown) or nitrogen atoms. The result is the formation of covalent bonds with proteins or carbohydrates on the cell surfaces. C4 is structurally homologous to C3 and has an identical thioester group.

Alternative pathway activation readily occurs on microbial cell surfaces and not on mammalian cells. If the C3bBb complex is formed on mammalian cells, it is rapidly degraded and the reaction is terminated by the action of several regulatory proteins present on these cells (discussed later). Lack of the regulatory proteins on microbial cells allows binding and activation of the alternative pathway C3 convertase. In addition, another protein of the alternative pathway, called properdin, can bind to and stabilize the C3bBb complex, and the attachment of properdin is favored on microbial as opposed to normal host cells. Properdin is the only known positive regulator of complement.

Some of the C3b molecules generated by the alternative pathway C3 convertase bind to the convertase itself. This results in the formation of a complex containing one Bb moiety and two molecules of C3b, which functions as the alternative pathway C5 convertase, which will cleave C5 and initiate the late steps of complement activation.

The Classical Pathway

The classical pathway is initiated by binding of the complement protein C1 to the C_H2 domains of IgG or the C_H3 domains of IgM molecules that have bound antigen (Fig. 13-9 and Table 13-5). Among IgG antibodies, IgG3 and IgG1 (in humans) are more efficient activators of complement than are other subclasses. C1 is a large, multimeric protein complex composed of C1q, C1r, and C1s subunits; C1q binds to the antibody, and C1r and C1s are proteases. The C1q subunit is made up of an umbrella-like radial array of six chains, each of which has a globular head connected by a collagen-like arm to a central stalk (Fig. 13-10). This hexamer performs the recognition function of the molecule and binds specifically to the Fc regions of μ and some γ heavy chains.

Only antibodies bound to antigens, and not free circulating antibodies, can initiate classical pathway activation (Fig. 13-11). The reason for this is that each C1q molecule must bind to at least two Ig heavy chains to be activated and each Ig Fc region has only a single C1q-binding site. Therefore, two or more Fc regions have to be accessible to C1 in order to initiate classical pathway activation. Because each IgG molecule has only one Fc region, multiple IgG molecules must be brought close together before C1q can bind, and multiple IgG antibodies are brought together only when they bind to a multivalent antigen. Even though free (circulating) IgM is pentameric, it does not bind C1q because the Fc regions of free IgM are in a configuration that is inaccessible to C1q. Binding of the IgM to an antigen induces a conformational change that exposes the C1q binding sites in the Fc regions and allows C1q to bind. Because of its pentameric structure, a single molecule of IgM can bind two C1q molecules, and this is one reason that IgM is a more efficient complement-binding (also called complement-fixing) antibody than IgG is.

C1r and C1s are serine proteases that form a tetramer containing two molecules of each protein. Binding of two or more of the globular heads of C1q to the Fc regions of IgG or IgM leads to enzymatic activation of the associated C1r, which cleaves and activates C1s

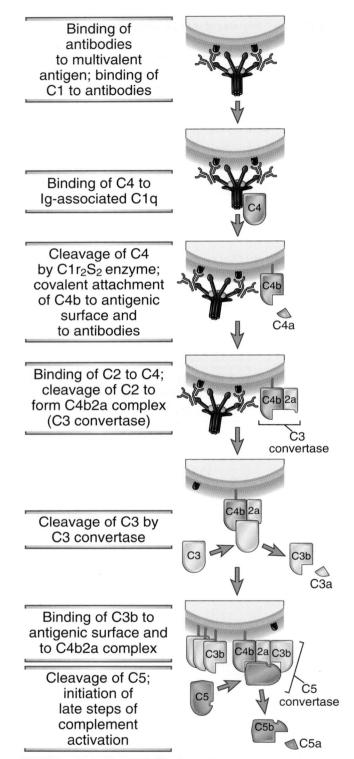

Binding of antibodies to multivalent antigen; binding of C1 to antibodies

Binding of C4 to Ig-associated C1q

Cleavage of C4 by $C1r_2S_2$ enzyme; covalent attachment of C4b to antigenic surface and to antibodies

Binding of C2 to C4; cleavage of C2 to form C4b2a complex (C3 convertase)

Cleavage of C3 by C3 convertase

Binding of C3b to antigenic surface and to C4b2a complex

Cleavage of C5; initiation of late steps of complement activation

FIGURE 13-9 The classical pathway of complement activation. Antigen-antibody complexes that activate the classical pathway may be soluble, fixed on the surface of cells (as shown), or deposited on extracellular matrices. The classical pathway is initiated by the binding of C1 to antigen-complexed antibody molecules, which leads to the production of C3 and C5 convertases attached to the surfaces where the antibody was deposited. The C5 convertase cleaves C5 to begin the late steps of complement activation.

TABLE 13-5 Proteins of the Classical Pathway of Complement

Protein	Structure	Serum Concentration (µg/mL)	Function
C1 (C1qr2s2)	750 kD		Initiates the classical pathway
C1q	460 kD; hexamer of three pairs of chains (22, 23, 24 kD)	75-150	Binds to the Fc portion of antibody that has bound antigen, to apoptotic cells, and to cationic surfaces
C1r	85-kD dimer	50	Serine protease, cleaves C1s to make it an active protease
C1s	85-kD dimer	50	Serine protease, cleaves C4 and C2
C4	210 kD, trimer of 97-, 75-, and 33-kD chains	300-600	C4b covalently binds to the surface of a microbe or cell, where antibody is bound and complement is activated. C4b binds C2 for cleavage by C1s. C4a stimulates inflammation (anaphylatoxin).
C2	102-kD monomer	20	C2a is a serine protease and functions as the active enzyme of C3 and C5 convertases to cleave C3 and C5.
C3	See Table 13-4		

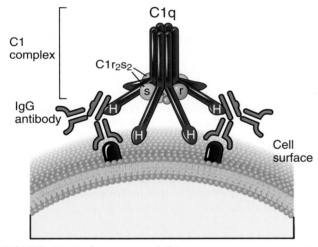

FIGURE 13-10 Structure of C1. C1q consists of six identical subunits arranged to form a central core and symmetrically projecting radial arms. The globular heads at the end of each arm, designated H, are the contact regions for immunoglobulin. C1r and C1s form a tetramer composed of two C1r and two C1s molecules. The ends of C1r and C1s contain the catalytic domains of these proteins. One C1r2s2 tetramer wraps around the radial arms of the C1q complex in a manner that juxtaposes the catalytic domains of C1r and C1s.

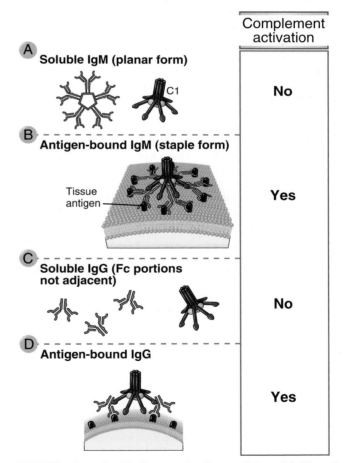

FIGURE 13-11 C1 binding to the Fc portions of IgM and IgG. C1 must bind to two or more Fc portions to initiate the complement cascade. The Fc portions of soluble pentameric IgM are not accessible to C1 **(A)**. After IgM binds to surface-bound antigens, it undergoes a shape change that permits C1 binding and activation **(B)**. Soluble IgG molecules will also not activate C1 because each IgG has only one Fc region **(C)**, but after binding to cell surface antigens, adjacent IgG Fc portions can bind and activate C1 **(D)**.

(see Fig. 13-9). Activated C1s cleaves the next protein in the cascade, C4, to generate C4b. (The smaller C4a fragment is released and has biologic activities that are described later.) C4 is homologous to C3, and C4b contains an internal thioester bond, similar to that in C3b, that forms covalent amide or ester linkages with the antigen-antibody complex or with the adjacent surface of a cell to which the antibody is bound. This attachment of C4b ensures that classical pathway activation proceeds on a cell surface or immune complex. The next complement protein, C2, then complexes with the cell surface–bound C4b and is cleaved by a nearby C1s molecule to generate a soluble C2b fragment of unknown importance and a larger C2a fragment that remains physically associated with C4b on the cell surface. (Note that the nomenclature of C2 fragments is different from that of the other complement proteins because the attached, larger fragment is called the *a* piece and the released part is the *b* fragment.) The resulting C4b2a complex is the classical pathway C3 convertase; it has the ability to bind to and proteolytically cleave C3. Binding of this enzyme complex to C3 is mediated by the C4b component, and proteolysis is catalyzed by the C2a component. Cleavage of C3 results in the removal of the small C3a fragment, and C3b can form covalent bonds with cell surfaces or with the antibody where complement activation was initiated. Once C3b is deposited, it can bind Factor B and generate more C3 convertase by the alternative pathway, as discussed earlier. The net effect of the multiple enzymatic steps and amplification is that a single molecule of C3 convertase can lead to the deposition of hundreds or thousands of molecules of C3b on the cell surface where complement is activated. The key early steps of the alternative and classical pathways are analogous: C3 in the alternative pathway is homologous to C4 in the classical pathway, and Factor B is homologous to C2.

Some of the C3b molecules generated by the classical pathway C3 convertase bind to the convertase (as in the alternative pathway) and form a C4b2a3b complex. This complex functions as the classical pathway C5 convertase; it cleaves C5 and initiates the late steps of complement activation.

An unusual antibody-independent but C1-dependent form of the classical pathway, which is activated by carbohydrates binding to a cell surface lectin, occurs in pneumococcal infections. Splenic marginal zone macrophages express a cell surface C-type lectin called SIGN-R1 that can recognize the pneumococcal polysaccharide and can also bind C1q. Multivalent binding of whole bacteria or the polysaccharide to SIGN-R1 activates the classical pathway and permits the eventual coating of the pneumococcus with C3b. This is an example of a cell surface lectin that mediates activation of the classical pathway but without a requirement for antibody.

The Lectin Pathway

The lectin pathway of complement activation is triggered in the absence of antibody by the binding of microbial polysaccharides to circulating lectins, such as plasma mannose (or mannan)–binding lectin (MBL), or to ficolins (Table 13-6). These soluble lectins are collagen-like proteins that structurally resemble C1q (see Fig. 4-10). MBL, L-ficolin, and H-ficolin are plasma proteins; M-ficolin is mainly secreted by activated macrophages in tissues. MBL is a member of the collectin family and has an N-terminal collagen-like domain and a C-terminal carbohydrate recognition (lectin) domain. The ficolins have a similar structure with an N-terminal collagen-like domain and a C-terminal fibrinogen-like domain. The collagen-like domains help assemble basic triple-helical structures that can form higher-order oligomers. MBL binds to mannose residues on polysaccharides; the ficolin fibrinogen-like domain binds N-acetylglucosamine–containing glycans. MBL and ficolins associate with MBL-associated serine proteases (MASPs) including MASP1, MASP2, and MASP3 (see Table 13-6). The MASP proteins are structurally homologous to the C1r and C1s proteases and serve a similar function, namely, the cleavage of C4 and C2 to activate the complement pathway. Higher-order oligomers of MBL associate with MASP1 and MASP2, although MASP3/MASP2 complexes may also be found. MASP1 (or MASP3) can form a tetrameric complex with MASP2 similar to the one formed by C1r and C1s, and MASP2 is the protease that cleaves C4 and C2. Subsequent events in this pathway are identical to those that occur in the classical pathway.

TABLE 13-6	Proteins of the Lectin Pathway of Complement		
Protein	**Structure**	**Serum Concentration (µg/mL)**	**Function**
Mannose-binding lectin	Helical trimer of 32-kD chain and dimers to hexamers of this triple helix	1-8	Agglutinin, opsonin, complement fixing
M-ficolin (ficolin-1)	Helical trimer of 34-kD chain and a tetramer of this triple helix	Undetectable	Agglutinin, opsonin, complement fixing
L-ficolin (ficolin-2)	Helical trimer of 34-kD chain and a tetramer of this triple helix	1-7	Agglutinin, opsonin, complement fixing
H-ficolin (ficolin-3)	Helical trimer of 34-kD chain and a tetramer of this triple helix	6-83	Agglutinin, opsonin, complement fixing
MASP1	90-kD homodimer; homology to C1r/C1s	2-13*	Forms complex with MASP2 and collectins or ficolins and activates MASP3
MASP2	110-kD homodimer; homology to C1r/C1s	2-13	Forms complex with lectins, especially ficolin-3
MASP3	76-kD homodimer; homology to C1r/C1s	0.02-1.0	Associates with collectins or ficolins and MASP1 and cleaves C4

*Published concentrations may have been influenced by cross-reactivity of antibodies with MASP3; concentrations of the latter are derived by use of specific monoclonal antibodies. Most of these are plasma proteins, except M-ficolin, which is secreted by activated macrophages.

TABLE 13-7 Proteins of the Late Steps of Complement Activation

Protein	Structure	Serum Concentration (µg/mL)	Function
C5	190-kD dimer of 115- and 75-kD chains	80	C5b initiates assembly of the MAC.
			C5a stimulates inflammation (anaphylatoxin).
C6	110-kD monomer	45	Component of the MAC: binds to C5b and accepts C7.
C7	100-kD monomer	90	Component of the MAC: binds to C5b,6 and inserts into lipid membranes.
C8	155-kD trimer of 64-, 64-, and 22-kD chains	60	Component of the MAC: binds to C5b,6,7 and initiates the binding and polymerization of C9.
C9	79-kD monomer	60	Component of the MAC: binds to C5b,6,7,8 and polymerizes to form membrane pores.

MAC, membrane attack complex.

Late Steps of Complement Activation

C5 convertases generated by the alternative, classical, or lectin pathway initiate activation of the late components of the complement system, which culminates in formation of the cytocidal membrane attack complex (MAC) (Table 13-7 and Fig. 13-12). C5 convertases cleave C5 into a small C5a fragment that is released and a two-chain C5b fragment that remains bound to the complement proteins deposited on the cell surface. C5a has potent biologic effects on several cells that are discussed later in this chapter. The remaining components of the complement cascade, C6, C7, C8, and C9, are structurally related proteins without enzymatic activity.

C5b transiently maintains a conformation capable of binding the next proteins in the cascade, C6 and C7. The C7 component of the resulting C5b,6,7 complex is hydrophobic, and it inserts into the lipid bilayer of cell membranes, where it becomes a high-affinity receptor for the C8 molecule. The C8 protein is a trimer composed of three distinct chains, one of which binds to the C5b,6,7 complex and forms a covalent heterodimer with the second chain; the third chain inserts into the lipid bilayer of the membrane. This stably inserted C5b,6,7,8 complex (C5b-8) has a limited ability to lyse cells. The formation of a fully active MAC is accomplished by the binding of C9, the final component of the complement cascades,

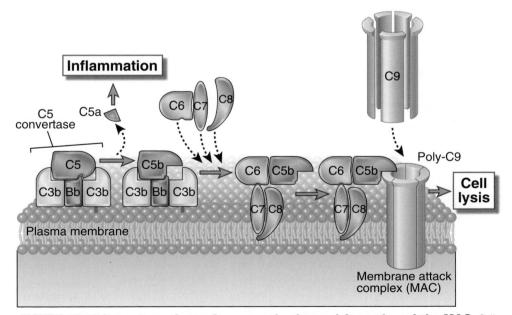

FIGURE 13-12 Late steps of complement activation and formation of the MAC. Cell-associated C5 convertase cleaves C5 and generates C5b, which becomes bound to the convertase. C6 and C7 bind sequentially, and the C5b,6,7 complex inserts into the plasma membrane, followed by insertion of C8. Up to 15 C9 molecules may then polymerize around the complex to form the MAC, which creates pores in the membrane and induces cell lysis. C5a released on proteolysis of C5 stimulates inflammation.

to the C5b-8 complex. C9 is a serum protein that polymerizes at the site of the bound C5b-8 to form pores in plasma membranes. These pores are about 100 Å in diameter, and they form channels that allow free movement of water and ions. The entry of water results in osmotic swelling and rupture of the cells on whose surface the MAC is deposited. The pores formed by polymerized C9 are similar to the membrane pores formed by perforin, the cytolytic granule protein found in cytotoxic T lymphocytes and NK cells (see Chapter 11), and C9 is structurally homologous to perforin.

Receptors for Complement Proteins

Many of the biologic activities of the complement system are mediated by the binding of complement fragments to membrane receptors expressed on various cell types. The best characterized of these receptors are specific for fragments of C3 and are described here (Table 13-8). Other receptors include those for C3a, C4a, and C5a, which stimulate inflammation, and some that regulate complement activation.

- *The type 1 complement receptor (CR1, or CD35) functions mainly to promote phagocytosis of C3b- and C4b-coated particles and clearance of immune complexes from the circulation.* CR1 is a high-affinity receptor for C3b and C4b. It is expressed mainly on bone marrow–derived cells, including erythrocytes, neutrophils, monocytes, macrophages, eosinophils, and T and B lymphocytes; it is also found on follicular dendritic cells in the follicles of peripheral lymphoid organs. Phagocytes use this receptor to bind and internalize particles opsonized with C3b or C4b. The binding of C3b- or C4b-coated particles to CR1 also transduces signals that activate the microbicidal mechanisms of the phagocytes, especially when the Fcγ receptor is simultaneously engaged by antibody-coated particles.

CR1 on erythrocytes binds circulating immune complexes with attached C3b and C4b and transports the complexes to the liver and spleen. Here, phagocytes remove the immune complexes from the erythrocyte surface, and the erythrocytes continue to circulate. CR1 is also a regulator of complement activation (discussed in the section that follows).

- *The type 2 complement receptor (CR2, or CD21) functions to stimulate humoral immune responses by enhancing B cell activation by antigen and by promoting the trapping of antigen-antibody complexes in germinal centers.* CR2 is present on B lymphocytes, follicular dendritic cells, and some epithelial cells. It specifically binds the cleavage products of C3b, called C3d, C3dg, and iC3b (*i* referring to inactive), which are generated by Factor I–mediated proteolysis (discussed later). On B cells, CR2 is expressed as part of a trimolecular complex that includes two other non-covalently attached proteins called CD19 and CD81 (or TAPA-1, target of antiproliferative antibody 1). This complex delivers signals to B cells that enhance the responses of B cells to antigen (see Fig. 7-20). On follicular dendritic cells, CR2 serves to trap iC3b- and C3dg-coated antigen-antibody complexes in germinal centers. The functions of complement in B cell activation are described later.

In humans, CR2 is the cell surface receptor for Epstein-Barr virus, a herpesvirus that causes infectious mononucleosis and is also linked to several malignant tumors. Epstein-Barr virus enters B cells via CR2, infects these cells, and can remain latent in infected cells for life.

- *The type 3 complement receptor, also called Mac-1 (CR3, CD11bCD18), is an integrin that functions as a receptor for the iC3b fragment generated by proteolysis of C3b.* Mac-1 is expressed on neutrophils, mononuclear phagocytes, mast cells, and NK cells. It is a member of the integrin family of cell surface receptors (see Chapter 3) and consists of an α chain (CD11b) non-covalently

---

TABLE 13-8   Receptors for Fragments of C3

Receptor	Structure	Ligands	Cell Distribution	Function
Type 1 complement receptor (CR1, CD35)	160-250 kD; multiple CCPRs	C3b > C4b > iC3b	Mononuclear phagocytes, neutrophils, B and T cells, erythrocytes, eosinophils, FDCs	Phagocytosis Clearance of immune complexes Promotes dissociation of C3 convertases by acting as cofactor for cleavage of C3b, C4b
Type 2 complement receptor (CR2, CD21)	145 kD; multiple CCPRs	C3d, C3dg > iC3b	B lymphocytes, FDCs, nasopharyngeal epithelium	Coreceptor for B cell activation Trapping of antigens in germinal centers Receptor for EBV
Type 3 complement receptor (CR3, Mac-1, CD11bCD18)	Integrin, with 165-kD α chain and 95-kD β2 chain	iC3b, ICAM-1; also binds microbes	Mononuclear phagocytes, neutrophils, NK cells	Phagocytosis Leukocyte adhesion to endothelium (via ICAM-1)
Type 4 complement receptor (CR4, p150,95, CD11cCD18)	Integrin, with 150-kD α chain and 95-kD β2 chain	iC3b	Mononuclear phagocytes, neutrophils, NK cells	Phagocytosis, cell adhesion?

CCPRs, complement control protein repeats; *EBV,* Epstein-Barr virus; *FDCs,* follicular dendritic cells; *ICAM-1,* intercellular adhesion molecule 1.

linked to a β chain (CD18) that is identical to the β chains of two closely related integrin molecules, leukocyte function-associated antigen 1 (LFA-1) and p150,95. Mac-1 on neutrophils and monocytes promotes phagocytosis of microbes opsonized with iC3b. In addition, Mac-1 may directly recognize bacteria for phagocytosis by binding to some unknown microbial molecules (see Chapter 4). It also binds to intercellular adhesion molecule 1 (ICAM-1) on endothelial cells and promotes stable attachment of the leukocytes to endothelium, even without complement activation. This binding leads to the recruitment of leukocytes to sites of infection and tissue injury (see Chapter 3).

- *The type 4 complement receptor (CR4, p150,95, CD11c/CD18) is another integrin with a different α chain (CD11c) and the same β chain as Mac-1.* It also binds iC3b, and the function of this receptor is probably similar to that of Mac-1. CD11c is abundantly expressed on dendritic cells and is used as a marker for this cell type.
- *The complement receptor of the immunoglobulin family (CRIg) is expressed on the surface of macrophages in the liver known as Kupffer cells.* CRIg is an integral membrane protein with an extracellular region made up of Ig domains. It binds the complement fragments C3b and iC3b and is involved in the clearance of opsonized bacteria and other blood-borne pathogens.

Regulation of Complement Activation

Activation of the complement cascade and the stability of active complement proteins are tightly regulated to prevent complement activation on normal host cells and to limit the duration of complement activation even on microbial cells and antigen-antibody complexes. Regulation of complement is mediated by several circulating and cell membrane proteins (Table 13-9). Many of these proteins as well as several proteins of the classical and alternative pathways belong to a family called regulators of complement activity (RCA) and are encoded by homologous genes that are located adjacent to one another in the genome.

Complement activation needs to be regulated for two reasons. First, low-level complement activation goes on spontaneously, and if such activation is allowed to proceed, the result can be damage to normal cells and tissues. Second, even when complement is activated where needed, such as on microbial cells or antigen-antibody complexes, it needs to be controlled because degradation products of complement proteins can diffuse to adjacent cells and injure them. Different regulatory mechanisms inhibit the formation of C3 convertases in the early steps of complement activation, break down and inactivate C3 and C5 convertases, and inhibit formation of the MAC in the late steps of the complement pathway.

- *The proteolytic activity of C1r and C1s is inhibited by a plasma protein called C1 inhibitor (C1 INH).* C1 INH is a serine protease inhibitor (serpin) that mimics the normal substrates of C1r and C1s. If C1q binds to an antibody and begins the process of complement activation, C1 INH becomes a target of the enzymatic activity of the bound $C1r_2$-$C1s_2$. C1 INH is cleaved by and becomes covalently attached to these complement proteins, and, as a result, the $C1r_2$-$C1s_2$ tetramer dissociates from C1q, thus stopping activation by the

TABLE 13-9 Regulators of Complement Activation

Receptor	Structure	Distribution	Interacts with	Function
C1 inhibitor (C1 INH)	104 kD	Plasma protein; conc. 200 µg/mL	C1r, C1s	Serine protease inhibitor; binds to C1r and C1s and dissociates them from C1q
Factor I	88-kD dimer of 50- and 38-kD subunits	Plasma protein; conc. 35 µg/mL	C4b, C3b	Serine protease; cleaves C3b and C4b by using factor H, MCP, C4BP, or CR1 as cofactors
Factor H	150 kD; multiple CCPRs	Plasma protein; conc. 480 µg/mL	C3b	Binds C3b and displaces Bb; Cofactor for factor I–mediated cleavage of C3b
C4-binding protein (C4BP)	570 kD; multiple CCPRs	Plasma protein; conc. 300 µg/mL	C4b	Binds C4b and displaces C2; Cofactor for factor I–mediated cleavage of C4b
Membrane cofactor protein (MCP, CD46)	45-70 kD; four CCPRs	Leukocytes, epithelial cells, endothelial cells	C3b, C4b	Cofactor for factor I–mediated cleavage of C3b and C4b
Decay-accelerating factor (DAF)	70 kD; GPI linked, four CCPRs	Blood cells, endothelial cells, epithelial cells	C4b2a, C3bBb	Displaces C2a from C4b and Bb from C3b (dissociation of C3 convertases)
CD59	18 kD; GPI linked	Blood cells, endothelial cells, epithelial cells	C7, C8	Blocks C9 binding and prevents formation of the MAC

CCPRs, complement control protein repeats; *conc.,* concentration; *GPI,* glycophosphatidylinositol; *MAC,* membrane attack complex.

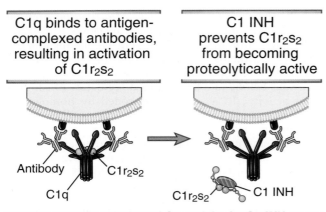

C1q binds to antigen-complexed antibodies, resulting in activation of C1r$_2$s$_2$	C1 INH prevents C1r$_2$s$_2$ from becoming proteolytically active

FIGURE 13-13 Regulation of C1 activity by C1 INH. C1 INH displaces C1r2s2 from C1q and terminates classical pathway activation.

classical pathway (Fig. 13-13). In this way, C1 INH prevents the accumulation of enzymatically active C1r$_2$-C1s$_2$ in the plasma and limits the time for which active C1r$_2$-C1s$_2$ is available to activate subsequent steps in the complement cascade. An autosomal dominant inherited disease called **hereditary angioneurotic edema** is due to a deficiency of C1 INH. Clinical manifestations of the disease include intermittent acute accumulation of edema fluid in the skin and mucosa, which causes abdominal pain, vomiting, diarrhea, and potentially life-threatening airway obstruction. In these patients, the plasma levels of C1 INH protein are sufficiently reduced (<20% to 30% of normal) that activation of C1 by immune complexes is not properly controlled and increased breakdown of C4 and C2 occurs. The mediators of edema formation in patients with hereditary angioneurotic edema include a proteolytic fragment of C2, called C2 kinin, and bradykinin. C1 INH is an inhibitor of other plasma serine proteases besides C1, including kallikrein and coagulation factor XII, and both activated kallikrein and factor XII can promote increased formation of bradykinin. Recombinant C1 INH is now used to treat patients with this deficiency.

- *Assembly of the components of C3 and C5 convertases is inhibited by the binding of regulatory proteins to C3b and C4b deposited on cell surfaces* (Fig. 13-14). If C3b is deposited on the surfaces of normal mammalian cells, it may be bound by several membrane proteins, including membrane cofactor protein (MCP, or CD46), type 1 complement receptor (CR1), decay-accelerating factor (DAF), and a plasma protein called Factor H. C4b deposited on cell surfaces is similarly bound by DAF, CR1, MCP, and another plasma protein called C4-binding protein (C4BP). By binding to C3b or C4b, these proteins competitively inhibit the binding of other components of the C3 convertase, such as Bb of the alternative pathway and C2a of the classical pathway, thus blocking further progression of the complement cascade. (Factor H inhibits binding of only Bb to C3b and is thus a regulator of the alternative but not the classical pathway.) MCP, CR1, and DAF are produced by mammalian cells but not

by microbes. Therefore, these regulators of complement selectively inhibit complement activation on host cells and allow complement activation to proceed on microbes. In addition, cell surfaces rich in sialic acid favor binding of the regulatory protein Factor H over the alternative pathway protein Factor B. Mammalian cells express higher levels of sialic acid than most microbes do, which is another reason that complement activation is prevented on normal host cells and permitted on microbes.

DAF is a glycophosphatidylinositol-linked membrane protein expressed on endothelial cells and erythrocytes. A deficiency in hematopoietic stem cells of the enzyme required to form such protein-lipid linkages results in the failure to express many glycophosphatidylinositol-linked membrane proteins, including DAF and CD59 (see following), and causes a disease called **paroxysmal nocturnal hemoglobinuria.** This disease is characterized by recurrent bouts of intravascular hemolysis, at least partly attributable to unregulated complement activation on the surface of erythrocytes. Recurrent intravascular hemolysis in turn leads to chronic hemolytic anemia and venous thrombosis. An unusual feature of this disease is that the causative gene mutation is not inherited but is an acquired mutation in hematopoietic stem cells.

- *Cell-associated C3b is proteolytically degraded by a plasma serine protease called Factor I, which is active only in the presence of regulatory proteins* (Fig. 13-15). MCP, Factor H, C4BP, and CR1 all serve as cofactors for Factor I–mediated cleavage of C3b (and C4b). Thus, these regulatory host cell proteins promote proteolytic degradation of complement proteins; as discussed earlier, the same regulatory proteins cause dissociation of C3b (and C4b)–containing complexes. Factor I–mediated cleavage of C3b generates the fragments

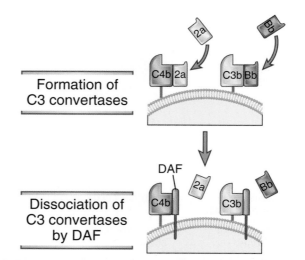

FIGURE 13-14 Inhibition of the formation of C3 convertases. The classical pathway C3 convertase, C4b2a, or the alternative pathway C3 convertase, C3bBb, can be dissociated by the replacement of one component with decay accelerating factor (DAF). Other regulatory proteins, such as MCP and CR1, function similarly to DAF (see text).

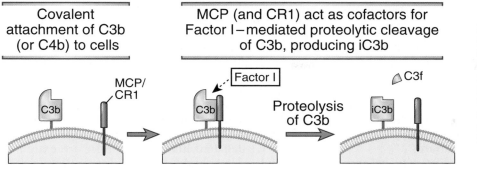

Covalent attachment of C3b (or C4b) to cells

MCP (and CR1) act as cofactors for Factor I–mediated proteolytic cleavage of C3b, producing iC3b

FIGURE 13-15 Factor I–mediated cleavage of C3b. In the presence of cell membrane–bound cofactors (MCP or CR1), plasma factor I proteolytically cleaves C3b attached to cell surfaces, leaving an inactive form of C3b (iC3b). Factor H and C4-binding protein can also serve as cofactors for factor I–mediated cleavage of C3b. The same process is involved in the proteolysis of C4.

called iC3b, C3d, and C3dg, which do not participate in complement activation but are recognized by receptors on phagocytes and B lymphocytes.

- ***Formation of the MAC is inhibited by a membrane protein called CD59.*** CD59 is a glycophosphatidylinositol-linked protein expressed on many cell types. It works by incorporating itself into assembling MACs after the membrane insertion of C5b-8, thereby inhibiting the subsequent addition of C9 molecules (Fig. 13-16). CD59 is present on normal host cells,

where it limits MAC formation, but it is not present on microbes. Formation of the MAC is also inhibited by plasma proteins such as S protein, which functions by binding to soluble C5b,6,7 complexes and thereby preventing their insertion into cell membranes near the site where the complement cascade was initiated. Growing MACs can insert into any neighboring cell membrane besides the membrane on which they were generated. Inhibitors of the MAC in the plasma and in host cell membranes ensure that lysis of

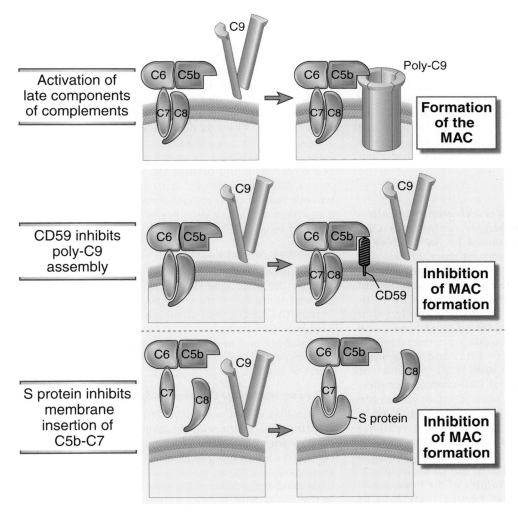

Activation of late components of complements

Formation of the MAC

CD59 inhibits poly-C9 assembly

Inhibition of MAC formation

S protein inhibits membrane insertion of C5b-C7

Inhibition of MAC formation

FIGURE 13-16 Regulation of formation of the MAC. The MAC is formed on cell surfaces as an end result of complement activation. The membrane protein CD59 and S protein in the plasma inhibit formation of the MAC.

innocent bystander cells does not occur near the site of complement activation.

Much of the analysis of the function of complement regulatory proteins has relied on in vitro experiments, and most of these experiments have focused on assays that measure MAC-mediated cell lysis as an endpoint. On the basis of these studies, a hierarchy of importance for inhibiting complement activation is believed to be CD59 > DAF > MCP; this hierarchy may reflect the relative abundance of these proteins on cell surfaces.

The function of regulatory proteins may be overwhelmed by excessive activation of complement pathways. We have emphasized the importance of these regulatory proteins in preventing complement activation on normal cells. However, complement-mediated phagocytosis and damage to normal cells are important pathogenic mechanisms in many immunologic diseases (see Chapter 19). In these diseases, large amounts of antibodies may be deposited on host cells, generating enough active complement proteins that the regulatory molecules are unable to control complement activation.

Functions of Complement

The principal effector functions of the complement system in innate immunity and adaptive humoral immunity are to promote phagocytosis of microbes on which complement is activated, to stimulate inflammation, and to induce the lysis of these microbes. In addition, products of complement activation facilitate the activation of B lymphocytes and the production of antibodies. Phagocytosis, inflammation, and stimulation of humoral immunity are all mediated by the binding of proteolytic fragments of complement proteins to various cell surface receptors, whereas cell lysis is mediated by the MAC. In the following section, we will describe these functions of the complement system and their roles in host defense.

Opsonization and Phagocytosis

Microbes on which complement is activated by the alternative or classical pathway become coated with C3b, iC3b, or C4b and are phagocytosed by the binding of these proteins to specific receptors on macrophages and neutrophils (Fig. 13-17, *A*). As discussed previously, activation of complement leads to the generation of C3b and iC3b covalently bound to cell surfaces. Both C3b and iC3b act as opsonins by virtue of the fact that they specifically bind to receptors on neutrophils and macrophages. C3b and C4b (the latter generated by the classical pathway only) bind to CR1, and iC3b binds to CR3 (Mac-1) and CR4. By itself, CR1 is inefficient at inducing the phagocytosis of C3b-coated microbes, but its ability to do so is enhanced if the microbes are coated with IgG antibodies that simultaneously bind to Fcγ receptors. Macrophage activation by the cytokine IFN-γ also enhances CR1-mediated phagocytosis. C3b- and iC3b-dependent phagocytosis of microorganisms is a major defense mechanism against infections in innate and adaptive immunity. One example of the importance of complement is host defense against bacteria with

polysaccharide-rich capsules, such as pneumococci and meningococci, which is mediated primarily by humoral immunity. IgM antibodies against capsular polysaccharides bind to the bacteria, activate the classical pathway of complement, and cause phagocytic clearance of the bacteria in the spleen. This is why individuals lacking the spleen (e.g., as a result of surgical removal after traumatic rupture or in patients with autoimmune hemolytic anemia or thrombocytopenia) are susceptible to disseminated pneumococcal and meningococcal septicemia. C3-deficient humans and mice are extremely susceptible to lethal bacterial infections.

Stimulation of Inflammatory Responses

The proteolytic complement fragments C5a, C4a, and C3a induce acute inflammation by activating mast cells, neutrophils and endothelial cells (Fig. 13-17, *B*). All three peptides bind to mast cells and induce degranulation, with the release of vasoactive mediators such as histamine. These peptides are also called **anaphylatoxins** because the mast cell reactions they trigger are characteristic of anaphylaxis (see Chapter 20). In neutrophils, C5a stimulates motility, firm adhesion to endothelial cells, and, at high doses, stimulation of the respiratory burst and production of reactive oxygen species. In addition, C5a may act directly on vascular endothelial cells and induce increased vascular permeability and the expression of P-selectin, which promotes neutrophil binding. This combination of C5a actions on mast cells, neutrophils, and endothelial cells contributes to inflammation at sites of complement activation. C5a is the most potent mediator of mast cell degranulation, C3a is about 20-fold less potent, and C4a is about 2500-fold less. The proinflammatory effects of C5a, C4a, and C3a are mediated by binding of the peptides to specific receptors on various cell types. The C5a receptor is the most thoroughly characterized. It is a member of the G protein–coupled receptor family. The C5a receptor is expressed on many cell types, including neutrophils, eosinophils, basophils, monocytes, macrophages, mast cells, endothelial cells, smooth muscle cells, epithelial cells, and astrocytes. The C3a receptor is also a member of the G protein–coupled receptor family.

Complement-Mediated Cytolysis

Complement-mediated lysis of foreign organisms is mediated by the MAC (Fig. 13-17, *C*). Most pathogens have evolved thick cell walls or capsules that impede access of the MAC to their cell membranes. Complement-mediated lysis appears to be critical for defense against only a few pathogens that are unable to resist MAC insertion, such as bacteria of the genus *Neisseria,* which have very thin cell walls.

Other Functions of the Complement System

By binding to antigen-antibody complexes, complement proteins promote the solubilization of these complexes and their clearance by phagocytes. Small numbers of immune complexes are frequently formed in the circulation when an individual mounts a vigorous antibody response to a circulating antigen. If the immune complexes accumulate in the blood, they may be deposited in vessel walls and

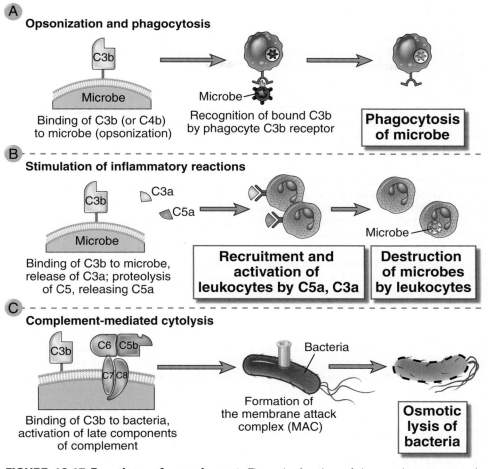

FIGURE 13-17 Functions of complement. The major functions of the complement system in host defense are shown. Cell-bound C3b is an opsonin that promotes phagocytosis of coated cells **(A)**; the proteolytic products C5a, C3a, and (to a lesser extent) C4a stimulate leukocyte recruitment and inflammation **(B)**; and the MAC lyses cells **(C)**.

lead to inflammatory reactions that damage the vessels and surrounding tissue. The formation of immune complexes may require not only the multivalent binding of Ig Fab regions to antigens but also non-covalent interactions of Fc regions of juxtaposed Ig molecules. Complement activation on Ig molecules can sterically block these Fc-Fc interactions, thereby promoting dissolution of the immune complexes. In addition, as discussed earlier, immune complexes with attached C3b are bound to CR1 on erythrocytes, and the complexes are cleared by phagocytes in the liver.

The C3d protein generated from C3 binds to CR2 on B cells and facilitates B cell activation and the initiation of humoral immune responses. C3d is generated when complement is activated by an antigen, either directly (e.g., when the antigen is a microbial polysaccharide) or after the binding of antibody. Complement activation results in the covalent attachment of C3b and its cleavage product C3d to the antigen. B lymphocytes can bind the antigen through their Ig receptors and simultaneously bind the attached C3d through CR2, the coreceptor for the B cell antigen receptor, thus enhancing antigen-induced signaling in B cells (see Chapter 12). Opsonized

antigens are also bound by follicular dendritic cells in the germinal centers of lymphoid organs. Follicular dendritic cells display antigens to B cells in the germinal centers, and this process is important for the selection of high-affinity B cells (see Fig. 12-19). The importance of complement in humoral immune responses is illustrated by the severe impairment in antibody production and germinal center formation seen in knockout mice lacking C3 or C4 or the CR2 protein.

Complement Deficiencies

Genetic deficiencies of complement proteins and regulatory proteins are the causes of various human diseases. Inherited and spontaneous deficiencies in many of the complement proteins have been described in humans.

- Genetic deficiencies in classical pathway components, including C1q, C1r, C4, C2, and C3, have been described; C2 deficiency is the most common human complement deficiency. More than 50% of patients with C1q, C2 and C4 deficiencies develop systemic lupus erythematosus. The reason for this association is unknown, but it may be related to the fact that defects in complement activation lead to failure to clear circulating immune complexes. If normally generated immune complexes are not cleared from the circulation, they may be deposited in blood vessel walls and tissues, where they activate leukocytes by Fc receptor–dependent pathways and produce local inflammation. Complement may also play an important role in the clearance of apoptotic bodies containing fragmented DNA. These apoptotic bodies are likely sources of the nuclear antigens that trigger autoantibody responses in lupus. In addition, complement proteins regulate antigen-mediated signals received by B cells; in their absence, self antigens may not induce B cell tolerance, and autoimmunity results. Somewhat surprisingly, C2 and C4 deficiencies are not usually associated with increased susceptibility to infections, which suggests that the alternative pathway and Fc receptor–mediated effector mechanisms are adequate for host defense against most microbes. Deficiency of C3 is associated with frequent serious pyogenic bacterial infections that may be fatal, illustrating the central role of C3 in opsonization, enhanced phagocytosis, and destruction of these organisms.

- Deficiencies in components of the alternative pathway, including properdin and Factor D, result in increased susceptibility to infection with pyogenic bacteria. A mutation of the gene encoding mannose-binding lectin (MBL) contributes to immunodeficiency in some patients; this is discussed in Chapter 21.
- Deficiencies in the terminal complement components, including C5, C6, C7, C8, and C9, have also been described. Interestingly, as mentioned earlier, the only consistent clinical problem in these patients is a propensity for disseminated infections by *Neisseria* bacteria, including *Neisseria meningitidis* and *Neisseria gonorrhoeae*, indicating that complement-mediated bacterial lysis is particularly important for defense against these organisms.
- Deficiencies in complement regulatory proteins are associated with abnormal complement activation and a variety of related clinical abnormalities. Deficiencies in C1 inhibitor and decay-accelerating factor were mentioned earlier. In patients with Factor I deficiency, plasma C3 is depleted as a result of the unregulated formation of fluid-phase C3 convertase (by the normal tickover mechanism). The clinical consequence is increased infections with pyogenic bacteria. Factor H deficiency is rare and is characterized by excess alternative pathway activation, consumption of C3, and glomerulonephritis caused by inadequate clearance of immune complexes and renal deposition of complement byproducts. An atypical form of hemolytic-uremic syndrome involves defective complement regulation, and the most common mutations in this condition are in the *Factor H* gene. Specific allelic variants of Factor H are strongly associated with age-related macular degeneration. The effects of a lack of Factor I or Factor H are similar to the effects of an autoantibody called C3 nephritic factor (C3NeF), which is specific for alternative pathway C3 convertase (C3bBb). C3NeF stabilizes C3bBb and protects the complex from Factor H–mediated dissociation, which results in unregulated consumption of C3. Patients with this antibody often have glomerulonephritis, possibly caused by inadequate clearing of circulating immune complexes.

- Deficiencies in complement receptors include the absence of CR3 and CR4, both resulting from rare mutations in the β chain (CD18) that is shared by the CD11CD18 family of integrin molecules. The congenital disease caused by this gene defect is called leukocyte adhesion deficiency (see Chapter 20). This disorder is characterized by recurrent pyogenic infections and is caused by inadequate adherence of neutrophils to endothelium at tissue sites of infection and perhaps by impaired iC3b-dependent phagocytosis of bacteria.

Pathologic Effects of the Complement System

Even when it is properly regulated and appropriately activated, the complement system can cause significant tissue damage. Some of the pathologic effects associated with bacterial infections may be due to complement-mediated acute inflammatory responses to infectious organisms. In some situations, complement activation is associated with intravascular thrombosis and can lead to ischemic injury to tissues. For instance, anti-endothelial antibodies against vascularized organ transplants and the immune complexes produced in autoimmune diseases may bind to vascular endothelium and activate complement, thereby leading to inflammation and generation of the MAC with damage to the endothelial surface, which favors coagulation. There is also evidence that some of the late complement proteins may activate prothrombinases in the circulation that initiate thrombosis independent of MAC-mediated damage to endothelium. In an autoantibody-mediated kidney disorder, membranous nephropathy, sub-lytic damage to glomerular epithelial cells can be mediated by the MAC that is generated after antibody binds to a glomerular autoantigen. In this disease, there is no inflammation or circulating immune complexes, and glomerular leakiness is a consequence of complement activation.

The clearest examples of complement-mediated pathology are immune complex–mediated diseases. Systemic vasculitis and immune complex glomerulonephritis result from the deposition of antigen-antibody complexes in the walls of vessels and kidney glomeruli (see Chapter 19). Complement activated by these deposited immune complexes initiates the acute inflammatory responses that destroy the vessel walls or glomeruli and lead to thrombosis, ischemic damage to tissues, and scarring. Studies with knockout mice lacking the complement proteins C3 or C4 or lacking Fcγ receptors suggest that Fc receptor–mediated leukocyte activation may also cause inflammation and tissue injury as a result of IgG deposition, even in the absence of complement activation.

Evasion of Complement by Microbes

Pathogens have evolved diverse mechanisms for evading the complement system. Some microbes express thick cell walls that prevent the binding of complement proteins, such as the MAC. Gram-positive bacteria and some fungi are examples of microbes that use this relatively nonspecific evasion strategy. A few of the more specific mechanisms employed by a small subset of pathogens will be considered here. These evasion mechanisms may be divided into three groups.

- *Microbes can evade the complement system by recruiting host complement regulatory proteins.* Many pathogens, in contrast to non–pathogenic microbes, express sialic acids, which can inhibit the alternative pathway of complement by recruiting Factor H, which displaces C3b from Bb. Some pathogens, like schistosomes, *Neisseria gonorrhoeae,* and certain *Haemophilus* species, scavenge sialic acids from the host and enzymatically transfer the sugar to their cell surfaces. Others, including *Escherichia coli K1* and some meningococci, have evolved special biosynthetic routes for sialic acid generation. Some microbes synthesize proteins that can recruit the regulatory protein Factor H to the cell surface. GP41 on human immunodeficiency virus (HIV) can bind to Factor H, and this property of the virus is believed to contribute to virion protection. Many other pathogens have evolved proteins that facilitate the recruitment of Factor H to their cell walls. These include bacteria such as *Streptococcus pyogenes, Borrelia burgdorferi* (the causative agent of Lyme disease), *Neisseria gonorrhoeae, Neisseria meningitidis,* the fungal pathogen *Candida albicans,* and nematodes such as *Echinococcus granulosus.* Other microbes, such as HIV, incorporate multiple host regulatory proteins into their envelopes. For instance, HIV incorporates the GPI-anchored complement regulatory proteins DAF and CD59 when it buds from an infected cell.
- *A number of pathogens produce specific proteins that mimic human complement regulatory proteins.* *Escherichia coli* makes a C1q-binding protein (C1qBP) that inhibits the formation of a complex between C1q, C1r and C1s. *Staphylococcus aureus* makes a protein called SCIN (staphylococcal complement inhibitor) that binds to and stably inhibits both the classical and alternative pathway C3 convertases and thus inhibits all three complement pathways. Glycoprotein C-1 of the herpes simplex virus destabilizes the alternative pathway convertase by preventing its C3b component from binding to properdin. GP160, a membrane protein on *Trypanosoma cruzi,* the causative agent of Chagas' disease, binds to C3b and prevents the formation of the C3 convertase and also accelerates its decay. VCP-1 (vaccinia virus complement inhibitory protein 1), a protein made by the vaccinia virus, structurally resembles human C4BP but can bind to both C4b and C3b and accelerate the decay of both C3 and C5 convertases.
- *Complement-mediated inflammation can also be inhibited by microbial gene products.* *Staphylococcus aureus* synthesizes a protein called CHIPS (chemokine inhibitory protein of staphylococci), which is an antagonist of the C5a anaphylatoxin.

These examples illustrate how microbes have acquired the ability to evade the complement system, presumably contributing to their pathogenicity.

NEONATAL IMMUNITY

Neonatal mammals are protected from infection by maternally produced antibodies transported across the placenta into the fetal circulation and by antibodies in ingested milk transported across the gut epithelium of newborns by a specialized process known as transcytosis. Neonates lack the ability to mount effective immune responses against microbes, and for several months after birth, their major defense against infection is passive immunity provided by maternal antibodies. Maternal IgG is transported across the placenta, and maternal IgA and IgG in breast milk are ingested by the nursing infant. The transepithelial transport of maternal IgA into breast milk depends on the poly-Ig receptor described in Chapter 14. Ingested IgA and IgG can neutralize pathogenic organisms that attempt to colonize the infant's gut, and ingested IgG antibodies are also transported across the gut epithelium into the circulation of the newborn. Thus, a newborn contains essentially the same IgG antibodies as the mother.

Transport of maternal IgG across the placenta and across the neonatal intestinal epithelium is mediated by an IgG-specific Fc receptor called the **neonatal Fc receptor** (FcRn). The FcRn is unique among Fc receptors in that it resembles a class I major histocompatibility complex (MHC) molecule containing a transmembrane heavy chain that is non-covalently associated with β2-microglobulin. However, the interaction of IgG with FcRn does not involve the portion of the molecule analogous to the peptide-binding cleft used by class I MHC molecules to display peptides for T cell recognition.

Adults also express the FcRn in the endothelium, macrophages, and many other cell types. This receptor functions to protect plasma IgG antibodies from catabolism. We described this process in Chapter 5.

SUMMARY

- Humoral immunity is mediated by antibodies and is the effector arm of the adaptive immune system responsible for defense against extracellular microbes and microbial toxins. The antibodies that provide protection against infection may be produced by long-lived antibody-secreting cells generated by the first exposure to microbial antigen or by reactivation of memory B cells by the antigen.
- Antibodies block, or neutralize, the infectivity of microbes by binding to the microbes and sterically hindering interactions of the microbes with cellular receptors. Antibodies similarly block the pathologic actions of toxins by preventing binding of the toxins to host cells.
- Antibody-coated (opsonized) particles are phagocytosed by binding of the Fc portions of the antibodies to phagocyte Fc receptors. There are several types of Fc receptors specific for different subclasses of IgG and for IgA and IgE antibodies, and different Fc receptors bind the antibodies with varying affinities. Attachment of antigen-complexed Ig

to phagocyte Fc receptors also delivers signals that stimulate the microbicidal activities of phagocytes.

* The complement system consists of serum and membrane proteins that interact in a highly regulated manner to produce biologically active products. The three major pathways of complement activation are the alternative pathway, which is activated on microbial surfaces in the absence of antibody; the classical pathway, which is activated by antigen-antibody complexes; and the lectin pathway, which is initiated by circulating lectins binding to carbohydrates on pathogens. These pathways generate enzymes that cleave the C3 protein, and cleaved products of C3 become covalently attached to microbial surfaces or antibodies, so subsequent steps of complement activation are limited to these sites. All pathways converge on a common pathway that involves the formation of a membrane pore after the proteolytic cleavage of C5.

* Complement activation is regulated by various plasma and cell membrane proteins that inhibit different steps in the cascades.

* The biologic functions of the complement system include opsonization of organisms and immune complexes by proteolytic fragments of C3, followed by binding to phagocyte receptors for complement fragments and phagocytic clearance, activation of inflammatory cells by proteolytic fragments of complement proteins called anaphylatoxins (C3a, C4a, C5a), cytolysis mediated by MAC formation on cell surfaces, solubilization and clearance of immune complexes, and enhancement of humoral immune responses.

* Protective immunity in neonates is a form of passive immunity provided by maternal antibodies transported across the placenta by a specialized neonatal Fc receptor.

SELECTED READINGS

Complement

Gros P, Milder FJ, Janssen BJ: Complement driven by conformational changes, *Nature Reviews Immunology* 8:48–58, 2008.

Holers VM: Complement and its receptors: new insights into human disease, *Annual Review of Immunology* 32:433–459, 2014.

Manderson AP, Botto M, Walport MJ: The role of complement in the development of systemic lupus erythematosus, *Annual Review of Immunology* 22:431–456, 2004.

Ricklin D, Lambris JD: Complement in immune and inflammatory disorders, *Journal of Immunology* 190:3831–3838, 2013.

Roozendaal R, Carroll MC: Emerging patterns in complement-mediated pathogen recognition, *Cell* 125:29–32, 2006.

Antibody Effector Functions and Fc Receptors

Nimmerjahn F, Ravetch JV: Fcγ receptors as regulators of immune responses, *Nature Reviews Immunology* 8:34–47, 2008.

Schwab I, Nimmerjahn F: Intravenous immunoglobulin therapy: how does IgG modulate the immune system? *Nature Reviews Immunology* 13:176–189, 2013.

Smith KG, Clatworthy MR: FcγRIIB in autoimmunity and infection: evolutionary and therapeutic implications, *Nature Reviews Immunology* 10:328–343, 2010.

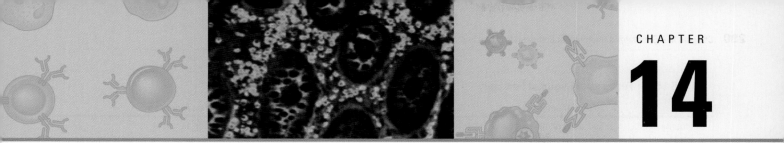

Specialized Immunity at Epithelial Barriers and in Immune Privileged Tissues

Most of our discussion of innate and adaptive immunity so far in this book has covered features and mechanisms of immune responses in any anatomic location in the mammalian body. However, the immune system has evolved specialized properties in different parts of the body, especially in epithelial barrier tissues. These features are essential for protection against the types of microbial challenges that are most often encountered at these locations, and they also ensure that we live in harmony with non-pathogenic commensal organisms that colonize epithelial surfaces and the lumens of mucosal organs (Table 14-1). The collection of the immune cells and molecules serving specialized functions at a particular anatomic location is called a regional immune system. Most of this chapter is

devoted to a discussion of these specialized immune systems. We end with a consideration of some tissues that do not normally support immune responses and are said to be immune privileged.

GENERAL FEATURES OF IMMUNITY AT EPITHELIAL BARRIERS

Regional immune systems include the mucosal immune systems, which protect the gastrointestinal, bronchopulmonary, and genitourinary mucosal barriers, and the cutaneous (skin) immune system. The gastrointestinal immune system is the largest and most complex. By two simple metrics—the number of lymphocytes located in the tissue and the amount of antibodies made there—the gastrointestinal system dwarfs all other parts of the immune system combined. The human intestinal mucosa is estimated to contain approximately 50×10^9 lymphocytes (Table 14-2). The dedication of so many immune system resources to the gut reflects the large surface area of the intestinal mucosa, which has evolved to maximize the primary absorptive function of the tissue but must also resist invasion by trillions of bacteria in the lumen. The skin is also a barrier tissue with vast surface area that must be protected from the environmental microbes that have ready access to the external lining. The total number of lymphocytes in the skin is estimated to be about 20×10^9, about twice the total number of circulating lymphocytes (see Table 14-2). The different physical features of the mucosa (soft, wet, and warm) and the skin (tough, dry, and cool) favor colonization and invasion by different types of microbes. Therefore, it is not surprising that the immune system is specialized in different ways in these two types of tissues.

The immune systems at epithelial barriers share a basic anatomic organization, with an outer epithelial layer that prevents microbial invasion, underlying connective tissue containing cells of various types that mediate immune responses to commensal or pathogenic organisms that do traverse the epithelium, and more distant draining lymph nodes where adaptive immune responses to invading microbes are initiated and amplified. The epithelial barrier may be several layers thick, as in the skin, or a single layer sitting on a basement membrane, as in the intestines. The

TABLE 14-1   Features of Regional Immunity

Region	Special Challenges	Special Anatomic Structures	Specialized Cells or Molecules: Functions
Gastrointestinal tract	Tolerance of food antigens Tolerance of commensal microbiota but responsive to rare pathogens Enormous surface area	Tonsils Peyer's patches, lamina, propria follicles	Intestinal epithelial cells: mucus secretion M cells: luminal antigen sampling Paneth cells: defensin production Secretory IgA, IgM: neutralization of microbes in the lumen Dendritic cell subsets: luminal antigen sampling; lamina propria antigen sampling; T cell tolerance induction; effector T cell activation; induction of B cell IgA class switching; imprinting gut-homing phenotypes of B and T cells
Respiratory system	Exposure to mix of airborne pathogens and innocuous microbes and particles	Tonsils Adenoids	Ciliated respiratory epithelial cells: mucus and defensin production and movement of mucus with trapped microbes and particles out of airways Secretory IgA, IgM, IgG: neutralization of microbes outside epithelial barrier
Cutaneous immune system	Large surface area	Keratinizing stratified squamous epithelial barrier	Keratinocytes: keratin production, cytokine and defensin secretion Langerhans cells: epidermal antigen sampling Dendritic cell subsets: dermal antigen sampling; T cell tolerance induction; effector T cell activation; imprinting skin-homing phenotype of T cells

underlying connective tissue, such as the dermis in the skin or the lamina propria in the gut, contains numerous scattered lymphocytes, dendritic cells, macrophages, and mast cells that mediate innate immune responses and the effector arm of adaptive immune responses. Mucosal tissues also contain unencapsulated but organized secondary lymphoid tissues just under the epithelial barrier, which include B and T lymphocytes, dendritic cells, and macrophages. These collections of immune cells, often called **mucosa-associated lymphoid tissue (MALT)**, are sites where some adaptive immune responses specialized for the particular mucosa are initiated. Adaptive immune responses in epithelial barrier immune systems are also induced in draining lymph nodes that are located outside the barrier tissues. In skin and mucosal tissues, antigens outside the epithelial barrier are sampled by specialized cells within the epithelium and are delivered to draining lymph nodes or MALT.

Regional immune systems contain specialized cell types and molecules that may not be abundant in other sites. The cell types that are restricted to one or more regional immune systems but are not present throughout the immune system include subsets of dendritic cells (e.g., Langerhans cells in the skin), antigen transport cells (e.g., M cells in the gut), T lymphocytes (e.g., $\gamma\delta$ T cells in epithelia), subsets of B lymphocytes (e.g., IgA producing B cells and plasma cells in mucosal tissues), and various innate lymphoid cells. The unique anatomic features and cell types in each tissue endow that tissue with special functional characteristics. For example, the sampling of antigens in the gut and their transport to secondary lymphoid tissues rely on cell types and routes of lymphatic drainage that are different from what takes place in the skin or internal organs. Furthermore, the MALT structures in different regions of the gut and in other mucosal organs have distinct features.

The effector lymphocytes that are generated in the draining lymph nodes or MALT of a particular regional immune system (e.g., skin, small bowel) will enter the blood and preferentially home back to the same organ (e.g., dermis, lamina propria). The migration and localization of subsets of lymphocytes to different tissues is in part due to tissue-specific homing mechanisms that direct these subsets from the blood into particular tissues, which we will discuss in detail later in this chapter.

Regional immune systems have important regulatory functions that serve to prevent unwanted responses to nonpathogenic microbes and foreign substances that are likely to be present at different barriers. The clearest example is the gut-associated immune system, which must suppress responses to commensal bacteria that colonize the intestinal mucosa as well as to foreign food substances but must respond to less frequent pathogenic bacteria. The suppression of immune responses to nonpathogenic organisms and harmless foreign substances is also important in other sites of the body, including the skin, lung, and genitourinary tract, which are not sterile and are constantly exposed to the environment.

With this introduction, we will discuss the details of these various features in different regional immune systems, beginning with the largest.

TABLE 14-2   Numbers of Lymphocytes in Different Tissues

Spleen	70×10^9
Lymph nodes	190×10^9
Bone marrow	50×10^9
Blood	10×10^9
Skin	20×10^9
Intestines	50×10^9
Liver	10×10^9
Lungs	30×10^9

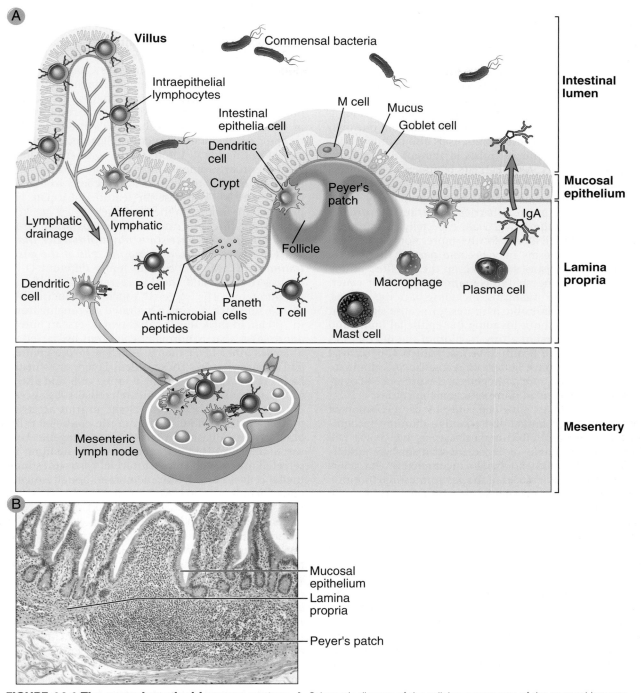

FIGURE 14-1 The gastrointestinal immune system. A, Schematic diagram of the cellular components of the mucosal immune system in the intestine. **B,** Photomicrograph of mucosal lymphoid tissue in the human intestine. Similar aggregates of lymphoid tissue are found throughout the gastrointestinal tract.

IMMUNITY IN THE GASTROINTESTINAL SYSTEM

The gastrointestinal system, like other mucosal tissues, is composed of a tube-like structure lined by a continuous epithelial cell layer sitting on a basement membrane that serves as a physical barrier to the external environment. Underlying the epithelium is a layer of loose connective tissue in the gut called the lamina propria that contains blood vessels, lymphatic vessels, and mucosa-associated lymphoid tissues (Fig. 14-1). The submucosa is a dense connective tissue layer that connects the mucosa with layers of smooth muscle.

From the perspective of the immunologist, the gastrointestinal tract has two remarkable properties. First, the combined mucosa of the small and large bowel has a total surface area of more than 200 m^2 (the size of a tennis court), made up mostly of small intestinal villi and microvilli. Second, the lumen of the gut is teeming with microbes, many of which are ingested along with food and most of which are continuously growing on the mucosal surface in healthy individuals as commensals. It is estimated that more than 500 different species of bacteria, amounting to approximately 10^{14} cells, live in the mammalian gut. This is 10 times more than the number of all the cells in the body, prompting some microbiologists to point out that we humans are actually only 10% human and 90% bacterial! We have evolved to depend on these commensals for several functions, including the degradation of components of our diet that our own cells cannot digest. These commensals also compete with potentially pathogenic microbes in the gut and prevent harmful infections. Although the commensal organisms are beneficial when they are contained on the outside of the gut mucosal barrier, they are potentially lethal if they cross the mucosal barrier and enter the circulation or traverse the bowel wall, especially in immune-compromised individuals. Furthermore, non-commensal pathogenic organisms may become part of the diverse mixture of organisms that make up the gut flora at any time if they are ingested in contaminated food or water. These pathogenic organisms, including bacteria, viruses, protozoa, and helminthic parasites, can cause significant disease, often without invading the epithelial lining and even if they represent a tiny fraction of the microbes in the gut lumen. For health to be maintained, the mucosal immune system must be able to recognize and eliminate these numerically rare pathogens in the presence of overwhelming numbers of non-pathogenic microbes.

These challenges have been met by the evolution of a complex set of innate and adaptive immune recognition strategies and effector mechanisms, which we will describe next. Some of these mechanisms we understand well, and others remain incompletely characterized. Many of the features of the gastrointestinal immune system are shared by other mucosal tissues, and we will point out these common features of mucosal immunity. Unfortunately, intestinal infections by pathogenic organisms are frequently not controlled by mucosal immunity and account for millions of deaths each year throughout the world.

Innate Immunity in the Gastrointestinal Tract

Intestinal epithelial cells lining the small and large bowel are an integral part of the gastrointestinal innate immune system, involved in responses to pathogens, tolerance to commensal organisms, and antigen sampling for delivery to the adaptive immune system in the gut. There are several different types of intestinal epithelial cells, all derived from a common precursor found in the crypts of intestinal glands. Among these are the mucus-secreting goblet cells, which reside at the top of the intestinal villi; cytokine-secreting absorptive epithelial cells; antigen-sampling M cells, found in specialized dome structures overlying lymphoid tissues; and anti-bacterial peptide–secreting Paneth cells, found at the bottom of the crypts. All of these cell types contribute in different ways to the barrier function of the mucosa, as we will discuss later.

Innate immune protection in the gut is mediated in part by the physical and chemical barrier provided by the mucosal epithelial cells and their mucus secretions. Adjacent intestinal epithelial cells are held together by

proteins that form tight junctions, including zonula occludens 1 and claudins, and these block the movement of microbes between the cells into the lamina propria. In addition, mucosal epithelial cells produce anti-microbial substances, including defensins (see Chapter 4). Several cell types located in the mucosa, including epithelial cells, dendritic cells, and macrophages, are capable of mounting inflammatory and anti-viral responses. Most of these responses are induced by pattern recognition receptor engagement by microbial ligands, which we discussed in Chapter 4. Interestingly, some innate immune receptors that promote inflammation in other parts of the body have anti-inflammatory actions in the gut. In this section, we will describe features of innate immunity that are unique to the intestines.

Several different extensively glycosylated proteins, called mucins, form a viscous physical barrier that prevents microbes from contacting the cells of the gastrointestinal tract. Mucins contain many different O-linked oligosaccharides and include secreted and cell surface glycoproteins. The secreted mucins, including MUC2, MUC5, and MUC6, form a hydrated gel ranging from 300 to 700 μm in thickness that has two layers: an outer less-dense layer that is normally colonized by bacteria, and a denser inner layer that is attached to the epithelium, and is bacteria-free. These mucus layers prevent microbial contact with the epithelial lining cells and also serve as a matrix for display of anti-microbial substances produced by the epithelial cells. Some mucins act as decoy molecules that can be shed from the epithelial cells and bind to the adhesin proteins that pathogenic bacteria use to attach to host cell membranes. In addition to the secreted mucus, the apical surface of gastrointestinal epithelial cells is coated with membrane-bound mucin proteins, including MUC1, MUC3A/b, MUC12, MUC13, and MUC17. These membrane-bound mucins combine with various glycolipids to form a dense macromolecular layer at the epithelial cell surface called the glycocalyx, which ranges from 30 to 500 nm in thickness in different locations in the gut. The glycocalyx, like the secreted mucus, serves as a physical barrier to prevent microbial contact.

The mucous barrier of the intestine undergoes turnover and chemical changes in response to various environmental and immune signals, which allows rapid increases in mucosal barrier function. Mucins are constitutively produced both by the surface epithelial cells in the gastrointestinal tract and by submucosal glands and are replaced by newly synthesized molecules every 6 to 12 hours. Several different environmental and immune stimuli can induce dramatic increases in mucin production. These stimuli include cytokines (IL-1, IL-4, IL-6, IL-9, IL-13, tumor necrosis factor [TNF], and type I interferons), neutrophil products (such as elastase), and microbial adhesive proteins. These stimuli not only increase mucin gene expression but also alter the glycosylation of the mucins because of induced changes in the expression of glycosyltransferase enzymes. The changes in quantity and glycosylation of mucins are thought to increase barrier function against pathogens.

Defensins produced by intestinal epithelial cells provide innate immune protection against luminal bacteria, and defects in their production are associated with bacterial invasion and inflammatory bowel disease. Defensins are peptides produced by various cell types in the body that exert lethal toxic effects on microbes by inserting into and causing loss of integrity of their outer phospholipid membranes (see Chapter 4). In the small bowel, the major defensins are the α-defensins, including human defensin 5 (HD5) and HD6, produced constitutively as inactive precursor proteins by Paneth cells located at the base of crypts between microvilli. Active HD5 and HD6 peptides are generated by proteolytic cleavage mediated by trypsin, also produced by Paneth cells. In the colon, β-defensins are produced by absorptive epithelial cells in the intestinal crypts, some constitutively and others in response to IL-1 or invasive bacteria. In addition, neutrophil granules are rich in α-defensins, which likely contribute to their anti-microbial functions in the setting of infections of the bowel wall. Several studies have identified defects in defensin production by epithelial cells in affected regions of bowel in Crohn's disease, a chronic inflammatory disease that can involve the entire gastrointestinal tract.

Paneth cells and other epithelial cells of the intestine also secrete a C-type lectin called regenerating islet-derived protein IIIγ (REGIIIγ), which blocks bacterial colonization of the epithelial surface. REGIIIγ and its human homolog REGIIIα bind to Gram-positive bacterial peptidoglycan. The expression of REGIIIγ by intestinal epithelial cells requires TLR signals in response to commensal organism and its production is increased after colonization and infection by pathogens.

Toll-like receptors (TLRs) and cytoplasmic NOD-like receptors (NLRs) expressed by intestinal epithelial cells promote immune responses to invasive pathogens but also limit inflammatory responses to commensal bacteria. As we discussed in Chapter 4, TLRs and NLRs are cellular receptors that recognize pathogen-associated molecular patterns (PAMPs) produced by microbes and generate signals that promote inflammatory and anti-viral responses by the cells. Most luminal bacteria of the gut are non-pathogenic if they are retained outside the epithelial barrier, yet they may express the same array of PAMPs that pathogenic bacteria express, such as lipopolysaccharide, peptidoglycans, CpG DNA, and flagellin. Because inflammatory responses that involve the intestinal epithelial cells can impair barrier function and can lead to bacterial invasion and pathologic inflammation, it is not surprising that stringent control mechanisms have evolved to limit TLR-induced proinflammatory responses to commensal bacteria. Intestinal epithelial cells express a wide range of TLRs, including TLRs 2, 4, 5, 6, 7, and 9, with different receptors expressed in different regions of the gut. Ligation of some TLRs results in the phosphorylation and reorganization of zona occludens 1 and increased strength of the tight junctions between epithelial cells, and TLR signaling also increases intestinal epithelial motility and proliferation. These functional responses to TLR signaling increase barrier function but not inflammation. TLR responses in the gut appear also to be regulated by levels of expression or compartmentalized expression in only certain sites (Fig. 14-2). For example, TLR5, which recognizes bacterial flagellins, is exclusively expressed on the basolateral surface of intestinal epithelial cells, where

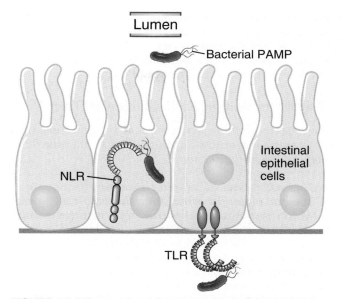

FIGURE 14-2 Expression of pattern recognition receptors in the intestinal mucosa. Pattern recognition receptors that recognize bacterial flagellin are concentrated in the cytosol (NLR) or basal membrane (TLR5) of intestinal epithelial cells but not on the apical/lumen membrane, and thus they do not recognize luminal microbes.

it will be accessible only to bacteria that have invaded through the barrier. Similarly, NLR family receptors for flagellins (e.g., NAIP and IPAF-1) are expressed in the cytosol of intestinal epithelial cells and will activate inflammatory responses only when pathogenic bacteria or their products gain access to the cytosol. There is also evidence that regulators of TLR signaling inside intestinal epithelial cells maintain a higher threshold for activation of inflammatory responses compared with epithelial cells and dendritic cells in other tissues.

In healthy individuals, dendritic cells and macrophages in the lamina propria of the gut inhibit inflammation and serve to maintain homeostasis. Some intestinal macrophages have a unique phenotype that enables them to phagocytose and kill microbes but at the same time to secrete anti-inflammatory cytokines, such as IL-10. This phenotype is apparently induced in the local mucosal environment by transforming growth factor-β (TGF-β). TLR4 expression on both macrophages and dendritic cells in the lamina propria is lower than in other tissues, and inflammatory gene expression in these cells is often inhibited by microbial products. This may be an evolved mechanism to prevent damaging inflammation in response to commensal bacteria and bacterial products that may traverse the epithelial barrier.

Innate lymphoid cells that produce IL-17 and IL-22 are found mainly in the intestinal mucosa and contribute to immune defense against some bacteria as well as to mucosal epithelial barrier function. Recall from Chapters 2 and 4 that innate lymphoid cells do not express TCRs, but subsets of these cells resemble helper T cell subsets because of the cytokines they secrete. The group 3 innate lymphoid cells secrete IL-17 and IL-22, similar to T_H17 cells. These cytokines enhance intestinal mucosal barrier function by stimulating production of mucus and defensins, and by enhancing epithelial tight junction function. The cytokines also enhance the transport of IgA into the intestinal lumen, which is a critical component of adaptive immunity in the gut, discussed later.

Adaptive Immunity in the Gastrointestinal Tract

The adaptive immune system in the gastrointestinal tract has features that are distinct from adaptive immune functions in other organ systems.

- *The major form of adaptive immunity in the gut is humoral immunity directed at microbes in the lumen*, which prevents commensals and pathogens from colonizing and invading through the mucosal epithelial barrier. This function is mediated by dimeric IgA antibodies that are secreted into the lumen of the gut or, in the case of breast-feeding infants, IgA that is secreted into colostrum and mother's milk and ingested by the infant. Significant quantities of IgG and IgM antibodies are also present in the gut lumen and contribute to humoral immunity in this location.
- *The dominant protective cell-mediated immune response consists of T_H17 effector cells*, which are the most numerous effector T cell subset found in the intestinal mucosa.
- *A major mechanism for controlling responses in the gut is the activation of regulatory T cells (Treg).* The adaptive immune system in the gut must continuously suppress potential immune responses to food antigens and commensal microbial antigens to prevent inflammatory reactions that would compromise the mucosal barrier. Nowhere else in the body is there such an extensive commitment of the immune system to maintaining tolerance to foreign antigens. Some subsets of Treg are more abundant in mucosa-associated lymphoid tissues (MALT) than in other lymphoid organs.

We will now discuss the special features of adaptive immunity in the gastrointestinal system, including anatomic organization, antigen sampling, lymphocyte homing and differentiation, and antibody delivery to the lumen.

The Functional Anatomy of the Adaptive Immune System in the Gastrointestinal Tract

In this section, we will discuss the anatomic organization of cells within the intestines and the relationship of this organization to how adaptive immune responses are initiated, carried out, and regulated. In general terms, the functional anatomy of the adaptive immune system in the gut has evolved to effectively deal with the conditions we emphasized earlier of abundant commensal microbes and rare pathogens just outside an epithelial barrier of enormous surface area.

Adaptive immune responses in the gut are initiated in discretely organized collections of lymphocytes and antigen-presenting cells closely associated with the mucosal epithelial lining of the bowel and in mesenteric lymph nodes (see Fig. 14-1). Naive lymphocytes are exposed to antigens in these sites and differentiate into effector cells. These gut-associated lymphoid tissues adjacent to the

mucosal epithelium are sometimes referred to as GALT, which is the gastrointestinal version of MALT, although the terms are often used interchangeably. The most prominent GALT structures are **Peyer's patches**, found mainly in the distal ileum and in smaller aggregates of lymphoid follicles or isolated follicles in the appendix and colon. Peyer's patches have the structure of lymphoid follicles, with germinal centers containing B lymphocytes, follicular helper T cells, follicular dendritic cells, and macrophages. The germinal centers in the follicles are surrounded by IgM- and IgD-expressing naive follicular B cells. A region called the dome is located between the follicles and the overlying epithelium and contains B and T lymphocytes, dendritic cells, and macrophages. Between the follicles are T cell–rich parafollicular areas, similar to lymph nodes, but overall, the ratio of B cells to T cells in GALT is about five times higher than in lymph nodes. Also in distinction from lymph nodes, GALT structures are not encapsulated, and there are routes of antigen delivery to these structures that are independent of lymphatics. Development of both specialized lymphoid structures, such as Peyer's patches, and isolated follicles in the gut lamina propria requires innate lymphoid tissue inducer cells, which are a subset of innate lymphoid cells that express the RORγT transcription factor and produce the cytokine lymphotoxin-β (LTβ).

A major pathway of antigen delivery from the lumen to the GALT is through specialized cells within the gut epithelium called microfold (M) cells (Fig. 14-3). M cells are located in regions of the gut epithelium called follicle-associated or dome epithelium that overlie the domes of Peyer's patches and other GALT structures. Although M cells and the more numerous epithelial cells with absorptive function likely arise from a common epithelial precursor, the M cells are distinguishable by a thin glycocalyx, their relatively short, irregular microvilli (referred to as microfolds), and large fenestrations in their membranes, all features that enhance the uptake of antigens from the gut lumen. The main function of M cells is transcellular transport of various substances from the lumen of the intestine across the epithelial barrier to underlying antigen-presenting cells. M cells take up luminal contents efficiently and in various ways, including phagocytosis in a manner similar to macrophages, and either clathrin-coated vesicular or fluid-phase endocytosis. These pathways enable uptake of whole bacteria, viruses, and soluble microbial products. Unlike macrophages or dendritic cells, M cells do not engage in extensive processing of the substances they take up, but rather they move the particles and molecules through endocytic vesicles across the cytosol and deliver them by exocytosis at the basolateral membrane to dendritic cells in the dome regions of underlying Peyer's patches and lamina propria lymphoid follicles. Although M cells play an important role in protective immunity to luminal microbes, some microbes have evolved to take advantage of M cells as a route of invasion through the mucosal barrier. The best described example of this is *Salmonella typhimurium*, which is similar to the human pathogen *S. typhi* that causes typhoid fever. M cells express lectins that allow these bacteria to specifically bind and be internalized. The bacteria are cytotoxic to the M cells, leading to gaps in the epithelium

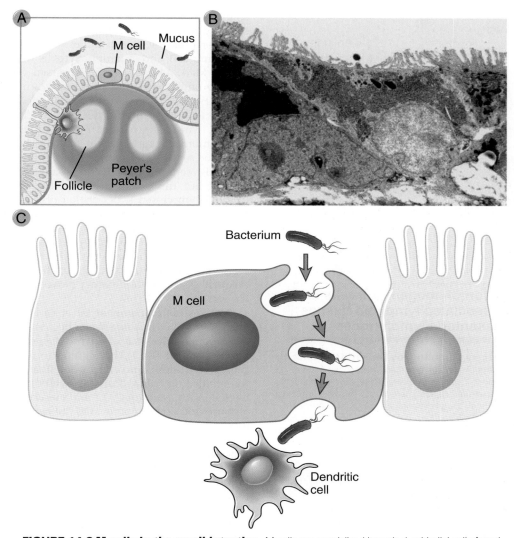

FIGURE 14-3 M cells in the small intestine. M cells are specialized intestinal epithelial cells found in the small bowel epithelium overlying Peyer's patches and lamina propria lymphoid follicles **(A)**. Unlike neighboring epithelial cells with tall microvillous borders and primary absorptive functions, M cells have shorter villi **(B)** and engage in transport of intact microbes or molecules across the mucosal barrier into gut-associated lymphoid tissues, where they are handed off to dendritic cells **(C)**. *(Electron micrograph from Corr SC, Gahan CC, Hill C: M-cells: origin, morphology and role in mucosal immunity and microbial pathogenesis, FEMS Immunology and Medical Microbiology 52:2-12, 2008.)*

that promote invasion of more organisms. M cell lectins may also be used by certain enteric viruses to breach the epithelial barrier.

Microbial antigens in the gut lumen can be sampled by lamina propria dendritic cells that extend cytoplasmic processes between the intestinal epithelial cells (Fig. 14-4). Antigen-sampling dendritic cells are numerous in certain regions of the intestine, especially the terminal ileum, where they extend dendrites through the junctions between adjacent epithelial cells, apparently without disrupting the tight junctions. These antigen-sampling dendritic cells may promote protective adaptive immune responses to pathogens in the lumen. Unlike M cells, these dendritic cells are capable of processing and presenting protein antigens to T cells within GALT. Dendritic cells resident in the lamina propria also capture antigens that enter between cells.

Mesenteric lymph nodes collect lymph-borne antigens from the small and large intestines and are sites of differentiation of effector and regulatory lymphocytes that home back to the lamina propria. There are 100 to 150 of these lymph nodes located between the membranous layers of the mesentery. Mesenteric lymph nodes serve some of the same functions as GALT, including differentiation of B cells into IgA–secreting plasma cells and the development of effector T cells as well as regulatory T cells. The cells that differentiate in the mesenteric lymph nodes in response to bowel wall invasion by pathogens or commensals often home to the lamina propria (discussed later).

Lingual and palatine tonsils are nonencapsulated lymphoid structures located beneath stratified squamous epithelial mucosa in the base of the tongue and oropharynx, respectively, and are sites of immune responses to

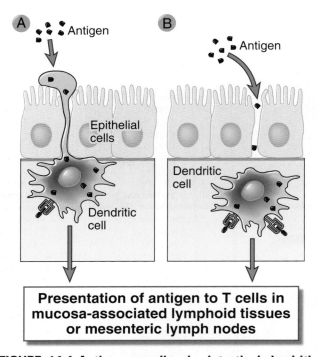

FIGURE 14-4 Antigen sampling by intestinal dendritic cells. Dendritic cells are present in the intestinal mucosa and sample antigens for presentation to T cells in GALT and mesenteric lymph nodes. **A,** Some dendritic cells extend dendritic processes between intestinal epithelial cells into the lumen to sample antigens. Macrophages may also sample luminal antigens in this manner. **B,** Other dendritic cells present in the lamina propria sample antigens that derived from lumina contents and have gotten through the epithelial barrier.

microbes in the oral cavity. These tonsils, together with nasopharyngeal tonsils, form a ring of lymphoid tissues called Waldeyer's ring. The bulk of the tonsillar tissue is composed of lymphoid follicles, usually with prominent germinal centers. There are multiple narrow and deep invaginations of the surface squamous epithelium, called crypts, which grow into the follicular tissue. Although these tonsils are often considered part of the GALT, they are distinct in that they are separated from the microbe-rich oral cavity by multiple layers of squamous epithelial cells rather than the single epithelial cell layer of the intestines. The mechanism of antigen sampling from oral cavity microbes is not well described; the crypts are possible sites where this may happen. Nonetheless, the lingual and palatine tonsils respond to infections of the epithelial mucosa by significant enlargement and vigorous, mainly IgA, antibody responses. Typical infections that are associated with tonsillar enlargement, usually in children, are caused by streptococci and the Epstein-Barr virus.

Effector lymphocytes that are generated in the GALT and mesenteric lymph nodes are imprinted with selective integrin- and chemokine receptor–dependent gut-homing properties, and they circulate from the blood back into the lamina propria of the gut (Fig. 14-5). The functions of the gastrointestinal immune system depend on a large number of T cells and antibody-secreting cells that are able to recirculate back into the lamina propria and respond rapidly to pathogens. Both effector T cells and IgA-secreting B cells acquire this gut-homing phenotype because of

changes in adhesion molecules and chemokine receptors that are acquired during lymphocyte activation in the GALT or draining lymph nodes. The major integrin on gut-homing B and T lymphocytes is $\alpha_4\beta_7$, which binds to the MadCAM-1 protein expressed on post-capillary venular endothelial cells in the gut lamina propria. Gut homing also requires the chemokine receptor CCR9 on the B and T lymphocytes and its chemokine ligand CCL25, which is produced by intestinal epithelial cells. The combined expression of MadCAM-1 and CCL25 is restricted to the gut. Homing of IgA-producing cells to the colon also requires CCR10 expression and the chemokine CCL28, but this is not a gut-specific pathway because CCL28 is expressed by epithelial cells in other mucosal tissues, such as the lung and genitourinary tract. Blocking monoclonal antibodies that are specific for the α_4 chain of $\alpha_4\beta_7$ has been used to treat patients with inflammatory bowel disease on the basis of the knowledge that effector T cells use this integrin to enter gut tissues in this disease. (We will discuss inflammatory bowel disease later in this chapter.)

The gut-homing phenotype of IgA-producing B cells and effector T cells is imprinted by dendritic cells through the action of retinoic acid during the process of T cell activation (see Fig. 14-5). In addition to promoting naive T cell differentiation into effector T cells and naive B cell differentiation into IgA antibody–secreting cells, discussed later, dendritic cells in GALT and mesenteric lymph nodes also provide signals that lead to the expression of the $\alpha_4\beta_7$ integrin and CCR9 on these effector cells. The induction of these homing molecules depends on secretion of retinoic acid by the dendritic cells, although the mechanisms are not well understood. The selective induction of gut-homing cells in the gut lymphoid tissues is explained by the fact that gut lymphoid tissues are exposed to dietary vitamin A, and dendritic cells in GALT and mesenteric lymph nodes express retinal dehydrogenases (RALDH), the enzyme needed for retinoic acid synthesis from vitamin A, whereas dendritic cells in other tissues do not. In addition, intestinal epithelial cells also express RALDH and can synthesize retinoic acid. Consistent with these properties of the intestinal immune system, it is known that oral vaccination not only favors the expansion of IgA-producing B cells, compared with intradermal immunization, but that oral vaccines also induce higher levels of $\alpha_4\beta_7$ on B cells.

The lamina propria contains diffusely distributed effector lymphocytes, dendritic cells, and macrophages and is the site of the effector phase of gastrointestinal adaptive immune responses. As discussed earlier, effector lymphocytes generated in Peyer's patches, other GALT structures, and mesenteric lymph nodes home back into the lamina propria. In this location, T cells can respond to invading pathogens, and B cells can secrete antibodies that are transported into the lumen and neutralize pathogens before they invade.

Humoral Immunity in the Gastrointestinal Tract

The major function of humoral immunity in the gastrointestinal tract is to neutralize luminal microbes, and this function is mediated mainly by IgA produced in the GALT and transported across the mucosal epithelium into the

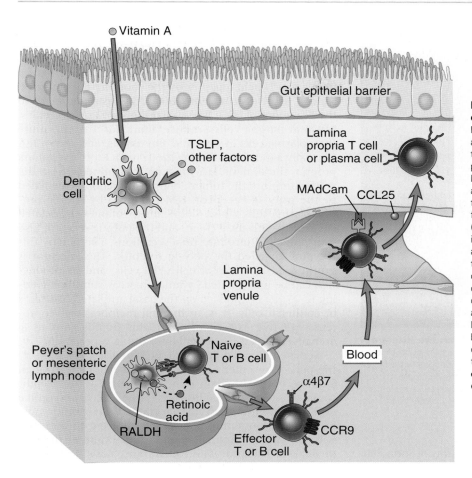

FIGURE 14-5 Homing properties of intestinal lymphocytes. The gut-homing properties of effector lymphocytes are imprinted in the lymphoid tissues, where they have undergone differentiation from naive precursors. Dendritic cells in gut-associated lymphoid tissues, including Peyer's patches and mesenteric lymph nodes, are induced by thymic stromal lymphopoietin (TSLP) and other factors to express retinaldehyde dehydrogenase (RALDH), which converts dietary vitamin A into retinoic acid. When naive B or T cells are activated by antigen in GALT, they are exposed to retinoic acid produced by the dendritic cells, and this induces the expression of the chemokine receptor CCR9 and the integrin $\alpha_4\beta_7$ on the plasma cells and effector T cells that arise from the naive lymphocytes. The effector lymphocytes enter the circulation and home back into the gut lamina propria because the chemokine CCL25 (the ligand for CCR9) and the adhesion molecule MadCAM (the ligand for $\alpha_4\beta_7$) are displayed on lamina propria venular endothelial cells.

lumen. Smaller but significant quantities of IgG and IgM are also secreted into the gut lumen. Within the lumen, IgA, IgG, and IgM antibodies bind to microbes and toxins and neutralize them by preventing their binding to receptors on host cells. This form of humoral immunity is sometimes called secretory immunity and has evolved to be particularly prominent in mammals. Antibody responses to antigens encountered by ingestion are typically dominated by IgA, and secretory immunity is the mechanism of protection induced by oral vaccines such as the polio vaccine. Several unique properties of the gut environment result in selective development of IgA-secreting cells that either stay in the gastrointestinal tract or, if they enter the circulation, home back to the lamina propria of the intestines. The result is that IgA-secreting cells efficiently accumulate next to the epithelium that will take up the secreted IgA and transport it into the lumen.

IgA is produced in larger amounts than any other antibody isotype. It is estimated that a normal 70-kg adult secretes about 2g of IgA per day, which accounts for 60% to 70% of the total production of antibodies. This tremendous output of IgA is because of the large number of IgA-producing plasma cells in the GALT, which by some estimates account for 80% of all the antibody-producing plasma cells in the body (Fig. 14-6). Because IgA synthesis occurs mainly in mucosal lymphoid tissue and most of the locally produced IgA is efficiently transported into the mucosal lumen, this isotype constitutes less than one

quarter of the antibody in plasma and is a minor component of systemic humoral immunity compared with IgG and IgM.

The dominance of IgA production by intestinal plasma cells is due in part to selective induction of IgA isotype switching in B cells in GALT and mesenteric lymph nodes. IgA class switching in the gut can occur by T-dependent and T-independent mechanisms (Fig. 14-7). In both cases, the molecules that drive IgA switching include a combination of soluble cytokines and membrane proteins on other cell types that bind to signaling receptors on B cells (see Chapter 12). TGF-β, the major cytokine required for IgA isotype switching in the gut as well as in other mucosal compartments, is produced by intestinal epithelial cells and dendritic cells in GALT. Furthermore, GALT dendritic cells express the $\alpha_v\beta_8$ integrin, which is required for activation of TGF-β. Several molecules that promote IgA class switching are expressed by intestinal epithelial cells or GALT dendritic cells in response to TLR signaling, and the commensal bacteria in the gut lumen produce ligands that bind to the relevant TLRs. For example, T-independent IgA and IgG switching requires binding of the TNF family cytokine APRIL to the TACI receptor on B cells, and intestinal epithelial cells produce APRIL in response to TLR ligands made by commensal bacteria. Intestinal epithelial cells also produce thymic stromal lymphopoietin (TSLP) in response to TLR signals, and TSLP stimulates additional APRIL production by GALT dendritic cells. TLR ligands made by commensal

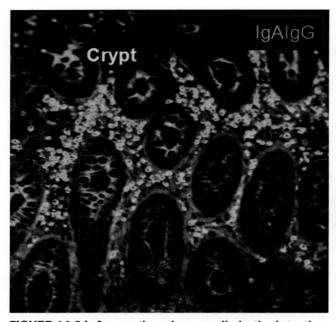

FIGURE 14-6 IgA-secreting plasma cells in the intestine.
The abundance of IgA-producing plasma cells (green) in colon mucosa compared with IgG-secreting cells (red) is shown by immunofluorescence staining. IgA that is being secreted can be seen as green cytoplasm in the crypt epithelial cells. *(From Brandtzaeg P. The mucosal immune system and its integration with the mammary glands.* The Journal of Pediatrics *156[Suppl 1]:S8-S16, 2010.)*

bacteria in the gut also increase expression of inducible nitric oxide synthase in dendritic cells, leading to nitric oxide production. Nitric oxide is thought to promote both T-dependent and T-independent IgA class switching, in part because nitric oxide enhances TGF-β signaling in B cells and also synthesis of APRIL by GALT dendritic cells. Finally, intestinal B cell IgA production is at least partly dependent on the vitamin A metabolite all-*trans* retinoic acid, which is made by intestinal epithelial cells and GALT dendritic cells, although the mechanisms by which retinoic acid promotes IgA production are not known. Retinoic acid is also important in B cell homing to the gut, as discussed earlier. There is an abundance of many of these molecules within the GALT and mesenteric lymph nodes compared with non-mucosal lymphoid tissues such as spleen and skin-draining lymph nodes, largely accounting for the propensity of B cells in the GALT to switch to IgA production.

The high level of IgA production by intestinal plasma cells is enhanced by selective gut-homing properties of IgA-producing cells that arise in GALT and mesenteric lymph nodes (see Fig. 14-5). Some of the IgA that is transported across the intestinal epithelium may be produced by plasma cells that differentiated and remained within underlying GALT follicles. However, IgA-secreting plasma cells are widely dispersed in the lamina propria of the gastrointestinal tract, not just in lymphoid follicles. As discussed earlier, activated B cells that undergo isotype switching into IgA-producing cells in the GALT and mesenteric lymph nodes may enter the systemic circulation and then selectively home back to the intestinal lamina propria, where they may reside as plasma cells.

Secreted IgA is transported through epithelial cells into the intestinal lumen by an IgA/IgM-specific Fc receptor called the poly-Ig receptor (Fig. 14-8). The IgA produced by plasma cells in the lamina propria is in the form of a dimer that is held together by the coordinately produced J chain, which is covalently bound by disulfide bonds to the Fc regions of the α heavy chains of two IgA molecules. Mucosal plasma cells produce abundant J chain, more than plasma cells in non-mucosal tissues, and serum IgA is usually a monomer lacking the J chain. From the lamina propria, the dimeric IgA must be transported across the epithelium into the lumen, and this function is mediated by the **poly-Ig receptor.** IgM produced by lamina propria plasma cells is also a polymer (pentamer) associated covalently with the J chain, and the poly-Ig receptor also transports IgM into intestinal secretions. This is why this receptor is called the poly-Ig receptor. This receptor is synthesized by mucosal epithelial cells, and its production can be upregulated by inflammatory stimuli, including IL-17. It is expressed on the basal and lateral surfaces of epithelial cells. It is an integral membrane glycoprotein with five extracellular domains homologous to Ig domains and is thus a member of the Ig superfamily.

Secreted dimeric IgA and pentameric IgM bind to the poly-Ig receptor on mucosal epithelial cells through a domain of the J chain (see Fig. 14-8). The Ig-receptor complex is endocytosed into the epithelial cell, and unlike other endosomes that typically traffic to lysosomes, poly Ig-receptor–containing vesicles are directed to and fuse with the apical (luminal) plasma membrane of the epithelial cell. This process is called transcytosis. On the cell surface, the poly-Ig receptor is proteolytically cleaved, its transmembrane and cytoplasmic domains are left attached to the epithelial cell, and the extracellular domain of the receptor, carrying the IgA molecule, is released into the intestinal lumen. The cleaved part of the poly-Ig receptor, called the secretory component, remains associated with the dimeric IgA in the lumen. It is believed that the bound secretory component protects IgA (and IgM) from proteolysis by enzymes present in the intestinal lumen, and these antibodies are therefore able to serve their function of neutralizing microbes and toxins in the lumen. The poly-Ig receptor is also responsible for the secretion of IgA into bile, milk, sputum, saliva, and sweat.

IgG is present in intestinal secretions at levels equal to IgM but lower than IgA. In some mucosal secretions (i.e., in the rectum, genitourinary tract, and airways), IgG levels are high and often exceed IgA. The transport of IgG into mucosal secretions is due to another transcytosing receptor, the neonatal Fc receptor (FcRn), which we discussed in Chapters 5 and 13. In contrast to the poly-Ig receptor, which transports IgA unidirectionally (from the basal side to the apical/lumen side), FcRn can mediate bidirectional transport of IgG. Therefore, FcRn-mediated IgG transport likely contributes to humoral immunity against luminal intestinal pathogens and may also contribute to uptake of antibody-coated microbes and other antigens from the lumen into the GALT.

IgA produced in lymphoid tissues in the mammary gland is secreted into colostrum and mature breast milk through poly-Ig receptor–mediated transcytosis and mediates passive mucosal immunity in breast-fed children.

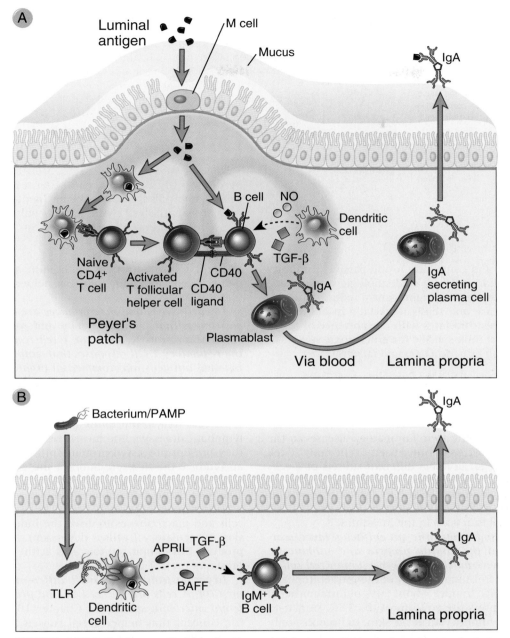

FIGURE 14-7 IgA class switching in the gut. IgA class switching in the gut occurs by both T-dependent and T-independent mechanisms. **A,** In T-dependent IgA class switching, dendritic cells in the subepithelial dome of Peyer's patches capture bacterial antigens delivered by M cells and migrate to the interfollicular zone, where they present antigen to naive CD4+ T cells. The activated T cells differentiate into helper T cells with a T follicular helper phenotype and engage in cognate interactions with antigen-presenting IgM+IgD+ B cells that have also taken up and processed the bacterial antigen. B cell class switching to IgA is stimulated through T cell CD40L binding to B cell CD40, together with the action of TGF-β. This T cell–dependent pathway yields high-affinity IgA antibodies. **B,** T-independent IgA class switching involves dendritic cell activation of IgM+IgD+ B cells, including B-1 cells. TLR ligand–activated dendritic cells secrete cytokines that induce IgA class switch, including BAFF, APRIL, and TGF-β. This T cell–independent pathway yields relatively low-affinity IgA antibodies to intestinal bacteria. The molecular mechanisms of class switching are described in Chapter 12.

The human lactating mammary gland contains a large number of IgA-secreting plasma cells, and the mammary gland epithelium can store large quantities of secretory IgA. The plasma cells in the breast originate from various mucosa-associated lymphoid tissues. They home to the breast because most IgA plasmablasts express CCR10, no matter which lymphoid tissues they were generated in, and the breast tissues express CCL28, the chemokine that binds CCR10. Therefore, during breast-feeding, a child ingests a significant quantity of maternal IgA, which provides broad polymicrobial protection in the infant's gut. Moderate amounts of IgG and IgM are also secreted

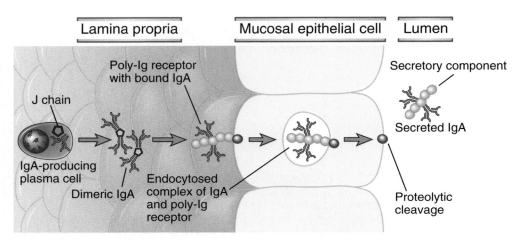

FIGURE 14-8 Transport of IgA across epithelial cells. IgA is produced by plasma cells in the lamina propria of mucosal tissue and binds to the poly-Ig receptor at the base of an epithelial cell. The complex is transported across the epithelial cell, and the bound IgA is released into the lumen by proteolytic cleavage. The process of transport across the cell, from the basolateral to the luminal surface in this case, is called transcytosis.

into breast milk and contribute to the passive immunity of breast-fed children. Many epidemiologic studies have shown that breast-feeding significantly reduces the risk of diarrheal disease and sepsis, especially in developing countries, and this correlates with the presence of secretory IgA in breast milk specific for enterotoxic species of bacteria including *Escherichia coli* and *Campylobacter*.

T Cell–Mediated Immunity in the Gastrointestinal Tract

T cells play important roles in protection against microbial pathogens in the gastrointestinal system and in regulating responses to food and commensal antigens. Furthermore, T cells contribute to inflammatory diseases in the gastrointestinal tract. As in other parts of the body, T cell immunity in the gut involves different subsets of T cells and is influenced in various ways by antigen-presenting dendritic cells, which also belong to different subsets. In this section, we will discuss important features of T cell and dendritic cell functions in the intestines.

T cells are found within the gut epithelial layer, scattered throughout the lamina propria and submucosa, and within Peyer's patches and other organized collections of follicles. In humans, most of the intraepithelial T cells are CD8+ cells. In mice, about 50% of intraepithelial lymphocytes express the γδ form of the TCR, similar to intraepidermal lymphocytes in the skin. In humans, only about 10% of intraepithelial lymphocytes are γδ cells, but this proportion is still higher than the proportions of γδ cells found among T cells in other tissues. Both the αβ and the γδ TCR–expressing intraepithelial lymphocytes show limited diversity of antigen receptors. These findings support the idea that mucosal intraepithelial lymphocytes have a limited range of specificity, distinct from that of most T cells, and this restricted repertoire may have evolved to recognize microbes that are commonly encountered at the epithelial surface. Lamina propria T cells are mostly CD4+, and most have the phenotype of activated effector or memory T cells, the latter with an effector memory phenotype (see Chapter 9). Recall that these lamina propria effector and memory T cells are generated from naive precursors in the GALT and mesenteric lymph nodes, enter the circulation, and preferentially home back into the lamina propria (see Fig. 14-5). T cells within Peyer's patches and in other follicles

adjacent to the intestinal epithelium are mostly CD4+ helper T cells, including follicular helper T cells, and regulatory T cells.

Dendritic cells and macrophages are abundant in the gastrointestinal immune system and can participate in stimulating protective effector T cell responses or inducing regulatory T cell responses that suppress immunity to ingested antigens and commensal organisms. In the gut and in other mucosal tissues, some dendritic cells and macrophages project dendrites between epithelial cells and sample luminal contents, as discussed earlier. Dendritic cells that have captured antigens migrate, through lymphatic drainage, into mesenteric lymph nodes, where they present processed protein antigens to naive T cells and induce the differentiation of these T cells into IFN-γ–, IL-17– or IL-4–producing effector cells or into FoxP3+ Treg. Gut tissue macrophages can also promote the local expansion of regulatory T cells. The ability of dendritic cells and macrophages to drive the induction or expansion of regulatory T cells is dependent on their ability to produce TGF-β and retinoic acid at the time of antigen presentation to T cells.

In the gastrointestinal tract, different subsets of effector CD4+ T cells are induced by and protect against different microbial species. In Chapter 10, we introduced the concept that helper T cell subsets that secrete different cytokines are specialized for protection against different types of microbes. This fundamental concept is highly relevant to the mucosal immune system. The commensal bacterial microflora of the gut lumen exerts profound influences on T cell phenotypes, even during homeostasis.

- $T_H 17$ *cells.* Studies in mice have shown that certain classes of bacteria, or in some cases individual species of bacteria, can shift the dominant pattern of T cell cytokine production. For example, the lamina propria of the small bowel in healthy mice is particularly rich in IL-17–producing cells, whereas the colon is not, and the presence of the $T_H 17$ cells depends on colonization of the gut with a certain phylum of bacteria (segmented filamentous bacteria) in the postnatal period. This steady-state presence of $T_H 17$ cells is required for protection against pathogenic species of bacteria (e.g., *Citrobacter rodentium*). Another example of bacterial microflora–induced changes in gut T cell phenotypes is the finding that colonization of the bowel with either polysaccharide A non-expressing or expressing strains of *Bacteroides fragilis* induces IL-17–producing T cells or IL-10–producing regulatory T cells, respectively. T_H17 cells appear to play a special role in maintaining mucosal epithelial barrier function because of the actions of the two signature cytokines they produce, IL-17 and IL-22, which, as discussed earlier, are also products of innate lymphoid cells in the gut. The receptors for both these cytokines are expressed on intestinal epithelial cells, and both induce the expression of proteins important for barrier function, such as mucins and β-defensins, which protect the epithelial cells against microbe-induced injury. The mechanisms underlying these microbe-induced changes in T cell responses are not well understood but likely involve microbe-induced signals in both intestinal epithelial cells and dendritic cells. These signals change the phenotype and cytokine secretion profile of dendritic cells, which in turn influence T cell subset differentiation when the dendritic cells present antigen to microbial antigen-specific naive T cells.

- T_H2 *cells.* Intestinal helminthic infections induce strong T_H2 responses, which are effective in eliminating the worms because the T_H2 cytokines IL-4 and IL-13 cooperate in enhancing fluid and mucus secretions and inducing smooth muscle contraction and bowel motility.

Regulation of Immunity in the Gastrointestinal Tract by Regulatory T Cells and Cytokines

Regulatory T cells are abundant in GALT and prevent inflammatory reactions against intestinal commensal microbes. It is estimated that the proportion of FoxP3+ Treg among CD4+ cells is about 2-fold greater in the lamina propria than in other peripheral lymphoid tissues. Many of these Treg are likely induced in the gut in response to antigens encountered locally and thus belong to the category of peripheral Treg (see Chapter 15). The factors that contribute to the generation of these Treg include CD103+ dendritic cells, local production of retinoic acid (which promotes FoxP3 expression), and local production of TGF-β (which also promotes FoxP3 expression and inhibits the generation of T_H1 and T_H2 cells). As discussed in Chapter 15, Treg are thought to suppress immune responses by several mechanisms. Of these, the dominant mechanism in the gut seems to be production of the immunosuppressive cytokine IL-10, as discussed below.

Several cytokines, including TGF-β, IL-10, and IL-2, appear to play crucial roles in maintaining homeostasis in the gut immune system, and deficiencies in these cytokines or their receptors result in pathologic bowel inflammation. Much of our knowledge of cytokine-mediated regulation in the gut comes from studies with cytokine or cytokine receptor gene knockout mice. A major feature of the phenotype of mice with engineered deficiencies in TGF-β, IL-10, IL-10 receptor, IL-2, and IL-2 receptor is uncontrolled inflammation in the bowel.

Mutations in the IL-10 and IL-10 receptor genes are also associated with severe colitis in children, confirming the importance of IL-10 in preventing pathologic intestinal inflammation in humans. The uncontrolled inflammation observed in the gut in the absence of these cytokines or their receptors is most likely caused by innate and adaptive immune responses to commensal gut flora because the inflammation does not occur in mice raised in germ-free conditions.

The cellular sources of the cytokines and the relevant receptor-expressing target cells that are critical for prevention of bowel inflammation are not completely understood. Mouse models in which cytokines, cytokine receptors, and cytokine receptor signaling are genetically ablated only in specific cell types have been used to address the question of which cell types are important. In the case of TGF-β– and IL-10–dependent regulation of gut inflammation, evidence indicates that Treg are an important source of these cytokines. For example, selective deletion of the *Il10* gene in FoxP3+ cells leads to severe colitis but no other manifestations of inflammatory disease, consistent with the critical role of Treg-produced IL-10 in maintaining homeostasis in the gastrointestinal tract. It is possible that macrophages, which produce IL-10, are another important source of IL-10. The target cells that express receptors for and are regulated by TGF-β and IL-10 likely include dendritic cells, effector T cells, innate effector cells such as macrophages, and epithelial cells. Inflammatory bowel disease in mice lacking IL-2 or its receptor is a consequence of defects in the development and function of Treg, which require IL-2 (see Chapter 15).

Oral Tolerance and Oral Vaccines

Oral tolerance is systemic adaptive immune tolerance to antigens that are ingested or otherwise administered orally. Oral tolerance has been most clearly demonstrated in experimental rodent models. Mice fed high doses of a protein antigen may subsequently show impaired humoral and T cell–mediated responses to the same antigen administered by other routes, such as through the skin. A similar phenomenon can be demonstrated when antigens are administered through the nasal passages into the respiratory mucosa, and the more general term mucosal tolerance is used to describe tolerance induced by either oral or nasal antigen administration. The physiologic role of oral tolerance is speculated to be the prevention of potentially harmful immune responses to food proteins and commensal bacteria. The underlying mechanisms of oral tolerance are not well understood but likely include the mechanisms of peripheral tolerance discussed in Chapter 15, such as anergy, deletion, and Treg-mediated suppression. The propensity of the immune system in the gut to suppress local immune responses to antigens in the intestinal lumen could be manifested in other parts of the body because of circulation of Treg to other tissues and deletion or anergy of effector T cells in the gut, which are no longer available to respond to antigens at other sites. Attempts to treat autoimmune disease or allergies by oral or nasal administration of relevant self antigens or allergens have so far been unsuccessful.

Oral administration of antigen in the setting of concomitant stimulation of innate immunity can lead to productive adaptive immune responses, as in the use of oral viral vaccines to induce protective antibody responses to viruses. These vaccines are live attenuated viruses that may infect dendritic cells in the intestine and stimulate strong innate responses that then promote T and B cell activation.

The Role of the Commensal Microbiome in Immune Regulation

The human intestinal microbiome includes all of the commensal bacteria that normally reside in the intestines, discussed earlier, as well as thousands of species of viruses, fungi, and protozoans. Humans and their intestinal microbiome have coevolved mechanisms for mutual benefit, including mechanisms to defend against invasion by these organisms together with mechanisms to maintain equilibrium by minimizing unneeded proinflammatory immune responses to the commensal organisms. One consequence of this coevolution is a profound influence of the microbiome on the immune system. The microbiome changes with age, diet, and disease, and mouse studies indicate that these changes have impacts on immune function both locally in the gut, and systemically.

Commensal organisms in the intestines are required for and regulate innate immune responses in the gut, and also influence systemic innate immunity. Studies in mice have shown that commensal bacteria are needed for proliferation and repair of the intestinal epithelial barrier after injury, an effect mediated by bacterial cell wall PAMPs and the TLRs they bind to on the epithelial cells. As mentioned earlier, microflora in the gut stimulate the expression of mucins and anti-microbial peptides (including the C-type lectin REGIIIγ) that prevent Gram-positive bacterial colonization. In addition, several studies in mice have shown that products of commensal bacteria in the gut influence the way circulating neutrophils and macrophages function systemically. For example, short-chain fatty acids from gut bacteria dampen neutrophil inflammatory responses, while fragments of intestinal bacteria peptidoglycan enhance the ability of circulating neutrophils to kill Gram-positive bacteria. Likewise, gut bacteria appear to be required for systemic anti-viral functions of macrophages, dendritic cells, and NK cells.

Intestinal commensal organisms influence local and systemic adaptive immune responses. The production of IgA in the intestinal mucosa, which is the major adaptive immune mechanism for protection against microbial invasion through the intestinal epithelial barrier, is dependent on the presence of luminal flora. Commensal bacterial antigens activate T-dependent IgA responses specific for these antigens. Furthermore, commensal organisms induce the expression of IgA switch factors, including BAFF, APRIL, and retinoic acid, which are required for T-dependent and T-independent B cell class switching to IgA (discussed earlier). By preventing commensals from reaching the barrier epithelium, IgA in the gut reduces innate responses to these organisms, and also limits B cell activation and antibody responses, both locally and systemically. For example, serum IgE levels,

blood basophil numbers, and mast-cell dependent allergic reactions outside the gut are all elevated in germ-free mice. Certain species of commensal organisms in the gut are also required for accumulation of T_H17 cells in the gut, and the presence of these species reduces resistance to some gut pathogens but may increase susceptibility to autoimmune disease outside the gut. Other commensal species contribute to the development of Tregs.

In humans, the impact of gut microflora on local and systemic immune responses is inferred from many clinical observations and experimental therapies. Normal flora appears to be required to prevent harmful intestinal innate responses and inflammation induced by pathogenic bacteria. For example, antibiotic treatment for infections outside the gut will invariably alter the makeup of the gut microflora, and this is associated with increased risk for pathologic bacterial infections in the colon, especially with *Clostridium difficile* (*C. difficile*). Patients with chronic *C. difficile* infection benefit from orally administered fecal transplants, which repopulate the gut with flora from healthy individuals. Patients with inflammatory bowel disease (discussed later) have abnormal gut flora, and both antibiotic treatment and fecal transplants have been successful in treating some of these patients.

The way human commensal gut flora influences systemic immunologic health is largely unknown. The risk for developing allergic disease, including asthma, has been linked to variations in microflora during early childhood as a consequence of mode of birth (vaginal vs. cesarean section), breast feeding, and antibiotic use. Currently, the microbiomes of various normal and patient populations are being characterized by genetic approaches, and the data generated may lead to a better understanding of how the human immune system is regulated by gut bacteria.

Diseases Related to Immune Responses in the Gut

Given the abundance of immune cells and their constant activity in the intestinal mucosa, it is not surprising that there are many intestinal diseases related to abnormal immune responses. These diseases are generally caused by unregulated responses to commensal organisms or to antigens in food. We will now discuss selected examples of these diseases; they are more thoroughly described in medical textbooks.

Inflammatory Bowel Disease

Inflammatory bowel disease (IBD) is a heterogeneous group of disorders characterized by chronic remitting inflammation in the small or large bowel, likely due to poorly regulated responses to commensal bacteria. The two main types of inflammatory bowel disease are **Crohn's disease,** which can affect the entire thickness of the bowel wall tissue in any part of the gastrointestinal tract but most frequently involves the terminal ileum, and **ulcerative colitis,** which is restricted to the colonic mucosa. Symptoms include abdominal pain, vomiting, diarrhea, and weight loss. Treatments include various anti-inflammatory drugs, such as sulfasalazine, corticosteroids, TNF antagonists, and antimetabolites. Although the etiology of Crohn's disease and ulcerative colitis is poorly understood, several types of evidence suggest that these disorders are a result of defects in the regulation of immune responses to commensal organisms in the gut in genetically susceptible individuals. A number of immunologic abnormalities may contribute to the development of inflammatory bowel disease.

- *Defects in innate immunity to gut commensals.* Earlier we discussed the possibility that inflammatory bowel disease results from either or both of two types of innate immune defects. First, there may be defective expression of molecules such as defensins, leading to increased commensal bacterial invasion through the intestinal epithelium. Second, there may be inadequate negative regulation of innate immune responses to commensal organisms. Polymorphisms in the gene encoding the NOD2 cytoplasmic innate immune sensor are associated with a subset of Crohn's disease and may lead to either of these two types of abnormalities in innate immunity.
- *Abnormal T_H17 and T_H1 responses.* Analysis of T cell responses in animal models and patients with inflammatory bowel disease indicates that there is an active T_H17 response in the affected parts of the bowel. Crohn's disease is also characterized by granulomatous inflammation driven by IFN-γ–producing T_H1 cells (see Chapter 19). These findings are the basis for treating inflammatory bowel disease patients with a monoclonal antibody that binds a polypeptide (p40) shared by IL-23 and IL-12. IL-23 is required for T_H17-mediated immune responses, as mentioned earlier, and IL-12 is required for T_H1 responses. Clinical trials of IL-17 antagonist treatment for inflammatory bowel disease have not shown efficacy, suggesting that excessive production of IL-17 may not, by itself, be responsible for these disorders.
- *Defective function of regulatory T cells.* It is possible that inflammatory bowel disease may be caused by inadequate Treg-mediated suppression of immune responses to commensal organisms. The evidence supporting this hypothesis comes from mouse models in which an absence of Treg leads to inflammatory bowel disease. In fact, one of the first experiments demonstrating the existence of Treg was the development of gastrointestinal inflammation in immunodeficient mice injected with naive $CD4^+CD25^-$ T cells, which we now know contain precursors of effector T cells but lack $CD4^+CD25^+$ Treg. Mice deficient in Treg because of deletion of *Il2* or *Il2r* genes, as mentioned earlier, or knockout of the *Foxp3* gene, also develop colitis. In humans, *FOXP3* mutations result in a failure to develop Treg and cause the disease called immune dysregulation, polyendocrinopathy, enteropathy, X-linked (IPEX), which includes severe gut inflammation as well as autoimmunity in many other tissues. Although all these observations are consistent with a need for Treg to maintain intestinal homeostasis, as discussed earlier, it is not known if Treg defects underlie most cases of human inflammatory bowel disease.
- *Polymorphisms of genes that are associated with macroautophagy and the unfolded protein response*

to endoplasmic reticulum stress are risk factors for inflammatory bowel disease. Experimental evidence suggests that the connection between inflammatory bowel disease and variants in the unfolded protein response and autophagy genes relates to diminished Paneth cell secretion of anti-microbial enzymes and defensins. Macroautophagy is a process by which cells sequester cytoplasmic organelles within autophagosomes, which then fuse with lysosomes, promoting the destruction of the organelles. Genetic variations of autophagy genes (including *ATG16L1* and *IRGM*) that are associated with Crohn's disease impair autophagy in Paneth cells, and, for unclear reasons, this reduces secretion of lysozyme and defensins into the intestinal lumen. Endoplasmic reticulum stress occurs when misfolded proteins accumulate in the endoplasmic reticulum. This leads to the activation of a series of proteins, including the transcription factor XBP-1, that work together to block protein translation and increase expression of chaperones that promote proper protein folding. Paneth cells, like other secretory cells, depend on the unfolded protein response to maintain protein secretory function.

Celiac Disease

Celiac disease (gluten-sensitive enteropathy or non-tropical sprue) is an inflammatory disease of the small bowel mucosa caused by immune responses against ingested gluten proteins present in wheat. Celiac disease is characterized by chronic inflammation in the small bowel mucosa, leading to atrophy of villi, malabsorption, and various nutritional deficiencies that lead to extraintestinal manifestations. The disease is treated by diets restricted to gluten-free foods. Patients produce IgA and IgG antibodies specific for gluten as well as autoantibodies specific for transglutaminase 2A, an enzyme that modifies the gluten protein gliadin. These autoantibodies are thought to arise when transglutaminase-specific B cells endocytose host transglutaminase covalently bound to gliadin and present gliadin peptides to helper T cells, which then provide help for the anti-transglutaminase antibody response. Whether these antibodies contribute to disease development is not known, but they are a sensitive diagnostic marker for the disease. There is strong evidence that $CD4^+$ T cell responses to gliadin are involved in disease pathogenesis. T cells specific for gliadin peptides are found in celiac patients, and the inflammatory process in the bowel includes T cells and T cell cytokines. There is a high relative risk for development of gluten enteropathy among people who carry the two class II HLA alleles HLA-DQ2 and HLA-DQ8, and gliadin peptides bind strongly to the MHC molecules encoded by these alleles. We will discuss the association of autoimmune diseases with MHC alleles in Chapter 15. In addition to $CD4^+$ T cell responses, $CD8^+$ cytotoxic T lymphocyte (CTL) killing of intestinal epithelial cells may also contribute to celiac disease, although the source of the peptides recognized by the CTLs is not clear.

Other Diseases

Food allergies are caused by T_H2 responses to many different food proteins and cause acute inflammatory *reactions locally in the gut and systemically on ingestion of these proteins.* Allergies result from T_H2-dependent IgE responses to environmental antigens (allergens), which are either proteins or chemicals that modify (haptenate) self proteins. In the case of food allergies, the environmental antigens are ingested, and this is another example of a failure of adaptive immune tolerance to food antigens. The anti-allergen antibodies bind to Fc receptors on mast cells, and subsequent exposure to the allergen will cause cross-linking of the Fc receptors, activation of the mast cells, and release of potent proinflammatory amine and lipid mediators and cytokines. There are abundant mast cells in the lamina propria of the bowel. Therefore, reingestion of a food allergen by a person who has previously mounted a T_H2 and IgE response to the allergen will trigger mast cell activation, with its pathologic consequences. Cytokines produced by T_H2 cells also directly stimulate peristalsis and may trigger symptoms of food allergies even without the participation of IgE. These reactions may cause gastrointestinal symptoms like nausea, vomiting, diarrhea, and abdominal pain, but the allergen can be absorbed into the blood and end up activating mast cells in many different tissues, producing systemic manifestations. We will discuss allergic reactions in more detail in Chapter 20.

Prolonged immune responses to gastrointestinal microbes can lead to tumors arising in the gastrointestinal tract. The best documented example of this is the so-called MALT lymphomas in the stomach of people with chronic *Helicobacter pylori* infection. These lymphomas are tumors arising from malignantly transformed follicular B cells in lymphoid follicles of the gastric lamina propria. It is believed that *H. pylori* sets up an inflammatory reaction that promotes the development and growth of tumors induced by B cell intrinsic oncogenic events. Remarkably, if gastric MALT lymphomas are diagnosed before they spread beyond the stomach wall, patients can be cured by antibiotic treatment of the *H. pylori* infection.

IMMUNITY IN OTHER MUCOSAL TISSUES

Like the gastrointestinal mucosa, the mucosae of the respiratory system, the genitourinary system, and the conjunctiva must maintain a barrier against invasion of diverse microbes in the environment and balance effective protective responses to invading microbes and suppression of responses to commensal organisms. Many of the features we described for gastrointestinal immunity are shared by mucosal immunity in these different locations. These shared features include relatively impermeable mucus- and defensin-secreting epithelial barriers; localized collections of lymphoid tissues just beneath the epithelium; the constant sampling of antigens located outside the barriers by immune cells within the barrier; the constant integration of proinflammatory and regulatory signals generated by microbial products binding to epithelial and dendritic cell TLRs; the strong reliance on secretory IgA–mediated humoral immunity to prevent microbial invasion; and the presence of

effector and regulatory dendritic cell populations that stimulate particular types of effector and regulatory T cell responses. In addition to these shared features, each different mucosal tissue has unique features that reflect the distinct functions and anatomy of the organs it is part of and the distinct range of environmental antigens and microbes that are present at each site. We will now discuss some of the major features of mucosal immunity in these organs, focusing mainly on the respiratory system.

Immunity in the Respiratory System

The mucosa of the respiratory system lines the nasal passages, nasopharynx, trachea, and bronchial tree. Alveoli, the epithelium-lined sac-like termini of the bronchial airways, may also be considered part of the respiratory mucosa. Inhalation of air exposes the respiratory mucosa to a wide variety of foreign substances, including airborne infectious organisms, plant pollens, dust particles, and various other environmental antigens. The microbial flora of the airways is far less dense and less diverse than that in the gut, and the deep airways and alveoli have less organisms than the upper airways. Nonetheless, similar mechanisms have evolved in the respiratory mucosal immune system to achieve a balance between immune activation to protect against pathogens and immune regulation to avoid unnecessary or excessive responses that might impair the physiologic functions. Failure of the immune system to control bronchopulmonary infections and excessive immune or inflammatory responses to infections are major causes of morbidity and mortality worldwide.

Innate Immunity in the Respiratory System

The pseudostratified, ciliated columnar epithelium that lines most of the respiratory mucosa, including the nasal passages, nasopharynx, and bronchial tree, performs similar physical and chemical barrier functions as gut epithelium, by virtue of tight junctions between cells and secretion of mucus, defensins, and cathelicidins. The mucus in the airways traps foreign substances including microbes, and the cilia move the mucus and trapped microbes up and out of the lungs. The importance of mucus and cilia in innate immune protection in the lung is illustrated by the greatly increased frequency of serious bronchopulmonary infections in people with decreased cilia function, such as heavy smokers, or impaired mucus production, such as patients with cystic fibrosis.

Innate responses in alveoli serve anti-microbial functions but are tightly controlled to prevent inflammation, which would impair gas exchange. The alveoli are susceptible to infection spreading from bronchopneumonia, and alveolar lining cells can be directly infected by viruses. Surfactant proteins A (SP-A) and D (SP-D), which are secreted into the alveolar spaces, are members of the collectin family (see Chapter 4) and bind to carbohydrate PAMPs on the surface of many pathogens. These surfactants are involved in viral neutralization and clearance of microbes from the airspaces, but they also suppress inflammatory and allergic responses in the lung. For example, SP-A inhibits TLR2 and TLR4 signaling and inflammatory cytokine expression in alveolar macrophages, and SP-A also binds to TLR4 and inhibits lipopolysaccharide binding. SP-A and SP-D reduce the phagocytic activity of alveolar macrophages.

Alveolar macrophages represent the majority of free cells within the alveolar spaces. These cells are functionally distinct from macrophages in most other tissues in that they maintain an anti-inflammatory phenotype. They express IL-10, nitric oxide, and TGF-β and are poorly phagocytic compared with resident macrophages in other tissues, such as the spleen and liver. Alveolar macrophages inhibit T cell responses as well as the antigen presentation function of CD103$^+$ airway dendritic cells.

Adaptive Immunity in the Respiratory System

Protective humoral immunity in the airways is dominated by secretory IgA, as in other mucosal tissues, although the amount of IgA secreted is much less than in the gastrointestinal tract. Secretory IgA plays an important role in the upper airway. The anatomic sites of naive B cell activation, differentiation, and IgA class switching may vary but include tonsils and adenoids in the nasopharynx and lymph nodes in the mediastinum and adjacent to bronchi in the lungs. There are relatively few aggregated or isolated lymphoid follicles in the lamina propria in the lower airways compared with the gut and likely less initiation of humoral immune responses in these locations. The homing of IgA-secreting plasma cells back into the airway tissue in proximity to respiratory mucosal epithelium depends on the chemokine CCL28 secreted by respiratory epithelium and its receptor CCR10 on the plasma cells. IgA and IgG are transported into the airway lumen by the same poly-Ig receptor and FcRn mechanism of transcellular transport as in the gut. IgE responses to airway antigens occur frequently and are involved in allergic diseases of the respiratory system, including hay fever and asthma. IgE performs its inflammatory effector functions when bound to mast cells, which are abundant in the airways.

T cell responses in the lung are initiated by dendritic cell sampling of airway antigens and presentation of these antigens to naive T cells in peribronchial and mediastinal lymph nodes. A network of dendritic cells is present in the mucosa of the airways, and one subset of these bronchial dendritic cells extend dendrites between the bronchial epithelial cells into the airway lumen. These dendritic cells sample airway antigens, migrate to draining lymph nodes, present the processed antigens to naive T cells, and have a propensity to drive differentiation of these T cells to the T_H2 subset. The T_H2 cells home back into the bronchial mucosa, where they may be reactivated by allergens presented by dendritic cells in lamina propria. This pathway is considered central to the development of allergic asthma (see Chapter 20). Other dendritic cells are found in the lamina propria beneath the epithelial cells.

Immunity in the Genitourinary System

Innate immune defense against microbial invasion and infection in the genitourinary mucosa relies mainly on the epithelial lining, as in other mucosal barriers. Stratified squamous epithelium lines the vaginal mucosa and terminal male urethra, and a single layer of mucus-secreting columnar epithelium lines the upper female genital tract. The vaginal epithelium contains Langerhans cells, and a variety of dendritic cells and macrophages have been described beneath the epithelium in vagina, endocervix, and urethra. There are also resident B and T cells in the genital mucosa. Differences in the phenotype of the dendritic cells and macrophages in the female genital mucosa from those in the gastrointestinal tract may underlie the greater susceptibility of the former to HIV infection. There is little regional specialization of the adaptive immune system in the genitourinary mucosa, which lacks prominent mucosa-associated lymphoid tissues. Unlike other mucosa, in which IgA is the dominant antibody isotype, most of the antibodies in genital secretions are IgGs, about half of which are produced by plasma cells in genital tract mucosa; the rest are from the circulation.

THE CUTANEOUS IMMUNE SYSTEM

The skin includes two main layers, the outer epidermis composed mainly of epithelial cells and, separated by a thin basement membrane, the underlying dermis composed of connective tissue and specialized adnexal structures such as hair follicles and sweat glands. Within both of these layers, a variety of different cell types and their products, comprising the cutaneous immune system (Fig. 14-9), provide physical barrier and active immune defense functions against microbes. The skin of an adult is about 2m^2 in area and is the second largest barrier of the body against environmental microbes and other foreign materials. Nonetheless, given its outermost location, the skin is normally colonized by many microbes and is frequently breached by trauma and burns. Therefore, the skin is a common portal of entry for a wide variety of microbes and other foreign substances and is the site of many immune responses.

Innate and Adaptive Immune Reponses in the Skin

The epidermis provides a physical barrier to microbial invasion. The epidermis consists of multiple layers of stratified squamous epithelium, made up almost entirely of specialized epithelial cells called keratinocytes. The basal layer of keratinocytes, anchored onto the basement membrane, continuously proliferate, and their maturing progeny cells are displaced upward and differentiate to form several different layers. In the top layer, called the stratum corneum, the cells undergo programmed death, thereby forming a keratin- and lipid-rich permeability barrier that is important for protection against microbes as well as harmful physical and chemical agents.

In addition to forming a physical barrier, keratinocytes actively respond to pathogens and injury by producing anti-microbial peptides, which kill microbes, and various cytokines, which promote and regulate immune responses. The anti-microbial peptides that keratinocytes

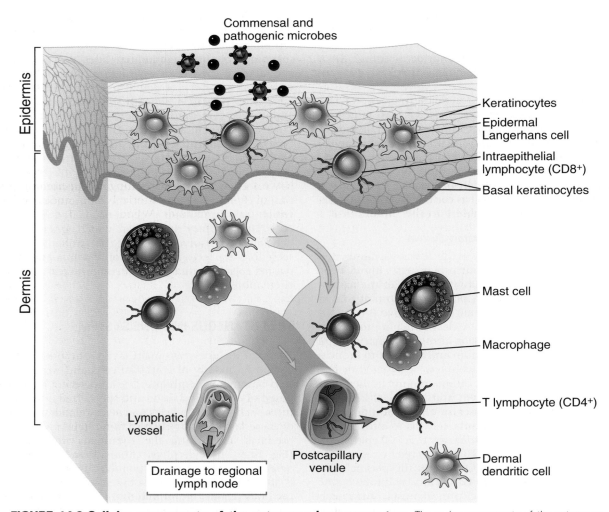

FIGURE 14-9 Cellular components of the cutaneous immune system. The major components of the cutaneous immune system shown in this schematic diagram include keratinocytes, Langerhans cells, and intraepithelial lymphocytes, all located in the epidermis, and T lymphocytes, dendritic cells, and macrophages, located in the dermis.

produce include defensins, S100, and cathelicidins (see Chapter 4). The cytokines made by keratinocytes include TNF, thymic stromal lymphopoietin (TSLP), IL-1, IL-6, IL-18, and IL-33, which promote inflammation; GM-CSF, which induces differentiation and activation of dendritic cells in the epidermis, discussed later; and IL-10, which controls immune responses. Keratinocytes produce the chemokine CCL27, which participates in recruitment of lymphocytes expressing CCR10. The induced expression of defensins, cytokines, and chemokines by keratinocytes depends on innate immune receptors including TLRs and NLRs. Keratinocytes express most of the TLRs and NLRP3, which is a component of the IL-1–processing inflammasome (see Chapter 4). Keratinocytes in normal skin constitutively synthesize pro–IL-1β and pro–IL-18. Stimuli such as UV irradiation activate the inflammasome to process these pro-cytokines to the active forms, which explains the inflammatory response to sunburn. When signal transduction pathways linked to inflammatory responses, such as the NF-κB and STAT3 pathways, are genetically activated only in keratinocytes, mice develop inflammatory skin diseases, showing the potential of keratinocytes to act as central players of cutaneous immune responses.

Several dendritic cell populations are normally present in the skin and contribute both to innate immune responses and to initiation of T cell responses to microbial and environmental antigens that enter the body through the skin. In the epidermis, the most abundant dendritic cells are the Langerhans cells, which express a C-type lectin receptor called langerin (CD207) and have numerous Birbeck granules in the cytoplasm (see Fig. 6-4). The dendrites of Langerhans cells form a dense meshwork between the keratinocytes of the epidermis. In the dermis, there are relatively sparse langerin-expressing CD103+ dendritic cells, which are a distinct lineage from Langerhans cells, and langerin-negative dendritic cells, such as plasmacytoid dendritic cells. Each of these dendritic cell populations express innate pattern recognition receptors for PAMPs expressed on microbes and for damage-associated molecular patterns (DAMPs) expressed on injured cells. The dendritic cells respond to these ligands by secreting inflammatory cytokines.

Skin dendritic cells take up foreign proteins, transport them to draining lymph nodes, and present processed peptides from these proteins to T cells or pass the protein antigens to other lymph node–resident dendritic cells. When Langerhans cells encounter pathogens they are activated by engagement of Toll-like receptors and other microbial sensors (see Chapter 6). The cells lose their adhesiveness for the epidermis, enter lymphatic vessels, begin to express the CCR7 chemokine receptor, and migrate to the T cell zones of draining lymph nodes in response to chemokines produced in that location. The Langerhans cells also mature into efficient antigen-presenting cells. What remains unclear is the relative contribution of the different skin dendritic cell subsets to the initiation of T cell responses. Mouse models have been developed in which langerin-expressing dendritic cells can be selectively eliminated, and under the proper conditions, the mice lack Langerhans cells but have dermal dendritic cells. Using these models, investigators have shown that some T cell responses to chemically modified self proteins, a model for contact hypersensitivity, occur in the absence of Langerhans cells. Furthermore, T cell responses to certain viruses, including herpes viruses, depend on dermal langerin$^+$ CD103$^+$ dendritic cells but not on Langerhans cells. Langerhans cells do appear to be required for T$_H$2 responses that contribute to atopic dermatitis (contact hypersensitivity and atopic dermatitis will be discussed later). The role of the different skin dendritic cell populations could vary with the antigen dose and type and likely will differ between mice and humans.

Normal human skin contains many T cells, 95% of which have a memory phenotype. Human skin contains about 1 million T cells/cm^2, which is about 2×10^{10} total T cells in the skin. About 98% of these T cells are present in the dermis, and 2% are intraepidermal lymphocytes. Dermal T lymphocytes (both CD4$^+$ and CD8$^+$ cells) are predominantly in perivascular and perifollicular locations and usually express phenotypic markers typical of activated or memory cells. It is not clear whether these cells reside permanently within the dermis or are merely in transit between blood and lymphatic capillaries as part of memory T cell recirculation. CD4$^+$ T cells of each major subset, T$_H$1, T$_H$2, T$_H$17, and Treg, are found in the skin. T$_H$1 and T$_H$17 cells are important for microbial defense against intracellular and extracellular microbes, respectively, as in other tissues. The two signature T$_H$17 cytokines, IL-17 and IL-22, are known to induce expression of defensins and cathelicidins by keratinocytes and epidermal cell proliferation. In contrast, the T$_H$2 cytokines IL-4 and IL-13 suppress production of defensins and cathelicidin, which can result in infections in T$_H$2 driven skin diseases. Dermal γδ T cells may be a source of IL-17 in some chronic inflammatory skin diseases. Intraepidermal T cells, most of which are CD8$^+$ cells, may express a more restricted set of antigen receptors than do T lymphocytes in most extracutaneous tissues. In mice (and some other species), many intraepidermal lymphocytes are T cells that express γδ T cell antigen receptors with limited diversity.

T cells in the skin express homing molecules that direct their migration out of dermal microvessels (Fig. 14-10). Migration of effector or memory T cells into the skin depends on T cell expression of cutaneous lymphocyte antigen (CLA), which is an E-selectin–binding carbohydrate moiety displayed on various glycoproteins on the endothelial cell plasma membrane. In addition, T cell expression of CCR4, CCR8, and CCR10, which bind the chemokines CCL17, CCL1, and CCL27, respectively, is also required for T cell trafficking to skin. The skin-homing properties of T cells are imprinted during activation in skin-draining lymph nodes, by a process analogous to imprinting of gut-homing properties of T cells in mesenteric lymph nodes, discussed earlier in the chapter. When naive T cells recognize antigens presented by dendritic cells in skin-draining lymph nodes, they receive signals from the dendritic cells that not only induce proliferation and differentiation into effector cells but also induce expression of the skin-homing molecules CLA, CCR4, CCR8, and CCR10. Interestingly, sunlight and vitamin D appear to play an important role in T cell migration to the skin, analogous to the role of vitamin A and its metabolite retinoic acid in lymphocyte migration to the gut. UVB rays in sunlight act on 7-dehydrocholesterol made in the basal layer of the epidermis, converting it to previtamin D$_3$. Dermal dendritic cells express vitamin D$_3$ hydroxylases that convert previtamin D$_3$ to the active form, 1,25(OH)$_2$D$_3$, which may be transported in free form or within migrating dendritic cells to skin-draining lymph nodes. Within the node, 1,25(OH)$_2$D$_3$ enters T cells that have been activated by antigen-presenting dendritic cells, translocates to the nucleus, and induces transcription of CCR10. IL-12 made by the dendritic cells participates in induction of CLA. CCR4 and CCR8 are also upregulated, and the gut-homing integrin $\alpha_4\beta_7$ is downregulated, by unknown signals, during T cell activation in skin-draining lymph nodes. Thus, naive T cells activated in skin-draining lymph nodes will differentiate into effector T cells that preferentially home back into the skin. 1,25(OH)$_2$D$_3$ may also act locally within the dermis on effector and memory T cells to upregulate CCR10 and promote migration of the T cells into the epidermis because the CCR10 ligand CCL27 is made by keratinocytes.

Diseases Related to Immune Responses in the Skin

There are many different inflammatory diseases that are caused by dysregulated or inappropriately targeted immune responses in the skin. We will discuss only two illustrative examples of these diseases. In addition to these inflammatory diseases, there are several malignant lymphomas that primarily affect the skin. Most of these are derived from skin-homing T cells.

Psoriasis, a chronic inflammatory disorder of the skin characterized by red scaly plaques, is caused by dysregulated innate and T cell–mediated immune responses triggered by various environmental stimuli. There is evidence that psoriasis is initiated when trauma or infection induces production of the cathelicidin LL-37 by keratinocytes, which forms complexes with host DNA and then

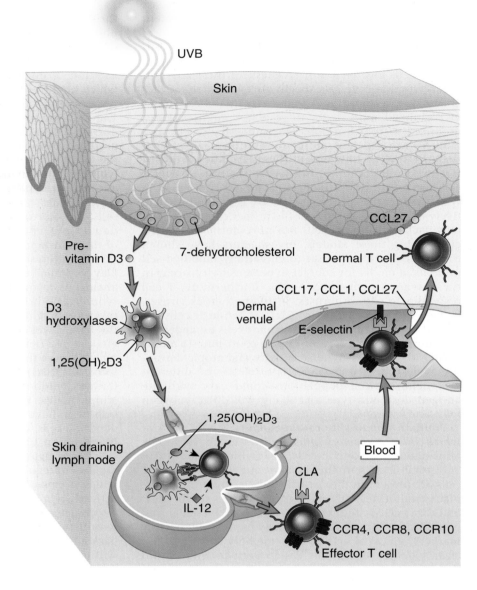

FIGURE 14-10 Homing properties of skin lymphocytes. The skin-homing properties of effector lymphocytes are imprinted in skin-draining lymph nodes where they have undergone differentiation from naive precursors. Ultraviolet rays in sunlight (UVB) stimulate production of vitamin D, which induces expression of CCR10, IL-12 induces expression of the E-selectin ligand cutaneous lymphocyte antigen (CLA), and other signals induce CCR4, CCR8, and CCR10 expression. These homing molecules direct migration of the effector T cells into the skin.

activates plasmacytoid dendritic cells in the skin through TLR9. Activated plasmacytoid dendritic cells produce abundant IFN-α, and psoriatic skin has a strong type I interferon signature (i.e., expression of many interferon-induced genes). One of the effects of IFN-α is activation of other dendritic cells that are induced to migrate to lymph nodes, activate helper T cells of unknown antigen specificity, and induce their differentiation into skin-homing effector cells. These T cells circulate to the dermis and further promote an inflammatory cascade and persistent keratinocyte proliferation. Both T_H1 and T_H17 cells have been implicated in this phase of the disease. Clinical trials of IL-17 antagonists have shown impressive efficacy in psoriasis, as have TNF inhibitors. A central unanswered question about this disease is the identity of the antigens recognized by the T cells.

Atopic dermatitis is a chronic inflammatory disease of the skin characterized by itchy rashes, which is driven by T_H2 responses to environmental antigens in genetically susceptible individuals. There is evidence that atopic dermatitis develops when there are underlying defects in epidermal barrier function, leading to increased antigen entry into the skin and accentuated T_H2-mediated immune responses to otherwise innocuous antigens. Mutations in a structural protein involved in keratinocyte differentiation and barrier function, called filaggrin, are often associated with atopic dermatitis. Secondarily, T_H2 responses stimulate B cell production of IgE specific for environmental antigens, as well as IgE-dependent mast cell activation in response to those antigens (see Chapter 20) contributes to the clinical manifestations of the disease.

IMMUNE PRIVILEGED TISSUES

Immune responses and associated inflammation in certain parts of the body, including brain, eye, testes, placenta, and fetus, carry a high risk of lethal organ dysfunction or reproductive failure. These tissues, which have evolved to be protected, to a variable degree, from immune responses, are called **immune privileged sites**. Peter Medawar coined the term *immune privilege* in the 1940s to describe the lack of immune responses to tissue transplanted into the brain or the anterior chamber of the eye of experimental animals. Foreign antigens that would evoke an immune response in most tissues are often tolerated in these immune privileged sites. The mechanisms underlying immune privilege vary between these tissues and are not fully understood. Some of the mechanisms are similar to mechanisms of regulation in gut and skin (discussed earlier) and mechanisms of self-tolerance (discussed in Chapter 15). In the sections that follow, we will discuss some of the distinguishing features of immune privilege in different tissues.

Immune Privilege in the Eye, Brain, and Testis

The Eye

Vision, which is essential to survival to most mammals, can be easily impaired by inflammation within the eye. Evolved mechanisms that minimize the likelihood of immune responses and inflammation in the eye have been most thoroughly described in the anterior chamber, a fluid-filled space between the transparent cornea in front and the iris and lens behind. Inflammation in this chamber could lead to opacification of the transparent cornea and lens, with loss of sight. At least some of the properties of immune privilege studied in the anterior chamber also apply to other ocular sites, such as the vitreous cavity and the subretinal space. Anatomic features of the anterior chamber that contribute to immune privilege include the tight junctions and resistance to leakiness of blood vessels in the tissues adjacent to the anterior chamber (the so-called blood-eye barrier), the avascular nature of the cornea, and the absence of lymphatics draining the anterior chamber, which limits access of the adaptive immune system to antigens in the eye. There are several soluble factors with immunosuppressive/anti-inflammatory properties in the aqueous humor that fills the anterior chamber, including neuropeptides (α-melanocyte–stimulating hormone, vasointestinal peptide, somatostatin), TGF-β, and indolamine 2,3-dioxygenase. Cells lining the anterior chamber, including the epithelium of the iris and the endothelium, constitutively express Fas ligand and PD-L1, which can induce death or inactivation of T cells, respectively.

Anterior chamber–associated immune deviation is a phenomenon in which introduction of foreign protein antigen into the anterior of the eye actively induces systemic tolerance to that antigen. This phenomenon presumably reduces the chance that adaptive immune responses will be mounted to foreign antigens that may be located in the eye. The tolerance is detectable as a diminished inflammatory T cell or antibody response to the same antigen when it is later introduced at extraocular sites compared with the response in individuals who were not given intraocular antigen. Anterior chamber–associated immune deviation may be mediated by Treg. Studies in mice show that the antigen introduced in the anterior chamber is transported by macrophages or dendritic cells, through the blood, to the spleen, and presented by splenic B cells to naive T cells, inducing the generation of regulatory T cells specific for the antigen.

In contrast to induced tolerance to foreign antigens introduced into the anterior chamber, self antigens in the eye are isolated from the immune system, and systemic tolerance to these antigens is not induced. This lack of tolerance becomes a problem only when eye trauma exposes the eye antigens to the immune system. A striking example of this is sympathetic ophthalmia, in which trauma to one eye causes release of eye antigens leading to autoimmune disease in both the injured eye and the uninjured eye. Presumably, although self antigens in the normal eye are inaccessible to the extraocular immune system to induce tolerance, activated immune effector cells and antibodies that are generated in the periphery when one eye is injured have access to and cause injury to the normal eye.

The Brain

Inflammation in the brain can lead to functional derangement and death of neurons, with disastrous consequences. Anatomic features of the brain that impair initiation of adaptive immunity to antigens include an absence of conventional lymphatic drainage and a scarcity of dendritic cells. Delivery of immune cells and inflammatory mediators into the brain is impaired by the nature of the tight junctions between brain microvascular endothelial cells (the so-called blood-brain barrier). Some of the mechanisms operative in the eye may also apply to the brain, including the action of neuropeptides. The brain is rich in resident macrophages, called microglia, which become activated in response to tissue damage or infections in the brain. The threshold for their activation, however, may be higher than that of macrophages in other tissues. One putative mechanism for maintaining this high threshold is inhibitory signaling by the CD200 receptor, which is expressed by microglia. CD200 serves as its own ligand, and, is highly expressed in the brain on neurons and other cell types.

Contrary to previously common assumptions based on classic experiments, there is evidence that immune surveillance against microbes does occur in the central nervous system. For example, the frequency of some opportunistic infections within the brain increases significantly in immunosuppressed patients. Patients treated with certain monoclonal antibodies that block lymphocyte and monocyte adhesion to endothelial cells have a significantly increased although still small risk for activation of latent JC virus, leading to a uniformly fatal central nervous system disease called progressive multifocal leukoencephalopathy. This finding suggests that T cell or monocyte trafficking into the brain is necessary to keep latent viruses in check and argues that the brain is not a stringently immune privileged site.

The Testis

Immune privilege in the testis serves to limit inflammation that may impair male fertility. Many self antigens in the adult testis are first expressed at the time of puberty, well after the development of a competent immune system, which may include testis antigen–specific precursor T and B cells. Therefore, immune privilege in the testis may also serve to prevent autoimmunity. The testis, like the eye and brain, has a blood-tissue barrier that limits delivery of cells and molecules to the sites of spermatogenesis. This barrier is not formed by endothelial cells but rather by Sertoli cells that line the outer layer of the seminiferous tubules where spermatogenesis takes place. The hormonal milieu of the testis, which is rich in androgens, has an anti-inflammatory influence on macrophages. TGF-β is produced by Leydig, Sertoli, and peritubular cells and likely contributes to local immune suppression.

Immune Privilege of the Mammalian Fetus

The mammalian fetus expresses paternally inherited genes that are allogeneic to the mother, but fetuses are not normally rejected by the mother. In essence, the fetus is a naturally occurring allograft, but one that is protected from graft rejection. (Allograft rejection is discussed in Chapter 17.) It is clear that the mother is exposed to fetal antigens during pregnancy because maternal antibodies against paternal MHC molecules are easily detectable. Obviously, there has been very strong selective pressure that has led to the evolution of mechanisms that protect the fetus from the maternal immune system, yet these mechanisms remain poorly understood. Probably several different special molecular and barrier features of the placenta and local immunosuppression contribute.

Several experimental observations indicate that the anatomic location of the fetus is a critical factor in the absence of rejection. For example, pregnant animals are able to recognize and reject allografts syngeneic to the fetus placed at extrauterine sites without compromising fetal survival. Wholly allogeneic fetal blastocysts that lack maternal genes can successfully develop in a pregnant or pseudopregnant mother. Thus, neither specific maternal nor paternal genes are necessary for survival of the fetus. Hyperimmunization of the mother with cells bearing paternal antigens does not compromise placental and fetal growth.

The failure to reject the fetus has focused attention on the region of physical contact between the mother and fetus. The fetal tissues of the placenta that most intimately contact the mother are composed of either vascular trophoblast, which is exposed to maternal blood for purposes of mediating nutrient exchange, or implantation site trophoblast, which diffusely infiltrates the uterine lining (decidua) for purposes of anchoring the placenta to the mother.

One simple explanation for fetal survival is that trophoblast cells fail to express paternal MHC molecules. Class II molecules have not been detected on trophoblast cells. In mice, cells of implantation trophoblast, but not of vascular trophoblast, do express paternal class I MHC molecules. In humans, the situation may be more complex in that trophoblast cells express only a non-polymorphic class IB molecule called HLA-G. This molecule may be involved in protecting trophoblast cells from maternal NK cell–mediated lysis. A specialized subset of NK cells called uterine NK cells are the major type of lymphocyte present at implantation sites, and IFN-γ production by these cells is essential for decidual development. The way in which uterine NK cells are stimulated and their role in maternal responses to fetal alloantigens are not known. Even if trophoblast cells do express classical MHC molecules, they may lack costimulator molecules and fail to act as antigen-presenting cells.

The uterine decidua may be a site where immune responses are functionally inhibited. In support of the idea is the observation that mouse decidua is highly susceptible to infection by *Listeria monocytogenes* and cannot support a delayed-type hypersensitivity response. The basis of immunologic privilege is clearly not a simple anatomic barrier because maternal blood is in extensive contact with trophoblast cells. Rather, the barrier is likely to be created by functional inhibition, attributable to multiple mechanisms.

Maternal tolerance of the fetus may be mediated by Treg. Experimental evidence suggests that regulatory T cells prevent immune reactions against paternally derived antigens that are not expressed in the mother. Fetal antigens induce long-lived FoxP3+ Treg in mice, and depletion of these cells results in fetal loss. During pregnancy, systemic and decidual Treg increase in mothers, and abundant Treg are found in the fetus. Indeed, Eutherian mammals (mammals with placentae) have evolved a transposon-mediated change in a regulatory sequence of the *FoxP3* gene that allows these mammals to generate peripheral Treg. This regulatory region of *FoxP3* is not found in earlier vertebrates or even in Metatherian mammals such as kangaroos and wallabies that carry their young. The contribution of Treg in human pregnancy is under active investigation, as is the possibility of Treg defects as the basis for recurrent spontaneous abortions.

Immune responses to the fetus may be regulated by local concentrations of tryptophan and its metabolites in the decidua. The enzyme indolamine 2,3-dioxygenase (IDO) catabolizes tryptophan, and the IDO-inhibiting drug 1-methyl-tryptophan induces abortions in mice in a T cell–dependent manner. These observations led to the hypothesis that T cell responses to the fetus are normally blocked because decidual tryptophan levels are kept low or the levels of toxic metabolites produced by IDO are high.

Several other mechanisms may also dampen maternal immune response of the fetus, including FasL expression by fetal trophoblast cells that promote apoptosis of activated Fas-expressing maternal lymphocytes, generation of tolerogenic dendritic cells in response to galectin-1 expressed in the decidua, and impaired dendritic cell migration from the uterus to lymph nodes.

Trophoblasts and decidua may also be resistant to complement-mediated damage. In mice, these tissues express a C3 and C4 inhibitor called Crry. Crry-deficient embryos die before birth and show evidence of complement activation on trophoblast cells. Thus, this inhibitor may block maternal alloantibody- and complement-mediated damage. However, Crry or equivalent molecules have not been found in humans.

SUMMARY

* Regional immune systems, including those in the gastrointestinal tract and skin, are specialized collections of innate and adaptive immune cells at particular anatomic locations, which perform protective and regulatory functions that are unique to those sites.
* The gastrointestinal immune system must cope with the presence of trillions of commensal bacteria in the gut lumen by preventing their invasion and tolerating their presence in the lumen, while also identifying and responding to numerically rare pathogenic organisms.
* Innate immunity in the gastrointestinal system is mediated by mucosal epithelial lining cells, which impede microbial invasion by tight intercellular junctions, secretion of mucus and production of anti-microbial molecules, such as defensins. Innate immune effector cells in the lamina propria include macrophages, dendritic cells, and mast cells. Intraepithelial lymphocytes, including γδ T cells, provide defense against commonly encountered microbes at the intestinal epithelial barrier.
* The adaptive immune system in the intestinal tract includes subepthelial collections of lymphoid tissues called gut-associated lymphoid tissues (GALT), such as the oropharyngeal tonsils, Peyer's patches in the ileum, and similar collections in the colon. M cells in the epithelial lining sample lumen antigens and transport them to antigen-presenting cells in the GALT. Lamina propria dendritic cells extend processes through intestinal epithelial lining cells to sample luminal antigens. There are also diffuse effector lymphocytes in the lamina propria of the gut and in mesenteric lymph nodes.
* Effector B and T lymphocytes that differentiate from naive T cells in the GALT or mesenteric lymph nodes enter the circulation, and selectively migrate back to the intestinal lamina propria.
* Humoral immunity in the gastrointestinal tract is dominated by IgA secretion into the lumen, where the antibodies neutralize potentially invading pathogens. B cells in the GALT and mesenteric lymph nodes differentiate into IgA-secreting plasma cells through both T-dependent and T-independent mechanisms, and the plasma cells migrate to the lamina propria beneath the epithelial barrier and secrete IgA. Dimerized IgA is transported across the epithelium by the poly-Ig-receptor and released into the lumen. IgA is also secreted into breast milk, and mediates passive immunity in the gut of breastfeeding infants.
* T_H17 cells in the intestinal tract secrete IL-17 and IL-22, which enhance epithelial barrier function. T_H2 cells are important in defense against intestinal parasites. Changes in bacterial flora influence the balance between different helper T cell subset responses, both in the gut and systemically.
* Immune responses to commensal organisms and food antigens in the lumen of the intestinal tract are minimized by a selective expression of pattern recognition receptors in the cytoplasm and basolateral surfaces of the epithelial lining cells, and the generation of regulatory T cells that suppress adaptive immune responses. TGF-β, IL-10, and IL-2 are essential to maintain immune homeostasis in the bowel wall. Systemic tolerance to some antigens can be induced by feeding the antigens to mice, a phenomenon called oral tolerance.
* Several intestinal diseases are related to abnormal immune responses, including inflammatory bowel diseases (Crohn's disease and ulcerative colitis), in which innate and adaptive immune responses to normal gut flora are not adequately regulated, and celiac disease, in which humoral and cell-mediated responses to dietary wheat glutens occur.
* Mucosal immunity in the respiratory system defends against airborne pathogens, and is the cause of allergic airway diseases, such as asthma. Innate immunity in the bronchial tree depends on the mucus-producing, ciliated epithelial lining, which moves the mucus with entrapped microbes out of the lungs. Defensins and surfactant proteins and alveolar macrophages provide both anti-microbial and anti-inflammatory functions. Treg and immunosuppressive cytokines are important for prevention of harmful responses to nonpathogenic organisms or other inhaled antigens.
* The cutaneous immune system defends against microbial invasion through the skin and suppresses responses against numerous commensal organisms. The multilayered keratinized squamous epithelial layer, called the epidermis, performs innate immune defense functions, providing a physical barrier to microbial invasion. Keratinocytes secrete defensins and inflammatory cytokines in response to microbial products. The dermis contains a mixed population of mast cells, macrophages, and dendritic cells that respond to microbes and injury and mediate inflammatory responses.
* Skin dendritic cells mediate innate immune responses, and also transport microbial and environmental antigens that enter through the skin to

draining lymph nodes, where they initiate T cell responses. T cells activated in skin-draining lymph nodes express chemokine receptors and adhesion molecules that favor homing back to the skin.

* CD4+ or CD8+ effector cells or memory cells are present in the dermis. T_H1, T_H2, and T_H17 cells are important for defense against different types of skin-invading pathogens, and may contribute to inflammatory dermatoses such as psoriasis (T_H1 and T_H17 cells) and atopic dermatitis (T_H2 cells).

* Immune privileged sites, which are tissues where immune responses are not readily initiated, include the brain, anterior chamber of the eye, and testis. The mechanisms of immune privilege include the tight junctions of endothelial cells in blood vessels, local production of immunosuppressive cytokines, and expression of cell surface molecules that inactivate or kill lymphocytes.

* Maternal immunological tolerance to the developing mammalian fetus, which expresses allogeneic paternal antigens, depends on mechanisms that act locally at the placental maternal-fetal interface. Possible mechanisms include lack of MHC expression on fetal trophoblasts, the actions of Treg, and local indolamine 2,3-dioxygenase–mediated depletion of tryptophan needed for lymphocyte growth.

SELECTED READINGS

Mucosal Immunity, General

Brandtzaeg P: Mucosal immunity: induction, dissemination, and effector functions, *Scandinavian Journal of Immunology* 70:505–515, 2009.

Doss M, White MR, Tecle T, Hartshorn KL: Human defensins and LL-37 in mucosal immunity, *Journal of Leukocyte Biology* 87:79–92, 2010.

Dubin PJ, Kolls JK: Th17 cytokines and mucosal immunity, *Immunological Reviews* 226:160–171, 2008.

Sheridan BS, Lefrancois L: Regional and mucosal memory T cells, *Nature immunology* 12:485–491, 2011.

Gastrointestinal Immune System

Abreu MT: Toll-like receptor signaling in the intestinal epithelium: how bacterial recognition shapes intestinal function, *Nature Reviews Immunology* 10:131–144, 2010.

Barnes MJ, Powrie F: Regulatory T cells reinforce intestinal homeostasis, *Immunity* 31:401–411, 2009.

Brestoff JR, Artis D: Commensal bacteria at the interface of host metabolism and the immune system, *Nature Immunology* 14:676–684, 2013.

Brown EM, Sadarangani M, Finlay BB: The role of the immune system in governing host-microbe interactions in the intestine, *Nature Immunology* 14:660–667, 2013.

Dommett R, Zilbauer M, George JT, Bajaj-Elliott M: Innate immune defense in the human gastrointestinal tract, *Molecular Immunology* 42:903–912, 2005.

Duerkop BA, Vaishnava S, Hooper LV: Immune responses to the microbiota at the intestinal mucosal surface, *Immunity* 31:368–376, 2009.

Eberl G, Lochner M: The development of intestinal lymphoid tissues at the interface of self and microbiota, *Mucosal Immunology* 2:478–485, 2009.

Hooper LV, Macpherson AJ: Immune adaptations that maintain homeostasis with the intestinal microbiota, *Nature Reviews Immunology* 10:159–169, 2010.

Johansson-Lindbom B, Agace WW: Generation of gut-homing T cells and their localization to the small intestinal mucosa, *Immunological Reviews* 215:226–242, 2007.

Maynard CL, Elson CO, Hatton RD, Weaver CT: Reciprocal interactions of the intestinal microbiota and immune system, *Nature* 489:231–241, 2012.

Maynard CL, Weaver CT: Intestinal effector T cells in health and disease, *Immunity* 31:389–400, 2009.

Rescigno M, Di Sabatino A: Dendritic cells in intestinal homeostasis and disease, *The Journal of Clinical Investigation* 119:2441–2450, 2009.

Varol C, Zigmond E, Jung S: Securing the immune tightrope: mononuclear phagocytes in the intestinal lamina propria, *Nature Reviews Immunology* 10:415–426, 2010.

Antibody Production in the Gastrointestinal Immune System

Cerutti A, Rescigno M: The biology of intestinal immunoglobulin A responses, *Immunity* 28:740–750, 2008.

Fagarasan S, Kawamoto S, Kanagawa O, Suzuki K: Adaptive immune regulation in the gut: T cell–dependent and T cell–independent IgA synthesis, *Annual Review of Immunology* 28:243–273, 2010.

Macpherson AJ, McCoy KD, Johansen FE, Brandtzaeg P: The immune geography of IgA induction and function, *Mucosal Immunology* 1:11–22, 2008.

Mora JR, von Andrian UH: Differentiation and homing of IgA-secreting cells, *Mucosal Immunology* 1:96–109, 2008.

Respiratory Mucosal Immune System

Chen K, Kolls JK: T cell-mediated host immune defenses in the lung, *Annual Review of Immunology* 31:605–633, 2013.

Holt PG, Strickland DH, Wikstrom ME, Jahnsen FL: Regulation of immunological homeostasis in the respiratory tract, *Nature Reviews Immunology* 8:142–152, 2008.

Lambrecht BN, Hammad H: Lung dendritic cells in respiratory viral infection and asthma: from protection to immunopathology, *Annual Reviews of Immunology* 30:243–270, 2012.

Wissinger E, Goulding J, Hussell T: Immune homeostasis in the respiratory tract and its impact on heterologous infection, *Seminars in Immunology* 21:147–155, 2009.

Skin Immune System

Clark RA: Skin-resident T cells: the ups and downs of on site immunity, *Journal of Investigative Dermatology* 130:362–370, 2010.

DiMeglio P, Perera GK, Nestle FO: The multitasking organ: recent insights into skin immune function, *Immunity* 35:857–870, 2011.

Heath WR, Carbone FR: The skin-resident and migratory immune system in steady state and memory: innate lymphocytes, dendritic cells and T cells, *Nature Immunology* 14:978–985, 2013.

Jabri B, Sollid LM: Tissue-mediated control of immunopathology in coeliac disease, *Nature Reviews Immunology* 9:858–870, 2009.

Kaser A, Zeissig S, Blumberg RS: Inflammatory bowel disease, *Annual Review of Immunology* 28:573–621, 2010.

Kaplan DH, Igyártó BZ, Gaspari AA: Early immune events in the induction of allergic contact dermatitis, *Nature Reviews Immunology* 12:570–580, 2012.

Khor B, Gardet A, Xavier RJ: Genetics and pathogenesis of inflammatory bowel disease, *Nature* 474:307–317, 2011.

Metz M, Maurer M: Innate immunity and allergy in the skin, *Current Opinion in Immunology* 21:687–693, 2009.

Nestle FO, Di Meglio P, Qin JZ, Nickoloff BJ: Skin immune sentinels in health and disease, *Nature Reviews Immunology* 9:679–691, 2009.

Romani N, Clausen BE, Stoitzner P: Langerhans cells and more: langerin-expressing dendritic cell subsets in the skin, *Immunological Reviews* 234:120–141, 2010.

Weaver CT, Elson CO, Fouser LA, Kolls JK: The Th17 pathway and inflammatory diseases of the intestines, lungs, and skin, *Annual Review of Pathology* 24:477–512, 2013.

Other Specialized Immune Systems

Erlebacher A: Mechanisms of T cell tolerance towards the allogeneic fetus, *Nature Reviews Immunology* 13:23–33, 2013.

Streilein JW: Ocular immune privilege: the eye takes a dim but practical view of immunity and inflammation, *Journal of Leukocyte Biology* 74:179–185, 2003.

von Rango U: Fetal tolerance in human pregnancy—a crucial balance between acceptance and limitation of trophoblast invasion, *Immunology Letters* 115:21–32, 2008.

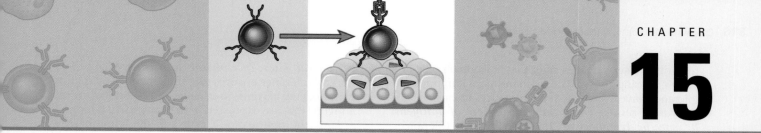

Immunologic Tolerance and Autoimmunity

Immunologic tolerance is defined as unresponsiveness to an antigen that is induced by previous exposure to that antigen. The term arose from the experimental observation that animals that had encountered an antigen under particular conditions would not respond to, or would tolerate, subsequent exposures to the same antigen. When specific lymphocytes encounter antigens, the lymphocytes may be activated, leading to immune responses, or the cells may be inactivated or eliminated, leading to tolerance. Different forms of the same antigen may induce an immune response or tolerance. Antigens that induce tolerance are called tolerogens, or tolerogenic antigens, to distinguish them from immunogens, which generate immunity. A single antigen may be an immunogen or a tolerogen, depending on whether it is displayed to specific lymphocytes in the presence or absence, respectively, of inflammation and innate immune responses. Tolerance to self antigens, also called **self-tolerance**, is a fundamental property of the normal immune system, and failure of self-tolerance results in immune reactions against self (autologous) antigens. Such reactions are called **autoimmunity**, and the diseases they cause are called **autoimmune diseases**. The importance of self-tolerance for the health of individuals was appreciated from the early days of immunology. In Chapter 1, we introduced the concept of self–non-self discrimination, which is the ability of the immune system to recognize and respond to foreign antigens but not to self antigens. Macfarlane Burnet added to his clonal selection hypothesis the corollary that lymphocytes specific for self antigens are eliminated to prevent immune reactions against one's own tissues. Elucidating the mechanisms of self-tolerance is the key to understanding the pathogenesis of autoimmunity.

In this chapter, we will discuss immunologic tolerance mainly in the context of self-tolerance and how self-tolerance may fail, resulting in autoimmunity. We will also consider tolerance to foreign antigens and the potential of tolerance induction as a therapeutic strategy for allergic and autoimmune diseases and to prevent the rejection of cell and organ transplants.

OVERVIEW OF IMMUNOLOGIC TOLERANCE

There are several characteristics of tolerance in T and B lymphocyte populations. It is important to appreciate the general principles before we discuss the specific mechanisms of tolerance in these lymphocytes.

- *Normal individuals are tolerant of their own (self) antigens because the lymphocytes that recognize self antigens are killed or inactivated or the specificity of these lymphocytes is changed.* All individuals inherit essentially the same antigen receptor gene segments, and these recombine and are expressed in lymphocytes as the cells arise from precursor cells. The specificities of the receptors encoded by the recombined genes are random, and are not influenced by what is foreign or self for each individual (see Chapter 8). It is not surprising that during this process of generating a large and diverse repertoire, some developing T and B cells in every individual may express receptors capable of recognizing normal molecules in that individual (i.e., self antigens). Therefore, there is a risk for lymphocytes to react against that individual's cells and tissues, causing disease. The mechanisms of immunologic tolerance have evolved to prevent such reactions.

- **Tolerance results from the recognition of antigens by specific lymphocytes.** In other words, tolerance, by definition, is antigen specific. This contrasts with therapeutic immunosuppression, which affects lymphocytes of many specificities. The key advance that allowed immunologists to study tolerance was the ability to induce this phenomenon in animals by exposure to defined antigens under various conditions and to then analyze the survival and functions of the lymphocytes that had encountered the antigens. Peter Medawar and colleagues showed in the 1950s that neonatal mice of one strain exposed to cells from other strains became unresponsive to subsequent skin grafts from the donor strain. Later studies showed that tolerance could be induced not only to foreign cells but also to proteins and other antigens.

- **Self-tolerance may be induced in immature self-reactive lymphocytes in the generative lymphoid organs (central tolerance) or in mature lymphocytes in peripheral sites (peripheral tolerance)** (Fig. 15-1). Central tolerance ensures that the repertoire of mature lymphocytes becomes incapable of responding to self antigens that are expressed in the generative lymphoid organs (the thymus for T cells and the bone marrow for B lymphocytes, also called central lymphoid organs). However, central tolerance is not perfect, and some self-reactive lymphocytes do complete their maturation. Therefore, the mechanisms of peripheral tolerance are needed to prevent activation of these potentially dangerous lymphocytes.

- **Central tolerance occurs during a stage in the maturation of lymphocytes when encounter with antigen may lead to cell death or replacement of a self-reactive antigen receptor with one that is not self-reactive.** The generative lymphoid organs contain mostly self antigens and not foreign antigens because foreign (e.g., microbial) antigens that enter from the external environment are typically captured and taken to peripheral lymphoid organs, such as the lymph nodes, spleen, and mucosal lymphoid tissues, and are not concentrated in the thymus or bone

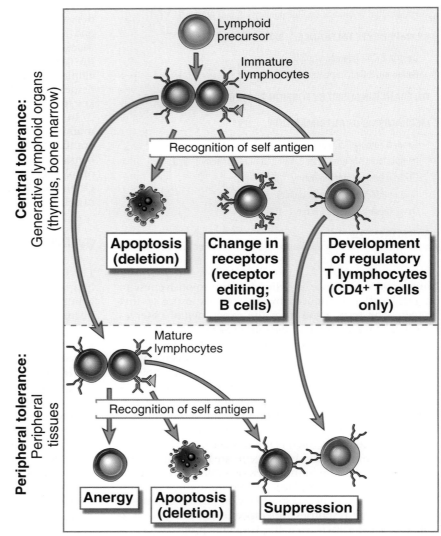

FIGURE 15-1 Central and peripheral tolerance to self antigens. Immature lymphocytes specific for self antigens may encounter these antigens in the generative (central) lymphoid organs and are deleted, change their specificity (B cells only), or (in the case of CD4+ T cells) develop into regulatory lymphocytes (central tolerance). Some self-reactive lymphocytes may mature and enter peripheral tissues and may be inactivated or deleted by encounter with self antigens in these tissues or are suppressed by the regulatory T cells (peripheral tolerance). Note that T cells recognize antigens presented by antigen-presenting cells (not shown).

marrow. The antigens normally present in the thymus and bone marrow include ubiquitous, or widely disseminated, self antigens including those bought in by the blood. In addition, many peripheral tissue–specific antigens are expressed in the thymus by a special mechanism that is described later. Therefore, in the generative lymphoid organs, the immature lymphocytes that specifically recognize antigens are typically cells specific for self, and not foreign, antigens. The fates of immature lymphocytes that recognize self antigens with high affinity are described later (see Fig. 15-1).

- *Peripheral tolerance is induced when mature lymphocytes recognize self antigens and die by apoptosis, or become incapable of activation by re-exposure to that antigen.* Peripheral tolerance is important for maintaining unresponsiveness to self antigens that are expressed in peripheral tissues and not in the generative lymphoid organs and for tolerance to self antigens that are expressed only in adult life, after many mature lymphocytes specific for these antigens may have already been generated. As mentioned earlier, peripheral mechanisms may also serve as a backup for the central mechanisms, which do not eliminate all self-reactive lymphocytes.
- *Peripheral tolerance is also maintained by regulatory T cells (Treg) that actively suppress self antigen-specific lymphocytes.* Treg suppression occurs in secondary lymphoid organs and in nonlymphoid tissues.
- *Some self antigens are sequestered from the immune system, and other antigens are ignored.* Antigens may be sequestered from the immune system by anatomic barriers, such as in the testes and eyes, and thus cannot engage antigen receptors (see Chapter 14). In experimental models, some self antigens are available for recognition by lymphocytes but, for unknown reasons, fail to elicit any response and are functionally ignored. The importance of this phenomenon of ignorance for the maintenance of self-tolerance is not established.
- *Foreign antigens in the absence of costimulatory signals may inhibit immune responses by inducing tolerance in specific lymphocytes.* Many of the mechanisms of tolerance to foreign antigens are similar to those of self-tolerance in mature lymphocytes (peripheral tolerance). Some microbes and tumors also evade immune attack by inducing unresponsiveness in specific lymphocytes.
- *The induction of immunologic tolerance has been exploited as a therapeutic approach for preventing harmful immune responses.* A great deal of effort is being devoted to the development of strategies for inducing tolerance to treat autoimmune and allergic diseases and to prevent the rejection of organ transplants. Tolerance induction may also be useful for preventing immune reactions to the products of newly expressed genes in gene therapy protocols, for preventing reactions to injected proteins in patients with deficiencies of these proteins (e.g., hemophiliacs treated with factor VIII), and for promoting acceptance of stem cell transplants.

Experimental approaches, especially the creation of genetically modified mice, have provided valuable models for analysis of self-tolerance, and many of our current concepts are based on studies with such models. Furthermore, by identifying genes that may be associated with autoimmunity in mice and humans, it has been possible to deduce some of the critical mechanisms of self-tolerance. However, we do not know which self antigens induce central or peripheral tolerance (or are ignored). More importantly, it is also not known which tolerance mechanisms might fail in common human autoimmune diseases, and this remains a major challenge in understanding autoimmunity.

In the sections that follow, we will discuss central and peripheral tolerance first in T cells and then in B lymphocytes, but many aspects of the processes are common to both lineages.

T LYMPHOCYTE TOLERANCE

Tolerance in CD4+ helper T lymphocytes is an effective way of preventing both cell-mediated and humoral immune responses to protein antigens because helper T cells are necessary inducers of all such responses. This realization has been the impetus for a large amount of work on the mechanisms of tolerance in CD4+ T cells. Immunologists have developed experimental models for studying tolerance in CD4+ T cells that have proved to be informative. Also, many of the therapeutic strategies that are being developed to induce tolerance to transplants and autoantigens are aimed at inactivating or eliminating these T cells. Therefore, much of the following discussion, especially of peripheral tolerance, focuses on CD4+ T cells. Less is known about peripheral tolerance in CD8+ T cells, and this is summarized at the end of the section.

Central T Cell Tolerance

During their maturation in the thymus, many immature T cells that recognize antigens with high avidity are deleted, and some of the surviving cells in the CD4+ lineage develop into regulatory T cells (Fig. 15-2). The process of **deletion**, or **negative selection**, of T lymphocytes in the thymus was described in Chapter 8, in the discussion of T cell maturation. This process affects both class I and class II MHC–restricted T cells and is therefore important for tolerance in both CD8+ and CD4+ lymphocyte populations. Negative selection of thymocytes is responsible for the fact that the repertoire of mature T cells that leave the thymus and populate peripheral lymphoid tissues is unresponsive to many self antigens that are present in the thymus. The two main factors that determine if a particular self antigen will induce negative selection of self-reactive thymocytes are the presence of that antigen in the thymus, either by local expression or delivery by the blood, and the affinity of the thymocyte T cell receptors (TCRs) that recognize the antigen. Thus, the important questions that are relevant to negative selection are what self antigens are present in the thymus and how immature T cells that recognize these antigens are deleted.

Negative selection occurs in double-positive T cells in the thymic cortex and newly generated single-positive T cells in the medulla. In both locations, immature thymocytes with

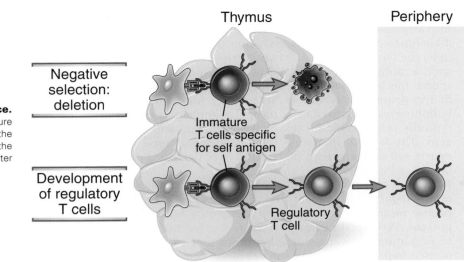

Thymus   Periphery

Negative selection: deletion

Immature T cells specific for self antigen

Development of regulatory T cells

Regulatory T cell

FIGURE 15-2 Central T cell tolerance. Recognition of self antigens by immature T cells in the thymus leads to the death of the cells (negative selection, or deletion) or to the development of regulatory T cells that enter peripheral tissues.

high-affinity receptors for self antigens that encounter these antigens die by apoptosis. T cell receptor (TCR) signaling in immature T cells triggers the mitochondrial pathway of apoptosis. The mechanisms of apoptosis are described later in this chapter, when we discuss deletion as a mechanism of peripheral T cell tolerance. Clearly, immature and mature lymphocytes interpret antigen receptor signals differently— the former die, and the latter are activated. The biochemical basis of this difference is not known.

The antigens that are present in the thymus include many circulating and cell-associated proteins that are widely distributed in tissues. The thymus also has a special mechanism for expressing many protein antigens that are typically present only in certain peripheral tissues, so that immature T cells specific for these antigens can be deleted from the developing T cell repertoire. These peripheral tissue antigens are expressed in thymic medullary epithelial cells under the control of the **autoimmune regulator (AIRE)** protein. Mutations in the *AIRE* gene are the cause of a multiorgan autoimmune disease called **autoimmune polyendocrine syndrome type 1 (APS1).** This group of diseases is characterized by antibody- and lymphocyte-mediated injury to multiple endocrine organs, including the parathyroids, adrenals, and pancreatic islets. A mouse model of APS1 has been developed by knockout of the *AIRE* gene, and it recapitulates many of the features of the human disease. Studies with mice have shown that several proteins that are produced in peripheral organs (such as pancreatic insulin) are also expressed at low levels in medullary thymic epithelial cells, and immature T cells that recognize these antigens are deleted in the thymus. In the absence of functional AIRE (as in APS1 patients and knockout mice) these antigens are not displayed in the thymus, and T cells specific for the antigens escape deletion, mature, and enter the periphery, where they attack the target tissues in which the antigens are expressed independent of AIRE (Fig. 15-3). The AIRE protein may function as a transcriptional regulator to promote the expression of selected tissue-restricted antigens in the thymus. It is a component of a multiprotein complex that is involved in transcriptional elongation and

chromatin unwinding and remodeling. How AIRE drives expression of a wide range of tissue antigens in one cell population in the thymus is still not known.

Some self-reactive CD4+ T cells that see self antigens in the thymus are not deleted but instead differentiate into regulatory T cells specific for these antigens (see Fig. 15-2). The regulatory cells leave the thymus and inhibit responses against self antigens in the periphery. What determines the choice between deletion and development of regulatory T cells is not known. Possible factors include the affinity of antigen recognition, the types of antigen-presenting cells (APCs) presenting the antigen, and the availability of certain cytokines locally in the thymus. We will describe the characteristics and functions of regulatory T cells later in the context of peripheral tolerance because these cells suppress immune responses in the periphery.

Peripheral T Cell Tolerance

The mechanisms of peripheral tolerance are anergy (functional unresponsiveness), suppression by regulatory T cells, and deletion (cell death) (Fig. 15-4). These mechanisms may be responsible for T cell tolerance to tissue-specific self antigens, especially those that are not abundant in the thymus. We do not know if tolerance to different self antigens is maintained by one or another mechanism or if all of these mechanisms function cooperatively to prevent autoimmunity. The same mechanisms may induce unresponsiveness to tolerogenic forms of foreign antigens.

Anergy (Functional Unresponsiveness)

Exposure of mature CD4+ T cells to an antigen in the absence of costimulation or innate immunity may make the cells incapable of responding to that antigen. In this process, which is called anergy, the self-reactive cells do not die but become unresponsive to the antigen. We previously introduced the concept that full activation of T cells requires the recognition of antigen by the TCR (which provides signal 1) and recognition of costimulators, mainly B7-1 and B7-2, by CD28 (signal 2) (see Chapter 9). Prolonged signal 1

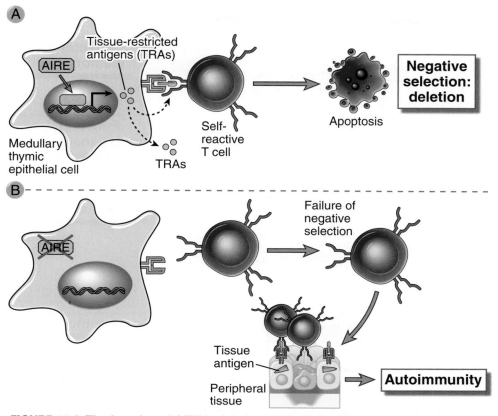

FIGURE 15-3 The function of AIRE in deletion of T cells in the thymus. A, The AIRE protein is part of a complex that regulates the expression of tissue-restricted antigens (TRAs) in medullary thymic epithelial cells (MTEC). Peptides derived from these antigens are displayed on the MTEC and recognized by immature antigen-specific T cells, leading to the deletion of many self-reactive T cells. **B,** In the absence of functional AIRE, these self-reactive T cells are not eliminated; they can enter tissues where the antigens continue to be produced and cause injury.

(i.e., antigen recognition) alone may lead to anergy. It is likely that self antigens are continuously displayed to specific T cells in the absence of innate immunity and strong costimulation. Antigen-induced anergy has been demonstrated in a variety of experimental models, including studies with T cell clones exposed to antigens in vitro (which were the basis for the original definition of anergy), experiments in which antigens are administered to mice without adjuvants, and studies with transgenic mice in which particular protein antigens are expressed throughout life and are recognized by T cells in the absence of the inflammation and innate immune responses that normally accompany exposure to microbes. In many of these situations, the T cells that recognize the antigens become functionally unresponsive and survive for days or weeks in a quiescent state.

Anergy results from biochemical alterations that reduce the ability of lymphocytes to respond to signals from their antigen receptors (Fig. 15-5). It is believed that several biochemical pathways cooperate to maintain this unresponsive state.

- *TCR-induced signal transduction is blocked in anergic cells.* The mechanisms of this signaling block are not fully known. In different experimental models, it is attributable to decreased TCR expression (perhaps because of increased degradation; see later) and recruitment

to the TCR complex of inhibitory molecules such as tyrosine phosphatases.

- *Self antigen recognition may activate cellular ubiquitin ligases, which ubiquitinate TCR-associated proteins and target them for proteolytic degradation in proteasomes or lysosomes.* The net result is loss of these signaling molecules and defective T cell activation (see Chapter 7, Fig. 7-22). One ubiquitin ligase that is important in T cells is called Cbl-b. Mice in which Cbl-b is knocked out show spontaneous T cell proliferation and manifestations of autoimmunity, suggesting that this enzyme is involved in maintaining T cell unresponsiveness to self antigens. It is not known why self antigen recognition, which occurs typically without strong costimulation, activates these ubiquitin ligases, whereas foreign antigens that are recognized with costimulation do so much less or not at all.

- *When T cells recognize self antigens, they may engage inhibitory receptors of the CD28 family, whose function is to terminate T cell responses.* The functions of the best known inhibitory receptors of T cells are described in the section that follows.

Regulation of T Cell Responses by Inhibitory Receptors

In Chapter 9, we introduced the general concept that the outcome of antigen recognition by T cells, particularly CD4+ cells, is determined by a balance between engagement of

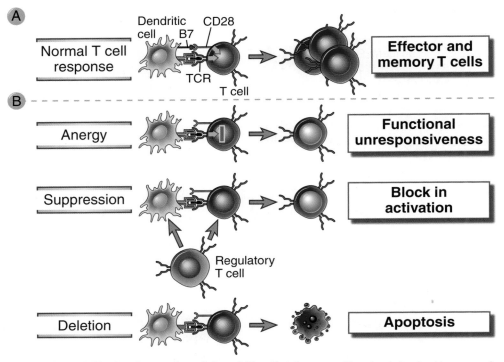

FIGURE 15-4 Mechanisms of peripheral T cell tolerance. The signals involved in a normal immune response **(A)** and the three major mechanisms of peripheral T cell tolerance **(B)** are illustrated.

activating and inhibitory receptors. Although many inhibitory receptors have been described, the two whose physiologic role in self-tolerance is best established are CTLA-4 and PD-1. Studies of these inhibitory receptors have increased our understanding of tolerance mechanisms and led to new therapeutic approaches for manipulating immune responses. The functions and mechanisms of action of these receptors are discussed next.

CTLA-4. CTLA-4 is a member of the CD28 receptor family (see Fig. 9-5) and, like the activating receptor CD28, it binds to B7 molecules. The importance of CTLA-4 in tolerance induction is illustrated by the finding that knockout mice lacking CTLA-4 develop uncontrolled lymphocyte activation with massively enlarged lymph nodes and spleen and fatal multiorgan lymphocytic infiltrates suggestive of systemic autoimmunity. In other words, elimination of this one control mechanism results in failure of peripheral tolerance and a severe T cell–mediated disease. Blocking of CTLA-4 with antibodies also enhances autoimmune diseases in animal models, such as encephalomyelitis induced by immunization with myelin antigens and diabetes induced by T cells reactive with antigens in the β cells of pancreatic islets. Polymorphisms in the *CTLA4* gene are associated with several autoimmune diseases in humans, including type 1 diabetes and Graves' disease. All of these findings, as well as results of clinical trials discussed below, indicate that CTLA-4 functions continuously to keep self-reactive T cells in check.

CTLA-4 has two important actions:

- CTLA-4 expression is low on most T cells until the cells are activated by antigen, and once expressed CTLA-4 terminates continuing activation of these responding T cells.

- CTLA-4 is expressed on regulatory T cells, described later, and mediates the suppressive function of these cells by inhibiting the activation of naive T cells.

CTLA-4 is thought to mediate its inhibitory activity by two main mechanisms (Fig. 15-6):

- *Signaling block.* Engagement of CTLA-4 by B7 activates a phosphatase, which removes phosphates from TCR- and CD28-associated signaling molecules and thus terminates responses.
- *Reducing the availability of B7.* CTLA-4, especially on regulatory T cells, binds to B7 molecules on APCs and blocks them from binding to CD28. It also captures B7 molecules and endocytoses them, thus reducing their expression on APCs. The net result is that the level of B7 on APCs available to bind CD28 is reduced, and the deficiency of costimulation results in a reduced T cell response.

It is still not clear what determines if CD28 will engage B7 molecules to activate T cells (as in infections or immunization with adjuvants) or if CTLA-4 will bind to B7 to block T cell responses (e.g., when self antigens are being presented). In Chapter 9, we discussed the hypothesis that CTLA-4, having a higher affinity for B7 than CD28, is preferentially engaged when APCs are presenting self antigens and expressing little B7. In contrast, microbes increase B7 expression and tilt the balance towards CD28 engagement and T cell activation. Other possibilities are that CD28, which is expressed on naive cells, binds B7 at the initiation of a T cell response, whereas CTLA-4, which is expressed after T cells are activated, functions to terminate these responses.

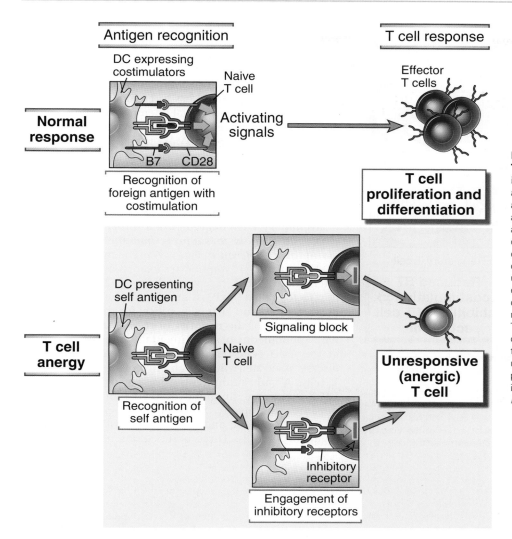

Antigen recognition

DC expressing costimulators

Naive T cell

Normal response

Activating signals

B7   CD28

Recognition of foreign antigen with costimulation

T cell response

Effector T cells

T cell proliferation and differentiation

T cell anergy

DC presenting self antigen

Naive T cell

Recognition of self antigen

Signaling block

Inhibitory receptor

Engagement of inhibitory receptors

Unresponsive (anergic) T cell

FIGURE 15-5 Mechanisms of T cell anergy. T cell responses are induced when the cells recognize an antigen presented by a professional antigen-presenting cell (APC) and activating receptors on the T cells (such as CD28) recognize costimulators on the APCs (such as B7). If the T cell recognizes a self antigen without costimulation, the T cell becomes unresponsive to the antigen because of a block in signaling from the TCR complex or engagement of inhibitory receptors (such as CTLA-4 and PD-1). The signaling block may be the result of recruitment of phosphatases to the TCR complex or the activation of ubiquitin ligases that degrade signaling proteins. The T cell remains viable but is unable to respond to the self antigen. *DC,* dendritic cell.

The realization that CTLA-4 sets checkpoints in immune responses has led to the idea that lymphocyte activation can be promoted by reducing inhibition, a process known as checkpoint blockade. Blocking CTLA-4 with antibodies results in increased immune responses to tumors (see Chapter 18). Anti-CTLA-4 antibody is now approved for the treatment of advanced melanomas, and it is effective in other cancers as well. Predictably, some of the treated patients develop manifestations of autoimmunity with inflammation in various organs.

PD-1. Another inhibitory receptor of the CD28 family is PD-1 (programmed cell death 1, so called because it was originally thought to be involved in programmed cell death but now is known not to have a role in T cell apoptosis). PD-1 recognizes two ligands, called PD-L1 and PD-L2; PD-L1 is expressed on APCs and many other tissue cells, and PD-L2 is expressed mainly on APCs. Engagement of PD-1 by either ligand leads to inactivation of the T cells. Mice in which PD-1 is knocked out develop autoimmune diseases, including a lupus-like kidney disease and arthritis in different inbred strains. The autoimmune disorders in PD-1 knockout mice are less severe than in CTLA-4 knockouts. PD-1 inhibits T cell responses to antigen stimulation,

presumably by inducing inhibitory signals in the T cells. Checkpoint blockade with anti-PD-1 and anti-PD-L1 antibodies is showing even more efficacy and less toxicity than with anti-CTLA-4 in several cancers (see Chapter 18).

Although CTLA-4 and PD-1 are both inhibitory receptors of the same family, their functions may not overlap. CTLA-4 may be more important for controlling the initial activation of CD4+ T cells in lymphoid organs and is a mediator of the suppressive function of regulatory T cells, whereas PD-1 is clearly important in terminating the peripheral responses of effector T cells, especially CD8+ cells, and may not be required for the function of regulatory T cells. Also, several other inhibitory receptors have been identified, including some belonging to the TNF-receptor family and others to the TIM family. There is great interest in defining the role of these receptors in self-tolerance and the regulation of immune responses and the potential of targeting these molecules therapeutically.

Suppression by Regulatory T Cells

The concept that some lymphocytes could control the responses of other lymphocytes was proposed many years

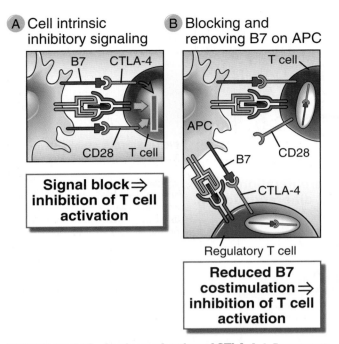

A Cell intrinsic inhibitory signaling

Signal block⇒ inhibition of T cell activation

B Blocking and removing B7 on APC

Reduced B7 costimulation⇒ inhibition of T cell activation

FIGURE 15-6 Mechanisms of action of CTLA-4. A, Engagement of CTLA-4 on a T cell may deliver inhibitory signals that terminate further activation of that cell (cell-intrinsic function of CTLA-4). **B,** CTLA-4 on regulatory or responding T cells binds to B7 molecules on APCs or removes these molecules from the surface of the APCs, making the B7 costimulators unavailable to CD28 and blocking T cell activation. CTLA-4–mediated inhibition by regulatory T cells is a cell-extrinsic action of this inhibitory receptor (since the responding T cells are suppressed by another cell).

ago and was soon followed by experimental demonstrations of populations of T lymphocytes that suppressed immune responses. These initial findings led to enormous interest in the topic, and *suppressor T cells* became one of the dominant topics of immunology research in the 1970s. However, this field has had a somewhat checkered history, mainly because initial attempts to define populations of suppressor cells and their mechanisms of action were largely unsuccessful. More than 20 years later, the idea had an impressive rebirth, with the application of better approaches to define, purify, and analyze populations of T lymphocytes that inhibit immune responses. These cells are called *regulatory T lymphocytes*; their properties and functions are described next.

Regulatory T lymphocytes are a subset of CD4+ T cells whose function is to suppress immune responses and maintain self-tolerance (Fig. 15-7). The majority of these CD4+ regulatory T lymphocytes express high levels of the interleukin-2 (IL-2) receptor α chain (CD25). A transcription factor called FoxP3, a member of the forkhead family of transcription factors, is critical for the development and function of the majority of regulatory T cells. Mice with spontaneous or experimentally induced mutations in the *foxp3* gene develop a multisystem autoimmune disease associated with an absence of CD25+ regulatory T cells. A rare autoimmune disease in humans called **IPEX** syndrome (immune dysregulation, polyendocrinopathy, enteropathy, X-linked) is caused by mutations in the *FOXP3* gene and is associated with deficiency of regulatory T cells. These observations have established

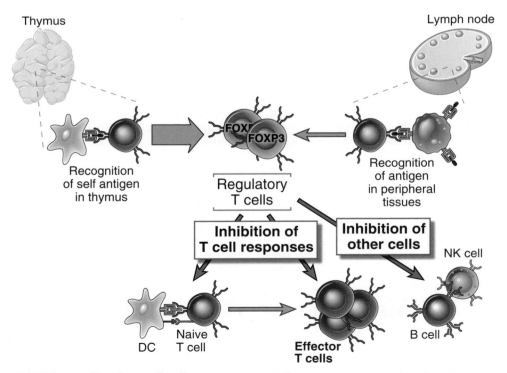

FIGURE 15-7 Regulatory T cells. Regulatory T cells are generated by self antigen recognition in the thymus (sometimes called natural regulatory cells) and (probably to a lesser extent) by antigen recognition in peripheral lymphoid organs (called inducible or adaptive regulatory cells). The development and survival of these regulatory T cells require IL-2 and the transcription factor FoxP3. In peripheral tissues, regulatory T cells suppress the activation and effector functions of other self-reactive and potentially pathogenic lymphocytes.

the importance of regulatory T cells for maintaining self-tolerance. The recent surge of interest in regulatory T cells is because of an increasing appreciation of their physiologic roles, as well as the possibility that defects in these cells may result in various autoimmune diseases and, conversely, that regulatory T cells can be used to treat inflammatory diseases.

Phenotypic Markers and Heterogeneity of Regulatory T Cells

Although numerous T cell populations have been described as possessing suppressive activity, the cell type whose regulatory role is best established is CD4$^+$ FoxP3$^+$ CD25^{high}. Both FoxP3 and CD25 are essential for the generation, maintenance, and function of these cells. These cells typically express low levels of receptors for IL-7 (CD127), and as predicted from this pattern of receptor expression, they use IL-2 but not IL-7 as their growth and survival factor. FoxP3$^+$ regulatory T cells typically express high levels of CTLA-4, which is also required for their function (discussed earlier). Demethylation of the *FOXP3* gene locus as well as of other loci containing genes that are expressed in these cells serves to maintain a stable regulatory T cell phenotype, and these epigenetic changes are now used to identify regulatory T cells in basic and clinical research.

Generation and Maintenance of Regulatory T Cells

Regulatory T cells are generated mainly by self antigen recognition in the thymus and by recognition of self and foreign antigens in peripheral lymphoid organs. In the thymus, development of regulatory T cells is one of the fates of T cells committed to the CD4 lineage that recognize self antigens; these thymic regulatory T cells (tTreg) have also been called natural regulatory T cells. In peripheral lymphoid organs, antigen recognition in the absence of strong innate immune responses favors the generation of regulatory cells from naive CD4$^+$ T lymphocytes; regulatory T cells can also develop after inflammatory reactions. These peripheral regulatory T cells (pTreg) have been called adaptive or inducible because they may be induced to develop from naive CD4$^+$ T cells in the peripheral lymphoid tissues as an adaptation of the immune system in response to certain types of antigen exposure. Predictably, thymic regulatory cells are specific for self antigens because these are the antigens mainly encountered in the thymus. Peripheral regulatory cells may be specific for self or foreign antigens.

The generation of some regulatory T cells requires the cytokine TGF-β. Culture of naive T cells with activating anti-TCR antibodies together with TGF-β (and IL-2, discussed next) can induce the development of regulatory cells in vitro. In mice, elimination of TGF-β or blocking of TGF-β signals in T cells leads to a systemic inflammatory disease because of uncontrolled leukocyte activation and deficiency of functional regulatory T cells. TGF-β stimulates expression of FoxP3, the transcription factor that is required for the development and function of regulatory T cells.

The survival and functional competence of regulatory T cells are dependent on the cytokine IL-2. Mice in which the gene for IL-2 or for the α or β chain of the IL-2 receptor is knocked out develop autoimmunity, manifested by inflammatory bowel disease, autoimmune hemolytic anemia, and multiple autoantibodies (including anti-erythrocyte and anti-DNA). These mice lack a full complement of CD25$^+$ FoxP3$^+$ regulatory T cells, and their disease can be corrected by restoring these cells. IL-2 promotes differentiation of T cells into the regulatory subset and is also required for the maintenance of this cell population. IL-2 activates the transcription factor STAT5, which may enhance expression of FoxP3 as well as other genes that are involved in the function of regulatory T cells. These results are the basis for ongoing clinical trials testing the ability of IL-2 to promote regulatory T cells in humans, for the control of graft-versus-host disease, autoimmune inflammation, and graft rejection.

Particular populations or subsets of dendritic cells may be especially important for stimulating the development of regulatory T cells in peripheral tissues. There is some evidence that dendritic cells exposed to retinoic acid, the vitamin A analogue, are inducers of regulatory T cells, especially in mucosal lymphoid tissues (see Chapter 14).

Mechanisms of Action of Regulatory T Cells

Regulatory T cells appear to suppress immune responses at multiple steps—at the induction of T cell activation in lymphoid organs as well as the effector phase of these responses in tissues. They may also directly suppress B cell activation and inhibit the proliferation and differentiation of natural killer (NK) cells. Although several mechanisms of suppression have been proposed, the following are the best supported by available data.

- ***Production of the immunosuppressive cytokines IL-10 and TGF-β.*** The biology of these cytokines is described in more detail later.
- ***Reduced ability of APCs to stimulate T cells.*** One proposed mechanism of this action is dependent on binding of CTLA-4 on regulatory cells to B7 molecules on APCs, described earlier (see Fig. 15-6).
- ***Consumption of IL-2.*** Because of the high level of expression of the IL-2 receptor, these cells may absorb IL-2 and deprive other cell populations of this growth factor, resulting in reduced proliferation and differentiation of other IL-2–dependent cells.

It is not established if all regulatory cells work by all of these mechanisms or if there are subpopulations that use different mechanisms to control immune responses. In fact, there is some evidence in humans that two different populations of regulatory T cells can be distinguished by the expression of FoxP3 or production of IL-10, but this separation may not be absolute.

Inhibitory Cytokines Produced by Regulatory T Cells

TGF-β and IL-10 are involved in both the generation and the functions of regulatory T cells. These cytokines are produced by and act on many other cell types besides regulatory cells. Here we describe the properties and actions of these cytokines.

Transforming Growth Factor-β. TGF-β was discovered as a tumor product that promoted the survival of tumor cells in vitro. It is actually a family of closely related molecules encoded by distinct genes, commonly designated TGF-β1, TGF-β2, and TGF-β3. Cells of the immune system synthesize mainly TGF-β1. TGF-β1 is produced by CD4+ regulatory T cells, activated macrophages, and many other cell types. It is synthesized as an inactive precursor that is proteolytically cleaved in the Golgi complex and forms a homodimer. Mature TGF-β1 is secreted in a latent form in association with other polypeptides, which must be removed extracellularly by enzymatic digestion before the cytokine can bind to receptors and exert biologic effects. The TGF-β1 receptor consists of two different proteins, TGF-βRI and TGF-βRII, both of which phosphorylate transcription factors called SMADs. On cytokine binding, a serine/threonine kinase domain of TGF-βRI phosphorylates SMAD2 and SMAD3, which in complex with SMAD4 translocate to the nucleus, bind to promoters of target genes, and regulate their transcription.

TGF-β has many important and quite diverse roles in the immune system.

- *TGF-β inhibits the proliferation and effector functions of T cells and the activation of macrophages.* TGF-β inhibits classical macrophage activation but is one of the cytokines secreted by alternatively activated macrophages (see Chapter 10). TGF-β also suppresses the activation of other cells, such as neutrophils and endothelial cells. By these inhibitory actions, TGF-β functions to control immune and inflammatory responses.
- *TGF-β regulates the differentiation of functionally distinct subsets of T cells.* As described earlier, TGF-β stimulates the development of peripheral FoxP3+ regulatory T cells. In combination with cytokines produced during innate immune responses, such as IL-1 and IL-6, TGF-β promotes the development of the T_H17 subset of CD4+ T cells by virtue of its ability to induce the transcription factor RORγt (see Chapter 10). The ability of TGF-β to suppress immune and inflammatory responses, in part by generating regulatory T cells, and also to promote the development of proinflammatory T_H17 cells in the presence of other cytokines, is an interesting example of how a single cytokine can have diverse and sometimes opposing actions depending on the context in which it is produced. TGF-β can also inhibit development of T_H1 and T_H2 subsets.
- *TGF-β stimulates production of IgA antibodies by inducing B cells to switch to this isotype.* IgA is the major antibody isotype required for mucosal immunity (see Chapter 14).
- *TGF-β promotes tissue repair after local immune and inflammatory reactions subside.* This function is mediated mainly by the ability of TGF-β to stimulate collagen synthesis and matrix-modifying enzyme production by macrophages and fibroblasts and by promotion of angiogenesis. This cytokine may play a pathologic role in diseases in which fibrosis is an important component, such as pulmonary fibrosis and systemic sclerosis.

Interleukin-10. IL-10 is an inhibitor of activated macrophages and dendritic cells and is thus involved in the control of innate immune reactions and cell-mediated immunity. It is a member of a family of heterodimeric cytokines that includes IL-22, IL-27, and others. The IL-10 receptor belongs to the type II cytokine receptor family (similar to the receptor for interferons) and consists of two chains, which associate with JAK1 and TYK2 Janus family kinases and activate STAT3. IL-10 is produced by many immune cell populations, including activated macrophages and dendritic cells, regulatory T cells, and T_H1 and T_H2 cells. Because it is both produced by and inhibits macrophage and dendritic cell functions, it functions as a negative feedback regulator. IL-10 is also produced by some B lymphocytes, which have been shown to have immune suppressive functions and have been called **regulatory B cells**.

The biologic effects of IL-10 result from its ability to inhibit many of the functions of activated macrophages and dendritic cells.

- *IL-10 inhibits the production of IL-12 by activated dendritic cells and macrophages.* Because IL-12 is a critical stimulus for IFN-γ secretion, which plays an important role in innate and adaptive cell-mediated immune reactions against intracellular microbes, IL-10 functions to suppress all such reactions. In fact, IL-10 was first identified as a protein that inhibited IFN-γ production.
- *IL-10 inhibits the expression of costimulators and class II MHC molecules on dendritic cells and macrophages.* Because of these actions, IL-10 serves to inhibit T cell activation and terminate cell-mediated immune reactions.

A rare inherited autoimmune disease has been described in which mutations in the IL-10 receptor cause severe colitis that develops early in life, before 1 year of age. Knockout mice lacking IL-10 either in all cells or only in regulatory T cells also develop colitis, probably as a result of uncontrolled activation of lymphocytes and macrophages reacting to enteric microbes. Because of these findings, it is believed that this cytokine is especially important for controlling inflammatory reactions in mucosal tissues, particularly in the gastrointestinal tract (see Chapter 14).

The Epstein-Barr virus contains a gene homologous to human IL-10, and viral IL-10 has the same activities as the natural cytokine. This raises the intriguing possibility that acquisition of the IL-10–like gene during the evolution of the virus has given it the ability to inhibit host immunity and thus a survival advantage in the infected host.

Roles of Regulatory T Cells in Self-Tolerance and Autoimmunity

The elucidation of the genetic basis of IPEX syndrome and the similar disease in mice caused by mutations in the *Foxp3* gene, described earlier, is convincing proof of the importance of regulatory T cells in maintaining self-tolerance and homeostasis in the immune system. Numerous attempts are being made to identify defects in the development or function of regulatory T cells in more common autoimmune diseases in humans, such as inflammatory bowel disease, type 1 diabetes, and multiple sclerosis, as well as in allergic disorders. It appears likely that defects in regulatory T cells or resistance of effector cells to suppression contribute to the pathogenesis of autoimmune and allergic diseases. There is also potential for expanding regulatory cells in culture and injecting them back into patients to control pathologic immune responses. Clinical trials of regulatory T cell transfer are ongoing in attempts to treat transplant rejection, graft-vs-host disease, and autoimmune and other inflammatory disorders. Attempts are also under way to induce these cells in patients by administering self peptides that are the targets of autoimmunity or low doses of the cytokine IL-2, either separately or in combination.

Deletion of T Cells by Apoptotic Cell Death

T lymphocytes that recognize self antigens with high affinity or are repeatedly stimulated by antigens may die by apoptosis. There are two major pathways of apoptosis in various cell types (Fig. 15-8), both of which have been implicated in peripheral deletion of mature T cells.

- The **mitochondrial** (or **intrinsic**) **pathway** is regulated by the Bcl-2 family of proteins, named after the founding member, Bcl-2, which was discovered as an

oncogene in a B cell lymphoma and shown to inhibit apoptosis. Some members of this family are pro-apoptotic and others are anti-apoptotic. The pathway is initiated when cytoplasmic proteins of the Bcl-2 family that belong to the BH3-only subfamily (so called because they contain one domain that is homologous to the third conserved domain of Bcl-2) are induced or activated as a result of growth factor deprivation, noxious stimuli, DNA damage, or certain types of receptor-mediated signaling (such as strong signals delivered by self antigens in immature lymphocytes). BH3-only proteins are sensors of cell stress that bind to and influence death effectors and regulators. In lymphocytes, the most important of these sensors is a protein called Bim. Activated Bim binds to two pro-apoptotic effector proteins of the Bcl-2 family called Bax and Bak, which oligomerize and insert into the outer mitochondrial membrane, leading to increased mitochondrial permeability. Growth factors and other survival signals induce the expression of anti-apoptotic members of the Bcl-2 family, such as Bcl-2 and Bcl-X_L, which function as inhibitors of apoptosis by blocking Bax and Bak and thus maintaining intact mitochondria. BH3-only proteins also antagonize Bcl-2 and Bcl-X_L. When cells are deprived of survival signals, the

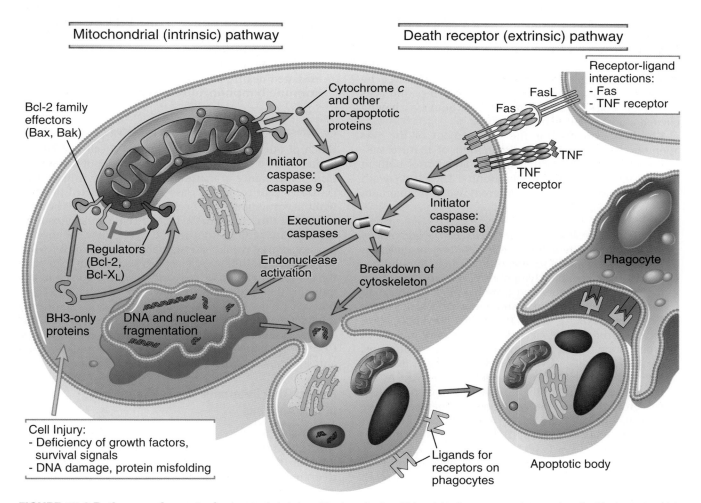

FIGURE 15-8 Pathways of apoptosis. Apoptosis is induced by the mitochondrial and death receptor pathways, described in the text, which culminate in fragmentation of the dead cell and phagocytosis of apoptotic bodies.

mitochondria become leaky because of the actions of the BH3-only protein sensors and Bax and Bak effectors and the relative deficiency of anti-apoptotic proteins such as Bcl-2 and Bcl-X$_L$. The result is that many mitochondrial components, including cytochrome c, leak out into the cytosol. These proteins activate cytosolic enzymes called **caspases**, initially caspase-9, which in turn cleaves downstream caspases that lead to nuclear DNA fragmentation and other changes that culminate in apoptotic death.

- In the **death receptor** (or **extrinsic**) **pathway**, cell surface receptors homologous to tumor necrosis factor (TNF) receptors are engaged by their ligands, which are homologous to the cytokine TNF. The receptors oligomerize and activate cytoplasmic adaptor proteins, which assemble procaspase-8, which cleaves itself when oligomerized to yield active caspase-8. The active caspase-8 then cleaves downstream caspases, again resulting in apoptosis. In many cell types, caspase-8 cleaves and activates a BH3-only protein called Bid that binds to Bax and Bak and induces apoptosis via the mitochondrial pathway. Thus, the mitochondrial pathway may serve to amplify death receptor signaling.

Cells undergoing apoptosis develop membrane blebs, and fragments of the nucleus and cytoplasm break off in membrane-bound structures called apoptotic bodies. There are also biochemical changes in the plasma membrane, including the exposure of lipids such as phosphatidylserine, which is normally on the inner face of the plasma membrane. These alterations are recognized by receptors on phagocytes, and apoptotic bodies and cells are rapidly engulfed and eliminated, without ever having elicited a host inflammatory response.

The best evidence for the involvement of the two apoptotic pathways in the elimination of mature self-reactive lymphocytes is that genetic ablation of both in mice results in systemic autoimmunity. These two death pathways may function in different ways to maintain self-tolerance.

- *T cells that recognize self antigens in the absence of costimulation may activate Bim, resulting in apoptosis by the mitochondrial pathway.* In normal immune responses, the responding lymphocytes receive signals from the TCR, costimulators, and growth factors. These signals stimulate the expression of anti-apoptotic proteins of the Bcl-2 family (Bcl-2, Bcl-X$_L$) and thus prevent apoptosis and promote cell survival, the necessary prelude to proliferation. When T cells avidly recognize self antigens, they may directly activate Bim, which triggers death by the mitochondrial pathway, as described earlier. At the same time, because of the relative lack of costimulation and growth factors, the anti-apoptotic members of the Bcl-2 family, Bcl-2 and Bcl-X$_L$, are expressed at low levels, and the actions of Bim, Bax, and Bak are thus not counteracted.

The Bim-dependent mitochondrial pathway of apoptosis is also involved in negative selection of self-reactive T cells in the thymus (described earlier) and in the contraction phase (decline) of immune responses after the initiating antigen has been eliminated (see Chapter 9).

- *Repeated stimulation of T cells results in the coexpression of death receptors and their ligands, and engagement of the death receptors triggers apoptotic death.* In CD4$^+$ T cells, the most important death receptor is Fas (CD95), and its ligand is Fas ligand (FasL). Fas is a member of the TNF receptor family, and FasL is homologous to TNF. When T cells are repeatedly activated, FasL is expressed on the cell surface, and it binds to surface Fas on the same or adjacent T cells. This activates a cascade of caspases, which ultimately cause the apoptotic death of the cells. The same pathway of apoptosis may be involved in the elimination of self-reactive B lymphocytes also in the periphery (discussed later).

Mice carrying mutations of the genes encoding Fas or Fas ligand provided the first clear evidence that failure of apoptotic cell death results in autoimmunity. These mice develop a systemic autoimmune disease with multiple autoantibodies and nephritis, resembling human systemic lupus erythematosus (see Chapter 19). The lpr (for lymphoproliferation) mouse strain produces low levels of Fas protein, and the gld (for generalized lymphoproliferative disease) strain produces FasL with a point mutation that interferes with its signaling function. The cause of autoimmunity is believed to be defective peripheral deletion and accumulation of autoreactive B and helper T cells. Children with a phenotypically similar disease have been identified and shown to carry mutations in the gene encoding Fas or in genes encoding proteins in the Fas-mediated death pathway. This disease is called **autoimmune lymphoproliferative syndrome (ALPS)**.

Peripheral Tolerance in CD8$^+$ T Lymphocytes

Much of our knowledge of peripheral T cell tolerance is limited to CD4$^+$ T cells, and less is known about the mechanisms of tolerance in mature CD8$^+$ T cells. It is likely that if CD8$^+$ T cells recognize class I MHC–associated peptides without costimulation or T cell help, the CD8$^+$ cells become anergic. In this situation, the CD8$^+$ T cells would encounter signal 1 (antigen) without second signals, and the mechanism of anergy would be essentially the same as for CD4$^+$ T lymphocytes. Inhibitory receptors such as PD-1 suppress the activation of CD8$^+$ T cells and may be involved in terminating their responses, in a phenomenon called exhaustion (see Chapter 11). CD25$^+$ regulatory T cells can directly inhibit the activation of CD8$^+$ T cells or suppress CD4$^+$ helper cells that are required for full CD8$^+$ T cell responses. CD8$^+$ T cells that are exposed to high concentrations of self antigens may also undergo apoptotic cell death.

Factors That Determine the Tolerogenicity of Self Antigens

Studies with a variety of experimental models have shown that many features of protein antigens determine whether these antigens will induce T cell activation or tolerance (Table 15-1). Self antigens have several properties that make them tolerogenic. These antigens are expressed in generative lymphoid organs, where they are recognized by immature lymphocytes. In peripheral

TABLE 15-1   Factors That Determine the Immunogenicity and Tolerogenicity of Protein Antigens

	Features That Favor Stimulation of Immune Responses	Features That Favor Tolerance
Persistence	Short-lived (eliminated by immune response)	Prolonged
Portal of entry; location	Subcutaneous, intradermal; absence from generative organs	Intravenous, mucosal; presence in generative organs
Presence of adjuvants	Antigens with adjuvants: stimulate helper T cells	Antigens without adjuvants: non-immunogenic or tolerogenic
Properties of antigen-presenting cells	High levels of costimulators	Low levels of costimulators and cytokines

tissues, self antigens engage antigen receptors of specific lymphocytes for prolonged periods and without inflammation or innate immunity.

The nature of the dendritic cell that displays antigens to T lymphocytes is an important determinant of the subsequent response. Dendritic cells that are resident in lymphoid organs and nonlymphoid tissues may present self antigens to T lymphocytes and maintain tolerance. Tissue dendritic cells are normally in a resting (immature) state and express few or no costimulators. Such APCs may be constantly presenting self antigens without providing activating signals, and T cells that recognize these antigens become anergic or differentiate into regulatory T lymphocytes instead of effector and memory lymphocytes. By contrast, dendritic cells that are activated by microbes are the principal APCs for initiation of T cell responses (see Chapter 6). As we will discuss later, local infections and inflammation may activate resident dendritic cells, leading to increased expression of costimulators, breakdown of tolerance, and autoimmune reactions against tissue antigens. The characteristics of dendritic cells that make them tolerogenic are not defined but presumably include low expression of costimulators. There is great interest in manipulating the properties of dendritic cells as a way of enhancing or inhibiting immune responses for therapeutic purposes.

Our understanding of the mechanisms that link the signals that a T cell receives at the time of antigen recognition with the fate of that T cell remains incomplete. These concepts are based largely on experimental models in which antigens are administered to mice or are produced by transgenes expressed in mice. One of the continuing challenges in this field is to define the mechanisms by which various normally expressed self antigens induce tolerance, especially in humans.

B LYMPHOCYTE TOLERANCE

Tolerance in B lymphocytes is necessary for maintaining unresponsiveness to thymus-independent self antigens, such as polysaccharides and lipids. B cell tolerance also plays a role in preventing antibody responses to protein antigens. Experimental studies have revealed multiple mechanisms by which encounter with self antigens may abort B cell maturation and activation.

Central B Cell Tolerance

Immature B lymphocytes that recognize self antigens in the bone marrow with high affinity either change their specificity or are deleted. The mechanisms of central B cell tolerance have been best described in experimental models (Fig. 15-9).

- *Receptor editing.* If immature B cells recognize self antigens that are present at high concentration in the bone marrow and especially if the antigen is displayed in multivalent form (e.g., on cell surfaces), many antigen receptors on each B cell are cross-linked, thus delivering strong signals to the cells. As discussed in Chapter 8, one consequence of such signaling is that the B cells reactivate their *RAG1* and *RAG2* genes and initiate a new round of VJ recombination in the immunoglobulin (Ig) κ light chain gene locus. A V_κ segment upstream of the already rearranged $V_\kappa J_\kappa$ unit is joined to a downstream J_κ. As a result, the previously rearranged $V_\kappa J_\kappa$ exon in the self-reactive immature B cell is deleted, and a new Ig light chain is expressed, thus creating a B cell receptor with a new specificity. This process is called **receptor editing** (see Chapter 8) and is an important mechanism for eliminating self-reactivity from the mature B cell repertoire. If the edited light chain rearrangement is non-productive, rearrangement may proceed at the κ locus on the other chromosome, and if that is non-productive, rearrangements at the λ light chain loci may follow. A B cell expressing a λ light chain is frequently a cell that has undergone receptor editing.
- *Deletion.* If editing fails, the immature B cells may die by apoptosis. The mechanisms of deletion are not well defined.
- *Anergy.* If developing B cells recognize self antigens weakly (e.g., if the antigen is soluble and does not cross-link many antigen receptors or if the B cell receptors recognize the antigen with low affinity), the cells become functionally unresponsive (anergic) and exit the bone marrow in this unresponsive state. Anergy is due to downregulation of antigen receptor expression as well as a block in antigen receptor signaling.

Peripheral B Cell Tolerance

Mature B lymphocytes that recognize self antigens in peripheral tissues in the absence of specific helper T cells may be rendered functionally unresponsive or die by apoptosis

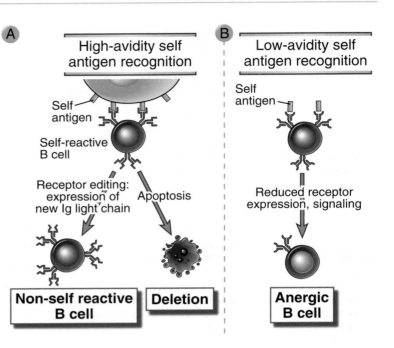

FIGURE 15-9 Central tolerance in B cells. Immature B cells that recognize self antigens in the bone marrow with high avidity (e.g., multivalent arrays of antigens on cells) die by apoptosis or change the specificity of their antigen receptors (receptor editing). Weak recognition of self antigens in the bone marrow may lead to anergy (functional inactivation) of the B cells.

(Fig. 15-10). Signals from helper T cells may be absent if these T cells are deleted or anergic or if the self antigens are non-protein antigens. Since self antigens usually do not elicit innate immune responses, B cells will also not be activated via complement receptors or pattern recognition receptors. Thus, as in T cells, antigen recognition without additional stimuli results in tolerance. Peripheral tolerance mechanisms also eliminate autoreactive B cell clones that may be generated as an unintended consequence of somatic mutation in germinal centers.

- *Anergy and deletion.* Some self-reactive B cells that are repeatedly stimulated by self antigens become

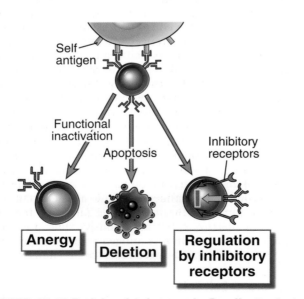

FIGURE 15-10 Peripheral tolerance in B cells. B cells that encounter self antigens in peripheral tissues become anergic or die by apoptosis. In some situations, recognition of self antigens may trigger inhibitory receptors that prevent B cell activation.

unresponsive to further activation. These cells require high levels of the growth factor BAFF/BLys for survival (see Chapter 11) and cannot compete efficiently with less BAFF–dependent normal naive B cells for survival in lymphoid follicles. As a result, the B cells that have encountered self antigens have a shortened life span and are eliminated more rapidly than cells that have not recognized self antigens. B cells that bind with high avidity to self antigens in the periphery may also undergo apoptotic death by the mitochondrial pathway.

The high rate of somatic mutation of Ig genes that occurs in germinal centers has the risk of generating self-reactive B cells (see Chapter 12). These B cells may be actively eliminated by the interaction of FasL on helper T cells with Fas on the activated B cells. The same interaction was described earlier as a mechanism for the death of self-reactive T cells. Failure of this pathway of peripheral B cell tolerance may contribute to the autoimmunity that is caused by mutations in the *Fas* and *FasL* genes in mice, and in patients with ALPS, discussed earlier.

- *Signaling by inhibitory receptors.* B cells that recognize self antigens with low affinity may be prevented from responding by the engagement of various inhibitory receptors. The function of these inhibitory receptors is to set a threshold for B cell activation, which allows responses to foreign antigens with T cell help but does not allow responses to self antigens. This mechanism of peripheral tolerance was revealed by studies showing that mice with defects in the SHP-1 tyrosine phosphatase, the Lyn tyrosine kinase, and the CD22 inhibitory receptor develop autoimmunity. ITIM motifs in the cytoplasmic tail of CD22 are phosphorylated by Lyn, and this inhibitory receptor then recruits SHP-1, thus attenuating B cell receptor signaling. However, it is not known when inhibitory receptors such as CD22 are engaged and what ligands they recognize.

Much has been learned about the mechanisms of tolerance in T and B lymphocytes, largely from the use of animal models such as genetically modified mice. Application of this knowledge to understanding the mechanisms of tolerance to different self antigens in normal individuals and to defining why tolerance fails, giving rise to autoimmune diseases, is an area of active investigation.

TOLERANCE INDUCED BY FOREIGN PROTEIN ANTIGENS

Foreign antigens may be administered in ways that preferentially induce tolerance rather than immune responses. Understanding how to induce tolerance by antigen administration is the key to developing antigen-specific tolerance as a treatment strategy for immunologic diseases. In general, protein antigens administered cutaneously with adjuvants favor immunity, whereas high doses of antigens administered without adjuvants tend to induce tolerance. The likely reason for this is that adjuvants stimulate innate immune responses and the expression of costimulators on APCs, and in the absence of these second signals, T cells that recognize the antigen may become anergic or die or may differentiate into regulatory cells. Many other features of antigens, and how they are administered, may influence the balance between immunity and tolerance (see Table 15-1).

The oral administration of a protein antigen often leads to suppression of systemic humoral and cell-mediated immune responses to immunization with the same antigen. This phenomenon, called **oral tolerance**, was discussed in Chapter 14.

MECHANISMS OF AUTOIMMUNITY

The possibility that an individual's immune system may react against autologous antigens and cause tissue injury was appreciated by immunologists from the time that the specificity of the immune system for foreign antigens was recognized. In the early 1900s, Paul Ehrlich coined the rather melodramatic phrase *horror autotoxicus* for harmful (toxic) immune reactions against self. Autoimmunity is an important cause of disease in humans and is estimated to affect at least 2% to 5% of the U.S. population. The term *autoimmunity* is often erroneously used for any disease in which immune reactions accompany tissue injury, even though it may be difficult or impossible to establish a role for immune responses against self antigens in causing these disorders. Because inflammation is a prominent component of these disorders, they are sometimes grouped under *immune-mediated inflammatory diseases,* which does not imply that the pathologic response is directed against self antigens (see Chapter 19).

The fundamental questions about autoimmunity are how self-tolerance fails and how self-reactive lymphocytes are activated. Answers to these questions are needed to understand the etiology and pathogenesis of autoimmune diseases, which is a major challenge in immunology. Our understanding of autoimmunity has improved greatly during the past two decades, mainly because of the development of informative animal models of these diseases, the identification of genes that may predispose to autoimmunity, and improved methods for analyzing immune responses in humans. Several important general concepts have emerged from studies of autoimmunity.

The factors that contribute to the development of autoimmunity are genetic susceptibility and environmental triggers, such as infections and local tissue injury. Susceptibility genes may disrupt self-tolerance mechanisms, and infection or necrosis in tissues promotes the influx of autoreactive lymphocytes and activation of these cells, resulting in tissue injury (Fig. 15-11). Infections and tissue injury may also alter the way in which self antigens are displayed to the immune system, leading to failure of self-tolerance and activation of self-reactive lymphocytes. The roles of these factors in the development of autoimmunity are discussed later. Other factors such as changes in the host microbiome and epigenetic alterations in immune cells may play important roles in pathogenesis, but studies on these topics are in their infancy.

General Features of Autoimmune Disorders

Autoimmune diseases have several general characteristics that are relevant to defining their underlying mechanisms.

- *Autoimmune diseases may be either systemic or organ specific, depending on the distribution of the autoantigens that are recognized.* For instance, the formation of circulating immune complexes composed of self nucleoproteins and specific antibodies typically produces systemic diseases, such as systemic lupus erythematosus (SLE). In contrast, autoantibody or T cell responses against self antigens with restricted tissue distribution lead to organ-specific diseases, such as myasthenia gravis, type 1 diabetes, and multiple sclerosis.
- *Various effector mechanisms are responsible for tissue injury in different autoimmune diseases.* These mechanisms include immune complexes, circulating autoantibodies, and autoreactive T lymphocytes and are discussed in Chapter 19. The clinical and pathologic features of the disease are usually determined by the nature of the dominant autoimmune response.
- *Autoimmune diseases tend to be chronic, progressive, and self-perpetuating.* The reasons for these features are that the self antigens that trigger these reactions are persistent, and once an immune response starts, many amplification mechanisms are activated that perpetuate the response. In addition, a response initiated against one self antigen that injures tissues may result in the release and alterations of other tissue antigens, activation of lymphocytes specific for these other antigens, and exacerbation of the disease. This phenomenon is called epitope spreading, and it may explain why once an autoimmune disease has developed, it may become prolonged and self-perpetuating.

Immunologic Abnormalities Leading to Autoimmunity

Autoimmunity results from some combination of three main immunologic aberrations.

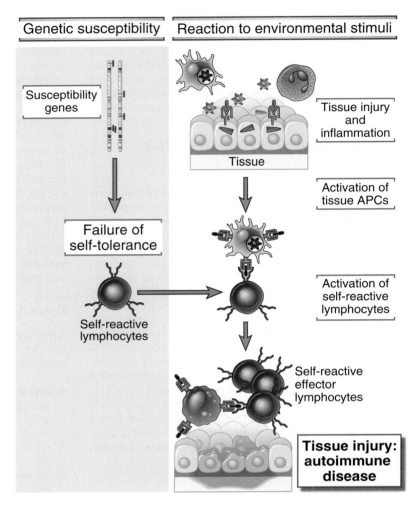

FIGURE 15-11 Postulated mechanisms of autoimmunity. In this proposed model of an organ-specific T cell–mediated autoimmune disease, various genetic loci may confer susceptibility to autoimmunity, in part by influencing the maintenance of self-tolerance. Environmental triggers, such as infections and other inflammatory stimuli, promote the influx of lymphocytes into tissues and the activation of self-reactive T cells, resulting in tissue injury.

• *Defective tolerance or regulation. Failure of the mechanisms of self-tolerance in T or B cells, leading to an imbalance between lymphocyte activation and control, is the underlying cause of all autoimmune diseases.* The potential for autoimmunity exists in all individuals because some of the randomly generated specificities of clones of developing lymphocytes may be for self antigens, and many self antigens are readily accessible to lymphocytes. As discussed earlier, tolerance to self antigens is normally maintained by selection processes that prevent the maturation of some self antigen–specific lymphocytes and by mechanisms that inactivate or delete self-reactive lymphocytes that do mature. Loss of self-tolerance may result if self-reactive lymphocytes are not deleted or inactivated during or after their maturation and if APCs are activated so that self antigens are presented to the immune system in an immunogenic manner. Experimental models and limited studies in humans have shown that any of the following mechanisms may contribute to the failure of self-tolerance:
  ○ Defects in deletion (negative selection) of T or B cells or receptor editing in B cells during the maturation of these cells in the generative lymphoid organs
  ○ Defective numbers and functions of regulatory T lymphocytes

  ○ Defective apoptosis of mature self-reactive lymphocytes
  ○ Inadequate function of inhibitory receptors
• *Abnormal display of self antigens.* Abnormalities may include increased expression and persistence of self antigens that are normally cleared, or structural changes in these antigens resulting from enzymatic modifications or from cellular stress or injury. If these changes lead to the display of antigenic epitopes that are not present normally, the immune system may not be tolerant to these epitopes, thus allowing anti-self responses to develop.
• *Inflammation or an initial innate immune response.* As we have discussed in previous chapters, the innate immune response is a strong stimulus for the subsequent activation of lymphocytes and the generation of adaptive immune responses. Infections or cell injury may elicit local innate immune reactions with inflammation. These may contribute to the development of autoimmune disease, perhaps by activating APCs, which overcomes regulatory mechanisms and results in excessive T cell activation.

Much recent attention has focused on the role of T cells in autoimmunity for two main reasons. First, helper T cells are the key regulators of all immune responses to proteins, and most self antigens implicated in autoimmune diseases are proteins. Second, several autoimmune diseases are genetically linked to the MHC (the HLA complex in humans), and the function of MHC molecules is to present peptide antigens to T cells. Failure of self-tolerance in T lymphocytes may result in autoimmune diseases in which tissue damage is caused by cell-mediated immune reactions. Helper T cell abnormalities may also lead to autoantibody production because helper T cells are necessary for the production of high-affinity antibodies against protein antigens.

In the following section, we describe the general principles of the pathogenesis of autoimmune diseases, with an emphasis on susceptibility genes, infections, and other factors that contribute to the development of autoimmunity. We will describe the pathogenesis and features of some illustrative autoimmune diseases in Chapter 19.

Genetic Basis of Autoimmunity

From the earliest studies of autoimmune diseases in patients and experimental animals, it has been appreciated that these diseases have a strong genetic component. For instance, type 1 diabetes shows a concordance of 35% to 50% in monozygotic twins and 5% to 6% in dizygotic twins, and other autoimmune diseases show similar evidence of a genetic contribution. Linkage analyses in families, genome-wide association studies, and large-scale sequencing efforts are revealing new information about the genes that may play causal roles in the development of autoimmunity and chronic inflammatory disorders. From these studies, several general features of genetic susceptibility have become apparent.

Most autoimmune diseases are complex polygenic traits in which affected individuals inherit multiple genetic polymorphisms that contribute to disease susceptibility, and these genes act with environmental factors to cause the diseases. Some of these polymorphisms are associated with several autoimmune diseases, suggesting that the causative genes influence general mechanisms of immune regulation and self-tolerance. Other loci are associated with particular diseases, suggesting that they may affect organ damage or autoreactive lymphocytes of particular specificities. Each genetic polymorphism makes a small contribution to the development of particular autoimmune diseases and is also found in healthy individuals but at a lower frequency than in patients with the diseases. It is postulated that in individual patients, multiple such polymorphisms are coinherited and together account for development of the disease. Understanding the interplay of multiple genes with one another and with environmental factors is one of the continuing challenges in the field.

The best-characterized genes associated with autoimmune diseases and our current understanding of how they may contribute to loss of self-tolerance are described here.

Association of MHC Alleles with Autoimmunity

Among the genes that are associated with autoimmunity, the strongest associations are with MHC genes. In fact, in

TABLE 15-2   Association of HLA Alleles with Autoimmune Disease

Disease	HLA Allele	Odds Ratio[1]
Rheumatoid arthritis (anti-CCP Ab positive)[2]	DRB1, 1 SE allele[3]	4
	DRB1, 2 SE alleles	12
Type 1 diabetes	DRB1*0301-DQA1*0501-DQB1*0201 haplotype	4
	DRB1*0401-DQA1*0301-DQB1*0302 haplotype	8
	DRB1*0301/0401 heterozygotes	35
Multiple sclerosis	DRB1*1501	3
Systemic lupus erythematosus	DRB1*0301	2
	DRB1*1501	1.3
Ankylosing spondylitis	B*27 (mainly B*2705 and B*2702)	100-200
Celiac disease	DQA1*0501-DQB1*0201 haplotype	7

[1]The odds ratio approximates values of increased risk of the disease associated with inheritance of particular HLA alleles. The data are from populations of European ancestry. Alleles of individual MHC genes (e.g., DRB1) are indicated by 4 numbers (e.g., 0301), based on serologic and molecular typing.
[2]Anti-CCP Ab, antibodies directed against cyclic citrullinated peptides. Data are from patients who test positive for these antibodies in the serum.
[3]SE refers to shared epitope, so called because it is a consensus sequence in the DRB1 protein (positions 70-74) present in multiple DRB1 alleles.
(Courtesy of Dr. Michelle Fernando, Kings College, London.)

many autoimmune diseases, such as type 1 diabetes, 20 or 30 disease-associated genes have been identified; in most of these diseases, the HLA locus alone contributes half or more of the genetic susceptibility. HLA typing of large groups of patients with various autoimmune diseases has shown that some HLA alleles occur at higher frequency in these patients than in the general population. From such studies, one can calculate the odds ratio for development of a disease in individuals who inherit various HLA alleles (often referred to as the relative risk) (Table 15-2). The strongest such association is between ankylosing spondylitis, an inflammatory, presumably autoimmune, disease of vertebral joints, and the class I HLA allele B27. Individuals who are HLA-B27 positive are over 100 times more likely to develop ankylosing spondylitis than individuals who are B27-negative. Neither the mechanism of this disease nor the basis of its association with HLA-B27 is known. The association of class II HLA-DR and HLA-DQ alleles with autoimmune diseases has received great attention, mainly because class II MHC molecules are involved in the selection and activation of CD4+ T cells, and CD4+ T cells regulate both humoral and cell-mediated immune responses to protein antigens.

Several features of the association of HLA alleles with autoimmune diseases are noteworthy.

● An HLA-disease association may be identified by serologic typing of one HLA locus, but the actual association may be with other alleles that are linked to the typed allele and inherited together. For instance, individuals with a particular HLA-DR allele (hypothetically DR1) may show a higher probability of inheriting a particular HLA-DQ allele (hypothetically DQ2) than the probability of inheriting these alleles separately and randomly (i.e., at equilibrium) in the population. Such inheritance is an example of linkage disequilibrium. A disease may be found to be DR1 associated by HLA typing, but the causal association may actually be with the coinherited DQ2. This realization has emphasized the concept of extended HLA haplotypes, which refers to sets of linked genes, both classical HLA and adjacent non-HLA genes, that tend to be inherited together as a single unit.

- In many autoimmune diseases, the disease-associated nucleotide polymorphisms encode amino acids in the peptide-binding clefts of the MHC molecules. This observation is not surprising because polymorphic residues of MHC molecules are located within and adjacent to the clefts, and the structure of the clefts is the key determinant of both functions of MHC molecules, namely, antigen presentation and recognition by T cells (see Chapter 6).

- Disease-associated HLA sequences are found in healthy individuals. In fact, if all individuals bearing a particular disease-associated HLA allele are monitored prospectively, most will never develop the disease. Therefore, expression of a particular HLA gene is not by itself the cause of any autoimmune disease, but it may be one of several factors that contribute to autoimmunity.

The mechanisms underlying the association of different HLA alleles with various autoimmune diseases are still not clear. In diseases in which particular MHC alleles increase the risk of disease, the disease-associated MHC molecule may present a self peptide and activate pathogenic T cells, and this has been established in a few cases. When a particular allele is shown to be protective, it is hypothesized that this allele might induce negative selection of some potentially pathogenic T cells, or it might promote the development of regulatory T cells.

Polymorphisms in Non-HLA Genes Associated with Autoimmunity

Linkage analyses of autoimmune diseases identified a few disease-associated genes and many chromosomal regions in which the identity of the associated genes was suspected but not established. The technique of genome-wide association studies led to the putative identification of nucleotide polymorphisms (variants) of several genes that are associated with autoimmune diseases, and this has been greatly extended by more recent genome sequencing efforts (Table 15-3). Before the genes that are most clearly validated are discussed, it is important to summarize some of the general features of these genes.

- It is likely that combinations of multiple inherited genetic polymorphisms interacting with environmental factors induce the immunologic abnormalities that lead to autoimmunity. There are, however, examples of rare gene variants that make much larger individual contributions to particular diseases.

- Many of the polymorphisms associated with various autoimmune diseases are in genes that influence the

TABLE 15-3 Selected Non-HLA Genetic Polymorphisms Associated with Autoimmune Diseases

Gene of Interest	Function	Diseases
Genes Involved in Immune Regulation		
PTPN22	Protein tyrosine phosphatase; role in T and B cell receptor signaling	RA, T1D, IBD
CD2/CD58	Costimulation of T cells	RA, MS
IL23R	Component of IL-23 receptor; role in generation and maintenance of T$_H$17 cells	IBD, PS, AS
IL10	Downregulates expression of costimulators, MHC molecules, IL-12 in dendritic cells; inhibits T$_H$1 responses	IBD, SLE, T1D
CTLA4	Inhibitory receptor of T cells, effector molecule of regulatory T cells	T1D, RA
IL2/IL21	Growth and differentiation factors for T cells; IL-2 is involved in maintenance of functional Tregs	IBD, CeD, RA, T1D, MS
IL12B	p40 subunit of IL-12 (T$_H$1-inducing cytokine) and IL-23 (T$_H$17-inducing cytokine)	IBD, PS
BLK	B lymphocyte tyrosine kinase, involved in B cell activation	SLE, RA
IL2RA	IL-2 receptor α chain (CD25); role in T cell activation and maintenance of regulatory T cells	MS, T1D
Genes Involved in Responses to Microbes		
NOD2	Cytoplasmic sensor of bacteria	IBD
ATG16	Autophagy (destruction of microbes, maintenance of epithelial cell integrity)	IBD
IRF5, IFIH1	Type I interferon responses to viruses	SLE

AS, ankylosing spondylitis; *CeD*, celiac disease; *IBD*, inflammatory bowel disease; *MS*, multiple sclerosis; *PS*, psoriasis; *RA*, rheumatoid arthritis; *SLE*, systemic lupus erythematosus; *T1D*, type 1 diabetes.
Data from Zenewicz L, Abraham C, Flavell RA, Cho J: Unraveling the genetics of autoimmunity, *Cell* 140:791-797, 2010, with permission of the publisher.

development and regulation of immune responses. Although this conclusion appears predictable, it has reinforced the utility of the approaches being used to identify disease-associated genes.

- Different polymorphisms may either protect against disease development or increase the incidence of the disease. The statistical methods used for genome-wide association studies have revealed both types of associations.

- Disease-associated polymorphisms are often located in noncoding regions of the genes. This suggests that many of the polymorphisms may affect the expression of the encoded proteins.

Some of the genes associated with human autoimmune diseases, which have been defined by linkage analyses, genome-wide association studies, and whole genome sequencing, are briefly described next.

- ***PTPN22.*** A variant of the protein tyrosine phosphatase PTPN22, in which arginine at position 620 is replaced

TABLE 15-4   Examples of Single-Gene Mutations That Cause Autoimmune Diseases

Gene	Phenotype of Mutant or Knockout Mouse	Mechanism of Failure of Tolerance	Human Disease?
AIRE	Destruction of endocrine organs by antibodies, lymphocytes	Failure of central tolerance	Autoimmune polyendocrine syndrome (APS)
C4	SLE	Defective clearance of immune complexes; failure of B cell tolerance	SLE
CTLA4	Lymphoproliferation; T cell infiltrates in multiple organs, especially heart; lethal by 3-4 weeks	Failure of anergy in CD4$^+$ T cells; defective function of regulatory T cells	CTLA-4 polymorphisms associated with several autoimmune diseases
FAS/FASL	Anti-DNA and other autoantibodies; immune complex nephritis; arthritis; lymphoproliferation	Defective deletion of anergic self-reactive B cells; reduced deletion of mature CD4$^+$ T cells	Autoimmune lymphoproliferative syndrome (ALPS)
FOXP3	Multiorgan lymphocytic infiltrates, wasting	Deficiency of functional regulatory T cells	IPEX
IL2, IL2Rα/β	Inflammatory bowel disease; anti-erythrocyte and anti-DNA autoantibodies	Defective development, survival, or function of regulatory T cells	None known
SHP1	Multiple autoantibodies	Failure of negative regulation of B cells	None known

AIRE, autoimmune regulator gene; IL-2, interleukin-2; IPEX, immune dysregulation, polyendocrinopathy, enteropathy, X-linked syndrome; SHP-1, SH2-containing phosphatase 1; SLE, systemic lupus erythematosus.

with a tryptophan, is associated with rheumatoid arthritis, type 1 diabetes, autoimmune thyroiditis, and other autoimmune diseases. The disease-associated variant causes complex signaling alterations in multiple immune cell populations. Precisely how these changes lead to autoimmunity is not known.

- **NOD2.** Polymorphisms in this gene are associated with Crohn's disease, one type of inflammatory bowel disease. NOD2 is a cytoplasmic sensor of bacterial peptidoglycans (see Chapter 4) and is expressed in multiple cell types, including intestinal epithelial cells. It is thought that the disease-associated polymorphism reduces the function of NOD2, which cannot provide effective defense against certain intestinal microbes. As a result, these microbes are able to traverse the epithelium and initiate a chronic inflammatory reaction in the intestinal wall, which is a hallmark of inflammatory bowel disease (see Chapter 14).

- **Insulin.** Polymorphisms in the insulin gene that encode variable numbers of repeat sequences are associated with type 1 diabetes. These polymorphisms may affect the thymic expression of insulin. It is postulated that if the protein is expressed at low levels in the thymus because of a genetic polymorphism, developing T cells specific for insulin may not be negatively selected. These cells survive in the mature immune repertoire and are capable of attacking insulin-producing islet β cells and causing diabetes.

- **CD25.** Polymorphisms affecting the expression or function of CD25, the α chain of the IL-2 receptor, are associated with multiple sclerosis, type 1 diabetes, and other autoimmune diseases. These changes in CD25 likely affect the generation or function of regulatory T cells, although there is no definitive evidence for a causal link between the CD25 abnormality, regulatory T cell defects, and the autoimmune disease.

- **IL-23 receptor (IL-23R).** Some polymorphisms in the receptor for IL-23 are associated with increased susceptibility

to inflammatory bowel disease and the skin disease psoriasis, while other polymorphisms protect against development of these diseases. IL-23 is one of the cytokines involved in the development of T_H17 cells, which stimulate inflammatory reactions (see Chapter 10).

- **ATG16L1.** A loss of function polymorphism in this gene that replaces a threonine in position 300 with an alanine is associated with inflammatory bowel disease. ATG16L1 is one of a family of proteins involved in autophagy, a cellular response to infection, nutrient deprivation and other forms of stress. In this process, the stressed cell eats its own organelles to provide substrates for energy generation and metabolism or an infected cell captures intracellular microbes and targets them to lysosomes. Autophagy may play a role in the maintenance of intact intestinal epithelial cells or the destruction of microbes that have entered the cytoplasm. It is also a mechanism for delivering cytosolic contents to the class II MHC pathway in antigen-presenting cells. A susceptibility allele of *ATG16L1* encodes a protein that is more rapidly destroyed in conditions of stress, and this results in defective autophagic clearance of intracellular microbes. How this polymorphism contributes to inflammatory bowel disease is not known.

Although many genetic associations with autoimmune diseases have been·reported, a continuing challenge is to correlate the genetic polymorphisms with the pathogenesis of the diseases. It is also possible that epigenetic changes may regulate gene expression and thus contribute to disease onset. This possibility remains to be established.

Inherited Single-Gene (Mendelian) Abnormalities That Cause Autoimmunity

Studies with mouse models and patients have identified several genes that strongly influence the maintenance of tolerance to self antigens (Table 15-4). Unlike the complex polymorphisms described previously, these single-gene defects are examples of Mendelian disorders in which the mutation is rare but has a high penetrance, so that most individuals carrying the mutation are affected. We mentioned many of these genes earlier in the chapter, when we discussed the mechanisms of self-tolerance. Although these genes are associated with rare autoimmune diseases, their identification has provided valuable information about the importance of various molecular pathways in the maintenance of self-tolerance. The known genes contribute to the established mechanisms of central tolerance *(AIRE)*, generation of regulatory T cells *(FOXP3, IL2, IL2R)*, anergy and the function of regulatory T cells *(CTLA4)*, and peripheral deletion of T and B lymphocytes *(FAS, FASL)*. Here we describe two other genes that are associated with autoimmune diseases in humans.

- ***Genes encoding complement proteins.*** Genetic deficiencies of several complement proteins, including C1q, C2, and C4 (see Chapter 13), are associated with lupus-like autoimmune diseases. The postulated mechanism of this association is that complement activation promotes the clearance of circulating immune complexes and apoptotic cell bodies, and in the absence of complement proteins, these complexes accumulate in the blood and are deposited in tissues and the antigens of dead cells persist.
- ***FcγRIIB.*** A polymorphism altering an isolecine to a threonine in the transmembrane domain of this inhibitory Fc receptor (see Chapter 12) impairs inhibitory signaling and is associated with SLE in humans. Genetic deletion of this receptor in mice also results in a lupus-like autoimmune disease. The likely mechanism of the disease is a failure to control antibody-mediated feedback inhibition of B cells.

Role of Infections in Autoimmunity

Viral and bacterial infections may contribute to the development and exacerbation of autoimmunity. In patients and in some animal models, the onset of autoimmune diseases is often associated with or preceded by infections. In most of these cases, the infectious microorganism is not present in lesions and is not even detectable in the individual when autoimmunity develops. Therefore, the lesions of autoimmunity are not due to the infectious agent itself but result from host immune responses that may be triggered or dysregulated by the microbe.

Infections may promote the development of autoimmunity by two principal mechanisms (Fig. 15-12).

- Infections of particular tissues may induce local innate immune responses that recruit leukocytes into the tissues and result in the activation of tissue APCs. These APCs begin to express costimulators and secrete T cell–activating cytokines, resulting in the breakdown of T cell tolerance. Thus, the infection results in the activation of T cells that are not specific for the infectious pathogen; this type of response is called **bystander activation**. The importance of aberrant expression of costimulators is suggested by experimental evidence that immunization of mice with self antigens together

with strong adjuvants (which mimic microbes) results in the breakdown of self-tolerance and the development of autoimmune disease. In other experimental models, viral antigens expressed in tissues such as islet β cells induce T cell tolerance, but systemic infection of the mice with the virus results in the failure of tolerance and autoimmune destruction of the insulin-producing cells.

Microbes may also engage Toll-like receptors (TLRs) on dendritic cells, leading to the production of lymphocyte-activating cytokines, and on autoreactive B cells, leading to autoantibody production. A role of TLR signaling in autoimmunity has been demonstrated in mouse models of SLE.

- Infectious microbes may contain antigens that cross-react with self antigens, so immune responses to the microbes may result in reactions against self antigens. This phenomenon is called **molecular mimicry** because the antigens of the microbe cross-react with, or mimic, self antigens. One example of an immunologic cross-reaction between microbial and self antigens is rheumatic fever, which develops after streptococcal infections and is caused by anti-streptococcal antibodies that cross-react with myocardial proteins. These antibodies are deposited in the heart and cause myocarditis. Molecular sequencing has revealed numerous short stretches of homologies between myocardial proteins and streptococcal proteins. However, the significance of limited homologies between microbial and self antigens in common autoimmune diseases remains to be established.

Some infections may protect against the development of autoimmunity. Epidemiologic studies suggest that reducing infections increases the incidence of type 1 diabetes and multiple sclerosis, and experimental studies show that diabetes in NOD mice is greatly retarded if the mice are infected. It seems paradoxical that infections can be triggers of autoimmunity and also inhibit autoimmune diseases. How they may reduce the incidence of autoimmune diseases is unknown.

The intestinal and cutaneous microbiome may influence the development of autoimmune diseases. As we discussed in Chapter 14, there is great interest in the idea that humans are colonized by commensal microbes that have significant effects on the maturation and activation of the immune system. It is not surprising that alterations in the microbiome also affect the incidence and severity of autoimmune diseases in experimental models. How this idea can be exploited to treat autoimmunity is a topic of great interest.

Other Factors in Autoimmunity

The development of autoimmunity is related to several factors in addition to susceptibility genes and infections.

- ***Anatomic alterations in tissues, caused by inflammation (possibly secondary to infections), ischemic injury, or trauma, may lead to the exposure of self antigens that are normally concealed from the immune system.*** Such sequestered antigens may not have induced self-tolerance. Therefore, if previously hidden self an-

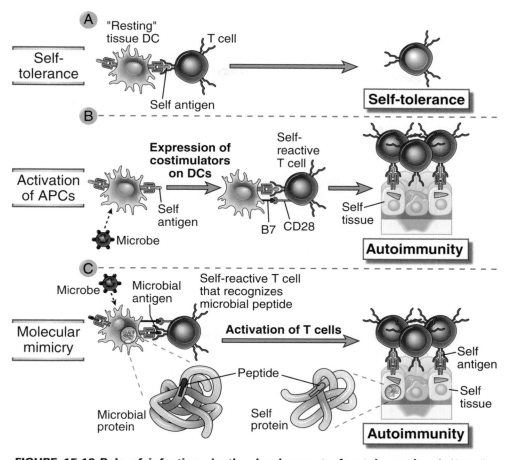

FIGURE 15-12 Role of infections in the development of autoimmunity. A, Normally, encounter of a mature self-reactive T cell with a self antigen presented by a costimulator-deficient resting tissue antigen-presenting cell (APC) results in peripheral tolerance by anergy. (Other possible mechanisms of self-tolerance are not shown.) **B,** Microbes may activate the APCs to express costimulators, and when these APCs present self antigens, the self-reactive T cells are activated rather than rendered tolerant. **C,** Some microbial antigens may cross-react with self antigens (molecular mimicry). Therefore, immune responses initiated by the microbes may activate T cells specific for self antigens.

tigens are released, they can interact with immuno-competent lymphocytes and induce specific immune responses. Examples of anatomically sequestered antigens include intraocular proteins and sperm. Post-traumatic uveitis and orchitis are thought to be due to autoimmune responses against self antigens that are released from their normal locations by trauma.

- *Hormonal influences play a role in some autoimmune diseases.* Many autoimmune diseases have a higher incidence in women than in men. For instance, SLE affects women about 10 times more frequently than men. The SLE-like disease of (NZB × NZW)F$_1$ mice develops only in females and is retarded by androgen treatment. Whether this female predominance results from the influence of sex hormones or other gender-related factors is not known.

Autoimmune diseases are among the most challenging scientific and clinical problems in immunology. The current knowledge of pathogenic mechanisms remains incomplete, so theories and hypotheses continue to outnumber facts. The application of new technical advances and the rapidly improving understanding of self-tolerance will, it is hoped, lead to clearer and more definitive answers to the enigmas of autoimmunity.

SUMMARY

- Immunologic tolerance is unresponsiveness to an antigen induced by the exposure of specific lymphocytes to that antigen. Tolerance to self antigens is a fundamental property of the normal immune system, and the failure of self-tolerance leads to autoimmune diseases. Antigens may be administered in ways that induce tolerance rather than immunity, and this may be exploited for the prevention and treatment of transplant rejection and autoimmune and allergic diseases.

- Central tolerance is induced in the generative lymphoid organs (thymus and bone marrow) when immature lymphocytes encounter self antigens present in these organs. Peripheral tolerance occurs when mature lymphocytes recognize self antigens in peripheral tissues under particular conditions.

* In T lymphocytes, central tolerance occurs when immature thymocytes with high-affinity receptors for self antigens recognize these antigens in the thymus. Some immature T cells that encounter self antigens in the thymus die (negative selection), and others develop into FoxP3+ regulatory T lymphocytes that function to control responses to self antigens in peripheral tissues.

* Several mechanisms account for peripheral tolerance in mature T cells. In CD4+ T cells, anergy is induced by antigen recognition without adequate costimulation or by engagement of inhibitory receptors such as CTLA-4 and PD-1. Regulatory T cells inhibit immune responses by multiple mechanisms. T cells that encounter self antigens without other stimuli or that are repeatedly stimulated may die by apoptosis.

* In B lymphocytes, central tolerance is induced when immature B cells recognize multivalent self antigens in the bone marrow. The result is the acquisition of a new specificity, called receptor editing, or apoptotic death of the immature B cells. Mature B cells that recognize self antigens in the periphery in the absence of T cell help may be rendered anergic and ultimately die by apoptosis or become functionally unresponsive because of the activation of inhibitory receptors.

* Autoimmunity results from a failure of self-tolerance. Autoimmune reactions may be triggered by environmental stimuli, such as infections, in genetically susceptible individuals.

* Most autoimmune diseases are polygenic, and numerous susceptibility genes contribute to disease development. The greatest contribution is from MHC genes; other genes are believed to influence the selection or regulation of self-reactive lymphocytes.

* Infections may predispose to autoimmunity by several mechanisms, including enhanced expression of costimulators in tissues and cross-reactions between microbial antigens and self antigens. Some infections may protect individuals from autoimmunity, by unknown mechanisms.

SELECTED READINGS

Immunologic Tolerance, General Mechanisms

Baxter AG, Hodgkin PD: Activation rules: the two-signal theories of immune activation, *Nature Reviews Immunology* 2:439–446, 2002.

Goodnow CC, Sprent J, Fazekas de St Groth B, Vinuesa CG: Cellular and genetic mechanisms of self tolerance and autoimmunity, *Nature* 435:590–597, 2005.

Mueller DL: Mechanisms maintaining peripheral tolerance, *Nature Immunology* 11:21–27, 2010.

Parish IA, Heath WR: Too dangerous to ignore: self-tolerance and the control of ignorant autoreactive T cells, *Immunology Cell Biology* 86:146–152, 2008.

Probst HC, Muth S, Schild H: Regulation of tolerogenic function of steady-state DCs, *European Journal of Immunology*, 44:927-933, 2014.

Redmond WL, Sherman LA: Peripheral tolerance of CD8 T lymphocytes, *Immunity* 22:275–284, 2005.

Schwartz RH: Historical overview of immunological tolerance, *Cold Spring Harbor Perspectives in Biology* 4:a006908, 2012.

Shlomchik MJ: Sites and stages of autoreactive B cell activation and regulation, *Immunity* 28:18–28, 2008.

Steinman RM, Hawiger D, Nussenzweig MC: Tolerogenic dendritic cells, *Annual Review of Immunology* 21:685–711, 2003.

Von Boehmer H, Melchers F: Checkpoints in lymphocyte development and autoimmune disease, *Nature Immunology* 11:14–20, 2010.

Central Tolerance

Hogquist KA, Baldwin TA, Jameson SC: Central tolerance: learning self-control in the thymus, *Nature Reviews Immunology* 5:772–782, 2005.

Kyewski B, Klein L: A central role for central tolerance, *Annual Review of Immunology* 24:571–606, 2006.

Laan M, Peterson P: The many faces of Aire in central tolerance, *Frontiers in Immunology* 4:1–6, 2013.

Mathis D, Benoist C: *Aire. Annual Review of Immunology* 27: 287–312, 2009.

Nemazee D: Receptor editing in lymphocyte development and central tolerance, *Nature Reviews Immunology* 6:728–740, 2006.

Anergy; Inhibitory Receptors

Mueller DL: E3 ubiquitin ligases as T cell anergy factors, *Nature Immunology* 5:883–890, 2004.

Okazaki T, Chikuma S, Iwai Y, Fagarasan S, Honjo T: A rheostat for immune responses: the unique properties of PD-1 and their advantages for clinical applications, *Nature Immunology* 14:1212–1218, 2013.

Walker LS, Sansom DM: The emerging role of CTLA-4 as a cell-extrinsic regulator of T cell responses, *Nature Reviews Immunology* 11:852–863, 2011.

Wells AD: New insights into the molecular basis of T cell anergy: anergy factors, avoidance sensors, and epigenetic imprinting, *Journal of Immunology* 182:7331–7341, 2009.

Apoptosis

Bidere N, Su HC, Lenardo MJ: Genetic disorders of programmed cell death in the immune system, *Annual Review of Immunology* 24:321–352, 2006.

Griffith TS, Ferguson TA: Cell death in the maintenance and abrogation of tolerance: the five Ws of dying cells, *Immunity* 35:456–466, 2011.

Strasser A, Jost PJ, Nagata S: The many roles of FAS receptor signaling in the immune system, *Immunity* 30:321–326, 2009.

Strasser A, Puthalakath H, O'Reilly LA, Bouillet P: What do we know about the mechanisms of elimination of autoreactive T and B cells and what challenges remain, *Immunology and Cell Biology* 86:57–66, 2008.

Regulatory T Cells

Bilate AM, Lafaille JJ: Induced CD4+Foxp3+ regulatory T cells in immune tolerance, *Annual Review of Immunology* 30: 733–758, 2012.

Burzyn D, Benoist C, Mathis D: Regulatory T cells in nonlymphoid tissues, *Nature Immunology* 14:1007–1013, 2013.

Campbell DJ, Koch MA: Phenotypic and functional specialization of FoxP3+ regulatory T cells, *Nature Reviews Immunology* 11:119–130, 2011.

Curotto MA, Lafaille JL: Natural and adaptive Foxp3+ regulatory T cells: more of the same or a division of labor? *Immunity* 30:626–635, 2009.

Hsieh C-S, Lee M-H, Lio C-WJ: Selection of regulatory T cells in the thymus, *Nature Reviews Immunology* 12:157–167, 2012.

Josefowicz SZ, Lu L-F, Rudensky Y: Regulatory T cells: mechanisms of differentiation and function, *Annual Review of Immunology* 30:531–564, 2012.

Li MO, Flavell RA: TGF-β: a master of all T cell trades, *Cell* 134:392–404, 2008.

Liston A, Gray DHD: Homeostatic control of regulatory T cell diversity, *Nature Reviews Immunology* 14:154–165, 2014.

Liston A, Piccirillo CA: Developmental plasticity of murine and human Foxp3+ regulatory T cells, *Advances in Immunology* 119:85–106, 2013.

Ohkura N, Kitagawa Y, Sakaguchi S: Development and maintenance of regulatory T cells, *Immunity* 38:414–423, 2013.

Riley JL, June CH, Blazar BR: Human T regulatory cell therapy: take a billion or so and call me in the morning, *Immunity* 30:656–665, 2009.

Sakaguchi S, Miyara M, Costantino CM, Hafler DA: FOXP3+ regulatory T cells in the human immune system, *Nature Reviews Immunology* 10:490–500, 2010.

Sakaguchi S, Yamaguchi T, Nomura T, Ono M: Regulatory T cells and immune tolerance, *Cell* 133:775–787, 2008.

Tang Q, Bluestone JA: The Foxp3+ regulatory T cell: a jack of all trades, master of regulation, *Nature Immunology* 9:239–244, 2008.

Wing K, Sakaguchi S: Regulatory T cells exert checks and balances on self tolerance and autoimmunity, *Nature Immunology* 11:7–13, 2010.

Ziegler SF: FoxP3: of mice and men, *Annual Review of Immunology* 6:209–226, 2006.

Mechanisms of Autoimmunity: Genetics

Cheng MH, Anderson MS: Monogenic autoimmunity, *Annual Review of Immunology* 30:393–427, 2012.

Deitiker P, Atassi MZ: Non-MHC genes linked to autoimmune disease, *Crticial Reviews of Immunology* 32:193–285, 2012.

Fernando MM, Stevens CR, Walsh EC, De Jager PL, Goyette P, Plenge RM, Vyse TJ, Rioux JD: Defining the role of the MHC in autoimmunity: a review and pooled analysis, *PLoS Genetics* 4, 2008. e1000024.

Gregersen PK, Olsson LM: Recent advances in the genetics of autoimmune disease, *Annual Review of Immunology* 27:363–391, 2009.

Pascual V, Chaussubel D, Banchereau J: A genomic approach to human autoimmune diseases, *Annual Review of Immunology* 28:535–571, 2010.

Voight BF, Cotsapas C: Human genetics offers an emerging picture of common pathways and mechanisms in autoimmunity, *Current Opinion in Immunology* 24:552–557, 2012.

Zenewicz L, Abraham C, Flavell RA, Cho J: Unraveling the genetics of autoimmunity, *Cell* 140:791–797, 2010.

Mechanisms of Autoimmunity: Environmental Factors

Belkaid Y, Hand TW: Role of the microbiota in immunity and inflammation, *Cell* 157:121–141, 2014.

Chervonsky A: Influence of microbial environment on autoimmunity, *Nature Immunology* 11:28–35, 2010.

Fourneau JM, Bach JM, van Endert PM, Bach JF: The elusive case for a role of mimicry in autoimmune diseases, *Molecular Immunology* 40:1095–1102, 2004.

Mathis D, Benoist C: Microbiota and autoimmune disease: the hosted self, *Cell Host Microbes* 10:297–301, 2011.

Immunity to Microbes

In the preceding chapters, we have described the components of the immune system and the development and functions of immune responses. Throughout, we have referred to protection against infections as the major physiologic function of the immune system, and discussed immune responses in the context of responses to microbes. In this chapter, we will integrate this information and discuss the main features of immunity to different types of pathogenic microorganisms as well as the mechanisms microbes use to resist immune defenses.

The development of an infectious disease in an individual involves complex interactions between the microbe and the host. The key events during infection include entry of the microbe, invasion and colonization of host tissues, evasion of host immunity, and tissue injury or functional impairment. Microbes produce disease by directly killing the host cells they infect, or by liberating toxins that can cause tissue damage and functional derangements in neighboring or distant cells and tissues that are not infected. In addition, microbes often cause disease by stimulating immune responses that injure both the infected tissues and normal tissues. Many features of microorganisms determine their virulence, and many diverse mechanisms contribute to the pathogenesis of infectious diseases. The topic of microbial pathogenesis is beyond the scope of this book and will not be discussed here. Rather, our discussion will focus on host immune responses to pathogenic microorganisms.

OVERVIEW OF IMMUNE RESPONSES TO MICROBES

Although anti-microbial host defense reactions are numerous and varied, there are several important general features of immunity to microbes.

- *Defense against microbes is mediated by the effector mechanisms of innate and adaptive immunity.* The innate immune system provides early defense, and the adaptive immune system provides a more sustained and stronger response. Many pathogenic microbes have evolved to resist innate immunity, and protection against such infections is critically dependent on adaptive immune responses. In adaptive responses, large numbers of effector cells and antibody molecules are generated that function to eliminate the microbes and memory cells that protect the individual from repeated infections.

- *The immune system responds in specialized and distinct ways to different types of microbes to most effectively combat these infectious agents.* Different microbes require different mechanisms for elimination, and the adaptive immune system has evolved to respond in the optimal way to microbes. The generation of T_H1, T_H2, and T_H17 subsets of effector CD4+ T cells and the production of different isotypes of antibodies are excellent examples of the specialization of adaptive immunity. Both have been described in earlier chapters; in this chapter, we will discuss their importance in defense against different types of microbes.

- *The survival and pathogenicity of microbes in a host are critically influenced by the ability of the microbes to evade or resist the effector mechanisms of immunity.* Infectious microbes and the immune system have coevolved and are engaged in a constant struggle for survival. The balance between host immune responses and microbial strategies for resisting immunity often determines the outcome of infections. As we will see later in this chapter, microorganisms have developed a variety of mechanisms for surviving in the face of powerful immunologic defenses.

- *Many microbes establish latent, or persistent, infections in which the immune response controls but does not eliminate the microbe and the microbe survives without propagating the infection.* Latency is a feature of infections by several viruses, especially DNA viruses of the herpesvirus and poxvirus families, and some intracellular bacteria. In latent viral infections, the viral DNA may be integrated into the DNA of infected cells, but no infectious virus is produced. In persistent bacterial infections such as tuberculosis, the bacteria may survive within the endosomal vesicles of infected cells. In all of these situations, if the host's immune system becomes defective for any reason (e.g., cancer or cancer therapy, immunosuppression to treat transplant rejection, or HIV infection), the latent microbe may be reactivated, resulting in an infection that causes significant clinical problems.

- *In many infections, tissue injury and disease may be caused by the host response to the microbe rather than by the microbe itself.* Immunity is necessary for host survival but also has the potential for causing injury to the host.

- *Inherited and acquired defects in innate and adaptive immunity are important causes of susceptibility to infections.* Many of these are well recognized, including acquired disorders such as acquired immunodeficiency syndrome (AIDS) caused by the human immunodeficiency virus (HIV), and other less common inherited immunodeficiency syndromes. In addition, subtle and poorly defined defects in host defenses may underlie many common infections. We will describe immunodeficiencies in detail in Chapter 21.

In this chapter, we will consider the main features of immunity to five major categories of pathogenic microorganisms: extracellular bacteria, intracellular bacteria, fungi, viruses, and protozoan as well as multicellular parasites (Table 16-1; also see Table 16-4). Our discussion of the immune responses to these microbes illustrates the diversity of anti-microbial immunity and the physiologic significance of the effector functions of lymphocytes discussed in earlier chapters.

IMMUNITY TO EXTRACELLULAR BACTERIA

Extracellular bacteria are capable of replicating outside host cells, for example, in the blood, in connective tissues, and in tissue spaces such as the lumens of the airways and gastrointestinal tract. Many different species of extracellular bacteria are pathogenic, and disease is caused by two principal mechanisms. First, these bacteria induce inflammation, which results in tissue destruction at the site of infection. Second, bacteria produce toxins, which have diverse pathologic effects. The toxins may be endotoxins, which are components of bacterial cell walls, or exotoxins, which are secreted by the bacteria. The endotoxin of gram-negative bacteria, also called lipopolysaccharide (LPS), has been mentioned in Chapter 4 as a potent activator of macrophages, dendritic cells, and endothelial cells. Many exotoxins are cytotoxic, and others cause disease by various mechanisms. For instance, diphtheria toxin shuts down protein synthesis in infected cells, cholera toxin interferes with ion and water transport, tetanus toxin inhibits neuromuscular transmission, and anthrax toxin disrupts several critical biochemical signaling pathways in infected cells. Other exotoxins interfere with normal cellular functions without killing cells, and yet other exotoxins stimulate the production of cytokines that cause disease.

Innate Immunity to Extracellular Bacteria

The principal mechanisms of innate immunity to extracellular bacteria are complement activation, phagocytosis, and the inflammatory response.

- *Complement activation.* Peptidoglycans in the cell walls of Gram-positive bacteria and LPS in Gram-negative bacteria activate complement by the alternative pathway (see Chapter 13). Bacteria that express mannose on their surface may bind mannose-binding lectin, which activates complement by the lectin pathway. One result of complement activation is opsonization and enhanced phagocytosis of the bacteria. In addition, the membrane attack complex generated by complement activation lyses bacteria, especially *Neisseria* species that are particularly susceptible to lysis because of their thin cell walls, and complement byproducts stimulate inflammatory responses by recruiting and activating leukocytes.

- *Activation of phagocytes and inflammation.* Phagocytes (neutrophils and macrophages) use surface receptors, including mannose receptors and scavenger receptors, to recognize extracellular bacteria, and they use Fc receptors and complement receptors to recognize bacteria opsonized with antibodies and

TABLE 16-1   Examples of Pathogenic Microbes

Microbe	Examples of Human Diseases	Mechanisms of Pathogenicity
Extracellular Bacteria		
Staphylococcus aureus	Skin and soft-tissue infections, lung abscess Systemic: toxic shock syndrome, food poisoning	Skin infections: acute inflammation induced by toxins; cell death caused by pore-forming toxins Systemic: enterotoxin ("superantigen")-induced cytokine production by T cells causing skin necrosis, shock, diarrhea
Streptococcus pyogenes (group A)	Pharyngitis Skin infections: impetigo, erysipelas; cellulitis Systemic: scarlet fever	Acute inflammation induced by various toxins (e.g., streptolysin O damages cell membranes)
Streptococcus pyogenes (pneumococcus)	Pneumonia, meningitis	Acute inflammation induced by cell wall constituents; pneumolysin is similar to streptolysin O
Escherichia coli	Urinary tract infections, gastroenteritis, septic shock	Toxins act on intestinal epithelium chloride and water secretion; endotoxin (LPS) stimulates cytokine secretion by macrophages
Vibrio cholerae	Diarrhea (cholera)	Cholera toxin ADP ribosylates G protein subunit, which leads to increased cyclic AMP in intestinal epithelial cells and results in chloride secretion and water loss
Clostridium tetani	Tetanus	Tetanus toxin binds to the motor end plate at neuromuscular junctions and causes irreversible muscle contraction
Neisseria meningitidis (meningococcus)	Meningitis	Acute inflammation and systemic disease caused by potent endotoxin
Corynebacterium diphtheriae	Diphtheria	Diphtheria toxin ADP-ribosylates elongation factor 2 and inhibits protein synthesis
Intracellular Bacteria		
Mycobacteria	Tuberculosis, leprosy	Macrophage activation resulting in granulomatous inflammation and tissue destruction
Listeria monocytogenes	Listeriosis	Listeriolysin damages cell membranes
Legionella pneumophila	Legionnaires' disease	Cytotoxin lyses cells and causes lung injury and inflammation
Fungi		
Candida albicans	Candidiasis	Acute inflammation; binds complement proteins
Aspergillus fumigatus	Aspergillosis	Invasion and thrombosis of blood vessels causing ischemic necrosis and cell injury
Histoplasma capsulatum	Histoplasmosis	Lung infection caused by granulomatous inflammation
Viruses		
Polio	Poliomyelitis	Inhibits host cell protein synthesis (tropism for motor neurons in the anterior horn of the spinal cord)
Influenza	Influenza pneumonia	Inhibits host cell protein synthesis (tropism for ciliated epithelium)
Rabies	Rabies encephalitis	Inhibits host cell protein synthesis (tropism for peripheral nerves)
Herpes simplex	Various herpes infections (skin, systemic)	Inhibits host cell protein synthesis; functional impairment of immune cells
Hepatitis B	Viral hepatitis	Host CTL response to infected hepatocytes
Epstein-Barr virus	Infectious mononucleosis; B cell proliferation, lymphomas	Acute infection: cell lysis (tropism for B lymphocytes) Latent infection: stimulates B cell proliferation
Human immunodeficiency virus (HIV)	Acquired immunodeficiency syndrome (AIDS)	Multiple: killing of CD4$^+$ T cells, functional impairment of immune cells (see Chapter 20)

Examples of pathogenic microbes of different classes are listed, with brief summaries of known or postulated mechanisms of tissue injury and disease. Examples of parasites are listed in Table 16-4.

ADP, adenosine diphosphate; *AMP*, adenosine monophosphate; *CTL*, cytotoxic T lymphocyte; *LPS*, lipopolysaccharide.

This table was compiled with the assistance of Dr. Arlene Sharpe, Department of Pathology, Harvard Medical School and Brigham and Women's Hospital, Boston, Massachusetts.

complement proteins, respectively. Microbial products activate Toll-like receptors (TLRs) and various cytoplasmic sensors in phagocytes and other cells. Some of these receptors function mainly to promote the phagocytosis of the microbes (e.g., mannose receptors, scavenger receptors); others stimulate the microbicidal activities of the phagocytes (mainly TLRs); and yet others promote both phagocytosis and activation of the phagocytes (Fc and complement receptors) (see Chapter 4). In addition, dendritic cells and phagocytes that are activated by the microbes secrete cytokines, which induce leukocyte infiltration into sites of infection (inflammation). The recruited leukocytes ingest and destroy the bacteria.

Adaptive Immunity to Extracellular Bacteria

Humoral immunity is a major protective immune response against extracellular bacteria, and it functions to block infection, to eliminate the microbes, and to neutralize their toxins (Fig. 16-1, *A*). Antibody responses against extracellular bacteria are directed against cell wall antigens and secreted and cell-associated toxins, which

may be polysaccharides or proteins. The polysaccharides are prototypic T-independent antigens, and humoral immunity is the principal mechanism of defense against polysaccharide-rich encapsulated bacteria. The effector mechanisms used by antibodies to combat these infections include neutralization, opsonization and phagocytosis, and activation of complement by the classical pathway (see Chapter 13). Neutralization is mediated by high-affinity IgG, IgM, and IgA isotypes, the latter mainly in the lumens of mucosal organs. Opsonization is mediated by some subclasses of IgG, and complement activation is initiated by IgM and subclasses of IgG.

The protein antigens of extracellular bacteria also activate CD4+ helper T cells, which produce cytokines that induce local inflammation, enhance the phagocytic and microbicidal activities of macrophages and neutrophils, and stimulate antibody production (Fig. 16-1, *B*). T_H17 responses induced by these microbes recruit neutrophils and monocytes and thus promote local inflammation at sites of bacterial infection. Genetic defects in T_H17 development and patients who make neutralizing autoantibodies specific for interleukin-17 (IL-17) have increased susceptibility to bacterial and fungal infections, with

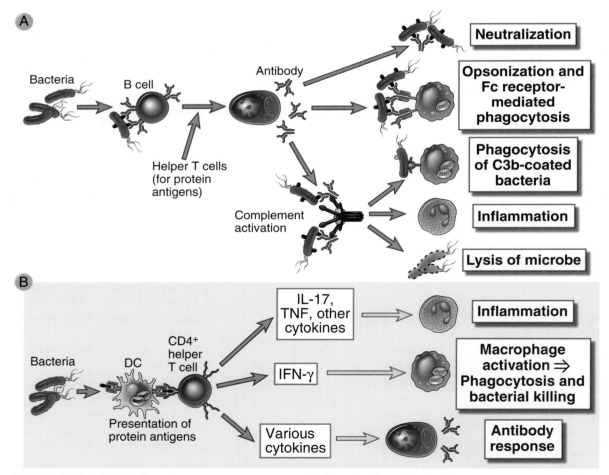

FIGURE 16-1 Adaptive immune responses to extracellular microbes. Adaptive immune responses to extracellular microbes such as bacteria and their toxins consist of antibody production **(A)** and the activation of CD4+ helper T cells **(B)**. Antibodies neutralize and eliminate microbes and toxins by several mechanisms. Helper T cells produce cytokines that stimulate inflammation, macrophage activation, and B cell responses. *DC,* dendritic cell.

formation of multiple skin abscesses. Bacteria also induce T_H1 responses, and interferon-γ (IFN-γ) produced by the T_H1 cells activates macrophages to destroy phagocytosed microbes. This cytokine may also stimulate production of opsonizing and complement-binding antibody isotypes.

Injurious Effects of Immune Responses to Extracellular Bacteria

The principal injurious consequences of host responses to extracellular bacteria are inflammation and septic shock. The same reactions of neutrophils and macrophages that function to eradicate the infection also cause tissue damage by local production of reactive oxygen species and lysosomal enzymes. These inflammatory reactions are usually self-limited and controlled. Cytokines secreted by leukocytes in response to bacterial products also stimulate the production of acute-phase proteins and cause the systemic manifestations of the infection (see Chapter 4). **Septic shock** is a severe pathologic consequence of disseminated infection by some Gram-negative and Gram-positive bacteria. It is a syndrome characterized by circulatory collapse and disseminated intravascular coagulation. The early phase of septic shock is caused by cytokines produced by macrophages that are activated by bacterial cell wall components, including LPS and peptidoglycans. Tumor necrosis factor (TNF), IL-6, and IL-1 are the principal cytokine mediators of septic shock, but IFN-γ and IL-12 may also contribute (see Chapter 4). This early burst of large amounts of cytokines is sometimes called a cytokine storm. There is some evidence that the progression of septic shock is associated with defective immune responses, perhaps related to depletion or suppression of T cells, resulting in unchecked microbial spread.

Certain bacterial toxins stimulate all T cells in an individual that express a particular family of V$_\beta$ T cell receptor (TCR) genes. Such toxins are called **superantigens** because they resemble antigens in that they bind to TCRs and to class II MHC molecules (although not to the peptide-binding clefts) but activate many more T cells than do conventional peptide antigens (Fig. 16-2). Their importance lies in their ability to activate many T cells, with the subsequent production of large amounts of cytokines that can also cause a systemic inflammatory syndrome.

A late complication of the humoral immune response to bacterial infection may be the generation of disease-producing antibodies. The best defined examples are two rare sequelae of streptococcal infections of the throat or skin that are manifested weeks or even months after the infections are controlled. Rheumatic fever is a sequel to pharyngeal infection with some serologic types of β-hemolytic streptococci. Infection leads to the production of antibodies against a bacterial cell wall protein (M protein). Some of these antibodies cross-react with myocardial proteins and are deposited in the heart, where they cause inflammation (carditis). Post-streptococcal glomerulonephritis is a sequel to infection of the skin or throat with other serotypes of β-hemolytic streptococci. Antibodies produced against these bacteria form complexes with bacterial antigen, which may be deposited in kidney glomeruli and cause nephritis.

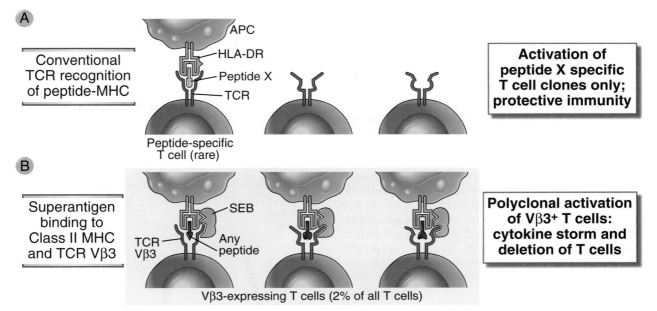

FIGURE 16-2 Polyclonal activation of T cells by bacterial superantigens. A, Conventional microbial T cell antigens, composed of a peptide bound to the peptide-binding groove of an MHC molecule, are recognized by a very small fraction of T cells in any one individual, and only these T cells are activated to become effector T cells that protect against the microbe. **B,** In contrast, a superantigen binds to class II MHC molecules outside the peptide-binding groove and simultaneously binds to the variable region of different TCR β chains, regardless of the peptide specificity of the TCR. Different superantigens bind to TCRs of different Vβ families. Because many T cells express a TCR β chain from a particular Vβ family, superantigens can activate a large number of T cells. In the example shown, the superantigen staphylococcal enterotoxin B (SEB) binds to HLA-DR and the V regions of TCRs belonging to the Vβ3 family. *APC,* antigen-presenting cell.

TABLE 16-2   Mechanisms of Immune Evasion by Bacteria

Mechanism of Immune Evasion	Examples
Extracellular Bacteria	
Antigenic variation	*Neisseria gonorrhoeae, Escherichia coli, Salmonella typhimurium*
Inhibition of complement activation	Many bacteria
Resistance to phagocytosis	Pneumococcus, *Neisseria meningitidis*
Scavenging of reactive oxygen species	Catalase-positive staphylococci
Intracellular Bacteria	
Inhibition of phagolysosome formation	*Mycobacterium tuberculosis, Legionella pneumophila*
Inactivation of reactive oxygen and nitrogen species	*Mycobacterium leprae* (phenolic glycolipid)
Disruption of phagosome membrane, escape into cytoplasm	*Listeria monocytogenes* (hemolysin protein)

Immune Evasion by Extracellular Bacteria

The virulence of extracellular bacteria has been linked to a number of mechanisms that enable the microbes to resist innate immunity (Table 16-2). Bacteria with polysaccharide-rich capsules resist phagocytosis and are therefore much more virulent than homologous strains lacking a capsule. The capsules of many pathogenic Gram-positive and Gram-negative bacteria contain sialic acid residues that inhibit complement activation by the alternative pathway.

A mechanism used by bacteria to evade humoral immunity is variation of surface antigens (Fig. 16-3). Some surface antigens of bacteria such as gonococci and *Escherichia coli* are contained in their pili, which are the structures responsible for bacterial adhesion to host cells. The major antigen of the pili is a protein called pilin. The pilin genes of gonococci undergo extensive gene conversion, because of which the progeny of one organism can produce up to 10^6 antigenically distinct pilin molecules. This ability to alter antigens helps the bacteria evade attack by pilin-specific antibodies, although its principal significance for the bacteria may be to select for pili that are more adherent to host cells so that the bacteria are more virulent. Changes in the production of glycosidases lead to chemical alterations in surface LPS and other polysaccharides, which enable the bacteria to evade humoral immune responses against these antigens. Bacteria can also alter the production of surface antigens over time, or release these antigens in membrane blebs.

IMMUNITY TO INTRACELLULAR BACTERIA

A characteristic of facultative intracellular bacteria is their ability to survive and even to replicate within phagocytes. Because these microbes are able to find a niche where they are inaccessible to circulating antibodies, their elimination requires the mechanisms of cell-mediated immunity (Fig. 16-4). As we will discuss later in this section, in many intracellular bacterial infections the host response also causes tissue injury.

Innate Immunity to Intracellular Bacteria

The innate immune response to intracellular bacteria is mediated mainly by phagocytes and natural killer (NK) cells. Phagocytes, initially neutrophils and later macrophages, ingest and attempt to destroy these microbes, but pathogenic intracellular bacteria are resistant to degradation within phagocytes. Products of these bacteria are recognized by TLRs and cytoplasmic proteins of the NOD-like receptor (NLR) family, resulting in activation of the phagocytes (see Chapter 4). Bacterial DNA in the cytosol stimulates type I interferon responses through the STING pathway.

Intracellular bacteria activate NK cells by inducing expression of NK cell–activating ligands on infected cells and by stimulating dendritic cell and macrophage production of IL-12 and IL-15, both of which are NK cell–activating cytokines. The NK cells produce IFN-γ, which in turn activates macrophages and promotes killing of the phagocytosed bacteria. Thus, NK cells provide an early defense against these microbes, before the development of adaptive immunity. In fact, mice with severe combined immunodeficiency, which lack T and B cells, are able to transiently control infection with the intracellular

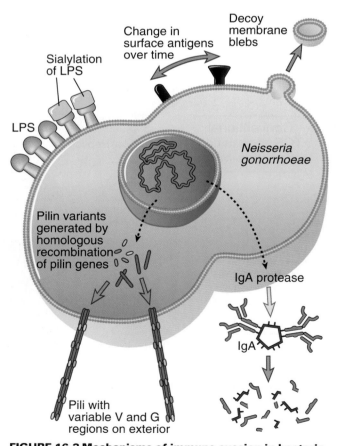

FIGURE 16-3 Mechanisms of immune evasion in bacteria.
Shown are the multiple mechanisms used by one bacterial species, *Neisseria*, to evade humoral immunity.

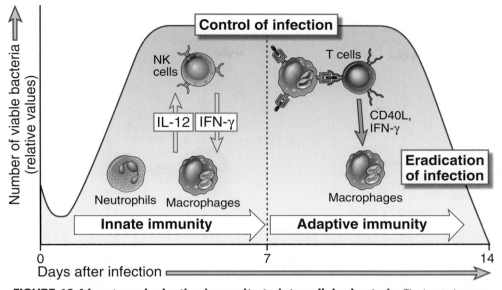

FIGURE 16-4 Innate and adaptive immunity to intracellular bacteria. The innate immune response to intracellular bacteria consists of phagocytes and NK cells, interactions among which are mediated by cytokines (IL-12 and IFN-γ). The typical adaptive immune response to these microbes is cell-mediated immunity, in which T cells activate phagocytes to eliminate the microbes. Innate immunity may control bacterial growth, but elimination of the bacteria requires adaptive immunity. These principles are based largely on analysis of *Listeria monocytogenes* infection in mice; the numbers of viable bacteria shown on the y-axis are relative values of bacterial colonies that can be grown from the tissues of infected mice.

bacterium *Listeria monocytogenes* by NK cell–derived IFN-γ production. However, innate immunity usually fails to eradicate these infections, and eradication requires adaptive cell-mediated immunity.

Adaptive Immunity to Intracellular Bacteria

The major protective immune response against intracellular bacteria is T cell–mediated recruitment and activation of phagocytes (cell-mediated immunity). Individuals with deficient cell-mediated immunity, such as patients with AIDS, are extremely susceptible to infections with intracellular bacteria (as well as intracellular fungi and viruses). Many of the important features of cell-mediated immunity were established in the 1950s based on studies of immune responses to the intracellular bacterium *Listeria monocytogenes* in mice. This form of immunity could be adoptively transferred to naive animals with lymphoid cells but not with serum from infected or immunized animals (see Fig. 10-2).

As we discussed in Chapters 10 and 11, T cells provide defense against infections by two types of reactions: CD4+ T cells activate phagocytes through the actions of CD40 ligand and IFN-γ, resulting in killing of microbes that are ingested by and survive within phagocytes, and CD8+ cytotoxic T lymphocytes (CTLs) kill infected cells, eliminating microbes that escape the killing mechanisms of phagocytes. CD4+ T cells differentiate into T_H1 effectors under the influence of IL-12, which is produced by macrophages and dendritic cells. The T cells express CD40 ligand and secrete IFN-γ, and these two stimuli activate macrophages to produce several microbicidal substances, including reactive oxygen species, nitric oxide, and lysosomal enzymes. In mice, IFN-γ also stimulates

the production of antibody isotypes that activate complement and opsonize bacteria for phagocytosis, thus aiding the effector functions of macrophages. The stimuli for the production of these antibodies in humans are not as well defined. The importance of IL-12 and IFN-γ in immunity to intracellular bacteria has been demonstrated in experimental models and in congenital immunodeficiencies. For instance, individuals with inherited mutations in receptors for IFN-γ or IL-12 are highly susceptible to infections with atypical mycobacteria.

Phagocytosed bacteria stimulate CD8+ T cell responses if bacterial antigens are transported from phagosomes into the cytosol or if the bacteria escape from phagosomes and enter the cytoplasm of infected cells. In the cytosol, the microbes are no longer susceptible to the microbicidal mechanisms of phagocytes, and for eradication of the infection, the infected cells have to be killed by CTLs. Thus, the effectors of cell-mediated immunity, namely, CD4+ T cells that activate macrophages and CD8+ CTLs, function cooperatively in defense against intracellular bacteria (Fig. 16-5).

The macrophage activation that occurs in response to intracellular microbes is capable of causing tissue injury. This injury may be the result of delayed-type hypersensitivity (DTH) reactions to microbial protein antigens (see Chapter 19). Because intracellular bacteria have evolved to resist killing within phagocytes, they often persist for long periods and cause chronic antigenic stimulation and T cell and macrophage activation, which may result in the formation of granulomas surrounding the microbes (see Fig. 19-8). The histologic hallmark of infection with some intracellular bacteria is granulomatous inflammation. This type of inflammatory reaction may serve to localize and prevent spread of the microbes, but it is also

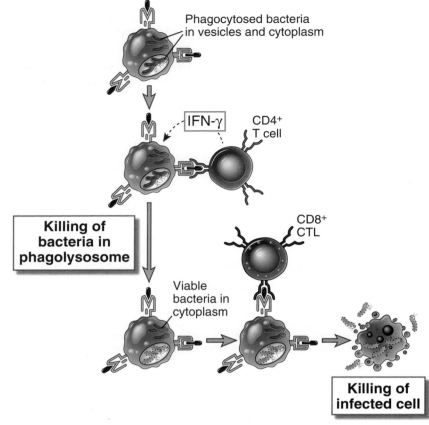

Phagocytosed bacteria
in vesicles and cytoplasm

IFN-γ

CD4+
T cell

**Killing of
bacteria in
phagolysosome**

CD8+
CTL

Viable
bacteria in
cytoplasm

**Killing of
infected cell**

FIGURE 16-5 Cooperation of CD4+ and CD8+ T cells in defense against intracellular microbes. Intracellular bacteria such as *L. monocytogenes* are phagocytosed by macrophages and may survive in phagosomes and escape into the cytoplasm. CD4+ T cells respond to class II MHC–associated peptide antigens derived from the intravesicular bacteria. These T cells produce IFN-γ, which activates macrophages to destroy the microbes in phagosomes. CD8+ T cells respond to class I–associated peptides derived from cytosolic antigens and kill the infected cells.

associated with severe functional impairment caused by tissue necrosis and fibrosis.

Tuberculosis is an example of an infection with an intracellular bacterium in which protective immunity and pathologic hypersensitivity coexist, and the host response contributes significantly to the pathology. In a primary infection with *M. tuberculosis,* bacilli multiply slowly in the lungs and cause only mild inflammation. The infection is contained by alveolar macrophages (and probably dendritic cells). More than 90% of infected patients remain asymptomatic, but bacteria survive in the lungs, mainly in macrophages. By 6 to 8 weeks after infection, the macrophages have traveled to the draining lymph nodes, and CD4+ T cells are activated; CD8+ T cells may also be activated later. These T cells produce IFN-γ, which activates macrophages and enhances their ability to kill phagocytosed bacilli. TNF produced by T cells and macrophages also plays a role in local inflammation and macrophage activation. The T cell reaction is adequate to control bacterial spread. However, *M. tuberculosis* is capable of surviving within macrophages because components of its cell wall inhibit the fusion of phagocytic vacuoles with lysosomes. As a result, the bacteria continue to elicit T cell responses. Prolonged T cell activation leads to the formation of granulomas, which may wall off the bacteria and are often associated with central necrosis, called caseous necrosis, which is caused by macrophage products such as lysosomal enzymes and reactive oxygen species. Necrotizing granulomas and the fibrosis (scarring) that accompanies granulomatous inflammation are important

causes of tissue injury and clinical disease in tuberculosis. Previously infected persons show cutaneous DTH reactions to skin challenge with a bacterial antigen preparation (purified protein derivative, or PPD). Bacilli may survive for many years and are contained without any pathologic consequences but may be reactivated at any time, especially if the immune response becomes unable to control the infection.

Differences among individuals in the patterns of T cell responses to intracellular microbes are important determinants of disease progression and clinical outcome (Fig. 16-6). The role of T_H1- and T_H2-derived cytokines in determining the outcome of infection has been most clearly demonstrated in infection by the protozoan parasite *Leishmania major* in different strains of inbred mice (discussed later in this chapter). An example of this relationship between the type of T cell response and disease outcome in humans is leprosy, which is caused by *Mycobacterium leprae*. There are two polar forms of leprosy, the lepromatous and tuberculoid forms, although many patients fall into less clear intermediate groups. In lepromatous leprosy, patients have high specific antibody titers but weak cell-mediated responses to *M. leprae* antigens. Mycobacteria proliferate within macrophages and are detectable in large numbers. The bacterial growth and persistent but inadequate macrophage activation result in destructive lesions in the skin and underlying tissue. In contrast, patients with tuberculoid leprosy have strong cell-mediated immunity but low antibody levels. This pattern of immunity is reflected in granulomas that form

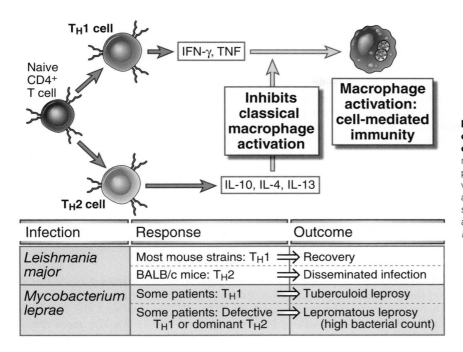

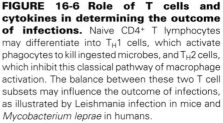

FIGURE 16-6 Role of T cells and cytokines in determining the outcome of infections. Naive CD4+ T lymphocytes may differentiate into T_H1 cells, which activate phagocytes to kill ingested microbes, and T_H2 cells, which inhibit this classical pathway of macrophage activation. The balance between these two T cell subsets may influence the outcome of infections, as illustrated by Leishmania infection in mice and *Mycobacterium leprae* in humans.

Infection	Response	Outcome
Leishmania major	Most mouse strains: T_H1	Recovery
	BALB/c mice: T_H2	Disseminated infection
Mycobacterium leprae	Some patients: T_H1	Tuberculoid leprosy
	Some patients: Defective T_H1 or dominant T_H2	Lepromatous leprosy (high bacterial count)

around nerves and produce peripheral sensory nerve defects and secondary traumatic skin lesions but with less tissue destruction and a paucity of bacteria in the lesions. One possible reason for the differences in these two forms of disease caused by the same organism may be that there are different patterns of T cell differentiation and cytokine production in individuals. Some studies indicate that patients with the tuberculoid form of the disease produce IFN-γ and IL-2 in lesions (indicative of T_H1 cell activation), whereas patients with lepromatous leprosy produce less IFN-γ and may exhibit weak cell-mediated immunity and failure to control bacterial spread.

Immune Evasion by Intracellular Bacteria

Intracellular bacteria have developed various strategies to resist elimination by phagocytes (see Table 16-2). These include inhibiting phagolysosome fusion or escaping into the cytosol, thus hiding from the microbicidal mechanisms of lysosomes, and directly scavenging or inactivating microbicidal substances such as reactive oxygen species. The outcome of infection by these organisms often depends on whether the T cell–stimulated anti-microbial mechanisms of macrophages or microbial resistance to killing gain the upper hand. Resistance to phagocyte-mediated elimination is also the reason that such bacteria tend to cause chronic infections that may last for years, often recur after apparent cure, and are difficult to eradicate.

IMMUNITY TO FUNGI

Fungal infections, also called mycoses, are important causes of morbidity and mortality in humans. Some fungal infections are endemic, and these infections are usually caused by fungi that are present in the environment and whose spores enter humans. Other fungal infections are said to be opportunistic because the causative agents

cause mild or no disease in healthy individuals but may infect and cause severe disease in immunodeficient persons. Compromised immunity is the most important predisposing factor for clinically significant fungal infections. Neutrophil deficiency as a result of bone marrow suppression or damage is frequently associated with such infections. Opportunistic fungal infections are also associated with immunodeficiency caused by HIV and by therapy for disseminated cancer and transplant rejection. A serious opportunistic fungal infection associated with AIDS is *Pneumocystis jiroveci* pneumonia, but many others contribute to the morbidity and mortality caused by immune deficiencies.

Different fungi infect humans and may live in extracellular tissues and within phagocytes. Therefore, the immune responses to these microbes are often combinations of the responses to extracellular and intracellular bacteria. However, less is known about antifungal immunity than about immunity against bacteria and viruses. This lack of knowledge is partly due to the paucity of animal models for mycoses and partly due to the fact that these infections typically occur in individuals who are incapable of mounting effective immune responses.

Innate and Adaptive Immunity to Fungi

The principal mediators of innate immunity against fungi are neutrophils and macrophages. Patients with neutropenia are extremely susceptible to opportunistic fungal infections. Phagocytes and dendritic cells sense fungal organisms by TLRs and lectin-like receptors called **dectins** (see Chapter 4). Neutrophils presumably liberate fungicidal substances, such as reactive oxygen species and lysosomal enzymes, and phagocytose fungi for intracellular killing. Virulent strains of *Cryptococcus neoformans* inhibit the production of cytokines such as TNF and IL-12 by macrophages and stimulate production of IL-10, thus inhibiting macrophage activation.

Cell-mediated immunity is the major mechanism of adaptive immunity against fungal infections. *Histoplasma capsulatum,* a facultative intracellular parasite that lives in macrophages, is eliminated by the same cellular mechanisms that are effective against intracellular bacteria. CD4⁺ and CD8⁺ T cells cooperate to eliminate the yeast forms of *C. neoformans,* which tend to colonize the lungs and brain in immunodeficient hosts. *Pneumocystis jiroveci* is another fungus that causes serious infections in individuals with defective cell-mediated immunity.

Many extracellular fungi elicit strong T_H17 responses, which are driven in part by the activation of dendritic cells by fungal glucans binding to dectin-1, a receptor for this fungal polysaccharide. Dendritic cells activated via this lectin receptor produce T_H17-inducing cytokines, such as IL-6 and IL-23 (see Chapter 10). The T_H17 cells stimulate inflammation, and the recruited neutrophils and monocytes destroy the fungi. Individuals with defective T_H17 responses are susceptible to chronic mucocutaneous *Candida* infections. T_H1 responses are protective in intracellular fungal infections, such as histoplasmosis, but these responses may elicit granulomatous inflammation, which is an important cause of host tissue injury in these infections. Fungi also elicit specific antibody responses that may be of protective value.

IMMUNITY TO VIRUSES

Viruses are obligatory intracellular microorganisms that use components of the nucleic acid and protein synthetic machinery of the host to replicate and spread. Viruses typically infect various cell types by using normal cell surface molecules as receptors to enter the cells. After entering cells, viruses can cause tissue injury and disease by any of several mechanisms. Viral replication interferes with normal cellular protein synthesis and function and leads to injury and ultimately death of the infected cell. This result is one type of cytopathic effect of viruses, and the infection is said to be lytic because the infected cell is lysed. Viruses may also cause latent infections, discussed later.

Innate and adaptive immune responses to viruses are aimed at blocking infection and eliminating infected cells (Fig. 16-7). Infection is prevented by type I interferons as part of innate immunity and neutralizing antibodies contributing to adaptive immunity. Once infection is established, infected cells are eliminated by NK cells in the innate response and CTLs in the adaptive response.

Innate Immunity to Viruses

The principal mechanisms of innate immunity against viruses are inhibition of infection by type I interferons and NK cell–mediated killing of infected cells. Infection by many viruses is associated with production of type I interferons by infected cells, especially dendritic cells of the plasmacytoid type (see Chapter 4). Several biochemical pathways trigger interferon production (see Fig. 4-16). These include recognition of viral RNA and DNA by endosomal TLRs and activation of cytoplasmic RIG-like receptors and the STING pathway by viral RNA

and DNA, respectively. These pathways converge on the activation of protein kinases, which in turn activate the IRF transcription factors that stimulate interferon gene transcription. Type I interferons function to inhibit viral replication in both infected and uninfected cells. The mechanisms by which interferons block viral replication were discussed in Chapter 4 (see Fig. 4-17).

NK cells kill other cells infected with a variety of viruses and are an important mechanism of immunity against viruses early in the course of infection, before adaptive immune responses have developed. Class I MHC expression is often shut off in virally infected cells as an escape mechanism from CTLs. This enables NK cells to kill the infected cells because the absence of class I releases NK cells from a normal state of inhibition (see Fig. 4-7).

Adaptive Immunity to Viruses

Adaptive immunity against viral infections is mediated by antibodies, which block virus binding and entry into host cells, and by CTLs, which eliminate the infection by killing infected cells (see Fig. 16-7). The most effective antibodies are high-affinity antibodies produced in T-dependent germinal center reactions (see Chapter 12). Antibodies are effective against viruses only during the extracellular stage of the lives of these microbes. Viruses may be extracellular early in the course of infection, before they infect host cells, or when they are released from infected cells by virus budding or if the infected cells die. Antiviral antibodies bind to viral envelope or capsid antigens and function mainly as neutralizing antibodies to prevent virus attachment and entry into host cells. Thus, antibodies prevent both initial infection and cell-to-cell spread. Secreted antibodies of the IgA isotype are important for neutralizing viruses within the respiratory and intestinal tracts. Oral immunization against polio virus works by inducing mucosal immunity. In addition to neutralization, antibodies may opsonize viral particles and promote their clearance by phagocytes. Complement activation may also participate in antibody-mediated viral immunity, mainly by promoting phagocytosis and possibly by direct lysis of viruses with lipid envelopes.

The importance of humoral immunity in defense against viral infections is supported by the observation that resistance to a particular virus, induced by either infection or vaccination, is often specific for the serologic (antibody-defined) type of the virus. An example is influenza virus, in which exposure to one serologic type does not confer resistance to other serotypes of the virus. Neutralizing antibodies block viral infection of cells and spread of viruses from cell to cell, but once the viruses enter cells and begin to replicate intracellularly, they are inaccessible to antibodies. Therefore, humoral immunity induced by previous infection or vaccination is able to protect individuals from viral infection but cannot by itself eradicate established infection.

Elimination of viruses that reside within cells is mediated by CTLs, which kill the infected cells. As we have mentioned in previous chapters, the principal physiologic function of CTLs is surveillance against viral infection. Most virus-specific CTLs are CD8⁺ T cells that recognize cytosolic, usually endogenously synthesized,

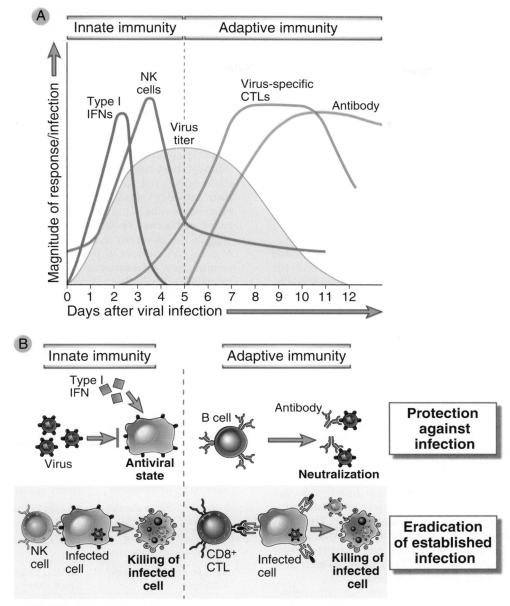

FIGURE 16-7 Innate and adaptive immune responses against viruses. A, Kinetics of innate and adaptive immune responses to a virus infection. **B,** Mechanisms by which innate and adaptive immunity prevent and eradicate virus infections. Innate immunity is mediated by type I interferons, which prevent infection, and NK cells, which eliminate infected cells. Adaptive immunity is mediated by antibodies and CTLs, which block infection and kill infected cells, respectively.

viral peptides presented by class I MHC molecules. If the infected cell is a tissue cell and not a professional antigen-presenting cell (APC), such as a dendritic cell, the infected cell may be phagocytosed by the dendritic cell, which processes the viral antigens and presents them to naive CD8+ T cells. We described this process of cross-presentation, or cross-priming, in Chapter 6 (see Fig. 6-20). Full differentiation of CD8+ CTLs often requires cytokines produced by CD4+ helper cells or costimulators expressed on infected cells (see Chapter 11). As discussed in Chapters 9 and 11, CD8+ T cells undergo massive proliferation during viral infection, and most of the proliferating cells are specific for a few viral peptides. Some of the activated T cells differentiate into effector CTLs, which can kill any

infected nucleated cell. The antiviral effects of CTLs are mainly due to killing of infected cells, but other mechanisms include activation of nucleases within infected cells that degrade viral genomes and secretion of cytokines such as IFN-γ, which activates phagocytes and may have some antiviral activity.

The importance of CTLs in defense against viral infection is demonstrated by the increased susceptibility to such infections seen in patients and animals deficient in T lymphocytes and by the experimental observation that mice can be protected against some virus infections by adoptive transfer of virus-specific, class I–restricted CTLs. Furthermore, many viruses are able to alter their surface antigens, such as envelope glycoproteins, and thus escape attack by antibodies. However, infected cells may produce some viral proteins that are invariant, so that CTL-mediated defense remains effective against such viruses.

In latent infections, viral DNA persists in host cells, but the virus does not replicate or kill infected cells. Latency is often a state of balance between infection and the immune response. CTLs are generated in response to the virus that can control the infection but not eradicate it. As a result, the virus persists in infected cells, sometimes for the life of the individual. Any deficiency in the host immune response can result in reactivation of the latent infection, with expression of viral genes that are responsible for cytopathic effects and for spread of the virus. These cytopathic effects may include lysis of infected cells or uncontrolled proliferation of the cells. Such latent infections are common with Epstein-Barr virus and several other DNA viruses of the herpesvirus family.

In some viral infections, tissue injury may be caused by CTLs. An experimental model of a disease in which the pathology is due to the host immune response is lymphocytic choriomeningitis virus (LCMV) infection in mice, which induces inflammation of the spinal cord meninges. LCMV infects meningeal cells, but it is non-cytopathic and does not injure the infected cells directly. The virus stimulates the development of virus-specific CTLs that kill infected meningeal cells during a physiologic attempt to eradicate the infection. Therefore, meningitis develops in normal mice with intact immune systems, but T cell–deficient mice do not develop disease and instead become carriers of the virus. This observation appears to contradict the usual situation, in which immunodeficient individuals are more susceptible to infectious diseases than normal individuals are. Hepatitis B virus infection in humans shows some similarities to murine LCMV in that immunodeficient persons who become infected do not develop the disease but become carriers who can transmit the infection to otherwise healthy persons. The livers of patients with acute and chronic active hepatitis contain large numbers of CD8[+] T cells, and hepatitis virus–specific, class I MHC–restricted CTLs can be isolated from liver biopsy specimens and propagated in vitro.

Immune responses to viral infections may be involved in producing disease in other ways. A consequence of persistent infection with some viruses, such as hepatitis B, is the formation of circulating immune complexes composed of viral antigens and specific antibodies (see Chapter 19). These complexes are deposited in blood vessels and lead to systemic vasculitis. Some viral proteins contain amino acid sequences that are also present in some self antigens. It has been postulated that because of this molecular mimicry, antiviral immunity can lead to immune responses against self antigens.

Immune Evasion by Viruses

Viruses have evolved numerous mechanisms for evading host immunity (Table 16-3).

- *Viruses can alter their antigens and are thus no longer targets of immune responses.* The antigens affected are most commonly surface glycoproteins that are recognized by antibodies, but T cell epitopes may also un-

dergo variation. The principal mechanisms of antigenic variation are point mutations and reassortment of RNA genomes (in RNA viruses), leading to antigenic drift and antigenic shift. These processes are of great importance in the spread of influenza virus. The two major antigens of the virus are the trimeric viral hemagglutinin (the viral spike protein) and neuraminidase. Viral genomes undergo mutations in the genes that encode these surface proteins, and the variation that occurs as a result is called **antigenic drift.** The segmented RNA genomes of influenza viruses that normally inhabit different host species can recombine in host cells, and these reassorted viruses can differ quite dramatically from prevalent strains (Fig. 16-8). Reassortment of viral genes results in major changes in antigenic structure called **antigenic shift**, which creates distinct viruses such as the avian flu or the swine flu viruses. Because of antigenic variation, a virus may become resistant to immunity generated in the population by previous infections. The influenza pandemics that occurred in 1918, 1957, and 1968 were due to different strains of the virus, and the H1N1 pandemic of 2009 was due to a strain in which the strands of the RNA genome were reassorted among strains endemic in pigs, fowl, and humans. Subtler viral variants arise more frequently. There are so many serotypes of rhinovirus that

TABLE 16-3	Mechanisms of Immune Evasion by Viruses
Mechanism of Immune Evasion	**Examples**
Antigenic variation	Influenza, rhinovirus, HIV
Inhibition of antigen processing	
Blockade of TAP transporter	Herpes simplex virus (HSV)
Removal of class I molecules from the ER	Cytomegalovirus (CMV)
Production of "decoy" MHC molecules to inhibit NK cells	Cytomegalovirus (murine)
Production of cytokine receptor homologues	Vaccinia, poxviruses (IL-1, IFN-γ) Cytomegalovirus (chemokine)
Production of immunosuppressive cytokine	Epstein-Barr (IL-10)
Infection and death or functional impairment of immune cells	HIV
Inhibition of complement activation	
Recruitment of factor H	HIV
Incorporation of CD59 in viral envelope	HIV, vaccinia, human CMV
Inhibition of innate immunity	
Inhibition of access to RIG-I RNA sensor	Vaccinia, HIV
Inhibition of PKR (signaling by IFN receptor)	HIV, HCV, HSV, polio

Representative examples of different mechanisms used by viruses to resist host immunity are listed.

ER, endoplasmic reticulum; *HCV,* hepatitis C virus; *HIV,* human immunodeficiency virus; *TAP,* transporter associated with antigen processing.

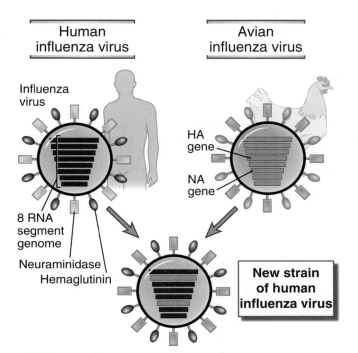

Human influenza virus

Avian influenza virus

Influenza virus

HA gene

NA gene

8 RNA segment genome

Neuraminidase

Hemaglutinin

New strain of human influenza virus

FIGURE 16-8 Generation of new influenza virus strains by genetic recombination (antigenic shift). The genome of the influenza virus is composed of eight separate RNA strands, which allows genetic recombination by reassortment of the segments in various hosts, such as a pig (not shown), bird, or humans, that are simultaneously infected with two different strains. These genetic reassortments create new viruses that are antigenically distinct from their precursors and thus are able to evade immune detection in large numbers of newly infected hosts. The H1N1 influenza virus, which was responsible for the pandemic of 2009, was generated by reassortment of swine, avian, and human viruses in pigs and then passed back to humans.

vaccination against the common cold may not be a feasible preventive strategy. Human immunodeficiency virus 1 (HIV-1), which causes AIDS, is also capable of tremendous antigenic variation due to a high error rate in reverse transcription of its RNA genome during viral reproduction (see Chapter 21). In these situations, prophylactic vaccination may have to be directed against invariant viral proteins.

- **Some viruses inhibit class I MHC–associated presentation of cytosolic protein antigens.** Viruses make a variety of proteins that block different steps in antigen processing, transport, and presentation (Fig. 16-9). Inhibition of antigen presentation blocks the assembly and expression of stable class I MHC molecules and the display of viral peptides. As a result, cells infected by such viruses cannot be recognized or killed by CD8+ CTLs. As discussed earlier, NK cells are activated by infected cells, especially in the absence of class I MHC molecules. Some viruses may produce proteins that act as ligands for NK cell inhibitory receptors and thus inhibit NK cell activation.

- **Some viruses produce molecules that inhibit the immune response.** Poxviruses encode molecules that are secreted by infected cells and bind to several cytokines, including IFN-γ, TNF, IL-1, IL-18, and chemokines. The secreted cytokine-binding proteins may function as competitive antagonists of the cytokines. Epstein-Barr virus produces a protein that is homologous to the cytokine IL-10, which inhibits activation of macrophages and dendritic cells and may thus suppress cell-mediated immunity. These examples probably represent a small fraction of immunosuppressive viral molecules. Identification of these molecules raises the intriguing possibility that viruses have acquired genes

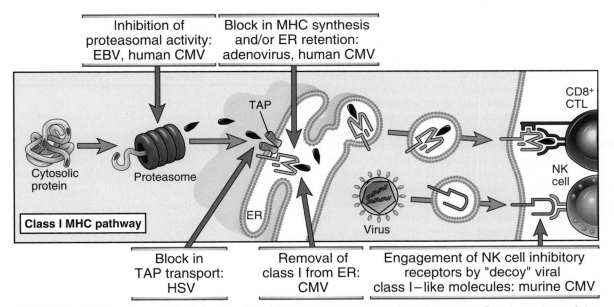

Inhibition of proteasomal activity: EBV, human CMV

Block in MHC synthesis and/or ER retention: adenovirus, human CMV

TAP

CD8+ CTL

NK cell

Cytosolic protein

Proteasome

ER

Virus

Class I MHC pathway

Block in TAP transport: HSV

Removal of class I from ER: CMV

Engagement of NK cell inhibitory receptors by "decoy" viral class I–like molecules: murine CMV

FIGURE 16-9 Mechanisms by which viruses inhibit antigen processing and presentation. The pathway of class I MHC–associated antigen presentation is shown, with examples of viruses that block different steps in this pathway. In addition to interfering with recognition by CD8+ T cells, some viruses produce "decoy" MHC molecules that engage inhibitory receptors of natural killer (NK) cells. *CMV*, cytomegalovirus; *EBV*, Epstein-Barr virus; *ER*, endoplasmic reticulum; *HSV*, herpes simplex virus; *TAP*, transporter associated with antigen processing.

encoding endogenous inhibitors of immune responses during their passage through human hosts and have thus evolved to infect and colonize humans.

- **Some chronic viral infections are associated with failure of CTL responses,** which allows viral persistence. Studies of a chronic infection with lymphocytic choriomeningitis in mice have shown that this type of immune deficit may result from signaling by T cell inhibitory receptors, such as PD-1, which normally functions to maintain T cell tolerance to self antigens (see Fig. 11-3). Thus, viruses may have evolved to exploit normal mechanisms of immune regulation and to activate these pathways in T cells. This phenomenon has been called exhaustion, implying that immune responses against the virus are initiated but then shut off prematurely. There is evidence for CD8+ T cell exhaustion in chronic human viral infections, including HIV and hepatitis virus infection.

- **Viruses may infect and either kill or inactivate immunocompetent cells.** The obvious example is HIV, which survives by infecting and eliminating CD4+ T cells, the key inducers of immune responses to protein antigens.

IMMUNITY TO PARASITES

In infectious disease terminology, parasitic infection refers to infection with animal parasites such as protozoa, helminths, and ectoparasites (e.g., ticks and mites). Such parasites currently account for greater morbidity and mortality than any other class of infectious organisms, particularly in developing countries. It is estimated that about 30% of the world's population suffers from parasitic infestations. Malaria alone affects more than 100 million people worldwide and is responsible for about 500,000 deaths annually. The magnitude of this public health problem is the principal reason for the great interest in immunity to parasites and for the development of immunoparasitology as a distinct branch of immunology.

Most parasites go through complex life cycles, part of which occurs in humans (or other vertebrates) and part of which occurs in intermediate hosts, such as flies, ticks, and snails. Humans are usually infected by bites from infected intermediate hosts or by sharing a particular habitat with an intermediate host. For instance, malaria and trypanosomiasis are transmitted by insect bites, and schistosomiasis is transmitted by exposure to water in which infected snails reside. Most parasitic infections are chronic because of weak innate immunity and the ability of parasites to evade or resist elimination by adaptive immune responses. Furthermore, many anti-parasitic drugs are not effective at killing the organisms. Individuals living in endemic areas require repeated chemotherapy because of continued exposure, and such treatment is often not possible because of expense and logistic problems.

Innate Immunity to Parasites

Although different protozoan and helminthic parasites have been shown to activate different mechanisms of innate immunity, these organisms are often able to survive and replicate in their hosts because they are well adapted to resisting host defenses. The principal innate immune response to protozoa is phagocytosis, but many of these parasites are resistant to phagocytic killing and may even replicate within macrophages. Some protozoa express surface molecules that are recognized by TLRs and activate phagocytes. *Plasmodium* species (the protozoa that are responsible for malaria), *Toxoplasma gondii* (the agent that causes toxoplasmosis), and *Cryptosporidium* species (the major parasite that causes diarrhea in HIV-infected patients) all express glycosyl phosphatidylinositol lipids that can activate TLR2 and TLR4. Phagocytes may also attack helminthic parasites and secrete microbicidal substances to kill organisms that are too large to be phagocytosed. However, many helminths have thick teguments that make them resistant to the cytocidal mechanisms of neutrophils and macrophages, and they are too large to be ingested by phagocytes. Some helminths may activate the alternative pathway of complement, although, as we will discuss later, parasites recovered from infected hosts appear to have developed resistance to complement-mediated lysis.

Adaptive Immunity to Parasites

Different protozoa and helminths vary greatly in their structural and biochemical properties, life cycles, and pathogenic mechanisms. It is therefore not surprising that different parasites elicit distinct adaptive immune responses (Table 16-4). Some pathogenic protozoa have evolved to survive within host cells, so protective immunity against these organisms is mediated by mechanisms similar to those that eliminate intracellular bacteria and viruses. In contrast, metazoa such as helminths survive in extracellular tissues, and their elimination is often dependent on special types of antibody responses.

TABLE 16-4	**Immune Responses to Disease-Causing Parasites**	
Parasite	**Diseases**	**Principal Mechanisms of Protective Immunity**
Protozoa		
Plasmodium species	Malaria	Antibodies and CD8+ CTLs
Leishmania donovani	Leishmaniasis (mucocutaneous disseminated)	CD4+ T$_H$1 cells activate macrophages to kill phagocytosed parasites
Trypanosoma brucei	African trypanosomiasis	Antibodies
Entamoeba histolytica	Amebiasis	Antibodies, phagocytosis
Metazoa		
Schistosoma species	Schistosomiasis	Killing by eosinophils, macrophages
Filaria (e.g., *Wuchereria bancrofti*)	Filariasis	Cell-mediated immunity; role of antibodies?

Selected examples of parasites and immune responses to them are listed.

The principal defense mechanism against protozoa that survive within macrophages is cell-mediated immunity, particularly macrophage activation by T_H1 cell–derived cytokines. Infection of mice with *Leishmania major*, a protozoan that survives within the endosomes of macrophages, is the best documented example of how dominance of T_H1 or T_H2 responses determines disease resistance or susceptibility (see Fig. 16-6). Resistance to the infection is associated with activation of Leishmania-specific CD4+ T_H1 cells, which produce IFN-γ and thereby activate macrophages to destroy intracellular parasites. Conversely, activation of T_H2 cells by the protozoa results in increased parasite survival and exacerbation of lesions because of the macrophage-suppressive actions of T_H2 cytokines. A good example of this difference is seen in *Leishmania* infections in different inbred mouse strains. Most inbred strains of mice are resistant to infection with *L. major*, but inbred BALB/c and some related strains of mice are highly susceptible and die if they are infected with large numbers of parasites. After infection, the resistant strains produce large amounts of IFN-γ in response to leishmanial antigens, whereas the strains that are susceptible to fatal leishmaniasis produce more IL-4 in response to the parasite. Promoting the T_H1 response or inhibiting the T_H2 response in susceptible strains increases their resistance to the infection. The mechanisms of this striking difference between strains of mice are not defined.

Protozoa that replicate inside various host cells and lyse these cells stimulate specific antibody and CTL responses, similar to cytopathic viruses. An example of such an organism is the malaria parasite, which resides mainly in red blood cells and in hepatocytes during its life cycle. It was thought for many years that antibodies were the major protective mechanism against malaria, and early attempts at vaccinating against this infection focused on generating antibodies. It is now apparent that the CTL response against parasites residing in hepatocytes is an important defense against the spread of this intracellular protozoan. The cytokine IFN-γ has been shown to be protective in many protozoal infections, including malaria, toxoplasmosis, and cryptosporidiosis.

Defense against many helminthic infections is mediated by the activation of T_H2 cells, which results in production of IgE antibodies and activation of eosinophils. Helminths stimulate differentiation of naive CD4+ T cells to the T_H2 subset of effector cells, which secrete IL-4 and IL-5. IL-4 stimulates the production of IgE, which binds to the Fcε receptor of eosinophils and mast cells, and IL-5 stimulates the development of eosinophils and activates eosinophils. IgE coats the parasites, and eosinophils bind to the IgE and are activated to release their granule contents, which destroy the helminths (see Chapter 20). The combined actions of mast cells and eosinophils also contribute to expulsion of the parasites from the intestine (see Fig. 10-9). The expulsion of some intestinal nematodes may be due to IL-4–dependent mechanisms that do not require IgE, such as increased peristalsis.

Adaptive immune responses to parasites can also contribute to tissue injury. Some parasites and their products induce granulomatous responses with concomitant fibrosis. *Schistosoma mansoni* eggs deposited in the liver stimulate CD4+ T cells, which in turn activate macrophages and induce DTH reactions. DTH reactions result in the formation of granulomas around the eggs; an unusual feature of these granulomas, especially in mice, is their association with T_H2 responses. (Granulomas are generally induced by T_H1 responses against persistent antigens; see Chapter 19.) Such T_H2-induced granulomas serve to contain the schistosome eggs, but severe fibrosis associated with this chronic cell-mediated immune response leads to cirrhosis, disruption of venous blood flow in the liver, and portal hypertension. In lymphatic filariasis, lodging of the parasites in lymphatic vessels leads to chronic cell-mediated immune reactions and ultimately to fibrosis. This results in lymphatic obstruction and severe lymphedema. Chronic and persistent parasitic infestations are often associated with the formation of complexes of parasite antigens and specific antibodies. The complexes can be deposited in blood vessels and kidney glomeruli and produce vasculitis and nephritis, respectively (see Chapter 19). Immune complex disease is a complication of schistosomiasis and malaria.

Immune Evasion by Parasites

Parasites evade protective immunity by reducing their immunogenicity and by inhibiting host immune responses. Different parasites have developed remarkably effective ways of resisting immunity (Table 16-5).

● Parasites change their surface antigens during their life cycle in vertebrate hosts. Two forms of antigenic variation are well defined. The first is a stage-specific change in antigen expression, such that the mature tissue stages of parasites produce antigens different from those of the infective stages. For example, the infective sporozoite stage of malaria parasites is antigenically distinct from the merozoites that reside in the host and are responsible for chronic infection. By the time the immune system has responded to infection by sporozoites, the parasite has differentiated, expresses new antigens, and is no longer a target for immune elimination. The second and more remarkable example of antigenic variation in parasites is the continuous variation of major surface antigens seen in African trypanosomes such as *Trypanosoma brucei* and *Trypanosoma rhodesiense*. Continuous antigenic variation in trypanosomes is mainly due to changes in expression of the genes encoding the major surface antigen. Infected patients show waves of blood

TABLE 16-5	Mechanisms of Immune Evasion by Parasites
Mechanism of Immune Evasion	**Examples**
Antigenic variation	Trypanosomes, *Plasmodium*
Acquired resistance to complement, CTLs	Schistosomes
Inhibition of host immune responses	Filaria (secondary to lymphatic obstruction), trypanosomes
Antigen shedding	Entamoeba
CTL, cytotoxic T lymphocyte.	

parasitemia, and each wave consists of parasites expressing a surface antigen that is different from the previous wave. Thus, by the time the host produces antibodies against the parasite, an antigenically different organism has grown out. More than 100 such waves of parasitemia can occur in a single infection. One consequence of antigenic variation in parasites is that it is difficult to effectively vaccinate individuals against these infections.

- Parasites become resistant to immune effector mechanisms during their residence in vertebrate hosts. Perhaps the best examples are schistosome larvae, which travel to the lungs of infected animals and during this migration develop a tegument that is resistant to damage by complement and by CTLs. The biochemical basis of this change is not known.
- Protozoan parasites may conceal themselves from the immune system either by living inside host cells or by developing cysts that are resistant to immune effectors. Some helminthic parasites reside in intestinal lumens and are sheltered from cell-mediated immune effector mechanisms. Parasites may also shed their antigenic coats, either spontaneously or after binding specific antibodies. Shedding of antigens renders the parasites resistant to subsequent antibody-mediated attack. *Entamoeba histolytica* is a protozoan parasite that sheds antigens and can also convert to a cyst form in the lumen of the large intestine.
- Parasites inhibit host immune responses by multiple mechanisms. T cell anergy to parasite antigens has been observed in severe schistosomiasis involving the liver and spleen and in filarial infections. The mechanisms of immunologic unresponsiveness in these infections are not well understood. In lymphatic filariasis, infection of lymph nodes with subsequent architectural disruption may contribute to deficient immunity. Some parasites, such as *Leishmania,* stimulate the development of regulatory T cells, which suppress the immune response enough to allow persistence of the parasites. More non-specific and generalized immunosuppression is observed in malaria and African trypanosomiasis. This immune deficiency has been attributed to the production of immunosuppressive cytokines by activated macrophages and T cells and defects in T cell activation.

The consequences of parasitic infestations for health and economic development are devastating. Attempts to develop effective vaccines against these infections have been actively pursued for many years. Although the progress has been slower than one would have hoped, elucidation of the fundamental mechanisms of immune responses to and immune evasion by parasites holds promise for the future.

STRATEGIES FOR VACCINE DEVELOPMENT

The birth of immunology as a science dates from Edward Jenner's successful vaccination against smallpox in 1796. The importance of prophylactic immunization against infectious diseases is best illustrated by the fact that worldwide programs of vaccination have led to the complete or nearly complete eradication of many of these diseases in developed countries (see Table 1-1). The fundamental principle of vaccination is to administer a killed or attenuated form of an infectious agent, or a component of a microbe, that does not cause disease but elicits an immune response that provides protection against infection by the live, pathogenic microbe.

The success of vaccination in eradicating infectious disease is dependent on several properties of the microbes. Vaccines are effective if the infectious agent does not establish latency, if it does not undergo much or any antigenic variation, and if it does not interfere with the host immune response. It is difficult to effectively vaccinate against microbes such as HIV, which establishes latent infection, and is highly variable. Vaccines are also most effective against infections that are limited to human hosts and do not have animal reservoirs.

Most vaccines in use today work by inducing humoral immunity. Antibodies are the only immune mechanism that prevents infections, by neutralizing and clearing microbes before they gain their foothold in the host. The best vaccines are those that stimulate the development of long-lived plasma cells that produce high-affinity antibodies as well as memory B cells. These aspects of humoral immune responses are best induced by the germinal center reaction (see Chapter 12), which requires help provided by protein antigen–specific CD4+ T cells.

In the following section, we will summarize the approaches to vaccination that have been tried (Table 16-6) and their major value and limitations.

Attenuated and Inactivated Bacterial and Viral Vaccines

Vaccines composed of intact non-pathogenic microbes are made by treating the microbes in such a way that they can no longer cause disease (i.e., their virulence is attenuated) or by killing the microbes while retaining their immunogenicity. The great advantage of attenuated microbial vaccines is that they elicit all the innate and adaptive immune responses (both humoral and cell mediated) that the pathogenic microbe would, and they are therefore the ideal way of inducing protective immunity. Live, attenuated bacteria were first shown by

TABLE 16-6   Vaccine Approaches

Type of Vaccine	Examples
Live attenuated or killed bacteria	Bacillus Calmette-Guérin, cholera
Live attenuated viruses	Polio, rabies
Subunit (antigen) vaccines	Tetanus toxoid, diphtheria toxoid
Conjugate vaccines	*Haemophilus influenzae,* pneumococcus
Synthetic vaccines	Hepatitis (recombinant proteins)
Viral vectors	Clinical trials of HIV antigens in canarypox vector
DNA vaccines	Clinical trials ongoing for several infections

Louis Pasteur to confer specific immunity. The attenuated or killed bacterial vaccines in use today generally induce limited protection and are effective for only short periods. Live, attenuated viral vaccines are usually more effective; polio, measles, and yellow fever are three good examples. The most frequently used approach for producing such attenuated viruses is repeated passage in cell culture. More recently, temperature-sensitive and gene deletion mutants have been generated to achieve the same goal. Viral vaccines often induce long-lasting specific immunity, so immunization of children is sufficient for lifelong protection. The major concern with attenuated viral or bacterial vaccines is safety. The live-attenuated oral polio vaccine has nearly eradicated the disease, but in rare cases the virus in the vaccine is reactivated and itself causes paralytic polio. In fact, the success of worldwide vaccination is creating the problem that the vaccine-induced disease, although rare, could become more frequent than the naturally acquired disease. This potential problem may have to be tackled by reverting to the killed virus vaccine in order to complete the eradication program.

A widely used inactivated vaccine of considerable public health importance is the influenza vaccine. Influenza viruses grown in chicken eggs are used in two types of vaccines. The most common vaccine is a trivalent inactivated (killed) vaccine that is used in the flu shot that is given intramuscularly. Three of the most frequently encountered influenza strains are selected every year and incorporated in this vaccine. A second type of influenza vaccine involves the same three strains, but the vaccine is made up of live attenuated viruses and is used as a nasal spray.

Purified Antigen (Subunit) Vaccines

Subunit vaccines are composed of antigens purified from microbes or inactivated toxins and are usually administered with an adjuvant. One effective use of purified antigens as vaccines is for the prevention of diseases caused by bacterial toxins. Toxins can be rendered harmless without loss of immunogenicity, and such toxoids induce strong antibody responses. Diphtheria and tetanus are two infections whose life-threatening consequences have been largely controlled because of immunization of children with toxoid preparations. Vaccines composed of bacterial polysaccharide antigens are used against pneumococcus and *H. influenzae*. Because polysaccharides are T-independent antigens, they tend to elicit low-affinity antibody responses and may be poorly immunogenic in infants (who do not mount strong T cell–independent antibody responses). High-affinity antibody responses may be generated against polysaccharide antigens even in infants by coupling the polysaccharides to proteins to form **conjugate vaccines**. Such vaccines work like hapten-carrier conjugates and are a practical application of the principle of T-B cell cooperation (see Chapter 12). The currently used *H. influenzae*, pneumococcal, and meningococcal vaccines are conjugate vaccines. Purified protein vaccines stimulate helper T cells and antibody responses, but they do not generate potent CTLs. The reason for poor CTL development is that exogenous proteins (and peptides) are inefficient at entering the class I MHC pathway of antigen presentation. As a result, protein vaccines are not recognized efficiently by class I–restricted CD8+ T cells.

Synthetic Antigen Vaccines

A goal of vaccine research has been to identify the most immunogenic microbial antigens or epitopes, to synthesize these in the laboratory, and to use the synthetic antigens as vaccines. It is possible to deduce the protein sequences of microbial antigens from nucleotide sequence data and to prepare large quantities of proteins by recombinant DNA technology. Vaccines made of recombinant DNA–derived antigens are now in use for hepatitis virus, herpes simplex virus, foot-and-mouth disease virus (a major pathogen for livestock), human papillomavirus, and rotavirus. In the case of the most widely used human papillomavirus vaccine, which was developed to prevent virally induced cancers, recombinant viral proteins from four viral strains (HPV 6, 11, 16, and 18) are made in yeast and combined with an adjuvant. HPV 6 and 11 are common causes of warts, and HPV 16 and 18 are the most common HPV strains linked to cervical cancer.

Live Viral Vaccines Involving Recombinant Viruses

Another approach for vaccine development is to introduce genes encoding microbial antigens into a non-cytopathic virus and to infect individuals with this virus. Thus, the virus serves as a source of the antigen in an inoculated individual. The great advantage of viral vectors is that they, like other live viruses, induce the full complement of immune responses, including strong CTL responses. This technique has been used most commonly with vaccinia virus vectors. Inoculation of such recombinant viruses into many species of animals induces both humoral and cell-mediated immunity against the antigen produced by the foreign gene (and, of course, against vaccinia virus antigens as well). A potential problem with recombinant viruses is that the viruses may infect host cells, and even though they are not pathogenic, they may produce antigens that stimulate CTL responses that kill the infected host cells. These and other safety concerns have limited widespread use of viral vectors for vaccine delivery.

DNA Vaccines

An interesting method of vaccination was developed on the basis of an unexpected observation. Inoculation of a plasmid containing complementary DNA (cDNA) encoding a protein antigen leads to humoral and cell-mediated immune responses to the antigen. It is likely that APCs, such as dendritic cells, are transfected by the plasmid and the cDNA is transcribed and translated into immunogenic protein that elicits specific responses. Bacterial plasmids are rich in unmethylated CpG nucleotides and are recognized by a TLR (TLR9) in dendritic cells and other cells, thereby eliciting an innate immune response that enhances adaptive immunity (see Chapter 4). Therefore, plasmid DNA vaccines could be effective even when administered without adjuvants. The ability to store DNA without refrigeration for use in the field also makes this technique promising. However, DNA vaccines have not been as effective as hoped in clinical trials, and the factors that determine the efficacy of these vaccines, especially in humans, are still not fully defined.

Adjuvants and Immunomodulators

The initiation of T cell–dependent immune responses against protein antigens requires that the antigens be administered with adjuvants. Most adjuvants elicit innate immune responses, with increased expression of costimulators and production of cytokines such as IL-12 that stimulate T cell growth and differentiation. Heat-killed bacteria are powerful adjuvants that are commonly used in experimental animals. However, the severe local inflammation that such adjuvants trigger precludes their use in humans. Much effort is currently being devoted to development of safe and effective adjuvants for use in humans. Only two are approved for patients–aluminum hydroxide gel (which appears to promote B cell responses) and a lipid formulation called Squalene that may activate phagocytes. An alternative to adjuvants is to administer natural substances that stimulate T cell responses together with antigens. For instance, IL-12 incorporated in vaccines promotes strong cell-mediated immunity. As mentioned, plasmid DNA has intrinsic adjuvant-like activities, and it is possible to incorporate costimulators (e.g., B7 molecules) or cytokines into plasmid DNA vaccines. These interesting ideas remain experimental.

Passive Immunization

Protective immunity can also be conferred by passive immunization, for instance, by transfer of specific antibodies. In the clinical situation, passive immunization is most commonly used for rapid treatment of potentially fatal diseases caused by toxins, such as tetanus, and for protection from rabies and hepatitis. Antibodies against snake venom can be lifesaving when administered after poisonous snakebites. Passive immunity is short-lived because the host does not respond to the immunization, and protection lasts only as long as the injected antibody persists. Moreover, passive immunization does not induce memory, so an immunized individual is not protected against subsequent exposure to the toxin or microbe.

SUMMARY

* The interaction of the immune system with infectious organisms is a dynamic interplay of host mechanisms aimed at eliminating infections and microbial strategies designed to permit survival in the face of powerful defenses. Different types of infectious agents stimulate distinct types of immune responses and have evolved unique mechanisms for evading immunity. In some infections, the immune response is the cause of tissue injury and disease.

* Innate immunity against extracellular bacteria is mediated by phagocytes and the complement system (the alternative and lectin pathways).

* The principal adaptive immune response against extracellular bacteria consists of specific antibodies that opsonize the bacteria for phagocytosis and activate the complement system. Toxins produced by such bacteria are neutralized by specific antibodies. Some bacterial toxins are powerful inducers of cytokine production, and cytokines account for much of the systemic disease associated with severe, disseminated infections with these microbes.

* Innate immunity against intracellular bacteria is mediated mainly by macrophages. However, intracellular bacteria are capable of surviving and replicating within host cells, including phagocytes, because they have developed mechanisms for resisting degradation within phagocytes.

* Adaptive immunity against intracellular bacteria is principally cell mediated and consists of activation of macrophages by CD4+ T cells as well as killing of infected cells by CD8+ CTLs. The characteristic pathologic response to infection by intracellular bacteria is granulomatous inflammation.

* Protective responses to fungi consist of innate immunity, mediated by neutrophils and macrophages, and adaptive cell-mediated and humoral immunity. Fungi are usually readily eliminated by phagocytes and a competent immune system, because of which disseminated fungal infections are seen mostly in immunodeficient persons.

* Innate immunity against viruses is mediated by type I interferons and NK cells. Neutralizing antibodies protect against virus entry into cells early in the course of infection and later if the viruses are released from killed infected cells. The major defense mechanism against established infection is CTL-mediated killing of infected cells. CTLs may contribute to tissue injury even when the infectious virus is not harmful by itself. Viruses evade immune responses by antigenic variation, inhibition of antigen presentation, and production of immunosuppressive molecules.

* Parasites such as protozoa and helminths give rise to chronic and persistent infections because innate immunity against them is weak and parasites have evolved multiple mechanisms for evading and resisting specific immunity. The structural and antigenic diversity of pathogenic parasites is reflected in the heterogeneity of the adaptive immune responses that they elicit. Protozoa that live within host cells are destroyed by cell-mediated immunity, whereas helminths are eliminated by IgE antibody and eosinophil-mediated killing as well as by other leukocytes. Parasites evade the immune system by varying their antigens during residence in vertebrate hosts, by acquiring resistance to immune effector mechanisms, and by masking and shedding their surface antigens.

⁕ Vaccination is a powerful strategy for preventing infections. The most effective vaccines are those that stimulate the production of high-affinity antibodies and memory cells. Many approaches for vaccinating are in clinical use and being tried for various infections.

SELECTED READINGS

General Principles

Alcais A, Abel L, Casanova J-L: Human genetics of infectious diseases: between proof of principle and paradigm, *Journal of Clinical Investigation* 119:2506–2514, 2009.

Dorhol A, Kaufmann SH: Fine-tuning T cell responses during infection, *Current Opinion in Immunology* 21:367–377, 2009.

Finlay BB, McFadden G: Anti-immunology: evasion of the host immune system by bacterial and viral pathogens, *Cell* 124:767–782, 2006.

Immunity to Extracellular and Intracellular Bacteria

Baxt LA, Garza-Mayers AC, Goldberg MB: Bacterial subversion of host immune pathways, *Science* 340:697–701, 2013.

Brodsky IE, Medzhitov R: Targeting of immune signaling networks by bacterial pathogens, *Nature Cell Biology* 11:521–526, 2009.

Curtis MM, Way SS: Interleukin-17 in host defence against bacterial, mycobacterial and fungal pathogens, *Immunology* 126:177–185, 2009.

O'Garra A, Redford PS, McNab FW, et al.: The immune response in tuberculosis, *Annual Review of Immunology* 31:475–527, 2013.

Immunity to Viruses

Antoniou AN, Powis SJ: Pathogen evasion strategies for the major histocompatibility complex class I assembly pathway, *Immunology* 124:1–12, 2008.

Klenerman P, Hill A: T cells and viral persistence: lessons from diverse infections, *Nature Immunology* 6:873–879, 2005.

Perry AK, Chen G, Zheng D, Tang H, Cheng G: The host type I interferon response to viral and bacterial infections, *Cell Research* 15:407–422, 2005.

Rouse BT, Seherwat S: Immunity and immunopathology to viruses: what decides the outcome? *Nature Reviews Immunology* 10:514–526, 2010.

Virgin HW, Wherry EJ, Ahmed R: Redefining chronic viral infection, *Cell* 138:30–50, 2009.

Yan N, Chen ZJ: Intrinsic antiviral immunity, *Nature Immunology* 13:214–222, 2012.

Immunity to Fungi

Romani L: Immunity to fungal infections, *Nature Reviews Immunology* 11:275–288, 2011.

Wuthrich M, Deepe GS, Klein B: Adaptive immunity to fungi, *Annual Review of Immunology* 30:115–148, 2012.

Immunity to Parasites

Good MF, Xu H, Wykes M, Engwerda CR: Development and regulation of cell-mediated immune responses to the blood stages of malaria: implications for vaccine research, *Annual Review of Immunology* 23:69–99, 2005.

Langhorne J, Ndungu FM, Sponaas A-M, Marsh K: Immunity to malaria: more questions than answers, *Nature Immunology* 9:725–732, 2008.

Maizels RM, Pearce EJ, Artis D, Yazdanbaksh M, Wynn TA: Regulation of pathogenesis and immunity in helminth infections, *Journal of Experimental Medicine* 201:2059–2066, 2009.

McCulloch R: Antigenic variation in African trypanosomes: monitoring progress, *Trends in Parasitology* 20:117–121, 2004.

Vaccines and Adjuvants

Brunner R, Jensen-Jarolim E, Pali-Scholl I: The ABC of clinical and experimental adjuvants—a brief overview, *Immunology Letters* 128:29–35, 2010.

Donnelly JJ, Wahren B, Liu MA: DNA vaccines: progress and challenges, *Journal of Immunology* 175:633–639, 2005.

Harris J, Sharp FA, Lavelle EC: The role of inflammasomes in the immunostimulatory effects of particulate vaccine adjuvants, *European Journal of Immunology* 40:634–638, 2010.

Koff WC, Burton DR, Johnson PR, et al.: Accelerating next-generation vaccine development for global disease prevention, *Science* 340:1232910, 2013.

Transplantation Immunology

Transplantation is a widely used treatment for replacement of non-functioning organs and tissues with healthy organs or tissues. Technically, transplantation is the process of taking cells, tissues, or organs, called a **graft**, from one individual and placing them into a (usually) different individual. The individual who provides the graft is called the **donor**, and the individual who receives the graft is called either the **recipient** or the **host**. If the graft is placed into its normal anatomic location, the procedure is called orthotopic transplantation; if the graft is placed in a different site, the procedure is called heterotopic transplantation. **Transfusion** refers to the transfer of circulating blood cells or plasma from one individual to another. Clinical transplantation to treat human diseases has increased steadily during the past 45 years. Transplantation of hematopoietic stem cells, kidneys, livers, and hearts is widely used today, and transplantation of other organs such as lung and pancreas is becoming more frequent (Fig. 17-1). More than 30,000 kidney, heart, lung, and liver transplants are currently performed in the United States each year. In addition, transplantation of many other organs or cells, including tissue stem cells, is now being attempted.

Once the technical challenge of surgically transplanting organs was overcome, it soon became clear that the immune response against grafted tissues was the major barrier to transplantation. Conversely, controlling this immune response is the key to successful transplantation. These realizations have led to the development of transplantation immunology as a discipline within the broader topic of immunology, and this is the theme of the chapter.

GENERAL PRINCIPLES OF TRANSPLANTATION IMMUNOLOGY

Based on experimental studies and clinical observations, several principles are now established that apply to reactions to transplants and to no other immune responses. These are summarized next.

Transplantation of cells or tissues from one individual to a genetically non-identical individual invariably leads to rejection of the transplant due to an adaptive immune response. This problem was first appreciated when attempts to replace damaged skin on burn patients with skin from unrelated donors proved to be uniformly unsuccessful. During a matter of 1 to 2 weeks, the transplanted skin would undergo necrosis and fall off. The failure of the grafts led Peter Medawar and other investigators to study skin transplantation in animal models. These experiments established that the failure of skin grafting was caused by an inflammatory reaction, which they called **rejection**. The conclusion that graft rejection is the result of an adaptive immune response

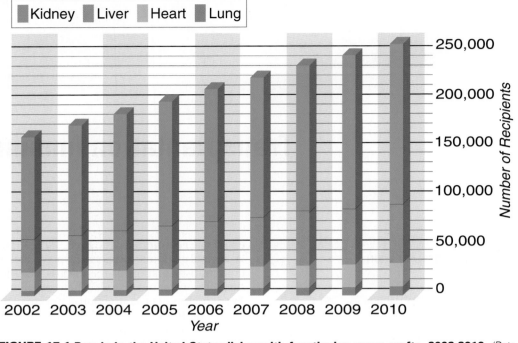

FIGURE 17-1 People in the United States living with functioning organ grafts, 2002-2010. *(Data from* SRTR annual report 2012. *Available at* http://www.srtr.org/. *Accessed April 2013.)*

came from experiments demonstrating that the process had characteristics of memory and specificity and was mediated by lymphocytes (Fig. 17-2). For instance, rejection occurs 10 to 14 days after the first transplant from a donor to a non-identical recipient (called first-set rejection) and more rapidly after the second transplant from the same donor to this recipient (called second-set rejection), implying that the recipient developed memory for the grafted tissue. Individuals who have rejected a graft from one donor show accelerated rejection of another graft from the same donor but not from a different donor, demonstrating that the rejection process is immunologically specific. These experimental results were recapitulated in clinical transplantation. Perhaps the most compelling evidence showing that allograft rejection is an adaptive immune response was the finding that the ability to rapidly reject a transplant can be transferred with lymphocytes from a sensitized to a naive host.

Transplant immunologists have developed a special vocabulary to describe the kinds of cells and tissues encountered in the transplant setting. A graft transplanted from one individual to the same individual is called an **autologous graft**. A graft transplanted between two genetically identical individuals is called a **syngeneic graft**. A graft transplanted between two genetically different individuals of the same species is called an **allogeneic graft** (or **allograft**). A graft transplanted between individuals of different species is called a **xenogeneic graft** (or **xenograft**). The molecules that are recognized as foreign on allografts are called **alloantigens**, and those on xenografts are called **xenoantigens**. The lymphocytes and antibodies that react with alloantigens or xenoantigens are described as being **alloreactive** or **xenoreactive**, respectively.

Most of this chapter focuses on allogeneic transplantation because it is far more commonly practiced and better understood than xenogeneic transplantation, which is discussed briefly at the end of the chapter. We will consider both the basic immunology and some aspects of the clinical practice of transplantation. We will conclude the chapter with a discussion of hematopoietic stem cell transplantation, which raises special issues not usually encountered with solid organ transplants.

ADAPTIVE IMMUNE RESPONSES TO ALLOGRAFTS

Alloantigens elicit both cellular and humoral immune responses. In this section, we will discuss the molecular and cellular mechanisms of allorecognition, with emphasis on the nature of graft antigens that stimulate allogeneic responses and the properties of the responding lymphocytes.

The Nature of Alloantigens

The antigens that stimulate adaptive immune responses against allografts are histocompatibility proteins, encoded by polymorphic genes that differ among individuals. As we discussed in Chapter 6, all of the animals of an inbred strain are genetically identical, and they are homozygous for all genes (except the sex chromosomes in males). In contrast, inbred animals of different strains, and individuals in an outbred species (except identical twins), differ in the genes they inherit, including histocompatibilty genes. The basic rules of transplantation immunology, which were first established from experiments largely with genetically defined mice, are the following (Fig. 17-3).

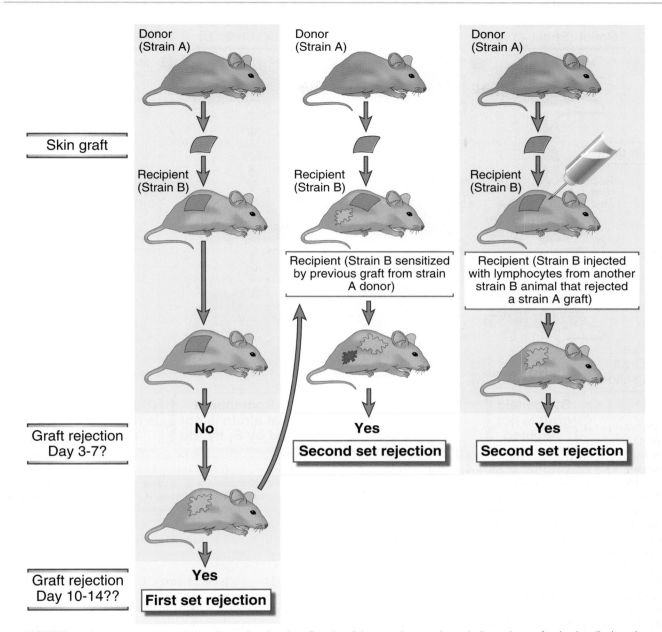

FIGURE 17-2 First- and second-set allograft rejection. Results of the experiments shown indicate that graft rejection displays the features of adaptive immune responses, namely, memory and mediation by lymphocytes. An inbred strain B mouse will reject a graft from an inbred strain A mouse with first-set kinetics *(left panel)*. An inbred strain B mouse sensitized by a previous graft from an inbred strain A mouse will reject a second graft from an inbred strain A mouse with second-set kinetics *(middle panel)*, demonstrating memory. An inbred strain B mouse injected with lymphocytes from another strain B mouse that has rejected a graft from a strain A mouse will reject a graft from a strain A mouse with second-set kinetics *(right panel)*, demonstrating the role of lymphocytes in mediating rejection and memory. An inbred strain B mouse sensitized by a previous graft from a strain A mouse will reject a graft from a third unrelated strain with first-set kinetics, thus demonstrating another feature of adaptive immunity, specificity *(not shown)*. Syngeneic grafts are never rejected *(not shown)*.

- Cells or organs transplanted between genetically identical individuals (identical twins or members of the same inbred strain of animals) are never rejected.
- Cells or organs transplanted between genetically nonidentical people or members of two different inbred strains of a species are always rejected.
- The offspring of a mating between two different inbred strains of animal will not reject grafts from either parent. In other words, an (A × B) F₁ animal will not reject grafts from an A or B strain animal. (This rule is violated by bone marrow transplantation, when NK cells in an [A x B] F1 recipient do reject bone marrow cells from either parent, as we will discuss later in this chapter.)
- A graft derived from the offspring of a mating between two different inbred strains of animal will be rejected by either parent. In other words, a graft from an (A × B) F₁ animal will be rejected by either an A or a B strain animal.

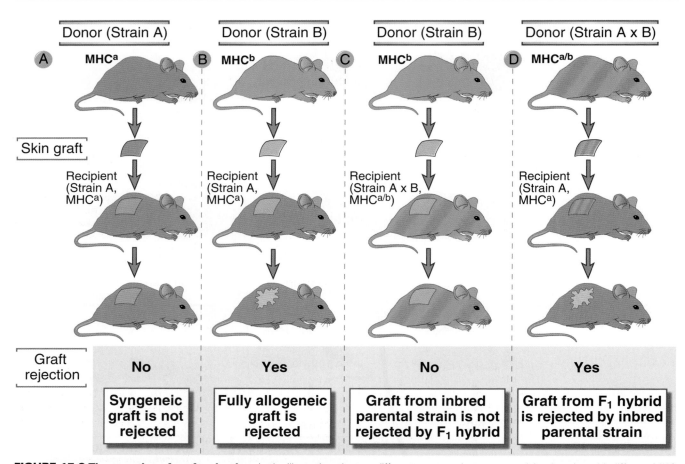

FIGURE 17-3 The genetics of graft rejection. In the illustration, the two different mouse colors represent inbred strains with different MHC haplotypes. Inherited MHC alleles from both parents are codominantly expressed in the skin of an A × B offspring, and therefore these mice are represented by both colors. Syngeneic grafts are not rejected **(A)**. Allografts are always rejected **(B)**. Grafts from an A or B parent will not be rejected by an (A × B)F1 offspring **(C)**, but grafts from the offspring will be rejected by either parent **(D)**. These phenomena are due to the fact that *MHC* gene products are responsible for graft rejection; grafts are rejected only if they express an MHC type (represented by green or orange) that is not expressed by the recipient mouse.

Such results suggested that the molecules in the grafts that are responsible for eliciting rejection must be polymorphic and their expression is codominant. **Polymorphic** refers to the fact that these graft antigens differ among the individuals of a species (other than identical twins) or between different inbred strains of animals. Codominant expression means that every individual inherits genes encoding these molecules from both parents, and both parental alleles are expressed. Therefore, (A × B) F_1 animals express both A and B alleles and see both A and B tissues as self, whereas inbred A or B animals express only one allele and see (A × B) F_1 tissues as partly foreign. This is why an (A × B) F_1 animal does not reject either A or B strain grafts and why both A and B strain recipients reject an (A × B) F_1 graft.

The molecules responsible for strong (rapid) rejection reactions are called major histocompatibility complex (MHC) molecules. George Snell and colleagues produced pairs of congenic strains of inbred mice that were bred to be genetically identical to each other except for genes needed for graft rejection. They used these mice to identify the polymorphic genes that

encode the molecular targets of allograft rejection, which were called MHC genes. Transplants of most tissues between any pair of individuals, except identical twins, will be rejected because MHC molecules are so polymorphic that no two individuals inherit the same ones. As discussed in Chapter 6, the normal function of MHC molecules is to present peptides derived from protein antigens in a form that can be recognized by T cells. The role of MHC molecules as the antigens that cause graft rejection is a consequence of the nature of T cell antigen recognition, as we will discuss later. Recall that human MHC molecules are called human leukocyte antigens (HLA), and in the context of human transplantation, the terms *MHC* and *HLA* are used interchangeably.

In the setting of any transplant between genetically non-identical donor and recipient, there will be polymorphic antigens other than MHC molecules against which the recipient may mount an immune response. These antigens typically induce weak or slower (more gradual) rejection reactions than do MHC molecules and are therefore called **minor histocompatibility antigens**. Most minor histocompatibility antigens are

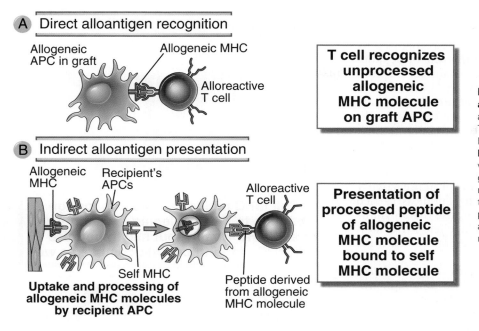

A Direct alloantigen recognition

Allogeneic APC in graft — Allogeneic MHC

Alloreactive T cell

T cell recognizes unprocessed allogeneic MHC molecule on graft APC

B Indirect alloantigen presentation

Allogeneic MHC — Recipient's APCs

Alloreactive T cell

Self MHC

Uptake and processing of allogeneic MHC molecules by recipient APC

Peptide derived from allogeneic MHC molecule

Presentation of processed peptide of allogeneic MHC molecule bound to self MHC molecule

FIGURE 17-4 **Direct and indirect alloantigen recognition.** **A,** Direct alloantigen recognition occurs when T cells bind directly to an intact allogeneic MHC molecule on a graft (donor) APC. **B,** Indirect alloantigen recognition occurs when allogeneic MHC molecules from graft cells are taken up and processed by recipient APCs and peptide fragments of the allogeneic MHC molecules containing polymorphic amino acid residues are bound and presented by recipient (self) MHC molecules. *APC,* antigen-presenting cell.

proteins that are processed and presented to host T cells in association with self MHC molecules on host antigen-presenting cells (APCs), similar to any protein antigen. The relevance of minor histocompatibility antigens in clinical solid organ transplantation is uncertain, mainly because there has been little success in identifying the relevant antigens. In mice, the male H-Y antigen appears to be a target of immune recognition by female recipients of grafts from male donors. Although in humans there is a slightly higher risk of rejection of heart transplants from male donor to female recipient, compared with sex-matched transplants, given the scarcity of donor hearts, sex matching is not practical. Minor histocompatibility antigens play a more significant role in stimulating graft-versus-host responses after hematopoietic stem cell transplantation, discussed later, but the nature of the relevant antigens in that setting is also not defined.

Recognition of Alloantigens by T Cells

Allogeneic MHC molecules of a graft can be presented for recognition by the recipient's T cells in two fundamentally different ways, called the direct and indirect pathways (Fig. 17-4). Initial studies showed that the T cells of a graft recipient recognize intact, unprocessed MHC molecules in the graft, and this is called **direct recognition of alloantigens**. Subsequent studies showed that sometimes the recipient T cells recognize graft MHC molecules only in the context of the recipient's MHC molecules, implying that the recipient's MHC molecules must be presenting allogeneic graft MHC proteins to recipient T cells. This process is called **indirect recognition**, and it is essentially the same as the recognition of any foreign (e.g., microbial) protein antigen. Not only MHC molecules but minor histocompatibility antigens can also be presented to host T cells by the indirect pathway. Either direct or indirect T cell recognition of alloantigens is an initial step in most

forms of allograft rejection. It is likely that, regardless of which pathway and graft antigens are recognized by host T cells, the initial response occurs in lymph nodes draining the graft, as we will discuss later. In this case, the APCs carrying the antigen must be capable of migrating from the graft to the lymph nodes.

Direct Recognition of MHC Alloantigens on Donor Cells

In the case of direct recognition, intact MHC molecules displayed by cells in the graft are recognized by recipient T cells without a need for processing by host APCs (see Fig. 17-5, *A*). It may seem puzzling that T cells that are normally selected during their maturation to be self MHC restricted are capable of recognizing foreign (allogeneic or xenogeneic) MHC molecules. A likely explanation is that T cell receptors (TCRs) have an inherent specificity for MHC molecules, regardless of whether they are self or foreign. In other words, TCR genes have evolved to encode a receptor structure that has some intrinsic affinity for MHC molecules. Furthermore, during T cell development in the thymus, positive selection promotes survival of T cells with weak self MHC reactivity, and among these T cells, there may be many with strong reactivity to allogeneic MHC molecules. Although negative selection in the thymus efficiently eliminates T cells with high affinity for self MHC (see Chapters 8 and 15), it will not necessarily eliminate T cells that bind strongly to allogeneic MHC molecules, simply because these molecules are not present in the thymus. The result is that the mature repertoire has an intrinsic weak affinity for self MHC molecules and includes many T cells that bind allogeneic MHC molecules with high affinity. Therefore, one can think of direct allorecognition as an example of an immunologic cross-reaction in which a T cell that was selected to be self MHC restricted is able to bind structurally similar allogeneic MHC molecules with high enough affinity to permit activation of the T cell.

MHC molecules that are expressed on cell surfaces normally contain bound peptides, and in some cases, the peptide contributes to the structure recognized by the alloreactive T cell, exactly like the role of peptides in the normal recognition of foreign antigens by self MHC–restricted T cells (Fig. 17-5, *B*). Even though these peptides may be derived from proteins that are present in both donor and recipient, on the graft cells, they are displayed by allogeneic MHC molecules. Therefore the complexes of peptides (self or foreign) with allogeneic MHC molecules will appear different from self peptide–self MHC complexes. In other cases, direct recognition and activation of an alloreactive T cell may occur regardless of which peptide is carried by the allogeneic MHC molecule, because the polymorphic amino acid residues of the allogeneic MHC molecule alone form a structure that resembles self MHC plus peptide (Fig. 17-5, *C*).

T cell responses to directly presented allogeneic MHC molecules are very strong because there is a high frequency of T cells that can directly recognize any single allogeneic MHC. It is estimated that up to 1% to 2% of all T cells in an individual will directly recognize an allogeneic MHC molecule on a donor cell, which is 100 to 1000 times greater than the frequency of T cells specific for any microbial peptide displayed by self MHC molecules. There are several explanations for this high frequency of T cells that can directly recognize allo-MHC.

- Many different peptides derived from donor cellular proteins may combine with a single allogeneic MHC molecule, and each of these peptide-MHC combinations can theoretically activate a different clone of recipient T cells. This is because the peptide-binding groove of MHC molecules can accommodate many different peptides, and each peptide in combination with the same MHC molecule will look different to TCRs and will bind to different clones of T cells.
- Every APC expresses thousands of copies of different MHC molecules on its surface, and if these are foreign MHC molecules, many or all of them can be recognized by alloreactive T cells. In contrast, in the case of an infection, less than 1% (and perhaps as few as 0.1%) of the self MHC molecules on an APC normally present any microbial peptide at one time, and only these can be recognized by T cells specific for the microbial antigen.
- Many of the T cells that respond to an allogeneic MHC molecule, even on first exposure, are memory T cells. It is likely that these memory cells were generated during previous exposure to other foreign (e.g., microbial) antigens and cross-react with allogeneic MHC molecules. These memory cells not only are expanded populations of antigen-specific cells but also are more rapid and powerful responders than are naive lymphocytes, and thus contribute to the greater strength of the alloreactive T cell response.

Direct allorecognition can generate both CD4+ and CD8+ T cells that recognize graft antigens and contribute to rejection. The role of the alloreactive T cell response in rejection is described later.

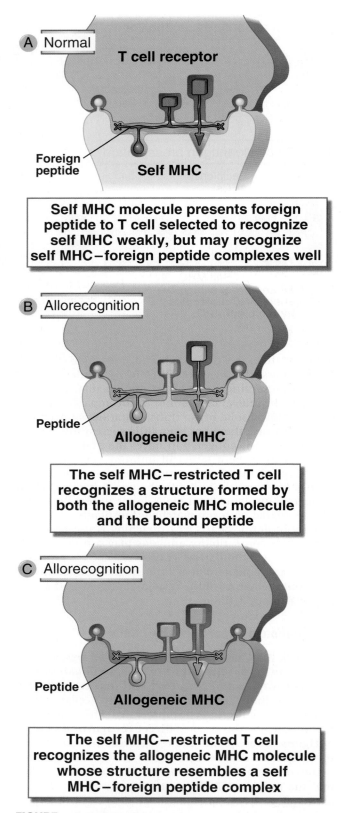

FIGURE 17-5 Molecular basis of direct recognition of allogeneic MHC molecules. Direct recognition of allogeneic MHC molecules may be thought of as a cross-reaction in which a T cell specific for a self MHC molecule–foreign peptide complex **(A)** also recognizes an allogeneic MHC molecule **(B, C)**. Peptides that bind to MHC molecules in the graft may contribute to allorecognition **(B)** or they may not **(C)**.

Indirect Recognition of Alloantigens

In the indirect pathway, donor (allogeneic) MHC molecules are captured and processed by recipient APCs, and peptides derived from the allogeneic MHC molecules are presented in association with self MHC molecules (see Fig. 17-4, *B*). Thus, peptides from the allogeneic MHC molecules are displayed by host APCs and recognized by T cells like conventional foreign protein antigens. Because allogeneic MHC molecules have amino acid sequences different from those of the host, they can generate foreign peptides associated with self MHC molecules on the surface of host APCs. In fact, MHC molecules are the most polymorphic proteins in the genome; therefore, each allogeneic MHC molecule may give rise to multiple peptides that are foreign for the host, each recognized by different T cells. Indirect presentation may result in allorecognition by CD4$^+$ T cells because alloantigen is acquired by host APCs primarily through the endosomal vesicular pathway (i.e., as a consequence of phagocytosis) and is therefore presented by class II MHC molecules. Some antigens of phagocytosed graft cells appear to enter the class I MHC pathway of antigen presentation and are indirectly recognized by CD8$^+$ T cells. This phenomenon is an example of cross-presentation or cross-priming (see Fig. 6-20), in which dendritic cells ingest antigens of another cell, from the graft, and present these antigens on class I MHC molecules to activate (prime) CD8$^+$ T lymphocytes.

Evidence that indirect recognition of allogeneic MHC molecules plays a significant role in graft rejection comes from studies with knockout mice lacking class II MHC expression. For example, skin grafts from donor mice lacking class II MHC are able to induce recipient CD4$^+$ (i.e., class II MHC–restricted) T cell responses to peptides derived from donor class I MHC molecules. In these experiments, the donor class I MHC molecules are processed and presented by class II molecules on the recipient's APCs and stimulate the recipient's helper T cells. Evidence has also been obtained that indirect antigen presentation may contribute to late rejection of human allografts. CD4$^+$ T cells from heart and liver allograft recipients recognize and are activated by peptides derived from donor MHC when presented by the patient's own APCs.

The relative importance of direct and indirect allorecognition in graft rejection is a matter of continuing debate. It is often stated that acute graft rejection is mediated mostly by direct recognition of alloantigens, primarily by CD8$^+$ T cells that directly destroy the graft, whereas chronic graft rejection has a larger component of indirect recognition, resulting in activation of CD4$^+$ T cells that induce rejection mainly by triggering cytokine-mediated inflammation, and by helping B cells to make antibodies against alloantigens.

Activation and Effector Functions of Alloreactive T Lymphocytes

When lymphocytes recognize alloantigens, they become activated to proliferate, differentiate, and perform effector functions that can damage grafts. The activation steps are similar to those we have described for lymphocytes reacting to microbial antigens.

Activation of Alloreactive T Lymphocytes

The T cell response to an organ graft may be initiated in the lymph nodes that drain the graft (Fig. 17-6). Most organs contain resident APCs such as dendritic cells, and therefore transplantation of these organs into an allogeneic recipient provides APCs that express donor MHC molecules as well as costimulators. It is believed that these donor APCs migrate to regional lymph nodes and present, on their surface, unprocessed allogeneic MHC molecules to the recipient's T cells (the direct pathway of allorecognition). Host dendritic cells from the recipient may also migrate into the graft, pick up graft alloantigens, and transport these back to the draining lymph nodes, where they are displayed (the indirect pathway). The connection between lymphatic vessel in allografts and the recipient's lymph nodes is not made surgically, and is likely established by growth of new lymphatic channels in response to inflammatory stimuli produced during grafting. Naive lymphocytes that normally traffic through the lymph node encounter these alloantigens and are induced to proliferate and differentiate into effector cells. This process is sometimes called sensitization to alloantigens. Effector T cells migrate back into the graft and mediate rejection.

As discussed earlier, many of the T cells that respond to the allogeneic MHC antigens in a new graft are cross-reactive memory T cells previously generated to environmental antigens before transplantation. Unlike naive T cells, memory T cells may not need to see antigens presented by dendritic cells in lymph nodes in order to be activated, and they may migrate directly into grafts where they can be activated by APCs or tissue cells displaying alloantigen.

Role of Costimulation in T Cell Responses to Alloantigens

In addition to recognition of alloantigen, costimulation of T cells primarily by B7 molecules on APCs is important for activating alloreactive T cells. Rejection of allografts, and stimulation of alloreactive T cells in a mixed lymphocyte reaction (described later), can be inhibited by agents that block B7 molecules. Allografts survive for longer periods when they are transplanted into knockout mice lacking B7-1 (CD80) and B7-2 (CD86) compared with transplants into normal recipients. As we will discuss later, blocking of B7 costimulation is a therapeutic strategy to inhibit graft rejection in humans as well.

The requirement for costimulation leads to the interesting question of why these costimulators are expressed by graft APCs in the absence of infection, which we have previously discussed as the physiologic stimulus for the expression of costimulators (see Chapter 9). One possibility is that the process of organ transplantation is associated with ischemic damage and death of some cells in the graft, during the time the organ is removed from the donor and before it is surgically connected to the circulatory system of the recipient. Several molecules expressed by or released from ischemically damaged cells (so-called damage-associated molecular patterns, discussed in Chapter 4) stimulate innate immune responses that result in increased expression of costimulators on

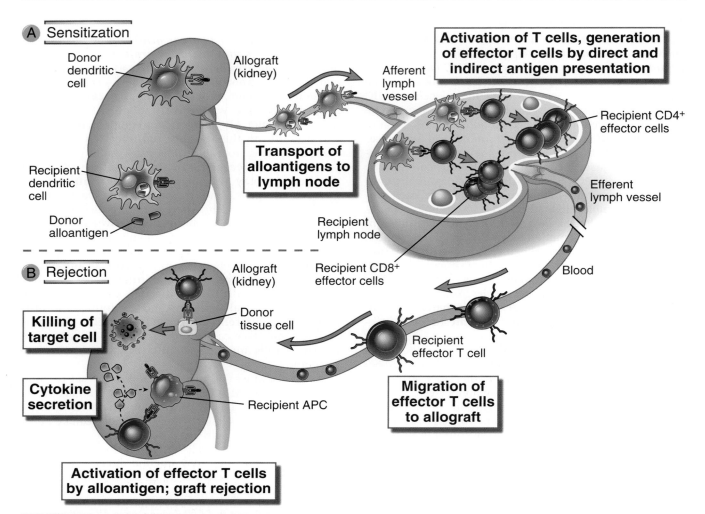

FIGURE 17-6 Activation of alloreactive T cells. A, In the case of direct allorecognition, donor dendritic cells in the allograft migrate to secondary lymphoid tissues, where they present allogeneic MHC molecules to host T cells. In the case of indirect allorecognition, recipient dendritic cells that have entered the allograft transport donor MHC proteins to secondary lymphoid tissues and present peptides derived from these MHC proteins to alloreactive host T cells. In both cases, the T cells become activated and differentiate into effector cells. **B,** The alloreactive effector T cells migrate into the allograft, become reactivated by alloantigen, and mediate damage.

APCs. In fact, the clinical experience is that the ischemia time of an organ is a determinant of the frequency and severity of rejection, and one reason for this may be that death of graft cells during ischemia stimulates subsequent anti-graft immune responses.

The Mixed Lymphocyte Reaction

The response of alloreactive T cells to foreign MHC molecules can be analyzed in an in vitro reaction called the **mixed lymphocyte reaction** (MLR). The MLR was used clinically in the past as a predictive test of T cell–mediated graft rejection, and as an in vitro model of graft rejection. Studies of the MLR were among the first to establish the role of class I and class II MHC molecules in activating distinct populations of T cells (CD8+ and CD4+, respectively).

The MLR is induced by culturing mononuclear leukocytes (which include T cells, B cells, natural killer [NK] cells, mononuclear phagocytes, and dendritic cells) from one individual with mononuclear leukocytes derived from another individual. In clinical practice, these cells

were typically isolated from peripheral blood; in mouse or rat experiments, mononuclear leukocytes are usually purified from the spleen or lymph nodes. If the two individuals differ in MHC alleles, a large proportion of the lymphocytes in these cultures will proliferate during a period of 4 to 7 days. This proliferative response is called the allogeneic MLR (Fig. 17-7). If cells from two MHC-disparate individuals are mixed, each can react against the other and both will proliferate, thus resulting in a two-way MLR. To simplify the analysis, one of the two leukocyte populations can be rendered incapable of proliferation before culture, either by γ-irradiation or by treatment with the anti-mitotic drug mitomycin C. In this one-way MLR, the treated cells serve exclusively as stimulators, and the untreated cells, still capable of proliferation, serve as the responders. Among the T cells that respond in an MLR, the CD4+ cells are specific for allogeneic class II MHC molecules and the CD8+ cells for class I molecules.

Because of the high frequency of T cells that can directly recognize allogeneic MHC, responses to

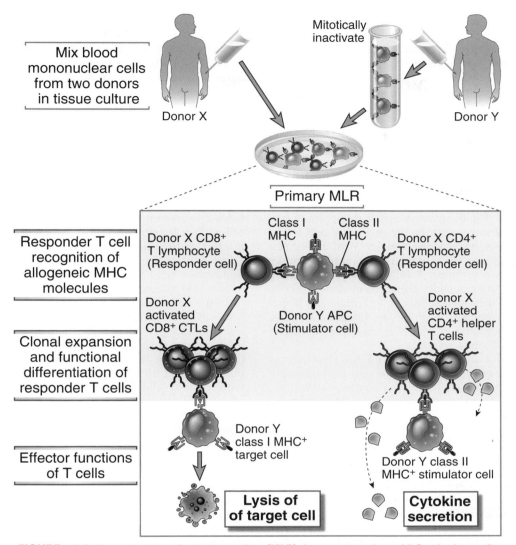

FIGURE 17-7 The mixed lymphocyte reaction (MLR). In a one-way primary MLR, stimulator cells (from donor Y) activate and cause the expansion of two types of responder T cells (from donor X). CD4+ T cells from donor X react to donor Y class II molecules, and CD8+ T lymphocytes from donor X react to donor Y class I MHC molecules. The CD4+ T cells differentiate into cytokine-secreting helper T cells, and the CD8+ T cells differentiate into CTLs. *APC*, antigen-presenting cell.

alloantigens are the only primary T cell responses (i.e., responses to an antigen by an individual who has not previously encountered the antigen) that can readily be detected in vitro. Responses of T cells to a non-MHC protein antigen in vitro can be detected only if the T cells are from an individual who has previously been immunized with that antigen (e.g., by infection or vaccination), because there are too few naive antigen-specific T cells to mount a detectable response in vitro.

Effector Functions of Alloreactive T Cells

Alloreactive CD4+ and CD8+ T cells that are activated by graft alloantigens cause rejection by distinct mechanisms (see Fig. 17-6). The CD4+ helper T cells differentiate into cytokine-producing effector cells that damage grafts by cytokine-mediated inflammation, similar to a delayed-type hypersensitivity (DTH) reaction (see Chapters 10 and 19). Alloreactive CD8+ T cells differentiate into cytotoxic

T lymphocytes (CTLs), which kill cells in the graft that express the allogeneic class I MHC molecules. CTLs also secrete inflammatory cytokines, which can contribute to graft damage.

Only CTLs that are generated by direct allorecognition can kill graft cells, whereas both CTLs and helper T cells generated by either direct or indirect alloantigen recognition can cause cytokine-mediated damage to grafts. CD8+ CTLs that are generated by direct allorecognition of donor MHC molecules on donor APCs can recognize the same MHC molecules on parenchymal cells in the graft and kill those cells. In contrast, any CD8+ CTLs that are generated by the indirect pathway are self MHC restricted, and they will not be able to kill the foreign graft cells because these cells do not express self MHC alleles displaying allogeneic peptides. Therefore, when alloreactive T cells are stimulated by the indirect pathway, the principal mechanism of rejection is not CTL-mediated killing of graft cells but inflammation caused by the cytokines produced by the effector T cells. Presumably, these effector cells infiltrate the graft and recognize graft alloantigens being displayed by host APCs that have also entered the graft.

Activation of Alloreactive B Cells and Production and Functions of Alloantibodies

Antibodies against graft antigens also contribute to rejection. Most high-affinity alloantibodies are produced by helper T cell–dependent activation of alloreactive B cells, much like antibodies against other protein antigens (see Chapter 12). The antigens most frequently recognized by alloantibodies are donor HLA molecules, including both class I and class II MHC proteins. The likely sequence of events leading to the generation of these alloantibody-producing cells is that naive B lymphocytes recognize foreign MHC molecules, internalize and process these proteins, and present peptides derived from them to helper T cells that were previously activated by the same peptides presented by dendritic cells. This is essentially the same sequence of events for any helper T cell-dependent antibody response (see Chapter 12). Thus, activation of alloreactive B cells is an example of indirect presentation of alloantigens.

The alloreactive antibodies produced in graft recipients engage the same effector mechanisms that antibodies use to combat infections, including complement activation, and targeting and activation of neutrophils, macrophages, and NK cells through Fc receptor binding. Because HLA antigens are expressed on endothelial cells, much of the alloantibody-mediated damage is targeted at the graft vasculature, as discussed in the section that follows.

PATTERNS AND MECHANISMS OF ALLOGRAFT REJECTION

Thus far, we have described the molecular basis of allo-antigen recognition and the cells involved in the recognition of and responses to allografts. We now turn to a consideration of the effector mechanisms responsible for the immunologic rejection of allografts. In different experimental models and in clinical transplantation, alloreactive CD4+ and CD8+ T cells and alloantibodies all have been shown to be capable of mediating allograft rejection. These different immune effectors cause graft rejection by different mechanisms, and all three effectors may contribute to rejection concurrently.

For historical reasons, graft rejection is classified on the basis of histopathologic features and the time course of rejection after transplantation rather than on the basis of immune effector mechanisms. Based on the experience of renal transplantation, the histopathologic patterns are called hyperacute, acute, and chronic (Fig. 17-8). These patterns are associated with different dominant immune effector mechanisms. We will describe these patterns of rejection with an emphasis on the underlying immune mechanisms.

Hyperacute Rejection

Hyperacute rejection is characterized by thrombotic occlusion of the graft vasculature that begins within minutes to hours after host blood vessels are anastomosed to graft vessels and is mediated by preexisting antibodies in the host circulation that bind to donor endothelial antigens (Fig. 17-8, *A*). Binding of antibody to endothelium activates complement, and antibody and complement products together induce a number of changes in the graft endothelium that promote intravascular thrombosis. Complement activation leads to endothelial cell injury and exposure of subendothelial basement membrane proteins that activate platelets. The endothelial cells are stimulated to secrete high–molecular-weight forms of von Willebrand factor, which cause platelet adhesion and aggregation. Both endothelial cells and platelets undergo membrane vesiculation, leading to shedding of lipid particles that promote coagulation. Endothelial cells lose the cell surface heparan sulfate proteoglycans that normally interact with antithrombin III to inhibit coagulation. These processes contribute to thrombosis and vascular occlusion (Fig. 17-9, *A*), and the grafted organ suffers irreversible ischemic necrosis.

In the early days of transplantation, hyperacute rejection was often mediated by preexisting IgM alloantibodies, which are present at high titer before transplantation. Such natural antibodies are believed to arise in response to carbohydrate antigens expressed by bacteria that normally colonize the intestine, and happen to cross-react with various alloantigens. The best known examples of such alloantibodies are those directed against the ABO blood group antigens expressed on red blood cells, described later in this chapter. ABO antigens are also expressed on vascular endothelial cells. Today, hyperacute rejection by anti-ABO antibodies is extremely rare because all donor and recipient pairs are selected so that they have compatible ABO types. As we will discuss later in this chapter, hyperacute rejection caused by natural antibodies is a major barrier to xenotransplantation and limits the use of animal organs for human transplantation.

Currently, hyperacute rejection of allografts, when it occurs, is usually mediated by IgG antibodies directed against protein alloantigens, such as donor MHC molecules, or against less well defined alloantigens expressed on vascular endothelial cells. Such antibodies generally arise as a result of previous exposure to alloantigens through blood transfusion, previous transplantation, or multiple pregnancies. If the level of these alloreactive antibodies is low, hyperacute rejection may develop slowly, during several days, but the onset is still earlier than that typical for acute rejection. As we will discuss later in this chapter, patients in need of allografts are routinely screened before grafting for the presence of antibodies that bind to cells of a potential organ donor to avoid hyperacute rejection.

In rare cases in which grafts have to be done between ABO-incompatible donors and recipients, graft survival may be improved by rigorous depletion of antibodies and B cells. Sometimes, if the graft is not rapidly rejected, it survives even in the presence of anti-graft antibody. One possible mechanism of this resistance to hyperacute rejection is increased expression of complement regulatory proteins on graft endothelial cells, a beneficial adaptation of the tissue that has been called accommodation.

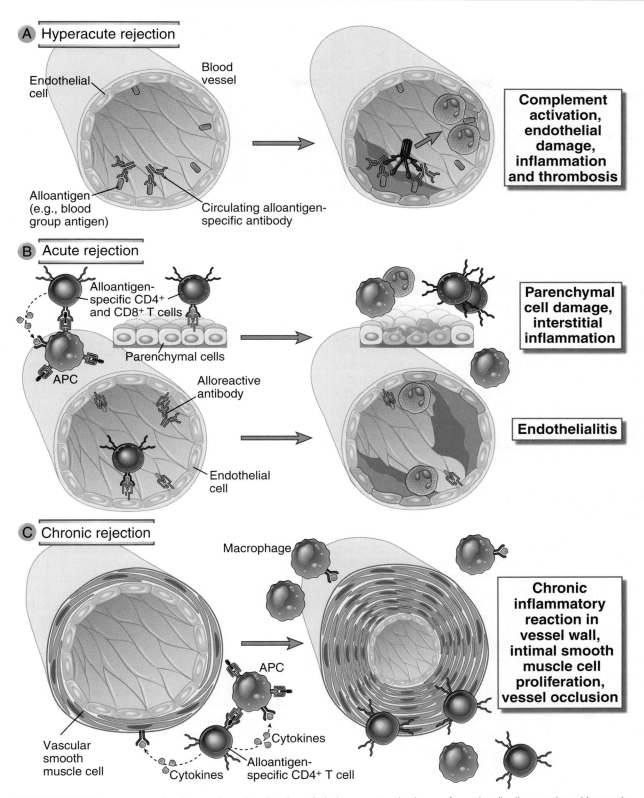

FIGURE 17-8 Immune mechanisms of graft rejection. A, In hyperacute rejection, preformed antibodies reactive with vascular endothelium activate complement and trigger rapid intravascular thrombosis and necrosis of the vessel wall. **B,** In acute rejection, CD4+ and CD8+ T lymphocytes reactive with alloantigens on endothelial cells and parenchymal cells mediate damage to these cell types. Alloreactive antibodies formed after engraftment may also contribute to parenchymal and vascular injury. **C,** In chronic rejection with graft arteriosclerosis, injury to the vessel wall leads to intimal smooth muscle cell proliferation and luminal occlusion. This lesion may be caused by a chronic inflammatory reaction to alloantigens in the vessel wall.

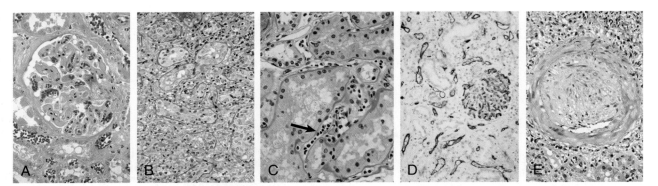

FIGURE 17-9 Histopathology of different forms of graft rejection. A, Hyperacute rejection of a kidney allograft with endothelial damage, platelet and thrombin thrombi, and early neutrophil infiltration in a glomerulus. **B,** Acute cellular rejection of a kidney with inflammatory cells in the connective tissue around the tubules and between epithelial cells of the tubules. **C,** Acute antibody-mediated rejection of a kidney allograft with inflammatory cells in peritubular capillaries (arrow). **D,** Complement C4d deposition in vessels in acute antibody-mediated rejection, revealed by immunohistochemistry as brown staining. **E,** Chronic rejection in a kidney allograft with graft arteriosclerosis. The vascular lumen is replaced by an accumulation of smooth muscle cells and connective tissue in the vessel intima. *(A, B, and E, Courtesy of Dr. Helmut Rennke, Department of Pathology, Brigham and Women's Hospital. C and D, Courtesy of Dr. Zoltan Laszik, Department of Pathology, University of California, San Francisco.)*

Acute Rejection

Acute rejection is a process of injury to the graft parenchyma and blood vessels mediated by alloreactive T cells and antibodies. Before modern immunosuppression, acute rejection would often begin several days to a few weeks after transplantation. The time of onset of acute rejection reflects the time needed to generate alloreactive effector T cells and antibodies in response to the graft. In current clinical practice, episodes of acute rejection may occur at much later times, even years after transplantation, if immunosuppression is reduced for any number of reasons. Although the patterns of acute rejection are divided into cellular (mediated by T cells) and humoral (mediated by antibodies), both typically coexist in an organ undergoing acute rejection.

Acute Cellular Rejection

The principal mechanisms of acute cellular rejection are inflammation caused by cytokines produced by helper T cells and CTL-mediated killing of graft parenchymal cells and endothelial cells (see Fig. 17-8, *B*). On histologic examination of kidney allografts, where this type of rejection is best characterized, there are infiltrates of lymphocytes and macrophages (Fig. 17-9, *B*). The infiltrates may involve the tubules (called tubulitis), with associated tubular necrosis, and blood vessels (called endothelialitis), with necrosis of vascular walls of capillaries and small arteries. The cellular infiltrates present in grafts undergoing acute cellular rejection include both CD4+ helper T cells and CD8+ CTLs specific for graft alloantigens, and both types of T cells may contribute to parenchymal cell and endothelial injury. The helper T cells include IFNγ- and TNF-secreting T_H1 cells and IL-17–secreting T_H17 cells, both of which contribute to macrophage and endothelial activation and inflammatory damage to the organ. Experimentally, adoptive transfer of alloreactive CD4+ helper T cells or CD8+ CTLs can cause acute cellular graft rejection in recipient mice.

Acute Antibody-Mediated Rejection

Alloantibodies cause acute rejection by binding to alloantigens, mainly HLA molecules, on vascular endothelial cells, causing endothelial injury and intravascular thrombosis that results in graft destruction (see Fig. 17-8, *B*). The binding of the alloantibodies to the endothelial cell surface triggers local complement activation, which leads to lysis of the cells, recruitment and activation of neutrophils, and thrombus formation. Alloantibodies may also engage Fc receptors on neutrophils and NK cells, which then kill the endothelial cells. In addition, alloantibody binding to the endothelial surface may directly alter endothelial function by inducing intracellular signals that enhance surface expression of proinflammatory and procoagulant molecules.

The histologic hallmarks of acute antibody-mediated rejection of renal allografts are acute inflammation of glomeruli and peritubular capillaries with focal capillary thrombosis (Fig. 17-9, *C*). Immunohistochemical identification of the C4d complement fragment in capillaries of renal allografts is used clinically as an indicator of activation of the classical complement pathway and humoral rejection (Fig. 17-9, *D*). In a significant fraction of cases of antibody-mediated rejection, there is no C4d deposition detectable, suggesting that damage is caused by the complement-independent effects of alloantibody binding to endothelial cells, as mentioned earlier.

Chronic Rejection and Graft Vasculopathy

As therapy for acute rejection has improved, the major cause of the failure of vascularized organ allografts has become chronic rejection. Since 1990, 1-year survival of kidney allografts has been better than 90%, but the 10-year survival has remained about 60% despite advances in immunosuppressive therapy. Chronic rejection develops insidiously during months or years and may or may not be preceded by clinically recognized episodes of acute rejection. Chronic rejection of different transplanted organs is associated with distinct pathologic changes. In the kidney and heart, chronic rejection results in vascular occlusion and interstitial fibrosis. Lung transplants undergoing chronic rejection show thickened small airways (called bronchiolitis obliterans), and liver transplants show fibrotic and non-functional bile ducts.

A dominant lesion of chronic rejection in vascularized grafts is arterial occlusion as a result of the proliferation of intimal smooth muscle cells, and the grafts eventually fail mainly because of the resulting ischemic damage (see Fig. 17-8, *C*). The arterial changes are called graft vasculopathy or accelerated graft arteriosclerosis (Fig. 17-9, *E*). Graft vasculopathy is frequently seen in failed cardiac and renal allografts and can develop in any vascularized organ transplant within 6 months to a year after transplantation. The likely mechanisms underlying the occlusive vascular lesions of chronic rejection are activation of alloreactive T cells and secretion of cytokines that stimulate proliferation of vascular smooth muscle cells. As the arterial lesions of graft arteriosclerosis progress, blood flow to the graft parenchyma is compromised, and the parenchyma is slowly replaced by non-functioning fibrous tissue. The interstitial fibrosis seen in chronic rejection may also be a repair response to parenchymal cell damage caused by repeated bouts of acute antibody-mediated or cellular rejection, perioperative ischemia, toxic effects of immunosuppressive drugs, and even chronic viral infections. Chronic rejection leads to congestive heart failure or arrhythmias in cardiac transplant patients or loss of glomerular and tubular function and renal failure in kidney transplant patients.

PREVENTION AND TREATMENT OF ALLOGRAFT REJECTION

If the recipient of an allograft has a fully functional immune system, transplantation almost invariably results in some form of rejection. The strategies used in clinical practice and in experimental models to avoid or to delay rejection are general immunosuppression and minimizing the strength of the specific allogeneic reaction. An important goal in transplantation research is to find ways of inducing donor-specific tolerance, which would allow grafts to survive without non-specific immunosuppression.

Methods to Reduce the Immunogenicity of Allografts

In human transplantation, the major strategy to reduce graft immunogenicity has been to minimize alloantigenic differences between the donor and recipient. Several clinical laboratory tests are routinely performed to reduce the risk for immunologic rejection of allografts. These include ABO blood typing; the determination of HLA alleles expressed on donor and recipient cells, called tissue typing; the detection of preformed antibodies in the recipient that recognize HLA and other antigens representative of the donor population; and the detection of preformed antibodies in the recipient that bind to antigens of an identified donor's leukocytes, called cross-matching. Not all of these tests are done in all types of transplantation. We will now summarize each of these tests and discuss their significance.

To avoid hyperacute rejection, the ABO blood group antigens of the graft donor are selected to be compatible with the recipient. This test is uniformly used in renal and cardiac transplantation because kidney and heart grafts will typically not survive if there are ABO incompatibilities between the donor and recipient. Natural IgM antibodies specific for allogeneic ABO blood group antigens will cause hyperacute rejection. Blood typing is performed by mixing a patient's red blood cells with standardized sera containing anti-A or anti-B antibodies. If the patient expresses either blood group antigen, the serum specific for that antigen will agglutinate the red blood cells. The biology of the ABO blood group system is discussed later in this chapter in the context of blood transfusion.

In kidney transplantation, the larger the number of MHC alleles that are matched between the donor and recipient, the better the graft survival (Fig. 17-10). HLA matching had a more profound influence on graft survival before modern immunosuppressive drugs were routinely used, but current data still show significantly greater survival of grafts when donor and recipient have fewer HLA allele mismatches. Past clinical experience with older typing methods showed that of all class I and class II MHC loci, matching at HLA-A, HLA-B, and HLA-DR is most important for predicting survival of kidney allografts. (HLA-C is not as polymorphic as HLA-A or HLA-B, and HLA-DR and HLA-DQ are in linkage disequilibrium, so matching at the DR locus often also matches at the DQ locus.) Although current typing protocols in many centers include HLA-C, DQ, and DP loci, most of the available data in predicting graft outcome refer only to HLA-A, HLA-B, and HLA-DR mismatches. Because two codominantly expressed alleles are inherited for each of these HLA genes, it is possible to have zero to six HLA mismatches of these three loci between the donor and recipient. Zero-antigen mismatches predict the best survival of living related donor grafts, and grafts with one-antigen mismatches do slightly worse. The survival of grafts with two to six HLA mismatches is significantly worse than that of grafts with zero- and one-antigen mismatches. Mismatching of two or more HLA genes has an even greater impact on non-living (unrelated) donor renal allografts. Therefore, attempts are made to reduce the number of differences in HLA alleles expressed on donor and recipient cells, which will have a modest effect in reducing the chance of rejection.

HLA matching in renal transplantation is possible because donor kidneys can be stored for up to 72 hours before being transplanted, and patients needing a kidney allograft can be maintained on dialysis until a well-matched organ is available. In the case of heart and liver transplantation, organ preservation is more difficult, and potential recipients are often in critical condition. For these reasons, HLA typing is not considered in pairing of potential donors and recipients, and the choice of donor and recipient is based on ABO blood group matching, other measures of immunologic compatibility described later, and anatomic compatibility. The paucity of heart donors, the emergent need for transplantation, and the success of immunosuppression override the possible benefit of reducing HLA mismatches between donor and recipient. As we will discuss later, in bone marrow transplantation, HLA matching is essential to reduce the risk of graft-versus-host disease.

Most HLA haplotype determinations are now performed by polymerase chain reaction (PCR), replacing

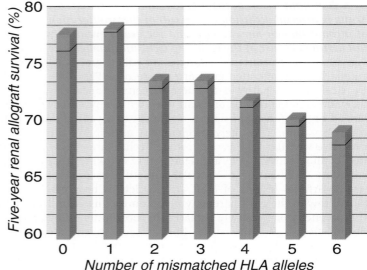

FIGURE 17-10 Influence of MHC matching on graft survival. Matching of *MHC* alleles between the donor and recipient significantly improves renal allograft survival. The data shown are for deceased donor (cadaver) grafts. HLA matching has less of an impact on survival of renal allografts from live donors, and some *MHC* alleles are more important than others in determining outcome. (*Data from* SRTR annual report 2012. *Available at* http://www.srtr.org/. *Accessed July 2013.*)

older serologic methods. MHC genes can be amplified by PCR with use of primers that bind to nonpolymorphic sequences within the 5′ and 3′ ends of exons encoding the polymorphic regions of class I and class II MHC molecules. The amplified segment of DNA can then be sequenced. Thus, the actual nucleotide sequence, and therefore the predicted amino acid sequence, can be directly determined for the MHC alleles of any cell, providing precise molecular tissue typing. On the basis of these DNA sequencing efforts, the nomenclature of HLA alleles has changed to reflect the identification of many alleles not distinguished by previous serologic methods. Each allele defined by sequence has at least a four-digit number, but some alleles require six or eight digits for precise definition. The first two digits usually correspond to the older serologically defined allotype, and the third and fourth digits indicate the subtypes. Alleles with differences in the first four digits encode proteins with different amino acids. For example, HLA-DRB1*1301 is the sequence-defined 01 allele of the serologically defined HLA-DR13 family of genes encoding the HLA-DR β1 protein.

Patients in need of allografts are also tested for the presence of preformed antibodies against donor MHC molecules or other cell surface antigens. Two types of tests are done to detect these antibodies. In the panel reactive antibody test, patients waiting for organ transplants are screened for the presence of preformed antibodies reactive with allogeneic HLA molecules prevalent in the population. These antibodies, which may be produced as a result of previous pregnancies, transfusions, or transplantation, can identify risk for hyperacute or acute vascular rejection. Small amounts of the patient's serum are mixed with multiple fluorescently labeled beads coated with defined MHC molecules, representative of the MHC alleles that may be present in an organ donor population. Each MHC allele is attached to a bead with a differently colored fluorescent label. Binding of the patient's antibodies to beads is determined by flow cytometry. The results are reported as percent reactive antibody (PRA), which is the percentage of the MHC allele pool with which the patient's serum reacts. The PRA is determined

on multiple occasions while a patient waits for an organ allograft. This is because the PRA can vary, as each panel is chosen at random and the patient's serum antibody titers may change over time.

If a potential donor is identified, the cross-matching test will determine if the patient has antibodies that react specifically with that donor's cells. The test is performed by mixing the recipient's serum with the donor's blood lymphocytes. Complement-mediated cytotoxicity tests or flow cytometric assays can then be used to determine if antibodies in the recipient serum have bound to the donor cells. For example, complement is added to the mixture of cells and serum, and if preformed antibodies, usually against donor MHC molecules, are present in the recipient's serum, the donor cells are lysed. This would be a positive cross-match, which indicates that the donor is not suitable for that recipient.

Immunosuppression to Prevent or to Treat Allograft Rejection

Immunosuppressive drugs that inhibit or kill T lymphocytes are the principal agents used to treat or prevent graft rejection. Several methods of immunosuppression are commonly used (Fig. 17-11).

Inhibitors of T Cell Signaling Pathways

The calcineurin inhibitors cyclosporine and FK506 (tacrolimus) inhibit transcription of certain genes in T cells, most notably genes encoding cytokines such as IL-2. Cyclosporine is a fungal peptide that binds with high affinity to a ubiquitous cellular protein called cyclophilin. The complex of cyclosporine and cyclophilin binds to and inhibits the enzymatic activity of the calcium/calmodulin-activated serine/threonine phosphatase calcineurin (see Chapter 7). Because calcineurin is required to activate the transcription factor NFAT (nuclear factor of activated T cells), cyclosporine inhibits NFAT activation and the transcription of IL-2 and other cytokine genes. The net result is that cyclosporine blocks the IL-2–dependent

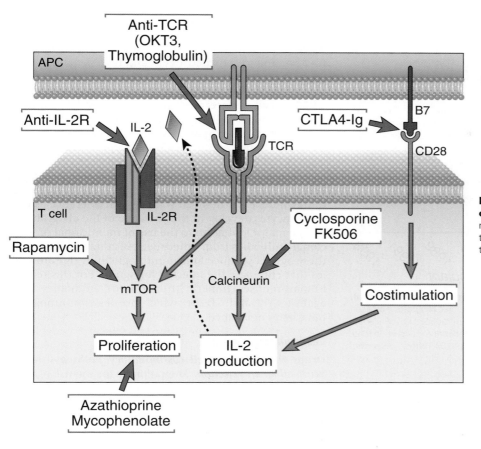

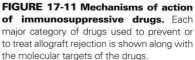

FIGURE 17-11 Mechanisms of action of immunosuppressive drugs. Each major category of drugs used to prevent or to treat allograft rejection is shown along with the molecular targets of the drugs.

proliferation and differentiation of T cells. FK506 is a macrolide made by a bacterium that functions like cyclosporine. FK506 and its binding protein (called FKBP) share with the cyclosporine-cyclophilin complex the ability to bind calcineurin and inhibit its activity.

The introduction of cyclosporine into clinical practice ushered in the modern era of transplantation. Before the use of cyclosporine, the majority of transplanted hearts and livers were rejected. Now as a result of the use of cyclosporine, FK506, and other more recently introduced drugs, the majority of these allografts survive for more than 5 years (Fig. 17-12). Nevertheless, these drugs have limitations. For example, at doses needed for optimal immunosuppression, cyclosporine causes kidney damage, and some rejection episodes are refractory to cyclosporine treatment. FK506 was initially used for liver transplant recipients, but it is now used widely for immunosuppression of kidney allograft recipients, including those who are not adequately controlled by cyclosporine.

The immunosuppressive drug rapamycin (sirolimus) inhibits growth factor–mediated T cell proliferation. Like FK506, rapamycin binds to FKBP, but the rapamycin-FKBP complex does not inhibit calcineurin. Instead, this complex binds to and inhibits a cellular enzyme called mammalian target of rapamycin (mTOR), which is a serine/threonine protein kinase required for translation of proteins that promote cell survival and proliferation. mTOR is negatively regulated by a protein complex

called tuberous sclerosis complex 1 (TSC1)–TSC2 complex. Phosphatidylinositol 3-kinase (PI3K)–Akt signaling results in phosphorylation of TSC2 and release of mTOR regulation. Several growth factor receptor signaling pathways, including the IL-2 receptor pathway in T cells, as well as TCR and CD28 signals, activate mTOR through PI3K-Akt, leading to translation of proteins needed for cell cycle progression. Thus, by inhibiting mTOR function, rapamycin blocks T cell proliferation. Combinations of cyclosporine (which blocks IL-2 synthesis) and rapamycin (which blocks IL-2–driven proliferation) are potent inhibitors of T cell responses. Interestingly, rapamycin inhibits the generation of effector T cells but does not impair the survival and functions of regulatory T cells as much, which may promote immune suppression of allograft rejection. mTOR is involved in dendritic cell functions, and therefore rapamycin may suppress T cell responses by its effects on dendritic cells as well. mTOR is also involved in B cell proliferation and antibody responses, and therefore rapamycin may also be effective in preventing or treating antibody-mediated rejection.

Other molecules involved in cytokine and T cell receptor signaling are also targets of immunosuppressive drugs that are in early trials for treatment or prevention of allograft rejection. One of these target molecules is JAK3, a kinase linked to signaling of various cytokine receptors, including IL-2, and protein kinase C, an essential kinase in T cell receptor signaling.

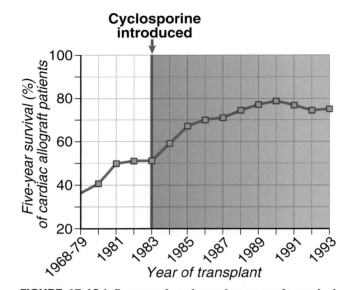

FIGURE 17-12 Influence of cyclosporine on graft survival. Five-year survival rates for patients receiving cardiac allografts increased significantly beginning when cyclosporine was introduced in 1983. *(Data from Transplant Patient DataSource, United Network for Organ Sharing, Richmond, Virginia. Available at http://207.239.150.13/tpd/. Accessed February 17, 2000.)*

Antimetabolites

Metabolic toxins that kill proliferating T cells are used in combination with other drugs to treat graft rejection. These agents inhibit the proliferation of lymphocyte precursors during their maturation and also kill proliferating mature T cells that have been stimulated by alloantigens. The first such drug to be developed for the prevention and treatment of rejection was azathioprine. This drug is still used, but it is toxic to precursors of leukocytes in the bone marrow and enterocytes in the gut. The most widely used drug in this class is **mycophenolate mofetil (MMF).** MMF is metabolized to mycophenolic acid, which blocks a lymphocyte-specific isoform of inosine monophosphate dehydrogenase, an enzyme required for de novo synthesis of guanine nucleotides. Because MMF selectively inhibits the lymphocyte-specific isoform of this enzyme, it has relatively few toxic effects on other cells. MMF is now routinely used, often in combination with cyclosporine or FK506, to prevent acute allograft rejection.

Function-Blocking or Depleting Anti-Lymphocyte Antibodies

Antibodies that react with T cell surface structures and deplete or inhibit T cells are used to treat acute rejection episodes. The first anti-T cell antibody used in transplant patients was a mouse monoclonal antibody called OKT3 that is specific for human CD3. (OKT3 was the first monoclonal antibody used as a drug in humans, but it is no longer being produced.) Polyclonal rabbit or horse antibodies specific for a mixture of human T cell surface proteins, so-called **anti-thymocyte globulin,** have also been in clinical use for many years to treat acute allograft rejection. These anti–T cell antibodies deplete circulating T cells either by activating the complement system to eliminate T cells or by opsonizing them for phagocytosis.

Monoclonal antibodies are now in clinical use that are specific for CD25, the α subunit of the IL-2 receptor. These reagents presumably prevent T cell activation by blocking IL-2 binding to activated T cells and IL-2 signaling.

Another monoclonal antibody in use in clinical transplantation is a rat IgM monoclonal antibody specific for CD52, a cell surface protein expressed widely on most mature B and T cells whose function is not understood. Anti-CD52 was originally developed to treat B cell malignant neoplasms, and it was found to profoundly deplete most peripheral B and T cells for many weeks after injection into patients. In current trials, it is administered just before and early after transplantation, with the hope that it may induce a prolonged state of graft tolerance as new lymphocytes develop in the presence of the allograft.

The major limitation to the use of monoclonal or polyclonal antibodies from other species is that humans given these agents produce anti-immunoglobulin (Ig) antibodies that eliminate the injected foreign Ig. For this reason, human-mouse chimeric (humanized) antibodies (e.g., against CD3 and CD25), which are less immunogenic, have been developed.

Costimulatory Blockade

Drugs that block T cell costimulatory pathways reduce acute allograft rejection. The rationale for the use of these types of drugs is to prevent the delivery of costimulatory signals required for activation of T cells (see Chapter 9). Recall that CTLA4-Ig is a recombinant protein composed of the extracellular portion of CTLA-4 fused to an IgG Fc domain. A high affinity form of CTLA4-Ig, which binds to B7 molecules on APCs and prevents them from interacting with T cell CD28 (see Fig. 9-7), is approved for use in allograft recipients. Clinical studies have shown that CTLA-4–Ig can be as effective as cyclosporine in preventing acute rejection, but its high cost and other factors have limited widespread use of this biologic agent. An antibody that binds to T cell CD40 ligand and prevents its interactions with CD40 on APCs (see Chapter 9) has also proved beneficial for preventing graft rejection in experimental animals. In some experimental protocols, simultaneous blockade of both B7 and CD40 appears to be more effective than either alone in promoting graft survival. However, the anti-CD40L antibody has a serious side effect of thrombotic complications, apparently related to the expression of CD40L on platelets.

Drugs Targeting Alloantibodies and Alloreactive B Cells

As we have learned more about the importance of alloantibodies in mediating acute and perhaps chronic rejection, therapies targeting antibodies and B cells that were developed for other diseases are now being used in transplant patients. For example, plasmapheresis is sometimes used to treat acute antibody-mediated rejection. In this procedure, a patient's blood is pumped through a machine that removes the plasma but returns the blood cells to the circulation. In this way, circulating antibodies, including pathogenic alloreactive antibodies, can be removed. Intravenous immune globulin (IVIG) therapy, which is used to treat several, often antibody-mediated, inflammatory diseases, is also being applied in the setting of acute antibody-mediated rejection. In IVIG therapy, pooled IgG from normal donors is injected intravenously into a patient. The mechanisms of action are not fully understood but likely involve binding of the injected IgG to the patient's Fc receptors on various cell types, thereby reducing allo-antibody production and blocking effector functions of the patient's own antibodies. IVIG also enhances degradation of the patient's antibodies by competitively inhibiting their binding to the neonatal Fc receptor (see Chapter 5). B cell depletion by administration of rituximab, an anti-CD20 antibody which is approved for treatment of B cell lymphomas and for autoimmune diseases, is used in some cases of acute antibody-mediated rejection.

Anti-Inflammatory Drugs

Anti-inflammatory agents, specifically corticosteroids, are frequently used to reduce the inflammatory reaction to organ allografts. The proposed mechanism of action of these natural hormones and their synthetic analogues is to block the synthesis and secretion of cytokines, including tumor necrosis factor (TNF) and IL-1, and other inflammatory mediators, such as prostaglandins, reactive oxygen species, and nitric oxide, produced by macrophages and other inflammatory cells. The net result of this therapy is reduced leukocyte recruitment, inflammation, and graft damage.

Current immunosuppressive protocols have dramatically improved graft survival. Before the use of calcineurin inhibitors, the 1-year survival rate of unrelated cadaveric kidney grafts was between 50% and 60%, with a 90% rate for grafts from living related donors (which are better matched with the recipients). Since cyclosporine, FK506, rapamycin, and MMF have been introduced, the survival rate of unrelated cadaveric kidney grafts has increased to about 90% at 1 year. Heart transplantation, for which HLA matching is not practical, has also significantly benefited from the use of the various classes of immunosuppressive drugs reviewed earlier, and now has a similar ~90% 1-year survival rate and ~75% 5-year survival rate (see Fig. 17-11). Experience with other organs is more limited, but survival rates have also improved with modern immunosuppressive therapy, with 10-year patient survival rates of approximately 60% and 75% for pancreas and liver recipients, respectively, and 3-year patient survival rates of 70% to 80% for lung recipients.

Strong immunosuppression is usually started in allograft recipients at the time of transplantation with a combination of drugs, and after a few days, the drugs are changed for long-term maintenance of immunosuppression. For example, in the case of adult kidney transplantation, a patient may be initially induced with an anti–IL-2R or anti–T cell depleting antibody and a high-dose corticosteroid, and then maintained on a calcineurin inhibitor, an antimetabolite, and maybe low-dose steroids. Acute rejection, when it occurs, is managed by rapidly intensifying immunosuppressive therapy. In modern transplantation, chronic rejection has become a more common cause of allograft failure, especially in cardiac transplantation. Chronic rejection is more insidious than acute rejection, and it is much less reversible by immunosuppression.

Immunosuppressive therapy leads to increased susceptibility to various types of intracellular infections and virus-associated tumors. The major goal of immunosuppression to treat graft rejection is to reduce the generation and function of helper T cells and CTLs, which mediate acute cellular rejection. It is therefore not surprising that defense against viruses and other intracellular pathogens, the physiologic function of T cells, is also compromised in immunosuppressed transplant recipients. Reactivation of latent herpesviruses is a frequent problem in immunosuppressed patients, including cytomegalovirus, herpes simplex virus, varicella-zoster virus, and Epstein-Barr virus. For this reason, transplant recipients are now given prophylactic anti-viral therapy for herpesvirus infections. Immunosuppressed allograft recipients are also at greater risk for a variety of so-called opportunistic infections, which normally do not occur in immunocompetent people, including fungal infections (*Pneumocystis jiroveci* pneumonia, histoplasmosis, coccidioidomycosis), protozoan infections (toxoplasmosis), and gastrointestinal parasitic infections (*Cryptosporidium* and *Microsporidium*). Immunosuppressed allograft recipients have a higher risk for development of cancer compared with the general population, including various forms of skin cancer. Some of the tumors that are more frequently found in allograft recipients are known to be caused by viruses, and therefore they may arise because of impaired anti-viral immunity. These include uterine cervical carcinoma, which is related to human papillomavirus infection, and lymphomas caused by Epstein-Barr virus infection. The lymphomas found in allograft recipients as a group are called post-transplantation lymphoproliferative disorders (PTLD), and most are derived from B lymphocytes.

Despite the risk for infections and neoplasias associated with the use of immunosuppressive drugs, the major limitation on the tolerated doses of most of these drugs, including calcineurin inhibitors, mTOR inhibitors, antimetabolites, and steroids, is direct toxicity to cells unrelated to immunosuppression. In some cases, the toxicities affect the same cells as rejection does, such as cyclosporine toxicity to renal tubular epithelial cells, which can complicate the interpretation of declining renal function in kidney allograft recipients.

Methods to Induce Donor-Specific Tolerance

Allograft rejection may be prevented by making the host tolerant to the alloantigens of the graft. Tolerance in this setting means that the host immune system does not injure the graft despite the absence or withdrawal of immunosuppressive and anti-inflammatory agents. It is presumed that tolerance to an allograft will involve the same mechanisms that are involved in tolerance to self antigens (see Chapter 15), namely, anergy, deletion, and active suppression of alloreactive T cells. Tolerance is desirable in transplantation because it is alloantigen specific and will therefore avoid the major problems associated with non-specific immunosuppression, namely, immune deficiency leading to increased susceptibility to infection and development of tumors and drug toxicity. In addition, achieving graft tolerance may reduce chronic rejection, which has to date been unaffected by the commonly used immunosuppressive agents that prevent and reverse acute rejection episodes.

Various experimental approaches and clinical observations have shown that it should be possible to achieve tolerance to allografts. In experiments in mice, Medawar and colleagues found that if neonatal mice of one strain (the recipient) are given spleen cells of another strain (the donor), the recipients will subsequently accept skin grafts from the donor. Such tolerance is alloantigen specific because the recipients will reject grafts from mouse strains that express MHC alleles that differ from the spleen cell donor's. Renal transplant patients who have received blood transfusions containing allogeneic leukocytes have a lower incidence of acute rejection episodes than do those who have not been transfused. The postulated explanation for this effect is that the introduction of allogeneic leukocytes by transfusion produces tolerance to alloantigens. One underlying mechanism for tolerance induction may be that the transfused donor cells contain immature dendritic cells, which induce unresponsiveness to donor alloantigens. Indeed, pretreatment of potential recipients with blood transfusions is now used as prophylactic therapy to reduce rejection. Some recipients of liver allografts are able to retain healthy grafts even after withdrawal of immunosuppression. The mechanism underlying this apparent spontaneous tolerance is not known, and it seems to be unique to liver grafts.

Several strategies are being tested to induce donor-specific tolerance in allograft recipients.

- *Costimulatory blockade.* It was postulated that recognition of alloantigens in the absence of costimulation would lead to T cell tolerance, and there is some experimental evidence in animals to support this. However, the clinical experience with agents that block costimulation is that they suppress immune responses to the allograft but do not induce long-lived tolerance, and patients have to be maintained on the therapy.
- *Hematopoietic chimerism.* We mentioned earlier that transfusion of donor blood cells into the graft recipient inhibits rejection. If the transfused donor cells or progeny of the cells survive for extended periods in the recipient, the recipient becomes a chimera. Long-term allograft tolerance by hematopoietic chimerism has been achieved in a small number of renal allograft recipients by doing a bone marrow cell transplant from the donor at the same time as the organ allograft, but the risks of bone marrow transplantation and the availability of appropriate donors may limit the applicability of this approach.
- *Transfer or induction of regulatory T cells.* Attempts to generate donor-specific regulatory T cells in culture and to transfer these into graft recipients are ongoing. There has been some success reported in recipients of hematopoietic stem cell transplants, in whom infusions of regulatory T cells reduce graft-versus-host disease. An alternative approach, which has been attempted in pancreatic islet transplanta-

tion, is to activate regulatory T cells in vivo by administration of a weakly stimulating anti-CD3 antibody, but the effectiveness of this therapy is not established.

XENOGENEIC TRANSPLANTATION

The use of solid organ transplantation as a clinical therapy is greatly limited by the inadequate numbers of donor organs available. For this reason, the possibility of transplantation of organs from other mammals, such as pigs, into human recipients has kindled great interest.

A major immunologic barrier to xenogeneic transplantation is the presence of natural antibodies in the human recipients that cause hyperacute rejection. More than 95% of primates have natural IgM antibodies that are reactive with carbohydrate determinants expressed by cells of species that are evolutionarily distant, such as the pig. The majority of human anti-pig natural antibodies are directed at one particular carbohydrate determinant formed by the action of a pig α-galactosyltransferase enzyme. This enzyme places an α-linked galactose moiety on the same substrate that in human and other primate cells is fucosylated to form the blood group H antigen. Natural antibodies are rarely produced against carbohydrate determinants of closely related species, such as humans and chimpanzees. Thus, organs from chimpanzees or other higher primates might theoretically be accepted in humans. However, ethical and logistic concerns have limited such procedures. For reasons of anatomic compatibility, pigs are the preferred xenogeneic species for organ donation to humans.

Natural antibodies against xenografts induce hyperacute rejection by the same mechanisms as those seen in hyperacute allograft rejection. These mechanisms include the generation of endothelial cell procoagulants and platelet-aggregating substances, coupled with the loss of endothelial anticoagulant mechanisms. However, the consequences of activation of human complement on pig cells are typically more severe than the consequences of activation of complement by natural antibodies on human allogeneic cells. This may be because some of the complement regulatory proteins made by pig cells, such as decay-accelerating factor, are not able to interact with human complement proteins and thus cannot limit the extent of complement-induced injury (see Chapter 13).

Even when hyperacute rejection is prevented, xenografts are often damaged by a form of acute vascular rejection that occurs within 2 to 3 days of transplantation. This form of rejection has been called delayed xenograft rejection, accelerated acute rejection, or acute vascular rejection, and is characterized by intravascular thrombosis and necrosis of vessel walls. The mechanisms of delayed xenograft rejection are incompletely understood; recent findings indicate that there may be incompatibilities between primate platelets and porcine endothelial cells that promote thrombosis independent of antibody-mediated damage.

Xenografts can also be rejected by T cell–mediated immune responses to xenoantigens. The mechanisms of cell-mediated rejection of xenografts are believed to be similar to those that we have described for allograft rejection, and T cell responses to xenoantigens can be as strong as or even stronger than responses to alloantigens.

BLOOD TRANSFUSION AND THE ABO AND Rh BLOOD GROUP ANTIGENS

Blood transfusion is a form of transplantation in which whole blood or blood cells from one or more individuals are transferred intravenously into the circulation of another individual. Blood transfusions are most often performed to replace blood lost by hemorrhage or to correct defects caused by inadequate production of blood cells, which may occur in a variety of diseases. The major barrier to successful blood transfusions is the immune response to cell surface molecules that differ between individuals. The most important alloantigen system in blood transfusion is the ABO system, which we will discuss in detail later. ABO antigens are expressed on virtually all cells, including red blood cells. Individuals lacking a particular blood group antigen produce natural IgM antibodies against that antigen. If such individuals are given blood cells expressing the target antigen, the preexisting antibodies bind to the transfused cells, activate complement, and cause **transfusion reactions,** which can be life-threatening. Transfusion across an ABO barrier may trigger an immediate hemolytic reaction, resulting in both intravascular lysis of red blood cells, probably mediated by the complement system, and extensive phagocytosis of antibody- and complement-coated erythrocytes by macrophages in the liver and spleen. Hemoglobin is liberated from the lysed red blood cells in quantities that may be toxic for kidney cells, causing acute renal tubular cell necrosis and kidney failure. High fever, shock, and disseminated intravascular coagulation may also develop, suggestive of release of massive amounts of cytokines (e.g., TNF or IL-1). The disseminated intravascular coagulation consumes clotting factors faster than they can be synthesized, and the patient may paradoxically die of bleeding in the presence of widespread clotting. More delayed hemolytic reactions may result from incompatibilities of minor blood group antigens. These result in progressive loss of the transfused red blood cells, leading to anemia and jaundice, the latter a consequence of overloading the liver with hemoglobin-derived pigments.

We will now discuss the ABO blood group antigens as well as other blood group antigens of clinical relevance.

ABO Blood Group Antigens

The ABO antigens are carbohydrates linked to cell surface proteins and lipids that are synthesized by polymorphic glycosyltransferase enzymes, which vary in activity depending on the inherited allele (Fig. 17-13).

The ABO antigens were the first alloantigen system to be defined in mammals. All normal individuals synthesize a common core glycan, which is attached mainly to plasma membrane proteins. Most individuals possess a fucosyltransferase that adds a fucose moiety to a nonterminal sugar residue of the core glycan, and the fucosylated glycan is called the H antigen. A single gene on chromosome 9 encodes a glycosyltransferase enzyme that may further modify the H antigen. There are three allelic variants of this gene. The O allele gene product is devoid of enzymatic activity. The A allele–encoded enzyme transfers a terminal *N*-acetylgalactosamine moiety onto the H antigen, and the B allele gene product transfers a terminal galactose moiety. Individuals who are homozygous for the O allele cannot attach terminal sugars to the H antigen and express only the H antigen. In contrast, individuals who possess an A allele (AA homozygotes, AO heterozygotes, or AB heterozygotes) form the A antigen by adding terminal *N*-acetylgalactosamine to some of their H antigens. Similarly, individuals who express a B allele (BB homozygotes, BO heterozygotes, or AB heterozygotes) form the B antigen by adding terminal galactose to some of their H antigens. AB heterozygotes form both A and B antigens from some of their H antigens. The terminology has been simplified so that OO individuals are said to be blood type O; AA and AO individuals are blood type A; BB and BO individuals are blood type B; and AB individuals are blood type AB. Mutations in the gene encoding the fucosyltransferase that produces the H antigen are rare; people who are homozygous for such a mutation are said to have the Bombay blood group and cannot produce H, A, or B antigens. and cannot receive type O, A, B, or AB blood.

Individuals who express a particular A or B blood group antigen are tolerant to that antigen, but individuals who do not express that antigen produce natural antibodies that recognize the antigen. Virtually all individuals express the H antigen, and therefore they are tolerant to this antigen and do not produce anti-H antibodies. Individuals who express A or B antigens are tolerant to these molecules and do not produce anti-A or anti-B antibodies, respectively. However, blood group O and A individuals produce anti-B IgM antibodies, and blood group O and B individuals produce anti-A IgM antibodies. Individuals who are unable to produce the core H antigens make antibodies against H, A, and B antigens. On face value, it seems paradoxical that individuals who do not express a blood group antigen make antibodies against it. The likely explanation is that the antibodies are produced against glycolipids of intestinal bacteria that happen to cross-react with the ABO antigens, unless the individual is tolerant to one or more of these. Predictably, the presence of any blood group antigen induces tolerance to that antigen.

In clinical transfusion, the choice of blood donors for a particular recipient is based on the expression of blood group antigens and the antibody responses to them. If a patient receives a transfusion of red blood cells from a donor who expresses the antigen not expressed on self red blood cells, a transfusion reaction may result (described earlier). It follows that AB individuals can

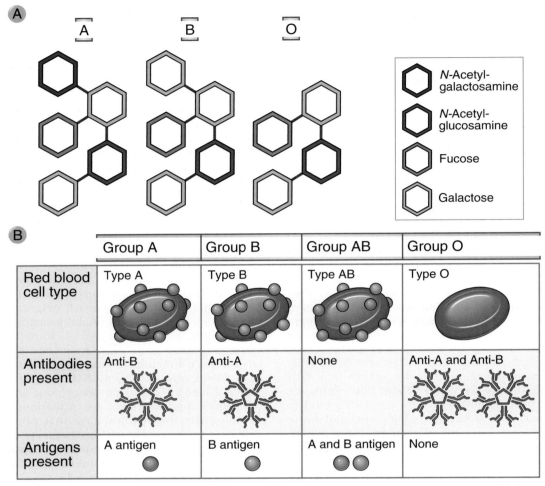

FIGURE 17-13 ABO blood group antigens. A, Blood group antigens are carbohydrate structures added onto cell surface proteins or lipids by the action of glycosyltransferases (see text). **B,** Different blood group antigens are produced by the addition of different sugars by different inherited glycosyltransferases. Individuals who express a particular blood group antigen are tolerant to that antigen but produce natural antibodies that react with other blood group antigens.

tolerate transfusions from all potential donors and are therefore called universal recipients; similarly, O individuals can tolerate transfusions only from O donors but can provide blood to all recipients and are therefore called universal donors. In general, differences in minor blood groups lead to red blood cell lysis only after repeated transfusions trigger a secondary antibody response.

A and B blood group antigens are expressed on many other cell types in addition to blood cells, including endothelial cells. For this reason, ABO typing is critical to avoid hyperacute rejection of certain solid organ allografts, as discussed earlier in the chapter. ABO incompatibility between mother and fetus generally does not cause problems for the fetus because most of the anti-carbohydrate antibodies are IgM and do not cross the placenta.

Other Blood Group Antigens

Lewis Antigen

The same glycoproteins that carry the A and B blood group determinants can be modified by other glycosyltransferases to generate minor blood group antigens. For

example, addition of fucose moieties at other non-terminal positions can be catalyzed by different fucosyltransferases and create epitopes of the Lewis antigen system. Lewis antigens have recently received much attention from immunologists because these carbohydrate groups serve as ligands for E-selectin and P-selectin and thus play a role in leukocyte migration (see Chapter 3).

Rhesus (Rh) Antigen

The Rhesus (Rh) antigens, named after the monkey species in which they were originally identified, are another clinically important set of blood group antigens. Rh antigens are non-glycosylated, hydrophobic cell surface proteins found in red blood cell membranes and are structurally related to other red blood cell membrane glycoproteins with transporter functions. Rh proteins are encoded by two tightly linked and highly homologous genes, but only one of them, called RhD, is commonly considered in clinical blood typing. This is because up to 15% of the population has a deletion or other alteration of the RhD allele. These people, called Rh negative, are not tolerant to the RhD antigen and will make antibodies to the antigen if they are exposed to Rh-positive blood cells.

The major clinical significance of anti-Rh antibodies is related to hemolytic reactions associated with pregnancy that are similar to transfusion reactions. Rh-negative mothers carrying an Rh-positive fetus can be sensitized by fetal red blood cells that enter the maternal circulation, usually during childbirth. Since the Rh antigen is a protein, as opposed to the carbohydrate ABO antigens, class-switched IgG antibodies are generated in Rh-negative mothers. Subsequent pregnancies in which the fetus is Rh positive are at risk because the maternal anti-Rh IgG antibodies can cross the placenta and mediate the destruction of the fetal red blood cells. This causes **erythroblastosis fetalis** (hemolytic disease of the newborn) and can be lethal for the fetus. This disease can be prevented by administration of anti-RhD antibodies to the mother within 72 hours of birth of the first Rh-positive baby. The treatment prevents the baby's Rh-positive red blood cells that entered the mother's circulation from inducing the production of anti-Rh antibodies in the mother. The exact mechanisms of action of the administered antibodies are not clear but may include phagocytic clearance or complement-mediated lysis of the baby's red blood cells or Fc receptor–dependent feedback inhibition of the mother's RhD-specific B cells (see Chapter 12).

HEMATOPOIETIC STEM CELL TRANSPLANTATION

The transplantation of pluripotent hematopoietic stem cells (HSCs) was done in the past using an inoculum of bone marrow cells collected by aspiration, and the procedure is often called bone marrow transplantation. In modern clinical practice, hematopoietic stem cells are more often obtained from the blood of donors, after treatment with colony-stimulating factors that mobilize stem cells from the bone marrow. The recipient is treated before transplantation with a combination of chemotherapy, immunotherapy or irradiation to deplete bone marrow cells to free up niches for the transferred stem cells. After transplantation, stem cells repopulate the recipient's bone marrow and differentiate into all of the hematopoietic lineages. We consider HSC transplantation separately from other forms of transplantation, because this type of grafting has several unique features that are not encountered with solid organ transplantation.

HSC transplantation is most often used clinically in the treatment of leukemias and pre-leukemic conditions. In fact, HSC transplantation is the only curative treatment for some of these diseases, including chronic lymphocytic leukemia and chronic myeloid leukemia. The mechanisms by which HSC transplantation cures hematopoietic neoplasms is the graft versus tumor effect, in which the reconstituted donor immune system recognizes residual tumor cells as foreign, and destroys them. HSC transplantation is also used clinically to treat diseases caused by inherited mutations in genes affecting only cells derived from hematopoietic stem cells, such as lymphocytes or red blood cells. Examples of such diseases that can be cured by HSC transfer are adenosine deaminase (ADA) deficiency, X-linked severe combined immunodeficiency disease, and hemoglobin mutations such as beta-thalassemia major and sickle cell disease.

Allogeneic hematopoietic stem cells are rejected by even a minimally immunocompetent host, and therefore the donor and recipient must be carefully matched at all MHC loci. The mechanisms of rejection of HSCs are not completely known, but in addition to adaptive immune mechanisms, HSCs may be rejected by NK cells. The role of NK cells in bone marrow rejection has been studied in experimental animals. Irradiated F_1 hybrid mice reject bone marrow donated by either inbred parent. This phenomenon, called hybrid resistance, appears to violate the classical laws of solid-organ transplantation. Hybrid resistance is seen in T cell–deficient mice, and depletion of recipient NK cells with anti–NK cell antibodies prevents the rejection of parental bone marrow. Hybrid resistance is probably due to host NK cells reacting against bone marrow precursors that lack class I MHC molecules expressed by the host. Recall that normally, recognition of self class I MHC inhibits the activation of NK cells, and if these self MHC molecules are missing, the NK cells are released from inhibition (see Fig. 4-8).

Even after successful engraftment, two additional problems are frequently associated with HSC transplantation, namely, graft-versus-host disease and immunodeficiency.

Graft-Versus-Host Disease

Graft-versus-host disease (GVHD) is caused by the reaction of grafted mature T cells in the HSC inoculum with alloantigens of the host. It occurs when the host is immunocompromised and therefore unable to reject the allogeneic cells in the graft. In most cases, the reaction is directed against minor histocompatibility antigens of the host because bone marrow transplantation is not performed when the donor and recipient have differences in MHC molecules. GVHD may also develop when solid organs that contain significant numbers of T cells are transplanted, such as the small bowel, lung, or liver.

GVHD is the principal limitation to the success of bone marrow transplantation. Immediately after HSC transplantation, immunosuppressive agents including the calcineurin inhibitors cyclosporine and tacrolimus, antimetabolites such as methotrexate, and the mTOR inhibitor sirolimus are given for prophylaxis against the development of GVHD. Despite these aggressive prophylactic strategies, GVHD is the principal cause of mortality among bone marrow transplant recipients. GVHD may be classified on the basis of histologic patterns into acute and chronic forms.

Acute GVHD is characterized by epithelial cell death in the skin (Fig. 17-14), liver (mainly the biliary epithelium), and gastrointestinal tract. It is manifested clinically by rash, jaundice, diarrhea, and gastrointestinal hemorrhage. When the epithelial cell death is extensive, the skin or the lining of the gut may slough off. In this circumstance, acute GVHD may be fatal.

Chronic GVHD is characterized by fibrosis and atrophy of one or more of the same organs, without evidence of acute cell death. Chronic GVHD may also involve the lungs and produce obliteration of small airways, called bronchiolitis obliterans, similar to what is seen in chronic rejection of lung allografts. When it is severe, chronic GVHD leads to complete dysfunction of the affected organ.

In animal models, acute GVHD is initiated by mature T cells transferred with HSCs, and elimination of mature

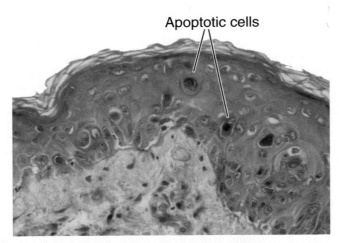

Apoptotic cells

FIGURE 17-14 Histopathology of acute GVHD in the skin.
A sparse lymphocytic infiltrate can be seen at the dermal-epidermal junction, and damage to the epithelial layer is indicated by spaces at the dermal-epidermal junction (vacuolization), cells with abnormal keratin staining (dyskeratosis), apoptotic keratinocytes, and disorganization of maturation of keratinocytes from the basal layer to the surface. *(Courtesy of Dr. Scott Grantor, Department of Pathology, Brigham and Women's Hospital and Harvard Medical School, Boston, Massachusetts.)*

donor T cells from the graft can prevent the development of GVHD. In clinical HSC transplantation, efforts to eliminate T cells from the inoculum have reduced the incidence of GVHD but also decreased the graft-versus-leukemia effect that is often critical in treating leukemias by this type of transplantation. T cell–depleted HSC preparations also tend to engraft poorly, perhaps because mature T cells produce colony-stimulating factors that aid in stem cell repopulation.

Although GVHD is initiated by grafted T cells recognizing host alloantigens, the effector cells that cause epithelial cell injury are less well defined. On histologic examination, NK cells are often attached to the dying epithelial cells, suggesting that NK cells are important effector cells of acute GVHD. CD8+ CTLs and cytokines also appear to be involved in tissue injury in acute GVHD.

The relationship of chronic GVHD to acute GVHD is not known and raises issues similar to those of relating chronic allograft rejection to acute allograft rejection. For example, chronic GVHD may represent the fibrosis of wound healing secondary to acute loss of epithelial cells. However, chronic GVHD can arise without evidence of prior acute GVHD. An alternative explanation is that chronic GVHD represents a response to ischemia caused by vascular injury.

Both acute and chronic GVHD are commonly treated with intense immunosuppression, such as high doses of steroids, but many patients do not respond favorably. Therapeutic failures may be because these treatments target only some of many effector mechanisms at play in GVHD, and some treatments may deplete regulatory T cells, which are important for preventing GVHD. With its high mortality, acute GVHD represents the major obstacle to successful HSC transplantation. Experimental therapies in development include anti-TNF antibodies, and regulatory T cell transfer.

Immunodeficiency After Hematopoietic Stem Cell Transplantation

HSC transplantation is often accompanied by clinical immunodeficiency. Several factors may contribute to defective immune responses in recipients. The transplant recipients may be unable to regenerate a complete new lymphocyte repertoire. Radiation therapy and chemotherapy used to prepare recipients for transplantation may deplete the patient's memory cells and long-lived plasma cells, and it can take a long time to regenerate these populations.

The consequence of immunodeficiency is that HSC transplant recipients are susceptible to viral infections, especially cytomegalovirus infection, and to many bacterial and fungal infections. They are also susceptible to Epstein-Barr virus–provoked B cell lymphomas. The immune deficiencies of HSC transplant recipients can be more severe than those of conventionally immunosuppressed patients. Therefore, the recipients commonly receive prophylactic antibiotics, antiviral prophylaxis to prevent cytomegalovirus infections, antifungal prophylaxis to prevent invasive *Aspergillus* infection, and maintenance intravenous immunoglobulin (IVIG) infusions. Recipients are also immunized against common infections, to restore the protective immunity that is lost upon transplantation.

There is great interest in the use of pluripotent stem cells to repair tissues that have little natural regenerative capacity, such as cardiac muscle, brain, and spinal cord. One approach is to use embryonic stem cells, which are pluripotent stem cells derived from the blastocyst stage of human embryos. Although embryonic stem cells have not yet been widely used clinically, it is likely that a major barrier to their successful grafting will be their alloantigenicity and rejection by the recipient's immune system. A possible solution to this may be to use induced pluripotent stem (iPS) cells, which can be derived from adult somatic tissues by transduction of certain genes. The immunologic advantage of the iPS cell approach is that these cells can be derived from somatic cells harvested from the patient, and therefore they will not be rejected.

SUMMARY

* Transplantation of tissues from one individual to a genetically non-identical recipient leads to a specific immune response called rejection that can destroy the graft. The major molecular targets in allograft rejection are allogeneic class I and class II MHC molecules.
* Intact allogeneic MHC molecules may be presented on donor APCs to recipient T cells (the direct pathway), or the alloantigens may be internalized by host APCs that enter the graft or reside in draining lymphoid organs and be processed and presented to T cells as peptides associated with self MHC molecules (the indirect pathway).
* The frequency of T cells capable of recognizing allogeneic MHC molecules is very high, explaining why the response to alloantigens is much stronger than the response to conventional foreign antigens.

* Graft rejection is mediated by T cells, including CTLs that kill graft cells and helper T cells that cause cytokine-mediated inflammation resembling DTH reactions, and by antibodies.
* Several effector mechanisms cause rejection of solid organ grafts. Preexisting antibodies specific for donor blood group or MHC antigens cause hyperacute rejection characterized by thrombosis of graft vessels. Alloreactive T cells and antibodies produced in response to the graft cause blood vessel wall damage and parenchymal cell death, called acute rejection. Chronic rejection is characterized by fibrosis and arterial stenosis (graft vasculopathy), which may be due to T cell– and cytokine-mediated inflammatory reactions.
* Graft rejection may be prevented or treated by immunosuppression of the host and by minimizing the immunogenicity of the graft (by limiting MHC allelic differences). Most immunosuppression is directed at T cell responses and entails the use of cytotoxic drugs, specific immunosuppressive agents, or anti–T cell antibodies. Widely used immunosuppressive agents target calcineurin, mTOR, and lymphocyte DNA synthesis. Immunosuppression is often combined with anti-inflammatory drugs such as corticosteroids that inhibit cytokine synthesis by macrophages and other cells.
* Patients receiving solid organ transplants may become immunodeficient because of their therapy and are susceptible to viral infections and malignant tumors.
* Xenogeneic transplantation of solid organs is limited by the presence of natural antibodies to carbohydrate antigens on the cells of discordant species that cause hyperacute rejection, antibody-mediated acute vascular rejection, T cell–mediated immune response to xenogeneic MHC molecules, and prothrombotic effects of xenogeneic endothelium on human platelets and coagulation proteins.
* The ABO blood group antigens are polymorphic carbohydrate structures present on blood cells and endothelium that limit transfusions and some solid organ transplantations between individuals. Preexisting natural anti-A or anti-B IgM antibodies are present in individuals who do not express A or B antigens on their cells, respectively, and these antibodies can cause transfusion reactions and hyperacute allograft rejection.
* Hematopoietic stem cell (HSC) transplants are preformed to treat leukemias and genetic defects restricted to hematopoietic cells. HSC transplants are susceptible to rejection, and recipients require intense preparatory immunosuppression. In addition, T lymphocytes in the HSC grafts may respond to alloantigens of the host and cause GVHD. Acute GVHD is characterized by epithelial cell death in the skin, intestinal tract, and liver; it may be fatal. Chronic GVHD is characterized by fibrosis and atrophy of one or more of these same target organs as well as the lungs and may also be fatal. Hematopoietic stem cell transplant recipients also often develop severe immunodeficiency, rendering them susceptible to infections.

SELECTED READINGS

Recognition and Rejection of Allogeneic Transplants

Baldwin WM, Valujskikh A, Fairchild RL: Antibody-mediated rejection: emergence of animal models to answer clinical questions, *American Journal of Transplantation* 10:1135–1142, 2010.

Colvin RB, Smith RN: Antibody-mediated organ-allograft rejection, *Nature Review Immunology* 5:807–817, 2005.

Gras S, Kjer-Nielsen L, Chen Z, Rossjohn J, McCluskey J: The structural bases of direct T-cell allorecognition: implications for T-cell-mediated transplant rejection, *Immunology and Cell Biology* 89:388–395, 2011.

Kinnear G, Jones ND, Wood KJ: Costimulation blockade: current perspectives and implications for therapy, *Transplantation* 95:527–535, 2013.

Lakkis FG, Lechler RI: Origin and biology of the allogeneic response, *Cold Spring Harbor Perspectives in Medicine* 3:1–10, 2013.

LaRosa DF, Rahman AH, Turka LA: The innate immune system in allograft rejection and tolerance, *Journal of Immunology* 178:7503–7509, 2007.

Li XC, Rothstein DM, Sayegh MH: Costimulatory pathways in transplantation: challenges and new developments, *Immunological Reviews* 229:271–293, 2009.

Nagy ZA: Alloreactivity: an old puzzle revisited, *Scandinavian Journal of Immunology* 75:463–470, 2012.

Nankivell BJ, Alexander SI: Rejection of the kidney allograft, *New England Journal of Medicine* 363:1451–1462, 2010.

Wood KJ, Goto R: Mechanisms of rejection: current perspectives, *Transplantation* 93:1–10, 2012.

Clinical Transplantation

Blazar BR, Murphy WJ, Abedi MM: Advances in graft-versus-host disease biology and therapy, *Nature Reviews Immunology* 12:443–458, 2012.

Chinen J, Buckley RH: Transplantation immunology: solid organ and bone marrow, *Journal of Allergy and Clinical Immunology* 125:S324–S335, 2010.

Li HW, Sykes M: Emerging concepts in haematopoietic cell transplantation, *Nature Reviews Immunology* 12:403–416, 2012.

McCall M, Shapiro AM: Update on islet transplantation, *Cold Spring Harbor Perspectives in Medicine* 2:a007823, 2012.

Immunosuppression and Tolerance Induction to Allografts

Chidgey AP, Layton D, Trounson A, Boyd RL: Tolerance strategies for stem-cell-based therapies, *Nature* 453:330–377, 2008.

Halloran PF: Immunosuppressive drugs for kidney transplantation, *New England Journal of Medicine* 351:2715–2729, 2004.

Safinia N, Sagoo P, Lechler R, Lombardi G: Adoptive regulatory T cell therapy: challenges in clinical transplantation, *Current Opinions in Organ Transplantation* 15:427–434, 2010.

Turka LA, Lechler RI: Towards the identification of biomarkers of transplantation tolerance, *Nature Reviews Immunology* 9:521–526, 2009.

Xenotransplantation

Yang YG, Sykes M: Xenotransplantation: current status and a perspective on the future, *Nature Reviews Immunology* 7:519–531, 2007.

Immunity to Tumors

Cancer is a major health problem worldwide and one of the most important causes of morbidity and mortality in children and adults. The lethality of malignant tumors is due to their uncontrolled growth within normal tissues, causing damage and functional impairment. The malignant phenotype of cancers reflects defects in regulation of cell proliferation, resistance of the tumor cells to apoptotic death, ability of the tumor cells to invade host tissues and metastasize to distant sites, and tumor evasion of host immune defense mechanisms. The possibility that cancers can be eradicated by specific immune responses has been the impetus for a large body of work in the field of tumor immunology. The concept **of immune surveillance** of cancer, which was proposed by Macfarlane Burnet in the 1950s, states that a physiologic function of the immune system is to recognize and destroy clones of transformed cells before they grow into tumors and to kill tumors after they are formed. The existence of immune surveillance has been demonstrated by the increased incidence of some types of tumors in immunocompromised experimental animals and humans. It is now clear that the innate and adaptive immune systems do react against many tumors, and exploiting these reactions to specifically destroy tumors remains an important goal of tumor immunologists. In this chapter, we will describe the types of antigens that are expressed by malignant tumors, how the immune system recognizes and responds to these antigens, how tumors evade the host immune system, and the application of immunologic approaches to the treatment of cancer.

OVERVIEW OF TUMOR IMMUNITY

Several characteristics of tumor antigens and immune responses to tumors are fundamental to an understanding of tumor immunity and for the development of strategies for cancer immunotherapy.

● *Tumors stimulate specific adaptive immune responses.* Clinical observations and animal experiments have established that although tumor cells are derived from host cells, the tumors elicit immune responses. Histopathologic studies show that many tumors are surrounded by mononuclear cell infiltrates composed of T lymphocytes, natural killer (NK) cells, and macrophages, and that activated lymphocytes and macrophages are present in lymph nodes draining the sites of tumor growth (Fig. 18-1). The presence of lymphocytic infiltrates in some types of melanoma and carcinomas of the colon and breast is predictive of a better prognosis. The first experimental demonstration that tumors can induce protective immune responses came from studies of transplanted tumors performed in the

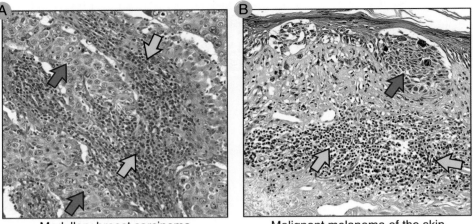

Medullary breast carcinoma

Malignant melanoma of the skin

FIGURE 18-1 Lymphocytic inflammation associated with certain tumors. A, Medullary breast carcinoma. **B,** Malignant melanoma. Red arrows indicate malignant cells. Yellow arrows indicate lymphocyte-rich inflammatory infiltrates.

1950s (Fig. 18-2). A sarcoma may be induced in an inbred mouse by painting its skin with the chemical carcinogen methylcholanthrene (MCA). If the MCA-induced tumor is excised and transplanted into other syngeneic mice, the tumor grows. In contrast, if cells from the original tumor are transplanted back into the original host, the mouse rejects this transplant and no tumor grows. The same mouse that had become immune to its tumor is incapable of rejecting MCA-induced tumors produced in other mice. Furthermore,

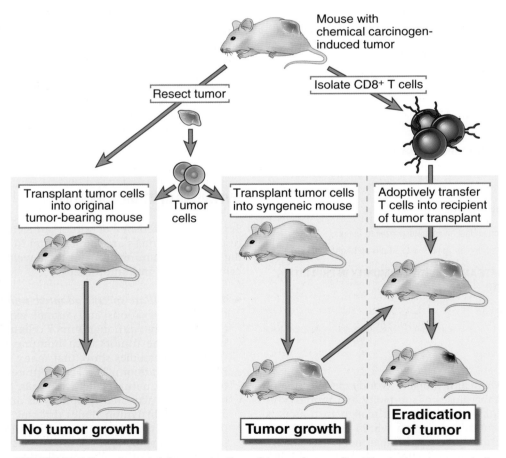

FIGURE 18-2 Experimental demonstration of tumor immunity. Mice that have been surgically cured of a chemical carcinogen (MCA)–induced tumor reject subsequent transplants of the same tumor, whereas the transplanted tumor grows in normal syngeneic mice. The tumor is also rejected in normal mice that are given adoptive transfer of T lymphocytes from the original tumor-bearing animal.

T cells from the tumor-bearing animal can transfer protective immunity against the tumor to a tumor-free animal. Thus, immune responses to tumors exhibit the defining characteristics of adaptive immunity, namely, specificity, memory, and the key role of lymphocytes. As predicted from these transplantation experiments, the most effective response against naturally arising tumors appears to be mediated mainly by T lymphocytes.

- *Immune responses frequently fail to prevent the growth of tumors.* There may be several reasons that anti-tumor immunity is unable to eradicate transformed cells. First, many tumors have specialized mechanisms for evading host immune responses. We will return to these mechanisms later in the chapter. Second, tumor cells are derived from host cells and resemble normal cells in many respects. Therefore, many tumors tend to be weakly immunogenic. Tumors that elicit strong immune responses include those induced by oncogenic viruses, in which the viral proteins are foreign antigens. Many spontaneous tumors induce weak or even undetectable immunity. This may be because the tumors that grow have undergone mutations that reduce their ability to stimulate strong immune responses. Thus, the importance of immune surveillance and tumor immunity varies with the type of tumor. Third, the rapid growth and spread of a tumor may overwhelm the capacity of the immune system to effectively control the tumor, which requires that all the malignant cells be eliminated.

- *The immune system can be activated to effectively kill tumor cells and eradicate tumors.* As we will see at the end of this chapter, this realization has spurred new directions in tumor immunotherapy in which augmentation of the host anti-tumor response is the goal of treatment.

The existence of specific anti-tumor immunity implies that tumors must express antigens that are recognized as foreign by the host. The nature and significance of these antigens are described next.

TUMOR ANTIGENS

The earliest classification of tumor antigens was based on their patterns of expression. Antigens that are expressed on tumor cells but not on normal cells are called **tumor-specific antigens**; some of these antigens are unique to individual tumors, whereas others are shared among tumors of the same type. Tumor antigens that are also expressed on normal cells are called **tumor-associated antigens**; in most cases, these antigens are normal cellular constituents whose expression is aberrant or dysregulated in tumors. The modern classification of tumor antigens is based on the molecular structure and source of antigens expressed by tumor cells that stimulate T cell or antibody responses in their hosts.

Various biochemical and molecular genetic approaches have been used to identify tumor antigens. For tumor antigens recognized by CD8+ cytotoxic T lymphocytes (CTLs), investigators have established cloned lines of tumor-reactive CTLs from cancer patients and used these as probes to specifically identify the relevant peptide antigens or the genes encoding the peptides. These tumor antigen–specific CTL clones can detect responses to tumor-derived peptides or responses to proteins made by complementary DNA (cDNA) libraries of the tumor. Such approaches were first employed to identify human melanoma antigens that stimulated CTL responses in patients with the tumor. The same methods have been used to identify antigens that are recognized by CD4+ helper cells, in which case the probes are helper T cell clones derived from patients' CD4+ T cells.

A method for identification of tumor antigens that stimulate humoral immune responses in patients is called the serologic analysis of recombinant cDNA expression (SEREX). In this method, expression libraries of cDNA derived from a patient's tumor RNA are transfected into a cell line, and assays are performed to detect binding of the cancer patient's serum immunoglobulins to the transfected cells. In this way, gene sequences for antibody-targeted proteins are obtained, and the encoded proteins that stimulated antibody responses in the patient are identified.

In the following section, we describe the main classes of tumor antigens (Table 18-1). We will include tumor antigens known to induce immune responses in humans with cancers as well as tumor-associated antigens that may not naturally induce host immune responses but are potential targets for immunotherapy or are useful markers for clinical diagnosis and for observation of patients.

Products of Mutated Genes

Oncogenes and mutated tumor suppressor genes produce proteins that differ from normal cellular proteins and, therefore, can induce immune responses. Many tumors express genes whose products are required for malignant transformation or for maintenance of the malignant phenotype. Often, these genes are produced by point mutations, deletions, chromosomal translocations, or viral gene insertions affecting cellular proto-oncogenes or tumor suppressor genes. The products of many of these mutant oncogenes and tumor suppressor genes are cytosolic or nuclear proteins that are degraded in proteasomes and can be presented on class I MHC molecules in tumor cells. These proteins may enter the MHC class I and class II antigen presentation pathways in dendritic cells that have phagocytosed dead tumor cells or apoptotic bodies derived from tumor cells. Because the mutated genes are not present in normal cells, peptides encoded by them do not induce self-tolerance and may stimulate T cell responses in the host. Some patients with cancer have circulating CD4+ and CD8+ T cells that can respond to the peptides encoded by mutated oncogenes such as *RAS*, or novel peptides derived from fusion proteins such as Bcr/Abl generated by tumor-related chromosomal translocations, as well as peptides encoded by mutated tumor suppressor genes such as *p53*. Furthermore, in animals, immunization with mutated Ras or p53 proteins induces CTLs and rejection responses against tumors expressing these mutants. However, these proteins do not appear to be major targets of tumor-specific CTLs in most patients with a variety of tumors.

TABLE 18-1   Tumor Antigens

Type of Antigen	Examples of Human Tumor Antigens
Products of mutated onco-genes, tumor suppressor genes	Oncogene products: Ras mutations (~10% of human carcinomas), p210 product of Bcr/Abl rearrange-ments (CML) Tumor suppressor gene products: mutated p53 (present in ~50% of human tumors)
Unmutated but overexpressed products of oncogenes	HER2/Neu (breast and other carci-nomas)
Mutated forms of cellular genes not involved in tumorigenesis	Various mutated proteins in melano-mas recognized by CTLs
Products of genes that are silent in most normal tis-sues	Cancer/testis antigens expressed in melanomas and many carcinomas; normally expressed mainly in the testis and placenta
Normal nononcogenic proteins overexpressed in tumor cells	Tyrosinase, gp100, MART in melanomas (normally expressed in melanocytes)
Products of oncogenic viruses	Papillomavirus E6 and E7 proteins (cervical carcinomas) EBNA-1 protein of EBV (EBV-associated lymphomas, nasopharyngeal carcinoma)
Oncofetal antigens	Carcinoembryonic antigen on many tumors, also expressed in liver and other tissues during inflammation α-Fetoprotein
Glycolipids and glycoproteins	GM_2, GD_2 on melanomas
Differentiation antigens normally present in tissue of origin	Prostate-specific antigen in prostate carcinomas CD20 on B cell lymphomas

CML, chronic myelogenous leukemia; *CTL*, cytotoxic T lymphocyte; *EBNA*, Epstein-Barr nuclear antigen; *EBV*, Epstein-Barr virus; *MART*, melanoma antigen recognized by T cells.

Tumor antigens may be produced by randomly mutated genes whose products are not related to the malignant phenotype. Tumor antigens that were defined by the transplantation of carcinogen-induced tumors in animals, called tumor-specific transplantation antigens, are mutants of various host cellular proteins. Stud-ies with chemically induced rodent sarcomas, such as those illustrated in Figure 18-2, established that differ-ent rodent tumors, all induced by the same carcinogen, expressed different transplantation antigens. The tumor antigens identified by such experiments are peptides derived from mutated self proteins and presented in the form of peptide–class I MHC complexes capable of stimulating CTLs. These antigens are extremely diverse because the carcinogens that induce the tumors may randomly mutagenize any host gene, and the class I MHC antigen-presenting pathway can display peptides from any mutated cytosolic protein in each tumor. More recently, sequencing of genes in common human cancers has revealed that many tumors carry large numbers of tumor-specific mutations, most of which

involve genes that are not believed to be related to the development and malignant phenotype of the tumor. Mutated proteins may serve as tumor antigens if they can yield peptides that bind to the MHC alleles of the affected individual. Recently, common tumors and matched normal cells from the same individual have been analyzed for all possible coding mutations by a Next Generation Sequencing approach. Such analyses have led to the identification of tumor-specific peptides.

Abnormally Expressed but Unmutated Cellular Proteins

Tumor antigens that elicit immune responses may be normal cellular proteins that are abnormally expressed in tumor cells. Many such antigens have been identified in human tumors, such as melanomas, by the molecu-lar cloning of antigens that are recognized by T cells and antibodies from tumor-bearing patients. One of the sur-prises that emerged from these studies was that some tumor antigens are unmutated proteins that are pro-duced at low levels in normal cells and overexpressed in tumor cells. One such antigen is tyrosinase, an enzyme involved in melanin biosynthesis that is expressed in normal melanocytes and melanomas. Both class I MHC–restricted $CD8^+$ CTL clones and class II MHC–restricted $CD4^+$ helper T cell clones from melanoma patients rec-ognize peptides derived from tyrosinase. On face value, it is surprising that these patients are able to respond to a normal self antigen. The likely explanation is that tyrosi-nase is normally produced in such small amounts and in so few cells that it is not recognized by the immune system and fails to induce tolerance. Therefore, the increased amount produced by melanoma cells is able to elicit immune responses. The finding of tyrosinase-spe-cific T cell responses in patients raises the possibility that vaccines that include tyrosinase peptides may stimulate such responses to melanomas; clinical trials with these vaccines are ongoing.

Cancer/testis antigens are proteins expressed in gametes and trophoblasts and in many types of cancers but not in normal somatic tissues. The first cancer/testis antigens were identified by cloning genes from human melanomas that encoded cellular protein antigens rec-ognized by melanoma-specific CTL clones derived from the melanoma-bearing patients. These were called MAGE proteins, and they were subsequently found to be expressed in other tumors in addition to mela-nomas, including carcinomas of the bladder, breast, skin, lung, and prostate and some sarcomas, as well as in normal testes. Subsequent to identification of the *MAGE* genes, several other unrelated gene fami-lies have been identified that encode melanoma anti-gens recognized by CTL clones derived from melanoma patients. Like the MAGE proteins, these other mela-noma antigens are silent in most normal tissues, except the testes or trophoblasts in the placenta, but they are expressed in a variety of malignant tumors. More than 40 different cancer/testis antigen families have been identified. About half are encoded by genes on the X chromosome; the rest are encoded by genes distrib-uted throughout the genome. Although some cancer/

testis antigens have been shown to regulate transcription or translation of other genes, the functions of most of these proteins are unknown. In general, they are not required for the malignant phenotype of the cells, and their sequences are identical to the corresponding genes in normal cells; that is, they are not mutated. Several X-linked cancer/testis antigens are currently being used in tumor vaccine trials.

Antigens of Oncogenic Viruses

The products of oncogenic viruses function as tumor antigens and elicit specific T cell responses that may serve to eradicate the tumors. DNA viruses are implicated in the development of a variety of tumors in humans and experimental animals. Examples in humans include the Epstein-Barr virus (EBV), which is associated with B cell lymphomas and nasopharyngeal carcinoma; human papillomavirus (HPV), which is associated with carcinomas of the uterine cervix, oropharynx, and other sites; and Kaposi sarcoma–associated herpesvirus (KSHV/HHV-8), which is associated with vascular tumors. Papovaviruses, including polyomavirus and simian virus 40 (SV40), and adenoviruses induce malignant tumors in neonatal or immunodeficient adult rodents. In most of these DNA virus–induced tumors, virus-encoded protein antigens are found in the nucleus, cytoplasm, or plasma membrane of the tumor cells. These endogenously synthesized viral proteins can be processed and presented by MHC molecules on the tumor cell surface. Because the viral peptides are foreign antigens, DNA virus–induced tumors are among the most immunogenic tumors known.

The ability of adaptive immunity to prevent the growth of DNA virus–induced tumors has been established by many observations. For instance, EBV-associated lymphomas and HPV-associated cervical cancers arise more frequently in immunosuppressed individuals, such as allograft recipients receiving immunosuppressive therapy and patients with acquired immunodeficiency syndrome (AIDS), than in healthy individuals, and Kaposi sarcoma occurs most commonly in AIDS patients. Tumor transplantation experiments of the kind illustrated in Figure 18-2 have shown that animals may be specifically immunized against DNA virus–induced tumors and will reject transplants of these tumors. Unlike MCA-induced tumor antigens, which are the products of randomly mutated cellular genes, virus-encoded tumor antigens are not unique for each tumor but are shared by all tumors induced by the same type of virus.

The realization that immune responses against viruses protect individuals from virus-induced cancers has led to the development of vaccines against oncogenic viruses. For example, a vaccine against HPV, which is now in use for women and men, has reduced the incidence of pre-cancerous cervical lesions in vaccinated women. The vaccine is composed of recombinant HPV capsid proteins from the most common oncogenic strains of HPV, which form virus-like particles free of viral genome. Vaccination against hepatitis B virus is reducing the incidence of liver cancer. In this case, the virus is not oncogenic, but it promotes the development of liver cancer probably by inducing chronic inflammation, which is a risk factor for cancer development (discussed later in this chapter).

RNA tumor viruses (retroviruses) are important causes of tumors in animals. Retroviral oncogene products theoretically have the same potential antigenic properties as mutated cellular oncogenes, and humoral and cell-mediated immune responses to retroviral gene products on tumor cells can be observed experimentally. The only well-defined human retrovirus that is known to cause tumors is human T cell lymphotropic virus 1 (HTLV-1), the etiologic agent of adult T cell leukemia/lymphoma (ATL), a malignant tumor of CD4+ T cells. Although immune responses specific for HTLV-1–encoded antigens have been demonstrated in individuals infected with the virus, it is not clear whether they play any role in protective immunity against the development of tumors. Furthermore, patients with ATL are often profoundly immunosuppressed, probably because the virus infects CD4+ T cells and induces functional abnormalities in these cells.

Oncofetal Antigens

Oncofetal antigens are proteins that are expressed at high levels in cancer cells and in normal developing fetal but not adult tissues. It is believed that the genes encoding these proteins are silenced during development and are derepressed with malignant transformation. Oncofetal antigens are identified with antibodies raised in other species, and their main importance is that they provide markers that aid in tumor diagnosis. However, their expression in adults is not limited to tumors, but is increased in tissues and in the circulation in various inflammatory conditions, and the antigens are found in small quantities even in normal tissues. There is no evidence that oncofetal antigens are important inducers or targets of antitumor immunity. The two most thoroughly characterized oncofetal antigens are carcinoembryonic antigen (CEA) and α-fetoprotein (AFP).

CEA (CD66) is a highly glycosylated membrane protein that is a member of the immunoglobulin (Ig) superfamily and functions as an intercellular adhesion molecule. High CEA expression is normally restricted to cells in the gut, pancreas, and liver during the first two trimesters of gestation, and low expression is seen in normal adult colonic mucosa and the lactating breast. CEA expression is increased in many carcinomas of the colon, pancreas, stomach, and breast, and serum levels are increased in these patients. The level of serum CEA is used to monitor the persistence or recurrence of the tumors after treatment, but it is not a diagnostic marker because serum CEA can also be elevated in the setting of non-neoplastic diseases, such as chronic inflammatory conditions of the bowel or liver.

AFP is a circulating glycoprotein normally synthesized and secreted in fetal life by the yolk sac and liver. Fetal serum concentrations can be as high as 2 to 3 mg/mL, but in adult life, the protein is replaced by albumin, and only low levels are present in serum. Serum levels of AFP can be significantly elevated in patients with hepatocellular carcinoma, germ cell tumors, and, occasionally, gastric and pancreatic cancers. An elevated serum AFP level is an indicator of advanced liver or germ cell tumors or of recurrence of these tumors after treatment. Furthermore, the detection of AFP in tissue sections by immunohistochemical techniques can help in the pathologic identification of tumor cells. As is the case for CEA, serum AFP is not a useful marker for tumor diagnosis because elevated levels are also found in non-neoplastic diseases, such as cirrhosis of the liver.

Altered Glycolipid and Glycoprotein Antigens

Most human and experimental tumors express higher than normal levels or abnormal forms of surface glycoproteins and glycolipids, which may be diagnostic markers and targets for therapy. These altered molecules include gangliosides, blood group antigens, and mucins. Some aspects of the malignant phenotype of tumors, including tissue invasion and metastatic behavior, may reflect altered cell surface properties that result from abnormal glycolipid and glycoprotein synthesis. Many antibodies have been raised in animals that recognize the carbohydrate groups or peptide cores of these molecules. Although most of the epitopes recognized by these antibodies are not specifically expressed on tumors, they are present at higher levels on cancer cells than on normal cells. This class of tumor-associated antigen is a target for cancer therapy with specific antibodies.

Gangliosides, including GM_2, GD_2, and GD_3, are glycolipids expressed at high levels in neuroblastomas, melanomas, and many sarcomas. Because of the tumor-selective expression of these molecules, they are attractive targets for tumor-specific therapies such as antibody therapy. Clinical trials of anti-ganglioside antibodies and immunization with ganglioside vaccines are under way in patients with melanoma. Mucins are high–molecular-weight glycoproteins containing numerous O-linked carbohydrate side chains on a core polypeptide. Tumors often have dysregulated expression of the enzymes that synthesize these carbohydrate side chains, which leads to the appearance of tumor-specific epitopes on the carbohydrate side chains or on the abnormally exposed polypeptide core. Several mucins have been the focus of diagnostic and therapeutic studies, including CA-125 and CA-19-9, expressed on ovarian carcinomas, and MUC-1, expressed on breast and colon carcinomas. Unlike many mucins, MUC-1 is an integral membrane protein that is normally expressed only on the apical surface of breast ductal epithelium, a site that is relatively sequestered from the immune system. In ductal carcinomas of the breast, however, the molecule is expressed in a non-polarized fashion and contains new, tumor-specific carbohydrate and peptide epitopes detectable by mouse monoclonal antibodies. The peptide epitopes induce both antibody and T cell responses in cancer patients, and efforts are under way to develop vaccines containing immunogenic forms of MUC-1 epitopes.

Tissue-Specific Differentiation Antigens

Tumors may express molecules that are normally expressed only on the cells of origin of the tumors and not on cells from other tissues. These antigens are called differentiation antigens because they are specific for particular lineages or differentiation stages of various cell types. Their importance is as potential targets for immunotherapy and for identification of the tissue of origin of tumors. For example, several melanoma antigens that are targets of CTLs in patients are melanocyte differentiation antigens, such as tyrosinase, mentioned earlier. Lymphomas may be diagnosed as B cell–derived tumors by the detection of surface markers characteristic of this lineage, such as CD10 (previously called common acute lymphoblastic leukemia antigen, or CALLA) and CD20. Antibodies against these molecules are also used for tumor immunotherapy; the most successful immunotherapy for non-Hodgkin's B cell lymphomas is an anti-CD20 antibody (rituximab). These differentiation antigens are normal self molecules, and therefore they do not usually induce strong immune responses in tumor-bearing hosts.

IMMUNE RESPONSES TO TUMORS

Adaptive immune responses, mainly mediated by T cells, have been shown to control the development and progression of malignant tumors. Both innate and adaptive immune responses can be detected in patients and experimental animals, and various immune mechanisms can kill tumor cells in vitro. The challenge for tumor immunologists is to determine which of these mechanisms may contribute significantly to protection against tumors and to enhance these effector mechanisms in ways that are tumor specific. In this section, we will review the evidence for tumor killing by various immune effector mechanisms and discuss which are the most likely to be relevant to human tumors.

T Lymphocytes

The principal mechanism of adaptive immune protection against tumors is killing of tumor cells by CD8+ CTLs. The ability of CTLs to provide effective anti-tumor immunity in vivo is clearly seen in animal experiments using carcinogen-induced and DNA virus–induced tumors. As discussed previously, CTLs may perform a surveillance function by recognizing and killing potentially malignant cells that express peptides that are derived from tumor antigens and are presented in association with class I MHC molecules. Tumor-specific CTLs can be isolated from animals and humans with established tumors, and there is evidence that the prognosis of human tumors, including common tumors such as colonic carcinomas, is more favorable when more CTLs are present within the tumor. Furthermore, mononuclear cells derived from the inflammatory infiltrate in human solid tumors, called tumor-infiltrating lymphocytes (TILs), contain CTLs with the capacity to kill the tumor from which they were derived. Importantly, the inability to detect tumor-specific CTLs in some patients may be because of regulatory mechanisms exploited by the tumor. One of the most impressive results of recent clinical trials is that blocking these inhibitory pathways, and thus removing the brakes on immune responses, leads to the development of strong T cell responses against the tumor. We will return to this idea later in this chapter.

CD8+ T cell responses specific for tumor antigens may require cross-presentation of the tumor antigens by dendritic cells. Most tumor cells are not derived from APCs and therefore do not express the costimulators needed to initiate T cell responses or the class II MHC molecules needed to stimulate helper T cells that promote the differentiation of CD8+ T cells. A likely explanation of how T cell responses to tumors are initiated is that tumor cells or their antigens are ingested by host APCs, particularly dendritic cells, and tumor antigens are processed inside the APCs. Peptides derived from these antigens are then displayed bound to class I MHC molecules for recognition by CD8+ T cells. The APCs express costimulators that provide the signals needed for differentiation of CD8+ T cells into anti-tumor CTLs. This process of cross-presentation, or cross-priming, has been described in earlier chapters (see Fig. 6-20). Once effector CTLs are generated, they are able to recognize and kill the tumor cells without a requirement for costimulation. A practical application of the concept of cross-priming is to grow dendritic cells from a patient with cancer, incubate the APCs with the cells or antigens from that patient's tumor, and use these antigen-pulsed APCs as vaccines to stimulate anti-tumor T cell responses.

The importance of CD4+ helper T cells in tumor immunity is less clear. CD4+ cells may play a role in anti-tumor immune responses by providing cytokines for differentiation of naive CD8+ T cells into effector and memory CTLs (see Chapter 11). In addition, helper T cells specific for tumor antigens may secrete cytokines, such as TNF and IFN-γ, that can increase tumor cell class I MHC expression and sensitivity to lysis by CTLs. IFN-γ may also activate macrophages to kill tumor cells. The importance of IFN-γ in tumor immunity is demonstrated by the finding of increased incidence of tumors in knockout mice lacking this cytokine, the IFN-γ receptor, or components of the IFN-γ receptor signaling cascade.

Antibodies

Tumor-bearing hosts may produce antibodies against various tumor antigens. For example, patients with EBV-associated lymphomas have serum antibodies against EBV-encoded antigens expressed on the surface of the lymphoma cells. Antibodies may kill tumor cells by activating complement or by antibody-dependent cell-mediated cytotoxicity, in which Fc receptor–bearing macrophages or NK cells mediate the killing. However, the ability of antibodies to eliminate tumor cells has been demonstrated largely in vitro, and there is little evidence for effective humoral immune responses against tumors. Some effective therapeutic anti-tumor antibodies that are passively administered to patients likely work by antibody-dependent cell-mediated cytotoxicity, as discussed later.

Natural Killer (NK) Cells

NK cells kill many types of tumor cells, especially cells that have reduced class I MHC expression and express ligands for NK cell–activating receptors. In vitro, NK cells can kill virally infected cells and certain tumor cell lines, especially hematopoietic tumors. NK cells also respond to the absence of class I MHC molecules because the recognition of class I MHC molecules delivers inhibitory signals to NK cells (see Fig. 4-8). As we will see later, some tumors lose expression of class I MHC molecules, perhaps as a result of selection against class I MHC–expressing cells by CTLs. This loss of class I MHC molecules makes the tumors particularly good targets for NK cells. Some tumors also express MIC-A, MIC-B, and ULB, which are ligands for the NKG2D activating receptor on NK cells. In addition, NK cells can be targeted to IgG antibody–coated tumor cells by Fc receptors (FcγRIII or CD16). The tumoricidal capacity of NK cells is increased by cytokines, including interferon-γ (IFN-γ), IL-15, and IL-12, and the anti-tumor effects of these cytokines are partly attributable to stimulation of NK cell activity. IL-2–activated NK cells, called lymphokine-activated killer (LAK) cells, are derived by culture of peripheral blood cells or tumor-infiltrating lymphocytes from tumor patients with high doses of IL-2. These cells are more potent killers of tumors than are unactivated NK cells. The use of LAK cells in adoptive immunotherapy for tumors is discussed later.

The importance of NK cells in tumor immunity in vivo is unclear. In some studies, T cell–deficient mice do not have a high incidence of spontaneous tumors, and this is attributed to the presence of normal numbers of NK cells that serve an immune surveillance function. A few patients have been described with deficiencies of NK cells and an increased incidence of EBV-associated lymphomas.

Macrophages

Macrophages are capable of both inhibiting and promoting the growth and spread of cancers, depending on their activation state. Classically activated M1 macrophages, discussed in Chapter 10, can kill many tumor cells. How macrophages are activated by tumors is not known. Possible mechanisms include recognition of damage-associated molecular patterns from dying tumor cells by macrophage TLRs and other innate immune receptors, and activation of macrophages by IFN-γ produced by tumor-specific T cells. M1 macrophages can kill tumor cells by mechanisms that they also use to kill infectious organisms. Prominent among these is production of nitric oxide (NO), which has been shown to kill tumors in vitro and in mouse models in vivo.

There is evidence that some macrophages in tumors contribute to tumor progression and have an M2 phenotype. These cells secrete vascular endothelial growth factor (VEGF), transforming growth factor-β (TGF-β), and other soluble factors that promote tumor angiogenesis. The role of these cells and other components of the host response in enhancing tumor growth is discussed at the end of this chapter.

EVASION OF IMMUNE RESPONSES BY TUMORS

Many cancers develop mechanisms that allow them to evade anti-tumor immune responses. These mechanisms can broadly be divided into those that are intrinsic to the

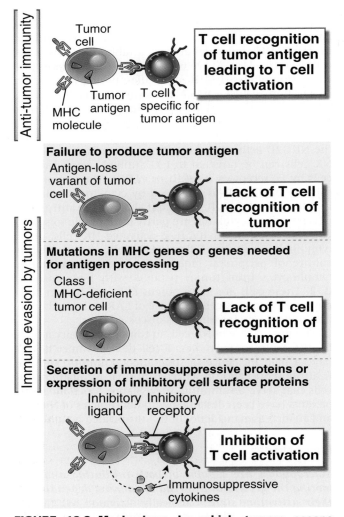

Anti-tumor immunity

Tumor cell

T cell recognition of tumor antigen leading to T cell activation

MHC molecule

Tumor antigen

T cell specific for tumor antigen

Immune evasion by tumors

Failure to produce tumor antigen

Antigen-loss variant of tumor cell

Lack of T cell recognition of tumor

Mutations in MHC genes or genes needed for antigen processing

Class I MHC-deficient tumor cell

Lack of T cell recognition of tumor

Secretion of immunosuppressive proteins or expression of inhibitory cell surface proteins

Inhibitory ligand

Inhibitory receptor

Inhibition of T cell activation

Immunosuppressive cytokines

FIGURE 18-3 Mechanisms by which tumors escape immune defenses. Anti-tumor immunity develops when T cells recognize tumor antigens and are activated. Tumor cells may evade immune responses by losing expression of antigens or MHC molecules or by producing ligands for T cell inhibitory receptors and immunosuppressive cytokines.

tumor cells and those that are mediated by other cells (Fig. 18-3). A major focus of tumor immunology is to understand the immune evasion mechanisms of tumors, with the hope that interventions to prevent immune evasion will increase the immunogenicity of tumors and maximize the responses of the host.

Escaping Immune Recognition by Loss of Antigen Expression

Immune responses to tumor cells impart selective pressures that result in the survival and outgrowth of variant tumor cells with reduced immunogenicity, a process that has been called tumor immunoediting. For example, when tumors are induced by carcinogen treatment in either immunodeficient or immunocompetent mice and the tumors are then transplanted into new immunocompetent mice, the tumors that were derived from the immunodeficient mice are more frequently rejected by the recipient animal's immune system than are the tumors derived from the

immunocompetent mice (Fig. 18-4). This result indicates that tumors developing in the setting of a normal immune system become less immunogenic over time, which is consistent with selection of less immunogenic variant cells. Given the high mitotic rate of tumor cells and their genetic instability, mutations or deletions in genes encoding tumor antigens are common. If these antigens are not required for growth of the tumors or maintenance of the transformed phenotype, the antigen-negative tumor cells will have a growth advantage in the face of the host immune system. Thus, tumor immunoediting is thought to underlie the emergence of tumors that escape immune surveillance.

In addition to loss of tumor-specific antigens, class I MHC expression may be downregulated on tumor cells so that they cannot be recognized by CTLs. Various tumors show decreased synthesis of class I MHC molecules, β_2-microglobulin, or components of the antigen-processing machinery, including the transporter associated with antigen processing and some subunits of the proteasome. These mechanisms are presumably adaptations of the tumors that arise in response to the selection pressures of host immunity, and they may allow tumor cells to evade T cell–mediated immune responses. However, there is no clear correlation between the level of MHC expression on a broad range of experimental or human tumor cells and the in vivo growth of these cells.

Active Inhibition of Immune Responses

Tumors may engage inhibitory mechanisms that suppress immune responses. There is strong experimental and clinical evidence that T cell responses to some tumors are inhibited by the involvement of CTLA-4 or PD-1, two of the best-defined inhibitory pathways in T cells (see Chapter 15). A possible reason for this role of CTLA-4 is that tumor antigens are presented by APCs in the absence of strong innate immunity and thus with low levels of B7 costimulators. These low levels may be enough to engage the high-affinity receptor CTLA-4. PD-L1, a B7 family protein that is a ligand for the T cell inhibitory receptor PD-1 (see Chapter 15), is expressed on many human tumors, and animal studies indicate that anti-tumor T cell responses are compromised by PD-L1 expression. PD-L1 on APCs may also be involved in inhibiting the activation of tumor-specific T cells. As we will discuss later, blockade of the CTLA-4 and PD-L1/PD-1 pathways is now being used in the clinic to enhance tumor immunity.

Secreted products of tumor cells may suppress anti-tumor immune responses. An example of an immunosuppressive tumor product is TGF-β, which is secreted in large quantities by many tumors and inhibits the proliferation and effector functions of lymphocytes and macrophages (see Chapter 15).

Regulatory T cells may suppress T cell responses to tumors. Evidence from mouse model systems and cancer patients indicates that the numbers of regulatory T cells are increased in tumor-bearing individuals, and these cells can be found in the cellular infiltrates in certain tumors. Depletion of regulatory T cells in tumor-bearing mice enhances anti-tumor immunity and reduces tumor growth.

Tumor-associated macrophages may promote tumor growth and invasiveness by altering the tissue microenvironment and by suppressing T cell responses. These macrophages have an M2 phenotype, as discussed briefly earlier,

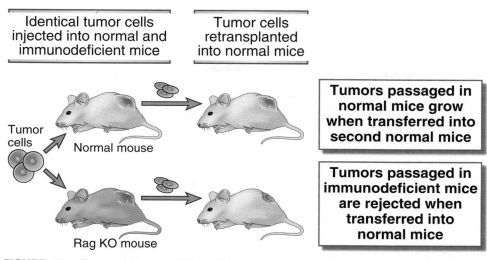

Identical tumor cells injected into normal and immunodeficient mice

Tumor cells retransplanted into normal mice

Tumor cells

Normal mouse

Rag KO mouse

Tumors passed in normal mice grow when transferred into second normal mice

Tumors passed in immunodeficient mice are rejected when transferred into normal mice

FIGURE 18-4 Tumor immunoediting. This experiment shows that tumor cells growing under the selection pressure of a normal immune system will be edited to yield tumor cells that can evade immunity. The cells will survive after transfer into a secondary host. In contrast, tumors removed from a RAG KO mouse, without an adaptive immune system, will not experience the same selection pressures, will remain immunogenic, and will be rejected after transfer to a normal mouse.

and they secrete mediators, such as IL-10 and prostaglandin E_2, that impair T cell activation and effector functions. Conversely, tumor-associated macrophages also secrete factors that promote angiogenesis, such as TGF-β and VEGF, which may enhance tumor growth.

Myeloid-derived suppressor cells (MDSCs) are immature myeloid precursors that are recruited from the bone marrow and accumulate in lymphoid tissues, blood, or tumors of tumor-bearing animals and cancer patients and suppress anti-tumor innate and T cell responses. MDSCs are a heterogeneous collection of cell types, including precursors of dendritic cells, monocytes, and neutrophils. They share some common surface markers, including Ly6C or Ly6G and CD11b in mice and CD33, CD11b, and CD15 in humans. Recruitment of MDSCs from the bone marrow into lymph nodes and other tissues is induced by various proinflammatory mediators produced by tumors. These mediators, which include prostaglandin E_2, IL-6, VEGF, and complement fragment C5a, are not specific to tumors, and, in fact, MDSCs accumulate at sites of chronic inflammation unrelated to tumors. MDSCs suppress innate immune responses by secreting IL-10, which inhibits various inflammatory functions of activated macrophages and dendritic cells. MDSCs also suppress T cell responses by a variety of mechanisms. They generate free radicals that inhibit T cell activation, such as peroxynitrite, and produce indolamine 2,3-dioxygenase, which catabolizes tryptophan needed for T cell proliferation. MDSCs indirectly impair anti-tumor T cell responses by inducing the development of regulatory T lymphocytes and skewing helper T cell differentiation toward T_H2 cells.

IMMUNOTHERAPY FOR TUMORS

The potential for treatment of cancer patients by immunologic approaches has held great promise for oncologists and immunologists for many years. The main reason for interest in an immunologic approach is that most current therapies for cancer rely on drugs that kill dividing cells or block cell division, and these treatments have harmful effects on normal proliferating cells. As a result, the treatment of cancers causes significant morbidity and mortality. Immune responses to tumors may be specific for tumor antigens and will not injure most normal cells. Therefore, immunotherapy has the potential of being the most tumor-specific treatment that can be devised. Advances in our understanding of the immune system and in defining antigens on tumor cells have encouraged many new strategies. Immunotherapy for tumors aims to augment the weak host immune response to the tumors (active immunity) or to administer tumor-specific antibodies or T cells, a form of passive immunity. In this section, we describe some of the modes of tumor immunotherapy that have been tried in the past or are currently being investigated.

Stimulation of Active Host Immune Responses to Tumors

The earliest attempts to boost anti-tumor immunity relied on non-specific immune stimulation. More recently, vaccines composed of killed tumor cells, tumor antigens, or dendritic cells incubated with tumor antigens have been administered to patients, and strategies to enhance immune responses against the tumor are being developed.

Vaccination with Tumor Antigens
Immunization of tumor-bearing individuals with tumor antigens may result in enhanced immune responses against the tumor. The identification of peptides recognized by tumor-specific CTLs and the cloning of genes that encode tumor-specific antigens recognized by CTLs have provided many candidate antigens to include in tumor vaccines (Table 18-2). For antigens that are unique to individual tumors, such as antigens produced by random point mutations in cellular genes, personalized

TABLE 18-2   Tumor Vaccines

Antigen Type	Examples	Features
Products of mutated genes	FNDC3B (for CLL), NeoVax	Epitopes generated from somatic tumor mutations; not present in normal cells
Overexpressed but unmutated cellular proteins	Gp100, Tyrosinase (melanoma)	Native proteins; preferentially over-expressed in tumors
Cancer/testis antigens	NY-ESO1	Aberrant expression in tumor cells; not present in normal differentiated tissue
Whole inactivated tumor cells/tumor cell lysates	GVAX, Can-avaxin	Complex mixtures of antigens generated from autologous whole tumor cells or human cancer cell lines
HSP-associated antigens	HSPPC-96	Misfolded proteins bound to HSPs destined for degradation by the proteasome
In situ tumor	OncoVAX	Infection of tumor cells in situ with an oncolytic virus that can intiate an immune reaction that extends systemically

CLL, chronic lymphocytic leukemia; *HSP,* heat shock protein.
This table was compiled with the assistance of Dr. Catherine Wu, Dana-Farber Cancer Institute and Harvard Medical School, Boston, Massachusetts.

vaccination approaches are now being attempted. An approach that has shown some success is the use of immunogenic long peptides that contain single amino acid changes corresponding to tumor mutations, along with selected adjuvants.

Tumor vaccination strategies employ a variety of adjuvants and delivery methods.

- Proinflammatory molecules are used to enhance the numbers of activated dendritic cells at the vaccination site. These adjuvants include TLR ligands, such as dsRNA, CpG DNA, and BCG, and cytokines such as GM-CSF and IL-12.
- The tumor antigens are delivered in the form of dendritic cell vaccines. In this approach, dendritic cells are purified from patients, incubated with tumor antigens, and then injected back into the patients. A cell-based vaccine is now approved to treat advanced prostate cancer. This vaccine is composed of a preparation of a patient's peripheral blood leukocytes that is enriched for dendritic cells, which are exposed to a recombinant fusion protein consisting of granulocyte-macrophage colony-stimulating factor (GM-CSF) and the tumor-associated antigen prostatic acid phosphatase. GM-CSF promotes the maturation of dendritic cells, which present the tumor antigen and stimulate anti-tumor T cell responses.
- Another approach is the use of DNA vaccines and viral vectors encoding tumor antigens; some of these are in active or planned clinical trials. The cell-based and DNA vaccines may be the best ways to induce CTL responses because the encoded antigens are synthesized in the

cytosol of cells, such as dendritic cells, that take up these antigens, plasmids and vectors, and peptides enter the class I MHC pathway of antigen presentation.

Overall, the results of trials with many different types of tumor vaccines have been inconsistent, and this likely reflects the fact that one of the hallmarks of cancer is to evade host immunity. Tumors often do this by inhibiting immune responses. Most tumor vaccines are therapeutic vaccines; they have to be given after the host has encountered the tumor (unlike preventive vaccines for infections), and in order to be effective, they have to overcome the immune regulation that cancers establish.

The development of virally induced tumors can be reduced by preventive vaccination with viral antigens or attenuated live viruses. As mentioned earlier, newly developed HPV vaccines have been effective in decreasing the incidence of HPV-induced premalignant lesions in the cervix. This approach has been extremely successful in reducing the incidence of feline leukemia virus–induced hematologic malignant tumors in cats and in preventing Marek's disease, a herpesvirus-induced lymphoma, in chickens.

Blocking Inhibitory Pathways to Promote Tumor Immunity

Blockade of T cell inhibitory molecules has emerged as one of the most promising methods for effectively enhancing patients' immune responses to their tumors. This approach is based on the idea that tumor cells exploit various normal pathways of immune regulation or tolerance to evade the host immune response, as discussed earlier. Because these inhibitors establish checkpoints in immune responses, the approach of stimulating immune responses by removing inhibition is often called **checkpoint blockade**. An antibody specific for CTLA-4, the inhibitory receptor on T cells for B7 (see Chapter 15), is an approved therapy for advanced melanoma, and it is effective in slowing tumor progression in many patients. This antibody may work not only by blocking the action of CTLA-4 but perhaps also by depleting regulatory T cells, which express high levels of CTLA-4. As discussed earlier, T cell responses against tumors may also be inhibited by the PD-L1/PD-1 pathway (Fig. 18-5). Antibody blockade of PD-1 or its ligand is effective in enhancing T cell killing of tumors in mice, and several human clinical trials have shown that PD-1 or PD-L1 blockade can limit tumor progression and reduce tumor burden in patients with advanced cancers. Trials of combined blockade of both PD-1 and CTLA-4 appear to be very effective. Common complications of these treatments have been autoimmune and inflammatory reactions, which is predictable in light of the known roles of CTLA-4 and PD-1 in maintaining self-tolerance and regulating T cell responses, but these reactions can be controlled with anti-inflammatory medications such as corticosteroids. Agents that block immune suppression and thereby boost anti-tumor immune responses may be most effective in combination with tumor vaccines or other drugs that target intrinsic molecular pathways that contribute to tumor growth.

Augmentation of Host Immunity to Tumors with Cytokines

Cell-mediated immunity to tumors can theoretically be enhanced by treating tumor-bearing individuals with

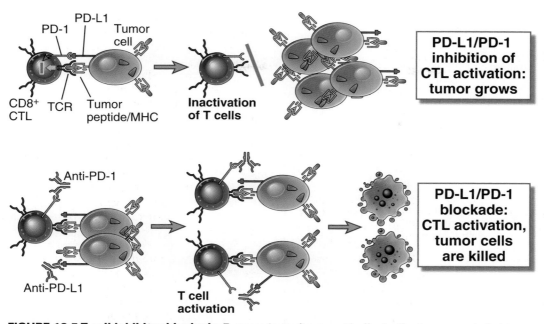

FIGURE 18-5 T cell inhibitor blockade. Tumor patients often mount ineffective T cell responses to their tumors because of the upregulation of inhibitory receptors such as PD-1 on the tumor-specific T cells and expression of the ligand PD-L1 on the tumor cells. Clinical trials using blocking anti-PD-1 or anti-PD-L1 antibodies have shown efficacy in treating several types of advanced tumors. A similar strategy using anti-CTLA-4 has been approved for treatment of melanomas, which may work by blocking CTLA-4 on effector T cells or Treg.

cytokines that stimulate the proliferation and differentiation of T lymphocytes and NK cells. One potential approach for boosting host responses to tumors is to artificially provide cytokines that can enhance the activation of dendritic cells and tumor-specific T cells, particularly CD8+ CTLs. Many cytokines also have the potential to induce non-specific inflammatory responses, which by themselves may have anti-tumor activity.

The largest clinical experience is with high-dose IL-2 given intravenously, which has been effective in inducing measurable tumor regression responses in about 10% of patients with advanced melanoma and renal cell carcinoma and is currently an approved therapy for these cancers. The use of high-dose IL-2 is, however, limited because it stimulates the production of toxic amounts of proinflammatory cytokines such as TNF and IFN-γ, which act on vascular endothelial and other cells and lead to a serious vascular leak syndrome.

IFN-α is approved for treatment of malignant melanoma, in combination with chemotherapy, and for carcinoid tumors. It is also used to treat certain lymphomas and leukemias. The mechanisms of the antineoplastic effects of IFN-α probably include inhibition of tumor cell proliferation, increased cytotoxic activity of NK cells, and increased class I MHC expression on tumor cells, which makes them more susceptible to killing by CTLs.

Other cytokines, such as TNF and IFN-γ, are effective anti-tumor agents in animal models, but their use in patients is limited by their toxic side effects. Hematopoietic growth factors, including GM-CSF and G-CSF, are used in cancer treatment protocols to shorten periods of neutropenia and thrombocytopenia after chemotherapy or autologous bone marrow transplantation.

Non-Specific Stimulation of the Immune System

Immune responses to tumors may be stimulated by the local administration of inflammatory substances or by systemic treatment with agents that function as polyclonal activators of lymphocytes. Non-specific immune stimulation of patients with tumors by injection of inflammatory substances such as killed bacillus Calmette-Guérin (BCG) at the sites of tumor growth has been tried for many years. The BCG mycobacteria activate macrophages and thereby promote macrophage-mediated killing of the tumor cells. In addition, the bacteria function as adjuvants and may stimulate T cell responses to tumor antigens. Intra-vesicular BCG is currently used to treat bladder cancer. Cytokine therapies, discussed earlier, represent another method of enhancing immune responses in a non-specific manner.

Passive Immunotherapy for Tumors with T Cells and Antibodies

Passive immunotherapy involves the transfer of immune effectors, including tumor-specific T cells and antibodies, into patients. Passive immunization against tumors is rapid but does not lead to long-lived immunity. Some anti-tumor antibodies are now approved for the treatment of certain cancers. Several other approaches to passive immunotherapy are being tried, with variable success.

Adoptive Cellular Therapy

Adoptive cellular immunotherapy is the transfer of cultured immune cells that have anti-tumor reactivity into a tumor-bearing host. The immune cells are derived from a cancer patient's blood or solid tumor, and then

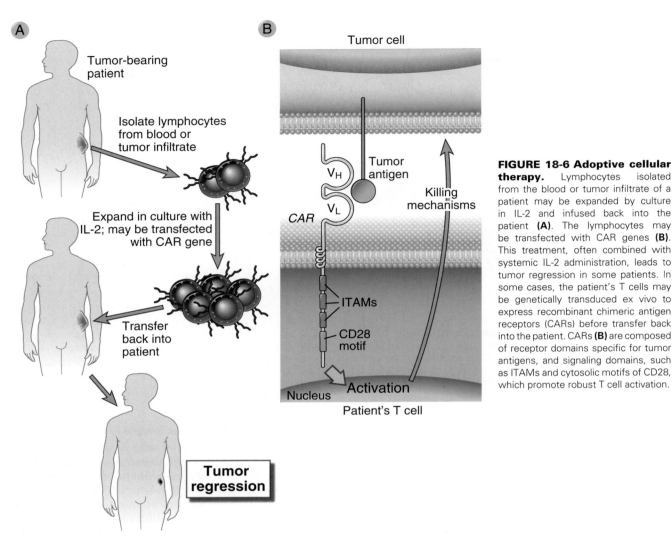

FIGURE 18-6 Adoptive cellular therapy. Lymphocytes isolated from the blood or tumor infiltrate of a patient may be expanded by culture in IL-2 and infused back into the patient **(A)**. The lymphocytes may be transfected with CAR genes **(B)**. This treatment, often combined with systemic IL-2 administration, leads to tumor regression in some patients. In some cases, the patient's T cells may be genetically transduced ex vivo to express recombinant chimeric antigen receptors (CARs) before transfer back into the patient. CARs **(B)** are composed of receptor domains specific for tumor antigens, and signaling domains, such as ITAMs and cytosolic motifs of CD28, which promote robust T cell activation.

are treated in various ways to expand their numbers and enhance their anti-tumor activity, before reinfusion back into the patient (Fig. 18-6, *A*).

Adoptive therapy using T cells expressing chimeric antigen receptors (CARs) has proven successful in some hematologic malignancies, and this approach is in trials for other tumors. CARs are genetically engineered receptors with tumor antigen–specific binding sites encoded by Ig-variable genes and cytoplasmic tails containing signaling domains of both antigen receptors and costimulatory molecules (Fig. 18-6, *B*). In current protocols, a patent's peripheral blood T cells are isolated, stimulated with anti-CD3 and/or anti-CD28 antibodies, and subjected to gene transduction with CAR-encoding vectors. The CAR-expressing T cells are then expanded in vitro and injected into the patient. The transferred T cells undergo further robust proliferation in the patient, in response to tumor antigen recognition by the CAR. Tumor killing is achieved by both direct cytotoxic and cytokine-mediated mechanisms. Patients with B cell malignancies, including chronic lymphocytic leukemia and acute lymphoblastic leukemia, have been effectively treated with CAR-expressing T cells

specific for CD19, a pan–B cell marker also expressed on the tumor cells. Killing of bystander normal B cells occurs, but patients can tolerate this because long-lived antibody-producing cells do not express CD19 and are not killed, and they continue to provide antibody-mediated immunity. A major roadblock to expanding the use of CAR-T cell therapy for tumors, such as carcinomas, is to identify target antigens that are relatively tumor specific.

Another, older protocol for adoptive cellular immunotherapy is to generate LAK cells by culturing peripheral blood leukocytes from patients with the tumor in high concentrations of IL-2, and injecting the LAK cells back into the patients. As discussed earlier, LAK cells are derived mainly from NK cells. Adoptive therapy with autologous LAK cells, in conjunction with in vivo administration of IL-2 or chemotherapeutic drugs, has yielded impressive results in mice, with regression of solid tumors. Human LAK cell therapy trials have thus far been largely restricted to cases of advanced metastatic tumors, and the efficacy of this approach appears to vary from patient to patient. A variation of this approach is to isolate TILs from the inflammatory infiltrate present in

TABLE 18-3 Anti-Tumor Monoclonal Antibodies in Trials or Approved for Clinical Use

Specificity of Antibody	Form of Antibody Used	Clinical Use
HER2/Neu (EGF receptor, oncogene)	Humanized mouse monoclonal	Breast cancer (approved)
CD20 (B cell marker)	Humanized mouse monoclonal	B cell lymphoma (approved)
CD52 (lymphocyte marker)	Humanized mouse monoclonal	B cell lymphoma (approved)
Carcinoembryonic antigen	Humanized mouse monoclonal	Gastrointestinal cancers (imaging)
CA-125 (tumor marker)	Mouse monoclonal	Ovarian cancer detection
GD$_3$ ganglioside (tumor antigen)	Humanized mouse monoclonal	Melanoma, neuroblastoma (trials)

and around solid tumors, obtained from surgical resection specimens, and to expand the TILs by culture in IL-2. The rationale for this approach is that TILs may be enriched for tumor-specific CTLs and for activated NK cells. TIL therapy for metastatic melanoma is used in several centers.

Graft-Versus-Leukemia Effect

In leukemia patients, administration of T cells and NK cells together with hematopoietic stem cells from an allogeneic donor can contribute to eradication of the tumor. The T cell–mediated graft-versus-leukemia effect is directed at the allogeneic MHC molecules present on the recipient's hematopoietic cells, including the leukemia cells. Donor NK cells respond to the tumor cells because tumors may express low levels of class I MHC molecules, which normally inhibit the activation of NK cells (see Chapter 4). The challenge in use of this treatment to improve clinical outcome is to minimize the dangerous graft-versus-host disease that may be mediated by the same donor T cells (see Chapter 17).

Therapy with Anti-Tumor Antibodies

Tumor-specific monoclonal antibodies may be useful for specific immunotherapy for tumors. The potential of using antibodies as magic bullets has been alluring to investigators for many years and is still an active area of research. Currently, there are more than 100 different monoclonal antibodies being considered as therapeutic agents for cancer, either in experimental animal studies or in human trials, and a few have been approved for clinical use (Table 18-3). Anti-tumor antibodies may eradicate tumors by the same effector mechanisms that are used to eliminate microbes, including opsonization and phagocytosis, activation of the complement system, and antibody-dependent cellular cytotoxicity (see Chapter 13). These mechanisms are likely at work in B cell lymphoma patients treated with anti-CD20, one of the most successful anti-tumor antibody treatments to date. In addition, some antibodies may directly activate intrinsic apoptosis pathways in tumor cells; this is the proposed mechanism for the use of anti-CD30 to treat lymphomas, currently in clinical trials. A monoclonal antibody specific for the oncogene product HER2/Neu is an approved treatment for breast cancer patients whose tumors express high levels of the protein. In addition to eliciting immune effector mechanisms, the anti–HER2/Neu antibody interferes with growth-signaling functions of the HER2/Neu molecule.

Because the anti-tumor antibodies used in the early human trials were mouse monoclonal antibodies, an immune response frequently occurred against the mouse Ig, resulting in anti–mouse Ig antibodies that caused increased clearance of the anti-tumor antibodies or blocked binding of the therapeutic agent to its target. This problem has been diminished by use of humanized antibodies consisting of the variable regions of a mouse monoclonal antibody specific for the tumor antigen combined with human Fc portions. One of the most difficult problems with the use of anti-tumor antibodies is the outgrowth of antigen loss variants of the tumor cells that no longer express the antigens that the antibodies recognize. One way to avoid this problem may be to use cocktails of antibodies specific for different antigens expressed on the same tumor.

Many variations on anti-tumor antibodies have been tried in attempts to improve their effectiveness. Tumor-specific antibodies may be coupled to toxic molecules, radioisotopes, and anti-tumor drugs to promote the delivery of these cytotoxic agents specifically to the tumor. Toxins such as ricin and diphtheria toxin are potent inhibitors of protein synthesis and can be effective at extremely low doses if they are carried to tumors attached to anti-tumor antibodies; such conjugates are called immunotoxins. This approach requires covalent coupling of the toxin (lacking its cell-binding component) to an anti-tumor antibody molecule without loss of toxicity or antibody specificity. The systemically injected immunotoxin is endocytosed by tumor cells, and the toxin part is delivered to its intracellular site of action. Several practical difficulties must be overcome for this technique to be successful. The specificity of the antibody must be such that it does not bind to non-tumor cells. A sufficient amount of antibody must reach the appropriate tumor target before it is cleared from the blood by Fc receptor–bearing phagocytic cells. The toxins, drugs, or radioisotopes attached to the antibody may have systemic effects as a result of circulation through normal tissues. For example, hepatotoxicity and vascular leak syndromes are common problems with immunotoxin therapy. Administration of immunotoxins may result in antibody responses against the toxins and the injected antibodies. Because of these practical difficulties, clinical trials of immunotoxins have had variable and modest success.

Tumor growth is usually dependent on growth factors, which are potential targets for therapy. Antibodies that block the epidermal growth factor receptor are approved for the treatment of colorectal tumors. Tumors depend on the formation of new blood vessels that supply the tumor with oxygen and nutrients. This process, called tumor angiogenesis, is dependent on other specialized growth factors, including VEGF. Various inhibitors of these angiogenic factors can block tumor growth. Anti-VEGF antibodies are now approved for clinical use, in combination with chemotherapeutic agents, to treat some metastatic tumors, although their efficacy is modest.

THE ROLE OF INNATE AND ADAPTIVE IMMUNITY IN PROMOTING TUMOR GROWTH

Although much of the emphasis in tumor immunology has been on the role of the immune system in eradicating tumors, it is clear that the immune system may also contribute to the development of some solid tumors. In fact, chronic inflammation has long been recognized as a risk factor for development of tumors in many different tissues, especially those affected by chronic inflammatory diseases such as Barrett's esophagus, Crohn's disease, and ulcerative colitis, for example. Some cancers associated with infections are also considered to be an indirect result of the carcinogenic effects of the chronic inflammatory states that are induced by the infectious organisms. These include gastric carcinoma and lymphoma in the setting of chronic *Helicobacter pylori* infection and hepatocellular carcinomas associated with chronic hepatitis B and C virus infections. Although the mechanisms by which chronic inflammation can promote tumor development are not well understood, there are several possibilities, supported by data in rodent models.

Cells of the innate immune system are considered the most direct tumor-promoting culprits among immune cells. Tumor-associated macrophages of the alternatively activated (M2) phenotype as well as other cells are sources of VEGF, which promotes angiogenesis, and matrix metalloproteinases, which modify the extracellular tissue. Therefore, chronic activation of some innate immune cells is characterized by angiogenesis and tissue remodeling, which favor tumor growth and spread. Innate immune cells may also contribute to malignant transformation of cells by generating free radicals that cause DNA damage and lead to mutations in tumor suppressor genes and oncogenes. Some data suggest that cells of the innate immune system, including mast cells, neutrophils, and macrophages, secrete soluble factors that promote cell cycle progression and survival of tumor cells. The transcription factor NF-κB, which is a key mediator of innate immune responses, may play an important role in inflammation-associated cancer progression.

The adaptive immune system can promote chronic activation of innate immune cells in several ways, including T cell–mediated activation of macrophages in the setting of persistent intracellular microbial infections as well as during early malignant disease even when infectious agents are not present. There is also experimental evidence that B lymphocytes may contribute to tumor progression by their secretion of factors that directly regulate proliferation of tumor cells as well as by their ability to chronically activate innate immune cells present in early tumors. The tumor-promoting effects of the immune system are paradoxical and a topic of active investigation at present. These effects of chronic inflammation are theoretically also targets for pharmacologic intervention because there are a large variety of effective anti-inflammatory drugs already available. The challenge for oncologists is to achieve a beneficial balance in which protective anti-tumor adaptive immune responses are not compromised while potentially harmful tumor-promoting inflammatory reactions are controlled.

SUMMARY

* Tumors express antigens that are recognized by the immune system, but most tumors suppress immune responses or are weakly immunogenic, and immune responses often fail to prevent the growth of tumors. The immune system can be stimulated to effectively kill tumors.

* Tumor antigens recognized by CTLs are the principal inducers of and targets for anti-tumor immunity. These antigens include mutants of oncogenes and other cellular proteins, normal proteins whose expression is dysregulated or increased in tumors, and products of oncogenic viruses.

* Antibodies specific for tumor cell antigens are used for diagnosis, and the antigens are potential targets for antibody therapy. These antigens include oncofetal antigens, which are expressed normally during fetal life and whose expression is dysregulated in some tumors; altered surface glycoproteins and glycolipids; and molecules that are normally expressed on the cells from which the tumors arise and are thus differentiation antigens for particular cell types.

* Immune responses that are capable of killing tumor cells are mediated by CTLs, NK cells, and activated macrophages. Among these immune effector mechanisms, the role of CTLs in protecting individuals from tumors is best defined.

* Tumors evade immune responses by several mechanisms, including downregulation of expression of MHC molecules, selective outgrowth of cells that do not express tumor antigens, production of soluble immunosuppressive substances, the engagement of inhibitory receptors on lymphocytes by their ligands expressed on the tumor cells, and the induction of regulatory T cells. Tumor-associated macrophages and myeloid-derived suppressor cells, found in most solid tumors, can suppress anti-tumor immunity.

* Immunotherapy for tumors is designed to augment active immune responses against these tumors or to administer tumor-specific immune effectors to patients. Anti-tumor immunity may be enhanced by blocking mechanisms of immune regulation. Immune responses may also be actively stimulated by vaccination with tumor cells or antigens, and by systemic administration of cytokines that stimulate immune responses. The most recent successful strategy is checkpoint blockade, in which antibodies against inhibitory

receptors on T cells or their ligands are administered to remove the brakes on lymphocyte activation and thus promote anti-tumor immunity.

* Approaches for passive immunotherapy include the administration of anti-tumor antibodies, antibodies conjugated with toxic drugs (immunotoxins), and tumor-reactive T cells and NK cells isolated from patients and expanded by culture with growth factors. A promising new approach is adoptive transfer of T cells transfected to express chimeric antigen receptors specific for tumor antigens.

SELECTED READINGS

Immune Responses to Tumors

Boon T, Coulie PG, Van den Eynde BJ, van der Bruggen P: Human T cell responses against melanoma, *Annual Review of Immunology* 24:175–208, 2006.

Burnet FM: The concept of immunological surveillance, *Progress in Experimental Tumor Research* 13:1–27, 1970.

Coussens LM, Zitvogel L, Palucka AK: Neutralizing tumor-promoting chronic inflammation: a magic bullet? *Science* 339:286–291, 2013.

Fridman WH, Pages F, Sautes-Fridman C, Galon J: The immune contexture in human tumors: impact on clinical outcome, *Nature Reviews Cancer* 12:298–306, 2012.

Gajewski TF, Schreiber H, Fu YX: Innate and adaptive immune cells in the tumor microenvironment, *Nature Immunology* 14:1014–1022, 2013.

Grivennikov SI, Greten FR, Karin M: Immunity, inflammation, and cancer, *Cell* 140:883–899, 2010.

Mantovani A, Allavena P, Sica A, Balkwill F: Cancer-related inflammation, *Nature* 454:436–444, 2008.

Schreiber RD, Old LJ, Smyth MJ: Cancer immunoediting: integrating immunity's roles in cancer suppression and promotion, *Science* 331:1565–1570, 2011.

Tumor Immunotherapy

Curiel TJ: Regulatory T cells and treatment of cancer, *Current Opinions in Immunology* 20:241–246, 2008.

Dranoff G: Cytokines in cancer pathogenesis and cancer therapy, *Nature Reviews Cancer* 4:11–22, 2004.

Farkas AM, Finn OJ: Vaccines based on abnormal self-antigens as tumor-associated antigens: immune regulation, *Seminars in Immunology* 22:125–131, 2010.

Gilboa E: DC-based cancer vaccines, *Journal of Clinical Investigation* 117:1195–1203, 2007.

Kalos M, June CH: Adoptive T cell transfer for cancer immunotherapy in the era of synthetic biology, *Immunity* 39:49–60, 2013.

Maus MV, Fraietta JA, Levine BL, Kalos m, Zhao Y, June CH: Adoptive immunotherapy for cancer and viruses, *Annual Review of Immunology* 32:189–225, 2014.

Mellman I, Coukos G, Dranoff G: Cancer immunotherapy comes of age, *Nature* 480:480–489, 2012.

Mougiakakos D, Choudhury A, Lladser A, Kiessling R, Johansson CC: Regulatory T cells in cancer, *Advances in Cancer Research* 107:57–117, 2010.

Page DB, Postow MA, Callahan MK, Allison JP, Wolchok JD: Immune modulation in cancer with antibodies, *Annual Review of Medicine* 65:185–202, 2014.

Palucka K, Banchereau J: Dendritic cell-based therapeutic cancer vaccines, *Immunity* 39:38–48, 2013.

Pardoll DM: The blockade of immune checkpoints in cancer immunotherapy, *Nature Reivews Cancer* 12:252–264, 2012.

Topalian SL, Weiner GJ, Pardoll DM: Cancer immunotherapy comes of age, *Journal of Clinical Oncology* 29:4828–4836, 2011.

Vanneman M, Dranoff GM: Combining immunotherapy and targeted therapies in cancer treatment, *Nature Reviews Cancer* 12:237–251, 2012.

Weiner LM, Surana R, Wang S: Monoclonal antibodies: versatile platforms for cancer immunotherapy, *Nature Reviews Immunology* 10:317–327, 2010.

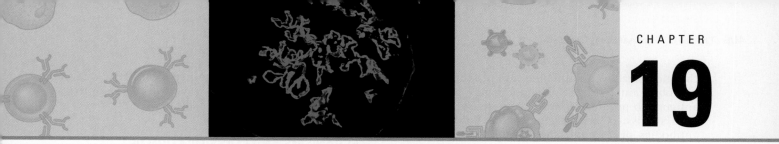

Hypersensitivity Disorders

Adaptive immunity serves the important function of host defense against microbial infections, but immune responses are also capable of causing tissue injury and disease. Disorders caused by immune responses are called **hypersensitivity diseases**. This term arose from the clinical definition of immunity as sensitivity, which is based on the observation that an individual who has been exposed to an antigen exhibits a detectable reaction, or is sensitive, to subsequent encounters with that antigen. Normally, immune responses eradicate infecting organisms without serious injury to host tissues. However, these responses are sometimes inadequately controlled, inappropriately targeted to host tissues, or triggered by commensal microorganisms or environmental antigens that are usually harmless. In these situations, the normally beneficial immune response is the cause of disease.

In this chapter, we will describe the pathogenesis of different types of hypersensitivity reactions, with an emphasis on the effector mechanisms that cause tissue injury. We will conclude with a brief consideration of the treatment of immunologic diseases and examples of diseases that illustrate important principles.

CAUSES OF HYPERSENSITIVITY DISEASES

Immune responses against antigens from different sources can be the underlying cause of hypersensitivity disorders.

- *Autoimmunity: reactions against self antigens.* Failure of the normal mechanisms of self-tolerance results in reactions against one's own cells and tissues that are called **autoimmunity** (see Chapter 15). The diseases caused by autoimmunity are referred to as **autoimmune diseases.** Autoimmune diseases are estimated to affect at least 2% to 5% of the population in developed countries, and the incidence of these disorders is rising. Many of these diseases are common in individuals in the 20- to 40-year age group. They are also more common in women than in men, for reasons that remain obscure. Autoimmune diseases are chronic and debilitating and an enormous medical and economic burden. Although these disorders have been refractory to treatment in the past, many new effective approaches were developed in the early twenty-first century based on scientific principles. The mechanisms of autoimmunity were described in Chapter 15. In this chapter, we will refer to various autoimmune diseases to illustrate how autoimmunity can cause disease.
- *Reactions against microbes.* Immune responses against microbial antigens may cause disease if the reactions are excessive or the microbes are unusually persistent. T cell responses against persistent microbes may give rise to severe inflammation, sometimes with the formation of granulomas; this is the cause of tissue injury in tuberculosis and some other

chronic infections. If antibodies are produced against microbial antigens, the antibodies may bind to the antigens to produce immune complexes, which deposit in tissues and trigger inflammation. Rarely, antibodies or T cells against a microbe will cross-react with a host tissue. In some diseases involving the intestinal tract, called inflammatory bowel disease, the immune response is directed against commensal bacteria that normally reside in the gut and cause no harm. Sometimes, the mechanisms that an immune response uses to eradicate a pathogenic microbe require killing infected cells and therefore cause host tissue injury. For example, in viral hepatitis, the virus that infects liver cells is not cytopathic, but it is recognized as foreign by the immune system. Cytotoxic T lymphocytes (CTLs) try to eliminate infected cells, and this normal immune response damages liver cells. This type of normal reaction is not considered hypersensitivity.

- **Reactions against environmental antigens.** Most healthy individuals do not react against common, generally harmless environmental substances, but almost 20% of the population is abnormally responsive to one or more of these substances. These individuals produce immunoglobulin E (IgE) antibodies that cause allergic diseases (see Chapter 20). Some individuals become sensitized to environmental antigens and chemicals that contact the skin and develop T cell reactions that lead to cytokine-mediated inflammation, resulting in contact sensitivity.

In all of these conditions, the mechanisms of tissue injury are the same as those that normally function to eliminate infectious pathogens. These mechanisms include innate and adaptive immune responses involving phagocytes, antibodies, T lymphocytes, mast cells, and various other effector cells, and mediators of inflammation. The problem in hypersensitivity diseases is that the immune response is not controlled appropriately. Because the stimuli for these abnormal immune responses are difficult or impossible to eliminate (e.g., self antigens, commensal microbes, and environmental antigens) and the immune system has many built-in positive feedback loops (amplification mechanisms), once a pathologic immune response starts, it is difficult to control or to terminate it. Therefore, these hypersensitivity diseases tend to be chronic and progressive and are major therapeutic challenges in clinical medicine.

MECHANISMS AND CLASSIFICATION OF HYPERSENSITIVITY REACTIONS

Hypersensitivity diseases are commonly classified according to the type of immune response and the effector mechanism responsible for cell and tissue injury (Table 19-1).

- Immediate hypersensitivity (type I hypersensitivity) caused by IgE antibodies specific for environmental antigens is the most prevalent type of hypersensitivity disease and will be described separately in Chapter 20. Immediate hypersensitivity diseases, commonly called allergic or atopic disorders, are the prototypes of diseases caused by activation of IL-4, IL-5 and IL-13 producing helper T cells, classically T_H2 cells, in which the T cells stimulate the production of IgE antibodies and inflammation.

- IgG and IgM antibodies can cause tissue injury by activating the complement system, by recruiting inflammatory cells, and by interfering with normal cellular functions. Some of these antibodies are specific for antigens of particular cells or the extracellular matrix and are found either attached to these cells or tissues or as unbound antibodies in the circulation; the diseases induced by such antibodies are called type II hypersensitivity disorders. Other antibodies may form immune complexes in the circulation, and the complexes are subsequently deposited in tissues, particularly in the walls of blood vessels, and cause injury. Immune complex diseases are also called type III hypersensitivity disorders.

- Tissue injury may be due to T lymphocytes that induce inflammation or directly kill target cells; such conditions are called type IV hypersensitivity disorders. They are caused mainly by the activation of CD4+ helper T cells, which secrete cytokines that promote inflammation and activate leukocytes, mainly neutrophils and macrophages. Helper T cells also stimulate the production of antibodies that damage tissues and induce inflammation. CTLs contribute to tissue injury in some diseases.

TABLE 19-1 Classification of Hypersensitivity Diseases		
Type of Hypersensitivity	**Pathologic Immune Mechanisms**	**Mechanisms of Tissue Injury and Disease**
Immediate: type I	IgE antibody, T_H2 cells	Mast cells, eosinophils, and their mediators (vasoactive amines, lipid mediators, cytokines)
Antibody–mediated: type II	IgM, IgG antibodies against cell surface or extracellular matrix antigens	Opsonization and phagocytosis of cells Complement- and Fc receptor–mediated recruitment and activation of leukocytes (neutrophils, macrophages) Abnormalities in cellular functions, e.g., hormone receptor signaling, neurotransmitter receptor blockade
Immune complex– mediated: type III	Immune complexes of circulating antigens and IgM or IgG antibodies	Complement- and Fc receptor–mediated recruitment and activation of leukocytes
T cell–mediated: type IV	1. CD4+ T cells (T_H1 and T_H17 cells) 2. CD8+ CTLs	1. Cytokine-mediated inflammation 2. Direct target cell killing, cytokine-mediated inflammation

This classification is useful because distinct types of pathologic immune responses show different patterns of tissue injury and may vary in their tissue specificity. As a result, the different immunologic mechanisms cause disorders with distinct clinical and pathologic features. However, immunologic diseases in humans are often complex and caused by combinations of humoral and cell-mediated immune responses and multiple effector mechanisms. This complexity is not surprising given that a single antigen may normally stimulate both humoral and cell-mediated immune responses in which several types of antibodies and effector T cells are produced. Because multiple mechanisms may be involved and repetitive bouts of inflammation are major components of the pathology and clinical manifestations of these disorders, they are sometimes grouped under the rubric **immune-mediated inflammatory diseases**. Considering these diseases together also has some clinical value because, as we will discuss later in this chapter, many of them are treated with the same or related biologic agents. In the discussion that follows, we will use descriptions that identify the pathogenic mechanisms rather than the less informative numerical designations for types of hypersensitivity. With this background, we will proceed to a discussion of antibody- and T cell-mediated diseases.

DISEASES CAUSED BY ANTIBODIES

Antibody-mediated diseases are produced either by antibodies that bind to antigens on particular cells or in extracellular tissues or by antigen-antibody complexes that form in the circulation and are deposited in vessel walls (Fig. 19-1). To prove that a disease is caused by antibodies, one would need to demonstrate that the lesions can be induced in a normal animal by the adoptive transfer of immunoglobulin purified from the blood or affected tissues of individuals with the disease. An experiment of nature is occasionally seen in children of mothers suffering from antibody-mediated diseases. These infants may be born with transient manifestations of such diseases because of transplacental passage of antibodies. However, in clinical situations, the diagnosis of diseases caused by antibodies or immune complexes is usually based on the demonstration of antibodies or immune complexes in the circulation or deposited in tissues as well as clinicopathologic similarities with experimental diseases that are proved to be antibody mediated by adoptive transfer.

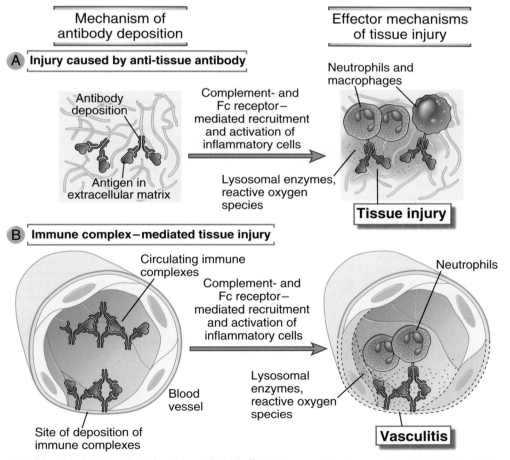

FIGURE 19-1 Types of antibody-mediated diseases. A, Antibodies may bind specifically to tissue antigens and the recruited leukocytes cause tissue injury. **B,** Complexes of antibodies and antigens may be formed in the circulation and deposited in blood vessels and other sites. These immune complexes induce vascular inflammation, and subsequent ischemic damage to the tissues. Antibodies against cellular proteins can also cause depletion of the cells and functional abnormalities *(not shown)*.

Diseases Caused by Antibodies Against Fixed Cell and Tissue Antigens

Antibodies against cellular or matrix antigens cause diseases that specifically affect the cells or tissues where these antigens are present, and these diseases are often not systemic. Antibodies against tissue antigens cause disease by three main mechanisms (Fig. 19-2).

- **Opsonization and phagocytosis.** Antibodies that bind to cell surface antigens may directly opsonize cells, or they may activate the complement system, resulting in the production of complement proteins that opsonize cells. These opsonized cells are phagocytosed and destroyed by phagocytes that express receptors for the Fc portions of IgG antibodies and receptors for complement proteins. This is the principal mechanism of

cell destruction in autoimmune hemolytic anemia and autoimmune thrombocytopenic purpura, in which antibodies specific for red blood cells or platelets, respectively, lead to the opsonization and removal of these cells from the circulation. The same mechanism is responsible for hemolysis in transfusion reactions (see Chapter 17).

- **Inflammation.** Antibodies deposited in tissues recruit neutrophils and macrophages, which bind to the antibodies or to attached complement proteins by IgG Fc and complement receptors. These leukocytes are activated by signaling from the receptors (particularly Fc receptors), and leukocyte products, including lysosomal enzymes and reactive oxygen species, are released and cause tissue injury. The mechanism of injury in antibody-mediated glomerulonephritis and many other diseases is inflammation and leukocyte activation.

FIGURE 19-2 Effector mechanisms of antibody-mediated disease. A, Antibodies opsonize cells and may activate complement, generating complement products that also opsonize cells, leading to phagocytosis of the cells through phagocyte Fc receptors or C3b receptors. **B,** Antibodies recruit leukocytes by binding to Fc receptors or by activating complement and thereby releasing byproducts that are chemotactic for leukocytes. **C,** Antibodies specific for cell surface receptors for hormones or neurotransmitters may stimulate the activity of the receptors even in the absence of the hormone, as in Graves' diseases (hyperthyroidism) *(left panel)*, or may inhibit binding of the neurotransmitter to its receptor, as in myasthenia gravis *(right panel). TSH,* thyroid-stimulating hormone.

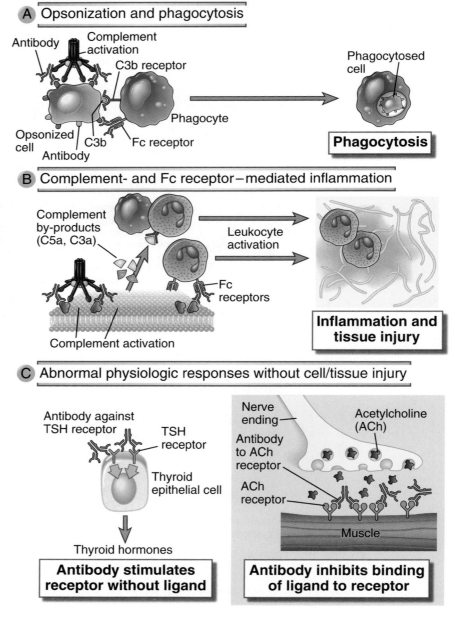

- *Abnormal cellular functions.* Antibodies that bind to normal cellular receptors or other proteins may interfere with the functions of these receptors or proteins and cause disease without inflammation or tissue damage. Antibodies specific for thyroid stimulating hormone receptor or the nicotinic acetylcholine receptor cause functional abnormalities that lead to Graves' disease and myasthenia gravis, respectively (Fig. 19-2, *C*). Antibodies specific for intrinsic factor, required for vitamin B_{12} absorption, cause pernicious anemia.

Antibodies that cause cell- or tissue-specific diseases are usually autoantibodies produced as part of an autoimmune reaction, but sometimes the antibodies are specific for microbes. Examples of autoantibodies against tissue antigens are listed in Table 19-2. Less commonly, the antibodies may be produced against a foreign (e.g., microbial) antigen that is immunologically cross-reactive with a component of self tissues. In a rare sequel of streptococcal infection called rheumatic fever, antibodies produced against the bacteria cross-react with antigens in the heart, deposit in this organ, and cause inflammation and tissue damage. Tissue deposits of antibodies may be detected by morphologic examination in some of these diseases, and the deposition of antibody is often associated with local complement activation, inflammation, and tissue injury (Fig. 19-3, *A*).

Immune Complex–Mediated Diseases

Immune complexes that cause disease may be composed of antibodies bound to either self antigens or foreign antigens. The pathologic features of diseases caused by immune complexes reflect the site of immune complex deposition and are not determined by the cellular source of the antigen. Therefore, immune complex–mediated diseases tend to be systemic and affect multiple tissues and organs, although some are particularly susceptible, such as kidneys and joints.

The occurrence of diseases caused by immune complexes was suspected in the early 1900s by an astute physician named Clemens von Pirquet. At the time, diphtheria infections were treated with serum from horses that had been immunized with the diphtheria toxin, which is an example of passive immunization against the toxin by the transfer of serum containing antitoxin antibodies. Von Pirquet astutely noted that joint inflammation (arthritis), rash, and fever developed in patients who were injected with the antitoxin-containing horse serum. Two clinical features of this reaction suggested that it was not due to the infection or a toxic component of the serum itself. First, these symptoms appeared even after the injection of horse serum not containing the antitoxin, so the lesions could not be attributed to the anti-diphtheria antibody. Second, the symptoms appeared at least 1 week after the first injection of horse serum and more rapidly with each repeated injection. von Pirquet concluded that this disease was due to a host response to some component of the serum. He suggested that the host made

---

TABLE 19-2   Examples of Diseases Caused by Cell- or Tissue-Specific Antibodies

Disease	Target Antigen	Mechanisms of Disease	Clinicopathologic Manifestations
Autoimmune hemolytic anemia	Erythrocyte membrane proteins	Opsonization and phagocytosis of erythrocytes, complement-mediated lysis	Hemolysis, anemia
Autoimmune thrombocytopenic purpura	Platelet membrane proteins (gpIIb-IIIa integrin)	Opsonization and phagocytosis of platelets	Bleeding
Pemphigus vulgaris	Proteins in intercellular junctions of epidermal cells (desmoglein)	Antibody-mediated activation of proteases, disruption of intercellular adhesions	Skin vesicles (bullae)
Vasculitis caused by ANCA	Neutrophil granule proteins, presumably released from activated neutrophils	Neutrophil degranulation and inflammation	Vasculitis
Goodpasture's syndrome	Non-collagenous NC1 protein of basement membrane in glomeruli and lung	Complement- and Fc receptor–mediated inflammation	Nephritis, lung hemorrhage
Acute rheumatic fever	Streptococcal cell wall antigen; antibody cross-reacts with myocardial antigen	Inflammation, macrophage activation	Myocarditis, arthritis
Myasthenia gravis	Acetylcholine receptor	Antibody inhibits acetylcholine binding, downmodulates receptors	Muscle weakness, paralysis
Graves' disease (hyperthyroidism)	TSH receptor	Antibody-mediated stimulation of TSH receptors	Hyperthyroidism
Insulin-resistant diabetes	Insulin receptor	Antibody inhibits binding of insulin	Diabetes mellitus
Pernicious anemia	Intrinsic factor of gastric parietal cells	Neutralization of intrinsic factor; decreased absorption of vitamin B_{12}	Abnormal erythropoiesis, anemia, neurologic symptoms

ANCA, anti-neutrophil cytoplasmic antibodies; *TSH,* thyroid-stimulating hormone.

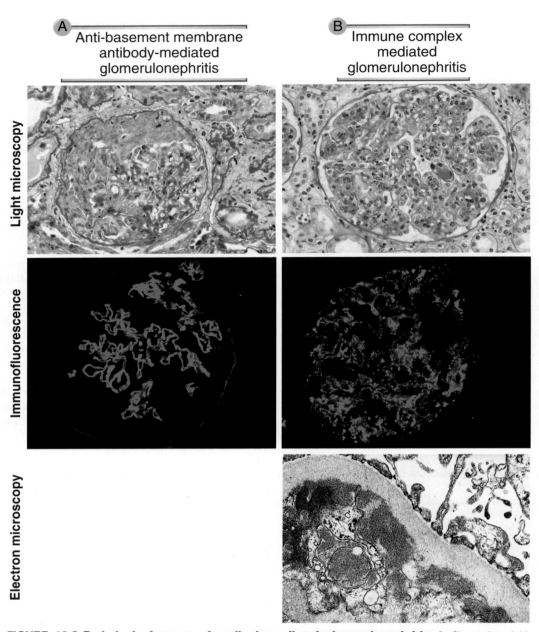

FIGURE 19-3 Pathologic features of antibody-mediated glomerulonephritis. A, Glomerulonephritis induced by an antibody against the glomerular basement membrane (Goodpasture's syndrome): the light micrograph shows glomerular inflammation and severe damage, and immunofluorescence shows smooth (linear) deposits of antibody along the basement membrane. **B,** Glomerulonephritis induced by the deposition of immune complexes (systemic lupus erythematosus): the light micrograph shows neutrophilic inflammation, and the immunofluorescence and electron micrograph show coarse (granular) deposits of antigen-antibody complexes along the basement membrane. *(Immunofluorescence micrographs are courtesy of Dr. Jean Olson, Department of Pathology, University of California, San Francisco, and the electron micrograph is courtesy of Dr. Helmut Rennke, Department of Pathology, Brigham and Women's Hospital, Boston, Massachusetts.)*

antibodies to horse serum proteins, these antibodies formed complexes with the injected proteins, and the disease was due to the antibodies or immune complexes. We now know that his conclusions were entirely accurate. He called this disease serum disease. The same reaction was also observed in humans receiving serum therapy for tetanus, and it is now more commonly known as serum sickness. It remains a clinical issue today in a proportion of subjects receiving therapeutic monoclonal antibodies derived in rodents or polyclonal human antisera to treat snake bites or rabies.

Systemic immune complex–mediated disorders unrelated to foreign protein injection share the same mechanisms of tissue injury as serum sickness.

Experimental Models of Immune Complex–Mediated Diseases
Serum Sickness

Much of our current knowledge of immune complex diseases is based on analyses of experimental models of serum sickness. Immunization of an animal such as a rabbit with a large dose of a foreign protein antigen leads

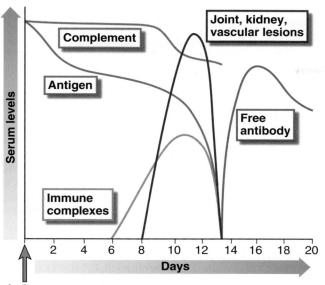

FIGURE 19-4 Sequence of immunologic responses in experimental acute serum sickness. Injection of bovine serum albumin into a rabbit leads to the production of specific antibody and the formation of immune complexes. These complexes are deposited in multiple tissues, activate complement (leading to a decrease in serum complement levels), and cause inflammatory lesions, which resolve as the complexes and the remaining antigen are removed and free antibody (not bound to antigen) appears in the circulation. *(Adapted from Cochrane CG: Immune complex–mediated tissue injury. In Cohen S, Ward PA, McCluskey RT [eds.]:* Mechanisms of immunopathology, *New York, 1979, Werbel & Peck, pp 29-48. Copyright © 1979, Wiley-Liss, Inc.)*

to the formation of antibodies against the antigen (Fig. 19-4). These antibodies bind to and form complexes with circulating antigen, and the complexes are initially cleared by macrophages in the liver and spleen. As more and more antigen-antibody complexes are formed, some of them are deposited in vascular beds. In these tissues, the complexes induce neutrophil-rich inflammation by activating the classical pathway of complement and engaging leukocyte Fc receptors. Because the complexes are often deposited in small arteries, renal glomeruli, and the synovia of joints, the most common clinical and pathologic manifestations are vasculitis, nephritis, and arthritis. The clinical symptoms are usually short-lived, and the lesions heal unless the antigen is injected again. This type of disease is an example of acute serum sickness. A more indolent and prolonged disease, called chronic serum sickness, is produced by multiple injections of antigen, which lead to the formation of smaller complexes that are deposited most often in the kidneys, arteries, and lungs.

Arthus Reaction

A localized form of experimental immune complex–mediated vasculitis is called the Arthus reaction. It is induced by subcutaneous injection of an antigen into a previously immunized animal or an animal that has been given an intravenous injection of antibody specific for the antigen. Circulating antibodies rapidly bind to the injected antigen and form immune complexes that are deposited in the walls of small arteries at the injection site. This deposition gives rise to a local cutaneous vasculitis, with thrombosis of

the affected vessels, leading to tissue necrosis. The clinical relevance of the Arthus reaction is limited; occasionally, a subject receiving a booster dose of a vaccine may develop inflammation at the site of injection because of local accumulation of immune complexes, as in an Arthus reaction.

Pathogenesis of Immune Complex–Mediated Diseases

The amount of immune complex deposition in tissues is determined by the nature of the complexes and the characteristics of the blood vessels. Antigen-antibody complexes are produced during normal immune responses, but they cause disease only when they are produced in excessive amounts, are not efficiently cleared, and become deposited in tissues. Small complexes are often not phagocytosed and tend to be deposited in vessels more than large complexes, which are usually cleared by phagocytes. Complexes containing cationic antigens bind avidly to negatively charged components of the basement membranes of blood vessels and kidney glomeruli. Such complexes typically produce severe and long-lasting tissue injury. Capillaries in the renal glomeruli and synovia are sites where plasma is ultrafiltered (to form urine and synovial fluid, respectively) by passing through specialized basement membranes, and these locations are among the most common sites of immune complex deposition. However, immune complexes may be deposited in small vessels in virtually any tissue. Deposits of antibody and complement may be detected in the vessels, and if the antigen is known, it is possible to identify antigen molecules in the deposits as well (Fig. 19-3, *B*).

Immune complexes deposited in vessel walls and tissues activate leukocytes and mast cells to secrete cytokines and vasoactive mediators. These mediators may cause more immune complex deposition in vessel walls by increasing vascular permeability and blood flow.

Many systemic immunologic diseases in humans are caused by the deposition of immune complexes in blood vessels (Table 19-3). Systemic lupus erythematosus (SLE) is an autoimmune disease in which complexes consisting of nuclear antigens and antibodies deposit in the kidneys, blood vessels, skin, and other tissues. In almost 50% of cases of one type of immune complex–mediated vasculitis involving medium-size muscular arteries, called polyarteritis nodosa, the complexes are made up of viral antigen and antibodies, and the disease is a late complication of viral infection, most often with hepatitis B virus. This also is the mechanism of a disease called post-streptococcal glomerulonephritis that develops in rare cases after streptococcal infection and is caused by complexes of streptococcal antigen and antibodies depositing in the glomeruli of the kidney. In some forms of glomerulonephritis, immune complexes are not detected in the circulation, leading to the postulate that the antigens are first planted in the kidney and the complexes form locally.

DISEASES CAUSED BY T LYMPHOCYTES

T lymphocytes injure tissues either by triggering inflammation or by directly killing target cells (Fig. 19-5). Inflammatory reactions are elicited mainly by CD4+ T cells of the T_H1 and T_H17 subsets, which secrete cytokines that

TABLE 19-3   Examples of Human Immune Complex–Mediated Diseases

Disease	Antigen Involved	Clinicopathologic Manifestations
Systemic lupus erythematosus	DNA, nucleoproteins, others	Nephritis, arthritis, vasculitis
Polyarteritis nodosa	Hepatitis B virus surface antigen (in some cases)	Vasculitis
Post-streptococcal glomerulonephritis	Streptococcal cell wall antigens	Nephritis
Serum sickness	Various proteins	Arthritis, vasculitis, nephritis

recruit and activate leukocytes. In some T cell–mediated disorders, CD8+ CTLs kill host cells. The T cells that cause tissue injury may be autoreactive, or they may be specific for foreign protein antigens that are present in or bound to cells or tissues. T lymphocyte–mediated tissue injury may also accompany strong protective immune responses against persistent microbes, especially intracellular microbes that resist eradication by phagocytes and antibodies.

A role for T cells in causing a particular immunologic disease is suspected largely on the basis of the demonstration of T cells in lesions and the detection of increased levels of cytokines in the blood or tissues that may be derived from T cells. Animal models have been very useful for elucidating the pathogenesis of these disorders.

Diseases Caused by Cytokine-Mediated Inflammation

In immune-mediated inflammation, T_H1 and T_H17 cells secrete cytokines that recruit and activate leukocytes. IL-17, produced by T_H17 cells, promotes neutrophil recruitment; interferon-γ (IFN-γ), produced by T_H1 cells, activates macrophages; and tumor necrosis factor (TNF) and chemokines, produced by T lymphocytes and other cells, are involved in the recruitment and activation of many types of leukocytes. Although we emphasize T_H1 and T_H17 cells as the sources of these cytokines, in lesions many other cells may produce the same cytokines. For instance, in some animal models of chronic skin inflammation, the source of IL-17 early in the course of the disease appears to be γδ T cells.

Tissue injury results from the products of the recruited and activated neutrophils and macrophages, such as lysosomal enzymes, reactive oxygen species, nitric oxide, and proinflammatory cytokines (see Chapter 10). Vascular endothelial cells in the lesions may express increased levels of cytokine-regulated surface proteins such as adhesion molecules and class II MHC molecules. The inflammation associated with T cell–mediated diseases is typically chronic, but bouts of acute inflammation may be superimposed on a background of chronic inflammation. Delayed-type hypersensitivity (DTH) is an example of such inflammatory reactions and

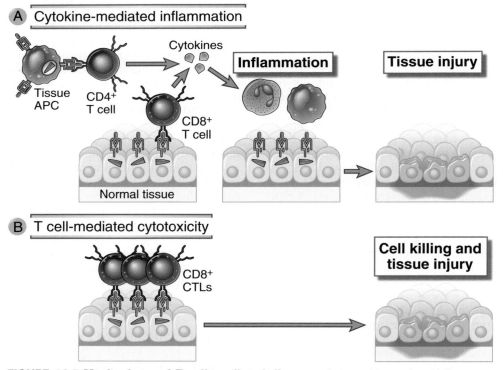

FIGURE 19-5 Mechanisms of T cell–mediated diseases. A, In cytokine-mediated inflammatory reactions, CD4+ T cells (and sometimes CD8+ cells) respond to tissue antigens by secreting cytokines that stimulate inflammation and activate phagocytes, leading to tissue injury. *APC,* antigen-presenting cell. **B,** In some diseases, CD8+ CTLs directly kill tissue cells.

TABLE 19-4 T Cell–Mediated Diseases

Disease	Specificity of Pathogenic T Cells	Principal Mechanisms of Tissue Injury
Rheumatoid arthritis	Collagen? Citrullinated self proteins?	Inflammation mediated by T_H1 and T_H17 cytokines Role of antibodies and immune complexes?
Multiple sclerosis	Protein antigens in myelin (e.g., myelin basic protein)	Inflammation mediated by T_H1 and T_H17 cytokines Myelin destruction by activated macrophages
Type 1 diabetes mellitus	Antigens of pancreatic islet β cells (insulin, glutamic acid decarboxylase, others)	T cell–mediated inflammation Destruction of islet cells by CTLs
Inflammatory bowel disease	Enteric bacteria Self antigens?	Inflammation mediated by T_H1 and T_H17 cytokines
Psoriasis	Unknown skin antigens	Inflammation mediated by T cell–derived cytokines

Examples of human T cell–mediated diseases are listed. In many cases, the specificity of the T cells and the mechanisms of tissue injury are inferred on the basis of the similarity with experimental animal models of the diseases. The roles of T_H1 and T_H17 cells have been inferred from experimental models and the presence of subset-specific cytokines in human lesions. The cytokines may be produced by cells other than CD4+ T lymphocytes. Ongoing clinical trials targeting these cytokines may provide new information about the contributions of the cytokines in different diseases.

is described later. Chronic inflammatory reactions often produce fibrosis as a result of the secretion of cytokines and growth factors by the macrophages and T cells.

Many organ-specific autoimmune diseases are caused by interaction of autoreactive T cells with self antigens, leading to cytokine release and inflammation. This is believed to be the major mechanism underlying rheumatoid arthritis (RA), multiple sclerosis, type 1 diabetes, psoriasis, and other autoimmune diseases (Table 19-4). Some of these are described in more detail at the end of this chapter.

T cell reactions specific for microbes and other foreign antigens may also lead to inflammation and tissue injury. Intracellular bacteria such as *Mycobacterium tuberculosis* induce strong T cell and macrophage responses that result in granulomatous inflammation and fibrosis (described later); the inflammation and fibrosis may cause extensive tissue destruction and functional impairment, typically in the lungs. Tuberculosis is a good example of an infectious disease in which tissue injury is mainly due to the host immune response (see Chapter 16). A variety of skin diseases that result from topical exposure to chemicals and environmental antigens, called **contact sensitivity**, are due to inflammatory reactions, presumably triggered by neoantigens formed by the binding of the chemicals to self proteins. Both CD4+ and CD8+ T cells may be the source of cytokines in contact sensitivity reactions. Examples of contact sensitivity include rashes induced by poison ivy and poison oak (in which T cells react against self proteins that are modified by chemicals made by the plants called urushiols), and rashes induced by contact with metals (nickel and beryllium) and a variety of chemicals, such as thiuram, which is used in the manufacture of latex gloves. Some of these reactions become chronic and clinically are called **eczema**. T cell responses against intestinal bacteria are believed to underlie some forms of inflammatory bowel disease.

The classical T cell–mediated inflammatory reaction is called **delayed-type hypersensitivity**, and is described next.

Delayed-Type Hypersensitivity

Delayed-type hypersensitivity (DTH) is an injurious cytokine-mediated inflammatory reaction resulting from the activation of T cells, particularly CD4+ T cells. The reaction is called delayed because it typically develops 24 to 48 hours after antigen challenge, in contrast to immediate hypersensitivity (allergic) reactions, which develop within minutes (described in Chapter 20).

In the classic animal model of DTH, a guinea pig is first immunized by the administration of a protein antigen in adjuvant; this step is called sensitization. About 2 weeks later, the animal is challenged subcutaneously with the same antigen, and the subsequent reaction is analyzed; this step is called the elicitation phase. Humans may be sensitized for DTH reactions by microbial infection, by contact sensitization with chemicals and environmental antigens, or by intradermal or subcutaneous injection of protein antigens (Fig. 19-6). Subsequent exposure to the same antigen (called challenge) elicits the reaction. For example, purified protein derivative (PPD), a protein antigen of *Mycobacterium tuberculosis,* elicits a DTH reaction, called the tuberculin reaction, when it is injected into individuals who have been exposed to *M. tuberculosis.* A positive tuberculin skin test response is a widely used clinical indicator for evidence of previous or active tuberculosis infection.

The characteristic response of DTH evolves during 24 to 48 hours. About 4 hours after the injection of antigen in a sensitized individual, neutrophils accumulate around the post-capillary venules at the injection site. By about 12 hours, the injection site becomes infiltrated by T cells and blood monocytes, also organized in a perivenular distribution (Fig. 19-7). The endothelial cells lining these venules become plump, show increased biosynthetic organelles, and become leaky to plasma macromolecules. Fibrinogen escapes from the blood vessels into the surrounding tissues, where it is converted into fibrin. The deposition of fibrin, edema, and the accumulation of T cells and monocytes within the extravascular tissue space around the injection site cause the tissue to swell and become firm (indurated). Induration, a diagnostic feature of DTH, is detectable by about 18 hours after the injection of antigen and is maximal by 24 to 48 hours. In clinical practice, loss of DTH responses to universally encountered antigens (e.g., *Candida* antigens) is an indication of deficient T cell function, a condition known as **anergy**. (This general loss of immune responsiveness is different from lymphocyte anergy, a mechanism for

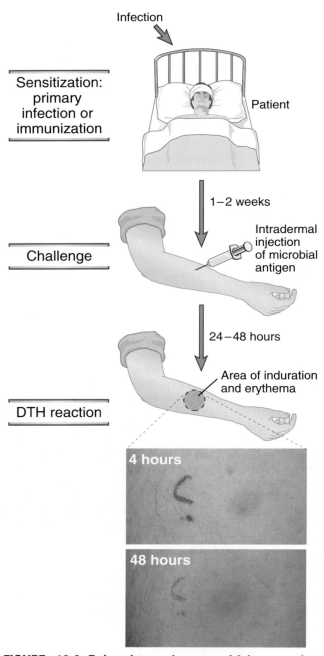

FIGURE 19-6 Delayed-type hypersensitivity reaction. Infection or immunization (vaccination) sensitizes an individual, and subsequent challenge with an antigen from the infectious agent elicits a DTH reaction. The reaction is manifested by induration with redness and swelling at the site of the challenge, which peaks at ~48 hours. *(Courtesy of Dr. J. Faix, Department of Pathology, Stanford University School of Medicine, Palo Alto, California.)*

maintaining tolerance to specific antigens, discussed in Chapter 15.)

Although DTH has traditionally been considered a T_H1-mediated injurious reaction, other T cells may contribute to the inflammation. In some DTH lesions, neutrophils are prominent, suggesting the involvement of T_H17 cells. In infections by some helminthic parasites, reactions against the parasite eggs elicit DTH with a strong component of eosinophils. In these cases, a role for T_H2 cytokines has

been demonstrated. CD8+ T cells also produce IFN-γ and contribute to DTH reactions, especially in the skin.

Chronic DTH reactions can develop if a T_H1 response to an infection activates macrophages but fails to eliminate phagocytosed microbes. If the microbes are localized in a small area, the reaction produces nodules of inflammatory tissue called granulomas (Fig. 19-8, *A*). Chronic DTH, as exemplified by granulomatous inflammation, is caused by prolonged cytokine signals (Fig. 19-8, *B*). In such reactions, the activated T cells and macrophages continue to produce cytokines and growth factors, which amplify the reactions of both cell types and progressively modify the local tissue environment. The result is a cycle of tissue injury and chronic inflammation followed by replacement with connective tissue (fibrosis). In chronic DTH reactions, activated macrophages also undergo changes in response to persistent cytokine signals. These macrophages develop increased cytoplasm and cytoplasmic organelles and histologically may resemble skin epithelial cells, because of which they are sometimes called epithelioid cells. Activated macrophages may fuse to form multinucleate giant cells. Granulomatous inflammation is an attempt to contain the infection but is also the cause of significant tissue injury and functional impairment. This type of inflammation is a characteristic response to some persistent microbes, such as *M. tuberculosis* and some fungi. Much of the respiratory difficulty associated with tuberculosis or chronic fungal infection of the lung is caused by replacement of normal lung with fibrotic tissue and is not directly attributable to the microbes.

Diseases Caused by Cytotoxic T Lymphocytes

CTL responses to viral infection can lead to tissue injury by killing infected cells, even if the virus itself has no cytopathic effects. The principal physiologic function of

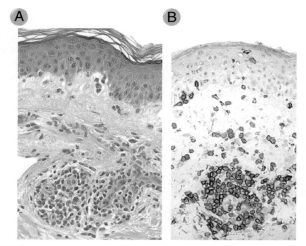

FIGURE 19-7 Morphology of a delayed-type hypersensitivity reaction. A, Histopathologic examination of the reaction in skin illustrated in Figure 19-6 shows perivascular mononuclear cell infiltrates in the dermis. At higher magnification (not shown), the infiltrate is seen to consist of activated lymphocytes and macrophages surrounding small blood vessels in which the endothelial cells are also activated. **B.** Immunohistochemical staining demonstrates the presence of many CD4+ T lymphocytes. *(Courtesy of Dr. J. Faix, Department of Pathology, Stanford University School of Medicine, Palo Alto, California.)*

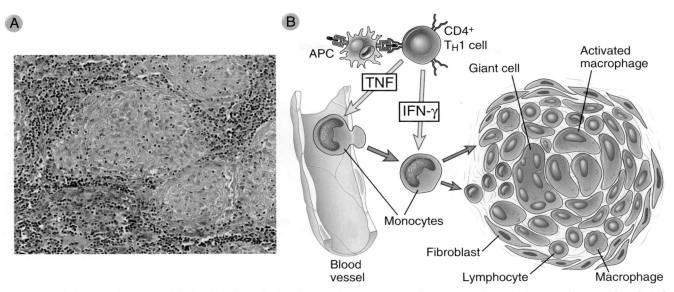

FIGURE 19-8 Granulomatous inflammation. A, Lymph node from a patient with tuberculosis containing granulomas with activated macrophages, multinucleate giant cells, and lymphocytes. In some granulomas, there may be a central area of necrosis. Immunohistochemical studies would identify the lymphocytes as T cells. **B,** Mechanisms of granuloma formation. Cytokines are involved in the generation of T_H1 cells, activation of macrophages, and recruitment of leukocytes. Prolonged reactions of this type lead to the formation of granulomas.

CTLs is to eliminate intracellular microbes, primarily viruses, by killing infected cells. Some viruses directly injure infected cells and are said to be cytopathic, whereas others are not. Because CTLs may not be able to distinguish between cytopathic and non-cytopathic viruses, they kill virally infected cells regardless of whether the infection itself is harmful to the host. Examples of viral infections in which the lesions are due to the host CTL response and not the virus itself include lymphocytic choriomeningitis in mice and certain forms of viral hepatitis in humans (see Chapter 16).

CTLs may contribute to tissue injury in autoimmune disorders in which destruction of particular host cells is a prominent component, such as type 1 diabetes, in which insulin-producing β cells in pancreatic islets are destroyed.

THERAPEUTIC APPROACHES FOR IMMUNOLOGIC DISEASES

One of the most impressive recent accomplishments of immunology has been the development of novel therapies for immunologic diseases based on the understanding of basic science (Fig. 19-9). The therapies can be divided into several broad groups.

Anti-Inflammatory Agents

The mainstay of therapy for hypersensitivity diseases for many years has been anti-inflammatory drugs, particularly corticosteroids. Such drugs inhibit the secretion of cytokines and other mediators of inflammation and thus reduce the inflammation associated with pathologic immune responses.

Depletion of Cells and Antibodies

Monoclonal antibodies that deplete all lymphoid cells, only B cells, or only T cells are used to treat severe

inflammatory diseases. In Chapter 5, we listed some of the depleting antibodies in clinical practice (see Table 5-3). A recent development is the successful use of anti-CD20 antibody (rituximab), which depletes only B cells, to treat diseases that were thought to be caused primarily by T cell–mediated inflammation. This treatment has shown efficacy in some patients with rheumatoid arthritis (RA), multiple sclerosis, and a host of other autoimmune disorders. The effectiveness of anti-CD20 may be related to a role of B cells in T cell responses, especially the generation and maintenance of memory T cells. Plasmapheresis has been used to eliminate circulating autoantibodies and immune complexes.

Anti-Cytokine Therapies

A large number of cytokines and their receptors involved in inflammation are being targeted by specific antagonists for the treatment of chronic T cell–mediated inflammatory diseases (Table 19-5). The first success with this class of biologic agents came with a soluble form of the TNF receptor and anti-TNF antibodies, which bind to and neutralize TNF. These agents are of great benefit in many patients with RA, Crohn's disease, and the skin disease psoriasis. Antibodies to the IL-6 receptor have been successfully used in trials for juvenile and adult rheumatoid arthritis. Antagonists of other proinflammatory cytokines, such as IL-1, the p40 chain that is present in both IL-12 and IL-23, IL-6, IL-17, and others, are in use or in clinical trials for inflammatory diseases.

Agents That Inhibit Cell-Cell Interactions and Leukocyte Migration

Agents that block B7 costimulators are approved for treatment of RA and graft rejection. Antibodies against integrins have been used to inhibit leukocyte migration into tissues, particularly the central nervous system (CNS) in multiple

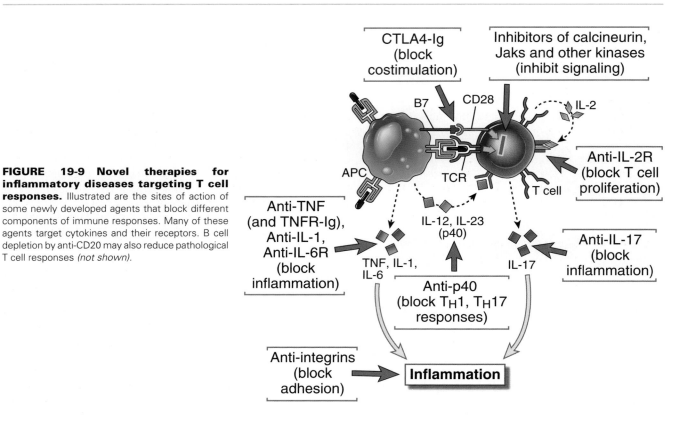

FIGURE 19-9 Novel therapies for inflammatory diseases targeting T cell responses. Illustrated are the sites of action of some newly developed agents that block different components of immune responses. Many of these agents target cytokines and their receptors. B cell depletion by anti-CD20 may also reduce pathological T cell responses (not shown).

sclerosis; a rare but serious complication of treatment with this antibody is described later in this chapter in the discussion of multiple sclerosis. Antibodies against CD40 ligand block T cell–mediated activation of B cells and macrophages and have been beneficial in patients with multiple sclerosis and inflammatory bowel disease, but some of the treated patients have developed thrombotic complications, apparently because this molecule is expressed on human platelets (where its function is unknown).

Intravenous IgG

Large doses of intravenous IgG (IVIG) have beneficial effects in some hypersensitivity diseases. It is not clear how this agent suppresses immune inflammation; one possibility is that the IgG binds to the inhibitory Fc receptor (FcγRIIB) on macrophages and B lymphocytes and thus attenuates inflammatory responses (see Chapter 12). IVIG may also compete with pathogenic antibodies for binding to the

---

TABLE 19-5 Examples of Cytokine Antagonists in Clinical Use or Trials

Cytokine or Receptor Targeted	Predicted Biologic Effects of Antagonist	Clinical Indications
TNF	Inhibits leukocyte migration into sites of inflammation	Rheumatoid arthritis, psoriasis, inflammatory bowel disease
IL-1	Inhibits leukocyte migration into sites of inflammation	Rare autoinflammatory syndromes, severe gout, rheumatoid arthritis
IL-6, IL-6 receptor	Inhibits inflammation, antibody responses?	Juvenile idiopathic arthritis, rheumatoid arthritis
IL-17	Inhibits leukocyte recruitment into sites of inflammation	Psoriasis; possibly rheumatoid arthritis (trials ongoing)
p40 chain of IL-12 and IL-23	Inhibits T_H1 and T_H17 responses	Inflammatory bowel disease, psoriasis
IL-2 receptor (CD25)	Inhibits IL-2–mediated T cell proliferation	Acute graft rejection
IFN-α	May be multiple effects on T_H1 differentiation, antibody production	Systemic lupus erythematosus
IL-4/IL-13	Inhibits T_H2 differentiation and function, IgE production	Asthma
BAFF	Reduces survival of B lymphocytes	Systemic lupus erythematosus

The table lists examples of antagonists against cytokines (antibodies or soluble receptors) that are approved for clinical use or in trials.
IFN, interferon; *IL*, interleukin; *TNF*, tumor necrosis factor.

neonatal Fc receptor (FcRn), which functions in adults to protect antibodies from catabolism (see Chapter 5), resulting in reduced half-lives of the pathogenic antibodies.

Regulatory T Cell-Based Therapies

There has been great interest recently in exploiting our knowledge of regulatory T cells (Tregs) to treat inflammatory diseases. Numerous clinical trials are ongoing to purify patients' Tregs, expand and activate them in culture, and transfer them back to the patients. Another approach is to treat patients with low doses of IL-2, which is expected to activate and maintain Tregs more than effector cells.

There are ongoing attempts at more specific treatment, such as inducing tolerance in disease-producing T cells. Multiple sclerosis and type 1 diabetes are two immune diseases in which the target antigens have been defined; in both diseases, clinical trials are under way in which the antigens (peptides of myelin basic protein and insulin, respectively) are administered to patients in ways that tolerize lymphocytes specific for the antigens. A risk of many treatments that block various components of the immune system is that these will interfere with the normal function of the immune system in combating microbes and thus make individuals susceptible to infections. Antigen-specific tolerance avoids this problem by selectively targeting the disease-causing lymphocytes. These general principles are similar to those on which treatment of transplant rejection is based (see Chapter 17).

SELECTED IMMUNOLOGIC DISEASES: PATHOGENESIS AND THERAPEUTIC STRATEGIES

In the following section, we will describe the pathogenesis of selected diseases that are caused by antibodies and T cells and the application of novel therapies for these diseases to illustrate the principles we discussed earlier.

Systemic Lupus Erythematosus (SLE): The Prototypic Immune Complex–Mediated Disease

SLE is a chronic, remitting and relapsing, multisystem autoimmune disease that affects predominantly women, with an incidence in the United States of 1 in 700 among women 20 to 60 years of age (about 1 in 250 among black women) and a female-to-male ratio of 10:1. The principal clinical manifestations are rashes, arthritis, and glomerulonephritis, but hemolytic anemia, thrombocytopenia, and CNS involvement are also common. Many different autoantibodies are found in patients with SLE. The most frequent are anti-nuclear, particularly anti-DNA, antibodies; others include antibodies against ribonucleoproteins, histones, and nucleolar antigens. Immune complexes formed from these autoantibodies and their specific antigens are responsible for glomerulonephritis, arthritis, and vasculitis involving small arteries throughout the body. Hemolytic

anemia and thrombocytopenia are due to autoantibodies against erythrocytes and platelets, respectively. The principal diagnostic test for the disease is the presence of anti-nuclear antibodies; antibodies against double-stranded native DNA are specific for SLE.

Pathogenesis of Systemic Lupus Erythematosus

SLE is a complex disease in which genetic and environmental factors contribute to a breakdown of tolerance in self-reactive B and T lymphocytes. Among the genetic factors is the inheritance of particular HLA alleles. The odds ratio (relative risk) for individuals with HLA-DR2 or HLA-DR3 is 2 to 3, and if both haplotypes are present, the odds ratio is about 5. Genetic deficiencies of classical pathway complement proteins, especially C1q, C2, or C4, are seen in about 5% of patients with SLE. The complement deficiencies may result in defective clearance of immune complexes and apoptotic cells and the failure of B cell tolerance. A polymorphism in the inhibitory Fc receptor FcγRIIB has been described in some patients; this may contribute to inadequate control of B cell activation or a failure to attenuate inflammatory responses in innate immune cells. Many other genes have been detected by genome-wide association studies, and the role of some of these like PTPN22 has been considered in Chapter 15. Mutations have also been identified in TREX1, discussed below. Environmental factors include exposure to ultraviolet (UV) light. It is postulated that this leads to apoptotic death of cells and release of nuclear antigens.

Two observations have led to new hypotheses of the pathogenesis of SLE. First, studies in patients have revealed that blood cells show a striking molecular signature (pattern of gene expression) that indicates exposure to IFN-α, a type I interferon that is produced mainly by plasmacytoid dendritic cells. Some studies have shown that plasmacytoid dendritic cells from SLE patients also produce abnormally large amounts of IFN-α. Second, studies in animal models have shown that Toll-like receptors (TLRs) that recognize DNA and RNA, notably the DNA-recognizing TLR9 and the RNA-recognizing TLR7, play a role in the activation of B cells specific for self nuclear antigens. On the basis of these studies, a model for the pathogenesis of SLE has been proposed (Fig. 19-10). According to this model, UV irradiation and other environmental insults lead to the apoptosis of cells. Inadequate clearance of the nuclei of these cells, in part because of defects in clearance mechanisms such as complement proteins and nucleases such as TREX1, results in a large burden of nuclear antigens. Polymorphisms in various susceptibility genes for lupus lead to defective ability to maintain self-tolerance in B and T lymphocytes, because of which self-reactive lymphocytes remain functional. Failure of B cell tolerance may be due to defects in receptor editing or in deletion of immature B cells in the bone marrow or in peripheral tolerance. Self-reactive B cells that are not rendered tolerant are stimulated by the self nuclear antigens, and antibodies are produced against the antigens. Complexes of the antigens and antibodies bind to Fc receptors on dendritic cells and to the antigen receptor on B cells and may be internalized into endosomes. The nucleic acid components engage endosomal TLRs and stimulate B cells to produce autoantibodies and activate

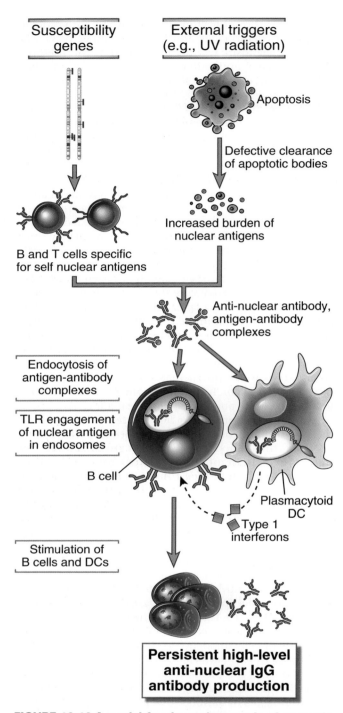

FIGURE 19-10 A model for the pathogenesis of systemic lupus erythematosus (SLE). In this hypothetical model, various susceptibility genes interfere with the maintenance of self-tolerance, and external triggers lead to persistence of nuclear antigens. The result is an antibody response against self nuclear antigens, which is amplified by the TLR-dependent activation of dendritic cells and B cells by nucleic acids, and the production of type I interferons.

dendritic cells, particularly plasmacytoid dendritic cells, to produce IFN-α, which further enhances the immune response and may cause more apoptosis. The net result is a cycle of antigen release and immune activation that leads to the production of high-affinity autoantibodies.

New Therapies for Systemic Lupus Erythematosus

The recent advances in our understanding of SLE are leading to novel therapeutic approaches. Clinical trials are under way to test the efficacy of anti–IFN-α antibodies in the disease, and attempts to inhibit TLR signals are being considered. There has been great interest in depleting B cells by use of an antibody against the B cell surface protein CD20. An antibody that blocks the B cell growth factor BAFF is now approved for the treatment of SLE. Clinical trials of B cell depletion using anti-CD20 or anti-BAFF have had limited success. While B cell depletion has not been abandoned, new therapeutic approaches are needed.

Rheumatoid Arthritis (RA)

RA is an inflammatory disease involving small and large joints of the extremities, including fingers and toes, wrists, shoulders, knees, and ankles. The disease is characterized by inflammation of the synovium associated with destruction of the joint cartilage and bone, with a morphologic picture indicative of a local immune response. Both cell-mediated and humoral immune responses may contribute to development of synovitis. CD4+ T_H1 and T_H17 cells, activated B lymphocytes, plasma cells, and macrophages as well as other inflammatory cells are found in the inflamed synovium, and, in severe cases, well-formed lymphoid follicles with germinal centers (so called tertiary lymphoid organs) may be present. Numerous cytokines, including IL-1, IL-8, TNF, IL-6, IL-17, and IFN-γ, have been detected in the synovial (joint) fluid. Cytokines are believed to recruit leukocytes whose products cause tissue injury and also to activate resident synovial cells to produce proteolytic enzymes, such as collagenase, that mediate destruction of the cartilage, ligaments, and tendons of the joints. Increased osteoclast activity in the joints contributes to the bone destruction in RA, and this may be caused by the production of the TNF family cytokine RANK (receptor activator of nuclear factor κB) ligand by activated T cells. RANK ligand binds to RANK, a member of the TNF receptor family that is expressed on osteoclast precursors, and induces their differentiation and activation. Systemic complications of RA include vasculitis, presumably caused by immune complexes, and lung injury.

Although much of the emphasis in studies of RA has been on the role of T cells, antibodies may also contribute to the joint destruction. Activated B cells and plasma cells are often present in the synovia of affected joints. Patients frequently have circulating IgM or IgG antibodies that react with the Fc (and rarely Fab) portions of their own IgG molecules. These autoantibodies are called rheumatoid factors, and their presence is used as a diagnostic test for RA. Rheumatoid factors may participate in the formation of injurious immune complexes, but their pathogenic role is not established. Another type of antibody that has been detected in at least 70% of patients is specific for cyclic citrullinated peptides (CCP), which are derived from certain proteins that are modified in an inflammatory environment by the enzymatic conversion of arginine residues to citrulline. These anti-CCP antibodies are a diagnostic marker for the disease and may be involved in tissue injury.

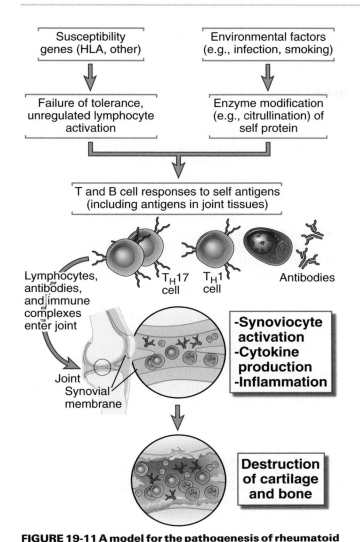

FIGURE 19-11 A model for the pathogenesis of rheumatoid arthritis. According to this model, citrullinated proteins induced by environmental stimuli elicit T cell and antibody responses in genetically susceptible individuals. The T cells and antibodies enter joints, respond to the self proteins, and cause tissue injury mainly by cytokine secretion and perhaps also by antibody-dependent effector mechanisms. Protein modifications other than citrullination may lead to the same result.

Pathogenesis of Rheumatoid Arthritis

Like other autoimmune diseases, RA is a complex disorder in which genetic and environmental factors contribute to the breakdown of tolerance to self antigens. The specificity of the pathogenic T and B cells remains unclear, although both B and T cells that recognize citrullinated peptides have been identified. Susceptibility to RA is linked to the HLA-DR4 haplotype. Recent linkage and genome-wide association studies have revealed a large number of genes in which polymorphisms are associated with RA. There is an association with the gene encoding a tyrosine phosphatase, PTPN22, discussed in Chapter 15.

The identification of anti-CCP immune responses has led to new ideas about the pathogenesis of RA (Fig. 19-11). According to one model, environmental insults, such as smoking and some infections, induce the citrullination

of self proteins, leading to the creation of new antigenic epitopes. In genetically susceptible individuals, tolerance to these epitopes fails, resulting in T cell and antibody responses against the proteins. If these modified self proteins are also present in joints, the T cells and antibodies attack the joints. T_H17 and perhaps T_H1 cells secrete cytokines that recruit leukocytes into the joint and activate synovial cells to produce collagenases and other enzymes. The net result is the progressive destruction of cartilage and bone. The chronic immune responses in the joints may lead to formation of tertiary lymphoid tissues in the synovium, and these may maintain and propagate the local inflammatory reaction.

New Therapies for Rheumatoid Arthritis

The realization of the central role of T cells and cytokines in the disease has led to remarkable advances in treatment, in which specific molecules have been targeted on the basis of scientific understanding. Chief among these new therapies are antagonists against TNF, which have transformed the course of the disease in many patients from one of progressive and inexorable joint destruction to one of smoldering but manageable chronic inflammation. A variety of other targeted therapies have been developed in the past 5 to 10 years; these have provided insight into disease pathogenesis. Blockade of cytokines other than TNF has been effective, including an antibody the blocks the IL-6 receptor, an IL-1 antagonist, and a small molecule that inhibits JAK signaling (an important intracellular signaling mediator of a variety of cytokine receptors). Inhibition of T cell activation has been accomplished by blockade of B7:CD28 costimulation with CTLA-4-Ig, a fusion protein made of the extracellular domain of CTLA-4 and the Fc portion of IgG that binds B7 (see Chapter 9). B cell depletion with anti-CD20 antibody has also proven to be efficacious, although the mechanisms underlying this effect are not well understood.

Multiple Sclerosis

Multiple sclerosis (MS) is an autoimmune disease of the CNS in which CD4+ T cells of the T_H1 and T_H17 subsets react against self myelin antigens, resulting in inflammation in the CNS with activation of macrophages around nerves in the brain and spinal cord, destruction of the myelin, abnormalities in nerve conduction, and neurologic deficits. It is the most common neurologic disease of young adults. On pathologic examination, there is inflammation in the CNS white matter with secondary demyelination. Multiple sclerosis is characterized clinically by weakness, paralysis, and ocular symptoms with exacerbations and remissions; CNS imaging suggests that in patients with active disease, there is frequent new lesion formation.

MS is modeled by experimental autoimmune encephalomyelitis (EAE) in mice, rats, guinea pigs, and non-human primates, and this is one of the best characterized experimental models of an organ-specific autoimmune disease mediated mainly by T lymphocytes. EAE is induced by immunizing animals with antigens normally present in CNS myelin, such as myelin basic protein, proteolipid protein, and myelin oligodendrocyte glycoprotein, with an adjuvant containing heat-killed mycobacteria, which is necessary to elicit a strong T cell response. About 1 to 2 weeks after immunization, animals develop encephalomyelitis, characterized by perivascular infiltrates composed of lymphocytes and macrophages in the CNS white matter, followed by demyelination. The neurologic lesions can be mild and self-limited or chronic and relapsing. These lesions result in progressive or remitting and relapsing paralysis. The disease can also be transferred to naive animals with T cells from diseased animals. Although antibodies against myelin antigens have been detected in patients as well as in the animal models, the pathogenic significance of these antibodies is not established.

Pathogenesis of Multiple Sclerosis

There is abundant evidence that in mice, EAE is caused by activated CD4+ T_H1 and T_H17 cells specific for protein antigens in myelin. By analogy with the experimental disease, MS is also thought to be caused by myelin-specific T_H1 and T_H17 cells, and these cells have been detected in patients and isolated from the blood and CNS. How these cells are activated in patients remains an enigma. It has been suggested that an infection, most likely a viral infection, activates self myelin–reactive T cells by the phenomenon of molecular mimicry (see Chapter 15). Self-tolerance may fail because of the inheritance of susceptibility genes. Identical twins have a 25% to 30% concordance rate for development of MS, whereas non-identical twins have a 6% concordance rate. These observations implicate genetic factors in the development of the disease but also indicate that genetics can only contribute part of the risk. Genetic polymorphisms associated with MS include the HLA locus, with HLA-DRB1*1501 being the strongest linkage. Genome-wide association studies and other genomic analyses have revealed over 100 genetic variants that contribute to disease risk; most of these map to genes involved in immune function. One interesting association is with a polymorphism in the non-coding region of the gene for the IL-2 receptor α chain, CD25. This polymorphism may alter the generation and maintenance of effector and/or regulatory T cells. Other studies have suggested that the peripheral maintenance of regulatory T cells is defective in MS patients, but how much this contributes to a failure of self-tolerance is not known. Once myelin-specific T cells are activated, they migrate into the CNS, where they encounter myelin proteins and release cytokines that recruit and activate macrophages and more T cells, leading to myelin destruction. Studies of EAE suggest that the disease is propagated by a process known as **epitope spreading** (see Chapter 15). The tissue breakdown results in release of new protein antigens and expression of new, previously sequestered epitopes that activate more autoreactive T cells.

New Therapies for Multiple Sclerosis

Immunotherapy for MS has, in the past, relied on approaches whose scientific basis is not well understood. These include administration of β-interferon, which may alter cytokine responses, and treatment with a random polymer of four amino acids, which is

postulated to bind to HLA molecules and block antigen presentation. Recently, however, several new immune-modifying therapies have been developed. One is an antibody against the VLA-4 integrin (see Chapter 3), which blocks leukocyte migration into the CNS and has shown benefit in patients. However, in a small number of patients this treatment resulted in reactivation of a latent JC virus infection that causes a severe and sometime fatal CNS disease. Another recently approved drug to treat MS also interferes with leukocyte migration. The drug, called fingolimod (FTY720), blocks the sphingosine 1-phosphate–mediated pathway of T cell egress from lymphoid tissues (see Chapter 3). In a large subset of patients, B cell depletion with anti-CD20 antibody is beneficial. These results suggest an important role of B cells, presumably as APCs, in the activation of pathogenic T cells. Because myelin basic protein (MBP) is known to be an important self antigen that is the target of the immune response in MS, there has been great hope that administration of MBP peptides will induce antigen-specific tolerance or generate regulatory T cells specific for the relevant antigen. It is also striking that most of the therapies are effective in early MS, which is characterized by inflammation, but not in progressive MS, which is characterized by neurodegeneration and is the major cause of permanent disability. This realization is leading to new attempts to restore myelination and repair of damaged axons and neurons.

Type 1 Diabetes Mellitus

Type 1 diabetes mellitus, previously called insulin-dependent diabetes mellitus, is a multisystem metabolic disease resulting from impaired insulin production that affects about 0.2% of the U.S. population, with a peak onset at 11 to 12 years of age. The incidence of the disease appears to be increasing in North America and Europe. The disease is characterized by hyperglycemia and ketoacidosis. Chronic complications of type 1 diabetes include progressive atherosclerosis of arteries, which can lead to ischemic necrosis of limbs and internal organs, and microvascular obstruction causing damage to the retina, renal glomeruli, and peripheral nerves. These patients have a deficiency of insulin resulting from immune-mediated destruction of the insulin-producing β cells of the islets of Langerhans in the pancreas, and continuous hormone replacement therapy is needed. There is usually a long lag of many years between the initiation of autoimmunity and overt clinical disease because 90% or more of the islets have to be destroyed before clinical manifestations are seen.

Pathogenesis of Type 1 Diabetes

Several mechanisms may contribute to β cell destruction, including inflammation mediated by CD4+ T_H1 cells reactive with islet antigens (including insulin), CTL-mediated lysis of islet cells, local production of cytokines (TNF and IL-1) that damage islet cells, and autoantibodies against islet cells. In the few cases in which the pancreatic lesions have been examined at the early active stages of the disease, the islets show cellular necrosis and lymphocytic infiltration consisting of both CD4+ and CD8+ T cells. This lesion is called insulitis. Autoantibodies against islet cells and insulin are also detected in the blood of these patients. In susceptible children who have not developed diabetes (such as relatives of patients), the presence of antibodies against islet cells is predictive of the development of type 1 diabetes. An informative animal model of the disease is the non-obese diabetic (NOD) mouse, which develops spontaneous diabetes. In this model, there is evidence for defective survival and function of regulatory T cells as well as resistance of effector T cells to suppression.

Multiple genes are associated with type 1 diabetes. A great deal of attention has been devoted to the role of HLA genes. Between 90% and 95% of Caucasians with type 1 diabetes have HLA-DR3, or DR4, or both, in contrast to about 40% of normal subjects, and 40% to 50% of patients are DR3/DR4 heterozygotes, in contrast to 5% of normal subjects. Several non-HLA genes also contribute to the disease. The first of these to be identified is insulin, with tandem repeats in the promoter region being associated with disease susceptibility. The mechanism of this association is unknown; it may be related to the level of expression of insulin in the thymus, which determines whether insulin-specific T cells will be deleted (negatively selected) during maturation. Several other polymorphisms have been identified in patients and in NOD mice, including in the *IL2* and *CD25* genes. The functional consequences of these polymorphisms are not known. Some studies have suggested that viral infections (e.g., with coxsackievirus B4) may precede the onset of type 1 diabetes, perhaps by initiating cell injury, inducing inflammation and the expression of costimulators, and triggering an autoimmune response. However, epidemiologic data suggest that repeated infections protect against type 1 diabetes, and this is similar to the NOD model. In fact, it has been postulated that one reason for the increased incidence of type 1 diabetes in developed countries is the control of infectious diseases.

New Therapies for Type 1 Diabetes

The most interesting new therapeutic strategies for type 1 diabetes are focused on inducing tolerance with diabetogenic peptides from islet antigens (such as insulin) or generating or giving regulatory T cells to patients. These clinical trials are in their infancy.

Inflammatory Bowel Disease

Inflammatory bowel disease consists of two disorders, Crohn's disease and ulcerative colitis, in which T cell–mediated inflammation causes intestinal injury. Crohn's disease is characterized by chronic inflammation and destruction of the intestinal wall, with frequent formation of fistulas. In ulcerative colitis, the lesions are largely confined to the mucosa and consist of ulcers with underlying foci of inflammation. The pathogenesis of inflammatory bowel disease was described in Chapter 14. New therapies for these diseases include antibodies against TNF and the p40 chain of IL-12 and IL-23.

SUMMARY

* Disorders caused by abnormal immune responses are called hypersensitivity diseases. Pathologic immune responses may be autoimmune responses directed against self antigens or uncontrolled and excessive responses to foreign (e.g., microbial) antigens.
* Hypersensitivity diseases may result from antibodies that bind to cells or tissues (type II hypersensitivity), circulating immune complexes that are deposited in tissues (type III), or T lymphocytes reactive with antigens in tissues (type IV). Immediate hypersensitivity (type I) reactions are the cause of allergic diseases and are described in Chapter 20.
* The effector mechanisms of antibody-mediated tissue injury are complement activation and Fc receptor–mediated inflammation. Some antibodies cause disease by interfering with normal cellular functions without producing tissue injury.
* The effector mechanisms of T cell–mediated tissue injury are inflammatory reactions induced by cytokines secreted mainly by CD4+ T_H1 and T_H17 cells and cell lysis by CTLs. The classical T cell–mediated reaction is delayed-type hypersensitivity, induced by activation of previously primed T cells and the production of cytokines that recruit and activate various leukocytes, predominantly macrophages.
* The current treatment of autoimmune diseases is targeted at reducing immune activation and the injurious consequences of the autoimmune reaction. Agents include those that block inflammation, such as antibodies against cytokines and integrins, and those that block lymphocyte activation or destroy lymphocytes. A future goal of therapy is to inhibit the responses of lymphocytes specific for self antigens and to induce tolerance in these cells.
* Autoimmune diseases such as systemic lupus erythematosus, rheumatoid arthritis, multiple sclerosis, and type 1 diabetes illustrate many of the effector mechanisms that cause tissue injury in hypersensitivity reactions and the roles of susceptibility genes and environmental factors in the development of autoimmunity.

SELECTED READINGS

General Principles

Goodnow CC: Multistep pathogenesis of autoimmune disease, *Cell* 130:25–35, 2007.

Nagata S, Hanayama R, Kawane K: Autoimmunity and the clearance of dead cells, *Cell* 140:619–630, 2010.

Antibody and Immune Complex–Mediated Disorders

Banchereau J, Pascual V: Type I interferon in systemic lupus erythematosus and other autoimmune diseases, *Immunity* 25:383–392, 2006.

Fairhurst AM, Wandstrat AE, Wakeland EK: Systemic lupus erythematosus: multiple immunological phenotypes in a complex genetic disease, *Advances in Immunology* 92:1–69, 2006.

Jancar S, Crespo MS: Immune complex–mediated tissue injury: a multistep paradigm, *Trends in Immunology* 26:48–55, 2005.

Munoz LE, Lauber K, Schiller M, Manfredi AA, Herrmann M: The role of defective clearance of apoptotic cells in systemic autoimmunity, *Nature Reviews Rheumatology* 6:280–289, 2010.

Plotz PH: The autoantibody repertoire: searching for order, *Nature Reviews Immunology* 3:73–78, 2003.

Tsokos GC: Systemic lupus erythematosus, *New England Journal of Medicine* 365:2110–2121, 2011.

T Cell–Mediated Disorders

Frohman EM, Racke MK, Raine CS: Multiple sclerosis—the plague and its pathogenesis, *New England Journal of Medicine* 354:942–955, 2006.

Klareskog L, Lundberg K, Malmstrom V: Autoimmunity in rheumatoid arthritis: citrulline immunity and beyond, *Advances in Immunology* 118:129–158, 2013.

Maddur MS, Miossec P, Kaveri SV, Bayry J: Th17 cells: biology, pathogenesis of autoimmune and inflammatory diseases, and therapeutic strategies, *American Journal of Pathology* 181:8–18, 2012.

McInnes IB, Schett G: The pathogenesis of rheumatoid arthritis, *New England Journal of Medicine* 365:2205–2219, 2011.

Palmer MT, Weaver CT: Autoimmunity: increasing suspects in the CD4+ T cell lineage, *Nature Immunology* 11:36–40, 2010.

Therapies for Immunologic Diseases

Burmester GR, Feist E, Dorner T: Emerging cell and cytokine targets in rheumatoid arthritis, *Nature Reviews Rheumatology* 10:77–88, 2014

Faurschou M, Jayne DRW: Anti-B cell antibody therapies for inflammatory rheumatic diseases, *Annual Review of Medicine* 65:263–278, 2014.

Hauser SL, Chan JR, Oksenberg JR: Multiple sclerosis: prospects and promise, *Annals of Neurology* 74:317–327, 2013

Shwab I, Nimmerjahn F: Intravenous immunoglobulin therapy: how does IgG modulate the immune system? *Nature Reviews Immunology* 13:176–189, 2013

Thanou A, Merrill JT: Treatment of systemic lupus erythematosus: new therapeutic avenues and blind alleys, *Nature Reviews Rheumatology* 10:23–34, 2014.

Allergy

A variety of human diseases are caused by immune responses to non-microbial environmental antigens that involve IL-4-, IL-5-, and IL-13–producing helper T cells, immunoglobulin E (IgE), mast cells, and eosinophils. In the effector phase of these responses, mast cells and eosinophils are activated to rapidly release mediators that cause increased vascular permeability, vasodilation, and bronchial and visceral smooth muscle contraction. This reaction is called **immediate hypersensitivity** because it begins rapidly, within minutes of antigen challenge (immediate), and has major pathologic consequences (hypersensitivity). Following the immediate response, there is a more slowly developing inflammatory component called the **late-phase reaction** characterized by the accumulation of neutrophils, eosinophils, and macrophages. The term immediate hypersensitivity is commonly used to describe the combined immediate and late-phase reactions. In clinical medicine, these reactions are called **allergy** or **atopy**, and the associated diseases are called allergic, atopic, or immediate hypersensitivity diseases. Repeated bouts of these reactions can lead to chronic allergic diseases, with tissue damage and remodeling. The antigens that elicit immediate hypersensitivity are called **allergens**. Most of them are common environmental proteins, animal products, and chemicals that can modify self proteins.

Although atopy originally meant unusual, we now realize that allergy is the most common disorder of immunity, affecting almost 20% of all individuals in the United States and Europe, and its prevalence is increasing worldwide. This chapter focuses on immune reactions underlying allergic diseases. We will describe the sequence of events that lead to mast cell activation and the roles of various mediators in immediate hypersensitivity. We will then describe selected clinical syndromes associated with IgE- and mast cell–dependent reactions and the principles of therapy for these diseases. We will conclude with a discussion of the physiologic role of IgE-mediated immune reactions in host defense.

OVERVIEW OF IgE-DEPENDENT ALLERGIC REACTIONS

All allergic reactions share common features, although they differ greatly in the types of antigens that elicit these reactions and their clinical and pathologic manifestations.

- *The hallmark of allergic diseases is the production of IgE antibody, which is dependent on the activation of IL-4–producing helper T cells.* Whereas healthy individuals either do not respond or have harmless T cell and

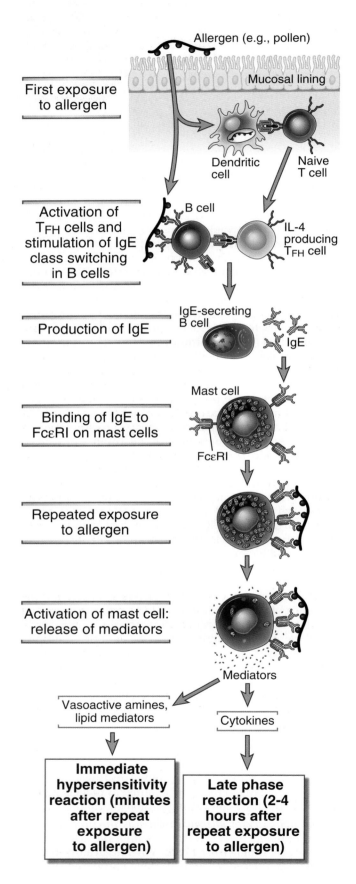

First exposure to allergen

Allergen (e.g., pollen)

Mucosal lining

Dendritic cell

Naive T cell

Activation of T$_{FH}$ cells and stimulation of IgE class switching in B cells

B cell

IL-4 producing T$_{FH}$ cell

Production of IgE

IgE-secreting B cell

IgE

Binding of IgE to FcεRI on mast cells

Mast cell

FcεRI

Repeated exposure to allergen

Activation of mast cell: release of mediators

Mediators

Vasoactive amines, lipid mediators

Cytokines

Immediate hypersensitivity reaction (minutes after repeat exposure to allergen)

Late phase reaction (2-4 hours after repeat exposure to allergen)

antibody responses to common environmental antigens, atopic individuals develop strong IL-4–producing helper T cell responses and produce IgE on exposure to these allergenic substances.

- *The typical sequence of events in immediate hypersensitivity consists of exposure to an antigen, activation of lymphocytes (T$_H$2 cells, IL-4–producing follicular helper T [T$_{FH}$] cells and B cells) specific for the antigen, production of IgE antibody, binding of the antibody to Fc receptors of mast cells, and triggering of the mast cells by re-exposure to the antigen, resulting in the release of mediators from the mast cells and the subsequent pathologic reaction* (Fig. 20-1). Binding of IgE to mast cells is also called **sensitization** because IgE-coated mast cells are ready to be activated on antigen encounter (i.e., they are sensitive to the antigen). We will describe each of these steps in the following sections.

- *Allergy is the prototypic T$_H$2-mediated disease. Many of the early events and pathologic features of the reaction are triggered by T$_H$2 cytokines, which may be produced by T$_{FH}$ cells in lymphoid organs and by classical T$_H$2 cells in tissues.* This contrasts with delayed type hypersensitivity, which is largely a T$_H$1-mediated immune reaction.

- *The clinical and pathologic manifestations of allergy consist of the vascular and smooth muscle reaction that develops rapidly after repeated exposure to the allergen (immediate hypersensitivity) and a delayed late phase inflammatory reaction.* These reactions may be initiated by IgE-mediated mast cell activation, but different mediators are responsible for the immediate versus late-phase reactions. Because mast cells are present in connective tissues and under epithelia, these tissues are the most common sites of immediate hypersensitivity reactions. Some immediate hypersensitivity reactions may be triggered by non-immunologic stimuli, such as exercise and exposure to cold. Such stimuli induce mast cell degranulation and the release of mediators without antigen exposure or IgE production. Such reactions are said to be non-atopic.

- *Allergic reactions are manifested in different ways, depending on the tissues affected, including skin rashes, sinus congestion, bronchial constriction, abdominal pain, diarrhea, and systemic shock.* In the most extreme systemic form, called **anaphylaxis**, mast cell–derived mediators can restrict airways to the point of asphyxiation and produce cardiovascular collapse leading to death. (The term *anaphylaxis* was coined to indicate that antibodies, especially IgE antibodies, could confer the opposite of protection [prophylaxis] on an unfortunate individual.) We will return to the pathogenesis of these reactions later in the chapter.

FIGURE 20-1 Sequence of events in immediate hypersensitivity reactions. Immediate hypersensitivity diseases are initiated by the introduction of an allergen, which stimulates IL-4 producing helper T cell responses and IgE production. IgE sensitizes mast cells by binding to FcεRI, and subsequent exposure to the allergen activates the mast cells to secrete the mediators that are responsible for the pathologic reactions of immediate hypersensitivity.

- *The development of allergies is the result of complex and poorly understood gene-environment interactions.* There is a genetic predisposition for the development of allergies, and relatives of allergic individuals are more likely to also have allergies than unrelated people, even when they do not share environments. Many susceptibility genes have been identified that we will discuss later in this chapter. Various environmental factors, especially in industrialized societies, including the presence of allergens and exposure to microbes, have a profound influence on the propensity to develop allergies.

With this introduction, we will proceed to a description of the steps in the development and reactions of immediate hypersensitivity.

PRODUCTION OF IgE

Atopic individuals produce high levels of IgE in response to environmental allergens, whereas normal individuals generally produce other Ig isotypes, such as IgM and IgG, and only small amounts of IgE. The quantity of IgE synthesized depends on the propensity of an individual to generate allergen-specific helper T cells that produce IL-4 and IL-13, because these cytokines stimulate B cell antibody class switching to IgE. The development of IL-4 and IL-13–expressing T cell responses against particular antigens may be influenced by a variety of factors, including inherited genes, the nature of the antigens, and the history of antigen exposure.

IgE antibody is responsible for sensitizing mast cells and provides recognition of antigen for immediate hypersensitivity reactions. IgE is the antibody isotype that contains the ε heavy chain (see Chapter 5). It binds to specific Fc receptors on mast cells and activates these cells.

The Nature of Allergens

Antigens that elicit immediate hypersensitivity reactions (allergens) are proteins or chemicals bound to proteins. Typical allergens include proteins in pollen, house dust mites, animal dander, foods, and chemicals like the antibiotic penicillin. It is not known why some antigens induce IL-4–producing helper T cell responses and allergic reactions whereas others do not. Two important characteristics of allergens are that individuals are exposed to them repeatedly and, unlike microbes, they do not generally stimulate the innate immune responses that are associated with macrophage and dendritic cell secretion of T_H1- and T_H17-inducing cytokines. Chronic or repeated cell activation in the absence of strong innate immunity may drive CD4+ T cells preferentially toward the T_H2 pathway (see Chapter 10).

The allergenicity of an antigen may also reside in its chemical nature. Although no structural characteristics of proteins can definitively predict whether they will be allergenic, some features are typical of many common allergens. These include low to medium molecular weight (5 to 70 kD), stability, glycosylation, and high solubility in body fluids. Anaphylactic responses to foods are typically induced by highly glycosylated small proteins. These structural features probably protect the antigens from denaturation and degradation in the gastrointestinal tract and allow them to be absorbed intact. Curiously, many allergens, such as the cysteine protease of the house dust mite *Dermatophagoides pteronyssinus* and phospholipase A_2 in bee venom, are enzymes, but the importance of the enzymatic activity in triggering immediate hypersensitivity reactions is not known.

Because immediate hypersensitivity reactions are dependent on CD4+ T cells, T cell–independent antigens such as polysaccharides cannot elicit these reactions unless they become attached to proteins. Some nonprotein substances, such as the antibiotic penicillin, can elicit strong IgE responses. These drugs react chemically with amino acid residues in self proteins to form hapten-carrier conjugates, which induce IL-4–producing helper T cell responses and IgE production.

The natural history of antigen exposure is an important determinant of the amount of specific IgE antibodies produced. Repeat exposure to a particular antigen is necessary for development of an allergic reaction to that antigen because switching to the IgE isotype and sensitization of mast cells with IgE must happen before an immediate hypersensitivity reaction to an antigen can occur. Individuals with allergic rhinitis or asthma often benefit from a geographic change of residence with a change in indigenous plant pollens, although environmental antigens in the new residence may trigger an eventual return of the symptoms. A dramatic example of the importance of repeated exposure to antigen in allergic disease is seen in cases of bee stings. The proteins in the insect venoms are not usually of concern on the first encounter because an atopic individual has no preexisting specific IgE antibodies. However, an IgE response may occur after a single encounter with antigen, and a second sting by an insect of the same species may induce fatal anaphylaxis! Similarly, exposures to small amounts of peanuts can trigger fatal reactions in previously sensitized individuals.

Activation of IL-4–Producing Helper T Cells

In allergic diseases, T_{FH} cells are required for differentiation of IgE-producing B cells, and T_H2 cells play a central role in the inflammatory reaction in tissues. It is likely that dendritic cells in epithelia through which allergens enter capture the antigens, transport them to draining lymph nodes, process them, and present peptides to naive CD4+ T cells. The T cells then differentiate into T_H2 cells or follicular helper T (T_{FH}) cells that secrete T_H2 cytokines. The major factors that stimulate the development of the T_H2 subset are cytokines, especially IL-4, which may be produced by various cell types (see Chapter 10). In addition, thymic stromal lymphopoietin, a cytokine secreted by epithelial cells in the skin, gut, and lungs, enhances the ability of tissue dendritic cells and innate lymphoid cells to promote T_H2 differentiation. The signals for differentiation of IL-4–producing T_{FH} cells are less well understood, but are likely to be similar to the signals for T_H2 differentiation.

The differentiated T_H2 cells migrate to tissue sites of allergen exposure, where they contribute to the inflammatory effector phase of allergic reactions, described later. T_{FH} cells, of course, remain in lymphoid organs, where they help B cells.

Activation of B Cells and Switching to IgE

B cells specific for allergens are activated by T_{FH} cells in lymphoid organs, as in other T cell–dependent B cell responses (see Chapter 12). In response to CD40 ligand and cytokines, mainly IL-4 and possibly IL-13, produced by these helper T cells, the B cells undergo heavy chain isotype switching and produce IgE. IgE circulates as a bivalent antibody and is normally present in plasma at a concentration of less than 1 µg/mL. In pathologic conditions such as helminthic infections and severe atopy, this level can rise to more than 1000 µg/mL. Allergen-specific IgE produced by plasmablasts and plasma cells enters the circulation and binds to Fc receptors on tissue mast cells, so that these cells are sensitized and poised to react to a subsequent encounter with the allergen. Circulating basophils are also capable of binding IgE.

ROLE OF T$_H$2 CELLS, MAST CELLS, BASOPHILS, AND EOSINOPHILS IN ALLERGIC REACTIONS

T$_H$2 cells, mast cells, basophils, and eosinophils are the major effector cells of immediate hypersensitivity reactions and allergic disease. Although each of these cell types has unique characteristics, all four secrete mediators of allergic reactions. Mast cells, basophils, and eosinophils, in distinction from T$_H$2 cells, have cytoplasmic granules that contain preformed amines and enzymes, and all three cell types produce lipid mediators and cytokines that induce inflammation (Table 20-1). T$_H$2 cells contribute to inflammation by secreting cytokines. In this section, we will discuss the roles of these cell types in allergic reactions.

Role of T$_H$2 Cells and Innate Lymphoid Cells in Allergic Disease

T$_H$2 cells secrete cytokines, including IL-4, IL-5, and IL-13, that work in combination with mast cells and eosinophils to promote inflammatory responses to allergens within tissues. The general properties of T$_H$2 cells and the signals that drive their differentiation from naive T cells were discussed in Chapter 10. IL-4 secreted by T$_H$2 cells induces expression of endothelial VCAM-1 that promotes the recruitment of eosinophils and additional T$_H$2 cells into tissues. IL-5 secreted by T$_H$2 cells activates eosinophils. IL-13 stimulates epithelial cells (e.g., in the airways) to secrete increased amounts of mucus, and excessive mucus production is also a common feature of these reactions. T$_H$2 cells also contribute to the inflammation of the late-phase reaction, described later.

Consistent with a central role of T$_H$2 cells in immediate hypersensitivity, larger numbers of allergen-specific IL-4–secreting T cells are found in the blood of atopic individuals than in non-atopic persons. In atopic patients, the allergen-specific T cells also produce more IL-4 per cell

than in normal individuals. In animal models, a disease resembling human asthma can be induced by generation of T$_H$2 cells specific for an inhaled antigen or by adoptive transfer of these cells into naive mice. Accumulations of T$_H$2 cells are found at sites of immediate hypersensitivity reactions in the skin and bronchial mucosa.

Group 2 innate lymphoid cells also secrete IL-5 and IL-13 (see Chapter 4), and animal models have shown that cytokines derived from these cells contribute to allergic airway inflammation.

Properties of Mast Cells and Basophils

All mast cells are derived from progenitors in the bone marrow. Normally, mature mast cells are not found in the circulation. Progenitors migrate to the peripheral tissues as immature cells and undergo differentiation in response to local microenvironmental biochemical cues, including stem-cell factor released by tissue cells, which binds to the c-Kit receptor on the mast cell progenitor. Mature mast cells are found throughout the body, predominantly near

TABLE 20-1 Properties of Mast Cells, Basophils, and Eosinophils

Characteristic	Mast Cells	Basophils	Eosinophils
Major site of maturation	Connective tissue	Bone marrow	Bone marrow
Cells in circulation	No	Yes (0.5% of blood leukocytes)	Yes (~2% of blood leukocytes)
Mature cells recruited into tissues from circulation	No	Yes	Yes
Mature cells residing in connective tissue	Yes	No	Yes
Proliferative ability of mature cells	Yes	No	No
Life span	Weeks to months	Days	Days to weeks
Major development factor (cytokine)	Stem cell factor, IL-3	IL-3	IL-5
Expression of FcεRI	High levels	High levels	Low levels (function not clear)
Major granule contents	Histamine, heparin and/or chondroitin sulfate, proteases	Histamine, chondroitin sulfate, protease	Major basic protein, eosinophil cationic protein, peroxidases, hydrolases, lysophospholipase

FcεRI, Fcε receptor type I; *IL,* interleukin.

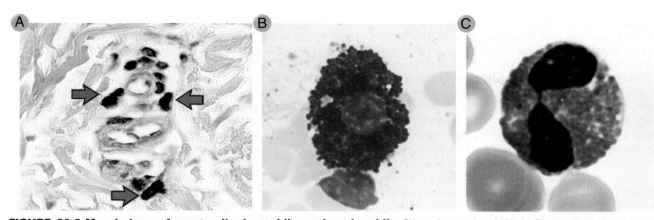

FIGURE 20-2 Morphology of mast cells, basophils, and eosinophils. Photomicrographs of Wright-Giemsa–stained perivascular dermal mast cells (**A,** *arrows*), peripheral blood basophil (**B**), and peripheral blood eosinophil (**C**) are presented. Note the characteristic blue-staining cytoplasmic granules of the basophil and red staining of the cytoplasmic granules in the eosinophil. (*A, Courtesy of Dr. George Murphy. **B** and **C** Courtesy of Dr. Jonathan Hecht, Department of Pathology, Brigham and Women's Hospital, Boston, Massachusetts.)*

blood vessels (Fig. 20-2, *A*) and nerves and beneath epithelia. They are also present in lymphoid organs. Human mast cells vary in shape and have round nuclei, and the cytoplasm contains membrane-bound granules and lipid bodies. The granules contain acidic proteoglycans that bind basic dyes.

Activated mast cells secrete a variety of mediators that are responsible for the manifestations of allergic reactions

(Table 20-2). These include substances that are stored in granules and rapidly released upon activation, and others that are synthesized upon activation. The production and actions of these mediators are described later.

Two major subsets of mast cells have been described, one found in the mucosa of the gastrointestinal tract and the other in connective tissues. Mucosal mast cells have abundant chondroitin sulfate and tryptase, and little

TABLE 20-2   Mediators Produced by Mast Cells, Basophils, and Eosinophils

Cell Type	Mediator Category	Mediator	Function/Pathologic Effects
Mast Cells and Basophils			
	Stored preformed in cytoplasmic granules	Histamine	Increase vascular permeability; stimulate smooth muscle cell contraction
		Enzymes: neutral proteases (tryptase and/or chymase), acid hydrolases, cathepsin G, carboxypeptidase	Degradation of microbial structures; tissue damage/remodeling
	Major lipid mediators produced on activation	Prostaglandin D$_2$	Vasodilation; bronchoconstriction; leukocyte chemotaxis
		Leukotrienes C$_4$, D$_4$, E$_4$	Prolonged bronchoconstriction; mucus secretion; increased vascular permeability
		Platelet-activating factor	Vasodilation; increased vascular permeability; leukocyte adhesion,chemotaxis, degranulation, oxidative burst
	Cytokines produced on activation	IL-3	Mast cell proliferation
		TNF, MIP-1α	Inflammation/late-phase reaction
		IL-4, IL-13	IgE production; mucus secretion
		IL-5	Eosinophil production and activation
Eosinophils			
	Stored preformed in cytoplasmic granules	Major basic protein, eosinophil cationic protein	Toxic to helminths, bacteria, host cells
		Eosinophil peroxidase, lysosomal hydrolases, lysophospholipase	Degradation of helminthic and protozoan cell walls; tissue damage/remodeling
	Major lipid mediators produced on activation	Leukotrienes C$_4$, D$_4$, E$_4$	Prolonged bronchoconstriction; mucus secretion; increased vascular permeability
	Cytokines produced on activation	IL-3, IL-5, GM-CSF	Eosinophil production and activation
		IL-8, IL-10, RANTES, MIP-1α, eotaxin	Chemotaxis of leukocytes

GM-CSF, granulocyte-monocyte colony-stimulating factor; *IL,* interleukin, *MIP-1α,* monocyte inflammatory protein 1α; *RANTES,* regulated by activation, normal T cell expressed and secreted; *TNF,* tumor necrosis factor.

histamine, in their granules, and in humans are found in intestinal mucosa and alveolar spaces in the lung. Connective tissue mast cells have abundant heparin and neutral proteases in their granules, produce large quantities of histamine, and are found in the skin and intestinal submucosa. Mucosal mast cells require T cells for their development, while connective tissue mast cells do not. The locations, granule contents, and relative T cell dependence of different mast cell populations suggest that each may be important in a different set of disease processes. It is likely that mucosal-type mast cells are involved in T cell– and IgE-dependent immediate hypersensitivity diseases involving the airways, such as bronchial asthma, and other mucosal tissues. Conversely, connective tissue–type mast cells mediate immediate hypersensitivity reactions in the skin. Although the idea of these subsets has provided a valuable framework for studies of mast cells, it is clear that the populations are neither fixed nor always clearly separable.

Basophils are blood granulocytes with structural and functional similarities to mast cells. Like other granulocytes, basophils are derived from bone marrow progenitors (a lineage different from that of mast cells), mature in the bone marrow, and circulate in the blood (Fig. 20-2, *B*). Basophils constitute less than 1% of blood leukocytes. Although they are normally not present in tissues, basophils may be recruited to some inflammatory sites. Basophils contain granules that bind basic dyes, and they are capable of synthesizing many of the same mediators as mast cells (see Table 20-2). Like mast cells, basophils express FcεRI, bind IgE, and can be triggered by antigen binding to the IgE. Therefore, basophils that are recruited into tissue sites where antigen is present may contribute to immediate hypersensitivity reactions.

Binding of IgE to Mast Cells and Basophils: The Fcε Receptor

Mast cells and basophils express a high-affinity Fc receptor specific for ε heavy chains, called FcεRI, which binds IgE. IgE, like all other antibodies, is made exclusively by B cells, yet IgE functions as an antigen receptor on the surface of mast cells and basophils. This function is accomplished by IgE binding to FcεRI on these cells. The affinity of FcεRI for IgE is very high (dissociation constant [K_d] of about 1×10^{-10} M), much higher than that of any other Fc receptor for its antibody ligand. Therefore, the normal serum concentration of IgE, although low in comparison to other Ig isotypes (less than 5×10^{-10} M), is sufficient to allow occupancy of FcεRI receptors. In addition to mast cells and basophils, FcεRI has been detected on eosinophils, epidermal Langerhans cells, some dermal macrophages, and activated monocytes. The function of the receptor on many of these cells is not established.

Each FcεRI molecule is composed of an α chain that binds the Fc region of IgE and a β chain and two γ chains that are responsible for signaling (Fig. 20-3). The amino-terminal extracellular portion of the α chain includes two Ig-like domains that form the binding site for IgE. The β chain of FcεRI contains a single immunoreceptor tyrosine-based activation motif (ITAM) in the

cytoplasmic carboxyl terminal domain. The two identical γ chain polypeptides are linked by a disulfide bond and are homologous to the ζ chain of the T cell antigen receptor complex (see Chapter 7). The cytoplasmic portion of each γ chain contains one ITAM. The same γ chain serves as the signaling subunit for FcγRI, FcγRIIIA, and FcαR and is called the FcR γ chain (see Chapter 13). Tyrosine phosphorylation of the ITAMs of the β and γ chains initiates the signaling cascade from the receptor that is required for mast cell activation, described next. The FcεRI on eosinophils and several other cell types lacks the β chain, so signaling is mediated only by the γ chain in these cells.

The importance of FcεRI in IgE-mediated immediate hypersensitivity reactions has been demonstrated in FcεRI α chain knockout mice. When these mice are given intravenous injections of IgE specific for a known antigen followed by that antigen, anaphylaxis does not develop or is mild, whereas it is a severe reaction in wild-type mice treated in the same way. FcεRI expression on the surface of mast cells and basophils is increased by IgE, thereby providing a mechanism for the amplification of IgE-mediated reactions.

Another IgE receptor called FcεRII, also known as CD23, is a protein related to C-type mammalian lectins whose affinity for IgE is much lower than that of FcεRI. The biologic role of FcεRII is not known.

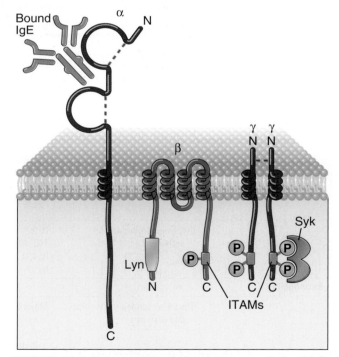

FIGURE 20-3 Polypeptide chain structure of the high-affinity IgE Fc receptor (FcεRI). IgE (not drawn to scale) binds to the Ig-like domains of the α chain. The β chain and the γ chains mediate signal transduction. The ITAMs in the cytoplasmic region of the β and γ chains are similar to those found in the T cell receptor complex (see Fig. 7-5). Lyn and Syk are tyrosine kinases that bind to the β and γ chains and participate in signaling events. A model structure of FcεRI is shown in Chapter 12.

Activation of Mast Cells

Mast cells are activated by cross-linking of FcεRI molecules, which occurs by binding of multivalent antigens to the IgE molecules that are attached to the Fc receptors (Fig. 20-4). In an individual allergic to a particular antigen, a large proportion of the IgE bound to FcεRI on the surface of mast cells is specific for that antigen. Exposure to the antigen will cross-link sufficient IgE molecules to trigger mast cell activation. In contrast, in non-atopic individuals, the IgE molecules bound to mast cells are specific for many different antigens, all of which may have induced low levels of IgE production. Therefore, no single antigen will cross-link enough of the IgE molecules to cause mast cell activation.

Activation of mast cells results in three types of biologic response: secretion of the preformed granule contents by exocytosis (degranulation), synthesis and secretion of lipid mediators, and synthesis and secretion of cytokines. The signaling cascades initiated by allergen-mediated FcεRI cross-linking are similar to the proximal signaling events initiated by antigen binding to lymphocytes (Fig. 20-5; also see Chapter 7). The Lyn tyrosine kinase is constitutively associated with the cytoplasmic tail of the FcεRI β chain. On cross-linking of FcεRI molecules by antigen, Lyn tyrosine kinase phosphorylates the ITAMs in the cytoplasmic domains of FcεRI β and γ chains. The Syk tyrosine kinase is then recruited to the ITAMs of the γ chain, becomes activated, and phosphorylates and activates other proteins in the signaling cascade, including several adaptor molecules and enzymes that participate in the formation of multicomponent signaling complexes, as described in T cells. Linker for activation of T cells (LAT) is one of the adaptor proteins required for mast cell activation, and one of the enzymes recruited to LAT is phospholipase Cγ (PLCγ). Once bound to LAT, PLCγ is phosphorylated and then catalyzes phosphatidylinositol bisphosphate breakdown to yield inositol trisphosphate (IP3) and diacylglycerol (DAG) (see Chapter 7). IP3 causes elevation of cytoplasmic calcium levels, and DAG activates protein kinase C (PKC). Another pathway of PKC activation in mast cells involves the tyrosine kinase Fyn, which phosphorylates the adaptor protein Grb-2–associated binder-like protein 2 (Gab2), which in turn binds phosphoinositide 3-kinase, leading to activation of PKC.

These signaling events lead to three major responses:

- **Degranulation.** Activated PKC phosphorylates the myosin light chain component of actin-myosin complexes located beneath the plasma membrane, leading to disassembly of the complex. This allows cytoplasmic granules to come in contact with the plasma membrane. The mast cell granule membrane then fuses with the plasma membrane, a process that is mediated by members of the SNARE protein family, which are involved in many other membrane fusion events. Different SNARE proteins present on the granule and plasma membranes interact to form a multimeric complex that catalyzes fusion. The formation of SNARE complexes is regulated by several accessory molecules, including Rab3 guanosine triphosphatases and Rab-associated kinases and phosphatases. In resting mast cells, these regulatory molecules inhibit mast cell granule membrane fusion with the plasma membrane. On FcεRI cross-linking, the resulting increase in cytoplasmic calcium concentrations and the activation of PKC block the regulatory functions of the accessory molecules. In addition, calcium sensor proteins respond to the elevated calcium concentrations by promoting SNARE complex formation and membrane fusion. Following membrane fusion, the contents of the mast cell granules are released into the extracellular environment. This process can occur within seconds of FcεRI cross-linking, and can be visualized morphologically by loss of the dense granules of mast cells (see Fig. 20-4).

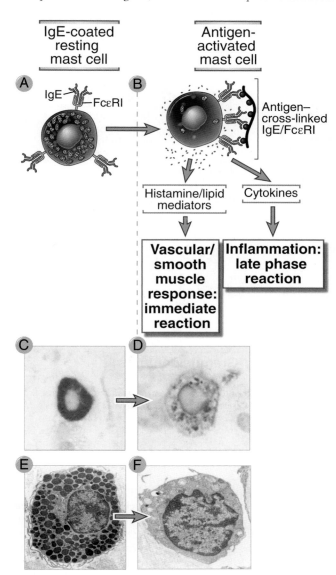

FIGURE 20-4 Mast cell activation. Antigen binding to IgE cross-links FcεRI molecules on mast cells, which induces the release of mediators that cause the hypersensitivity reaction **(A, B)**. Other stimuli, including the complement fragment C5a, can also activate mast cells. A light photomicrograph of a resting mast cell with abundant purple-staining cytoplasmic granules is shown in **C**. These granules are also seen in the electron micrograph of a resting mast cell shown in **E**. In contrast, the depleted granules of an activated mast cell are shown in the light photomicrograph **(D)** and electron micrograph **(F)**. *(Courtesy of Dr. Daniel Friend, Department of Pathology, Brigham and Women's Hospital and Harvard Medical School, Boston, Massachusetts.)*

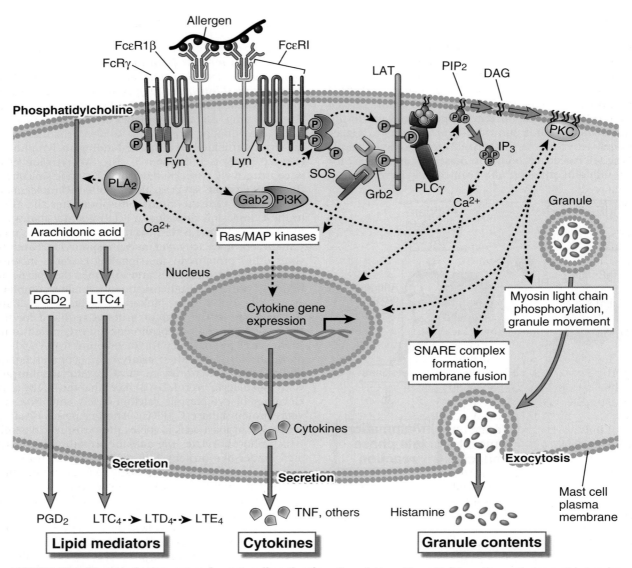

FIGURE 20-5 Biochemical events of mast cell activation. Cross-linking of bound IgE by antigen activates protein tyrosine kinases (Syk and Lyn), which in turn cause activation of a MAP kinase cascade and phospholipase Cγ (PLCγ). PLCγ catalyzes the release of IP3 and DAG from membrane PIP2. IP3 causes release of intracellular calcium from the endoplasmic reticulum. Calcium and DAG activate PKC, which phosphorylates substrates such as myosin light chain protein and thereby leads to the degradation and release of preformed mediators. Calcium and MAP kinases combine to activate the enzyme cytosolic phospholipase A_2 (PLA$_2$), which initiates the synthesis of lipid mediators, including prostaglandin D_2 (PGD$_2$) and leukotriene C_4 (LTC$_4$).

The biologic actions of the mediators released upon mast cell degranulation are described later.

- **Lipid mediator production.** Synthesis of lipid mediators is controlled by the cytosolic enzyme phospholipase A_2 (PLA$_2$) (see Fig. 20-5). This enzyme is activated by two signals: elevated cytoplasmic calcium and phosphorylation catalyzed by a mitogen-activated protein (MAP) kinase such as extracellular receptor-activated kinase (ERK). ERK is activated as a consequence of a kinase cascade initiated through the receptor ITAMs, probably using the same intermediates as in T cells (see Chapter 7). Once activated, PLA$_2$ hydrolyzes membrane phospholipids to release substrates that are converted further by enzyme cascades into the ultimate mediators. The major substrate is arachidonic acid, which is converted by cyclooxygenase or lipoxygenase into

different mediators (discussed later).
- **Cytokine production.** Cytokine secretion by activated mast cells is a consequence of newly induced cytokine gene transcription. The biochemical events that regulate cytokine gene transcription in mast cells appear to be similar to the events that occur in T cells. Recruitment and activation of various adaptor molecules and kinases in response to FcεRI cross-linking lead to nuclear translocation of nuclear factor of activated T cells (NFAT) and nuclear factor κB (NF-κB) as well as activation of activation protein 1 (AP-1) by protein kinases such as c-Jun N-terminal kinase. These transcription factors stimulate expression of several cytokines (IL-4, IL-5, IL-6, IL-13, and tumor necrosis factor [TNF], among others) but, in contrast to T cells, not IL-2.

Mast cell activation through the FcεRI pathway is regulated by various inhibitory receptors, which contain an immunoreceptor tyrosine-based inhibition motif (ITIM) within their cytoplasmic tails (see Chapter 7). One such inhibitory receptor is FcγRIIB, which coaggregates with FcεRI during mast cell activation. The ITIM of FcγRIIB is phosphorylated by Lyn, and this leads to recruitment of the phosphatase called SH2 domain–containing inositol 5-phosphatase (SHIP) and inhibition of FcεRI signaling. Experiments in mice indicate that FcγRIIB regulates mast cell degranulation in vivo. Several other inhibitory receptors are also expressed on mast cells, but their importance in vivo is not yet known.

Mast cells can be activated by a variety of biologic substances independent of allergen-mediated cross-linking of FcεRI, including polybasic compounds, peptides, chemokines, and complement-derived anaphylatoxins (C3a, C4a, C5a). These additional modes of mast cell activation may be important in non–immune-mediated immediate hypersensitivity reactions, or they may amplify IgE-mediated reactions. Certain types of mast cells or basophils may respond to macrophage-derived chemokines, such as macrophage inflammatory protein 1α (MIP-1α), produced as part of innate immunity, and to T cell–derived chemokines, produced as part of adaptive cell-mediated immunity. The complement-derived anaphylatoxins, especially C5a, bind to specific receptors on mast cells and stimulate degranulation. These chemokines and complement fragments that activate mast cells are likely to be produced at sites of inflammation. Therefore, mast cell activation and release of mediators may amplify IgE-independent inflammatory reactions. Polybasic compounds, such as compound 48/40 and mastoparan, are used experimentally as pharmacologic triggers for mast cells. These agents contain a cationic region adjacent to a hydrophobic moiety, and they work by activating G proteins.

Many neuropeptides, including substance P, somatostatin, and vasoactive intestinal peptide, induce mast cell histamine release and may mediate neuroendocrine-linked mast cell activation. The nervous system is known to modulate immediate hypersensitivity reactions, and neuropeptides may be involved in this effect. The flare produced at the edge of the wheal in elicited immediate hypersensitivity reactions is in part mediated by the nervous system, as shown by the observation that it is markedly diminished in skin sites lacking innervation. Cold temperatures and intense exercise may also trigger mast cell degranulation, but the mechanisms involved are not known.

Mast cells also express Fc receptors for IgG heavy chains, and the cells can be activated by cross-linking bound IgG. This IgG-mediated reaction is the likely explanation for the finding that Ig ε chain knockout mice are not completely resistant to antigen-induced mast cell–mediated anaphylaxis. However, IgE is the major antibody isotype involved in most immediate hypersensitivity reactions.

Mast cell activation is not an all-or-nothing phenomenon, and different types or levels of stimuli may elicit partial responses, with production of some mediators but not others. Such variations in activation and mediator release may account for variable clinical presentations.

Mediators Derived from Mast Cells

The effector functions of mast cells are mediated by soluble molecules released from the activated cells (Fig. 20-6 and Table 20-2). These mediators may be divided into preformed mediators, which include biogenic amines and granule macromolecules, and newly synthesized mediators, which include lipid mediators and cytokines.

Biogenic Amines

Many of the biologic effects of mast cell activation are mediated by biogenic amines that are released from cytoplasmic granules and act on blood vessels and smooth muscle. Biogenic amines, also called vasoactive amines, are low–molecular-weight compounds that contain an amine group. In human mast cells, the major mediator of this class is **histamine,** but in some rodents, serotonin may be of equal or greater import. Histamine acts by binding to target cell receptors, and different cell types express distinct classes of histamine receptors (e.g., H$_1$, H$_2$, H$_3$) that can be distinguished by their sensitivity to different pharmacologic inhibitors. The actions of histamine are short-lived because histamine is rapidly removed from the extracellular milieu by amine-specific transport systems. On binding to cellular receptors, histamine initiates intracellular events, such as phosphatidylinositol breakdown to IP3 and DAG, and these products cause different changes in different cell types. Binding of histamine to endothelium causes contraction of the endothelial cells, leading to increased interendothelial spaces, increased vascular permeability, and leakage of plasma into the tissues. Histamine also stimulates endothelial cells to synthesize vascular smooth muscle cell relaxants, such as prostacyclin (PGI$_2$) and nitric oxide, which cause vasodilation. These actions of histamine produce the wheal-and-flare response of immediate hypersensitivity (described later). H$_1$ receptor antagonists (commonly called antihistamines) can inhibit the wheal-and-flare response to intradermal allergen or anti-IgE antibody. Histamine also causes contraction of intestinal and bronchial smooth muscle. Thus, histamine may contribute to the increased peristalsis and bronchospasm associated with ingested and inhaled allergens, respectively. However, in some allergic disorders, and especially in asthma, antihistamines are not effective at suppressing the reaction. Moreover, bronchoconstriction in asthma is more prolonged than are the effects of histamine, suggesting that other mast cell–derived mediators are important in some forms of immediate hypersensitivity.

Granule Enzymes and Proteoglycans

Neutral serine proteases, including tryptase and chymase, are the most abundant protein constituents of mast cell secretory granules and contribute to tissue damage in immediate hypersensitivity reactions. Tryptase is present in all human mast cells and is not known to be present in any other cell type. Therefore, the presence of tryptase in human biologic fluids is interpreted as a marker of mast cell activation. Chymase is found in some human mast cells, and its presence or absence is one

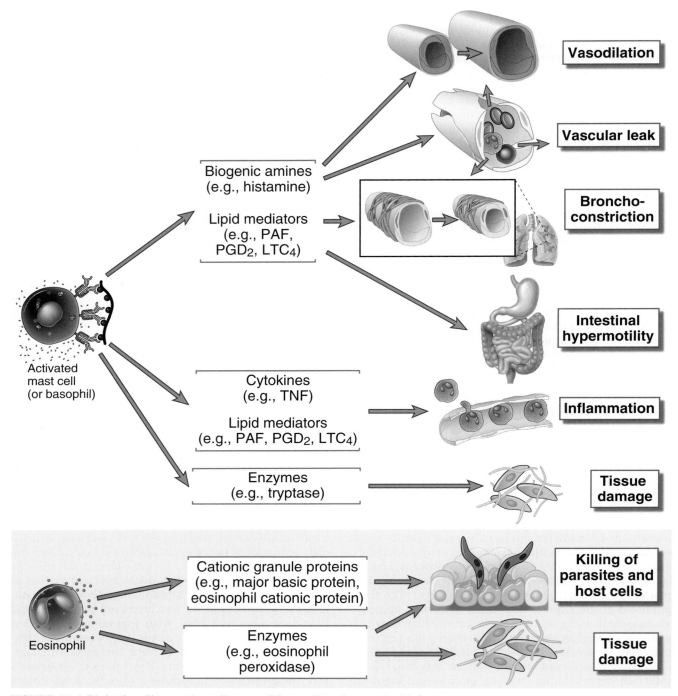

FIGURE 20-6 Biologic effects of mediators of immediate hypersensitivity. Mast cells and basophil mediators include biogenic amines and enzymes stored preformed in granules as well as cytokines and lipid mediators, which are largely newly synthesized on cell activation. The biogenic amines and lipid mediators induce vascular leakage, bronchoconstriction, and intestinal hypermotility, all components of the immediate response. Cytokines and lipid mediators contribute to inflammation, which is part of the late-phase reaction. Enzymes probably contribute to tissue damage. Activated eosinophils release preformed cationic proteins as well as enzymes that are toxic to parasites and host cells. Some eosinophil granule enzymes probably contribute to tissue damage in chronic allergic diseases.

criterion for characterizing human mast cell subsets, as discussed earlier. The functions of these enzymes in vivo are not known; however, several activities demonstrated in vitro suggest important biologic effects. For example, tryptase cleaves fibrinogen and activates collagenase, thereby causing tissue damage, whereas chymase can convert angiotensin I to angiotensin II, degrade epidermal basement membranes, and stimulate mucus secretion. Other enzymes found within mast cell granules include carboxypeptidase A and cathepsin G. Basophil granules also contain several enzymes, some of which are the same as those in mast cell granules, such as neutral proteases. Other enzymes, such as major basic protein and lysophospholipase, are found in eosinophil granules.

Proteoglycans, including heparin and chondroitin sulfate, are also major constituents of both mast cell and basophil granules. These molecules are composed of a polypeptide core and multiple unbranched glycosaminoglycan side chains that impart a strong net negative charge to the molecules. Within the granules, proteoglycans serve as storage matrices for positively charged biogenic amines, proteases, and other mediators and prevent their accessibility to the rest of the cell. The mediators are released from the proteoglycans at different rates after granule exocytosis, with biogenic amines dissociating much more rapidly than tryptase or chymase. In this way, the proteoglycans may control the kinetics of immediate hypersensitivity reactions.

Lipid Mediators

Mast cell activation results in the rapid de novo synthesis and release of lipid mediators that have a variety of effects on blood vessels, bronchial smooth muscle, and leukocytes. The most important of these mediators are derived from arachidonic acid, which is generated by PLA$_2$-mediated hydrolysis of membrane phospholipids, as discussed earlier. Arachidonic acid is then metabolized by either the cyclooxygenase or lipoxygenase pathways to produce mediators of allergic reactions.

The major arachidonic acid–derived mediator produced by the cyclooxygenase pathway in mast cells is **prostaglandin D$_2$** (PGD$_2$). Released PGD$_2$ binds to receptors on smooth muscle cells and acts as a vasodilator and a bronchoconstrictor. PGD$_2$ also promotes neutrophil chemotaxis and accumulation at inflammatory sites. PGD$_2$ synthesis can be prevented by cyclooxygenase inhibitors, such as aspirin and other non-steroidal anti-inflammatory agents. These drugs may paradoxically exacerbate asthmatic bronchoconstriction because they shunt arachidonic acid toward production of leukotrienes, discussed next.

The major arachidonic acid–derived mediators produced by the lipoxygenase pathway are the **leukotrienes**, especially LTC$_4$ and its degradation products LTD$_4$ and LTE$_4$. LTC$_4$ is made by mucosal mast cells and basophils, but not by connective tissue mast cells. Mast cell–derived leukotrienes bind to specific receptors on smooth muscle cells, different from the receptors for PGD$_2$, and cause prolonged bronchoconstriction. Collectively, LTC$_4$, LTD$_4$, and LTE$_4$ constitute what was once called slow-reacting substance of anaphylaxis (SRS-A) and are thought to be important mediators of asthmatic bronchoconstriction. When injected into the skin, these leukotrienes produce a characteristic long-lived wheal-and-flare reaction. Pharmacologic inhibitors of 5-lipoxygenase also block anaphylactic reactions in experimental systems.

A third type of lipid mediator produced by mast cells is **platelet-activating factor** (PAF), named for its discovery as an inducer of rabbit platelet aggregation. In mast cells and basophils, PAF is synthesized by acylation of lysoglyceryl ether phosphorylcholine, a derivative of PLA$_2$-mediated hydrolysis of membrane phospholipids. PAF has direct bronchoconstricting actions. It also causes retraction of endothelial cells and can relax vascular smooth muscle. However, PAF is hydrophobic and is rapidly destroyed by a plasma enzyme called PAF hydrolase, which limits its biologic actions. Pharmacologic inhibitors of PAF receptors ameliorate some aspects of immediate hypersensitivity in the rabbit lung. Recent genetic evidence has pointed to PAF as a mediator of asthma. Asthma develops in early childhood in individuals with an inherited deficiency of PAF hydrolase. PAF may also be important in late-phase reactions, in which it can activate inflammatory leukocytes. In this situation, the source of PAF may be basophils or vascular endothelial cells (stimulated by histamine or leukotrienes), in addition to mast cells.

Cytokines

Mast cells produce many different cytokines that contribute to allergic inflammation (the late-phase reaction). These cytokines include TNF, IL-1, IL-4, IL-5, IL-6, IL-13, CCL3, CCL4, and various colony-stimulating factors such as IL-3 and granulocyte-monocyte colony-stimulating factor (GM-CSF). As mentioned earlier, mast cell activation induces transcription and synthesis of these cytokines, but preformed TNF may also be stored in granules and rapidly released on FcεRI cross-linking. T$_H$2 cells that are recruited into the sites of allergic reactions also produce some of these cytokines. The cytokines that are released from activated mast cells and T$_H$2 cells are mainly responsible for the inflammation associated with the late-phase reaction. TNF activates endothelial expression of adhesion molecules and together with chemokines accounts for neutrophil and monocyte infiltrates (see Chapter 3). In addition to allergic inflammation, mast cell cytokines also apparently contribute to innate immune responses to infections. For example, as we will discuss later, mouse models indicate that mast cells are required for effective defense against some bacterial infections, and this effector function is mediated largely by TNF.

Properties of Eosinophils

Eosinophils are bone marrow–derived granulocytes that are abundant in the inflammatory infiltrates of late-phase reactions and are involved in many of the pathologic processes in allergic diseases. Eosinophils develop in the bone marrow, and after maturation they circulate in the blood. GM-CSF, IL-3, and IL-5 promote eosinophil maturation from myeloid precursors. Eosinophils are normally present in peripheral tissues, especially in mucosal linings of the respiratory, gastrointestinal, and genitourinary tracts, and their numbers can increase by recruitment in the setting of inflammation. The granules of eosinophils contain basic proteins that bind acidic dyes such as eosin (see Table 20-2 and Fig. 20-2, *C*).

Cytokines produced by T$_H$2 cells promote the activation of eosinophils and their recruitment to late-phase reaction inflammatory sites. Both T$_H$2 cells and group 2 innate lymphoid cells are sources of IL-5. IL-5 is a potent eosinophil-activating cytokine that enhances the ability of eosinophils to release granule contents. IL-5 also increases maturation of eosinophils from bone marrow precursors, and in the absence of this cytokine (e.g., in IL-5 knockout mice), there is a deficiency of eosinophil numbers and functions. Eosinophils are recruited into late-phase reaction sites as well as sites of helminthic infection, and their recruitment is mediated by a combination of adhesion molecule interactions and chemokines. Eosinophils bind to endothelial cells expressing E-selectin and VCAM-1, the ligand for the VLA-4 integrin. IL-4 produced by T_H2 cells may enhance expression of adhesion molecules for eosinophils. Eosinophil recruitment and infiltration into tissues also depend on the chemokine eotaxin (CCL11), which is produced by epithelial cells at sites of allergic reactions and binds to the chemokine receptor CCR3, which is expressed constitutively by eosinophils. In addition, the complement product C5a and the lipid mediators PAF and LTB_4, which are produced by mast cells, also function as chemoattractants for eosinophils.

Eosinophils release granule proteins that are toxic to helminthic parasites and may injure normal tissue. Eosinophils express Fc receptors for IgG, IgA, and IgE, and are presumably able to respond to cross-linking of these receptors by binding of antigen to the receptor-associated antibodies. FcεRI on human eosinophils lacks the β chain, a signaling component of the receptor, and it is unclear how efficiently these cells degranulate in response to IgE cross-linking. The granule contents of eosinophils include lysosomal hydrolases found in other granulocytes as well as eosinophil-specific proteins that are particularly toxic to helminthic organisms, including major basic protein and eosinophil cationic protein. These two cationic polypeptides have no known enzymatic activities, but they are toxic to helminths and bacteria, as well as normal tissue. In addition, eosinophilic granules contain eosinophil peroxidase, which is distinct from the myeloperoxidase found in neutrophils and catalyzes the production of hypochlorous or hypobromous acid. These products are also toxic to helminths, protozoa, and host cells.

Activated eosinophils, like mast cells and basophils, produce and release lipid mediators, including PAF, prostaglandins, and the leukotrienes LTC_4, LTD_4 and LTE_4.

These eosinophil-derived lipid mediators may contribute to the pathologic processes of allergic diseases. Eosinophils also produce a variety of cytokines that may promote inflammatory responses and tissue repair, but the biologic significance of eosinophil cytokine production is not known.

IgE- AND MAST CELL–DEPENDENT REACTIONS

The cells and mediators we have discussed are responsible for the immediate vascular changes and later inflammatory responses that occur in allergic reactions. In the following sections, we will describe these immediate and late-phase reactions (Fig. 20-7).

The Immediate Reaction

The early vascular changes that occur during immediate hypersensitivity reactions are demonstrated by the wheal-and-flare reaction to the intradermal injection of an allergen (Fig. 20-8). When an individual who has previously encountered an allergen and produced IgE antibody is challenged by intradermal injection of the same antigen, the injection site becomes red from locally dilated blood vessels engorged with red blood cells. The site then rapidly swells as a result of leakage of plasma from the venules. This soft swelling is called a **wheal** and can involve an area of skin as large as several centimeters in diameter. Subsequently, blood vessels at the margins of the wheal dilate and become engorged with red blood cells and produce a characteristic red rim called a **flare**. The full wheal-and-flare reaction can appear within 5 to 10 minutes after administration of antigen and usually subsides in less than 1 hour.

The wheal-and-flare reaction is dependent on IgE and mast cells. Histologic examination shows that mast cells in the area of the wheal-and-flare have released preformed mediators; that is, their cytoplasmic granules have been

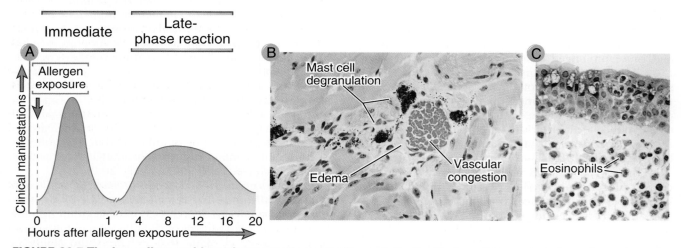

FIGURE 20-7 The immediate and late-phase reactions of allergy. A, Kinetics. The immediate vascular and smooth muscle reaction to allergen develops within minutes after challenge (allergen exposure in a previously sensitized individual), and the late-phase reaction develops 2 to 24 hours later. **B, C,** Morphology. The immediate reaction **(B)** is characterized by vasodilation, congestion, and edema, and the late-phase reaction **(C)** is characterized by an inflammatory infiltrate rich in eosinophils, neutrophils, and T cells. *(Courtesy of Dr. Daniel Friend, Department of Pathology, Brigham and Women's Hospital, Boston, Massachusetts.)*

discharged. A causal association of IgE and mast cells with immediate hypersensitivity was first deduced from experiments involving the passive transfer of IgE antibodies from an allergic individual into a normal recipient. For example, immediate hypersensitivity reactions against an allergen can be elicited in unresponsive individuals if the

local skin site is first injected with IgE from an allergic individual. Such adoptive transfer experiments were first performed with serum from immunized individuals, and the serum factor responsible for the reaction was originally called reagin. For this reason, IgE molecules are still sometimes called reaginic antibodies. The antigen-initiated skin reaction that follows adoptive transfer of IgE is called passive cutaneous anaphylaxis.

The wheal-and-flare reaction results from sensitization of dermal mast cells by IgE that binds to FcεRI, cross-linking of IgE by the antigen, and activation of mast cells with release of mediators, notably histamine. Histamine binds to histamine receptors on venular endothelial cells; the endothelial cells synthesize and release PGI$_2$, nitric oxide, and PAF; and these mediators cause vasodilation and vascular leak, as described earlier. Skin mast cells appear to produce only small amounts of long-acting mediators such as leukotrienes, so the wheal-and-flare response subsides rapidly. Allergists often test patients for allergies to different antigens by examining the ability of these antigens applied in skin patches or administered through small needle pricks to elicit wheal-and-flare reactions.

The Late-Phase Reaction

The immediate wheal-and-flare reaction is followed 2 to 4 hours later by a late-phase reaction consisting of the accumulation of inflammatory leukocytes, including neutrophils, eosinophils, basophils, and helper T cells (see Fig. 20-7). The inflammation is maximal by about 24 hours and then gradually subsides. Like the immediate wheal-and-flare reaction, the capacity to mount a late-phase reaction also can be adoptively transferred with IgE, and the reaction can be mimicked with anti-IgE antibodies that cross-link FcεR1 receptors on mast cells with bound IgE, or with mast cell–activating agents. Cytokines produced by mast cells, including TNF, upregulate endothelial expression of leukocyte adhesion molecules, such as E-selectin and intercellular adhesion molecule 1 (ICAM-1), and chemokines recruit blood leukocytes. Thus, mast cell activation promotes the influx of leukocytes into tissues. The types of leukocytes that are typical of late-phase reactions are eosinophils and helper T cells. Although T$_H$2 cells are the dominant subset in uncomplicated late-phase reactions, the T cells found in chronic atopic dermatitis and asthma include T$_H$1 and T$_H$17 cells, as well as T cells that produce both IL-17 and IFNγ. Neutrophils are also often present in these reactions. Eosinophils and T$_H$2 cells both express CCR4 and CCR3, and the chemokines that bind to these receptors are produced by many cell types at sites of immediate hypersensitivity reactions, including epithelial cells.

The late-phase reaction may occur without a detectable preceding immediate hypersensitivity reaction. Bronchial asthma is a disease in which there may be repeated bouts of inflammation with accumulations of eosinophils and T$_H$2 cells without the vascular changes that are characteristic of the immediate response. In such disorders, there may be little mast cell activation, and the cytokines that sustain the late-phase reaction may be produced mainly by T cells.

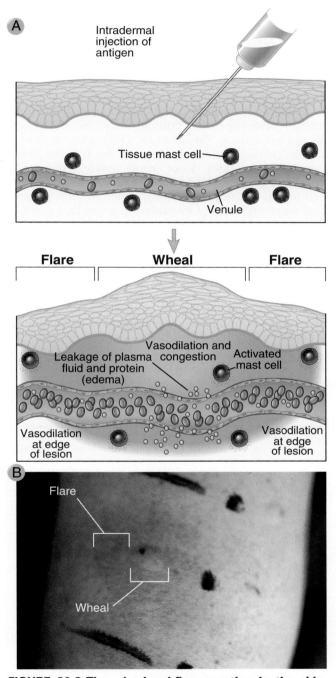

FIGURE 20-8 The wheal-and-flare reaction in the skin. A, In response to antigen-stimulated release of mast cell mediators, local blood vessels first dilate and then become leaky to fluid and macromolecules, which produces redness and local swelling (a wheal). Subsequent dilation of vessels on the edge of the swelling produces the appearance of a red rim (the flare). **B,** Photograph of a typical wheal-and-flare reaction in the skin in response to injection of an allergen. *(Courtesy of Dr. James D. Faix, Department of Pathology, Stanford University School of Medicine, Palo Alto, California.)*

GENETIC SUSCEPTIBILITY TO ALLERGIC DISEASE

The propensity to develop allergies is influenced by the inheritance of several genes. Abnormally high levels of IgE synthesis and associated atopy often run in families. Family studies have shown clear autosomal transmission of atopy, although the full inheritance pattern is multigenic. Within the same family, the target organ of atopic disease is variable. Thus, hay fever, asthma, and eczema can be present to various degrees in different members of the same kindred. All these individuals, however, will show higher than average plasma IgE levels.

Various approaches have been taken to identify allelic variations of genes that carry a risk for allergic diseases, including positional cloning, candidate gene studies, and genome-wide association studies. These approaches have identified many different genes associated with increased susceptibility for asthma and other atopic diseases (Table 20-3). Based on the known functions of the proteins encoded by many of these genes, rational speculations can be made about how altered expression or activity of these proteins might impact the development or severity of allergic diseases. Nonetheless, we still know very little about whether or not the genetic polymorhisms that are associated with increased risk for allergy actually alter expression or function of the encoded proteins, and, in many cases, it is not clear how the function of the encoded proteins could impact the development of allergy.

One of the first significant findings from genetic studies of allergy was the identification of a susceptibility locus for atopy on chromosome 5q, near the site of the gene cluster encoding the cytokines IL-4, IL-5, IL-9, and IL-13 and the IL-4 receptor. This region is of great interest because of the connection between several genes located there and the mechanisms of IgE regulation and mast cell and eosinophil growth and differentiation. Among the genes in this cluster, polymorphisms in the *IL13* gene appear to have the strongest association with asthma. The loci containing the *IL33* gene and its receptor (IL1R1) were identified in a genome-wide association study of asthma susceptibility genes. IL-33 induces T_H2 cytokine production in various cell types, including innate lymphoid cells. Hypomorphic mutations in the gene encoding filaggrin, a known barrier protein in the skin and esophagus, increase the risk of sensitization to allergens and consequent IgE responses and atopic disease.

Some genes whose products regulate the innate immune response to infections have been associated with allergy and asthma. These include CD14, a component of the lipopolysaccharide receptor, and the Toll-like receptors TLR2 and TLR4. Since strong innate responses to infections generally favor development of T_H1 responses and inhibit T_H2 responses (see Chapter 10), it is possible that polymorphisms or mutations in genes that result in enhanced or diminished innate responses to common infectious organisms may influence the risk for development of atopy. Other genome-wide association studies have found significant associations of common variants of numerous other genes with asthma and other atopic diseases. However, either the products of these genes are of unknown function, or the connection between their known functions and the development of atopic disease is not known.

TABLE 20-3 Examples of Genes Associated with Atopy and Asthma

Candidate Genes or Encoded Protein	Chromosomal Location	Disease Association	Putative Role of Gene Products in Disease
Genes in cytokine gene cluster (IL-4, IL-5, IL-13), CD14, β_2-adrenergic receptor	5q	Asthma	IL-4 and IL-13 promote IgE switching, IL-5 promotes eosinophil growth and activation; CD14 is a component of the LPS receptor that, through interaction with TLR4, may influence the balance between T_H1 and T_H2 responses to antigens; β_2-adrenergic receptor regulates bronchial smooth muscle contraction
Class II MHC	6p	Asthma	Some alleles may regulate T cell responses to allergens
FcεRI β chain	11q	Asthma	Mediates mast cell activation
Stem cell factor, interferon-γ, STAT6	12q	Asthma	Stem cell factor regulates mast cell growth and differentiation; interferon-γ opposes actions of IL-4; STAT6 mediates IL-4 signal transduction
IL-4 receptor α chain	16	Asthma	Subunit of both IL-4 and IL-13 receptors
ADAM33	20p	Asthma	Metalloproteinase involved in airway remodeling
DPP10	2q14	Asthma	Peptidase that may regulate chemokine and cytokine activity
PHF11	13q	Asthma	Transcriptional regulator involved in B cell clonal expansion and Ig expression
ORMDL3	17q	Asthma	ER stress inflammatory response
IL-1 receptor–like 1 (IL-33 receptor)	2q	Asthma	IL-33 induces T_H2 cytokines in T cells, mast cells, eosinophils, innate lymphoid cells
Phosphodiesterase 4D	5q	Asthma	Degrades cAMP and regulates airway smooth muscle contractility
Filaggrin	1q	Atopic dermatitis	Component of terminally differentiated keratinocytes important for epithelial barrier function

Environmental Factors in Allergy

It is clear that environmental influences have a significant impact on the development of allergy, and they synergize with genetic risk factors. Environmental influences include exposure to allergens themselves, to infectious organisms, and possibly other factors that impact mucosal barrier function, such as air pollution. Furthermore, the time of life when exposure to these environmental factors occurs, especially early-life exposure, appears to be important.

Exposure to microbes during early childhood may reduce the risk for developing allergies. One possible explanation for the increased prevalence of asthma and other atopic diseases in industrialized countries is that the frequency of infections in these countries is generally lower. A variety of epidemiologic data show that early childhood exposure to environmental microbes, such as those found on farms but not in cities, is associated with decreased prevalence of allergic disease. Based on these data, the **hygiene hypothesis** was proposed, which states that early-life exposure to gut commensals and infections leads to a regulated maturation of the immune system, and perhaps early development of regulatory T cells. As a result, later in life these individuals are less likely to mount T_H2 responses to non-infectious environmental antigens, and less likely to develop allergic diseases.

Respiratory viral and bacterial infections are a predisposing factor in the development of asthma or exacerbations of preexisting asthma. For example, it is estimated that respiratory viral infections precede up to 80% of asthma attacks in children. How such infections stimulate T_H2 and mast cell responses is not understood.

ALLERGIC DISEASES IN HUMANS: PATHOGENESIS AND THERAPY

Mast cell degranulation is a central component of many allergic diseases, and the clinical and pathologic manifestations of the diseases depend on the tissues in which the mast cell mediators have effects as well as the chronicity of the resulting inflammatory process. Atopic individuals may have one or more manifestations of allergic disease. The most common forms of these diseases are allergic rhinitis (hay fever), bronchial asthma, atopic dermatitis (eczema), and food allergies. The clinical and pathologic features of allergic reactions vary with the anatomic site of the reaction, for several reasons. The point of contact with the allergen can determine the organs or tissues that are involved. For example, inhaled antigens cause rhinitis or asthma, ingested antigens often cause vomiting and diarrhea (but can also produce skin and respiratory symptoms if larger doses are ingested), and injected antigens cause systemic effects on the circulation. The concentration of mast cells in various target organs influences the severity of responses. Mast cells are particularly abundant in the skin and the mucosa of the respiratory and gastrointestinal tracts, and these tissues frequently suffer the most injury in immediate hypersensitivity reactions. The local mast cell phenotype may influence the characteristics of the immediate hypersensitivity reaction. For example, connective

tissue mast cells produce abundant histamine and are responsible for wheal-and-flare reactions in the skin.

In the following section, we will discuss the major features of allergic diseases manifested in different tissues.

Systemic Anaphylaxis

Anaphylaxis is a systemic immediate hypersensitivity reaction characterized by edema in many tissues and a decrease in blood pressure, secondary to vasodilation. These effects usually result from the systemic presence of antigen introduced by injection, an insect sting, or absorption across an epithelial surface such as gut mucosa. The allergen activates mast cells in many tissues, resulting in the release of mediators that gain access to vascular beds throughout the body. The decrease in vascular tone and leakage of plasma caused by mast cell mediators can lead to a significant decrease in blood pressure or shock, called anaphylactic shock, which is often fatal. The cardiovascular effects are accompanied by constriction of the upper and lower airways, laryngeal edema, hypermotility of the gut, outpouring of mucus in the gut and respiratory tract, and urticarial lesions (hives) in the skin. It is not known which mast cell mediators are the most important in anaphylactic shock. The mainstay of treatment is systemic epinephrine, which can be lifesaving by reversing the bronchoconstrictive and vasodilatory effects of mast cell mediators. Epinephrine also improves cardiac output, further aiding survival from threatened circulatory collapse. Antihistamines may also be beneficial in anaphylaxis, suggesting a role for histamine in this reaction.

Bronchial Asthma

Asthma is an inflammatory disease caused by repeated immediate-type hypersensitivity and late-phase allergic reactions in the lung leading to the clinicopathologic triad of intermittent and reversible airway obstruction, chronic bronchial inflammation with eosinophils, and bronchial smooth muscle cell hypertrophy and hyperreactivity to bronchoconstrictors (Fig. 20-9). Patients suffer paroxysms of bronchoconstriction and increased production of thick mucus, which leads to bronchial obstruction and exacerbates respiratory difficulties. Asthma frequently coexists with chronic obstructive pulmonary disease, and the combination of these diseases can cause severe irreversible airflow obstruction. Affected individuals may suffer considerable morbidity, and asthma can be fatal. Asthma affects about 20 million people in the United States, and the frequency of this disease has increased significantly in recent years. The prevalence rate is similar to that in other industrialized countries, but it may be lower in less developed areas of the world.

About 70% of cases of asthma are associated with IgE-mediated reactions reflecting atopy. In the remaining 30% of patients, asthma may not be associated with atopy and may be triggered by non-immune stimuli such as drugs, cold, and exercise. Even among non-atopic asthmatics, the pathophysiologic process of airway constriction is similar, which suggests that alternative mechanisms of mast cell degranulation (e.g., by locally produced neurotransmitters) may underlie the disease.

The pathophysiologic sequence in atopic asthma is probably initiated by mast cell activation in response to allergen

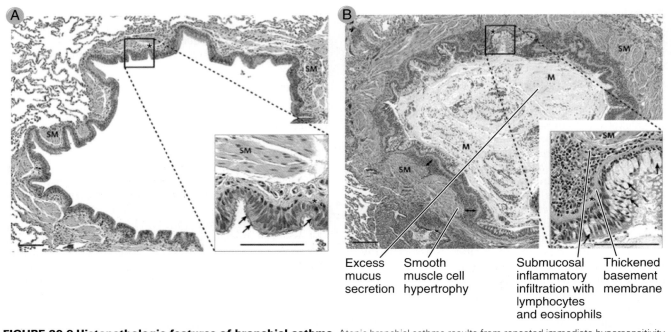

FIGURE 20-9 Histopathologic features of bronchial asthma. Atopic bronchial asthma results from repeated immediate hypersensitivity reactions in the lungs with chronic late-phase reactions. A cross-section of a normal bronchus **(A)** and a cross-section of a bronchus from a patient with asthma **(B)** are shown. The diseased bronchus has excessive mucus (M) production, many submucosal inflammatory cells (including eosinophils), and smooth muscle (SM) hypertrophy, and many more goblet cells than in the normal bronchus *(black arrows in insets)*. *(From Galli SJ, Tsai M, Piliponsky AM: The development of allergic inflammation,* Nature *454:445-454, 2008. Courtesy of G. J. Berry, Stanford University, California.)*

binding to IgE as well as by T_H2 cells reacting to allergens (Fig. 20-10). The lipid mediators and cytokines produced by the mast cells and T cells lead to the recruitment of eosinophils, basophils, and more T_H2 cells. The chronic inflammation in this disease may continue without mast cell activation. There is experimental evidence that other T cell subsets, including T_H1 and T_H17 cells, as well as IL-9–secreting T cells, contribute to the pathology of established disease. Smooth muscle cell hypertrophy and hyperreactivity are thought to result from leukocyte-derived mediators and cytokines. Mast cells, basophils, and eosinophils all produce mediators that constrict airway smooth muscle. The most important of the bronchoconstricting mediators are LTC_4, LTD_4, and LTE_4. In some clinical studies, antagonists of LTC_4 synthesis or leukotriene receptor antagonists have reduced allergen-induced airway constriction. Increased mucus secretion results from the action of cytokines, mainly IL-13, on bronchial epithelial cells.

Current therapy for asthma has two major targets: prevention and reversal of inflammation and relaxation of airway smooth muscle (see Fig. 20-10). In recent years, the balance of therapy has shifted toward anti-inflammatory agents as the primary mode of treatment. Several classes of drugs are in current use to treat asthma. Inhaled corticosteroids block the production of inflammatory cytokines. Corticosteroids may also be given systemically, especially once an attack is under way, to reduce inflammation. Bronchial smooth muscle cell relaxation is achieved principally by drugs that elevate intracellular cyclic adenosine monophosphate (cAMP) levels in smooth muscle cells, which inhibits contraction. The major drugs used are activators of adenylate cyclase, which work through binding to β_2-adrenergic receptors. Oral theophylline,

which inhibits phosphodiesterase enzymes that degrade cAMP, was once widely used but is less so now because it is less effective and more toxic than the inhaled long-acting β_2-agonists. Leukotriene inhibitors block the binding of bronchoconstricting leukotrienes to airway smooth muscle cells. Humanized monoclonal anti-IgE antibody is an approved therapy that effectively reduces serum IgE levels in patients. Because histamine has little role in airway constriction, antihistamines (H_1 receptor antagonists) are not useful in the treatment of asthma. Indeed, because many antihistamines are also anticholinergics, these drugs may worsen airway obstruction by causing thickening of mucus secretions.

Immediate Hypersensitivity Reactions in the Upper Respiratory Tract, Gastrointestinal Tract, and Skin

Allergic rhinitis, also called hay fever, is perhaps the most common allergic disease and is a consequence of immediate hypersensitivity reactions to common allergens such as plant pollen or house dust mites localized to the upper respiratory tract by inhalation. The pathologic and clinical manifestations include mucosal edema, leukocyte infiltration with abundant eosinophils, mucus secretion, coughing, sneezing, and difficulty in breathing. Allergic conjunctivitis with itchy eyes is commonly associated with the rhinitis. Focal protrusions of the nasal mucosa, called nasal polyps, filled with edema fluid and eosinophils may develop in patients who suffer frequent repetitive bouts of allergic rhinitis. Antihistamines are the most common drugs used to treat allergic rhinitis.

Food allergies are immediate hypersensitivity reactions to ingested foods that lead to the release of mediators

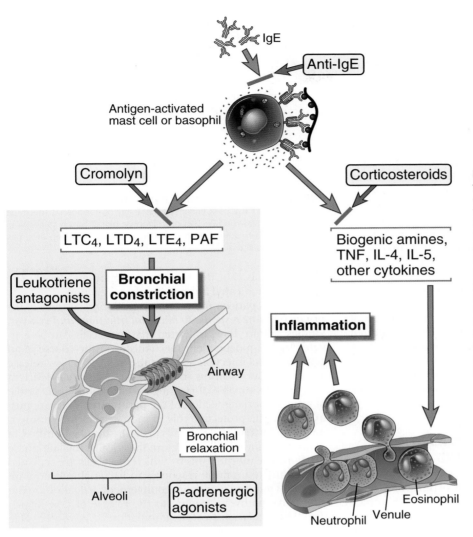

FIGURE 20-10 Mediators and treatment of asthma. Mast cell–derived leukotrienes and PAF are thought to be the major mediators of acute bronchoconstriction. Therapy is targeted both at reducing mast cell activation with inhibitors such as cromolyn and at countering mediator actions on bronchial smooth muscle by bronchodilators such as inhaled β-adrenergic receptor agonists. These drugs also inhibit mast cell activation. Mast cell–derived cytokines are thought to be the major mediators of sustained airway inflammation, which is an example of a late-phase reaction, and corticosteroid therapy is used to inhibit cytokine synthesis. Cytokines are also produced by helper T cells *(not shown)*.

from intestinal mucosal and submucosal mast cells of the GI tract, including the oropharynx. The resulting clinical manifestations include pruritis, tissue edema, enhanced peristalsis, increased epithelial fluid secretion, and associated symptoms of oropharyngeal swelling, vomiting and diarrhea. Rhinitis, urticaria and mild bronchospasm are also often associated with allergic reactions to food, suggestive of systemic antigen circulation, and systemic anaphylaxis may occasionally occur. Allergic reactions to many different types of food have been described, but some of the most common are peanuts and shellfish. Individuals may be sufficiently sensitive to these allergens that severe systemic reactions can occur in response to small accidental ingestions.

Common allergic reactions in the skin include **urticaria** and **atopic dermatitis**. Urticaria, or hives, is an acute wheal-and-flare reaction induced by mast cell mediators and occurs in response to direct local contact with an allergen or after an allergen enters the circulation. Because the reaction that ensues is mediated largely by histamine, antihistamines (H_1 receptor antagonists) can attenuate this response and are the mainstay of therapy. Urticaria may persist for several hours or days.

Atopic dermatitis (also commonly referred to as eczema) is part of the atopic triad (atopic dermatitis, allergic rhinitis and asthma) but can also occur in isolation. It is a common skin disorder that may be caused by a late-phase reaction to an allergen in the skin. In the cutaneous late-phase reaction, TNF, IL-4, and other cytokines, probably derived from T_H2 cells and mast cells, act on endothelial cells to promote inflammation. As may be expected for a cytokine-mediated response, the late-phase inflammatory reaction is not inhibited by antihistamines. It can be blocked by treatment with corticosteroids, which inhibit cytokine synthesis. Children with genetic alteration in skin barrier function, due to mutations in the gene encoding filaggrin, are highly susceptible to atopic dermatitis, and these children often also go on to develop asthma.

Immunotherapy for Allergic Diseases

In addition to therapy aimed at the consequences of immediate hypersensitivity, mentioned earlier, clinical immunologists often try to limit the onset of allergic reactions by treatments aimed at altering the allergen-specific immune response in the patient. Several empirical immunotherapy protocols have been developed which induce multiple changes associated with efficacy. In one approach, called **desensitization**, small quantities of antigen are repeatedly administered subcutaneously. As a result of this treatment, specific IgE levels decrease and IgG titers often rise, perhaps further inhibiting IgE production by neutralizing the antigen and by antibody feedback (see Chapter 12). It is possible that desensitization may work by inducing specific T cell tolerance or by changing the predominant phenotype of antigen-specific T cells from T_H2 to T_H1; however, there is no clear evidence to support any of these hypotheses. The beneficial effects of desensitization may occur in a matter of hours, much earlier than changes in IgE levels. The precise mechanism is not known, but this approach has been effective in preventing acute anaphylactic responses to protein antigens (e.g., insect venom) or vital drugs (e.g., penicillin). Although many people with more common chronic atopic conditions, such as hay fever and asthma, benefit from desensitization therapy, the overall effectiveness for allergic disorders is more variable.

Other approaches being used to alter the immune response to allergen include systemic administration of humanized monoclonal anti-IgE antibodies, mentioned earlier, and an antibody to the shared subunit of the IL-4 and IL-13 receptors, which has been shown to be effective in clinical trials in a subset of patients with asthma and atopic dermatitis. Antibodies against IL-4 and IL-5 are also in clinical trials.

THE PROTECTIVE ROLES OF IgE- AND MAST CELL–MEDIATED IMMUNE REACTIONS

Although most of our understanding of IgE- and mast cell–mediated reactions comes from analysis of immediate hypersensitivity, it is logical to assume that these responses have evolved because they provide protective functions. This assumption is supported by the correlation of certain types of infections with elevated IgE levels and eosinophilia. Studies in mice that were deficient in IgE, T_H2 cytokines, or mast cells have provided evidence showing that IgE- and mast cell–mediated responses are important for defense against certain types of infection.

A major protective function of IgE-initiated immune reactions is the eradication of helminthic parasites. Eosinophil-mediated killing of helminths is an effective defense against these organisms (Fig. 20-11 and see Chapter 10). The activities of IL-4 and IL-13 in IgE production and IL-5 in eosinophil activation contribute to a coordinated defense against helminths. In addition, IgE-dependent mast cell activation in the gastrointestinal tract promotes the expulsion of parasites by increasing peristalsis and by an outpouring of mucus. Studies in mice have highlighted the beneficial roles of IgE and mast cells. For example, mice treated with anti–IL-4 antibody and IL-4 knockout mice do not make IgE and appear to be more susceptible than normal animals to some helminthic infections. IL-5 knockout mice, which are unable to activate eosinophils, also show increased susceptibility to some helminths. Furthermore, genetically mast cell–deficient mice show increased susceptibility to infection by tick larvae, and immunity can be provided to these mice by adoptive transfer of specific IgE

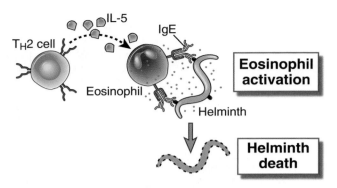

FIGURE 20-11 Activation of eosinophils to kill helminths. IL-5 secreted by T_H2 cells enhances the ability of eosinophils to kill the helminths. Cross-linking FcεR1 on eosinophils by IgE bound to helminth antigens may also induce eosinophil degranulation, releasing enzymes toxic to the parasites.

and mast cells (but not by either component alone). The larvae are eradicated by the late-phase reaction.

Mast cells play an important protective role as part of the innate immune response to bacterial infections and venoms. Studies in mice have indicated that mast cells can be activated by IgE-independent mechanisms in the course of an acute bacterial infection and that the mediators they release are critical for clearing the infection. Mast cell–deficient mice are less capable of clearing and are more likely to die of acute bacterial infection of the peritoneum than are normal mice. The protective role of mast cells in this setting is mediated by TNF and depends on TNF-stimulated influx of neutrophils into the peritoneum, specifically, the late-phase reaction. The mechanisms by which mast cells are activated during innate immune responses to bacterial infection are not known but may involve complement activation by the alternative pathway, leading to the release of C5a, which directly triggers mast cell degranulation. It is also possible that the classical pathway of complement could be activated by natural antibodies that are produced by B-1 cells and that recognize common microbial pathogens. Bacterial products may also activate mast cells by binding to Toll-like receptors expressed by the mast cells.

Mast cell–derived proteases have been shown to destroy some snake and insect venoms in mice and venom-specific IgE confers protection from envenomation. This is an unusual form of innate immunity against a potentially lethal encounter with non-microbial organisms.

SUMMARY

* Immediate hypersensitivity is an immune reaction triggered by antigen binding to IgE pre-bound to mast cells, which leads to the release of inflammatory mediators.
* The steps in the development of immediate hypersensitivity are exposure to an antigen (allergen) that stimulates T_H2 responses and IgE production, binding of the IgE to Fcε receptors on mast cells, cross-linking of the IgE and the Fcε receptors by the allergen, activation of mast cells, and release of mediators.

* Individuals who are susceptible to immediate hypersensitivity reactions are called atopic and often have more IgE in the blood and more IgE-specific Fc receptors per mast cell than do non-atopic individuals. IgE synthesis is induced by exposure to antigen and IL-4 secreted by T_{FH} cells.
* Mast cells are derived from bone marrow precursors that mature in tissues. They express high-affinity receptors for IgE (FcεRI) and contain cytoplasmic granules in which various inflammatory mediators are stored. Subsets of mast cells, including mucosal and connective tissue mast cells, may produce different mediators. Basophils are a type of circulating granulocyte that expresses high-affinity Fcε receptors and contains granules with contents similar to those of mast cells.
* Eosinophils are a special class of granulocyte; they are recruited into inflammatory reactions by chemokines and IL-4 and are activated by IL-5. Eosinophils are effector cells that are involved in killing parasites. In allergic reactions, eosinophils contribute to tissue injury.
* On binding of antigen to IgE on the surface of mast cells or basophils, the high-affinity Fcε receptors become cross-linked and activate intracellular second messengers that lead to granule release and new synthesis of mediators. Activated mast cells and basophils produce three important classes of mediators: biogenic amines, such as histamine; lipid mediators, such as prostaglandins, leukotrienes, and PAF; and cytokines, such as TNF, IL-4, IL-13, and IL-5.
* Biogenic amines and lipid mediators cause the rapid vascular and smooth muscle reactions of immediate hypersensitivity, such as vasodilation, vascular leakage and edema, bronchoconstriction, and gut hypermotility. Cytokines released by mast cells and T_H2 cells mediate the late-phase reaction, which is an inflammatory reaction involving neutrophil and eosinophil infiltration.
* Susceptibly to allergic diseases is inherited, and allelic variations of several genes have been associated with allergic asthma. Genetic susceptibly interacts with environmental factors to result in atopy.
* Various organs show distinct forms of immediate hypersensitivity involving different mediators and target cell types. The most severe form is a systemic reaction called anaphylactic shock. Asthma is a manifestation of immediate hypersensitivity and late-phase reactions in the lung. Allergic rhinitis (hay fever) is the most common allergic disease of the upper respiratory tract. Food allergens can cause diarrhea and vomiting. In the skin, immediate hypersensitivity is manifested as wheal-and-flare and late-phase reactions and may lead to chronic eczema.
* Drug therapy is aimed at inhibiting mast cell mediator production and at blocking or counteracting the effects of released mediators on target organs. The goal of immunotherapy is to prevent or to reduce T_H2 cell responses to specific allergens and the production of IgE.

* Immediate hypersensitivity reactions provide protection against helminthic infections by promoting IgE- and eosinophil-mediated antibody-dependent cell-mediated cytotoxicity and gut peristalsis. Mast cells may also play a role in innate immune responses to bacterial infections.

SELECTED READINGS

IgE and T_H2 Cells
Wu LC, Zarrin AA: The production and regulation of IgE by the immune system. *Nature Reviews Immunology* 14:247–260, 2014.

Mast Cells and Eosinophils
Abraham SN: St John AL: Mast cell–orchestrated immunity to pathogens, *Nature Reviews Immunology* 10:440–452, 2010.
Galli SJ, Tsai M: IgE and mast cells in allergic disease, *Nature Medicine* 18:693–704, 2012.
Gilfillan AM, Tkaczyk C: Integrated signalling pathways for mast-cell activation, *Nature Reviews Immunology* 6:218–230, 2006.
Gurish MF, Austen KF: Developmental origin and functional specialization of mast cell subsets, *Immunity* 37:25–33, 2012.
Kalesnikoff J, Galli SJ: New developments in mast cell biology, *Nature Immunology* 9:1215–1223, 2008.
Rivera J, Fierro NA, Olivera A, Suzuki R: New insights on mast cell activation via the high affinity receptor for IgE, *Advances in Immunology* 98:85–120, 2008.
Rothenberg ME, Hogan SP: The eosinophil, *Annual Review of Immunology* 24:147–174, 2006.
Stone KD, Prussin C, Metcalfe DD: IgE, mast cells, basophils, and eosinophils, *Journal of Allergy and Clinical Immunology* 125:S73–S80, 2010.

Allergic Diseases
Bossé Y: Genome-wide expression quantitative trait loci analysis in asthma, *Current Opinion in Allergy and Clinical Immunology* 3:443–452, 2013.
Bufford JD, Gern JE: The hygiene hypothesis revisited, *Immunology and Allergy Clinics of North America* 25:247–262, v-vi, 2005.
Galli SJ, Tsai M, Piliponsky AM: The development of allergic inflammation, *Nature* 454:445–454, 2008.
Gould HJ, Sutton BJ: IgE in allergy and asthma today, *Nature Reviews Immunology* 8:205–217, 2008.
Holgate ST: Innate and adaptive immune responses in asthma, *Nature Medicine* 18:673–683, 2012.
Holloway JW, Yang IA, Holgate ST: Genetics of allergic disease, *Journal of Allergy and Clinical Immunology* 125:S81–S94, 2010.
Kauffmann F, Demenais F: Gene-environment interactions in asthma and allergic diseases: challenges and perspectives, *Journal of Allergy and Clinical Immunology* 130:1229–1240, 2012.
Kim HY, DeKruyff RH, Umetsu DT: The many paths to asthma: phenotype shaped by innate and adaptive immunity, *Nature Immunology* 11:577–584, 2010.
Lambrecht BN, Hammad H: Biology of lung dendritic cells at the origin of asthma, *Immunity* 31:412–424, 2009.
Licona-Limon P, Kim LK, Flavell RA: T_H2, allergy and group 2 innate lymphoid cells, *Nature Immunology* 14:536–542, 2013.

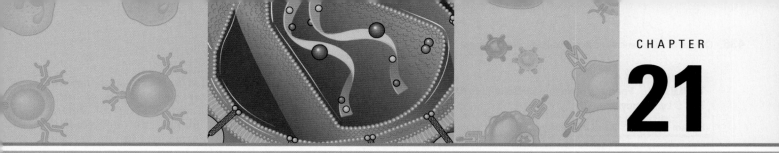

21

Congenital and Acquired Immunodeficiencies

Integrity of the immune system is essential for defense against infectious organisms and their toxic products and therefore for the survival of all individuals. Defects in one or more components of the immune system can lead to serious and often fatal disorders, which are collectively called **immunodeficiency diseases**. These diseases are broadly classified into two groups. The **congenital**, or **primary, immunodeficiencies** are genetic defects that result in an increased susceptibility to infection that is frequently manifested in infancy and early childhood but is sometimes clinically detected later in life. It is estimated that in the United States, approximately 1 in 500 individuals is born with a defect in some component of the immune system, although only a small proportion are affected severely enough for development of life-threatening complications. **Acquired,** or **secondary, immunodeficiencies** are not inherited diseases but develop as a consequence of malnutrition, disseminated cancer, treatment with immunosuppressive drugs, or infection of cells of the immune system, most notably with the human immunodeficiency virus (HIV), the etiologic agent of acquired immunodeficiency syndrome (AIDS). This chapter describes the major types of congenital and acquired immunodeficiencies, with an emphasis on their pathogenesis and the components of the immune system that are involved in these disorders.

OVERVIEW OF IMMUNODEFICIENCY DISEASES

Before beginning our discussion of individual diseases, it is important to summarize some general features of immunodeficiencies.

- *The principal consequence of immunodeficiency is an increased susceptibility to infection.* The nature of the infection in a particular patient depends largely on the component of the immune system that is defective (Table 21-1). Deficient humoral immunity usually results in increased susceptibility to infection by encapsulated, pus-forming bacteria and some viruses, whereas defects in cell-mediated immunity lead to infection by viruses and other intracellular microbes. Combined deficiencies in both humoral and cell-mediated immunity make patients susceptible to infection by all classes of microorganisms. Immunodeficient patients, especially those with defects in cellular immunity, often present with infections by microbes that are commonly encountered but effectively eliminated by healthy persons; such infections are said to be opportunistic. Defects in innate immunity can result in different categories of microbial infections, depending on the pathway or cell type affected. Complement deficiencies, for instance, resemble antibody deficiencies in their clinical presentation, while natural killer (NK) cell deficiencies result mainly in recurrent viral

TABLE 21-1 Features of Immunodeficiencies Affecting T or B Lymphocytes

Feature	B Cell Deficiency	T Cell Deficiency
Susceptibility to infection	Pyogenic bacteria (otitis, pneumonia, meningitis, osteomyelitis), enteric bacteria and viruses, some parasites	*Pneumocystis jiroveci,* many viruses, atypical mycobacteria, fungi
Diagnosis		
Serum Ig levels DTH reactions to common antigens	Reduced Normal	Normal or reduced Reduced
Morphology of lymphoid tissues	Absent or reduced follicles and germinal centers (B cell zones)	Usually normal follicles, may be reduced parafollicular cortical regions (T cell zones)

DTH, delayed-type hypersensitivity.

infections. There is growing evidence that adults with recurrent or severe infections often harbor mutations in genes that regulate immune function. The availability of new rapid and efficient DNA sequencing approaches has exponentially enhanced the ability to identify specific genetic loci that, when mutated, confer susceptibility to pathogens.

- *Patients with immunodeficiencies are also susceptible to certain types of cancer.* Many of these cancers appear to be caused by oncogenic viruses, such as the Epstein-Barr virus and human papilloma viruses. An increased incidence of cancer is most often seen in T cell immunodeficiencies because, as discussed in Chapter 18, T cells play an important role in surveillance against malignant tumors.
- *Paradoxically, certain immunodeficiencies are associated with an increased incidence of autoimmunity.* The mechanisms underlying this association are not fully understood.
- *Immunodeficiency may result from defects in lymphocyte development or activation or from defects in the effector mechanisms of innate and adaptive immunity.* Immunodeficiency diseases are clinically and pathologically heterogeneous, in part because different diseases involve different components of the immune system.

In this chapter, we will first describe congenital immunodeficiencies, including defects in components of the innate immune system and defects in the humoral and cell-mediated arms of the adaptive immune system. We will conclude with a discussion of acquired immunodeficiencies, with an emphasis on AIDS.

CONGENITAL (PRIMARY) IMMUNODEFICIENCIES

In different congenital immunodeficiencies, the causative abnormality may be in components of the innate system, *at different stages of lymphocyte development, or in the responses of mature lymphocytes to antigenic stimulation.* Inherited abnormalities of innate immunity most commonly involve the complement pathway or phagocytes. Abnormalities in lymphocyte development may be caused by mutations in genes encoding enzymes, adaptors, transport proteins, and transcription factors. These inherited defects, and the corresponding targeted disruptions in mice, have been instructive in elucidating mechanisms of lymphocyte development and function (see Chapter 8). Abnormalities in B lymphocyte development and function result in deficient antibody production and are diagnosed by reduced levels of serum immunoglobulin (Ig), defective antibody responses to vaccination, and, in some cases, reduced numbers of B cells in the circulation or lymphoid tissues or absent plasma cells in tissues (see Table 21-1). Abnormalities in T lymphocyte maturation and function lead to deficient cell-mediated immunity and may also result in reduced T cell–dependent antibody production. Primary T cell immunodeficiencies are diagnosed by reduced numbers of peripheral blood T cells, low proliferative responses of blood lymphocytes to polyclonal T cell activators such as phytohemagglutinin, and deficient cutaneous delayed-type hypersensitivity (DTH) reactions to ubiquitous microbial antigens, such as *Candida* antigens. Defects in both humoral and cell-mediated immunity are classified under severe combined immunodeficiencies. In the following sections, we will describe immunodeficiencies caused by inherited mutations in genes encoding components of the innate immune system or in genes required for lymphocyte development and activation. We will conclude with a brief discussion of therapeutic strategies for these diseases.

Defects in Innate Immunity

Innate immunity constitutes the first line of defense against infectious organisms. Two important components of innate immunity are phagocytes and complement, both of which also participate in the effector phases of adaptive immunity. Therefore, congenital disorders of phagocytes and the complement system result in recurrent infections. We described complement deficiencies in Chapter 13. Deficiencies have been described in the classical and alternative complement pathways as well as in the lectin pathway.

In this section of the chapter, we will discuss some examples of congenital phagocyte disorders (Table 21-2) and inherited defects in Toll-like receptor (TLR) pathways and in the IL-12/IFN-γ pathway. Phagocyte defects generally result in infections of the skin and respiratory tract with bacteria or fungi, the latter predominantly involving *Aspergillus* and *Candida* species. Deep-seated abscesses and oral stomatitis are also common. Defects in TLR signaling and in type I interferon signaling may contribute to recurrent pyogenic infections as well as to severe viral infections; defects in IL-12 and the IFN-γ pathway increase susceptibility to intracellular pathogens, particularly mycobacterial infections.

TABLE 21-2 Congenital Disorders of Innate Immunity

Disease	Functional Deficiencies	Mechanism of Defect
Chronic granulomatous disease	Defective production of reactive oxygen species by phagocytes; recurrent intracellular bacterial and fungal infections	Mutation in genes of phagocyte oxidase complex; phox-91 (cytochrome b_{558} α subunit) is mutated in X-linked form
Leukocyte adhesion deficiency type 1	Defective leukocyte adhesion to endothelial cells and migration into tissues linked to decreased or absent expression of β_2 integrins; recurrent bacterial and fungal infections	Mutations in gene encoding the β chain (CD18) of β_2 integrins
Leukocyte adhesion deficiency type 2	Defective leukocyte rolling and migration into tissues linked to decreased or absent expression of leukocyte ligands for endothelial E- and P-selectins, causing failure of leukocyte migration into tissues; recurrent bacterial and fungal infections	Mutations in gene encoding GDP-fucose transporter-1, required for transport of fucose into the Golgi and its incorporation into sialyl Lewis X
Leukocyte adhesion deficiency type 3	Defective leukocyte adhesion and migration into tissues linked to defective chemokine-stimulated inside-out signaling and therefore defective integrin activation	Mutations in gene encoding KINDLIN-3, a cytoskeletal protein linked to inside-out signaling
Chédiak-Higashi syndrome	Defective vesicle fusion and lysosomal function in neutrophils, macrophages, dendritic cells, NK cells, cytotoxic T cells, and many other cell types; recurrent infections by pyogenic bacteria	Mutation in LYST leading to defect in secretory granule exocytosis and lysosomal function
NK cell deficiencies	Reduced or absent NK cells	Mutations in the gene encoding the GATA-2 transcription factor and in the gene encoding the MCM-4 DNA helicase
Toll-like receptor signaling defects	Recurrent infections caused by defects in TLR and CD40 signaling and defective type I interferon production	Mutations in *TLR3*, *TRIF*, *TBK1*, *NEMO*, *UNC93B*, *MyD88*, *IκBα*, and *IRAK-4* compromise NF-κB activation downstream of Toll-like receptors
Mendelian Susceptibility to Mycobacterial Diseases	Severe disease caused by non-tuberculous environmental mycobacteria and BCG	Mutations in *IL-12p40*, *IL-12RB*, *IFNGR1*, *IFNGR2*, *STAT1*, *NEMO*, and *ISG15*

BCG, bacillus Calmette-Guérin; *IRAK-4*, IL-1 receptor–associated kinase 4; *LYST*, lysosomal trafficking protein; *NEMO*, NF-κB essential modulator.

Defective Microbicidal Activities of Phagocytes: Chronic Granulomatous Disease

Chronic granulomatous disease (CGD) is caused by mutations in components of the phagocyte oxidase (phox) enzyme complex. It is a rare disease, estimated to affect about 1 in a million individuals in the United States. About two thirds of cases show an X-linked recessive pattern of inheritance, and the remainder are autosomal recessive. In the most common, X-linked, form of the disease, there is a mutation in the gene encoding the 91-kD α subunit of cytochrome b_{558}, an integral membrane protein also known as phox-91. This mutation results in defective production of superoxide anion, one of several reactive oxygen species that constitute a major microbicidal mechanism of phagocytes, especially neutrophils (see Chapter 4). Mutations in other components of the phox complex contribute to autosomal recessive forms of CGD. Defective production of reactive oxygen species results in a failure to kill phagocytosed microbes.

CGD is characterized by recurrent infections with intracellular fungi and bacteria, such as *Staphylococcus*, usually from early childhood. Invasive infection with the fungus *Aspergillus* is the leading cause of death. Many of the organisms that are particularly troublesome in CGD patients produce catalase, which destroys the microbicidal hydrogen peroxide that may be produced by host cells from the residual reactive oxygen radical superoxide. Because the infections are not controlled by phagocytes,

they stimulate chronic cell-mediated immune responses, resulting in T cell–mediated macrophage activation and the formation of granulomas composed of activated macrophages. Presumably, these activated macrophages try to eliminate the microbes despite defective production of reactive oxygen species. This histologic appearance is the basis for the name of the disorder. The disease is often fatal, even with aggressive antibiotic therapy.

The cytokine interferon-γ (IFN-γ) enhances transcription of the gene encoding phox-91 and also stimulates other components of the phagocyte oxidase enzyme complex. Therefore, IFN-γ stimulates the production of superoxide by CGD neutrophils, especially in cases in which the coding portion of the phox-91 gene is intact but its transcription is reduced. Once neutrophil superoxide production is restored to about 10% of normal levels, resistance to infection is greatly improved. IFN-γ therapy is now commonly used for the treatment of X-linked CGD.

Leukocyte Adhesion Deficiencies

The leukocyte adhesion deficiencies are a group of autosomal recessive disorders caused by defects in leukocyte and endothelial adhesion molecules. These diseases are characterized by a failure of leukocyte, particularly neutrophil, recruitment to sites of infection, resulting in severe periodontitis and other recurrent infections starting early in life, and the inability to make pus. Different types of leukocyte adhesion deficiencies are caused by mutations in different genes.

- *Leukocyte adhesion deficiency type 1 (LAD-1)* is a rare autosomal recessive disorder characterized by recurrent bacterial and fungal infections and impaired wound healing. In these patients, most adhesion-dependent functions of leukocytes are defective, including adherence to endothelium, neutrophil aggregation and chemotaxis, phagocytosis, and cytotoxicity mediated by neutrophils, NK cells, and T lymphocytes. The molecular basis of the defect is absent or reduced expression of the β_2 integrins (heterodimers of CD18 and the CD11 family of glycoproteins) due to various mutations in the *CD18* gene. The β_2 integrins include leukocyte function–associated antigen 1 (LFA-1 or CD11aCD18), Mac-1 (CD11bCD18), and p150,95 (CD11cCD18). These proteins participate in the adhesion of leukocytes to other cells, notably endothelial cells, and the binding of T lymphocytes to antigen-presenting cells (APCs) (see Chapter 3).

- *Leukocyte adhesion deficiency type 2 (LAD-2)* is another rare disorder that is clinically similar to LAD-1 but is not due to integrin defects. LAD-2 results from an absence of sialyl Lewis X, the tetrasaccharide carbohydrate ligand on neutrophils and other leukocytes that is required for binding to E-selectin and P-selectin on cytokine-activated endothelium (see Chapter 3). This defect is caused by a mutation in a GDP-fucose transporter responsible for the transport of fucose into the Golgi, resulting in an inability to synthesize sialyl Lewis X. The absence of sialyl Lewis X results in defective binding of leukocytes to endothelium, the absence of leukocyte rolling, and therefore the defective recruitment of leukocytes to sites of infection. This abnormality in fucosylation seen in LAD-2 also contributes to a Bombay blood group phenotype, which is a lack of A or B blood group antigens due to the absence of the fucosylated precursor H core glycan. LAD-2 is also associated with mental retardation and other developmental defects.

- *Leukocyte adhesion deficiency type 3 (LAD-3)* involves a defect in the inside-out signaling pathway that mediates chemokine-induced integrin activation that is required for leukocytes to bind firmly to endothelium (see Chapter 3). In a subset of patients, it is caused by mutations in the gene encoding KINDLIN-3, a protein that binds to the cytoplasmic tail of some integrins and is involved in signaling. Increased bleeding is also observed in subjects with KINDLIN-3 mutations because of integrin dysfunction in platelets.

Defects in NK Cells and Phagocytes

Rare patients lack NK cells because of autosomal dominant mutations in the gene encoding the GATA-2 transcription factor. The loss of GATA-2 activity results in diminished precursor populations in the bone marrow and a resulting loss of NK cells as well as decreases in monocytes, dendritic cells, and B cells. Autosomal recessive mutations in MCM4 (minichromosome maintenance complex component 4), a DNA helicase, also results in the loss of NK cells accompanied by adrenal insufficiency and growth retardation. Autosomal recessive mutations in CD16 (FcγRIIIA), an Fc receptor that mediates ADCC, results in a loss of NK cell function that goes beyond the loss of ADCC activity. Why CD16 is required broadly for NK cell function is unclear. Patients present with severe infections with viruses mainly of the herpesvirus and papillomavirus families.

Chédiak-Higashi syndrome is a rare autosomal recessive disorder characterized by recurrent infections by pyogenic bacteria, partial oculocutaneous albinism, and infiltration of various organs by non-neoplastic lymphocytes. The neutrophils, monocytes and lymphocytes of these patients contain giant lysosomes. This disease is caused by mutations in the gene encoding the protein LYST, which regulates intracellular trafficking of lysosomes. The mutations result in defective phagosome-lysosome fusion in neutrophils and macrophages (causing reduced resistance to infection), defective melanosome formation in melanocytes (causing albinism), and lysosomal abnormalities in cells of the nervous system (causing nerve defects) and platelets (leading to bleeding disorders). Giant lysosomes form in neutrophils during the maturation of these cells from myeloid precursors. Some of these neutrophil precursors die prematurely, resulting in moderate leukopenia. Surviving neutrophils may contain reduced levels of the lysosomal enzymes that normally function in microbial killing. These cells are also defective in chemotaxis and phagocytosis, further contributing to their deficient microbicidal activity. NK cell function in these patients is impaired, probably because of an abnormality in the cytoplasmic granules that store proteins mediating cytotoxicity. The severity of the defect in cytotoxic T lymphocyte (CTL) function is variable among patients. A mutant mouse strain called the beige mouse is an animal model for Chédiak-Higashi syndrome. This strain is characterized by deficient NK cell function and giant lysosomes in leukocytes. The beige mutation has been mapped to the mouse *Lyst* locus.

Inherited Defects in TLR Pathways, Nuclear Factor-κB Signaling, and Type I Interferons

Inherited defects in TLR-dependent responses are rare and have been recognized only recently. Defects in TLR signaling tend to cause fairly circumscribed clinical phenotypes. The major signaling pathway downstream of most TLRs as well as of the interleukin-1 receptor (IL-1R) involves the MyD88 adaptor and the IRAK-4 and IRAK-1 kinases (see Chapter 4), and this pathway results in the nuclear factor-κB (NF-κB)–dependent induction of proinflammatory cytokines. Individuals with mutations in MyD88 and IRAK4 suffer from severe invasive bacterial infections early in life, especially pneumococcal pneumonia. Later in life, infections tend to be less severe. TLR3 signaling utilizes the TRIF adaptor protein instead of MyD88, and TBK1, a serine-threonine kinase that functions downstream of TRIF to activate IRF3 as well as NFκB in a non-canonical manner. Autosomal recessive mutations in TRIF and autosomal dominant mutations in the TRAF3 E3 ligase result in susceptibility to herpes simplex encephalitis. A similar phenotype is observed with autosomal dominant mutations in the gene encoding TBK1. TLR 3, 7, 8, and 9 recognize nucleic acids, are located in endosomes, and require a protein called UNC93B (Uncoordinated 93B) for their function. UNC93B is an endoplasmic reticulum membrane protein that interacts with endosomal TLRs when they are synthesized in the endoplasmic reticulum and helps deliver these TLRs to the endosomes. The UNC93B protein is also critical for signaling by nucleic acid–specific TLRs. Heterozygous mutations in TLR3 as well as homozygous mutations in UNC93B result in reduced type I interferon generation and also increase susceptibility to herpes simplex encephalitis.

Signaling downstream of the endosomal TLRs results in the synthesis and secretion of type I interferons, which bind to type I interferon receptors and activate the STAT1 transcription factor. In some patients, loss-of-function *STAT1* mutations are linked to severe viral infections, notably herpes simplex encephalitis.

Some immune deficiencies are caused by defects that specifically affect NF-κB activation. Point mutations in the inhibitor of κB kinase γ (IKKγ), also known as nuclear factor κB essential modulator (NEMO), a component of the IκB kinase complex that is required for NF-κB activation, contribute to the X-linked recessive condition known as anhidrotic ectodermal dysplasia with immunodeficiency (EDA-ID). In this disorder, differentiation of ectoderm-derived structures is abnormal, and immune function is impaired in a number of ways. Responses to TLR signals as well as CD40 signals are compromised. These patients suffer from infections with encapsulated pyogenic bacteria as well as with intracellular bacterial pathogens including mycobacteria, viruses, and fungi such as *Pneumocystis jiroveci* (see also discussion later in the section on hyper-IgM syndromes). An autosomal recessive form of EDA-ID has been described in which a hypermorphic point mutation in IκBα prevents the phosphorylation, ubiquitination, and degradation of IκBα, thus leading to impaired NF-κB activation.

Defects in the IL-12/IFN-γ Pathway

IL-12 is secreted by dendritic cells and macrophages, and IL-12R signaling stimulates the synthesis of IFN-γ by helper T cells, cytotoxic T cells, and NK cells (see Chapter 4). Mutations in the genes encoding IL-12p40, the IL-12Rβ1 chain, and both chains of the IFN-γ receptor, as well as some mutations in STAT1 and IKKγ/NEMO, result in susceptibility to environmental *Mycobacterium* species (often called atypical mycobacteria), such as *Mycobacterium avium*, *Mycobacterium kansasii*, and *Mycobacterium fortuitum*. The term Mendelian Susceptibility to Mycobacterial Disease (MSMD) is used for these disorders in which subjects are predisposed to severe disease caused by weakly virulent mycobacteria such as non-tuberculous environmental mycobacteria and BCG (Bacillis Calmette-Guérin). Autosomal recessive mutations in ISG15 (Interferon stimulated gene 15) also cause MSMD. ISG15 is an interferon-inducible factor that is released by phagocytic cells including neutrophils and induces IFN-γ secretion by other cells, mainly NK cells. ISG15 also has been shown to function intracellularly to modify proteins in a ubiquitin-like manner, but it is the secreted form of this protein that appears to be required for protection from mycobacterial infections.

Defects in Splenic Development

Splenic development may fail due to an autosomal dominant (and sometimes sporadic) condition called Isolated Congenital Asplenia. In these patients, heterozygous missense mutations have been found in *NBX2.5*, which encodes a protein involved in the transcriptional regulation of splenic development. Asplenia may also be caused by mutations in genes controlling left-right laterality, which also affects other organs. Congenitally asplenic patients have severe infections with encapsulated bacteria, especially *Streptococcus pneumoniae*.

Severe Combined Immunodeficiencies

Immunodeficiencies that affect both humoral and cell-mediated immunity are called severe combined immunodeficiencies (SCIDs) (Table 21-3). SCID results from impaired T lymphocyte development with or without defects in B cell maturation (Fig. 21-1). When there is no block in B cell development, the defect in humoral immunity is due to the absence of T cell help.

The clinical manifestation of SCID is dominated by severe infections that may be life threatening. These infections include pneumonia, meningitis, and disseminated bacteremia. Among the most dangerous organisms is a fungus called *Pneumocystis jiroveci*, which can cause a severe pneumonia. Many viruses cause serious disease in patients with SCID. Chicken pox (varicella) infection is usually limited to the skin and mucous membranes in healthy children and typically resolves in days, but in patients with SCID, it can progress to involve the lungs, liver, and brain. Cytomegalovirus (CMV), which is present as a latent infection in most people, may be reactivated and cause fatal pneumonia in patients with SCID. Children with SCID commonly develop gastrointestinal infections caused commonly by rotavirus, *Crytosporidium* species, *Giardia lamblia*, and *cytomegalovirus*, leading to persistent diarrhea and malabsorption.

Children with SCID may also develop infections caused by live attenuated vaccines, which are not harmful in children who have normal immunity. Vaccines for chicken pox, measles, mumps, rubella, and rotavirus are live virus vaccines, and children with SCID can contract infections from these vaccines.

SCID patients may also develop a chronic skin rash that is often mistaken for infection. The rash is actually caused by a graft-versus-host reaction in which maternal T cells enter the fetus but are not rejected (because the fetus lacks a competent immune system) and react against the baby's tissues.

Mutations in genes involved in different steps in lymphocyte development may cause SCID. The process of T and B lymphocyte maturation from hematopoietic stem cells to functionally competent mature lymphocytes involves proliferation of early lymphocyte progenitors, rearrangement of the locus encoding one chain of the antigen receptor followed by selection of cells that have made in-frame productive rearrangements at a pre-antigen receptor checkpoint, expression of both chains of the antigen receptor, and selection of cells with useful specificities (see Chapter 8). Defects in many of these steps have been described in different forms of SCID. About 50% of SCIDs are autosomal recessive; the rest are X-linked. The most common cause of autosomal recessive SCID is deficiency of the enzyme adenosine deaminase, required for purine metabolism. X-linked SCID is caused by mutations in the gene encoding a cytokine receptor component called the common γ chain.

TABLE 21-3   Severe Combined Immunodeficiencies

Disease	Functional Deficiencies	Mechanism of Defect
Defects in Cytokine Signaling		
X-linked SCID	Marked decrease in T cells; normal or increased B cells; reduced serum Ig	Cytokine receptor common γ chain mutations; defective T cell development in the absence of IL-7–derived signals
Autosomal recessive forms	Marked decrease in T cells; normal or increased B cells; reduced serum Ig	Mutations in *IL2RA, IL7RA, JAK3*
Defects in Nucleotide Salvage Pathways		
ADA deficiency	Progressive decrease in T cells, B cells, and NK cells; reduced serum Ig	Mutations in the *ADA* gene, leading to accumulation of toxic metabolites in lymphocytes
PNP deficiency	Progressive decrease in T cells, B cells, and NK cells; reduced serum Ig	Mutations in the *PNP* gene, leading to accumulation of toxic metabolites in lymphocytes
Defects in V(D)J Recombination		
RAG1 or RAG2 deficiency recombination*	Decreased T cells and B cells; reduced serum Ig; absence or deficiency of T and B cells	Cleavage defect during V(D)J recombination; mutations in *RAG1* or *RAG2*
Double-stranded break repair and checkpoint	Decreased T and B cells; reduced serum Ig; absence or deficiency of T cells and B cells	Failure to resolve hairpins during V(D)J recombination; mutations in *ARTEMIS*, DNA-PKcs, *CERNUNNOS, LIG4, NBS1, MRE11, ATM*
Defective Thymic Development		
Defective pre-TCR checkpoint	Decreased T cells; normal or reduced B cells; reduced serum Ig	Mutations in *CD45, CD3D, CD3E, ORAI1* (CRAC channel component), *STIM1*
DiGeorge syndrome	Decreased T cells; normal B cells; normal or reduced serum Ig	22q11 deletion; T-box 1 (*TBX1*) transcription factor mutations
FoxN1 deficiency	Thymic aplasia with defective T cell development	Recessive mutation in *FOXN1*
TCR α chain deficiency	No αβ T cells; γδ T cells normal; recurrent infections and autoimmunity	Autosomal recessive deletion in C region of *TCR* α chain
Defective T cell thymic egress and defective T cell signaling	Marked reduction in all peripheral T cells	Mutations in *RHOH* and *MST1*
Selective loss of CD4+ T cells and defective T cell signaling	Decreased CD4+ T cells	Mutations in *LCK* and *UNC119*
Other Defects		
Reticular dysgenesis	Decreased T cells, B cells, and myeloid cells	Mutation in *AK2*

ADA, adenosine deaminase; *AK2,* adenylate kinase 2; *ATM,* ataxia-telangiectasia mutated; *CRAC,* calcium release activated channel; *DNA-PKcs,* DNA-dependent protein kinase catalytic subunit; *LIG4,* DNA ligase 4; *MRE11,* meiotic recombination homologue 11; *NBS1,* Nijmegen breakpoint syndrome 1; *PNP,* purine nucleoside phosphorylase.
*Hypomorphic mutations in *RAG* genes and in *ARTEMIS* can contribute to Omenn's syndrome.

The DiGeorge Syndrome and Other Forms of SCID due to Defective Thymic Epithelial Development

Complete or partial failure of development of the thymic anlage can lead to defective T cell maturation. The most common defect in thymic development linked to SCID is seen in children with the ***DiGeorge syndrome***. This selective T cell deficiency is due to a congenital malformation that results in defective development of the thymus and the parathyroid glands as well as other structures that develop from the third and fourth pharyngeal pouches during fetal life. The congenital defect is manifested by hypoplasia or agenesis of the thymus leading to deficient T cell maturation, absent parathyroid glands causing abnormal calcium homeostasis and muscle twitching (tetany),

abnormal development of the great vessels, and facial deformities. Different patients may show varying degrees of these abnormalities. The disease is caused most frequently by a deletion in the chromosomal region 22q11. A mouse line that has a similar defect in thymic development carries a mutation in a gene encoding a transcription factor called T-box 1 (TBX1), which lies within the region deleted in DiGeorge syndrome. It is likely that the immunodeficiency associated with DiGeorge syndrome can be explained, at least in part, by the deletion of the *TBX1* gene. In this syndrome, peripheral blood T lymphocytes are absent or greatly reduced in number, and the cells do not respond to polyclonal T cell activators or in mixed leukocyte reactions. Antibody levels are usually normal

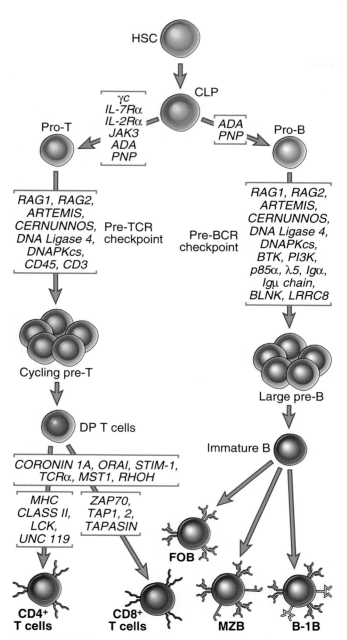

FIGURE 21-1 Immunodeficiency caused by defects in B and T cell maturation. Primary immunodeficiencies caused by genetic defects in lymphocyte maturation are shown. These defects may affect T cell maturation alone, B cell maturation alone, or both. *CLP,* common lymphoid progenitor; *DP,* double-positive; *FoB,* follicular B cells; *HSC,* hematopoietic stem cell; *MZB,* marginal zone B cells.

but may be reduced in severely affected patients. As in other severe T cell deficiencies, patients are susceptible to mycobacterial, viral, and fungal infections.

The immunodeficiency associated with DiGeorge syndrome can be corrected by fetal thymic transplantation or by bone marrow transplantation. Such treatment is usually not necessary, however, because T cell function tends to improve with age in a large fraction of patients with this syndrome and is often normal by 5 years. Improvement with age probably occurs because of the presence of some thymic tissue or because some as yet undefined extrathymic

sites assume the function of T cell maturation. It is also possible that as these patients grow older, thymus tissue develops at ectopic sites (i.e., other than the normal location).

An animal model of T cell immunodeficiency resulting from abnormal development of the thymus is the *nude (athymic) mouse.* These mice have an inherited defect of certain types of epithelial cells in the skin, leading to hairlessness, and in the lining of the third and fourth pharyngeal pouches, causing thymic hypoplasia. The disorder is caused by a mutation in the *FoxN1* gene, which encodes a Forkhead family transcription factor that is required for the normal development of certain ectoderm-derived cell types. Affected mice have rudimentary thymuses in which T cell maturation cannot occur normally. As a result, few or no mature T cells are present in peripheral lymphoid tissues, and cell-mediated immune reactions cannot occur. Autosomal recessive *FOXN1* mutations have been described in a small number of patients who present with SCID, alopecia (hair loss), and nail dystrophy.

An even rarer defect in the thymus has been described involving a mutation in *CORONIN1A,* which encodes a protein that regulates the actin cytoskeleton. The absence of functional CORONIN-1A results in defective egress of mature T cells from the thymus. Homozygous mutations in the *MST1* gene, which encodes a serine/threonine protein kinase, results in the loss of naive T cells in the circulation and the failure of T cells to emigrate from the thymus. Patients present with recurrent bacterial and viral infections, and some develop Epstein-Barr virus (EBV)-driven lymphomas. Some patients present with epidermodysplasia verruciformis, with HPV-infected warts and skin carcinomas. MST1 plays diverse roles in proliferation, cell survival, and cell migration. While the major defect is in emigration of T cells from the thymus, there are also humoral immune defects in some patients who present with diminished B cell numbers and hypogammaglobulinemia.

ADA Deficiency and Other Forms of SCID Caused by Defects in Nucleotide Metabolism

The most common cause of autosomal recessive SCID is deficiency of an enzyme called adenosine deaminase (ADA) due to mutations in the ADA gene. ADA functions in the salvage pathway of purine synthesis and catalyzes the irreversible deamination of adenosine and 2'-deoxyadenosine to inosine and 2'-deoxyinosine, respectively. Deficiency of the enzyme leads to the accumulation of deoxyadenosine and its precursors S-adenosylhomocysteine and deoxyadenosine triphosphate (dATP). These byproducts have many toxic effects, including inhibition of DNA synthesis. Although ADA is present in most cells, developing lymphocytes are less efficient than most other cell types at degrading dATP into 2'-deoxyadenosine, and therefore lymphocyte maturation is particularly sensitive to ADA deficiency. Other features of the disease can include deafness, costochondral abnormalities, liver damage, and behavioral problems. ADA deficiency leads to reduced numbers of B and T cells; lymphocyte cell numbers are usually normal at birth but fall off precipitously during the first year of life. A few patients may have a nearly normal number of T cells, but these cells do not proliferate in response to antigenic stimulation.

A rarer autosomal recessive form of SCID is due to the deficiency of purine nucleoside phosphorylase (PNP), an enzyme that is also involved in purine catabolism. PNP catalyzes the conversion of inosine to hypoxanthine and guanosine to guanine, and deficiency of PNP leads to the accumulation of deoxyguanosine and deoxyguanosine triphosphate, with toxic effects on immature lymphocytes, mainly T cells. Autoimmune hemolytic anemia and progressive neurologic deterioration are also features of this disorder.

A particularly severe form of SCID is seen in a disease called *reticular dysgenesis*. This rare disorder is characterized by the absence of T and B lymphocytes and most myeloid cells, including granulocytes, and is due to a defect in the development of lymphoid and myeloid progenitors. This autosomal recessive disease is due to a mutation in the *adenylate kinase 2 (AK2)* gene. The AK2 protein regulates the level of adenosine diphosphate, and in the absence of AK2 there is increased apoptosis of lymphoid and myeloid precursors.

X-Linked SCID

X-linked SCID is caused by mutations in the gene encoding the common γ ($γ_c$) chain shared by the receptors for the interleukins IL-2, IL-4, IL-7, IL-9, and IL-15 (see Chapters 4, 9, and 10). X-linked SCID is characterized by impaired maturation of T cells and NK cells and greatly reduced numbers of mature T cells and NK cells, but the number of B cells is usually normal or increased. The humoral immunodeficiency in this disease is due to a lack of T cell help for antibody production. This disease is a result of the inability of the lymphopoietic cytokine IL-7, whose receptor uses the $γ_c$ chain for signaling, to stimulate the growth of immature thymocytes. In addition, the receptor for IL-15, which is required for NK cell development, also uses the $γ_c$ signaling chain, and the failure of IL-15 function accounts for the deficiency of NK cells.

Heterozygous females are usually phenotypically normal carriers, whereas males who inherit the abnormal X chromosome manifest the disease. Because developing cells in females randomly inactivate one of the two X chromosomes, the normal allele encoding a functional $γ_c$ protein will not be expressed in half the lymphocyte precursors in a female carrier. These cells will fail to mature, and consequently, all the mature lymphocytes in a female carrier will have inactivated the same X chromosome (carrying the mutant allele). In contrast, half of all non-lymphoid cells will have inactivated one X chromosome, and half the other. A comparison of X chromosome inactivation in lymphoid cells versus non-lymphoid cells may be used to identify carriers of the mutant allele. The non-random use of X chromosomes in mature lymphocytes is also characteristic of female carriers of other mutated X-linked genes that affect lymphocyte development, as discussed later.

Autosomal Recessive Mutations in Cytokine Signaling Components

Some patients with a disease clinically identical to X-linked SCID show an autosomal recessive inheritance. These patients have mutations in the *IL-7 receptor α chain* or the *JAK3 kinase*, which associates with the $γ_c$ chain and is required for signaling by this receptor (see

Chapter 7). Patients with mutations in the gene encoding the IL-7Rα chain have a defect in T cell development but exhibit normal NK cell development, because IL-15 signaling is unaffected, and have normal numbers of B cells.

Severe Combined Immunodeficiency Caused by Defects in V(D)J Recombination and Pre-TCR Checkpoint Signaling

Absence of V(D)J recombination leads to a failure to express the pre–T cell receptor (TCR) and the pre–B cell receptor (BCR) and a block in T and B cell development. Mutations in the *RAG1* or *RAG2* genes, whose protein products mediate the cleavage step during V(D)J recombination, or the *ARTEMIS* gene, which encodes an endonuclease that resolves coding-end hairpins during V(D)J recombination, all result in a failure of V(D)J recombination. These diseases are rare, but they account for a large percentage of the autosomal recessive forms of SCID. The functions of these genes are discussed in Chapter 8. In children with these mutations, B and T lymphocytes are absent and immunity is severely compromised. Mutations in genes encoding proteins involved in double-stranded break repair/non-homologous end joining of DNA also lead to SCID because of defects in V(D)J recombination. Homozygous mutations in the gene encoding the catalytic subunit of the DNA-dependent protein kinase (DNA-PK), and DNA LIGASE 4 all lead to SCID. Genetic defects in this end-joining process also result in increased cellular sensitivity to radiation and can result in other manifestations, such as microcephaly, facial dysmorphisms, and defective tooth development.

Hypomorphic mutations (that only partially reduce function) in the *RAG* genes, in *ARTEMIS*, or in the *IL7RA* gene are the cause of a disorder called *Omenn's syndrome* characterized by reduced generation of T and B cells, immunodeficiency, and autoimmune and allergic manifestations. Omenn's syndrome is phenotypically different from the diseases described earlier because the immunodeficiency coexists with exaggerated immune activation and autoimmunity. This may be a result of an abnormally low ratio of regulatory T cells to effector T cells, or in cases with decreased V(D)J recombination, defective receptor editing in immature B cells.

Although most autosomal recessive forms of SCID are linked to mutations in *ADA, RAG1, RAG2, and ARTEMIS*, other forms of this syndrome are caused by mutations in the genes encoding the CD45 phosphatase (that is a positive regulator of Src family kinases, such as Fyn, Lck, and Lyn) and mutations in the CD3 δ or ε chains or in the CD3-associated ζ chain. These mutations contribute to defective pre-TCR signaling and result in a block in αβ T cell development.

Another disorder of naive T cell development is caused by homozygous mutations in RHOH (Ras homologous gene family member H), an atypical Rho family GTPase required for pre-TCR and TCR signaling. The failure of the pre-TCR checkpoint results in a block in αβ T cell development. The clinical presentation includes epidermodysplasia verruciformis, which is a diffuse HPV infection in the skin that causes the growth of macules and papules.

A specific defect in αβ T cell development and a clinical presentation that involves recurrent viral infections is caused by homozygous mutations in the gene encoding the T cell receptor α chain (TCRα) constant region. Affected individuals present with increased susceptibility to infections, including chronic varicella zoster and EBV infections, as well as autoimmunity and features of atopy. The immune dysregulation may reflect the absence of regulatory T cells; the only T cells present in infants with this disease are γδ T cells. Clinical features include eosinophilia, vitiligo, eczema, alopecia areata, autoimmune hemolytic anemia, and the presence of other autoantibodies.

Autosomal recessive mutations in LCK, a critical tyrosine kinase involved in pre-TCR and TCR signaling, also contribute to SCID with T cell deficiency, the lack of regulatory T cells, recurrent infections, and features of immune dysregulation.

The Bare Lymphocyte Syndrome and Other Defects in T Cell Positive Selection

The generation of single-positive CD4+ and CD8+ T cells from double-positive thymocytes depends on positive selection and lineage commitment events. Specific inherited mutations in genes that regulate the process of positive selection abrogate the development of CD4+ T cells or of CD8+ T cells.

Class II major histocompatibility complex (MHC) deficiency, also called **bare lymphocyte syndrome,** is a rare heterogeneous group of autosomal recessive diseases in which patients express little or no HLA-DP, HLA-DQ, or HLA-DR on B lymphocytes, macrophages, and dendritic cells and fail to express class II MHC molecules in response to IFN-γ. They express normal or only slightly reduced levels of class I MHC molecules and β_2-microglobulin. Most cases of bare lymphocyte syndrome are due to mutations in genes encoding proteins that regulate class II MHC gene transcription. For example, mutations affecting the constitutively expressed transcription factor RFX5 or the IFN-γ–inducible transcriptional activator CIITA lead to reduced class II MHC expression and a failure of APCs to activate CD4+ T lymphocytes. Failure of antigen presentation may result in defective positive selection of T cells in the thymus, with a reduction in the number of mature CD4+ T cells or defective activation of cells in the periphery. Affected individuals are deficient in DTH responses and in antibody responses to T cell–dependent protein antigens. The disease appears within the first year of life and is usually fatal unless it is treated by bone marrow transplantation.

Autosomal recessive class I MHC deficiencies have also been described and are characterized by decreased CD8+ T cell numbers and function. In some cases, the failure to express class I MHC molecules is due to mutations in the *TAP-1* or *TAP-2* genes, which encode the subunits of the TAP (transporter associated with antigen processing) complex, which normally transports peptides from the cytosol into the endoplasmic reticulum, where they are loaded onto class I MHC molecules (see Chapter 6). Because empty MHC molecules are degraded intracellularly, the level of cell surface class I MHC molecules is reduced in these TAP-deficient patients, a phenotype similar to *TAP* gene knockout mice. Such patients suffer mainly from necrotizing granulomatous skin lesions and respiratory tract bacterial infections, but not viral infections, which is surprising considering that a principal function of CD8+ T cells is defense against viruses. A similar deficiency of class I MHC expression has been observed in patients with mutations in the gene encoding the tapasin protein (see Chapter 6).

Patients with ZAP-70 deficiency have a lineage commitment defect resulting in reduced CD8+ T cells but normal numbers of CD4+ T cells; the reason for the selective loss is not clear. Although CD4+ T cell development or emigration to the periphery is not compromised, the cells fail to proliferate normally when challenged with antigens.

Heterozygous dominant negative mutations in the gene encoding UNC119 (Uncoordinated 119), a protein that delivers myristylated proteins, including LCK, to the plasma membrane, results in a CD4+ lymphopenia. LCK binds more strongly to CD4 than CD8, and in this disorder, deficiency of LCK at the cell surface presumably leads to a defect in the positive selection of CD4+ T cells. The clinical presentation includes recurrent viral and fungal infections.

SCID Caused by Defective T Cell Activation

Another rare form of SCID is caused by a mutation in the gene encoding Orai1, a component of the CRAC channel (see Chapter 7). Antigen receptor signaling leads to the activation of the γ isoform of phospholipase C (PLCγ) and the inositol trisphosphate (IP3)–dependent release of calcium ions from the endoplasmic reticulum and mitochondria (see Chapter 7). The released calcium is replenished by store-operated CRAC channels that facilitate an influx of extracellular calcium. This process is crucial for lymphocyte activation, and it is defective in cells with mutant *ORAI1*. A similar phenotype is observed in patients with mutations in *STIM1*, which encodes an endoplasmic reticulum protein that senses the depletion of calcium stores and contributes to the opening of the CRAC channel. Patients with *ORAI1* and *STIM1* mutations do not exhibit a defect in T cell development, but their T cells cannot be properly activated.

Antibody Deficiencies: Defects in B Cell Development and Activation

Whereas defects in T cell development or in both T and B cell development contribute to the SCID phenotype, more circumscribed defects in B cells result in disorders in which the primary abnormality is in antibody production (Table 21-4). Some of these disorders are caused by defects in B cell development (see Fig. 21-1), and others are caused by abnormal B cell activation and antibody synthesis (Fig. 21-2). However, in one subset of hyper-IgM syndromes, discussed later, antibody deficiencies are also accompanied by defects in macrophage and APC activation, which, in turn, result in attenuated cell-mediated immunity.

TABLE 21-4   Antibody Deficiencies

Disease	Functional Deficiencies	Mechanism of Defect
Agammaglobulinemias		
X-linked	Decrease in all serum Ig isotypes; reduced B cell numbers	Pre-B receptor checkpoint defect; Btk mutation
Autosomal recessive forms	Decrease in all serum Ig isotypes; reduced B cell numbers	Pre-B receptor checkpoint defect; mutations in IgM heavy chain (μ), surrogate light chains ($\lambda5$), Igα, BLNK, PI3K p85α
Hypogammaglobulinemias/Isotype Defects		
Selective IgA deficiency	Decreased IgA; may be associated with increased susceptibility to bacterial infections and protozoa such as *Giardia lamblia*	Mutations in *TACI* in some patients
Selective IgG2 deficiency	Increased susceptibility to bacterial infections	Small subset have deletion in IgH $\gamma2$ locus
Common variable immunodeficiency	Hypogammaglobulinemia; normal or decreased B cell numbers	Mutations in *ICOS* and *TACI* in some patients
ICF syndrome	Hypogammaglobulinemia, occasional mild T cell defects	Mutations in *DNMT3B*
Hyper-IgM Syndromes		
X-linked	Defects in T helper cell–mediated B cell, macrophage, and dendritic cell activation; defects in somatic mutation, class switching, and germinal center formation; defective cell-mediated immunity	Mutation in *CD40L*
Autosomal recessive with cell-mediated immune defects	Defects in T helper cell–mediated B cell, macrophage, and dendritic cell activation; defects in somatic mutation, class switching, and germinal center formation; defective cell-mediated immunity	Mutations in *CD40*, *NEMO*
Autosomal recessive with antibody defect only	Defects in somatic mutation and isotype switching	Mutations in *AID*, *UNG*

AID, activation-induced cytidine deaminase; *DNMT3B*, DNA methyltransferase 3B; *ICF*, immunodeficiencies-centromeric instability-facial anomalies; *ICOS*, inducible costimulator; *NEMO*, NF-κB essential modulator; *TACI*, transmembrane activator and calcium modulator and cyclophilin ligand interactor; *UNG*, uracil N-glycosylase.

X-Linked Agammaglobulinemia: An X-linked Pre-BCR Signaling Defect

X-linked agammaglobulinemia, also called Bruton's agammaglobulinemia, is caused by mutations or deletions in the gene encoding an enzyme called Bruton tyrosine kinase (Btk) that result in a failure of B cells to mature beyond the pre-B cell stage in the bone marrow (see Fig. 21-1). The disease is characterized by the absence of gamma globulin in the blood, as the name implies. It is one of the most common congenital immunodeficiencies and the prototype of a failure of B cell maturation. Btk is involved in transducing signals from the pre-BCR that are required for the survival and differentiation of pre–B cells (see Chapter 8). In female carriers of this disease, only B cells that have inactivated the X chromosome carrying the mutant allele mature. Patients with X-linked agammaglobulinemia usually have low or undetectable serum Ig, reduced or absent B cells in peripheral blood and lymphoid tissues, no germinal centers in lymph nodes, and no plasma cells in tissues. The maturation, numbers, and functions of T cells are generally normal, although some studies have revealed reduced numbers of activated T cells in patients, which may be a consequence of reduced antigen presentation caused by the lack of B cells. Autoimmune disorders develop in almost 20% of patients, for unknown reasons. The infectious complications of X-linked agammaglobulinemia are greatly reduced by periodic (e.g., weekly or monthly) injections of pooled gamma globulin preparations. Such preparations contain preformed antibodies against common pathogens and provide effective passive immunity.

Knockout mice lacking Btk, as well as naturally Btk mutant *Xid* mice, show a less severe defect in B cell maturation than humans do because a Btk-like tyrosine kinase called Tec is active in mouse pre-B cells that lack Btk and partially compensates for the mutant Btk. The main abnormalities in *Xid* mice are defective antibody responses to some polysaccharide antigens and a deficiency in mature follicular B cells and B-1 cells.

Autosomal Recessive Pre-BCR Checkpoint Defects

Autosomal recessive forms of agammaglobulinemia have been described, most of which can be linked to defects in pre-BCR signaling. Mutant genes that have been identified in this context include genes encoding the μ (IgM) heavy chain, the $\lambda5$ surrogate light chain, Igα (a signaling component of the pre-BCR and BCR), the p85α subunit of PI3Kinase, and BLNK (an adaptor protein downstream of the pre-BCR and BCR).

Selective Immunoglobulin Isotype Deficiencies

Many immunodeficiencies that selectively involve one or a few Ig isotypes have been described. The most common is *selective IgA deficiency,* which affects about 1 in 700 Caucasians and is thus the most common primary immunodeficiency known. IgA deficiency usually occurs sporadically, but many familial cases with either autosomal dominant or autosomal recessive patterns of inheritance are also known. The clinical features are variable. Many patients are entirely normal; others have occasional respiratory infections and diarrhea; and rarely, patients have

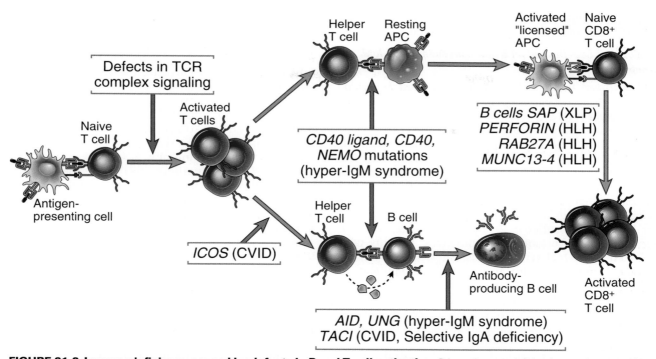

FIGURE 21-2 Immunodeficiency caused by defects in B and T cell activation. Primary immunodeficiencies may be caused by genetic defects in molecules required for T or B lymphocyte antigen receptor signaling, for helper T cell–mediated activation of B cells and APCs, or for activation of cytotoxic T lymphocytes and NK cells. *CVID,* common variable immunodeficiency; *HLH,* hemophagocytic lymphohistiocytosis.

severe, recurrent infections leading to permanent intestinal and airway damage, with associated autoimmune disorders. These manifestations reflect the importance of secretory IgA in protection of mucosal barriers from commensal and pathogenic microbes (see Chapter 14). IgA deficiency is characterized by low serum IgA, usually less than 50 μg/mL (normal, 2 to 4 mg/mL), with normal or elevated levels of IgM and IgG, and low IgA in mucosal secretions. The defect in these patients is a block in the differentiation of B cells to IgA antibody–secreting plasma cells. The α heavy chain genes and the expression of membrane-associated IgA are normal. No gross abnormalities in the numbers, phenotypes, or functional responses of T cells have been noted in these patients. In a small proportion of patients with selective IgA deficiency, mutations have been described in *TACI* (transmembrane activator and calcium modulator and cyclophilin ligand interactor), one of the three types of receptors for the cytokines BAFF (B cell–activating factor) and APRIL (a proliferation-inducing ligand), both of which stimulate B cell survival and proliferation, albeit at different stages of B cell differentiation. *TACI* mutations are also an important cause of common variable immunodeficiency, discussed later.

Selective IgG subclass deficiencies have been described in which total serum IgG levels are normal but concentrations of one or more subclasses are below normal. IgG3 deficiency is the most common subclass deficiency in adults, and IgG2 deficiency associated with IgA deficiency is most common in children. Some individuals with these deficiencies have recurrent bacterial infections, but many do not have any clinical problems. Selective IgG subclass deficiencies are usually due to abnormal B cell differentiation and rarely to homozygous deletions of various constant region (C_γ) genes.

Defects in B Cell Differentiation: Common Variable Immunodeficiency

Common variable immunodeficiency is a group of heterogeneous disorders defined by reduced levels of serum Ig, impaired antibody responses to infection and vaccines, and increased incidence of infections. The diagnosis is usually one of exclusion when other primary immunodeficiency diseases are ruled out. The presentation and pathogenesis are, as the name implies, highly variable. Although Ig deficiency and associated pyogenic infections, typically with *Haemophilus influenzae* and *Streptococcus pneumoniae,* are major components of these disorders, autoimmune diseases, including pernicious anemia, hemolytic anemia, inflammatory bowel disease, and rheumatoid arthritis, may be just as clinically significant. A high incidence of malignant tumors, particularly lymphomas, is also associated with common variable immunodeficiency. These disorders may be diagnosed early in childhood or late in life. Both sporadic and familial cases occur, the latter with both autosomal dominant and autosomal recessive inheritance patterns. Mature B lymphocytes are present in these patients, but plasma cells are absent in lymphoid tissues, which suggests a block in B cell differentiation to antibody-secreting cells.

The defective antibody production has been attributed to multiple abnormalities, including intrinsic B cell defects or deficient T cell help. A small proportion of patients with common variable immunodeficiency have a mutation in the *ICOS* (inducible T cell costimulator) gene. ICOS is required for T follicular helper cell generation (see Chapter 12). A more common cause of this syndrome is the existence of mutations in *TACI,* described earlier in the context of selective IgA deficiency. A few cases of common variable immunodeficiency are linked to mutations in the *CD19* gene. CD19 is a signaling component of the CR2 (CD21) coreceptor complex (see Chapter 7).

Defects in T Cell–Dependent B Cell Activation: Hyper-IgM Syndromes

The X-linked hyper-IgM syndrome is caused by mutations in the gene encoding the T cell effector molecule CD40 ligand (CD154). It is a rare disorder associated with defective switching of B cells to the IgG and IgA isotypes; production of these antibodies is therefore reduced, and the major isotype detected in the blood is IgM. The mutant forms of CD40 ligand produced in these patients do not bind to or transduce signals through CD40 and therefore do not stimulate B cells to undergo heavy chain isotype switching, which requires T cell help (see Chapter 12). Patients suffer from infections similar to those seen in other hypogammaglobulinemias. Patients with X-linked hyper-IgM syndrome also show defects in cell-mediated immunity, with an increased susceptibility to infection by the intracellular fungal microbe *Pneumocystis jiroveci*. This defective cell-mediated immunity occurs because CD40 ligand is also involved in T cell–dependent activation of macrophages and dendritic cells (see Chapter 10). Knockout mice lacking CD40 or CD40 ligand have a phenotype similar to that of the human disease.

Rare cases of hyper-IgM syndrome show an autosomal recessive inheritance pattern. In these patients, the genetic defects may be in CD40 or in the enzyme activation-induced deaminase (AID), which is involved in heavy chain isotype switching and affinity maturation (see Chapter 12). Mutations in *AID* are generally homozygous recessive. A small fraction of mutations in the region of the *AID* gene that corresponds to the C-terminal part of this enzyme exhibit an autosomal dominant inheritance pattern. One form of hyper-IgM syndrome is caused by autosomal recessive mutations in the gene encoding uracil N-glycosylase (UNG; see Chapter 12), an enzyme that removes U residues from Ig genes during class switching and somatic mutation. An inherited disorder, EDA-ID, in which hypomorphic *NEMO* mutations contribute to a hyper-IgM state as well as defects in ectodermal structures, is described earlier in the section on defects in innate immunity.

AID and *UNG* mutations affect class-switch recombination and somatic hypermutation in distinct ways. In the absence of AID, both switching and hypermutation are defective because AID is required for both processes. In the absence of UNG, isotype switching is defective but somatic hypermutation is largely preserved, although it exhibits less A:T mutations without the activity of UNG. The role of DNA repair gene mutations in class-switching defects will be considered when we discuss ataxia-telangiectasia later in this chapter.

Defects in T Lymphocyte Activation and Function

Congenital abnormalities in the activation of T lymphocytes are being increasingly recognized as our understanding of the molecular basis of lymphocyte activation improves (Table 21-5). Included in this broad category are some disorders of CTL and NK cell granule composition or exocytosis. Although we classify disorders linked to defective MHC expression with disorders of T cell development,

TABLE 21-5 Defects in T Cell Activation

Disease	Functional Deficiencies	Mechanism of Defect
Defects in MHC Expression		
Bare lymphocyte syndrome	Defective MHC class II expression and deficiency in CD4+ T cells; defective cell-mediated immunity and T-dependent humoral immune responses	Defects in transcription factors regulating MHC class II gene expression, including *CIITA*, *RFXANK*, *RFX5*, and *RFXAP*
MHC class I deficiency	Decreased MHC class I levels; reduced CD8+ T cells	Mutations in *TAP1*, *TAP2*, and *TAPASIN*
Defective T Cell Signaling		
Proximal TCR signaling defects	Defects in cell-mediated immunity and T-cell–dependent humoral immunity	Mutations in *CD3* genes, *CD45*, *STIM1*, *ORAI1*
Wiskott-Aldrich syndrome Autosomal recessive WAS-like disease	Defective T cell activation and leukocyte mobility Defective T cell activation and leukocyte mobility	TCR-dependent actin-cytoskeletal rearrangements are defective because of mutations in *WAS*, an X-linked gene mutation in *WIP*
Familial Hemophagocytic Lymphohistiocytoses		
X-linked lymphoproliferative syndrome	Uncontrolled EBV-induced B cell proliferation, uncontrolled macrophage and CTL activation, defective NK cell and CTL function	Mutations in *SAP* Mutations in *X-IAP*
Perforin deficiencies	Uncontrolled macrophage and CTL activation, defective NK cell and CTL function	Mutations in *PERFORIN*
Granule fusion	Uncontrolled macrophage and CTL activation, defective NK cell and CTL function	Defective cytotoxic granule exocytosis; mutations in *RAB27A*, *MUNC13-4*, *SYNTAXIN*, *AP3* (and in *LYST* in Chédiak-Higashi syndrome—see Table 21-2)

AP3, adaptor-related protein complex 3; *LYST*, lysosomal trafficking regulator protein; *SAP*, SLAM-associated protein; *TAP*, transporter associated with antigen processing; *WASP*, Wiskott-Aldrich syndrome protein.

these abnormalities also result in defective activation of T cells that do mature and emerge from the thymus.

Defects in TCR Signal Transduction

Many rare immunodeficiency diseases are caused by defects in the expression of molecules required for T cell activation and function. Biochemical and molecular analyses of affected individuals have revealed mutations in the genes encoding various T cell proteins (see Table 21-5). Examples include impaired TCR complex expression or function caused by mutations in the *CD3* ε or γ genes, defective TCR-mediated signaling caused by mutations in the *ZAP70* gene, reduced synthesis of cytokines such as IL-2 and IFN-γ (in some cases caused by defects in transcription factors), and lack of expression of IL-2 receptor chains. These defects are often found in only a few isolated cases or in a few families, and the clinical features and severity vary widely. Patients with these abnormalities may have deficiencies predominantly in T cell function or have mixed T cell and B cell immunodeficiencies despite normal or even elevated numbers of blood lymphocytes. We have previously considered the importance of the CD3 complex, RHOH, and LCK at the pre-TCR checkpoint; the role of *ZAP70* mutations in CD8$^+$ T cell development; the role of *LCK* and *UNC119* mutations in CD4$^+$ T cell development; and the relevance of *ORAI1* and *STIM1* mutations in T cell activation, all in the clinical context of SCID. Other syndromes involving the defective activation of mature T cells are considered here.

Wiskott-Aldrich Syndrome

Variable degrees of T and B cell immunodeficiency occur in certain congenital diseases with a wide spectrum of abnormalities involving multiple organ systems. One such disorder is Wiskott-Aldrich syndrome, an X-linked disease characterized by eczema, thrombocytopenia (reduced blood platelets), and susceptibility to bacterial infection. Some of the abnormalities in this disorder can be traced to defective T cell activation, although intrinsic loss of B cell function also contributes to the pathogenesis. In the initial stages of the disease, lymphocyte numbers are normal, and the principal defect is an inability to produce antibodies in response to T cell–independent polysaccharide antigens, because of which these patients are especially susceptible to infections with encapsulated bacteria. The lymphocytes (and platelets) are smaller than normal. With increasing age, the patients show reduced numbers of lymphocytes and more severe immunodeficiency.

The defective gene responsible for Wiskott-Aldrich syndrome encodes a cytoplasmic protein called WASP (Wiskott-Aldrich syndrome protein), which is expressed exclusively in bone marrow–derived cells. WASP interacts with several proteins, including adaptor molecules downstream of the antigen receptor such as Grb-2 (see Chapter 7), the Arp2/3 complex involved in actin polymerization, and small G proteins of the Rho family that regulate actin cytoskeletal rearrangement. Defective activation and synapse formation in lymphocytes and defective mobility of all leukocytes may account for the immunodeficiency observed in this syndrome.

An autosomal recessive disease that resembles Wiskott-Aldrich syndrome has been described. This disease is caused by mutations in the gene encoding WIP (WASP-Interacting Protein), a protein that binds to WASP and stabilizes it.

The X-Linked Lymphoproliferative Syndrome

X-linked lymphoproliferative (XLP) syndrome is a disorder characterized by an inability to eliminate EBV, eventually leading to fulminant infectious mononucleosis and the development of B cell tumors. In about 80% of cases, the disease is due to mutations in the gene encoding an adaptor molecule called SAP (SLAM-associated protein) that binds to a family of cell surface molecules involved in the activation of NK cells and T and B lymphocytes, including the signaling lymphocyte activation molecule (SLAM). SAP links the membrane proteins SLAM and 2B4 (see Chapter 7) to the Src family kinase Fyn. Defects in SAP contribute to attenuated NK and T cell activation and result in increased susceptibility to viral infections. As discussed in Chapter 12, SAP is required for follicular helper T (T$_{FH}$) cell development, and the inability of XLP patients to generate germinal centers and high-affinity antibodies also likely contributes to the associated hypogammaglobulinemia and susceptibility to viral infection. In about 20% of cases of XLP, the genetic defect resides not in SAP but in the gene encoding XIAP (X-linked inhibitor of apoptosis). The resulting enhanced apoptosis of T cells and NKT cells leads to a marked depletion of these cell types. This immunodeficiency is most commonly manifested by severe EBV infections, which probably arise opportunistically because of the ubiquitous nature of EBV.

Defective CTL and NK Cell Function: The Familial Hemophagocytic Lymphohistiocytosis Syndromes

Hemophagocytic lymphohistiocytosis (HLH) syndromes are a group of life-threatening immunodeficiency disorders in which NK cells and CTLs are defective in their ability to kill infected cells. As a result, viral infections are not held in check, and compensatory excessive macrophage activation is a feature of these syndromes. A late but striking feature of these disorders is the ingestion of red blood cells by activated macrophages (hemophagocytosis). Mutations in the *perforin* gene are the most common cause of HLH, but mutations in genes encoding the cellular machinery involved in granule exocytosis are found in some cases of this syndrome. Specifically, mutations in *RAB27A*, a small guanosine triphosphatase involved in vesicular fusion, and in *MUNC13-4*, which encodes an adaptor that participates in granule exocytosis, compromise the fusion of lytic granules with the plasma membrane and thus contribute to various subtypes of HLH. Similarly, mutations in the gene for one component of the AP-3 cytosolic adaptor protein complex can also disrupt intracellular transport and contribute to a form of HLH. It is believed that T cells and NK cells respond strongly to the persistent microbes by secreting IFN-γ, but in the absence of cytotoxic activity, the CTL and NK cells cannot clear the infections, and the excessive IFN-γ mediated macrophage activation is manifested by hemophagocytosis and lymphadenopathy in the context of immunodeficiency.

Multisystem Disorders with Immunodeficiency

Immunodeficiency is often one of a constellation of symptoms in a number of inherited disorders. Examples of such syndromes discussed earlier include Chédiak-Higashi syndrome, Wiskott-Aldrich syndrome, and DiGeorge syndrome.

Ataxia Telangectasia

Ataxia-telangiectasia is an autosomal recessive disorder characterized by abnormal gait (ataxia), vascular malformations (telangiectases), neurologic deficits, increased incidence of tumors, and immunodeficiency. The immunologic defects are of variable severity and may affect both B and T cells. The most common humoral immune defects are IgA and IgG2 deficiency, probably because of the crucial role a protein called ATM (ataxia-telangiectasia mutated) plays in class-switch recombination. The T cell defects, which are usually less pronounced, are associated with thymic hypoplasia. Patients experience upper and lower respiratory tract bacterial infections, multiple autoimmune phenomena, and increasingly frequent cancers with advancing age.

ATM is a protein kinase related structurally to phosphatidylinositol 3-kinase. This protein can activate cell cycle checkpoints and apoptosis in response to double-stranded DNA breaks. It has also been shown to contribute to the stability of DNA double-stranded break complexes during V(D)J recombination. In Wiskott-Aldrich syndrome, these abnormalities in DNA repair account for abnormal generation of antigen receptors. In addition, ATM contributes to DNA stability when double strand DNA breaks are generated in the course of isotype switch recombination, and mutations in ATM result in defective class switching and reduced levels of IgG, IgA and IgE.

Therapeutic Approaches for Congenital Immunodeficiencies

The current treatment for immunodeficiencies has two aims: to minimize and control infections, and to replace the defective or absent components of the immune system by adoptive transfer or transplantation. Passive immunization with pooled gamma globulin is very beneficial for agammaglobulinemic patients and has been lifesaving for many boys with X-linked agammaglobulinemia. Hematopoietic stem cell transplantation is currently the treatment of choice for many immunodeficiency diseases and has been successful in the treatment of SCID with ADA deficiency, Wiskott-Aldrich syndrome, bare lymphocyte syndrome, and leukocyte adhesion deficiencies. It is most successful with careful T cell depletion from the marrow and HLA matching to prevent graft-versus-host disease (see Chapter 17). Enzyme replacement therapy for ADA and PNP deficiencies has been attempted, with red blood cell transfusions used as a source of the enzymes. This approach has produced temporary clinical improvement in several patients with autosomal SCID. Injection of bovine ADA, conjugated to polyethylene glycol to prolong its serum half-life, has proved successful in some cases, but the benefits are usually short-lived.

In theory, the therapy of choice for congenital disorders of lymphocytes is to replace the defective gene in self-renewing stem cells. Gene replacement remains a distant goal for most human immunodeficiencies at present, despite considerable effort. The main obstacles to this type of gene therapy are difficulties in purifying self-renewing stem cells, which are the ideal target for introduction of the replacement gene, and in introducing genes into cells to achieve stable, long-lived, and high-level expression. In addition, transplant recipients have to be conditioned by depleting their bone marrow cells to allow transplanted stem cells to engraft, and this carries potential risks because of transient reduction of blood cells. Some progress has been made in gene therapy for ADA deficiency by use of a mild conditioning approach. A small number of patients with X-linked SCID have been successfully treated by transplantation of autologous bone marrow cells engineered to express a normal γ_c gene. However, a few of these treated patients have developed leukemia, apparently because the introduced γ_c gene inserted adjacent to an oncogene and activated this gene. The development of self-inactivating lentiviral vectors has reduced the risk of insertional mutagenesis, and there has recently been some success with gene therapy, especially for ADA-SCID.

ACQUIRED (SECONDARY) IMMUNODEFICIENCIES

Deficiencies of the immune system often develop because of abnormalities that are not genetic but acquired during life (Table 21-6). Acquired immunodeficiency diseases are caused by a variety of pathogenic mechanisms. First, immunosuppression may occur as a biologic complication of another disease process. Second, so-called iatrogenic immunodeficiencies may develop as complications of therapy for other diseases. Third, immunodeficiency may be acquired by an infection that target cells of the immune system. The most prominent of these is HIV infection, which is described separately later in the chapter.

Diseases in which immunodeficiency is a frequent complicating element include malnutrition, neoplasms, and infections. Protein-calorie malnutrition is common in developing countries and is associated with impaired

TABLE 21-6 Acquired Immunodeficiencies

Cause	Mechanism
HIV infection	Depletion of CD4+ T cells
Protein-calorie malnutrition	Metabolic derangements inhibit lymphocyte maturation and function
Irradiation and chemotherapy for cancer	Decreased bone marrow lymphocyte precursors
Cancer metastases and leukemia involving bone marrow	Reduced site of leukocyte development
Immunosuppression for transplants, autoimmune diseases	Reduced lymphocyte activation, cytokine blockade, impaired leukocyte trafficking
Removal of spleen	Decreased phagocytosis of microbes

cellular and humoral immunity to microorganisms. Much of the morbidity and mortality that afflict malnourished people is due to infections. The basis for the immunodeficiency is not well defined, but it is reasonable to assume that the global metabolic disturbances in these individuals, caused by deficient intake of protein, fat, vitamins, and minerals, will adversely affect maturation and function of the cells of the immune system.

Patients with advanced widespread cancer often are susceptible to infection because of impaired cell-mediated and humoral immune responses to a variety of organisms. Bone marrow tumors, including cancers metastatic to marrow and leukemias that arise in the marrow, may interfere with the growth and development of normal lymphocytes and other leukocytes. In addition, tumors may produce substances that interfere with lymphocyte development or function. An example of malignancy-associated immunodeficiency is the impairment in T cell function commonly observed in patients with a type of lymphoma called Hodgkin's disease. Patients are unable to mount DTH reactions on intradermal injection of various common antigens to which they were previously exposed, such as *Candida* or tetanus toxoid. Other in vitro measures of T cell function, such as proliferative responses to polyclonal activators, are also impaired in patients with Hodgkin's disease. Such a generalized deficiency in cell-mediated immune responses has been called anergy. The cause of these T cell abnormalities is not known.

Various types of infections lead to immunosuppression. Viruses other than HIV are known to impair immune responses; examples include the measles virus and human T cell lymphotropic virus 1 (HTLV-1). Both viruses can infect lymphocytes, which may be a basis for their immunosuppressive effects. Like HIV, HTLV-1 is a retrovirus with tropism for CD4+ T cells; however, instead of killing helper T cells, it transforms them and produces an aggressive malignant neoplasm called adult T cell leukemia/lymphoma (ATL). Patients with ATL typically have severe immunosuppression with multiple opportunistic infections. Chronic infections with *Mycobacterium tuberculosis* and various fungi frequently result in anergy to many antigens. Chronic parasitic infections may also lead to immunosuppression. For example, African children with chronic malarial infections have depressed T cell function, and this may be one reason why these children have an increased propensity to develop EBV-associated malignant tumors.

Iatrogenic immunosuppression is most often due to drug therapies that kill or functionally inactivate lymphocytes. Some drugs are given intentionally to immunosuppress patients, either for the treatment of inflammatory diseases or to prevent rejection of organ allografts. The most commonly used anti-inflammatory and immunosuppressive drugs are corticosteroids and cyclosporine, respectively, but many others are widely used now (see Chapters 17 and 19). Various chemotherapeutic drugs are administered to patients with cancer, and these drugs are usually cytotoxic to proliferating cells, including mature and developing lymphocytes as well as other leukocyte precursors. Thus, cancer chemotherapy is almost always accompanied by a period of immunosuppression and risk for infection. Iatrogenic immunosuppression and tumors involving the bone marrow are the most common causes of immunodeficiency in developed countries.

One other form of acquired immunodeficiency results from the absence of a spleen caused by surgical removal of the organ after trauma and as treatment of certain hematologic diseases, or by infarction in sickle cell disease. Patients without spleens are more susceptible to infection by some organisms, particularly encapsulated bacteria such as *Streptococcus pneumoniae*. This enhanced susceptibility is partly due to defective phagocytic clearance of opsonized blood-borne microbes, an important physiologic function of the spleen, and partly due to defective antibody responses resulting from the absence of marginal zone B cells.

HUMAN IMMUNODEFICIENCY VIRUS AND THE ACQUIRED IMMUNODEFICIENCY SYNDROME

AIDS is the disease caused by infection with HIV and is characterized by profound immunosuppression with associated opportunistic infections and malignant tumors, wasting, and central nervous system (CNS) degeneration. HIV infects a variety of cells of the immune system, including CD4+ helper T cells, macrophages, and dendritic cells. HIV evolved as a human pathogen very recently relative to most other known human pathogens, and the HIV epidemic was first identified only in the 1980s. However, the degree of morbidity and mortality caused by HIV and the global impact of this infection on health care resources and economics are already enormous and continue to grow. HIV has infected 50 to 60 million people and has caused the death of more than 25 million adults and children. Approximately 35 million people are living with HIV infection and AIDS, of which approximately 70% are in Africa and 20% in Asia, and almost 1-2 million die of the disease every year. The disease is especially devastating because about half of the approximately 3 million new cases every year occur in young adults (15 to 24 years of age). AIDS has left approximately 14 million orphans. Currently, there is no vaccine or permanent cure for AIDS, but quite effective antiretroviral drugs have been developed that are capable of controlling the infection. In this section of the chapter, we describe the properties of HIV, the pathogenesis of HIV-induced immunodeficiency, and the clinical and epidemiologic features of HIV-related diseases.

Molecular and Biologic Features of HIV

HIV is a member of the lentivirus family of animal retroviruses. Lentiviruses, including visna virus of sheep and the bovine, feline, and simian immunodeficiency viruses, are capable of long-term latent infection of cells and short-term cytopathic effects, and they all produce slowly progressive, fatal diseases that include wasting syndromes and CNS degeneration. Two closely related types of HIV, designated HIV-1 and HIV-2, have been identified. HIV-1 is by far the most common cause of AIDS; HIV-2, which differs in genomic structure and antigenicity, causes a form of AIDS with slower progression than HIV-1–linked disease.

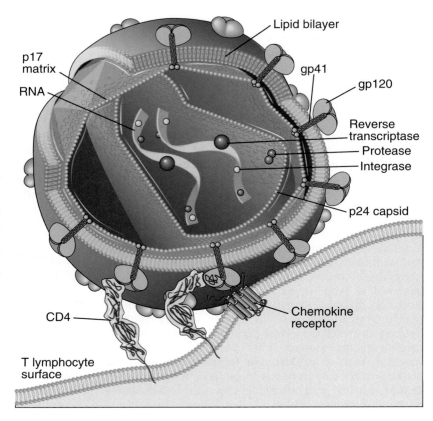

FIGURE 21-3 Structure of HIV-1. An HIV-1 virion is shown next to a T cell surface. HIV-1 consists of two identical strands of RNA (the viral genome) and associated enzymes, including reverse transcriptase, integrase, and protease, packaged in a cone-shaped core composed of p24 capsid protein with a surrounding p17 protein matrix, all surrounded by a phospholipid membrane envelope derived from the host cell. Virally encoded membrane proteins (gp41 and gp120) are bound to the envelope. CD4 and chemokine receptors on the host cell surface function as HIV-1 receptors. *(Copyright © 2000 Terese Winslow.)*

HIV Structure and Genes

An infectious HIV particle consists of two identical strands of RNA packaged within a core of viral proteins and surrounded by a phospholipid bilayer envelope derived from the host cell membrane but including virally encoded membrane proteins (Fig. 21-3). The RNA genome of HIV is approximately 9.2 kb long and has the basic arrangement of nucleic acid sequences characteristic of all known retroviruses (Fig. 21-4). Long terminal repeats (LTRs) at each end of the genome regulate viral gene expression, viral integration into the host genome, and viral replication. The *gag* sequence encodes core structural proteins. The *env* sequence encodes the envelope glycoproteins gp120 and gp41, which non-covalently associate with each other and are required for infection of cells. The *pol* sequence encodes reverse transcriptase, integrase, and viral protease enzymes, which are required for viral replication. In addition to these typical retrovirus genes, the HIV-1 genome contains six other regulatory genes, namely, the *tat, rev, vif, nef, vpr,* and *vpu* genes, whose products regulate viral replication and host immune evasion in various ways. The functions of these genes are summarized in Figure 21-4 and discussed later.

Viral Life Cycle

HIV infection of cells begins when the envelope glycoprotein gp120 of the virus binds to two proteins on host cells, CD4 and a coreceptor that is a member of the chemokine receptor family (Fig. 21-5). The viral particles that initiate infection are usually in the blood, semen, or other body fluids of one individual and are introduced into another individual by sexual contact, needle stick, or transplacental passage. The viral envelope glycoprotein complex, called Env, is composed of a transmembrane gp41 subunit and an external, non-covalently associated gp120 subunit. These subunits are produced by proteolytic cleavage of a gp160 precursor. The Env complex is expressed as a trimeric structure of three gp120/gp41 pairs. This complex mediates a multistep process of fusion of the virion envelope with the membrane of the target cell (Fig. 21-6). The first step of this process is the binding of gp120 subunits to CD4 molecules, which induces a conformational change that promotes secondary gp120 binding to a chemokine coreceptor. Coreceptor binding induces a conformational change in gp41 that exposes a hydrophobic region, called the fusion peptide, which inserts into the cell membrane and enables the viral membrane to fuse with the target cell membrane. After the virus completes its life cycle in the infected cell (described later), free viral particles are released from the infected cell and bind to an uninfected cell, thus propagating the infection. In addition, gp120 and gp41, which are expressed on the plasma membrane of infected cells before virus is released, can mediate cell-cell fusion with an uninfected cell that expresses CD4 and coreceptors, and HIV genomes can then be passed between the fused cells directly.

The most important chemokine receptors that act as coreceptors for HIV are CXCR4 and CCR5. More than seven different chemokine receptors have been shown to serve as coreceptors for HIV entry into cells, and several other proteins belonging to the seven-transmembrane–spanning G protein–coupled receptor family, such as the leukotriene B_4 receptor, can also

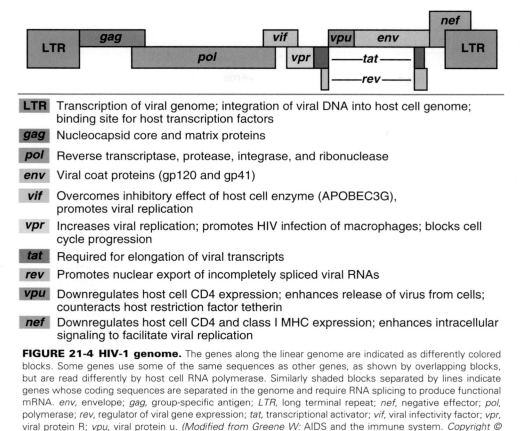

LTR Transcription of viral genome; integration of viral DNA into host cell genome; binding site for host transcription factors

gag Nucleocapsid core and matrix proteins

pol Reverse transcriptase, protease, integrase, and ribonuclease

env Viral coat proteins (gp120 and gp41)

vif Overcomes inhibitory effect of host cell enzyme (APOBEC3G), promotes viral replication

vpr Increases viral replication; promotes HIV infection of macrophages; blocks cell cycle progression

tat Required for elongation of viral transcripts

rev Promotes nuclear export of incompletely spliced viral RNAs

vpu Downregulates host cell CD4 expression; enhances release of virus from cells; counteracts host restriction factor tetherin

nef Downregulates host cell CD4 and class I MHC expression; enhances intracellular signaling to facilitate viral replication

FIGURE 21-4 HIV-1 genome. The genes along the linear genome are indicated as differently colored blocks. Some genes use some of the same sequences as other genes, as shown by overlapping blocks, but are read differently by host cell RNA polymerase. Similarly shaded blocks separated by lines indicate genes whose coding sequences are separated in the genome and require RNA splicing to produce functional mRNA. *env,* envelope; *gag,* group-specific antigen; *LTR,* long terminal repeat; *nef,* negative effector; *pol,* polymerase; *rev,* regulator of viral gene expression; *tat,* transcriptional activator; *vif,* viral infectivity factor; *vpr,* viral protein R; *vpu,* viral protein u. *(Modified from Greene W:* AIDS and the immune system. *Copyright © 1993 by Scientific American, Inc. All rights reserved.)*

mediate HIV infection of cells. Different isolates of HIV have distinct tropisms for different cell populations that are related to the expression of different chemokine receptors on these cells.

All HIV strains can infect and replicate in freshly isolated human CD4+ T cells that are activated in vitro. In contrast, some strains will infect primary cultures of human macrophages but not continuous T cell lines (and are called macrophage-tropic, or M-tropic, virus), whereas other strains will infect T cell lines but not macrophages (T-tropic virus), and some infect both T cell lines and macrophages (dual-tropic virus). Macrophage-tropic virus isolates express a gp120 that binds to CCR5, which is expressed on macrophages (and some memory T cells), whereas T cell–tropic viruses bind to CXCR4, which is expressed on T cell lines. HIV variants are described as X4 for CXCR4 binding, R5 for CCR5 binding, or R5X4 for the ability to bind to both chemokine receptors. In many HIV-infected individuals, there is a change from the production of virus that uses CCR5 and is predominantly macrophage-tropic early in the disease to virus that binds to CXCR4 and is T-tropic late in the disease. The T-tropic strains tend to be more virulent, presumably because they infect and deplete T cells more than do M-tropic strains. The importance of CCR5 in HIV infection in vivo is supported by the finding that individuals who do not express this receptor on the cell surface because of an inherited homozygous 32-bp deletion in the *CCR5* gene are resistant to HIV infection.

Once an HIV virion enters a cell, the enzymes within the nucleoprotein complex become active and begin the viral reproductive cycle (see Fig. 21-5). The nucleoprotein core of the virus becomes disrupted, the RNA genome of HIV is reverse-transcribed into a double-stranded DNA form by viral reverse transcriptase, and the viral DNA enters the nucleus. The viral integrase also enters the nucleus and catalyzes the integration of viral DNA into the host cell genome. The integrated HIV DNA is called the **provirus.** The provirus may remain transcriptionally inactive for months or years, with little or no production of new viral proteins or virions, and in this way HIV infection of an individual cell can be latent.

Transcription of the genes of the integrated DNA provirus is regulated by the LTR upstream of the viral structural genes, and cytokines and other stimuli that activate T cells and macrophages enhance viral gene transcription. The LTRs contain polyadenylation signal sequences, the TATA box promoter sequence, and binding sites for two host cell transcription factors, NF-κB and SP1. Initiation of HIV gene transcription in T cells is linked to activation of the T cells by antigen or cytokines. For example, polyclonal activators of T cells, such as phytohemagglutinin, and cytokines, such as IL-2, tumor necrosis factor (TNF) and lymphotoxin, stimulate HIV gene expression in infected T cells, and IL-1, IL-3, IL-6, TNF, lymphotoxin, IFN-γ, and granulocyte-macrophage colony-stimulating factor (GM-CSF) stimulate HIV gene expression and viral replication in infected monocytes and macrophages. TCR

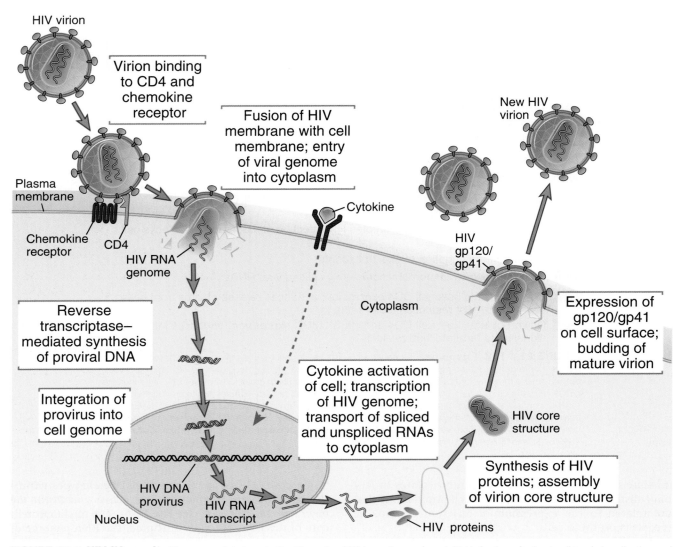

FIGURE 21-5 HIV life cycle. The sequential steps in the life cycle of HIV are shown, from initial infection of a host cell to viral replication and release of a new virion. For the sake of clarity, the production and release of only one new virion are shown. An infected cell actually produces many virions, each capable of infecting cells, thereby amplifying the infectious cycle.

and cytokine stimulation of HIV gene transcription probably involves the activation of NF-κB and its binding to sequences in the LTR. This phenomenon is significant to the pathogenesis of AIDS because the normal response of a latently infected T cell to a microbe may be the way in which HIV latency is ended and virus production begins. The multiple infections that AIDS patients acquire thus stimulate HIV production and infection of additional cells.

The Tat protein is required for HIV gene expression and acts by enhancing the production of complete viral mRNA transcripts. Even in the presence of optimal signals to initiate transcription, few if any HIV mRNA molecules are actually synthesized without the action of Tat because transcription of HIV genes by mammalian RNA polymerase is inefficient, and the polymerase complex usually stops before the mRNA is completed. Tat allows DNA-dependent RNA polymerase to remain bound to the viral DNA molecule long enough for transcription to be completed and to thus produce a functional viral mRNA.

Synthesis of mature infectious viral particles begins after full-length viral RNA transcripts are produced and the viral genes are expressed as proteins. The mRNAs encoding the various HIV proteins are derived from a single full-genome-length transcript by differential splicing events. HIV gene expression may be divided into an early stage, during which regulatory genes are expressed, and a late stage, during which structural genes are expressed and full-length viral genomes are packaged. The Rev, Tat, and Nef proteins are early gene products encoded by fully spliced mRNAs that are exported from the nucleus and translated into proteins in the cytoplasm soon after infection of a cell. Late genes include *env, gag,* and *pol,* which encode the structural components of the virus and are translated from singly spliced or unspliced RNA. The Rev protein initiates the switch from early to late gene expression by promoting the export of these incompletely spliced late gene RNAs out of the nucleus. The pol gene product is a precursor protein that is sequentially cleaved to form reverse transcriptase, protease,

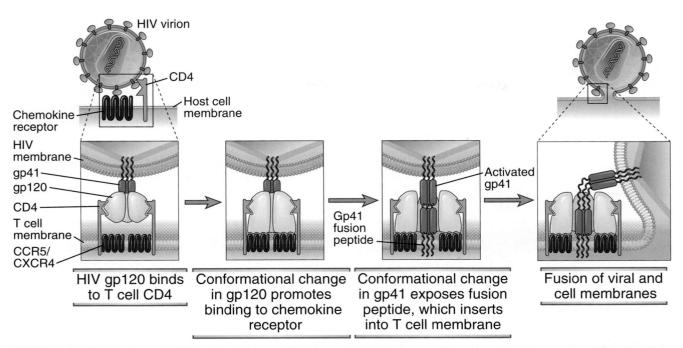

FIGURE 21-6 Mechanism of HIV entry into a cell. In the model depicted, sequential conformational changes in gp120 and gp41 are induced by binding to CD4. These changes promote binding of the virus to the coreceptor (a chemokine receptor) and fusion of the HIV-1 and host cell membranes. The fusion peptide of activated gp41 contains hydrophobic amino acid residues that mediate insertion into the host cell plasma membrane.

ribonuclease, and integrase enzymes. As mentioned earlier, reverse transcriptase and integrase proteins are required to produce a DNA copy of the viral RNA genome and to integrate it as a provirus into the host genome. The *gag* gene encodes a 55-kD protein that is proteolytically cleaved into p24, p17, and p15 polypeptides by the action of the viral protease encoded by the *pol* gene. These polypeptides are the core proteins that are required for assembly of infectious viral particles. The primary product of the *env* gene is a 160-kD glycoprotein (gp160) that is cleaved by cellular proteases within the endoplasmic reticulum into the gp120 and gp41 proteins required for HIV binding to cells, as discussed earlier. Current antiviral drug therapy for HIV disease includes inhibitors of the enzymes reverse transcriptase, protease, and integrase.

After transcription of various viral genes, viral proteins are synthesized in the cytoplasm. Assembly of infectious viral particles then begins by packaging full-length RNA transcripts of the proviral genome within a nucleoprotein complex that includes the *gag* core proteins and the *pol*-encoded enzymes required for the next cycle of integration. This nucleoprotein complex then buds from the plasma membrane, capturing Env and host glycoproteins as part of its envelope. The rate of virus production can reach sufficiently high levels to cause cell death, as discussed later.

Host restriction factors inhibit viral infection and many viral proteins have evolved to counter these restriction factors. A host factor that prevents virion release in certain cell types is a protein called tetherin. Tetherin prevents the pinching off of certain viruses including HIV, and its inhibition of the budding process can be antagonized by an HIV protein called Vpu. Host cells incorporate certain restriction factors into the virus particle including APOBEC3 (Apolipoprotein B mRNA editing enzyme catalytic polypeptide like 3) proteins. These host

proteins are cytidine deaminases that interfere with viral replication in infected cells. The HIV Vif protein helps target APOBEC3 proteins for ubiquitination and proteasomal degradation and thus promotes viral replication. In infected cells, another important host restriction factor is TRIM5α of the Tripartite Motif (TRIM) family of ubiquitin E3 ligases. TRIM5α interacts with HIV capsid proteins to cause premature uncoating of the virus and proteasomal degradation of the viral reverse transcriptase complex. It can also block nuclear translocation of the viral pre-integration complexes.

Pathogenesis of HIV Infection and AIDS

HIV disease begins with acute infection, which is only partly controlled by the host immune response, and advances to chronic progressive infection of peripheral lymphoid tissues (Fig. 21-7). The virus typically enters through mucosal epithelia. The subsequent events in the infection can be divided into several phases.

Acute (early) infection is characterized by infection of memory CD4+ T cells in mucosal lymphoid tissues and death of many infected cells. Because the mucosal tissues are the largest reservoir of T cells in the body and the major site of residence of memory T cells, this local loss is reflected in considerable depletion of lymphocytes. In fact, within 2 weeks of infection, a large fraction of CD4+ T cells may be destroyed.

The transition from the acute phase to the chronic phase of infection is accompanied by dissemination of the virus, viremia, and the development of host immune responses. Dendritic cells in epithelia at sites of virus entry capture the virus and then migrate into the lymph nodes. Dendritic cells express a protein with a mannose-binding lectin domain, called DC-SIGN, which may be particularly

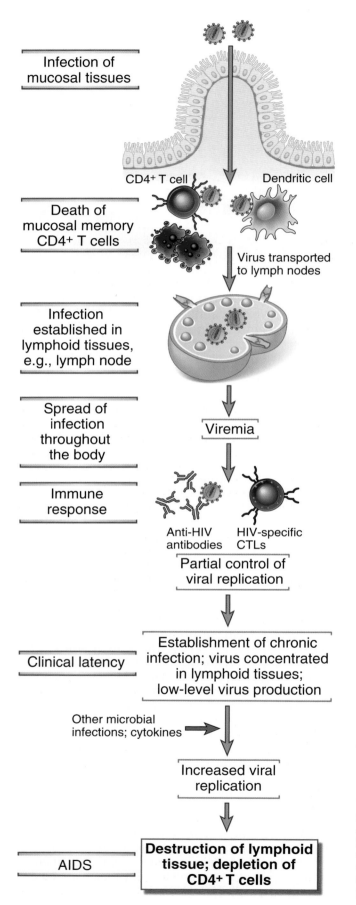

important in binding the HIV envelope and transporting the virus. Once in lymphoid tissues, dendritic cells may pass HIV on to CD4+ T cells through direct cell-cell contact. Within days after the first exposure to HIV, viral replication can be detected in the lymph nodes. This replication leads to viremia, during which large numbers of HIV particles are present in the patient's blood, accompanied by an acute HIV syndrome that includes a variety of nonspecific signs and symptoms typical of many viral infections (described later). The viremia allows the virus to disseminate throughout the body and to infect helper T cells, macrophages, and dendritic cells in peripheral lymphoid tissues. As the HIV infection spreads, the adaptive immune system mounts both humoral and cell-mediated immune responses directed at viral antigens, which we will describe later. These immune responses partially control the infection and viral production, and such control is reflected by a drop in viremia to low but detectable levels by approximately 12 weeks after the primary exposure.

In the next, chronic, phase of the disease, lymph nodes and the spleen are sites of continuous HIV replication and cell destruction (see Fig. 21-7). During this period of the disease, the immune system remains competent at handling most infections with opportunistic microbes, and few or no clinical manifestations of the HIV infection are present. Therefore, this phase of HIV disease is called the clinical latency period. Although the majority of peripheral blood T cells do not harbor the virus, destruction of CD4+ T cells within lymphoid tissues steadily progresses during the latent period, and the number of circulating blood CD4+ T cells steadily declines (Fig. 21-8). More than 90% of the body's approximately 10^{12} T cells are normally found in peripheral and mucosal lymphoid tissues, and it is estimated that HIV destroys up to 1 to 2×10^9 CD4+ T cells every day. Early in the course of the disease, the individual may continue to make new CD4+ T cells, and therefore these cells can be replaced almost as quickly as they are destroyed. At this stage, up to 10% of CD4+ T cells in lymphoid organs may be infected, but the number of circulating CD4+ T cells that are infected at any one time may be less than 0.1% of the total CD4+ T cells in an individual. Eventually, over a period of years, the continuous cycle of virus infection, T cell death, and new infection leads to a detectable loss of CD4+ T cells from the lymphoid tissues and the circulation.

Mechanisms of Immunodeficiency Caused by HIV

HIV infection ultimately results in impaired function of both the adaptive and innate immune systems. The most prominent defects are in cell-mediated immunity, and they can be attributed to several mechanisms, including direct cytopathic effects of the virus and indirect effects. The indirect effects may be especially important in the

FIGURE 21-7 Progression of HIV infection. The progression of HIV infection correlates with spread of the virus from the initial site of infection to lymphoid tissues throughout the body. The immune response of the host temporarily controls acute infection but does not prevent the establishment of chronic infection of cells in lymphoid tissues. Cytokine stimuli induced by other microbes serve to enhance HIV production and progression to AIDS.

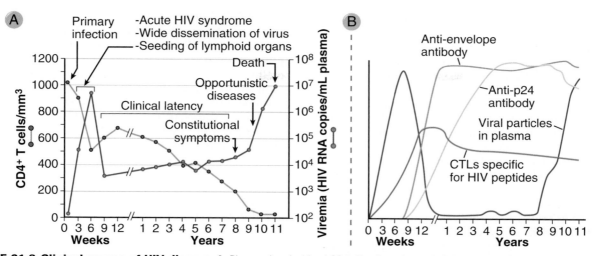

FIGURE 21-8 Clinical course of HIV disease. A, Plasma viremia, blood CD4+ T cell counts, and clinical stages of disease. About 12 weeks after infection, the blood-borne virus (plasma viremia) is reduced to very low levels (detectable only by sensitive reverse transcriptase–polymerase chain reaction assays) and stays this way for many years. Nonetheless, CD4+ T cell counts steadily decline during this clinical latency period because of active viral replication and T cell infection in lymph nodes. When CD4+ T cell counts drop below a critical level (about 200/mm3), the risk for infection and other clinical features of AIDS is high. **B,** Immune response to HIV infection. A CTL response to HIV is detectable by 2 to 3 weeks after the initial infection and peaks by 9 to 12 weeks. Marked expansion of virus-specific CD8+ T cells occurs during this time, and up to 10% of a patient's CTLs may be HIV specific at 12 weeks. The humoral immune response to HIV peaks at about 12 weeks. (**A,** *From Pantaleo G, Graziosi C, Fauci AS: New concepts in the immunopathogenesis of human immunodeficiency virus infection,* New England Journal of Medicine *328:327-335, 1993. Copyright © 1993 Massachusetts Medical Society. All rights reserved.)*

pathogenesis of HIV infection because many or even most infected T cells may be abortively infected, such that there is no virus production and no direct cytopathic effects.

An important cause of the loss of CD4+ T cells in HIV-infected individuals is the direct effect of infection of these cells by HIV. Death of CD4+ T cells is associated with production of virus in infected cells and is a major cause of the decline in the numbers of these cells, especially in the early (acute) phase of the infection. Several direct toxic effects of HIV on infected CD4+ cells have been described.

- The process of virus production, with expression of gp41 in the plasma membrane and budding of viral particles, may lead to increased plasma membrane permeability and the influx of lethal amounts of calcium, which induces apoptosis, or osmotic lysis of the cell caused by the influx of water.
- Viral production can interfere with cellular protein synthesis and thereby lead to cell death.
- Non-cytopathic (abortive) HIV infection activates the inflammasome pathway and leads to a form of cell death called pyroptosis. During this process, inflammatory cytokines and cellular contents are released, leading to recruitment of new cells and increasing the numbers of cells that can be infected. This form of cell death may play an important role not only in death of infected cells but also in spread of the infection.
- The plasma membranes of HIV-infected T cells fuse with uninfected CD4+ T cells by virtue of gp120-CD4 interactions, and multinucleated giant cells or syncytia are formed. The process of HIV-induced syncytia formation can be lethal to HIV-infected T cells as well as to uninfected CD4+ T cells that fuse to the infected cells. However, this phenomenon has largely been observed in vitro, and syncytia are rarely seen in the tissues of patients with AIDS.

Mechanisms in addition to virus-induced death of infected CD4+ T cells have been proposed for the depletion and functional impairment of these cells in HIV-infected individuals. One mechanism is related to chronic activation of uninfected cells by the infections that are common in patients infected with HIV and also by cytokines produced in response to these infections. Chronic activation of the T cells may predispose the cells to apoptosis; the molecular pathway involved in this type of activation-induced cell death is not yet defined. Apoptotic death of activated lymphocytes may account for the observation that the loss of T cells greatly exceeds the numbers of HIV-infected cells. HIV-specific CTLs are present in many patients with AIDS, and these cells can kill infected CD4+ T cells. In addition, antibodies against HIV envelope proteins may bind to HIV-infected CD4+ T cells and target the cells for antibody-dependent cell-mediated cytotoxicity. Binding of gp120 to newly synthesized intracellular CD4 may interfere with normal protein processing in the endoplasmic reticulum and block cell surface expression of CD4, making the cells incapable of responding to antigenic stimulation. It has also been suggested that the maturation of CD4+ T cells in the thymus becomes defective in infected individuals. The relative importance of these indirect mechanisms of CD4+ T cell depletion in HIV-infected patients is uncertain and controversial.

Functional defects in the immune system of HIV-infected individuals exacerbate the immune deficiency caused by depletion of CD4+ T cells. These functional defects include a decrease in T cell responses to antigens and weak humoral immune responses, even though total serum Ig levels may be elevated. The defects may be a result of the direct effects of HIV infection on CD4+ T cells, including the effects of soluble gp120 released from infected cells binding to uninfected cells. For example, CD4 that has bound gp120 may not be available to interact with class II MHC molecules on APCs, and thus T cell responses to antigens would be inhibited. Alternatively, gp120 binding to CD4 may deliver signals that downregulate helper T cell function. HIV-infected T cells are unable to form tight synapses with APCs, and this may also interfere with T cell activation. Some studies have demonstrated that patients with HIV infection have increased numbers of CD4+CD25+ regulatory T cells, but it is not yet clear if this is a consistent finding or if these cells actually contribute to defective immunity.

The Tat protein may play some role in the pathogenesis of immunodeficiency caused by HIV. Within T cells, Tat can interact with a variety of regulatory proteins, and these interactions can interfere with normal T cell functions such as cytokine synthesis. Remarkably, Tat not only enters the nucleus of infected T cells but can also escape across the plasma membrane and enter neighboring cells, thus interfering with activation of uninfected T cells in a paracrine fashion.

Macrophages, dendritic cells, and follicular dendritic cells may be infected or injured by HIV, and their abnormalities also contribute to the progression of immunodeficiency.

- Macrophages express much lower levels of CD4 than helper T lymphocytes do, but they do express CCR5 coreceptors and are susceptible to HIV infection. However, macrophages are relatively resistant to the cytopathic effects of HIV. Macrophages may also be infected by a gp120/gp41-independent route, such as phagocytosis of other infected cells or Fc receptor–mediated endocytosis of antibody-coated HIV virions. Because macrophages can be infected but are not generally killed by HIV, they may become a reservoir for the virus. In fact, the quantity of macrophage-associated HIV exceeds T cell–associated virus in most tissues from patients with AIDS, including the brain and lung. HIV-infected macrophages may be impaired in antigen presentation functions and cytokine secretion.
- Dendritic cells can also be infected by HIV. Like macrophages, dendritic cells are not directly injured by HIV infection. However, these cells form intimate contact with naive T cells during the course of antigen presentation. It is proposed that dendritic cells infect naive T cells during these encounters and this may be a pathway for spread of the infection.
- Follicular dendritic cells (FDCs) in the germinal centers of lymph nodes and the spleen trap large amounts of HIV on their surfaces, in part by Fc receptor–mediated binding of antibody-coated virus. Although FDCs are not efficiently infected, they contribute to the pathogenesis of HIV-associated immunodeficiency in at least two ways. First, the FDC surface is a reservoir for HIV that can infect macrophages and CD4+ T cells in the lymph nodes. Second, the normal functions of FDCs in immune responses are impaired, and they may eventually be destroyed by the virus. Although the mechanisms of HIV-induced death of FDCs are not understood, the net result of loss of the FDC network in the lymph nodes and spleen is a profound dissolution of the architecture of the peripheral lymphoid system.

HIV Reservoirs and Viral Turnover

The virus detected in patients' blood is produced mostly by short-lived infected CD4+ T cells and in smaller amounts by other infected cells. Three phases of decay of plasma viremia have been observed in patients treated with antiretroviral drugs or predicted by mathematical modeling, and these decay curves have been used to surmise the distribution of HIV in different cellular reservoirs. More than 90% of plasma virus is believed to be produced by short-lived cells (half-lives of ~1 day), which are most likely activated CD4+ T cells that are major reservoirs and sources of the virus in infected patients. About 5% of plasma virus is produced by macrophages, which have a slower turnover (half-life of about 2 weeks). It is hypothesized that a small fraction of the virus, perhaps as little as 1%, is present in latently infected memory T cells. Because of the long life span of memory cells, it could take decades for this reservoir of virus to be eliminated, even if all new rounds of infection were blocked.

Clinical Features of HIV Disease

A vast amount of information has accumulated about the epidemiology and clinical course of HIV infection. As antiretroviral drug therapy is improving, many of the clinical manifestations are changing. In the following section, we will describe the classical features of HIV infection and refer to the changing pictures when relevant.

Transmission of HIV and Epidemiology of AIDS

HIV is transmitted from one individual to another by three major routes:

- *Sexual contact is the most frequent mode of transmission,* either between heterosexual couples (the most frequent mode of transmission in Africa and Asia) or between homosexual male partners. In sub-Saharan Africa, where the infection rate is the highest in the world (estimated to be about 10,000 new cases every day), more than half the infected individuals are women.
- *Mother-to-child transmission* of HIV accounts for the majority of pediatric cases of AIDS. This type of transmission occurs most frequently in utero or during childbirth, although transmission through breast milk is also possible.
- *Inoculation of a recipient with infected blood or blood products* is also a frequent mode of HIV transmission. Needles shared by intravenous drug abusers account for most cases of this form of transmission. With the advent of routine laboratory screening, transfusion of blood or blood products in a clinical setting accounts for a small portion of HIV infections.

Clinical Course of HIV Infection

The course of HIV disease can be followed by measuring the amount of virus in the patient's plasma and by the blood CD4+ T cell count (see Fig. 21-8).

- *The acute phase* of the illness, also called acute HIV syndrome, is the period of viremia characterized by non-specific symptoms of infection. It develops in

50% to 70% of infected adults typically 3 to 6 weeks after infection. There is a spike of plasma virus and a modest reduction in CD4+ T cell counts, but the number of blood CD4+ T cells often returns to normal. In many patients, however, the infection is occult and there are no symptoms.

- *The chronic phase of clinical latency* may last for many years. During this time, the virus is contained within lymphoid tissues, and the loss of CD4+ T cells is corrected by replenishment from progenitors. Patients are asymptomatic or suffer from minor infections. Within 2 to 6 months after infection, the concentration of plasma virus stabilizes at a particular set-point, which differs among patients. The level of the viral set-point and the number of blood CD4+ T cells are clinically useful predictors of the progression of disease. As the disease progresses, patients become susceptible to other infections, and immune responses to these infections may stimulate HIV production and accelerate the destruction of lymphoid tissues. As discussed earlier, HIV gene transcription can be enhanced by stimuli that activate T cells, such as antigens and various cytokines. Cytokines, such as TNF, which are produced during the innate immune response to microbial infections, are particularly effective in boosting HIV production. Thus, as the immune system attempts to eradicate other microbes, it brings about its own destruction by HIV.

- *HIV disease progresses to the final and once almost invariably lethal phase, called AIDS, when the blood CD4+ T cell count drops below 200 cells/mm³.* HIV viremia may climb dramatically as viral replication accelerates unchecked in reservoirs other than T cells. Patients with AIDS suffer from combinations of opportunistic infections, neoplasms, cachexia (HIV wasting syndrome), kidney failure (HIV nephropathy), and CNS degeneration (AIDS encephalopathy) (Table 21-7). Because CD4+ helper T cells are essential for both cell-mediated and humoral immune responses to various microbes, the loss of these lymphocytes is the main reason that patients with AIDS become susceptible to many different types of infections. Furthermore, many of the tumors that arise in patients with AIDS have a viral etiology, and their prevalence in the setting of AIDS reflects an inability of the HIV-infected patient to mount an effective immune response against oncogenic viruses. Cachexia is often seen in patients with chronic inflammatory diseases and may result from effects of inflammatory cytokines (such as TNF) on appetite and metabolism. The CNS disease in AIDS may be due to neuronal damage by the virus or by shed viral proteins such as gp120 and Tat, as well as the effects of cytokines elaborated by infected microglial cells. Many of these devastating consequences of HIV infection, including opportunistic infections and tumors, have been significantly reduced by highly active antiretroviral therapy.

Although this summary of the clinical course is true for the most severe cases, the rate of progression of the disease is highly variable, and some individuals are long-term non-progressors. The immunologic correlates of variable progression remain unknown. Also, recent

TABLE 21-7	Clinical Features of HIV Infection
Phase of Disease	**Clinical Feature**
Acute HIV disease	Fever, headaches, sore throat with pharyngitis, generalized lymphadenopathy, rashes
Clinical latency period	Declining blood CD4+ T cell count

AIDS	Opportunistic infections
	  Protozoa *(Toxoplasma, Cryptosporidium)*
	  Bacteria *(Mycobacterium avium, Nocardia, Salmonella)*
	  Fungi *(Candida, Cryptococcus neoformans, Coccidioides immitis, Histoplasma capsulatum, Pneumocystis)*
	  Viruses (cytomegalovirus, herpes simplex, varicella-zoster)
	Tumors
	  Lymphomas (including EBV-associated B cell lymphomas)
	  Kaposi's sarcoma
	  Cervical carcinoma
	Encephalopathy
	Wasting syndrome

antiretroviral therapy has changed the course of the disease and greatly reduced the incidence of severe opportunistic infections (such as *Pneumocystis*) and tumors (such as Kaposi's sarcoma).

Immune Responses to HIV

HIV-specific humoral and cell-mediated immune responses develop after infection but generally provide limited protection. The early response to HIV infection is, in fact, similar in many ways to the immune response to other viruses and serves to clear most of the virus present in the blood and in circulating T cells. Nonetheless, it is clear that these immune responses fail to eradicate all virus, and the infection eventually overwhelms the immune system in most individuals. Despite the poor effectiveness of immune responses to the virus, it is important to characterize them for three reasons. First, the immune responses may be detrimental to the host, for example, by stimulating the uptake of opsonized virus into uninfected cells by Fc receptor–mediated endocytosis or by eradication of CD4+ T cells expressing viral antigens by CD8+ CTLs. Second, antibodies against HIV are diagnostic markers of HIV infection that are widely used for screening purposes. Third, the design of effective vaccines for immunization against HIV requires knowledge of the types of immune responses that are most likely to be protective (the correlates of protection).

Many innate immune responses against HIV have been described. These include production of antimicrobial peptides (defensins), and activation of NK cells, dendritic cells (particularly plasmacytoid dendritic cells producing type I interferons), and the complement system. The role of these responses in combating the infection is not established.

The initial adaptive immune response to HIV infection is characterized by expansion of CD8+ T cells specific for HIV peptides. As many as 10% or more of circulating

CD8$^+$ T cells may be specific for HIV during acute infection. These CTLs control infection in the early phase (see Fig. 21-8) but ultimately prove ineffective because of the emergence of viral escape mutants (variants with mutated antigens). CD4$^+$ T cells also respond to the virus, and these CD4$^+$ T cells may contribute to viral control in a number of ways. An effective CD4$^+$ T cell response is required as a source of help for the generation of CD8$^+$ memory T cells, but CD4$^+$ T cells have also been shown to mediate cytolytic responses against HIV-infected cells, perhaps using Fas ligand to target Fas on infected CD4$^+$ T cells.

The importance of CTL responses in HIV control is underscored by the evolution of the virus under immune pressure, resulting in viral isolates that have lost their original CTL epitopes. The evolution of the virus also results in the loss of epitopes recognized by CD4$^+$ T cells, indicating that both CD8$^+$ and CD4$^+$ cells contribute to host defense against the virus.

Antibody responses to a variety of HIV antigens are detectable within 6 to 9 weeks after infection. The most immunogenic HIV molecules that elicit antibody responses appear to be the envelope glycoproteins, and high titers of anti-gp120 and anti-gp41 antibodies are present in most HIV-infected individuals. Other anti-HIV antibodies found frequently in patients' sera include antibodies to p24, reverse transcriptase, and *gag* and *pol* products (see Fig. 20-8). The effect of these antibodies on the clinical course of HIV infection is uncertain. The early antibodies are generally not neutralizing and are thus poor inhibitors of viral infectivity or cytopathic effects. Neutralizing antibodies against gp120 develop 2 to 3 months after primary infection, but even these antibodies cannot cope with a virus that is able to rapidly change the most immunodominant epitopes of its envelope glycoproteins. Sequencing of antibody heavy- and light-chain genes from gp-140–specific B cells in subjects who have been infected with HIV-1 for a few years has revealed the presence of broadly neutralizing antibodies. These antibodies bind to a site on a viral protein that the virus cannot afford to mutate, for example, the CD4 binding site of gp140. They are, therefore, effective in clearing the virus. A striking feature of all of these antibodies is that they have been selected after extensive somatic hypermutation, implying helper T cell–dependent antibody responses. The implication is that the starting naive HIV-specific B cell repertoire primarily consists of B cells whose antigen receptors bind weakly to certain antigenic epitopes such as the CD4 binding site of gp140. Many rounds of somatic hypermutation and selection that may occur in a long-standing infection can eventually generate B cell populations that bind with high affinity to the original weakly recognized epitope. One of the goals of vaccination is to generate such high-affinity broadly neutralizing antibodies, but so far this has not been achieved with any consistency.

Mechanisms of Immune Evasion by HIV

HIV is the prototype of an infectious pathogen that evades host defenses by destroying the immune system. In addition, several features of HIV may help the virus to evade host immunity.

HIV has an extremely high mutation rate because of error-prone reverse transcription, and in this way it may evade detection by antibodies or T cells generated in response to viral proteins. It has been estimated that in an infected person, every possible point mutation in the viral genome occurs every day. A region of the gp120 molecule, called the V3 loop, is one of the most antigenically variable parts of the virus; it differs even in HIV isolates taken from the same individual at different times. Many epitopes of the virus that could potentially serve as targets for broadly neutralizing antibodies are also shielded by bulky N-linked sugars that make up what is known as the HIV-glycan shield.

HIV-infected cells may evade CTLs through down-regulation of class I MHC molecule expression. The HIV Nef protein inhibits expression of class I MHC molecules, mainly by promoting internalization of these molecules. Other mechanisms of inhibiting cell-mediated immunity have been demonstrated in some cases. As mentioned earlier, these include a preferential inhibition of T$_H$1 cytokines, activation of regulatory T cells, and suppression of dendritic cell functions. The mechanisms of these actions of the virus as well as their pathogenic significance are not established.

Elite Controllers and Long-Term Non-Progressors: A Possible Role for Host Genes

Although most individuals infected with HIV eventually develop AIDS, approximately 1% of individuals who are infected do not develop disease. Such individuals have high CD4$^+$ and CD8$^+$ T cell counts, do not require therapy, and have persistent viremia but no disease for at least 10 to 15 years. On the basis of the degree of viremia, this group can be divided into two subsets: long-term non-progressors have detectable viremia of around 5000 copies of HIV-1 RNA per milliliter of blood; and a much smaller subset of elite controllers present with viral loads of about 50 copies or less of HIV-1 RNA per milliliter of blood. There is considerable interest in understanding the genetic basis of HIV control by examining these cohorts of individuals in detail. So far, a strong role for the MHC locus in protecting individuals and preventing progression has been suggested by genetic association studies. Specific HLA class I and some HLA class II loci have been linked to the absence of disease progression. We have previously mentioned the importance of the inheritance of the CCR5 homozygous 32-bp deletion in protection from infection, and other genetic factors contributing to resistance are likely to be revealed in the coming years.

Treatment and Prevention of AIDS and Vaccine Development

Active research efforts have been aimed at developing reagents that interfere with the viral life cycle. Treatment of HIV infection and AIDS now typically involves the administration of three antiviral drugs, used in combination, that target viral molecules for which no human homologues exist. The first antiretroviral drugs to be widely used were nucleoside analogues that inhibit viral reverse transcriptase activity. These drugs include deoxythymidine nucleoside analogues such as 3′-azido-3′-deoxythymidine (AZT), deoxycytidine nucleoside analogues, and deoxyadenosine analogues. When these drugs are used alone, they are often effective in significantly reducing plasma HIV RNA levels for several months to years, but they usually do not halt progression of HIV-induced disease, largely because of the evolution of virus with mutated forms of reverse transcriptase that are resistant to the drugs. Non-nucleoside reverse transcriptase inhibitors directly bind to the enzyme and inhibit its function. Viral protease inhibitors have been developed that block the processing of precursor proteins into mature viral capsid and core proteins. When these protease inhibitors are used alone, mutant viruses resistant to their effects emerge. However, protease inhibitors are now a common component of a three-drug therapeutic regimen with two different reverse transcriptase inhibitors. This new triple-drug therapy, commonly referred to as HAART (highly active antiretroviral therapy) or ART (antiretroviral therapy), has proved to be effective in reducing plasma viral RNA to undetectable levels in most treated patients for years. An integrase inhibitor is now also available for antiviral therapy. Entry inhibitors, which prevent viral entry by targeting either CD4 or CCR5 on the host cell or gp41 or gp120 on the virus, are another novel category of therapeutics. Drugs that target gp41 include compounds that prevent fusion of the viral envelope with the host cell plasma membrane. Although antiretroviral therapy has reduced viral titers to below detection for up to 10 years in some patients, it is unlikely that such treatment can eliminate the virus from all reservoirs (especially long-lived infected cells), and resistance to the drugs may ultimately develop. Other formidable problems associated with these new drug therapies, which will impair their effective use in many parts of the world, include high expense, complicated administration schedules, and significant adverse effects.

The individual infections experienced by patients with AIDS are treated with the appropriate prophylaxis, antibiotics, and supportive measures. More aggressive antibiotic therapy is often required than for similar infections in less compromised hosts.

Efforts at prevention of HIV infection are extremely important and potentially effective in controlling the HIV epidemic. In the United States, the routine screening of blood products for evidence of donor HIV infection has already reduced the risk of this mode of transmission to negligible levels. Various public health measures to increase condom use and to reduce the use of contaminated needles by intravenous drug users are now widespread. Perhaps the most effective efforts at prevention are campaigns to increase public awareness of HIV. Recent clinical trials have shown that administration of antiretroviral drugs to pregnant mothers is effective at preventing infection of the newborns. Prophylactic use of these drugs in high-risk patients also reduces the rate of infection.

The development of an effective vaccine against HIV is a priority for biomedical research institutions worldwide. The task has been complicated by the ability of the virus to mutate and vary many of its immunogenic antigens. It is likely that an effective vaccine will have to stimulate both humoral and cell-mediated responses to viral antigens that are critical for the viral life cycle. To achieve this goal, several approaches are being tried for HIV vaccine development. Much of the preliminary work has involved simian immunodeficiency virus (SIV) infection of macaques, and effective vaccines against SIV have already been developed. This success is encouraging because SIV is molecularly closely related to HIV and causes a disease in macaques that is similar to AIDS in humans. Various live virus vaccines have been tested in the hope that they will induce strong CTL responses. Such vaccines include non-virulent recombinant hybrid viruses composed of part SIV and part HIV sequences or viruses that have been attenuated by deletions in one or more parts of the viral genome, such as the *nef* gene. One concern with live virus vaccines is their potential to cause disease if they are not completely attenuated and possibly to recombine with wild-type HIV to produce a pathogenic variant. Another approach that avoids this safety concern but retains efficacy in inducing CTL-mediated immunity is the use of live recombinant non-HIV viral vectors carrying HIV genes. Preliminary trials in human volunteers have shown that canarypox vaccines expressing several HIV-1 genes can induce strong CTL responses to the HIV antigens. Many DNA vaccines have also been studied; these vaccines are composed of combinations of structural and regulatory genes of SIV or HIV packaged in mammalian DNA expression vectors. Combinations of vaccines, such as initial immunization with a DNA vaccine followed by boosting with a canarypox vector expressing HIV genes, have yielded some of the most promising results to date. Recombinant protein or peptide subunit vaccines that elicit antibodies have so far been of limited value because the antibodies induced by these vaccines typically do not neutralize clinical isolates of HIV.

SUMMARY

* Immunodeficiency diseases are caused by congenital or acquired defects in lymphocytes, phagocytes, and other mediators of adaptive and innate immunity. These diseases are associated with an increased susceptibility to infection, the nature and severity of which depend largely on which component of the immune system is abnormal and the extent of the abnormality.
* Disorders of innate immunity include defects in microbial killing by phagocytes (e.g., CGD or Chédiak-Higashi syndrome), leukocyte migration and adhesion (e.g., leukocyte adhesion deficiency), TLR signaling, and complement.
* Severe combined immunodeficiencies include defects in lymphocyte development that affect both T and B cells and are caused by defective cytokine signaling, abnormal purine metabolism, defective V(D)J recombination, and mutations that affect T cell maturation.
* Antibody immunodeficiencies include diseases caused by defective B cell maturation or activation

and defects in T cell–B cell collaboration (X-linked hyper-IgM syndrome).

* T cell immunodeficiencies include diseases in which the expression of MHC molecules is defective, T cell signaling disorders, and rare diseases involving CTL and NK cell functions.

* Treatment of congenital immunodeficiencies involves transfusions of antibodies, bone marrow or stem cell transplantation, or enzyme replacement. Gene therapy may offer improved treatments in the future.

* Acquired immunodeficiencies are caused by infections, malnutrition, disseminated cancer, and immunosuppressive therapy for transplant rejection or autoimmune diseases.

* AIDS is a severe immunodeficiency caused by infection with HIV. This retrovirus infects CD4+ T lymphocytes, macrophages, and dendritic cells and causes progressive dysfunction of the immune system. Most of the immunodeficiency in AIDS can be attributed to the depletion of CD4+ T cells.

* HIV enters cells by binding to both the CD4 molecule and a coreceptor of the chemokine receptor family. Once it is inside the cell, the viral genome is reverse-transcribed into DNA and incorporated into the cellular genome. Viral gene transcription and viral reproduction are stimulated by signals that normally activate the host cell. Production of virus is accompanied by death of infected cells.

* The acute phase of infection is characterized by death of memory CD4+ T cells in mucosal tissues and dissemination of the virus to lymph nodes. In the subsequent latent phase, there is low-level virus replication in lymphoid tissues and slow, progressive loss of T cells. Persistent activation of T cells promotes their death, leading to rapid loss and immune deficiency in the chronic phase of the infection.

* CD4+ T cell depletion in HIV-infected individuals is due to direct cytopathic effects of the virus, toxic effects of viral products such as shed gp120, and indirect effects such as activation-induced cell death or CTL killing of infected CD4+ cells.

* Several reservoirs of HIV exist in infected individuals, including short-lived activated CD4+ T cells, longer-lived macrophages, and very long-lived, latently infected memory T cells.

* HIV-induced depletion of CD4+ T cells results in increased susceptibility to infection by a number of opportunistic microorganisms. In addition, HIV-infected patients have an increased incidence of tumors, particularly Kaposi's sarcoma and EBV-associated B cell lymphomas, and encephalopathy. The incidence of these complications has been greatly reduced by antiretroviral therapy.

* HIV has a high mutation rate, which allows the virus to evade host immune responses and become resistant to drug therapies. Genetic variability also poses a problem for the design of an effective vaccine against HIV. HIV infection can be treated by a combination of inhibitors of viral enzymes.

SELECTED READINGS

Congenital (Primary) Immunodeficiencies

Blackburn MR, Kellems RE: Adenosine deaminase deficiency: metabolic basis of immune deficiency and pulmonary inflammation, *Advances in Immunology* 86:1–4, 2005.

Casanova J-L, Abel L: The genetic theory of infectious diseases: a brief history and selected illustrations, *Annual Review of Genomics and Human Genetics* 14:215–243, 2013.

Castigli E, Geha RS: Molecular basis of common variable immunodeficiency, *Journal of Allergy and Clinical Immunology* 117:740–746, 2006.

Chen X, Jensen PE: MHC class II antigen presentation and immunological abnormalities due to deficiency of MHC class II and its associated genes, *Experimental and Molecular Pathology* 85:40–44, 2008.

Conley ME, Dobbs AK, Farmer DM, Kilic S, Paris K, Grigoriadou S, Coustan-Smith E, Howard V, Campana D: Primary B cell immunodeficiencies: comparisons and contrasts, *Annual Review of Immunology* 27:199–227, 2009.

Durandy A, Kracker S, Fischer A: Primary antibody deficiencies, *Nature Reviews Immunology* 13:519–533, 2013.

Janka GE: Hemophagocytic lymphohistiocytosis, *Hematology* 10(suppl 1):104–107, 2005.

Lavin MF: Ataxia-telangiectasia: from a rare disorder to a paradigm for cell signaling and cancer, *Nature Reviews Molecular and Cell Biology* 9:759–769, 2008.

Milner JD, Holland SM: The cup runneth over: lessons from the ever-expanding pool of primary immunodeficiency diseases, *Nature Reviews Immunology* 13:635–668, 2013.

Notarangelo LD: Functional T cell immunodeficiencies (with T cells present), *Annual Review of Immunology* 31:195–225, 2013.

Ochs HD, Thrasher AJ: The Wiskott-Aldrich syndrome, *Journal of Allergy and Clinical Immunology* 117:725–738, 2006.

Parvaneh N, Casanova JL, Notarangelo LD, Conley ME: Primary immunodeficiencies: a rapidly evolving story, *Journal of Allergy and Clinical Immunology* 131:314–323, 2013.

Puel A, Yang K, Ku CL, et al.: Heritable defects of the human TLR signaling pathways, *Journal of Endotoxin Research* 11:220–224, 2005.

HIV and AIDS

Barouch DH: Challenges in the development of an HIV-1 vaccine, *Nature* 455:613–619, 2008.

Brenchley JM, Price DA, Douek DC: HIV disease: fallout from a mucosal catastrophe? *Nature Immunology* 7:235–239, 2006.

Douek DC, Roederer M, Koup RA: Emerging concepts in the immunopathogenesis of AIDS, *Annual Review of Medicine* 60:471, 2009.

Haase AT: Perils at mucosal front lines for HIV and SIV and their hosts, *Nature Reviews Immunology* 5:783–792, 2005.

Hladik F, McElrath MJ: Setting the stage: host invasion by HIV, *Nature Reviews Immunology* 8:447–457, 2008.

Johnston MI, Fauci AS: An HIV vaccine—evolving concepts, *New England Journal of Medicine* 356:2073–2081, 2007.

Kwong PD, Mascola JR, Nabel GJ: Broadly neutralizing antibodies and the search for an HIV-1 vaccine: the end of the beginning, *Nature Reviews Immunology* 13:693–701, 2013.

Lusso P: HIV and the chemokine system: 10 years later, *EMBO Journal* 25:447–456, 2006.

Mascola JR, Montefiori DC: The role of antibodies in HIV vaccines, *Annual Review of Immunology* 28:413–444, 2010.

McMichael AJ, Borrow P, Tomaras GD, Goonetilleke N, Haynes BF: The immune response during acute HIV-1 infection: clues for vaccine development, *Nature Reviews Immunology* 10:11–23, 2010.

Nixon DF, Aandahl EM, Michaelsson J: CD4+CD25+ regulatory T cells in HIV infection, *Microbes and Infection* 7:1063–1065, 2005.

Walker B, McMichael A: The T-cell response to HIV, *Cold Spring Harb Perspect Med* 2:a007054, 2012.

Walker BD, Yu XG: Unraveling the mechanisms of durable control of HIV-1, *Nature Reviews Immunology* 13:487–498, 2013.

GLOSSARY

αβ T cell receptor (αβ TCR) The most common form of TCR, expressed on both CD4⁺ and CD8⁺ T cells. The αβ TCR recognizes peptide antigen bound to an MHC molecule. Both α and β chains contain highly variable (V) regions that together form the antigen-binding site as well as constant (C) regions. TCR V and C regions are structurally homologous to the V and C regions of Ig molecules.

ABO blood group antigens Carbohydrate antigens attached mainly to cell surface proteins or lipids that are present on many cell types, including red blood cells. These antigens differ among individuals, depending on inherited alleles encoding the enzymes required for synthesis of the carbohydrate antigens. The ABO antigens act as alloantigens that are responsible for blood transfusion reactions and hyperacute rejection of allografts.

Acquired immunodeficiency A deficiency in the immune system that is acquired after birth, usually because of infection (e.g., AIDS), and that is not related to a genetic defect. Synonymous with **secondary immunodeficiency.**

Acquired immunodeficiency syndrome (AIDS) A disease caused by human immunodeficiency virus (HIV) infection that is characterized by depletion of CD4⁺ T cells, leading to a profound defect in cell-mediated immunity. Clinically, AIDS includes opportunistic infections, malignant tumors, wasting, and encephalopathy.

Activation-induced cell death (AICD) Apoptosis of activated lymphocytes, generally used for T cells.

Activation-induced (cytidine) deaminase (AID) An enzyme expressed in B cells that catalyzes the conversion of cytosine into uracil in DNA, which is a step required for somatic hypermutation and affinity maturation of antibodies and for Ig class switching.

Activation protein 1 (AP-1) A family of DNA-binding transcription factors composed of dimers of two proteins that bind to one another through a shared structural motif called a leucine zipper. The best-characterized AP-1 factor is composed of the proteins Fos and Jun. AP-1 is involved in transcriptional regulation of many different genes that are important in the immune system, such as cytokine genes.

Active immunity The form of adaptive immunity that is induced by exposure to a foreign antigen and activation of lymphocytes and in which the immunized individual plays an active role in responding to the antigen. This type contrasts with passive immunity, in which an individual receives antibodies or lymphocytes from another individual who was previously actively immunized.

Acute-phase reactants Proteins, mostly synthesized in the liver in response to inflammatory cytokines such as IL-6 and IL-1, whose plasma concentrations increase shortly after infection as part of the systemic inflammatory response syndrome. Examples include C-reactive protein, fibrinogen, and serum amyloid A protein. The acute-phase reactants play various roles in the innate immune response to microbes.

Acute-phase response The increase in plasma concentrations of several proteins, called acute-phase reactants, that occurs as part of the early innate immune response to infections.

Acute rejection A form of graft rejection involving vascular and parenchymal injury mediated by T cells, macrophages, and antibodies that usually occurs days or weeks after transplantation, but may occur later if pharmacologic immunosuppression becomes inadequate.

Adaptive immunity The form of immunity that is mediated by lymphocytes and stimulated by exposure to infectious agents. In contrast to innate immunity, adaptive immunity is characterized by exquisite specificity for distinct macromolecules and by memory, which is the ability to respond more vigorously to repeated exposure to the same microbe. Adaptive immunity is also called specific immunity or acquired immunity.

Adaptor protein Proteins involved in intracellular signal transduction pathways by serving as bridge molecules or scaffolds for the recruitment of other signaling molecules. During lymphocyte antigen receptor or cytokine receptor signaling, adaptor molecules may be phosphorylated on tyrosine residues to enable them to bind other proteins containing Src homology 2 (SH2) domains. Adaptor molecules involved in T cell activation include LAT, SLP-76, and Grb-2.

Addressin Adhesion molecule expressed on endothelial cells in different anatomic sites that directs organ-specific lymphocyte homing. Mucosal addressin cell adhesion molecule 1 (MadCAM-1) is an example of an addressin expressed in Peyer's patches in the intestinal wall that binds to the integrin $\alpha_4\beta_7$ on gut-homing T cells.

Adhesion molecule A cell surface molecule whose function is to promote adhesive interactions with other cells or the extracellular matrix. Leukocytes express various types of adhesion molecules, such as selectins, integrins, and members of the Ig superfamily, and these molecules play crucial roles in cell migration and cellular activation in innate and adaptive immune responses.

Adjuvant A substance, distinct from antigen, that enhances T and B cell activation mainly by promoting the accumulation and activation of antigen-presenting cells (APCs) at the site of antigen exposure. Adjuvants stimulate expression of T cell–activating costimulators and cytokines by APCs and may also prolong the expression of peptide-MHC complexes on the surface of APCs.

Adoptive transfer The process of transferring cells from one individual into another or back into the same individual after in vitro expansion and activation. Adoptive transfer is used in research to define the role of a particular cell population (e.g., T cells) in an immune response. Clinically, adoptive transfer of tumor-reactive T lymphocytes and tumor antigen–presenting dendritic cells is used in experimental cancer therapy, and trials of adoptive transfer of regulatory T cells are ongoing.

Affinity The strength of the binding between a single binding site of a molecule (e.g., an antibody) and a ligand (e.g., an antigen). The affinity of a molecule X for a ligand Y is represented by the dissociation constant (K_d), which is the concentration of Y that is required to occupy the combining sites of half the X molecules present in a solution. A smaller K_d indicates a stronger or higher affinity interaction, and a lower concentration of ligand is needed to occupy the sites.

Affinity maturation The process that leads to increased affinity of antibodies for a particular antigen as a T cell–dependent antibody response progresses. Affinity maturation takes place in germinal centers of lymphoid tissues and is the result of somatic mutation of *Ig* genes, followed by selective survival of the B cells producing the highest affinity antibodies.

Allele One of different forms of the same gene present at a particular chromosomal locus. An individual who is heterozygous at a locus has two different alleles, each on a different member of a pair of chromosomes, one inherited from the mother and one from the father. If a particular gene in a population has different alleles, the gene or locus is said to be polymorphic. MHC genes have many alleles (i.e., they are highly polymorphic).

Allelic exclusion The exclusive expression of only one of two inherited alleles encoding Ig heavy and light chains and TCR β chains. Allelic exclusion occurs when the protein product of one productively recombined antigen receptor locus on one chromosome blocks rearrangement of the corresponding locus on the other chromosome. This property ensures that each lymphocyte will express a single antigen receptor and that all antigen receptors expressed by one clone of lymphocytes will have the identical specificity. Because the TCR α chain locus does not show allelic exclusion, some T cells do express two different types of TCR.

Allergen An antigen that elicits an immediate hypersensitivity (allergic) reaction. Allergens are proteins or chemicals bound to proteins that induce IgE antibody responses in atopic individuals.

Allergy A disorder caused by an immediate hypersensitivity reaction, often named according to the type of antigen (allergen) that elicits the disease, such as food allergy, bee sting allergy, and penicillin allergy. All of these conditions are the result of IgE production stimulated by IL-4–producing helper T cells, followed by allergen and IgE-dependent mast cell activation.

Alloantibody An antibody specific for an alloantigen (i.e., an antigen present in some individuals of a species but not in others).

Alloantigen A cell or tissue antigen that is present in some individuals of a species but not in others and that is recognized as foreign on an allograft. Alloantigens are usually products of polymorphic genes.

Alloantiserum The alloantibody-containing serum of an individual who has previously been exposed to one or more alloantigens.

Allogeneic graft An organ or tissue graft from a donor who is of the same species but genetically non-identical to the recipient (also called an allograft).

Alloreactive Reactive to alloantigens; describes T cells or antibodies from one individual that will recognize antigens on cells or tissues of another genetically non-identical individual.

Allotype The property of a group of antibody molecules defined by their sharing of a particular antigenic determinant found on the antibodies of some individuals but not others. Such determinants are called **allotopes**. Antibodies that share a particular allotope belong to the same allotype. *Allotype* is also often used synonymously with *allotope*.

Alternative macrophage activation Macrophage activation by IL-4 and IL-13 leading to an anti-inflammatory and tissue-reparative phenotype, in contrast to classical macrophage activation by interferon-γ and TLR ligands.

Alternative pathway of complement activation An antibody-independent pathway of activation of the complement system that occurs when the C3b protein binds to microbial cell surfaces. The alternative pathway is a component of the innate immune system and mediates inflammatory responses to infection as well as direct lysis of microbes.

Anaphylatoxins The C5a, C4a, and C3a complement fragments that are generated during complement activation. The anaphylatoxins bind specific cell surface receptors and promote acute inflammation by stimulating neutrophil chemotaxis and activating mast cells.

Anaphylaxis A severe form of immediate hypersensitivity in which there is systemic mast cell or basophil activation, and the released mediators cause bronchial constriction, tissue edema, and cardiovascular collapse.

Anchor residues The amino acid residues of a peptide whose side chains fit into pockets in the peptide-binding cleft of an MHC molecule. The side chains bind to complementary amino acids in the MHC molecule and therefore serve to anchor the peptide in the cleft of the MHC molecule.

Anergy A state of unresponsiveness to antigenic stimulation. Lymphocyte anergy (also called clonal anergy) is the failure of clones of T or B cells to react to antigen and is a mechanism of maintaining immunologic tolerance to self. Clinically, anergy describes the lack of T cell–dependent cutaneous delayed-type hypersensitivity reactions to common antigens.

Angiogenesis New blood vessel formation regulated by a variety of protein factors elaborated by cells of the innate and adaptive immune systems and often accompanying chronic inflammation.

Antibody A type of glycoprotein molecule, also called immunoglobulin (Ig), produced by B lymphocytes that binds antigens, often with a high degree of specificity and affinity. The basic structural unit of an antibody is composed of two identical heavy chains and two identical light chains. The N-terminal variable regions of the heavy and light chains form the antigen-binding sites, whereas the C-terminal constant regions of the heavy chains functionally interact with other molecules in the immune system. Every individual has millions of different antibodies, each with a unique antigen-binding site. Secreted antibodies perform various effector functions, including neutralizing antigens, activating complement, and promoting leukocyte-dependent destruction of microbes.

Antibody-dependent cell-mediated cytotoxicity (ADCC) A process by which NK cells are targeted to IgG-coated cells, resulting in lysis of the antibody-coated cells. A specific receptor for the constant region of IgG, called FcγRIII (CD16), is expressed on the NK cell membrane and mediates binding to the IgG.

Antibody feedback The downregulation of antibody production by secreted IgG antibodies that occurs when antigen-antibody complexes simultaneously engage B cell membrane Ig and one type of Fcγ receptor (FcγRIIb). Under these conditions, the cytoplasmic tail of FcγRIIb transduces inhibitory signals inside the B cell.

Antibody repertoire The collection of different antibody specificities expressed in an individual.

Antibody-secreting cell A B lymphocyte that has undergone differentiation and produces the secretory form of Ig. Antibody-secreting cells are generated from naive B cells in response to antigen and reside in the spleen and lymph nodes as well as in the bone marrow. Often used synonymously with plasma cells.

Antigen A molecule that binds to an antibody or a TCR. Antigens that bind to antibodies include all classes of molecules. Most TCRs bind only peptide fragments of proteins complexed with MHC molecules; both the peptide ligand and the native protein from which it is derived are called **T cell antigens**.

Antigen presentation The display of peptides bound by MHC molecules on the surface of an APC that permits specific recognition by TCRs and activation of T cells.

Antigen-presenting cell (APC) A cell that displays peptide fragments of protein antigens, in association with MHC molecules, on its surface and activates antigen-specific T cells. In addition to displaying peptide-MHC complexes, APCs also express costimulatory molecules to optimally activate T lymphocytes.

Antigen processing The intracellular conversion of protein antigens derived from the extracellular space or the cytosol into peptides and loading of these peptides onto MHC molecules for display to T lymphocytes.

Antigenic variation The process by which antigens expressed by microbes may change by various genetic mechanisms, and therefore allow the microbe to evade immune responses. One example of antigenic variation is the change in influenza virus surface proteins hemagglutinin and neuraminidase, which necessitates the use of new vaccines each year.

Antiserum Serum from an individual previously immunized with an antigen that contains antibody specific for that antigen.

Antiretroviral therapy (ART) Combination chemotherapy for HIV infection, usually consisting of two nucleoside reverse transcriptase inhibitors and either one viral protease inhibitor or one non-nucleoside reverse transcriptase inhibitor. ART can reduce plasma virus titers to below detectable levels for more than 1 year and slow the progression of HIV disease.

Apoptosis A process of cell death characterized by activation of intracellular caspases, DNA cleavage, nuclear condensation and fragmentation, and plasma membrane blebbing that leads to phagocytosis of cell fragments without inducing an inflammatory response. This type of cell death is important in development of lymphocytes, return to homeostasis after an immune response to an infection, maintenance of tolerance to self antigens, and killing of infected cells by cytotoxic T lymphocytes and natural killer cells.

Arthus reaction A localized form of experimental immune complex–mediated vasculitis induced by injection of an antigen subcutaneously into a previously immunized animal or into an animal that has been given intravenous antibody specific for the antigen. Circulating antibodies bind to the injected antigen and form immune complexes that are deposited in the walls of small arteries at the injection site and give rise to a local cutaneous vasculitis with necrosis.

Atopy The propensity of an individual to produce IgE antibodies in response to various environmental antigens and to develop strong immediate hypersensitivity (allergic) responses. People who have allergies to environmental antigens, such as pollen or house dust, are said to be atopic.

Autoantibody An antibody produced in an individual that is specific for a self antigen. Autoantibodies can cause damage to cells and tissues and are produced in excess in systemic autoimmune diseases, such as systemic lupus erythematosus.

Autocrine factor A molecule that acts on the same cell that produces the factor. For example, IL-2 is an autocrine T cell growth factor that stimulates mitotic activity of the T cell that produces it.

Autoimmune disease A disease caused by a breakdown of self-tolerance such that the adaptive immune system responds to self antigens and mediates cell and tissue damage. Autoimmune diseases can be caused by immune attack against one organ or tissue (e.g., multiple sclerosis, thyroiditis, or type 1 diabetes) or against multiple and systemically distributed antigens (e.g., systemic lupus erythematosus).

Autoimmune regulator (AIRE) A protein that functions to stimulate expression of peripheral tissue protein antigens in thymic medullary epithelial cells. Mutations in the *AIRE* gene in humans and mice lead to tissue-specific autoimmune disease because of defective expression of tissue antigens in the thymus and failure to delete T cells specific for these antigens.

Autoimmunity The state of adaptive immune system responsiveness to self antigens that occurs when mechanisms of self-tolerance fail.

Autologous graft A tissue or organ graft in which the donor and recipient are the same individual. Autologous bone marrow and skin grafts are performed in clinical medicine.

Autophagy The normal process by which a cell degrades its own components by lysosomal catabolism. Autophagy plays a role in innate immune defense against infections, and polymorphisms of genes that regulate autophagy are linked to risk for some autoimmune diseases.

Avidity The overall strength of interaction between two molecules, such as an antibody and antigen. Avidity depends on both the affinity and the valency of interactions. Therefore, the avidity of a pentameric IgM antibody, with 10 antigen-binding sites, for a multivalent antigen may be much greater than the avidity of a dimeric IgG molecule for the same antigen. Avidity can be used to describe the strength of cell-cell interactions, which are mediated by many binding interactions between cell surface molecules.

B-1 lymphocytes A subset of B lymphocytes that develop earlier during ontogeny than do conventional B cells, express a limited repertoire of V genes with little junctional diversity, and secrete IgM antibodies that bind T-independent antigens. Many B-1 cells express the CD5 (Ly-1) molecule.

B lymphocyte The only cell type capable of producing antibody molecules and therefore the mediator of humoral immune responses. B lymphocytes, or B cells, develop in the bone marrow, and mature B cells are found mainly in lymphoid follicles in secondary lymphoid tissues, in bone marrow, and in low numbers in the circulation.

Bare lymphocyte syndrome An immunodeficiency disease characterized by a lack of class II MHC molecule expression that leads to defects in antigen presentation and cell-mediated immunity. The disease is caused by mutations in genes encoding factors that regulate class II MHC gene transcription.

Basophil A type of bone marrow–derived circulating granulocyte with structural and functional similarities to mast cells that has granules containing many of the same inflammatory mediators as mast cells and expresses a high-affinity Fc receptor for IgE. Basophils that are recruited into tissue sites where antigen is present may contribute to immediate hypersensitivity reactions.

Bcl-6 A transcriptional repressor that is required for germinal center B cell development and for T_{FH} development.

Bcl-2 family proteins A family of partially homologous cytoplasmic and mitochondrial membrane proteins that regulate apoptosis by influencing mitochondrial outer membrane permeability. Members of this family can be pro-apoptotic (such as Bax, Bad, and Bak) or anti-apoptotic (such as Bcl-2 and Bcl-X_L).

BCR (B cell receptor) The cell surface antigen receptor on B lymphocytes, which is a membrane bound immunoglobulin molecule.

BCR (B cell receptor) complex A multiprotein complex expressed on the surface of B lymphocytes that recognizes antigen and transduces activating signals into the cell. The BCR complex includes membrane Ig, which is responsible for binding antigen, and Igα and Igβ proteins, which initiate signaling events.

Biogenic amines Low–molecular-weight non-lipid compounds, such as histamine, that all have an amine group, are stored in and released from the cytoplasmic granules of mast cells, and mediate many of the biologic effects of immediate hypersensitivity (allergic) reactions. (Biogenic amines are sometimes called vasoactive amines.)

BLIMP-1 A transcriptional repressor that is required for plasma cell generation.

Bone marrow The tissue within the central cavity of bone that is the site of generation of all circulating blood cells in adults, including immature lymphocytes, and the site of B cell maturation.

Bone marrow transplantation
See **hematopoietic stem cell transplantation.**

Bronchial asthma An inflammatory disease usually caused by repeated immediate hypersensitivity reactions in the lung that leads to intermittent and reversible airway obstruction, chronic bronchial inflammation with eosinophils, and bronchial smooth muscle cell hypertrophy and hyperreactivity.

Bruton's tyrosine kinase (Btk) A Tec family tyrosine kinase that is essential for B cell maturation. Mutations in the gene encoding Btk cause X-linked agammaglobulinemia, a disease characterized by failure of B cells to mature beyond the pre–B cell stage.

Burkitt's lymphoma A malignant B cell tumor that is diagnosed by histologic features but almost always carries a reciprocal chromosomal translocation involving *Ig* gene loci and the cellular *MYC* gene on chromosome 8. Many cases of Burkitt's lymphoma in Africa are associated with Epstein-Barr virus infection.

C (constant region) gene segments The DNA sequences in the *Ig* and *TCR* gene loci that encode the non-variable portions of Ig heavy and light chains and TCR α, β, γ, and δ chains.

C1 A serum complement system protein composed of several polypeptide chains that initiates the classical pathway of complement activation by attaching to the Fc portions of IgG or IgM antibody that has bound antigen.

C1 inhibitor (C1 INH) A plasma protein inhibitor of the classical pathway of complement activation. C1 INH is a serine protease inhibitor (serpin) that mimics the normal substrates of the C1r and C1s components of C1. A genetic deficiency in C1 INH causes the disease hereditary angioneurotic edema.

C3 The central and most abundant complement system protein; it is involved in both the classical and alternative pathway cascades. C3 is proteolytically cleaved during complement activation to generate a C3b fragment, which covalently attaches to cell or microbial surfaces, and a C3a fragment, which has various proinflammatory activities.

C3 convertase A multiprotein enzyme complex generated by the early steps of classical, lectin, and alternative pathways of complement activation. C3 convertase cleaves C3, which gives rise to two proteolytic products called C3a and C3b.

C5 convertase A multiprotein enzyme complex generated by C3b binding to C3 convertase. C5 convertase cleaves C5 and initiates the late steps of complement activation leading to formation of the membrane attack complex and lysis of cells.

Calcineurin A cytoplasmic serine/threonine phosphatase that dephosphorylates the transcription factor NFAT, thereby allowing NFAT to enter the nucleus. Calcineurin is activated by calcium signals generated through TCR signaling in response to antigen recognition, and the immunosuppressive drugs cyclosporine and FK506 work by blocking calcineurin activity.

Carcinoembryonic antigen (CEA, CD66) A highly glycosylated membrane protein; increased expression of CEA in many carcinomas of the colon, pancreas, stomach, and breast results in a rise in serum levels. The level of serum CEA is used to monitor the persistence or recurrence of metastatic carcinoma after treatment.

Caspases Intracellular proteases with cysteines in their active sites that cleave substrates at the C-terminal sides of aspartic acid residues. Most are components of enzymatic cascades that cause apoptotic death of cells, but caspase-1, which is part of the inflammasome, drives inflammation by processing inactive precursor forms of the cytokines IL-1 and IL-18 into their active forms.

Cathelicidins Polypeptides produced by neutrophils and various barrier epithelia that serve various functions in innate immunity, including direct toxicity to microorganisms, activation of leukocytes, and neutralization of lipopolysaccharide.

Cathepsins Thiol and aspartyl proteases with broad substrate specificities, which are abundant in the endosomes in APCs, and play an important role in generating peptide fragments from exogenous protein antigens that bind to class II MHC molecules.

CD molecules Cell surface molecules expressed on various cell types in the immune system that are designated by the "cluster of differentiation" or CD number. See Appendix III for a list of CD molecules.

Cell-mediated immunity (CMI) The form of adaptive immunity that is mediated by T lymphocytes and serves as the defense mechanism against various types of microbes that are taken up by phagocytes or infect non-phagocytic cells. Cell-mediated immune responses include CD4+ T cell–mediated activation of phagocytes and CD8+ CTL–mediated killing of infected cells.

Central tolerance A form of self-tolerance induced in generative (central) lymphoid organs as a consequence of immature self-reactive lymphocytes recognizing self antigens and subsequently leading to their death or inactivation. Central tolerance prevents the emergence of lymphocytes with high-affinity receptors for the self antigens that are expressed in the bone marrow or thymus.

Centroblasts Rapidly proliferating B cells in the dark zone of germinal centers of secondary lymphoid tissues, which give rise to thousands of progeny, express activation-induced deaminase (AID), and undergo somatic mutation of their *V* genes. Centroblasts become the centrocytes of the light zone of germinal centers.

Centrocytes B cells in the light zone of germinal centers of secondary lymphoid organs, which are the progeny of proliferating centroblasts of the dark zone. Centrocytes that express high-affinity Ig are positively selected to survive and undergo isotype switching and further differentiation into long-lived plasma cells and memory B cells.

Chédiak-Higashi syndrome A rare autosomal recessive immunodeficiency disease caused by a defect in the cytoplasmic granules of various cell types that affects the lysosomes of neutrophils and macrophages as well as the granules of CTLs and NK cells. Patients show reduced resistance to infection with pyogenic bacteria.

Chemokine receptors Cell surface receptors for chemokines that transduce signals stimulating the migration of leukocytes. There are at least 19 different mammalian chemokine receptors, each of which binds a different set of chemokines; all are members of the seven-transmembrane α-helical, G protein–coupled receptor family.

Chemokines A large family of structurally homologous low–molecular-weight cytokines that stimulate leukocyte chemotaxis, regulate the migration of leukocytes from the blood to tissues by activating leukocyte integrins, and maintain the spatial organization of different subsets of lymphocytes and antigen-presenting cells within lymphoid organs.

Chemotaxis Movement of a cell directed by a chemical concentration gradient. The movement of leukocytes within various tissues is often directed by gradients of low–molecular-weight cytokines called chemokines.

Chromosomal translocation A chromosomal abnormality in which a segment of one chromosome is transferred to another. Many malignant diseases of lymphocytes are associated with chromosomal translocations involving an Ig or TCR locus and a chromosomal segment containing a cellular oncogene.

Chronic granulomatous disease A rare inherited immunodeficiency disease caused by mutations in genes encoding components of the phagocyte oxidase enzyme complex that is needed for microbial killing by polymorphonuclear leukocytes and macrophages. The disease is characterized by recurrent intracellular bacterial and fungal infections, often accompanied by chronic cell-mediated immune responses and the formation of granulomas.

Chronic rejection A form of allograft rejection characterized by fibrosis with loss of normal organ structures occurring during a prolonged period. In many cases, the major pathologic event in chronic rejection is graft arterial occlusion caused by proliferation of intimal smooth muscle cells, which is called graft arteriosclerosis.

c-Kit ligand (stem cell factor) A protein required for hematopoiesis, early steps in T cell development in the thymus, and mast cell development. c-Kit ligand is produced in membrane-bound and soluble forms by stromal cells in the bone marrow and thymus, and it binds to the c-Kit tyrosine kinase membrane receptor on pluripotent stem cells.

Class I major histocompatibility complex (MHC) molecule One of two forms of polymorphic heterodimeric membrane proteins that bind and display peptide fragments of protein antigens on the surface of APCs for recognition by T lymphocytes. Class I MHC molecules usually display peptides derived from proteins in the cytosol of the cell, for recognition by CD8$^+$ T cells.

Class II–associated invariant chain peptide (CLIP) A peptide remnant of the invariant chain that sits in the class II MHC peptide-binding cleft and is removed by action of the HLA-DM molecule before the cleft becomes accessible to peptides produced from extracellular protein antigens.

Class II major histocompatibility complex (MHC) molecule One of two major classes of polymorphic heterodimeric membrane proteins that bind and display peptide fragments of protein antigens on the surface of APCs for recognition by T lymphocytes. Class II MHC molecules usually display peptides derived from extracellular proteins that are internalized into phagocytic or endocytic vesicles, for recognition by CD4$^+$ T cells.

Class II vesicle (CIIV) A membrane-bound organelle identified in murine B cells that is important in the class II MHC pathway of antigen presentation. The CIIV is similar to the MHC class II compartment (MIIC) identified in other cells and contains all of the components required for the formation of complexes of peptide antigens and class II MHC molecules, including the enzymes that degrade protein antigens, class II molecules, invariant chain, and HLA-DM.

Classical macrophage activation Macrophage activation by interferon-γ, T$_H$1 cells, and TLR ligands, leading to a proinflammatory and microbicidal phenotype. "Classically activated" macrophages are also called M1 macrophages.

Classical pathway of complement activation The pathway of activation of the complement system that is initiated by binding of antigen-antibody complexes to the C1 molecule and induces a proteolytic cascade involving multiple other complement proteins. The classical pathway is an effector arm of the humoral immune system that generates inflammatory mediators, opsonins for phagocytosis of antigens, and lytic complexes that destroy cells.

Clonal anergy A state of antigen unresponsiveness of a clone of T lymphocytes experimentally induced by recognition of antigen in the absence of additional signals (costimulatory signals) required for functional activation. Clonal anergy is considered a model for one mechanism of tolerance to self antigens and may be applicable to B lymphocytes as well.

Clonal deletion A mechanism of lymphocyte tolerance in which an immature T cell in the thymus or an immature B cell in the bone marrow undergoes apoptotic death as a consequence of recognizing a self antigen.

Clonal expansion The ~10,000- to 100,000-fold increase in number of lymphocytes specific for an antigen that results from antigen stimulation and proliferation of naive T cells. Clonal expansion occurs in lymphoid tissues and is required to generate enough antigen-specific effector lymphocytes from rare naive precursors to eradicate infections.

Clonal ignorance A form of lymphocyte unresponsiveness in which self antigens are ignored by the immune system even though lymphocytes specific for those antigens remain viable and functional.

Clonal selection hypothesis A fundamental tenet of the immune system (no longer a hypothesis) stating that every individual possesses numerous clonally derived lymphocytes, each clone having arisen from a single precursor, expresses one antigen receptor, and is capable of recognizing and responding to a distinct antigenic determinant. When an antigen enters, it selects a specific preexisting clone and activates it.

Clone A group of cells, all derived from a single common precursor, which maintain many of the genotypic and phenotypic features shared by the cell of origin. In adaptive immunity, all members of a clone of lymphocytes share the same clonally unique recombined *Ig* or *TCR* genes, although the rearranged *Ig V* genes of different cells within a clone of B cells may vary in sequence due to somatic hypermutation that occurs after VDJ recombination.

Coinhibitor A cell surface protein expressed by antigen-presenting cells, regulatory T or B cells, or tissue cells that binds to inhibitory receptors on effector T cells, inducing signals that block T cell activation by antigen. An example is PD-L1, a coinhibitor expressed on various cell types, which binds to PD-1 on effector T cells. The PD-L1/PD-1 pathway is being therapeutically targeted to enhance anti-tumor and anti-viral T cell responses.

Collectins A family of proteins, including mannose-binding lectin, that are characterized by a collagen-like domain and a lectin (i.e., carbohydrate-binding) domain. Collectins play a role in the innate immune system by acting as microbial pattern recognition receptors, and they may activate the complement system by binding to C1q.

Colony-stimulating factors (CSFs) Cytokines that promote the expansion and differentiation of bone marrow progenitor cells. CSFs are essential for the maturation of red blood cells, granulocytes, monocytes, and lymphocytes. Examples of CSFs include granulocyte-monocyte colony-stimulating factor (GM-CSF), granulocyte colony-stimulating factor (G-CSF), and IL-3.

Combinatorial diversity The diversity of Ig and TCR specificities generated by the use of many different combinations of different variable, diversity, and joining segments during somatic recombination of DNA in the Ig and TCR loci in developing B and T cells. Combinatorial diversity is one mechanism, which works together with junctional diversity, for the generation of large numbers of different antigen receptor genes from a limited number of DNA gene segments.

Complement A system of serum and cell surface proteins that interact with one another and with other molecules of the immune system to generate important effectors of innate and adaptive immune responses. The classical, alternative, and lectin pathways of the complement system are activated by antigen-antibody complexes, microbial surfaces, and plasma lectins binding to microbes, respectively, and consist of a cascade of proteolytic enzymes that generate inflammatory mediators and opsonins. All three pathways lead to the formation of a common terminal cell lytic complex that is inserted in cell membranes.

Complement receptor type 1 (CR1) A high-affinity receptor for the C3b and C4b fragments of complement. Phagocytes use CR1 to mediate internalization of C3b- or C4b-coated particles. CR1 on erythrocytes serves in the clearance of immune complexes from the circulation. CR1 is also a regulator of complement activation.

Complement receptor type 2 (CR2) A receptor expressed on B cells and follicular dendritic cells that binds proteolytic fragments of the C3 complement protein, including C3d, C3dg, and iC3b. CR2 functions to stimulate humoral immune responses by enhancing B cell activation by antigen and by promoting the trapping of antigen-antibody complexes in germinal centers. CR2 is also the receptor for Epstein-Barr virus.

Complementarity-determining region (CDR) Short segments of Ig and TCR proteins that contain most of the sequence differences between different antibodies or TCRs and make contact with antigen; also called **hypervariable regions.** Three CDRs are present in the variable domain of each antigen receptor polypeptide chain, and six CDRs are present in an intact Ig or TCR molecule. These hypervariable segments assume loop structures that together form a surface complementary to the three-dimensional structure of the bound antigen.

Congenic mouse strains Inbred mouse strains that are identical to one another at every genetic locus except the one for which they are selected to differ; such strains are created by repetitive back-crossbreeding and selection for a particular trait. Congenic strains that differ from one another only at a particular MHC allele have been useful in defining the function of MHC molecules.

Congenital immunodeficiency A genetic defect in which an inherited deficiency in some aspect of the innate or adaptive immune system leads to an increased susceptibility to infections. Congenital immunodeficiency is frequently manifested early in infancy and childhood but is sometimes clinically detected later in life. Synonymous with **primary immunodeficiency.**

Constant (C) region The portion of Ig or TCR polypeptide chains that does not vary in sequence among different clones and is not involved in antigen binding.

Contact hypersensitivity A state of immune responsiveness to certain chemical agents leading to T cell–mediated delayed-type hypersensitivity reactions upon skin contact. Substances that elicit contact hypersensitivity, including nickel ions and urushiols in poison ivy, bind to and modify self proteins on the surfaces of APCs, which are then recognized by CD4+ or CD8+ T cells.

Coreceptor A lymphocyte surface receptor that binds to an antigen complex at the same time that membrane Ig or TCR binds the antigen and delivers signals required for optimal lymphocyte activation. CD4 and CD8 are T cell coreceptors that bind non-polymorphic parts of an MHC molecule concurrently with the TCR binding to polymorphic residues and the bound peptide. CR2 is a coreceptor on B cells that binds to complement-opsonized antigens at the same time that membrane Ig binds another part of the antigen.

Costimulator A molecule expressed on the surface of APCs in response to innate immune stimuli, which provides a stimulus, in addition to antigen (the "second signal"), required for the activation of naive T cells. The best defined costimulators are the B7 molecules (CD80 and CD86) on APCs that bind to the CD28 receptor on T cells. Other costimulators bind to receptors that are expressed on activated T cells, leading to enhanced effector responses.

CpG nucleotides Unmethylated cytidine-guanine sequences found in microbial DNA that stimulate innate immune responses. CpG nucleotides are recognized by Toll-like receptor-9, and they have adjuvant properties in the mammalian immune system.

C-reactive protein (CRP) A member of the pentraxin family of plasma proteins involved in innate immune responses to bacterial infections. CRP is an acute-phase reactant, and it binds to the capsule of pneumococcal bacteria. CRP also binds to C1q and may thereby activate complement or act as an opsonin by interacting with phagocyte C1q receptors.

Cross-matching A screening test performed to minimize the chance of adverse transfusion reactions or graft rejection, in which a patient in need of a blood transfusion or organ allograft is tested for the presence of preformed antibodies against donor cell surface antigens (usually blood group antigens or MHC antigens). The test involves mixing the recipient serum with leukocytes or red blood cells from potential donors, and analyzing for agglutination or complement-dependent lysis of the cells.

Cross-presentation A mechanism by which a dendritic cell activates (or primes) a naive CD8+ CTL specific for the antigens of a third cell (e.g., a virus-infected or tumor cell). Cross-presentation occurs, for example, when an infected (often apoptotic) cell is ingested by a dendritic cell and the microbial antigens are processed and presented in association with class I MHC molecules, unlike the general rule for phagocytosed antigens, which are presented in association with class II MHC molecules. The dendritic cell also provides costimulation for the T cells. Also called **cross-priming.**

CTLA-4 An Ig superfamily protein expressed on the surface of activated effector T cells and Treg, which binds B7-1 and B7-2 with high affinity and plays an essential role in inhibiting T cell responses. CTLA-4 is essential for Treg function and T cell tolerance to self antigens.

C-type lectin A member of a large family of calcium-dependent carbohydrate-binding proteins, many of which play important roles in innate and adaptive immunity. For example, soluble C-type lectins bind to microbial carbohydrate structures and mediate phagocytosis or complement activation (e.g., mannose-binding lectin, dectins, collectins, ficolins).

Cutaneous immune system The components of the innate and adaptive immune system found in the skin that function together in a specialized way to detect and respond to pathogens on or in the skin and to maintain homeostasis with commensal microbes. Components of the cutaneous immune system include keratinocytes, Langerhans cells, dermal dendritic cells, intraepithelial lymphocytes, and dermal lymphocytes.

Cyclosporine A calcineurin inhibitor widely used as an immunosuppressive drug to prevent allograft rejection by blocking T cell activation. Cyclosporine (also called cyclosporin A) binds to a cytosolic protein called cyclophilin, and cyclosporine-cyclophilin complexes bind to and inhibit calcineurin, thereby inhibiting activation and nuclear translocation of the transcription factor NFAT.

Cytokines Proteins that are produced and secreted by many different cell types, and mediate inflammatory and immune reactions. Cytokines are principal mediators of communication between cells of the immune system (see Appendix II).

Cytotoxic (or cytolytic) T lymphocyte (CTL) A type of T lymphocyte whose major effector function is to recognize and kill host cells infected with viruses or other intracellular microbes. CTLs usually express CD8 and recognize microbial peptides displayed by class I MHC molecules. CTL killing of infected cells involves delivery of the contents of cytoplasmic granules into the cytosol of infected cells, leading to apoptotic death.

Damage-associated molecular patterns (DAMPs) Endogenous molecules that are produced by or released from damaged and dying cells that bind to pattern recognition receptors and stimulate innate immune responses. Examples include high-mobility group box 1 (HMGB1) protein, extracellular ATP, and uric acid.

Death receptors Plasma membrane receptors expressed on various cell types that, upon ligand binding, transduce signals that lead to recruitment of the Fas-Associated protein with Death Domain (FADD) adaptor protein, which activates caspase-8, leading to apoptotic cell death. All death receptors, including FAS, TRAIL, and TNFR, belong the TNF receptor superfamily.

Dectins Pattern recognition receptors expressed on dendritic cells that recognize fungal cell wall carbohydrates and induce signaling events that promote inflammation and enhance adaptive immune responses.

Defensins Cysteine-rich peptides produced by epithelial barrier cells in the skin, gut, lung, and other tissues and in neutrophil granules that act as broad-spectrum antibiotics to kill a wide variety of bacteria and fungi. The synthesis of defensins is increased in response to stimulation of innate immune system receptors such as Toll-like receptors and inflammatory cytokines such as IL-1 and TNF.

Delayed-type hypersensitivity (DTH) An immune reaction in which T cell–dependent macrophage activation and inflammation cause tissue injury. A DTH reaction to the subcutaneous injection of antigen is often used as an assay for cell-mediated immunity (e.g., the purified protein derivative skin test for immunity to *Mycobacterium tuberculosis*).

Dendritic cells Bone marrow–derived cells found in epithelial and lymphoid tissues that are morphologically characterized by thin membranous projections. Many subsets of dendritic cells exist with diverse functions. Classical dendritic cells function as innate sentinel cells and become APCs for naive T lymphocytes upon activation, and they are important for initiation of adaptive immune responses to protein antigen. Immature (resting) classical dendritic cells are important for induction of tolerance to self antigens. Plasmacytoid dendritic cells produce abundant type 1 interferons in response to exposure to viruses.

Desensitization A method of treating immediate hypersensitivity disease (allergies) that involves repetitive administration of low doses of an antigen to which individuals are allergic. This process often prevents severe allergic reactions on subsequent environmental exposure to the antigen, but the mechanisms are not well understood.

Determinant The specific portion of a macromolecular antigen to which an antibody binds. In the case of a protein antigen recognized by a T cell, the determinant is the peptide portion that binds to an MHC molecule for recognition by the TCR. Synonymous with **epitope.**

Diacylglycerol (DAG) A signaling molecule generated by phospholipase C (PLCγ1)–mediated hydrolysis of the plasma membrane phospholipid phosphatidylinositol 4,5-bisphosphate (PIP2) during antigen activation of lymphocytes. The main function of DAG is to activate an enzyme called protein kinase C that participates in the generation of active transcription factors.

DiGeorge syndrome A selective T cell deficiency caused by a congenital malformation that results in defective development of the thymus, parathyroid glands, and other structures that arise from the third and fourth pharyngeal pouches.

Direct antigen presentation (or direct allorecognition) Presentation of cell surface allogeneic MHC molecules by graft APCs to a graft recipient's T cells that leads to activation of the alloreactive T cells. In direct recognition of allogeneic MHC molecules, a TCR that was selected to recognize a self MHC molecule plus foreign peptide cross-reacts with the allogeneic MHC molecule plus peptide. Direct presentation is partly responsible for strong T cell responses to allografts.

Diversity The existence of a large number of lymphocytes with different antigenic specificities in any individual. Diversity is a fundamental property of the adaptive immune system and is the result of variability in the structures of the antigen-binding sites of lymphocyte receptors for antigens (antibodies and TCRs).

Diversity (D) segments Short coding sequences between the variable (V) and constant (C) gene segments in the Ig heavy chain and TCR β and γ loci that together with J segments are somatically recombined with V segments during lymphocyte development. The resulting recombined VDJ DNA codes for the carboxyl-terminal ends of the antigen receptor V regions, including the third hypervariable (CDR) regions. Random use of D segments contributes to the diversity of the antigen receptor repertoire.

DNA vaccine A vaccine composed of a bacterial plasmid containing a complementary DNA encoding a protein antigen. DNA vaccines presumably work because professional APCs are transfected in vivo by the plasmid and express immunogenic peptides that elicit specific responses. Furthermore, the plasmid DNA contains CpG nucleotides that act as potent adjuvants.

Double-negative thymocyte A subset of developing T cells in the thymus (thymocytes) that express neither CD4 nor CD8. Most double-negative thymocytes are at an early developmental stage and do not express antigen receptors. They will later express both CD4 and CD8 during the intermediate double-positive stage before further maturation to single-positive T cells expressing only CD4 or CD8.

Double-positive thymocyte A subset of developing T cells in the thymus (thymocytes) that express both CD4 and CD8 and are at an intermediate developmental stage. Double-positive thymocytes also express TCRs and are subject to selection processes, and they mature to single-positive T cells expressing only CD4 or CD8.

Ectoparasites Parasites that live on the surface of an animal, such as ticks and mites. Both the innate and adaptive immune systems may play a role in protection against ectoparasites, often by destroying the larval stages of these organisms.

Effector cells The cells that perform effector functions during an immune response, such as secreting cytokines (e.g., helper T cells), killing microbes (e.g., macrophages), killing microbe-infected host cells (e.g., CTLs), or secreting antibodies (e.g., differentiated B cells).

Effector phase The phase of an immune response in which a foreign antigen is destroyed or inactivated. For example, in a humoral immune response, the effector phase may be characterized by antibody-dependent complement activation and phagocytosis of antibody- and complement-opsonized bacteria.

Endosome An intracellular membrane-bound vesicle into which extracellular proteins are internalized during antigen processing. Endosomes have an acidic pH and contain proteolytic enzymes that degrade proteins into peptides that bind to class II MHC molecules. A subset of class II MHC–rich endosomes, called MIIC, play a special role in antigen processing and presentation by the class II pathway.

Endotoxin A component of the cell wall of Gram-negative bacteria, also called **lipopolysaccharide** (LPS), that is released from dying bacteria and stimulates innate immune inflammatory responses by binding to TLR4 on many different cell types, including phagocytes, endothelial cells, dendritic cells, and barrier epithelial cells. Endotoxin contains both lipid components and carbohydrate (polysaccharide) moieties.

Enhancer A regulatory nucleotide sequence in a gene that is located either upstream or downstream of the promoter, binds transcription factors, and increases the activity of the promoter. In cells of the immune system, enhancers are responsible for integrating cell surface signals that lead to induced transcription of genes encoding many of the effector proteins of an immune response, such as cytokines.

Envelope glycoprotein (Env) A membrane glycoprotein encoded by a retrovirus that is expressed on the plasma membrane of infected cells and on the host cell–derived membrane coat of viral particles. Env proteins are often required for viral infectivity. The Env proteins of HIV include gp41 and gp120, which bind to CD4 and chemokine receptors, respectively, on human T cells and mediate fusion of the viral and T cell membranes.

Enzyme-linked immunosorbent assay (ELISA) A method of quantifying an antigen immobilized on a solid surface by use of a specific antibody with a covalently coupled enzyme. The amount of antibody that binds the antigen is proportional to the amount of antigen present and is determined by spectrophotometrically measuring the conversion of a clear substrate to a colored product by the coupled enzyme (see Appendix IV).

Eosinophil A bone marrow–derived granulocyte that is abundant in the inflammatory infiltrates of immediate hypersensitivity late-phase reactions and contributes to many of the pathologic processes in allergic diseases. Eosinophils are important in defense against extracellular parasites, including helminths.

Epitope The specific portion of a macromolecular antigen to which an antibody binds. In the case of a protein antigen recognized by a T cell, an epitope is the peptide portion that binds to an MHC molecule for recognition by the TCR. Synonymous with **determinant.**

Epitope spreading In autoimmunity, the development of immune responses to multiple epitopes as an autoimmune disease originally targeting one epitope progresses, likely caused by further breakdown in tolerance and release of additional tissue antigens due to the inflammatory process stimulated by the initial response.

Epstein-Barr virus (EBV) A double-stranded DNA virus of the herpesvirus family that is the etiologic agent of infectious mononucleosis and is associated with some B cell malignant tumors and nasopharyngeal carcinoma. EBV infects B lymphocytes and some epithelial cells by specifically binding to CR2 (CD21).

Experimental autoimmune encephalomyelitis (EAE) An animal model of multiple sclerosis, an autoimmune demyelinating disease of the central nervous system. EAE is induced in rodents by immunization with components of the myelin sheath (e.g., myelin basic protein) of nerves, mixed with an adjuvant. The disease is mediated in large part by cytokine-secreting CD4+ T cells specific for the myelin sheath proteins.

Fab (fragment, antigen-binding) A proteolytic fragment of an IgG antibody molecule that includes one complete light chain paired with one heavy chain fragment containing the variable domain and only the first constant domain. Fab fragments retain the ability to monovalently bind an antigen but cannot interact with IgG Fc receptors on cells or with complement. Therefore, Fab preparations are used in research and therapeutic applications when antigen binding is desired without activation of effector functions. (The Fab′ fragment retains the hinge region of the heavy chain.)

F(ab′)₂ fragment A proteolytic fragment of an IgG molecule that includes two complete light chains but only the variable domain, first constant domain, and hinge region of the two heavy chains. F(ab′)₂ fragments retain the entire bivalent antigen-binding region of an intact IgG molecule but cannot bind complement or IgG Fc receptors. They are used in research and therapeutic applications when antigen binding is desired without antibody effector functions.

Fas (CD95) A death receptor of the TNF receptor family that is expressed on the surface of T cells and many other cell types and initiates a signaling cascade leading to apoptotic death of the cell. The death pathway is initiated when Fas binds to Fas ligand expressed on activated T cells. Fas-mediated killing of lymphocytes is important for the maintenance of self-tolerance. Mutations in the *FAS* gene cause systemic autoimmune disease (see also **death receptor**).

Fas ligand (CD95 ligand) A membrane protein that is a member of the TNF family of proteins expressed on activated T cells. Fas ligand binds to the death receptor Fas, thereby stimulating a signaling pathway leading to apoptotic cell death of the Fas-expressing cell. Mutations in the Fas ligand gene cause systemic autoimmune disease in mice.

Fc (fragment, crystalline) A proteolytic fragment of IgG that contains only the disulfide-linked carboxyl-terminal regions of the two heavy chains. Fc is also used to describe the corresponding region of an intact Ig molecule that mediates effector functions by binding to cell surface receptors or the C1q complement protein. (Fc fragments are so named because they tend to crystallize out of solution.)

Fc receptor A cell surface receptor specific for the carboxyl-terminal constant region of an Ig molecule. Fc receptors are typically multichain protein complexes that include signaling components and Ig-binding components. Several types of Fc receptors exist, including those specific for different IgG isotypes, IgE, and IgA. Fc receptors mediate many of the cell-dependent effector functions of antibodies, including phagocytosis of antibody-bound antigens, antigen-induced activation of mast cells, and targeting and activation of NK cells.

FcεRI A high-affinity receptor for the carboxyl-terminal constant region of IgE molecules that is expressed on mast cells, basophils, and eosinophils. FcεRI molecules on mast cells are usually occupied by IgE, and antigen-induced cross-linking of these IgE-FcεRI complexes activates the mast cell and initiates immediate hypersensitivity reactions.

Fcγ receptor (FcγR) A specific cell surface receptor for the carboxyl-terminal constant region of IgG molecules. There are several different types of Fcγ receptors, including a high-affinity FcγRI that mediates phagocytosis by macrophages and neutrophils, a low-affinity FcγRIIB that transduces inhibitory signals in B cells, and a low-affinity FcγRIIIA that mediates targeting and activation of NK cells.

Ficolins Hexameric innate immune system plasma proteins, containing collagen-like domains and fibrinogen-like carbohydrate-recognizing domains, which bind to cell wall components of Gram-positive bacteria, opsonizing them and activating complement.

First-set rejection Allograft rejection in an individual who has not previously received a graft or otherwise been exposed to tissue alloantigens from the same donor. First-set rejection usually takes about 7 to 14 days.

FK506 An immunosuppressive drug (also known as tacrolimus) used to prevent allograft rejection that functions blocking T cell cytokine gene transcription, similar to cyclosporine. FK506 binds to a cytosolic protein called FK506-binding protein, and the resulting complex binds to calcineurin, thereby inhibiting activation and nuclear translocation of the transcription factor NFAT.

Flow cytometry A method of analysis of the phenotype of cell populations requiring a specialized instrument (flow cytometer) that can detect fluorescence on individual cells in a suspension and thereby determine the number of cells expressing the molecule to which a fluorescent probe binds, as well as the relative amount of the molecule expressed. Suspensions of cells are incubated with fluorescently labeled antibodies or other probes, and the amount of probe bound by each cell in the population is measured by passing the cells one at a time through a fluorimeter with a laser-generated incident beam.

Fluorescence-activated cell sorter (FACS) An adaptation of the flow cytometer that is used for the purification of cells from a mixed population according to which and how much fluorescent probe the cells bind. Cells are first stained with fluorescently labeled probe, such as an antibody specific for a surface antigen of a cell population. The cells are then passed one at a time through a fluorimeter with a laser-generated incident beam and are deflected into different collection tubes by electromagnetic fields whose strength and direction are varied according to the measured intensity of the fluorescence signal.

Follicle
See **lymphoid follicle.**

Follicular dendritic cells (FDCs) Cells in lymphoid follicles of secondary lymphoid organs that express complement receptors, Fc receptors, and CD40 ligand and have long cytoplasmic processes that form a meshwork integral to the architecture of the follicles. Follicular dendritic cells display antigens on their surface for B cell recognition and are involved in the activation and selection of B cells expressing high-affinity membrane Ig during the process of affinity maturation. They are non-hematopoietic cells (not of bone marrow origin).

Follicular helper T cell (T_{FH})
See **T follicular helper (T_{FH}) cells.**

N-Formylmethionine An amino acid that initiates all bacterial proteins and no mammalian proteins (except those synthesized within mitochondria) and serves as a signal to the innate immune system of infection. Specific receptors for *N*-formylmethionine–containing peptides are expressed on neutrophils and mediate activation of the neutrophils.

FoxP3 A forkhead family transcription factor expressed by and required for the development of CD4+ regulatory T cells. Mutations in FoxP3 in mice and humans result in an absence of CD25+ regulatory T cells and multisystem autoimmune disease.

γδ T cell receptor (γδ TCR) A form of TCR that is distinct from the more common αβ TCR and is expressed on a subset of T cells found mostly in epithelial barrier tissues. Although the γδ TCR is structurally similar to the αβ TCR, the forms of antigen recognized by γδ TCRs are poorly understood; they do not recognize peptide complexes bound to polymorphic MHC molecules.

G protein–coupled receptor family A diverse family of receptors for hormones, lipid inflammatory mediators, and chemokines that use associated trimeric G proteins for intracellular signaling.

G proteins Proteins that bind guanyl nucleotides and act as exchange molecules by catalyzing the replacement of bound guanosine diphosphate (GDP) by guanosine triphosphate (GTP). G proteins with bound GTP can activate a variety of cellular enzymes in different signaling cascades. Trimeric GTP-binding proteins are associated with the cytoplasmic portions of many cell surface receptors, such as chemokine receptors. Other small soluble G proteins, such as Ras and Rac, are recruited into signaling pathways by adaptor proteins.

GATA-3 A transcription factor that promotes the differentiation of T_H2 cells from naive T cells.

Generative lymphoid organ An organ in which lymphocytes develop from immature precursors. The bone marrow and thymus are the major generative lymphoid organs in which B cells and T cells develop, respectively.

Germinal centers Specialized structures in lymphoid organs generated during T-dependent humoral immune responses, where extensive B cell proliferation, isotype switching, somatic mutation, affinity maturation, memory B cell generation, and induction of long-lived plasma cells take place. Germinal centers appear as lightly staining regions within a lymphoid follicle in spleen, lymph node, and mucosal lymphoid tissue.

Germline organization The inherited arrangement of variable, diversity, joining, and constant region gene segments of the antigen receptor loci in non-lymphoid cells or in immature lymphocytes. In developing B or T lymphocytes, the germline organization is modified by somatic recombination to form functional *Ig* or *TCR* genes.

Glomerulonephritis Inflammation of the renal glomeruli, often initiated by immunopathologic mechanisms such as deposition of circulating antigen-antibody complexes in the glomerular basement membrane or binding of antibodies to antigens expressed in the glomerulus. The antibodies can activate complement and phagocytes, and the resulting inflammatory response can lead to renal failure.

Graft A tissue or organ that is removed from one site and placed in another site, usually in a different individual.

Graft arteriosclerosis Occlusion of graft arteries caused by proliferation of intimal smooth muscle cells. This process is evident within 6 months to a year after transplantation and is responsible for chronic rejection of vascularized organ grafts. The mechanism is likely to be a chronic immune response to vessel wall alloantigens. Graft arteriosclerosis is also called accelerated arteriosclerosis.

Graft rejection A specific immune response to an organ or tissue graft that leads to inflammation, damage, and possibly graft failure.

Graft-versus-host disease A disease occurring in bone marrow transplant recipients that is caused by the reaction of mature T cells in the marrow graft with alloantigens on host cells. The disease most often affects the skin, liver, and intestines.

Granulocyte colony-stimulating factor (G-CSF) A cytokine made by activated T cells, macrophages, and endothelial cells at sites of infection that acts on bone marrow to increase the production of and mobilize neutrophils to replace those consumed in inflammatory reactions.

Granulocyte-monocyte colony-stimulating factor (GM-CSF) A cytokine made by activated T cells, macrophages, endothelial cells, and stromal fibroblasts that acts on bone marrow to increase the production of neutrophils and monocytes. GM-CSF is also a macrophage-activating factor and promotes the maturation of dendritic cells.

Granuloma A nodule of inflammatory tissue composed of clusters of activated macrophages and T lymphocytes, usually with associated fibrosis. Granulomatous inflammation is a form of chronic delayed-type hypersensitivity, often in response to persistent microbes, such as *Mycobacterium tuberculosis* and some fungi, or in response to particulate antigens that are not readily phagocytosed.

Granzyme A serine protease enzyme found in the granules of CTLs and NK cells that is released by exocytosis, enters target cells, and proteolytically cleaves and activates caspases, which in turn cleave several substrates and induce target cell apoptosis.

Gut-associated lymphoid tissue (GALT) Collections of lymphocytes and APCs within the mucosa of the gastrointestinal tract where adaptive immune responses to intestinal microbial flora and ingested antigens are initiated (see also **mucosa-associated lymphoid tissues**).

H-2 molecule An MHC molecule in the mouse. The mouse MHC was originally called the H-2 locus.

Haplotype The set of MHC alleles inherited from one parent and therefore on one chromosome.

Hapten A small chemical that can bind to an antibody but must be attached to a macromolecule (carrier) to stimulate an adaptive immune response specific for that chemical. For example, immunization with dinitrophenol (DNP) alone will not stimulate an anti-DNP antibody response, but immunization with a protein with covalently bonded DNP hapten will.

Heavy-chain class (isotype) switching The process by which a B lymphocyte changes the class, or isotype, of the antibodies that it produces, from IgM to IgG, IgE, or IgA, without changing the antigen specificity of the antibody. Heavy-chain class switching is stimulated by cytokines and CD40 ligand expressed by helper T cells and involves recombination of B cell VDJ segments with downstream heavy-chain gene segments.

Helminth A parasitic worm. Helminthic infections often elicit T_H2-dependent immune responses characterized by eosinophil-rich inflammatory infiltrates and IgE production.

Helper T cells The class of T lymphocytes whose main functions are to activate macrophages and to promote inflammation in cell-mediated immune responses and to promote B cell antibody production in humoral immune responses. These functions are mediated by secreted cytokines and by T cell CD40 ligand binding to macrophage or B cell CD40. Most helper T cells express the CD4 molecule.

Hematopoiesis The development of mature blood cells, including erythrocytes, leukocytes, and platelets, from pluripotent stem cells in the bone marrow and fetal liver. Hematopoiesis is regulated by several different cytokine growth factors produced by bone marrow stromal cells, T cells, and other cell types.

Hematopoietic stem cell An undifferentiated bone marrow cell that divides continuously and gives rise to additional stem cells and cells of multiple different lineages. A hematopoietic stem cell in the bone marrow will give rise to cells of the lymphoid, myeloid, and erythrocytic lineage.

Hematopoietic stem cell transplantation The transplantation of hematopoietic stem cells taken from the blood or bone marrow; it is performed clinically to treat hematopoietic or lymphopoietic disorders and malignant diseases and is also used in various immunologic experiments in animals.

High endothelial venules (HEVs) Specialized venules that are the sites of lymphocyte migration from the blood into the stroma of secondary lymphoid tissues. HEVs are lined by plump endothelial cells that protrude into the vessel lumen and express unique adhesion molecules involved in binding naive and central memory B and T cells.

Hinge region A region of Ig heavy chains between the first two constant domains that can assume multiple conformations, thereby imparting flexibility in the orientation of the two antigen-binding sites. Because of the hinge region, an antibody molecule can simultaneously bind two epitopes that are anywhere within a range of distances from one another.

Histamine A biogenic amine stored in the granules of mast cells that is one of the important mediators of immediate hypersensitivity. Histamine binds to specific receptors in various tissues and causes increased vascular permeability and contraction of bronchial and intestinal smooth muscle.

HLA
See **human leukocyte antigens.**

HLA-DM A peptide exchange molecule that plays a critical role in the class II MHC pathway of antigen presentation. HLA-DM is found in the specialized MIIC endosomal compartment and facilitates removal of the invariant chain–derived CLIP peptide and the binding of other peptides to class II MHC molecules. HLA-DM is encoded by a gene in the MHC and is structurally similar to class II MHC molecules, but it is not polymorphic.

Homeostasis In the adaptive immune system, the maintenance of a constant number and diverse repertoire of lymphocytes, despite the emergence of new lymphocytes and tremendous expansion of individual clones that may occur during responses to immunogenic antigens. Homeostasis is achieved by several regulated pathways of lymphocyte death and inactivation.

Homing receptor Adhesion molecules expressed on the surface of lymphocytes that are responsible for the different pathways of lymphocyte recirculation and tissue homing. Homing receptors bind to ligands (addressins) expressed on endothelial cells in particular vascular beds.

Human immunodeficiency virus (HIV) The etiologic agent of AIDS. HIV is a retrovirus that infects a variety of cell types, including CD4-expressing helper T cells, macrophages, and dendritic cells, and causes chronic progressive destruction of the immune system.

Human leukocyte antigens (HLA) MHC molecules expressed on the surface of human cells. Human MHC molecules were first identified as alloantigens on the surface of white blood cells (leukocytes) that bound serum antibodies from individuals previously exposed to other individuals' cells (e.g., mothers or transfusion recipients) (see also **major histocompatibility complex [MHC] molecule**).

Humanized antibody A monoclonal antibody encoded by a recombinant hybrid gene and composed of the antigen-binding sites from a murine monoclonal antibody and the constant region of a human antibody. Humanized antibodies are less likely than mouse monoclonal antibodies to induce an anti-antibody response in humans; they are used clinically in the treatment of inflammatory diseases, tumors, and transplant rejection.

Humoral immunity The type of adaptive immune response mediated by antibodies produced by B lymphocytes. Humoral immunity is the principal defense mechanism against extracellular microbes and their toxins.

Hybridoma A cell line derived by fusion, or somatic cell hybridization, between a normal lymphocyte and an immortalized lymphocyte tumor line. B cell hybridomas created by fusion of normal B cells of defined antigen specificity with a myeloma cell line are used to produce monoclonal antibodies. T cell hybridomas created by fusion of a normal T cell of defined specificity with a T cell tumor line are commonly used in research.

Hyperacute rejection A form of allograft or xenograft rejection that begins within minutes to hours after transplantation and that is characterized by thrombotic occlusion of the graft vessels. Hyperacute rejection is mediated by preexisting antibodies in the host circulation that bind to donor endothelial antigens, such as blood group antigens or MHC molecules, and activate the complement system.

Hypersensitivity diseases Disorders caused by immune responses. Hypersensitivity diseases include autoimmune diseases, in which immune responses are directed against self antigens, and diseases that result from uncontrolled or excessive responses against foreign antigens, such as microbes and allergens. The tissue damage that occurs in hypersensitivity diseases is due to the same effector mechanisms used by the immune system to protect against microbes.

Hypervariable region (hypervariable loop) Short segments of about 10 amino acid residues within the variable regions of antibody or TCR proteins that form loop structures that contact antigen. Three hypervariable loops, also called CDRs, are present in each antibody heavy chain and light chain and in each TCR chain. Most of the variability between different antibodies or TCRs is located within these loops.

Idiotype The property of a group of antibodies or TCRs defined by their sharing a particular idiotope; that is, antibodies that share a particular idiotope belong to the same idiotype. *Idiotype* is also used to describe the collection of idiotopes expressed by an Ig molecule, and it is often used synonymously with *idiotope*.

Igα and Igβ β proteins that are required for surface expression and signaling functions of membrane Ig on B cells. Igα and Igβ pairs are disulfide linked to one another, non-covalently associated with the cytoplasmic tail of membrane Ig, and form the BCR complex. The cytoplasmic domains of Igα and Igβ contain ITAMs that are involved in early signaling events during antigen-induced B cell activation.

IL-1 receptor antagonist (IL-1Ra) A natural inhibitor of IL-1 produced by mononuclear phagocytes that is structurally homologous to IL-1 and binds to the same receptors but is biologically inactive. IL-1RA is used as drug to treat autoinflammatory syndromes caused by dysregulated IL-1 production.

Immature B lymphocyte A membrane IgM⁺, IgD⁻ B cell, recently derived from marrow precursors, that does not proliferate or differentiate in response to antigens but rather may undergo apoptotic death or become functionally unresponsive. This property is important for the negative selection of B cells that are specific for self antigens present in the bone marrow.

Immediate hypersensitivity The type of immune reaction responsible for allergic diseases, which is dependent on antigen-mediated activation of IgE-coated tissue mast cells. The mast cells release mediators that cause increased vascular permeability, vasodilation, bronchial and visceral smooth muscle contraction, and local inflammation.

Immune complex A multimolecular complex of antibody molecules with bound antigen. Because each antibody molecule has a minimum of two antigen-binding sites and many antigens are multivalent, immune complexes can vary greatly in size. Immune complexes activate effector mechanisms of humoral immunity, such as the classical complement pathway and Fc receptor–mediated phagocyte activation. Deposition of circulating immune complexes in blood vessel walls or renal glomeruli can lead to inflammation and disease.

Immune complex disease An inflammatory disease caused by the deposition of antigen-antibody complexes in blood vessel walls, resulting in local complement activation and phagocyte recruitment. Immune complexes may form because of overproduction of antibodies against microbial antigens or as a result of autoantibody production in the setting of an autoimmune disease such as systemic lupus erythematosus. Immune complex deposition in the specialized capillary basement membranes of renal glomeruli can cause glomerulonephritis and impair renal function. Systemic deposition of immune complexes in arterial walls can cause vasculitis, with thrombosis and ischemic damage to various organs.

Immune deviation The conversion of a T cell response associated with one set of cytokines, such as T_H1 cytokines that stimulate inflammatory functions of macrophages, to a response associated with other cytokines, such as T_H2 cytokines that activate anti-inflammatory responses of macrophages.

Immune inflammation Inflammation that is a result of an adaptive immune response to antigen. The cellular infiltrate at the inflammatory site may include cells of the innate immune system such as neutrophils and macrophages, which are recruited as a result of the actions of T cell cytokines.

Immune-mediated inflammatory disease A broad group of disorders in which immune responses, either to self or foreign antigens, and chronic inflammation are major components.

Immune response A collective and coordinated response to the introduction of foreign substances in an individual mediated by the cells and molecules of the immune system.

Immune response (Ir) genes Originally defined as genes in inbred strains of rodents that were inherited in a dominant Mendelian manner and that controlled the ability of the animals to make antibodies against simple synthetic polypeptides. We now know that *Ir* genes are the polymorphic genes that encode class II MHC molecules, which display peptides to T lymphocytes and are therefore required for T cell activation and helper T cell–dependent B cell (antibody) responses to protein antigens.

Immune surveillance The concept that a physiologic function of the immune system is to recognize and destroy clones of transformed cells before they grow into tumors and to kill tumors after they are formed. The term *immune surveillance* is sometimes used in a general sense to describe the function of T lymphocytes to detect and destroy any cell, not necessarily a tumor cell, that is expressing foreign (e.g., microbial) antigens.

Immune system The molecules, cells, tissues, and organs that collectively function to provide immunity, or protection, against foreign organisms.

Immunity Protection against disease, usually infectious disease, mediated by the cells and tissues that are collectively called the immune system. In a broader sense, immunity refers to the ability to respond to foreign substances, including microbes and non-infectious molecules.

Immunoblot An analytical technique in which antibodies are used to detect the presence of an antigen bound to (i.e., blotted on) a solid matrix such as filter paper (also known as a Western blot).

Immunodeficiency
See **acquired immunodeficiency** and **congenital immunodeficiency**.

Immunodominant epitope The epitope of a protein antigen that elicits most of the response in an individual immunized with the native protein. Immunodominant epitopes correspond to the peptides of the protein that are proteolytically generated within APCs and bind most avidly to MHC molecules, and are most likely to stimulate T cells.

Immunofluorescence A technique in which a molecule is detected by use of an antibody labeled with a fluorescent probe. For example, in immunofluorescence microscopy, cells that express a particular surface antigen can be stained with a fluorescein-conjugated antibody specific for the antigen and then visualized with a fluorescent microscope.

Immunogen An antigen that induces an immune response. Not all antigens are immunogens. For example, low–molecular-weight compounds (haptens) can bind to antibodies but will not stimulate an immune response unless they are linked to macromolecules (carriers).

Immunoglobulin (Ig) Synonymous with antibody (see **antibody**).

Immunoglobulin domain A three-dimensional globular structural motif found in many proteins in the immune system, including Igs, TCRs, and MHC molecules. Ig domains are about 110 amino acid residues in length, include an internal disulfide bond, and contain two layers of β-pleated sheets, each layer composed of three to five strands of antiparallel polypeptide chain. Ig domains are classified as V-like or C-like on the basis of closest homology to either the Ig V or C domains.

Immunoglobulin heavy chain One of two types of polypeptide chains in an antibody molecule. The basic structural unit of an antibody includes two identical disulfide-linked heavy chains and two identical light chains. Each heavy chain is composed of a variable (V) Ig domain and three or four constant (C) Ig domains. The different antibody isotypes, including IgM, IgD, IgG, IgA, and IgE, are distinguished by structural differences in their heavy chain constant regions. The heavy chain constant regions also mediate effector functions, such as complement activation or engagement of phagocytes.

Immunoglobulin light chain One of two types of polypeptide chains in an antibody molecule. The basic structural unit of an antibody includes two identical light chains, each disulfide linked to one of two identical heavy chains. Each light chain is composed of one variable (V) Ig domain and one constant (C) Ig domain. There are two light chain isotypes, called κ and λ, both functionally identical. About 60% of human antibodies have κ light chains, and 40% have λ light chains.

Immunoglobulin superfamily A large family of proteins that contain a globular structural motif called an Ig domain, or Ig fold, originally described in antibodies. Many proteins of importance in the immune system, including antibodies, TCRs, MHC molecules, CD4, and CD8, are members of this superfamily.

Immunohistochemistry A technique to detect the presence of an antigen in histologic tissue sections by use of an enzyme-coupled antibody that is specific for the antigen. The enzyme converts a colorless substrate to a colored insoluble substance that precipitates at the site where the antibody and thus the antigen are localized. The position of the colored precipitate, and therefore the antigen, in the tissue section is observed by conventional light microscopy. Immunohistochemistry is a routine technique in diagnostic pathology and various fields of research.

Immunologic tolerance
See **tolerance.**

Immunologically privileged site A site in the body that is inaccessible to or constitutively suppresses immune responses. The anterior chamber of the eye, the testes, and the brain are examples of immunologically privileged sites.

Immunoperoxidase technique A common immunohistochemical technique in which a horseradish peroxidase–coupled antibody is used to identify the presence of an antigen in a tissue section. The peroxidase enzyme converts a colorless substrate to an insoluble brown product that is observable by light microscopy.

Immunoprecipitation A technique for the isolation of a molecule from a solution by binding it to an antibody and then rendering the antigen-antibody complex insoluble, either by precipitation with a second antibody or by coupling the first antibody to an insoluble particle or bead.

Immunoreceptor tyrosine-based activation motif (ITAM) A conserved protein motif composed of two copies of the sequence tyrosine-x-x-leucine (where x is an unspecified amino acid) found in the cytoplasmic tails of various membrane proteins in the immune system that are involved in signal transduction. ITAMs are present in the ζ and CD3 proteins of the TCR complex, in Igα and Igβ proteins in the BCR complex, and in several Ig Fc receptors. When these receptors bind their ligands, the tyrosine residues of the ITAMs become phosphorylated and form docking sites for other molecules involved in propagating cell-activating signal transduction pathways.

Immunoreceptor tyrosine-based inhibition motif (ITIM) A six–amino acid (isoleucine-x-tyrosine-x-x-leucine) motif found in the cytoplasmic tails of various inhibitory receptors in the immune system, including FcγRIIB on B cells and killer cell Ig-like receptors (KIRs) on NK cells. When these receptors bind their ligands, the ITIMs become phosphorylated on their tyrosine residues and form a docking site for protein tyrosine phosphatases, which in turn function to inhibit other signal transduction pathways.

Immunosuppression Inhibition of one or more components of the adaptive or innate immune system as a result of an underlying disease or intentionally induced by drugs for the purpose of preventing or treating graft rejection or autoimmune disease. A commonly used immunosuppressive drug is cyclosporine, which blocks T cell cytokine production.

Immunotherapy The treatment of a disease with therapeutic agents that promote or inhibit immune responses. Cancer immunotherapy, for example, involves promotion of active immune responses to tumor antigens or administration of anti-tumor antibodies or T cells to establish passive immunity.

Immunotoxins Reagents that may be used in the treatment of cancer and consist of covalent conjugates of a potent cellular toxin, such as ricin or diphtheria toxin, with antibodies specific for antigens expressed on the surface of tumor cells. It is hoped that such reagents can specifically target and kill tumor cells without damaging normal cells, but safe and effective immunotoxins have yet to be developed.

Inbred mouse strain A strain of mice created by repetitive mating of siblings that is characterized by homozygosity at every genetic locus. Every mouse of an inbred strain is genetically identical (syngeneic) to every other mouse of the same strain.

Indirect antigen presentation (or indirect allorecognition) In transplantation immunology, a pathway of presentation of donor (allogeneic) MHC molecules by recipient APCs that involves the same mechanisms used to present microbial proteins. The allogeneic MHC proteins are processed by recipient professional APCs, and peptides derived from the allogeneic MHC molecules are presented, in association with recipient (self) MHC molecules, to host T cells. In contrast to indirect antigen presentation, direct antigen presentation involves recipient T cell recognition of unprocessed allogeneic MHC molecules on the surface of graft cells.

Inflammasome A multiprotein complex in the cytosol of mononuclear phagocytes, dendritic cells, and other cell types that proteolytically generates the active form of IL-1β from the inactive pro-IL-1β precursor. The formation of the inflammasome complex, which includes NLRP3 (a NOD-like pattern recognition receptor) and caspase-1, is stimulated by a variety of microbial products, cell damage–associated molecules, and crystals.

Inflammation A complex reaction of vascularized tissue to infection or cell injury that involves extravascular accumulation of plasma proteins and leukocytes. Acute inflammation is a common result of innate immune responses, and local adaptive immune responses can also promote inflammation. Although inflammation serves a protective function in controlling infections and promoting tissue repair, it can also cause tissue damage and disease.

Inflammatory bowel disease (IBD) A group of disorders, including ulcerative colitis and Crohn's disease, characterized by chronic inflammation in the gastrointestinal tract. The etiology of IBD is not known, but some evidence indicates that it is caused by inadequate regulation of T cell responses, probably against intestinal commensal bacteria. IBD develops in gene knockout mice lacking IL-2, IL-10, or the TCR α chain.

Innate immunity Protection against infection that relies on mechanisms that exist before infection, are capable of a rapid response to microbes, and react in essentially the same way to repeated infections. The innate immune system includes epithelial barriers, phagocytic cells (neutrophils, macrophages), NK cells, the complement system, and cytokines, largely made by dendritic cells and mononuclear phagocytes, that regulate and coordinate many activities of the cells of innate immunity.

Integrins Heterodimeric cell surface proteins whose major functions are to mediate the adhesion of cells to other cells or to extracellular matrix. Integrins are important for T cell interactions with APCs and for migration of leukocytes from blood into tissues. The ligand-binding activity of leukocyte integrins depends on signals induced by chemokines binding to chemokine receptors. Two integrins important in the immune system are VLA-4 (very late antigen 4), and LFA-1 (leukocyte function-associated antigen 1).

Interferon regulatory factors (IRFs) A family of inducibly activated transcription factors that are important in expression of inflammatory and anti-viral genes. For example, IRF3 is activated by TLR signals and regulates expression of type I interferons, which are cytokines that protect cells from viral infection.

Interferons A subgroup of cytokines originally named for their ability to interfere with viral infections but that have other important immunomodulatory functions. Type I interferons include interferon-α and interferon-β, whose main function is to prevent viral replication in cells; type II interferon, also called interferon-γ, activates macrophages and various other cell types (see Appendix II).

Interleukins Any of a large number of cytokines named with a numerical suffix roughly sequentially in order of discovery or molecular characterization (e.g., interleukin-1, interleukin-2). Some cytokines were originally named for their biologic activities and do not have an interleukin designation (see Appendix II).

Intracellular bacterium A bacterium that survives or replicates within cells, usually in endosomes. The principal defense against intracellular bacteria, such as *Mycobacterium tuberculosis,* is T cell–mediated immunity.

Intraepithelial T lymphocytes T lymphocytes present in the epidermis of the skin and in mucosal epithelia that typically express a limited diversity of antigen receptors. Some of these lymphocytes, called invariant NKT cells, may recognize microbial products, such as glycolipids, associated with non-polymorphic class I MHC–like molecules. Others, called γδ T cells, recognize various non-peptide antigens, not bound to MHC molecules. Intraepithelial T lymphocytes may be considered effector cells of innate immunity and function in host defense by secreting cytokines and activating phagocytes and by killing infected cells.

Invariant chain (I$_i$) A non-polymorphic protein that binds to newly synthesized class II MHC molecules in the endoplasmic reticulum. The invariant chain prevents loading of the class II MHC peptide-binding cleft with peptides present in the endoplasmic reticulum, and such peptides are left to associate with class I molecules. The invariant chain also promotes folding and assembly of class II molecules and directs newly formed class II molecules to the specialized endosomal MIIC compartment, where peptide loading takes place.

Isotype One of five types of antibodies, determined by which of five different forms of heavy chain is present. Antibody isotypes include IgM, IgD, IgG, IgA, and IgE, and each isotype performs a different set of effector functions. Additional structural variations characterize distinct subtypes of IgG and IgA.

J chain A small polypeptide that is disulfide bonded to the tail pieces of multimeric IgM and IgA antibodies and contributes to the transepithelial transport of these immunoglobulins.

JAK-STAT signaling pathway A signaling pathway initiated by cytokine binding to type I and type II cytokine receptors. This pathway sequentially involves activation of receptor-associated Janus kinase (JAK) tyrosine kinases, JAK-mediated tyrosine phosphorylation of the cytoplasmic tails of cytokine receptors, docking of signal transducers and activators of transcription (STATs) to the phosphorylated receptor chains, JAK-mediated tyrosine phosphorylation of the associated STATs, dimerization and nuclear translocation of the STATs, and STAT binding to regulatory regions of target genes causing transcriptional activation of those genes.

Janus kinases (JAKs) A family of tyrosine kinases that associate with the cytoplasmic tails of several different cytokine receptors, including the receptors for IL-2, IL-3, IL-4, IFN-γ, IL-12, and others. In response to cytokine binding and receptor dimerization, JAKs phosphorylate the cytokine receptors to permit the binding of STATs, and then the JAKs phosphorylate and thereby activate the STATs. Different JAK kinases associate with different cytokine receptors.

Joining (J) chain A polypeptide that links IgA or IgM molecules to form multimers (e.g., dimeric IgA and pentameric IgM).

Joining (J) segments Short coding sequences between the variable (V) and constant (C) gene segments in all Ig and TCR loci, which together with D segments are somatically recombined with V segments during lymphocyte development. The resulting recombined VDJ DNA codes for the carboxyl-terminal ends of the antigen receptor V regions, including the third hypervariable (CDR) regions. Random use of different J segments contributes to the diversity of the antigen receptor repertoire.

Junctional diversity The diversity in antibody and TCR repertoires that is attributed to the random addition or removal of nucleotide sequences at junctions between V, D, and J gene segments.

Kaposi's sarcoma A malignant tumor of vascular cells that frequently arises in patients with AIDS. Kaposi's sarcoma is associated with infection by the Kaposi's sarcoma–associated herpesvirus (human herpesvirus 8).

Killer cell Ig-like receptors (KIRs) Ig superfamily receptors expressed by NK cells that recognize different alleles of HLA-A, HLA-B, and HLA-C molecules. Some KIRs have signaling components with ITIMs in their cytoplasmic tails, and these deliver inhibitory signals to inactivate the NK cells. Some members of the KIR family have short cytoplasmic tails without ITIMs but associate with other ITAM-containing polypeptides and function as activating receptors.

Knockout mouse A mouse with a targeted disruption of one or more genes that is created by homologous recombination techniques. Knockout mice lacking functional genes encoding cytokines, cell surface receptors, signaling molecules, and transcription factors have provided extensive information about the roles of these molecules in the immune system.

Lamina propria A layer of loose connective tissue underlying epithelium in mucosal tissues such as the intestines and airways, where dendritic cells, mast cells, lymphocytes, and macrophages mediate immune responses to invading pathogens.

Langerhans cells Immature dendritic cells found as a meshwork in the epidermal layer of the skin whose major function is to trap microbes and antigens that enter through the skin and transport the antigens to draining lymph nodes. During their migration to the lymph nodes, Langerhans cells differentiate into mature dendritic cells, which can efficiently present antigen to naive T cells.

Large granular lymphocyte Another name for an NK cell based on the morphologic appearance of this cell type in the blood.

Late-phase reaction A component of the immediate hypersensitivity reaction that ensues 2 to 4 hours after mast cell degranulation and that is characterized by an inflammatory infiltrate of eosinophils, basophils, neutrophils, and lymphocytes. Repeated bouts of this late-phase inflammatory reaction can cause tissue damage.

Lck A Src family non-receptor tyrosine kinase that noncovalently associates with the cytoplasmic tails of CD4 and CD8 molecules in T cells and is involved in the early signaling events of antigen-induced T cell activation. Lck mediates tyrosine phosphorylation of the cytoplasmic tails of CD3 and ζ proteins of the TCR complex.

Lectin pathway of complement activation A pathway of complement activation triggered by the binding of microbial polysaccharides to circulating lectins such as MBL. MBL is structurally similar to C1q and activates the C1r-C1s enzyme complex (like C1q) or activates another serine esterase, called mannose-binding protein–associated serine esterase. The remaining steps of the lectin pathway, beginning with cleavage of C4, are the same as the classical pathway.

Leishmania An obligate intracellular protozoan parasite that infects macrophages and can cause a chronic inflammatory disease involving many tissues. *Leishmania* infection in mice has served as a model system for study of the effector functions of several cytokines and the helper T cell subsets that produce them. T_H1 responses to *Leishmania major* and associated IFN-γ production control infection, whereas T_H2 responses with IL-4 production lead to disseminated lethal disease.

Lethal hit A term used to describe the events that result in irreversible damage to a target cell when a CTL binds to it. The lethal hit includes CTL granule exocytosis, and perforin-dependent delivery of apoptosis-inducing enzymes (granzymes) into the target cell cytoplasm.

Leukemia A malignant disease of bone marrow precursors of blood cells in which large numbers of leukemic cells usually occupy the bone marrow and often circulate in the blood stream. Lymphocytic leukemias are derived from B or T cell precursors, myelogenous leukemias are derived from granulocyte or monocyte precursors, and erythroid leukemias are derived from red blood cell precursors.

Leukocyte adhesion deficiency (LAD) One of a rare group of immunodeficiency diseases with infectious complications that is caused by defective expression of the leukocyte adhesion molecules required for tissue recruitment of phagocytes and lymphocytes. LAD-1 is due to mutations in the gene encoding the CD18 protein, which is part of β_2 integrins. LAD-2 is caused by mutations in a gene that encodes a fucose transporter involved in the synthesis of leukocyte ligands for endothelial selectins.

Leukotrienes A class of arachidonic acid–derived lipid inflammatory mediators produced by the lipoxygenase pathway in many cell types. Mast cells make abundant leukotriene C_4 (LTC$_4$) and its degradation products LTD_4 and LTE_4, which bind to specific receptors on smooth muscle cells and cause prolonged bronchoconstriction. Leukotrienes contribute to the pathologic processes of bronchial asthma. Collectively, LTC_4, LTD_4, and LTE_4 constitute what was once called slow-reacting substance of anaphylaxis.

Lipopolysaccharide
Synonymous with **endotoxin.**

Live virus vaccine A vaccine composed of a live but nonpathogenic (attenuated) form of a virus. Attenuated viruses carry mutations that interfere with the viral life cycle or pathogenesis. Because live virus vaccines actually infect the recipient cells, they can effectively stimulate immune responses, such as the CTL response, that are optimal for protecting against wild-type viral infection. A commonly used live virus vaccine is the Sabin poliovirus vaccine.

Lymph node Small nodular, encapsulated lymphocyte-rich organs situated along lymphatic channels throughout the body where adaptive immune responses to lymph-borne antigens are initiated. Lymph nodes have a specialized anatomic architecture that regulates the interactions of B cells, T cells, dendritic cells, and antigens to maximize the induction of protective immune responses.

Lymphatic system A system of vessels throughout the body that collects tissue fluid called lymph, originally derived from the blood, and returns it, through the thoracic duct, to the circulation. Lymph nodes are interspersed along these vessels and trap and retain antigens present in the lymph.

Lymphocyte homing The directed migration of subsets of circulating lymphocytes into particular tissue sites. Lymphocyte homing is regulated by the selective expression of endothelial adhesion molecules and chemokines, in different tissues. For example, some lymphocytes preferentially home to the intestinal mucosa, which is regulated by the chemokine CCL25 and the endothelial adhesion molecule MadCAM, both expressed in the gut, which bind respectively to the CCR9 chemokine receptor and the $\alpha_4\beta_1$ integrin on gut-homing lymphocytes.

Lymphocyte maturation The process by which pluripotent bone marrow stem cells develop into mature, antigen receptor–expressing naive B or T lymphocytes that populate peripheral lymphoid tissues. This process takes place in the specialized environments of the bone marrow (for B cells) and the thymus (for T cells). Synonymous with lymphocyte development.

Lymphocyte migration The movement of lymphocytes from the blood stream into peripheral tissues.

Lymphocyte recirculation The continuous movement of naive lymphocytes from the blood stream to secondary lymphoid organs, and back into the blood.

Lymphocyte repertoire The complete collection of antigen receptors and therefore antigen specificities expressed by the B and T lymphocytes of an individual.

Lymphoid follicle A B cell–rich region of a lymph node or the spleen that is the site of antigen-induced B cell proliferation and differentiation. In T cell–dependent B cell responses to protein antigens, a germinal center forms within the follicles.

Lymphoid tissue inducer cells A type of hematopoietically derived innate lymphoid cell that stimulates the development of lymph nodes and other secondary lymphoid organs, in part through production of the cytokines lymphotoxin-α (LTα) and lymphotoxin-β (LTβ).

Lymphokine An old name for a cytokine (soluble protein mediator of immune responses) produced by lymphocytes.

Lymphokine-activated killer (LAK) cells NK cells with enhanced cytolytic activity for tumor cells as a result of exposure to high doses of IL-2. LAK cells generated in vitro have been adoptively transferred back into patients with cancer to treat their tumors.

Lymphoma A malignant tumor of B or T lymphocytes usually arising in and spreading between lymphoid tissues but that may spread to other tissues. Lymphomas often express phenotypic characteristics of the normal lymphocytes from which they were derived.

Lymphotoxin (LT, TNF-β) A cytokine produced by T cells that is homologous to and binds to the same receptors as TNF. Like TNF, LT has proinflammatory effects, including endothelial and neutrophil activation. LT is also critical for the normal development of lymphoid organs.

Lysosome A membrane-bound, acidic organelle abundant in phagocytic cells that contains proteolytic enzymes that degrade proteins derived both from the extracellular environment and from within the cell. Lysosomes are involved in the class II MHC pathway of antigen processing.

M cells Specialized gastrointestinal mucosal epithelial cells overlying Peyer's patches in the gut that play a role in delivery of antigens to Peyer's patches.

M1 macrophages
See **classical macrophage activation.**

M2 macrophages
See a**lternative macrophage activation.**

Macrophage A tissue-based phagocytic cell derived from fetal hematopoietic organs or blood monocytes that plays important roles in innate and adaptive immune responses. Macrophages are activated by microbial products such as endotoxin and by T cell cytokines such as IFN-γ. Activated macrophages phagocytose and kill microorganisms, secrete proinflammatory cytokines, and present antigens to helper T cells. Macrophages may assume different morphologic forms in different tissues, including the microglia of the central nervous system, Kupffer cells in the liver, alveolar macrophages in the lung, and osteoclasts in bone.

Major histocompatibility complex (MHC) A large genetic locus (on human chromosome 6 and mouse chromosome 17) that includes the highly polymorphic genes encoding the peptide-binding molecules recognized by T lymphocytes. The MHC locus also includes genes encoding cytokines, molecules involved in antigen processing, and complement proteins.

Major histocompatibility complex (MHC) molecule A heterodimeric membrane protein encoded in the MHC locus that serves as a peptide display molecule for recognition by T lymphocytes. Two structurally distinct types of MHC molecules exist. Class I MHC molecules are present on most nucleated cells, bind peptides derived from cytosolic proteins, and are recognized by CD8+ T cells. Class II MHC molecules are restricted largely to dendritic cells, macrophages, and B lymphocytes, bind peptides derived from endocytosed proteins, and are recognized by CD4+ T cells.

Mannose-binding lectin (MBL) A plasma protein that binds to mannose residues on bacterial cell walls and acts as an opsonin by promoting phagocytosis of the bacterium by macrophages. Macrophages express a surface receptor for C1q that can also bind MBL and mediate uptake of the opsonized organisms.

Mannose receptor A carbohydrate-binding receptor (lectin) expressed by macrophages that binds mannose and fucose residues on microbial cell walls and mediates phagocytosis of the organisms.

Marginal zone A peripheral region of splenic lymphoid follicles containing macrophages that are particularly efficient at trapping polysaccharide antigens. Such antigens may persist for prolonged periods on the surfaces of marginal zone macrophages, where they are recognized by specific B cells, or they may be transported into follicles.

Marginal zone B lymphocytes A subset of B lymphocytes, found exclusively in the marginal zone of the spleen, that respond rapidly to blood-borne microbial antigens by producing IgM antibodies with limited diversity.

Mast cell The major effector cell of immediate hypersensitivity (allergic) reactions. Mast cells are derived from the marrow, reside in most tissues adjacent to blood vessels, express a high-affinity Fc receptor for IgE, and contain numerous mediator-filled granules. Antigen-induced cross-linking of IgE bound to the mast cell Fc receptors causes release of their granule contents as well as new synthesis and secretion of other mediators, leading to an immediate hypersensitivity reaction.

Mature B cell IgM- and IgD-expressing, functionally competent naive B cells that represent the final stage of B cell maturation in the bone marrow and that populate peripheral lymphoid organs.

Membrane attack complex (MAC) A lytic complex of the terminal components of the complement cascade, including multiple copies of C9, which forms in the membranes of target cells. The MAC causes lethal ionic and osmotic changes in cells.

Memory The property of the adaptive immune system to respond more rapidly, with greater magnitude, and more effectively to a repeated exposure to an antigen compared with the response to the first exposure.

Memory lymphocytes Memory B and T cells are produced by antigen stimulation of naive lymphocytes and survive in a functionally quiescent state for many years after the antigen is eliminated. Memory lymphocytes mediate rapid and enhanced (i.e., memory or recall) responses to second and subsequent exposures to antigens.

MHC class II (MIIC) compartment A subset of endosomes (membrane-bound vesicles involved in cell trafficking pathways) found in macrophages and human B cells that are important in the class II MHC pathway of antigen presentation. The MIIC contains all of the components required for formation of peptide–class II MHC molecule complexes, including the enzymes that degrade protein antigens, class II molecules, invariant chain, and HLA-DM.

MHC restriction The characteristic of T lymphocytes that they recognize a foreign peptide antigen only when it is bound to a particular allelic form of an MHC molecule.

MHC tetramer A reagent used to identify and enumerate T cells that specifically recognize a particular MHC-peptide complex. The reagent consists of four recombinant, biotinylated MHC molecules (usually class I) bound to a fluorochrome-labeled avidin molecule and loaded with a peptide. T cells that bind the MHC tetramer can be detected by flow cytometry.

β_2-Microglobulin The light chain of a class I MHC molecule. β_2-Microglobulin is an extracellular protein encoded by a non-polymorphic gene outside the MHC, is structurally homologous to an Ig domain, and is invariant among all class I molecules.

Mitogen-activated protein (MAP) kinase cascade A signal transduction cascade initiated by the active form of the Ras protein and involving the sequential activation of three serine/threonine kinases, the last one being MAP kinase. MAP kinase in turn phosphorylates and activates other enzymes and transcription factors. The MAP kinase pathway is one of several signal pathways activated by antigen binding to the TCR and BCR.

Mixed leukocyte reaction (MLR) An in vitro reaction of alloreactive T cells from one individual against MHC antigens on blood cells from another individual. The MLR involves proliferation of and cytokine secretion by both CD4+ and CD8+ T cells.

Molecular mimicry A postulated mechanism of autoimmunity triggered by infection with a microbe containing antigens that cross-react with self antigens. Immune responses to the microbe result in reactions against self tissues.

Monoclonal antibody An antibody that is specific for one antigen and is produced by a B cell hybridoma (a cell line derived by the fusion of a single normal B cell and an immortal B cell tumor line). Monoclonal antibodies are widely used in research, clinical diagnosis, and therapy.

Monocyte A type of bone marrow–derived circulating blood cell that is the precursor of tissue macrophages. Monocytes are actively recruited into inflammatory sites, where they differentiate into macrophages.

Mononuclear phagocytes Cells with a common bone marrow lineage whose primary function is phagocytosis. These cells function as accessory cells in the recognition and activation phases of adaptive immune responses and as effector cells in innate and adaptive immunity. Mononuclear phagocytes circulate in the blood in an incompletely differentiated form called monocytes, and once they settle in tissues, they mature into macrophages.

Mucosa-associated lymphoid tissue (MALT) Collections of lymphocytes, dendritic cells, and other cell types within the mucosa of the gastrointestinal and respiratory tracts that are sites of adaptive immune responses to antigens. Mucosa-associated lymphoid tissues contain intraepithelial lymphocytes, mainly

T cells, and organized collections of lymphocytes, often rich in B cells, below mucosal epithelia, such as Peyer's patches in the gut or pharyngeal tonsils.

Mucosal immune system A part of the immune system that responds to and protects against microbes that enter the body through mucosal surfaces, such as the gastrointestinal and respiratory tracts, but also maintains tolerance to commensal organisms that live on the outside of the mucosal epithelium. The mucosal immune system is composed of organized mucosa-associated lymphoid tissues, such as Peyer's patches, as well as diffusely distributed cells within the lamina propria.

Multiple myeloma A malignant tumor of antibody-producing B cells that often secretes Igs or parts of Ig molecules. The monoclonal antibodies produced by multiple myelomas were critical for early biochemical analyses of antibody structure.

Multivalency
See **polyvalency**.

Mycobacterium A genus of aerobic bacteria, many species of which can survive within phagocytes and cause disease. The principal host defense against mycobacteria such as *Mycobacterium tuberculosis* is cell-mediated immunity.

Myeloid-derived suppressor cells A heterogeneous group of immature myeloid precursors that suppress anti-tumor immune responses and are found in lymphoid tissues, blood, or tumors of tumor-bearing animals and cancer patients. The cells express Ly6C or Ly6G and CD11b in mice and CD33, CD11b, and CD15 in humans.

N nucleotides The name given to nucleotides randomly added to the junctions between V, D, and J gene segments in *Ig* or *TCR* genes during lymphocyte development. The addition of up to 20 of these nucleotides, which is mediated by the enzyme terminal deoxyribonucleotidyl transferase, contributes to the diversity of the antibody and TCR repertoires.

Naive lymphocyte A mature B or T lymphocyte that has not previously encountered antigen. When naive lymphocytes are stimulated by antigen, they differentiate into effector lymphocytes, such as antibody-secreting B cells or helper T cells and CTLs. Naive lymphocytes have surface markers and recirculation patterns that are distinct from those of previously activated lymphocytes. ("Naive" also refers to an unimmunized individual.)

Natural antibodies IgM antibodies, largely produced by B-1 cells, specific for bacteria that are common in the environment and gastrointestinal tract. Normal individuals contain natural antibodies without any evidence of infection, and these antibodies serve as a preformed defense mechanism against microbes that succeed in penetrating epithelial barriers. Some of these antibodies cross-react with ABO blood group antigens and are responsible for transfusion reactions.

Natural killer (NK) cells A subset of innate lymphoid cells that function in innate immune responses to kill microbe-infected cells by direct lytic mechanisms and by secreting IFN-γ. NK cells do not express clonally distributed antigen receptors like Ig receptors or TCRs, and their activation is regulated by a combination of cell surface stimulatory and inhibitory receptors, the latter recognizing self MHC molecules.

Natural killer T cells (NKT cells) A numerically small subset of lymphocytes that express T cell receptors and some surface molecules characteristic of NK cells. Some NKT cells, called invariant NKT (iNKT), express αβ T cell antigen receptors with very little diversity, recognize lipid antigens presented by CD1 molecules, and perform various effector functions typical of helper T cells.

Negative selection The process by which developing lymphocytes that express self-reactive antigen receptors are eliminated, thereby contributing to the maintenance of self-tolerance. Negative selection of developing T lymphocytes (thymocytes) is best understood and involves high-avidity binding of a thymocyte to self MHC molecules with bound peptides on thymic APCs, leading to apoptotic death of the thymocyte.

Neonatal Fc receptor (FcRn) An IgG-specific Fc receptor that mediates the transport of maternal IgG across the placenta and the neonatal intestinal epithelium and, in adults, promotes the long half-life of IgG molecules in the blood by protecting them from catabolism by phagocytes or endothelial cells.

Neonatal immunity Passive humoral immunity to infections in mammals in the first months of life, before full development of the immune system. Neonatal immunity is mediated by maternally produced antibodies transported across the placenta into the fetal circulation before birth or derived from ingested milk and transported across the gut epithelium.

Neutrophil (also polymorphonuclear leukocyte, PMN) A phagocytic cell characterized by a segmented lobular nucleus and cytoplasmic granules filled with degradative enzymes. PMNs are the most abundant type of circulating white blood cells and are the major cell type mediating acute inflammatory responses to bacterial infections.

Nitric oxide A biologic effector molecule with a broad range of activities that in macrophages functions as a potent microbicidal agent to kill ingested organisms.

Nitric oxide synthase A member of a family of enzymes that synthesize the vasoactive and microbicidal compound nitric oxide from L-arginine. Macrophages express an inducible form of this enzyme on activation by various microbial or cytokine stimuli.

NOD-like receptors (NLRs) A family of cytosolic multidomain proteins that sense cytoplasmic PAMPs and DAMPs and recruit other proteins to form signaling complexes that promote inflammation.

Notch 1 A cell surface signaling receptor that is proteolytically cleaved after ligand binding, and the cleaved intracellular portion translocates to the nucleus and regulates gene expression. Notch 1 signaling is required for commitment of developing T cell precursors to the alpha beta T cell lineage.

Nuclear factor κB (NF-κB) A family of transcription factors composed of homodimers or heterodimers of proteins homologous to the c-Rel protein. NF-κB proteins are required for the inducible transcription of many genes important in both innate and adaptive immune responses.

Nuclear factor of activated T cells (NFAT) A transcription factor required for the expression of IL-2, IL-4, TNF, and other cytokine genes. The four different NFATs are each encoded by separate genes; NFATp and NFATc are found in T cells. Cytoplasmic NFAT is activated by calcium/calmodulin-dependent, calcineurin-mediated dephosphorylation that permits NFAT to translocate into the nucleus and bind to consensus binding sequences in the regulatory regions of IL-2, IL-4, and other cytokine genes, usually in association with other transcription factors such as AP-1.

Nude mouse A strain of mice that lacks development of the thymus, and therefore T lymphocytes, as well as hair follicles. Nude mice have been used experimentally to define the role of T lymphocytes in immunity and disease.

Oncofetal antigen Proteins that are expressed at high levels on some types of cancer cells and in normal developing fetal (but not adult) tissues. Antibodies specific for these proteins are often used in histopathologic identification of tumors or to monitor the progression of tumor growth in patients. CEA (CD66) and α-fetoprotein are two oncofetal antigens commonly expressed by certain carcinomas.

Opsonin A molecule that becomes attached to the surface of a microbe and can be recognized by surface receptors of neutrophils and macrophages and that increases the efficiency of phagocytosis of the microbe. Opsonins include IgG antibodies, which are recognized by the Fcγ receptor on phagocytes, and fragments of complement proteins, which are recognized by CR1 (CD35) and by the leukocyte integrin Mac-1.

Opsonization The process of attaching opsonins, such as IgG or complement fragments, to microbial surfaces to target the microbes for phagocytosis.

Oral tolerance The suppression of systemic humoral and cell-mediated immune responses to an antigen after the oral administration of that antigen as a result of anergy of antigen-specific T cells or the production of immunosuppressive cytokines such as transforming growth factor-β. Oral tolerance is a possible mechanism for prevention of immune responses to food antigens and to bacteria that normally reside as commensals in the intestinal lumen.

P nucleotides Short inverted repeat nucleotide sequences in the VDJ junctions of rearranged *Ig* and *TCR* genes that are generated by RAG-1– and RAG-2–mediated asymmetric cleavage of hairpin DNA intermediates during somatic recombination events. P nucleotides contribute to the junctional diversity of antigen receptors.

Paracrine factor A molecule that acts on cells in proximity to the cell that produces the factor. Most cytokines act in a paracrine fashion.

Passive immunity The form of immunity to an antigen that is established in one individual by transfer of antibodies or lymphocytes from another individual who is immune to that antigen. The recipient of such a transfer can become immune to the antigen without ever having been exposed to or having responded to the antigen. An example of passive immunity is the transfer of human sera containing antibodies specific for certain microbial toxins or snake venom to a previously unimmunized individual.

Pathogen-associated molecular patterns (PAMPs) Structures produced by microorganisms but not mammalian (host) cells, which are recognized by and stimulate the innate immune system. Examples include bacterial lipopolysaccharide and viral double-stranded RNA.

Pathogenicity The ability of a microorganism to cause disease. Multiple mechanisms may contribute to pathogenicity, including production of toxins, stimulation of host inflammatory responses, and perturbation of host cell metabolism.

Pattern recognition receptors Signaling receptors of the innate immune system that recognize PAMPs and DAMPs, and thereby activate innate immune responses. Examples include Toll-like receptors (TLRs) and Nod-like receptors (NLRs).

PD-1 An inhibitory receptor homologous to CD28 that is expressed on activated T cells and binds to PD-L1 or PD-L2, members of the B7 protein family expressed on various cell types. PD-1 is upregulated on T cells in the setting of chronic infection or tumors, and blockade of PD-1 with monoclonal antibodies enhances antitumor immune responses.

Pentraxins A family of plasma proteins that contain five identical globular subunits; includes the acute-phase reactant C-reactive protein.

Peptide-binding cleft The portion of an MHC molecule that binds peptides for display to T cells. The cleft is composed of paired α helices resting on a floor made up of an eight-stranded β-pleated sheet. The polymorphic residues, which are the amino acids that vary among different MHC alleles, are located in and around this cleft.

Perforin A protein that is homologous to the C9 complement protein and is present in the granules of CTLs and NK cells. When perforin is released from the granules of activated CTLs or NK cells, it promotes entry of granzymes into the target cell, leading to apoptotic death of the cell.

Periarteriolar lymphoid sheath (PALS) A cuff of lymphocytes surrounding small arterioles in the spleen, adjacent to lymphoid follicles. A PALS contains mainly T lymphocytes, about two thirds of which are CD4+ and one third CD8+. In humoral immune responses to protein antigens, B lymphocytes are activated at the interface between the PALS and follicles and then migrate into the follicles to form germinal centers.

Peripheral lymphoid organs and tissues Organized collections of lymphocytes and accessory cells, including the spleen, lymph nodes, and mucosa-associated lymphoid tissues, in which adaptive immune responses are initiated.

Peripheral tolerance Unresponsiveness to self antigens that are present in peripheral tissues and not usually in the generative lymphoid organs. Peripheral tolerance is induced by the recognition of antigens without adequate levels of the costimulators required for lymphocyte activation or by persistent and repeated stimulation by these self antigens.

Peyer's patches Organized lymphoid tissue in the lamina propria of the small intestine in which immune responses to intestinal pathogens and other ingested antigens may be initiated. Peyer's patches are composed mostly of B cells, with smaller numbers of T cells and accessory cells, all arranged in follicles similar to those found in lymph nodes, often with germinal centers.

Phagocytosis The process by which certain cells of the innate immune system, including macrophages and neutrophils, engulf large particles (>0.5 μm in diameter) such as intact microbes. The cell surrounds the particle with extensions of its plasma membrane by an energy- and cytoskeleton-dependent process; this process results in the formation of an intracellular vesicle called a phagosome, which contains the ingested particle.

Phagosome A membrane-bound intracellular vesicle that contains microbes or particulate material from the extracellular environment. Phagosomes are formed during the process of phagocytosis. They fuse with other vesicular structures such as lysosomes, leading to enzymatic degradation of the ingested material.

Phosphatase (protein phosphatase) An enzyme that removes phosphate groups from the side chains of certain amino acid residues of proteins. Protein phosphatases in lymphocytes, such as CD45 or calcineurin, regulate the activity of various signal transduction molecules and transcription factors. Some protein phosphatases may be specific for phosphotyrosine residues and others for phosphoserine and phosphothreonine residues.

Phospholipase Cγ (PLCγ) An enzyme that catalyzes hydrolysis of the plasma membrane phospholipid PIP2 to generate two signaling molecules, IP3 and DAG. PLCγ becomes activated in lymphocytes by antigen binding to the antigen receptor.

Phytohemagglutinin (PHA) A carbohydrate-binding protein, or lectin, produced by plants that cross-links human T cell surface molecules, including the T cell receptor, thereby inducing polyclonal activation and agglutination of T cells. PHA is frequently used in experimental immunology to study T cell activation. In clinical medicine, PHA is used to assess whether a patient's T cells are functional or to induce T cell mitosis for the purpose of generating karyotypic data.

Plasmablast Circulating antibody-secreting cells that may be precursors of the plasma cells that reside in the bone marrow and other tissues.

Plasma cell A terminally differentiated antibody-secreting B lymphocyte with a characteristic histologic appearance, including an oval shape, eccentric nucleus, and perinuclear halo.

Platelet-activating factor (PAF) A lipid mediator derived from membrane phospholipids in several cell types, including mast cells and endothelial cells. PAF can cause bronchoconstriction and vascular dilation and leak, and it may be an important mediator in asthma.

Polyclonal activators Agents that are capable of activating many clones of lymphocytes, regardless of their antigen specificities. Examples of polyclonal activators include anti-IgM antibodies for B cells and anti-CD3 antibodies, bacterial superantigens, and PHA for T cells.

Poly-Ig receptor An Fc receptor expressed by mucosal epithelial cells that mediates the transport of IgA and IgM through the epithelial cells into the intestinal lumen.

Polymerase chain reaction (PCR) A rapid method of copying and amplifying specific DNA sequences up to about 1 kb in length that is widely used as a preparative and analytical technique in all branches of molecular biology. The method relies on the use of short oligonucleotide primers complementary to the sequences at the ends of the DNA to be amplified and involves repetitive cycles of melting, annealing, and synthesis of DNA.

Polymorphism The existence of two or more alternative forms, or variants, of a gene that are present at stable frequencies in a population. Each common variant of a polymorphic gene is called an allele, and one individual may carry two different alleles of a gene, each inherited from a different parent. The MHC genes are the most polymorphic genes in the mammalian genome, some of which have thousands of alleles.

Polyvalency The presence of multiple identical copies of an epitope on a single antigen molecule, cell surface, or particle. Polyvalent antigens, such as bacterial capsular polysaccharides, are often capable of activating B lymphocytes independent of helper T cells. Used synonymously with **multivalency**.

Positive selection The process by which developing T cells in the thymus (thymocytes) whose TCRs bind to self MHC molecules are rescued from programmed cell death, whereas thymocytes whose receptors do not recognize self MHC molecules die by default. Positive selection ensures that mature T cells are self MHC restricted and that CD8+ T cells are specific for complexes of peptides with class I MHC molecules and CD4+ T cells for complexes of peptides with class II MHC molecules.

Pre–B cell A developing B cell present only in hematopoietic tissues that is at a maturational stage characterized by expression of cytoplasmic Ig μ heavy chains and surrogate light chains but not Ig light chains. Pre–B cell receptors composed of μ chains and surrogate light chains deliver signals that stimulate further maturation of the pre–B cell into an immature B cell.

Pre–B cell receptor A receptor expressed on developing B lymphocytes at the pre–B cell stage that is composed of Ig μ heavy chains and invariant surrogate light chains. The pre–B cell receptor associates with the Igα and Igβ signal transduction proteins to form the pre–B cell receptor complex. Pre–B cell receptors are required for stimulating the proliferation and continued maturation of the developing B cell, serving as a checkpoint for productive μ heavy chain VDJ rearrangement. It is not known whether the pre–B cell receptor binds a specific ligand.

Pre–T cell A developing T lymphocyte in the thymus at a maturational stage characterized by expression of the TCR β chain but not the α chain or CD4 or CD8. In pre-T cells, the TCR β chain is found on the cell surface as part of the pre–T cell receptor.

Pre–T cell receptor A receptor expressed on the surface of pre–T cells that is composed of the TCR β chain and an invariant pre-Tα protein. This receptor associates with CD3 and ζ molecules to form the pre–T cell receptor complex. The function of this complex is similar to that of the pre–B cell receptor in B cell development, namely, the delivery of signals that stimulate further proliferation, antigen receptor gene rearrangements, and other maturational events. It is not known whether the pre–T cell receptor binds a specific ligand.

Pre-Tα An invariant transmembrane protein with a single extracellular Ig-like domain that associates with the TCR β chain in pre–T cells to form the pre–T cell receptor.

Primary immune response An adaptive immune response that occurs after the first exposure of an individual to a foreign antigen. Primary responses are characterized by relatively slow kinetics and small magnitude compared with the responses after a second or subsequent exposure.

Primary immunodeficiency
See **congenital immunodeficiency.**

Pro–B cell A developing B cell in the bone marrow that is the earliest cell committed to the B lymphocyte lineage. Pro–B cells do not produce Ig, but they can be distinguished from other immature cells by the expression of B lineage–restricted surface molecules such as CD19 and CD10.

Pro–T cell A developing T cell in the thymic cortex that is a recent arrival from the bone marrow and does not express TCRs, CD3, ζ chains, or CD4 or CD8 molecules. Pro–T cells are also called double-negative thymocytes.

Professional antigen-presenting cells (professional APCs) A term sometimes used to refer to APCs that activate T lymphocytes; includes dendritic cells, mononuclear phagocytes, and B lymphocytes, all of which are capable of expressing class II MHC molecules and costimulators. The most important professional APCs for initiation of primary T cell responses are dendritic cells.

Programmed cell death
See **apoptosis.**

Promoter A DNA sequence immediately 5′ to the transcription start site of a gene where the proteins that initiate transcription bind. The term *promoter* is often used to mean the entire 5′ regulatory region of a gene, including enhancers, that are additional sequences that bind transcription factors and interact with the basal transcription complex to increase the rate of transcriptional initiation. Other enhancers may be located at a significant distance from the promoter, either 5′ of the gene, in introns, or 3′ of the gene.

Prostaglandins A class of lipid inflammatory mediators that are derived from arachidonic acid in many cell types through the cyclooxygenase pathway and that have vasodilator, bronchoconstrictor, and chemotactic activities. Prostaglandins made by mast cells are important mediators of allergic reactions.

Proteasome A large multiprotein enzyme complex with a broad range of proteolytic activity that is found in the cytoplasm of most cells and generates from cytosolic proteins the peptides that bind to class I MHC molecules. Proteins are targeted for proteasomal degradation by covalent linkage of ubiquitin molecules.

Protein kinase C (PKC) Any of several isoforms of an enzyme that mediates the phosphorylation of serine and threonine residues in many different protein substrates and thereby serves to propagate various signal transduction pathways leading to transcription factor activation. In T and B lymphocytes, PKC is activated by DAG, which is generated in response to antigen receptor ligation.

Protein tyrosine kinases (PTKs) Enzymes that mediate the phosphorylation of tyrosine residues in proteins and thereby promote phosphotyrosine-dependent protein-protein interactions. PTKs are involved in numerous signal transduction pathways in cells of the immune system.

Protozoa Single-celled eukaryotic organisms, many of which are human parasites and cause diseases. Examples of pathogenic protozoa include *Entamoeba histolytica,* which causes amebic dysentery; *Plasmodium,* which causes malaria; and *Leishmania,* which causes leishmaniasis. Protozoa stimulate both innate and adaptive immune responses. It has proved difficult to develop effective vaccines against many of these organisms.

Provirus A DNA copy of the genome of a retrovirus that is integrated into the host cell genome and from which viral genes are transcribed and the viral genome is reproduced. HIV proviruses can remain inactive for long periods and thereby represent a latent form of HIV infection that is not accessible to immune defense.

Purified antigen (subunit) vaccine A vaccine composed of purified antigens or subunits of microbes. Examples of this type of vaccine include diphtheria and tetanus toxoids, pneumococcus and *Haemophilus influenzae* polysaccharide vaccines, and purified polypeptide vaccines against hepatitis B and influenza virus. Purified antigen vaccines may stimulate antibody and helper T cell responses, but they typically do not generate CTL responses.

Pyogenic bacteria Bacteria, such as Gram-positive staphylococci and streptococci, that induce inflammatory responses rich in polymorphonuclear leukocytes (giving rise to pus). Antibody responses to these bacteria greatly enhance the efficacy of innate immune effector mechanisms to clear infections.

Radioimmunoassay A highly sensitive and specific immunologic method of quantifying the concentration of an antigen in a solution that relies on a radioactively labeled antibody specific for the antigen. Usually, two antibodies specific for the antigen are used. The first antibody is unlabeled but attached to a solid support, where it binds and immobilizes the antigen whose concentration is being determined. The amount of the second, labeled antibody that binds to the immobilized antigen, as determined by radioactive decay detectors, is proportional to the concentration of antigen in the test solution.

Rapamycin An immunosuppressive drug (also called sirolimus) used clinically to prevent allograft rejection. Rapamycin inhibits the activation of a protein called molecular target of rapamycin (mTOR), which is a key signaling molecule in a variety of metabolic and cell growth pathways including the pathway required for interleukin-2–mediated T cell proliferation.

Ras A member of a family of 21-kD guanine nucleotide–binding proteins with intrinsic GTPase activity that are involved in many different signal transduction pathways in diverse cell types. Mutated *ras* genes are associated with neoplastic transformation. In T cell activation, Ras is recruited to the plasma membrane by tyrosine-phosphorylated adaptor proteins, where it is activated by GDP-GTP exchange factors. GTP·Ras then initiates the MAP kinase cascade, which leads to expression of the *fos* gene and assembly of the AP-1 transcription factor.

Reactive oxygen species (ROS) Highly reactive metabolites of oxygen, including superoxide anion, hydroxyl radical, and hydrogen peroxide, that are produced by activated phagocytes. Reactive oxygen species are used by the phagocytes to form oxyhalides that damage ingested bacteria. They may also be released from cells and promote inflammatory responses or cause tissue damage.

Reagin IgE antibody that mediates an immediate hypersensitivity reaction.

Receptor editing A process by which some immature B cells that recognize self antigens in the bone marrow may be induced to change their Ig specificities. Receptor editing involves reactivation of the *RAG* genes, additional light-chain VJ recombinations, and new Ig light-chain production, which allows the cell to express a different Ig receptor that is not self-reactive.

Recombination-activating genes 1 and 2 (*RAG1* and *RAG2*) The genes encoding RAG-1 and RAG-2 proteins, which make up the V(D)J recombinase and are expressed in developing B and T cells. RAG proteins bind to recombination signal sequences and are critical for DNA recombination events that form functional *Ig* and *TCR* genes. Therefore, RAG proteins are required for expression of antigen receptors and for the maturation of B and T lymphocytes.

Recombination signal sequences Specific DNA sequences found adjacent to the V, D, and J segments in the antigen receptor loci and recognized by the RAG-1/RAG-2 complex during V(D)J recombination. The recognition sequences consist of a highly conserved stretch of 7 nucleotides, called the heptamer, located adjacent to the V, D, or J coding sequence, followed by a spacer of exactly 12 or 23 non-conserved nucleotides and a highly conserved stretch of 9 nucleotides, called the nonamer.

Red pulp An anatomic and functional compartment of the spleen composed of vascular sinusoids, scattered among which are large numbers of erythrocytes, macrophages, dendritic cells, sparse lymphocytes, and plasma cells. Red pulp macrophages clear the blood of microbes, other foreign particles, and damaged red blood cells.

Regulatory T cells A population of T cells that inhibits the activation of other T cells and is necessary to maintain peripheral tolerance to self antigens. Most regulatory T cells are CD4+ and express the α chain of the IL-2 receptor (CD25), CTLA4, and the transcription factor FoxP3.

Respiratory burst The process by which reactive oxygen intermediates such as superoxide anion, hydroxyl radical, and hydrogen peroxide are produced in macrophages and polymorphonuclear leukocytes. The respiratory burst is mediated by the enzyme phagocyte oxidase and is usually triggered by inflammatory mediators, such as LTB$_4$, PAF, and TNF, or by bacterial products, such as *N*-formylmethionyl peptides.

Reverse transcriptase An enzyme encoded by retroviruses, such as HIV, that synthesizes a DNA copy of the viral genome from the RNA genomic template. Purified reverse transcriptase is used widely in molecular biology research for purposes of cloning complementary DNAs encoding a gene of interest from messenger RNA. Reverse transcriptase inhibitors are used as drugs to treat HIV-1 infection.

Rh blood group antigens A complex system of protein alloantigens expressed on red blood cell membranes that are the cause of transfusion reactions and hemolytic disease of the newborn. The most clinically important Rh antigen is designated D.

Rheumatoid arthritis An autoimmune disease characterized primarily by inflammatory damage to joints and sometimes inflammation of blood vessels, lungs, and other tissues. CD4+ T cells, activated B lymphocytes, and plasma cells are found in the inflamed joint lining (synovium), and numerous proinflammatory cytokines, including IL-1 and TNF, are present in the synovial (joint) fluid.

RIG-like receptors (RLRs) Cytosolic receptors of the innate immune system that recognize viral RNA and induce production of type I interferons. The two best characterized RLRs are RIG-I (retinoic acid–inducible gene I) and MDA5 (melanoma differentiation-associated gene 5).

RORγT (retinoid-related orphan receptor γ T) A transcription factor expressed in and required for differentiation of T$_H$17 cells and Type 3 innate lymphoid cells.

Scavenger receptors A family of cell surface receptors expressed on macrophages, originally defined as receptors that mediate endocytosis of oxidized or acetylated low-density lipoprotein particles but that also bind and mediate the phagocytosis of a variety of microbes.

SCID mouse A mouse strain in which B and T cells are absent because of an early block in maturation from bone marrow precursors. SCID mice carry a mutation in a component of the enzyme DNA-dependent protein kinase, which is required for double-stranded DNA break repair. Deficiency of this enzyme results in abnormal joining of Ig and TCR gene segments during recombination and therefore failure to express antigen receptors.

Secondary immune response An adaptive immune response that occurs on second exposure to an antigen. A secondary response is characterized by more rapid kinetics and greater magnitude relative to the primary immune response, which occurs on first exposure.

Secondary immunodeficiency.
See **acquired immunodeficiency.**

Second-set rejection Allograft rejection in an individual who has previously been sensitized to the donor's tissue alloantigens by having received another graft or transfusion from that donor. In contrast to first-set rejection, which occurs in an individual who has not previously been sensitized to the donor alloantigens, second-set rejection is rapid and occurs in 3 to 7 days as a result of immunologic memory.

Secretory component The proteolytically cleaved portion of the extracellular domain of the poly-Ig receptor that remains bound to an IgA molecule in mucosal secretions.

Selectin Any one of three separate but closely related carbohydrate-binding proteins that mediate adhesion of leukocytes to endothelial cells. Each of the selectin molecules is a single-chain transmembrane glycoprotein with a similar modular structure, including an extracellular calcium-dependent lectin domain. The selectins include L-selectin (CD62L), expressed on leukocytes; P-selectin (CD62P), expressed on platelets and activated endothelium; and E-selectin (CD62E), expressed on activated endothelium.

Selective immunoglobulin deficiency Immunodeficiencies characterized by a lack of only one or a few Ig classes or subclasses. IgA deficiency is the most common selective Ig deficiency, followed by IgG3 and IgG2 deficiencies. Patients with these disorders may be at increased risk for bacterial infections, but many are normal.

Self MHC restriction The limitation (or restriction) of T cells to recognize antigens displayed by MHC molecules that the T cell encountered during maturation in the thymus (and thus sees as self).

Self-tolerance Unresponsiveness of the adaptive immune system to self antigens, largely as a result of inactivation or death of self-reactive lymphocytes induced by exposure to these antigens. Self-tolerance is a cardinal feature of the normal immune system, and failure of self-tolerance leads to autoimmune diseases.

Septic shock A severe complication of bacterial infections that spread to the blood stream (sepsis), and is characterized by vascular collapse, disseminated intravascular coagulation, and metabolic disturbances. This syndrome is due to the effects of bacterial cell wall components, such as LPS or peptidoglycan, that bind to TLRs on various cell types and induce expression of inflammatory cytokines, including TNF and IL-12.

Seroconversion The production of detectable antibodies in the serum specific for a microorganism during the course of an infection or in response to immunization.

Serology The study of blood (serum) antibodies and their reactions with antigens. The term *serology* is often used to refer to the diagnosis of infectious diseases by detection of microbe-specific antibodies in the serum.

Serotype An antigenically distinct subset of a species of an infectious organism that is distinguished from other subsets by serologic (i.e., serum antibody) tests. Humoral immune responses to one serotype of microbes (e.g., influenza virus) may not be protective against another serotype.

Serum The cell-free fluid that remains when blood or plasma forms a clot. Blood antibodies are found in the serum fraction.

Serum amyloid A (SAA) An acute-phase protein whose serum concentration rises significantly in the setting of infection and inflammation, mainly because of IL-1– and TNF-induced synthesis by the liver. SAA activates leukocyte chemotaxis, phagocytosis, and adhesion to endothelial cells.

Serum sickness A disease caused by the injection of large doses of a protein antigen into the blood and characterized by the deposition of antigen-antibody (immune) complexes in blood vessel walls, especially in the kidneys and joints. Immune complex deposition leads to complement fixation and leukocyte recruitment and subsequently to glomerulonephritis and arthritis. Serum sickness was originally described as a disorder that occurred in patients receiving injections of serum containing antitoxin antibodies to prevent diphtheria.

Severe combined immunodeficiency (SCID) Immunodeficiency diseases in which both B and T lymphocytes do not develop or do not function properly, and therefore both humoral immunity and cell-mediated immunity are impaired. Children with SCID usually have infections during the first year of life and succumb to these infections unless the immunodeficiency is treated. SCID has several different genetic causes.

Shwartzman reaction An experimental model of the pathologic effects of bacterial LPS and TNF in which two intravenous injections of LPS are administered to a rabbit 24 hours apart. After the second injection, the rabbit suffers disseminated intravascular coagulation and neutrophil and platelet plugging of small blood vessels.

Signal transducer and activator of transcription (STAT) A member of a family of proteins that function as signaling molecules and transcription factors in response to binding of cytokines to type I and type II cytokine receptors. STATs are present as inactive monomers in the cytosol of cells and are recruited to the cytoplasmic tails of cross-linked cytokine receptors, where they are tyrosine phosphorylated by JAKs. The phosphorylated STAT proteins dimerize and move to the nucleus, where they bind to specific sequences in the promoter regions of various genes and stimulate their transcription. Different STATs are activated by different cytokines.

Simian immunodeficiency virus A lentivirus closely related to HIV-1 that causes disease similar to AIDS in monkeys.

Single-positive thymocyte A maturing T cell precursor in the thymus that expresses CD4 or CD8 molecules but not both. Single-positive thymocytes are found mainly in the medulla and have matured from the double-positive stage, during which thymocytes express both CD4 and CD8 molecules.

Smallpox A disease caused by variola virus. Smallpox was the first infectious disease shown to be preventable by vaccination and the first disease to be completely eradicated by a worldwide vaccination program.

Somatic hypermutation High-frequency point mutations in Ig heavy and light chains that occur in germinal center B cells in response to signals from T_{FH} cells. Mutations that result in increased affinity of antibodies for antigen impart a selective survival advantage to the B cells producing those antibodies and lead to affinity maturation of a humoral immune response.

Somatic recombination The process of DNA recombination by which the functional genes encoding the variable regions of antigen receptors are formed during lymphocyte development. A relatively limited set of inherited, or germline, DNA sequences that are initially separated from one another are brought together by enzymatic deletion of intervening sequences and re-ligation. This process occurs only in developing B or T lymphocytes, and is mediated by RAG-1 and RAG-2 proteins. This process is also called V(D)J recombination or somatic rearrangement.

Specificity A cardinal feature of the adaptive immune system, namely, that immune responses are directed toward and able to distinguish between distinct antigens or small parts of macromolecular antigens. This fine specificity is attributed to lymphocyte antigen receptors that may bind to one molecule but not to another, even closely related, molecule.

Spleen A secondary lymphoid organ in the left upper quadrant of the abdomen. The spleen is the major site of adaptive immune responses to blood-borne antigens. The red pulp of the spleen is composed of blood-filled vascular sinusoids lined by active phagocytes that ingest opsonized antigens and damaged red blood cells. The white pulp of the spleen contains lymphocytes and lymphoid follicles where B cells are activated.

Src homology 2 (SH2) domain A three-dimensional domain structure of about 100 amino acid residues present in many signaling proteins that permits specific non-covalent interactions with other proteins by binding to phosphotyrosines. Each SH2 domain has a unique binding specificity that is determined by the amino acid residues adjacent to the phosphotyrosine on the target protein. Several proteins involved in early signaling events in T and B lymphocytes interact with one another through SH2 domains.

Src homology 3 (SH3) domain A three-dimensional domain structure of about 60 amino acid residues present in many signaling proteins that mediates protein-protein binding. SH3 domains bind to proline residues and function cooperatively with the SH2 domains of the same protein. For instance, SOS, the guanine nucleotide exchange factor for Ras, contains both SH2 and SH3 domains, and both are involved in SOS binding to the adaptor protein Grb-2.

Stem cell An undifferentiated cell that divides continuously and gives rise to additional stem cells and to cells of multiple different lineages. For example, all blood cells arise from a common hematopoietic stem cell.

Superantigens Proteins that bind to and activate all of the T cells in an individual that express a particular set or family of V_β *TCR* genes. Superantigens are presented to T cells by binding to non-polymorphic regions of class II MHC molecules on APCs, and they interact with conserved regions of TCR V_β domains. Several staphylococcal enterotoxins are superantigens. Their importance lies in their ability to activate many T cells, which results in large amounts of cytokine production and a clinical syndrome that is similar to septic shock.

Suppressor T cells T cells that block the activation and function of other T lymphocytes. It has been difficult to clearly identify suppressor T cells, and the term is not widely used at this time. The much better defined T cells that function to control immune responses are **regulatory T cells**.

Surrogate light chains Two non-variable proteins that associate with Ig μ heavy chains in pre-B cells to form the pre-B cell receptor. The two surrogate light chain proteins include the V pre-B protein, which is homologous to a light-chain V domain, and λ5, which is covalently attached to the μ heavy chain by a disulfide bond.

Switch recombination The molecular mechanism underlying Ig isotype switching in which a rearranged VDJ gene segment in an antibody-producing B cell recombines with a downstream C gene and the intervening C gene or genes are deleted. DNA recombination events in switch recombination are triggered by CD40 and cytokines and involve nucleotide sequences called switch regions located in the introns at the 5′ end of each C_H locus.

Syk A cytoplasmic protein tyrosine kinase, similar to ZAP-70 in T cells, that is critical for early signaling steps in antigen-induced B cell activation. Syk binds to phosphorylated tyrosines in the cytoplasmic tails of the Igα and Igβ chains of the BCR complex and in turn phosphorylates adaptor proteins that recruit other components of the signaling cascade.

Syngeneic Genetically identical. All animals of an inbred strain and monozygotic twins are syngeneic.

Syngeneic graft A graft from a donor who is genetically identical to the recipient. Syngeneic grafts are not rejected.

Synthetic vaccine Vaccines composed of recombinant DNA–derived antigens. Synthetic vaccines for hepatitis B virus and herpes simplex virus are now in use.

Systemic inflammatory response syndrome (SIRS) The systemic changes observed in patients who have disseminated bacterial infections. In its mild form, SIRS consists of neutrophilia, fever, and a rise in acute-phase reactants in the plasma. These changes are stimulated by bacterial products such as LPS and are mediated by cytokines of the innate immune system. In severe cases, SIRS may include disseminated intravascular coagulation, adult respiratory distress syndrome, and septic shock.

Systemic lupus erythematosus (SLE) A chronic systemic autoimmune disease that affects predominantly women and is characterized by rashes, arthritis, glomerulonephritis, hemolytic anemia, thrombocytopenia, and central nervous system involvement. Many different autoantibodies are found in patients with SLE, particularly anti-DNA antibodies. Many of the manifestations of SLE are due to the formation of immune complexes composed of autoantibodies and their specific antigens, with deposition of these complexes in small blood vessels in various tissues. The underlying mechanism for the breakdown of self-tolerance in SLE is not understood.

T cell receptor (TCR) The clonally distributed antigen receptor on CD4+ and CD8+ T lymphocytes that recognizes complexes of foreign peptides bound to self MHC molecules on the surface of APCs. The most common form of TCR is composed of a heterodimer of two disulfide-linked transmembrane polypeptide chains, designated α and β, each containing one N-terminal Ig-like variable (V) domain, one Ig-like constant (C) domain, a hydrophobic transmembrane region, and a short cytoplasmic region. (Another less common type of TCR, composed of γ and δ chains, is found on a small subset of T cells and recognizes different forms of antigen.)

T cell receptor (TCR) transgenic mouse A mouse in a genetically engineered strain that expresses transgenically encoded functional TCR α and β genes encoding a TCR of a single defined specificity. Because of allelic exclusion of endogenous TCR genes, most or all of the T cells in a TCR transgenic mouse have the same antigen specificity, which is a useful property for various research purposes.

T follicular helper (T$_{FH}$) cells A heterogeneous subset of CD4$^+$ helper T cells present within lymphoid follicles that are critical in providing signals to B cells in the germinal center reaction that stimulate somatic hypermutation, isotype switching and the generation of memory B cells and long lived plasma cells. T$_{FH}$ cells express CXCR5, ICOS, IL-21, and Bcl-6.

T lymphocyte The key component of cell-mediated immune responses in the adaptive immune system. T lymphocytes mature in the thymus, circulate in the blood, populate secondary lymphoid tissues, and are recruited to peripheral sites of antigen exposure. They express antigen receptors (TCRs) that recognize peptide fragments of foreign proteins bound to self MHC molecules. Functional subsets of T lymphocytes include CD4$^+$ helper T cells and CD8$^+$ CTLs.

T-bet A T-box family transcription factor that promotes the differentiation of T$_H$1 cells from naive T cells.

T-dependent antigen An antigen that requires both B cells and helper T cells to stimulate an antibody response. T-dependent antigens are protein antigens that contain some epitopes recognized by T cells and other epitopes recognized by B cells. Helper T cells produce cytokines and cell surface molecules that stimulate B cell growth and differentiation into antibody-secreting cells. Humoral immune responses to T-dependent antigens are characterized by isotype switching, affinity maturation, and memory.

Tertiary lymphoid organ A collection of lymphocytes and antigen-presenting cells organized into B cell follicles and T cell zones that develop in sites of chronic immune-mediated inflammation, such as the joint synovium of rheumatoid arthritis patients.

T-independent antigen Non-protein antigens, such as polysaccharides and lipids, which can stimulate antibody responses without a requirement for antigen-specific helper T lymphocytes. T-independent antigens usually contain multiple identical epitopes that can cross-link membrane Ig on B cells and thereby activate the cells. Humoral immune responses to T-independent antigens show relatively little heavy-chain isotype switching or affinity maturation, two processes that require signals from helper T cells.

T$_H$1 cells A subset of CD4$^+$ helper T cells that secrete a particular set of cytokines, including IFN-γ, and whose principal function is to stimulate phagocyte-mediated defense against infections, especially with intracellular microbes.

T$_H$2 cells A functional subset of CD4$^+$ helper T cells that secrete a particular set of cytokines, including IL-4, IL-5, and IL-3 and whose principal function is to stimulate IgE and eosinophil/mast cell–mediated immune reactions.

T$_H$17 cells A functional subset of CD4$^+$ helper T cells that secrete a particular set of inflammatory cytokines, including IL-17 and IL-22, that are protective against bacterial and fungal infections and also mediate inflammatory reactions in autoimmune and other inflammatory diseases.

Thymic epithelial cells Epithelial cells abundant in the cortical and medullary stroma of the thymus that play a critical role in T cell development. In the process of positive selection, maturing T cells that weakly recognize self peptides bound to MHC molecules on the surface of thymic epithelial cells are rescued from programmed cell death.

Thymocyte A precursor of a mature T lymphocyte present in the thymus.

Thymus A bilobed organ situated in the anterior mediastinum that is the site of maturation of T lymphocytes from bone marrow–derived precursors. Thymic tissue is divided into an outer cortex and an inner medulla and contains stromal thymic epithelial cells, macrophages, dendritic cells, and numerous T cell precursors (thymocytes) at various stages of maturation.

Tissue typing The determination of the particular MHC alleles expressed by an individual for the purpose of matching allograft donors and recipients. Tissue typing, also called HLA typing, is usually done by molecular (PCR-based) sequencing of HLA alleles or by serologic methods (lysis of an individual's cells by panels of anti-HLA antibodies).

TNF receptor–associated factors (TRAFs) A family of adaptor molecules that interact with the cytoplasmic domains of various receptors in the TNF receptor family, including TNF-RII, lymphotoxin (LT)-β receptor, and CD40. Each of these receptors contains a cytoplasmic motif that binds different TRAFs, which in turn engage other signaling molecules, leading to activation of the transcription factors AP-1 and NF-κB.

Tolerance Unresponsiveness of the adaptive immune system to antigens, as a result of inactivation or death of antigen-specific lymphocytes, induced by exposure to the antigens. Tolerance to self antigens is a normal feature of the adaptive immune system, but tolerance to foreign antigens may be induced under certain conditions of antigen exposure.

Tolerogen An antigen that induces immunologic tolerance, in contrast to an immunogen, which induces an immune response. Many antigens can be either tolerogens or immunogens, depending on how they are administered. Tolerogenic forms of antigens include large doses of the proteins administered without adjuvants and orally administered antigens.

Toll-like receptors A family of pattern recognition receptors of the innate immune system that are expressed on the surface and in endosomes of many cell types and that recognize microbial structures, such as endotoxin and viral RNA, and transduce signals that lead to the expression of inflammatory and anti-viral genes.

Toxic shock syndrome An acute illness characterized by shock, skin exfoliation, conjunctivitis, and diarrhea that is associated with tampon use and caused by a *Staphylococcus aureus* superantigen.

Transfusion Transplantation of circulating blood cells, platelets, or plasma from one individual to another. Transfusions are performed to treat blood loss from hemorrhage or to treat a deficiency in one or more blood cell types resulting from inadequate production or excess destruction.

Transfusion reactions An immunologic reaction against transfused blood products, usually mediated by preformed antibodies in the recipient that bind to donor blood cell antigens, such as ABO blood group antigens or histocompatibility antigens. Transfusion reactions can lead to intravascular lysis of red blood cells and, in severe cases, kidney damage, fever, shock, and disseminated intravascular coagulation.

Transgenic mouse A mouse that expresses an exogenous gene that has been introduced into the genome by injection of a specific DNA sequence into the pronuclei of fertilized mouse eggs. Transgenes insert randomly at chromosomal break points and are subsequently inherited as simple Mendelian traits. By the design of transgenes with tissue-specific regulatory sequences, mice can be produced that express a particular gene only in certain tissues. Transgenic mice are used extensively in immunology research to study the functions of various cytokines, cell surface molecules, and intracellular signaling molecules.

Transplantation The process of transferring cells, tissues, or organs (i.e., grafts) from one individual to another or from one site to another in the same individual. Transplantation is used to treat a variety of diseases in which there is a functional disorder of a tissue or organ. The major barrier to successful transplantation between individuals is immunologic reaction (rejection) to the transplanted graft.

Transporter associated with antigen processing (TAP) An adenosine triphosphate (ATP)-dependent peptide transporter that mediates the active transport of peptides from the cytosol to the site of assembly of class I MHC molecules inside the endoplasmic reticulum. TAP is a heterodimeric molecule composed of TAP-1 and TAP-2 polypeptides, both encoded by genes in the MHC. Because peptides are required for stable assembly of class I MHC molecules, TAP-deficient animals express few cell surface class I MHC molecules, which results in diminished development and activation of $CD8^+$ T cells.

Tumor immunity Protection against the development or progression of tumors by the immune system. Although immune responses to naturally occurring tumors can frequently be demonstrated, tumors often escape these responses. New therapies that target T cell inhibitory molecules, such as PD-1, are proving effective in enhancing effective T cell mediated anti-tumor immunity.

Tumor-infiltrating lymphocytes (TILs) Lymphocytes isolated from the inflammatory infiltrates present in and around surgical resection samples of solid tumors that are enriched with tumor-specific CTLs and NK cells. In an experimental mode of cancer treatment, TILs are grown in vitro in the presence of high doses of IL-2 and are then adoptively transferred back into patients with the tumor.

Tumor necrosis factor receptor superfamily (TNFRSF) A large family of structurally homologous transmembrane proteins that bind TNFSF proteins and generate signals that regulate proliferation, differentiation, apoptosis, and inflammatory gene expression (see Appendix II).

Tumor necrosis factor superfamily (TNFSF) A large family of structurally homologous transmembrane proteins that regulate diverse functions in responding cells, including proliferation, differentiation, apoptosis, and inflammatory gene expression. TNFSF members typically form homotrimers, either within the plasma membrane or after proteolytic release from the membrane, and bind to homotrimeric TNF receptor superfamily (TNFRSF) molecules, which then initiate a variety of signaling pathways (see Appendix II).

Tumor-specific antigen An antigen whose expression is restricted to a particular tumor and is not expressed by normal cells. Tumor-specific antigens may serve as target antigens for anti-tumor immune responses.

Tumor-specific transplantation antigen (TSTA) An antigen expressed on experimental animal tumor cells that can be detected by induction of immunologic rejection of tumor transplants. TSTAs were originally defined on chemically induced rodent sarcomas and shown to stimulate CTL-mediated rejection of transplanted tumors.

Two-signal hypothesis A now proven hypothesis that states that the activation of lymphocytes requires two distinct signals, the first being antigen and the second either microbial products or components of innate immune responses to microbes. The requirement for antigen (so-called signal 1) ensures that the ensuing immune response is specific. The requirement for additional stimuli triggered by microbes or innate immune reactions (signal 2) ensures that immune responses are induced when they are needed, that is, against microbes and other noxious substances and not against harmless substances, including self antigens. Signal 2 is referred to as costimulation and is often mediated by membrane molecules on professional APCs, such as B7 proteins.

Type 1 diabetes mellitus A disease characterized by a lack of insulin that leads to various metabolic and vascular abnormalities. The insulin deficiency results from autoimmune destruction of the insulin-producing β cells of the islets of Langerhans in the pancreas, usually during childhood. $CD4^+$ and $CD8^+$ T cells, antibodies, and cytokines have been implicated in the islet cell damage. Also called insulin-dependent diabetes mellitus.

Ubiquitination Covalent linkage of one or several copies of a small polypeptide called ubiquitin to a protein. Ubiquitination frequently serves to target proteins for proteolytic degradation by lysosomes or by proteasomes, the later a critical step in the class I MHC pathway of antigen processing and presentation.

Urticaria Localized transient swelling and redness of the skin caused by leakage of fluid and plasma proteins from small vessels into the dermis during an immediate hypersensitivity reaction.

V gene segments A DNA sequence that encodes the variable domain of an Ig heavy chain or light chain or a TCR α, β, γ, or δ chain. Each antigen receptor locus contains many different V gene segments, any one of which may recombine with downstream D or J segments during lymphocyte maturation to form functional antigen receptor genes.

V(D)J recombinase The complex of RAG1 and RAG2 proteins that catalyzes lymphocyte antigen receptor gene recombination.

Vaccine A preparation of microbial antigen, often combined with adjuvants, which is administered to individuals to induce protective immunity against microbial infections. The antigen may be in the form of live but avirulent microorganisms, killed microorganisms, purified macromolecular components of a microorganism, or a plasmid that contains a complementary DNA encoding a microbial antigen.

Variable region The extracellular, N-terminal region of an Ig heavy or light chain or a TCR α, β, γ, or δ chain that contains variable amino acid sequences that differ between every clone of lymphocytes and that are responsible for the specificity for antigen. The antigen-binding variable sequences are localized to extended loop structures or hypervariable segments.

Virus A primitive obligate intracellular parasitic organism or infectious particle that consists of a simple nucleic acid genome packaged in a protein capsid, sometimes surrounded by a membrane envelope. Many pathogenic animal viruses cause a wide range of diseases. Humoral immune responses to viruses can be effective in blocking infection of cells, and NK cells and CTLs are necessary to kill cells already infected.

Western blot An immunologic technique to determine the presence of a protein in a biologic sample. The method involves separation of proteins in the sample by electrophoresis, transfer of the protein array from the electrophoresis gel to a support membrane by capillary action (blotting), and finally detection of the protein by binding of an enzymatically or radioactively labeled antibody specific for that protein.

Wheal-and-flare reaction Local swelling and redness in the skin at a site of an immediate hypersensitivity reaction. The wheal reflects increased vascular permeability, and the flare results from increased local blood flow, both changes resulting from mediators such as histamine released from activated dermal mast cells.

White pulp The part of the spleen that is composed predominantly of lymphocytes, arranged in periarteriolar lymphoid sheaths, and follicles and other leukocytes.

The remainder of the spleen contains sinusoids lined with phagocytic cells and filled with blood, called the **red pulp.**

Wiskott-Aldrich syndrome An X-linked disease characterized by eczema, thrombocytopenia (reduced blood platelets), and immunodeficiency manifested as susceptibility to bacterial infections. The defective gene encodes a cytosolic protein involved in signaling cascades and regulation of the actin cytoskeleton.

XBP-1 A transcription factor that is required for the unfolded protein response and plasma cell development.

Xenoantigen An antigen on a graft from another species.

Xenograft (xenogeneic graft) An organ or tissue graft derived from a species different from the recipient. Transplantation of xenogeneic grafts (e.g., from a pig) to humans is not yet practical because of special problems related to immunologic rejection.

Xenoreactive Describing a T cell or antibody that recognizes and responds to an antigen on a graft from another species (a xenoantigen). The T cell may recognize an intact xenogeneic MHC molecule or a peptide derived from a xenogeneic protein bound to a self MHC molecule.

X-linked agammaglobulinemia An immunodeficiency disease, also called Bruton's agammaglobulinemia, characterized by a block in early B cell maturation and an absence of serum Ig. Patients suffer from pyogenic bacterial infections. The disease is caused by mutations or deletions in the gene encoding Btk, an enzyme involved in signal transduction in developing B cells.

X-linked hyper-IgM syndrome A rare immunodeficiency disease caused by mutations in the CD40 ligand gene and characterized by failure of B cell heavy-chain isotype switching and cell-mediated immunity. Patients suffer from both pyogenic bacterial and protozoal infections.

ζ Chain A transmembrane protein expressed in T cells as part of the TCR complex that contains ITAMs in its cytoplasmic tail and binds the ZAP-70 protein tyrosine kinase during T cell activation.

Zeta-associated protein of 70 kD (ZAP-70) A cytoplasmic protein tyrosine kinase, similar to Syk in B cells, that is critical for early signaling steps in antigen-induced T cell activation. ZAP-70 binds to phosphorylated tyrosines in the cytoplasmic tails of the ζ chain and CD3 chains of the TCR complex and in turn phosphorylates adaptor proteins that recruit other components of the signaling cascade.

CYTOKINES

Cytokine and Subunits	Principal Cell Source	Cytokine Receptor and Subunits*	Principal Cellular Targets and Biologic Effects
Type I Cytokine Family Members			
Interleukin-2 (IL-2)	T cells	CD25 (IL-2Rα) CD122 (IL-2Rβ) CD132 (γc)	T cells: proliferation and differentiation into effector and memory cells; promotes regulatory T cell development, survival, and function NK cells: proliferation, activation B cells: proliferation, antibody synthesis (in vitro)
Interleukin-3 (IL-3)	T cells	CD123 (IL-3Rα) CD131 (βc)	Immature hematopoietic progenitors: induced maturation of all hematopoietic lineages
Interleukin-4 (IL-4)	CD4+ T cells (T$_H$2), mast cells	CD124 (IL-4Rα) CD132 (γc)	B cells: isotype switching to IgE T cells: T$_H$2 differentiation, proliferation Macrophages: alternative activation and inhibition of IFN-γ–mediated classical activation Mast cells: proliferation (in vitro)
Interleukin-5 (IL-5)	CD4+ T cells (T$_H$2), group 2 innate lymphoid cells	CD125 (IL-5Rα) CD131 (βc)	Eosinophils: activation, increased generation B cells: proliferation, IgA production (in vitro)
Interleukin-6 (IL-6)	Macrophages, endothelial cells, T cells	CD126 (IL-6Rα) CD130 (gp130)	Liver: synthesis of acute-phase protein B cells: proliferation of antibody-producing cells
Interleukin-7 (IL-7)	Fibroblasts, bone marrow stromal cells	CD127 (IL-7R) CD132 (γc)	Immature lymphoid progenitors: proliferation of early T and B cell progenitors T lymphocytes: survival of naive and memory cells
Interleukin-9 (IL-9)	CD4+ T cells	CD129 (IL-9R) CD132 (γc)	Mast cells, B cells, T cells, and tissue cells: survival and activation
Interleukin-11 (IL-11)	Bone marrow stromal cells	IL-11Rα CD130 (gp130)	Production of platelets
Interleukin-12 (IL-12): IL-12A (p35) IL-12B (p40)	Macrophages, dendritic cells	CD212 (IL-12Rβ1) IL-12Rβ2	T cells: T$_H$1 differentiation NK cells and T cells: IFN-γ synthesis, increased cytotoxic activity
Interleukin-13 (IL-13)	CD4+ T cells (T$_H$2), NKT cells, group 2 innate lymphoid cells, mast cells	CD213a1 (IL-13Rα1) CD213a2 (IL-13Rα2) CD132 (γc)	B cells: isotype switching to IgE Epithelial cells: increased mucus production Fibroblasts: increased collagen synthesis Macrophages: alternative activation
Interleukin-15 (IL-15)	Macrophages, other cell types	IL-15Rα CD122 (IL-2Rβ) CD132 (γc)	NK cells: proliferation T cells: survival and proliferation of memory CD8+ cells
Interleukin-16 (IL-16)	T cells, mast cells, eosinophils, epithelial cells	CD4	CD4+ T cells, monocytes, and eosinophils: chemoattractant
Interleukin-17A (IL-17A) Interleukin-17F (IL-17F)	CD4+ T cells (T$_H$17), group 3 innate lymphoid cells	CD217 (IL-17RA) IL-17RC	Endothelial cells: increased chemokine production Macrophages: increased chemokine and cytokine production Epithelial cells: GM-CSF and G-CSF production

Continued

Cytokine and Subunits	Principal Cell Source	Cytokine Receptor and Subunits*	Principal Cellular Targets and Biologic Effects
Interleukin-21 (IL-21)	T_H2 cells, T_H17 cells, T_{FH} cells	CD360 (IL-21R) CD132 (γc)	B cells: activation, proliferation, differentiation T_{FH} cells: development T_H17 cells: increased generation NK cells: functional maturation
Interleukin-23 (IL-23): IL-23A (p19) IL-12B (p40)	Macrophages, dendritic cells	IL-23R CD212 (IL-12Rβ1)	T cells: differentiation and expansion of T_H17 cells
Interleukin-25 (IL-25; IL-17E)	T cells, mast cells, eosinophils, macrophages, mucosal epithelial cells	IL-17RB	T cells and various other cell types: expression of IL-4, IL-5, IL-13
Interleukin-27 (IL-27): IL-27 (p28) EBI3 (IL-27B)	Macrophages, dendritic cells	IL-27Rα CD130 (gp130)	T cells: inhibition of T_H1 cells NK cells: IFN-γ synthesis?
Interleukin-31 (IL-31)	T_H2 cells	IL-31RA OSMR CD130 (gp130)	Not established
Stem cell factor (c-Kit ligand)	Bone marrow stromal cells	CD117 (KIT)	Pluripotent hematopoietic stem cells: induced maturation of all hematopoietic lineages
Granulocyte-monocyte CSF (GM-CSF)	T cells, macrophages, endothelial cells, fibroblasts	CD116 (GM-CSFRα) CD131 (βc)	Immature and committed progenitors, mature macrophages: induced maturation of granulocytes and monocytes, macrophage activation
Monocyte CSF (M-CSF, CSF1)	Macrophages, endothelial cells, bone marrow cells, fibroblasts	CD115 (CSF1R)	Committed hematopoietic progenitors: induced maturation of monocytes
Granulocyte CSF (G-CSF, CSF3)	Macrophages, fibroblasts, endothelial cells	CD114 (CSF3R)	Committed hematopoietic progenitors: induced maturation of granulocytes
Type II Cytokine Family Members			
IFN-α (multiple proteins)	Plasmacytoid dendritic cells, macrophages	IFNAR1 CD118 (IFNAR2)	All cells: anti-viral state, increased class I MHC expression NK cells: activation
IFN-β	Fibroblasts, plasmacytoid dendritic cells	IFNAR1 CD118 (IFNAR2)	All cells: anti-viral state, increased class I MHC expression NK cells: activation
Interferon-γ (IFN-γ)	T cells (T_H1, CD8$^+$ T cells), NK cells	CD119 (IFNGR1) IFNGR2	Macrophages: classical activation (increased microbicidal functions) B cells: isotype switching to opsonizing and complement-fixing IgG subclasses (established in mice) T cells: T_H1 differentiation Various cells: increased expression of class I and class II MHC molecules, increased antigen processing and presentation to T cells
Interleukin-10 (IL-10)	Macrophages, T cells (mainly regulatory T cells)	CD210 (IL-10Rα) IL-10Rβ	Macrophages, dendritic cells: inhibition of expression of IL-12, costimulators, and class II MHC
Interleukin-19 (IL-19)	Macrophages	IL-20Rα IL-10Rβ	Macrophages: stimulates IL-1 and TNF secretion Keratinocytes: proliferation
Interleukin-22 (IL-22)	T_H17 cells	IL-22Rα1 IL-10Rβ2 or IL-22α2 IL-10Rβ2	Epithelial cells: production of defensins, increased barrier function Hepatocytes: survival
Interleukin-26 (IL-26)	T cells, monocytes	IL-20R1 IL-10R2	Not established
Interferon-λs (type III interferons)	Dendritic cells	IFNLR1 (IL-28Rα) CD210B (IL-10Rβ2)	Epithelial cells: anti-viral state
Leukemia inhibitory factor (LIF)	Embryonic trophectoderm Bone marrow stromal cells	CD118 (LIFR) CD130 (gp130)	Stem cells: block in differentiation
Oncostatin M	Bone marrow stromal cells	OSMR CD130 (gp130)	Endothelial cells: regulation of hematopoietic cytokine production Cancer cells: inhibition of proliferation

Cytokine and Subunits	Principal Cell Source	Cytokine Receptor and Subunits[*]	Principal Cellular Targets and Biologic Effects
TNF Superfamily Cytokines[†]			
Tumor necrosis factor (TNF, TNFSF1)	Macrophages, NK cells, T cells	CD120a (TNFRSF1) *or* CD120b (TNFRSF2)	Endothelial cells: activation (inflammation, coagulation) Neutrophils: activation Hypothalamus: fever Muscle, fat: catabolism (cachexia)
Lymphotoxin-α (LTα, TNFSF1)	T cells, B cells	CD120a (TNFRSF1) *or* CD120b (TNFRSF2)	Same as TNF
Lymphotoxin-αβ (LTαβ)	T cells, NK cells, follicular B cells, lymphoid inducer cells	LTβR *or* HVEM	Lymphoid tissue stromal cells and follicular dendritic cells: chemokine expression and lymphoid organogenesis
BAFF (CD257, TNFSF13B)	Dendritic cells, monocytes, follicular dendritic cells B cells	BAFF-R (TNFRSF13C) *or* TACI (TNFRSF13B) *or* BCMA (TNFRSF17)	B cells: survival, proliferation
APRIL (CD256, TNFSF13)	T cells, dendritic cells, monocytes, follicular dendritic cells	TACI (TNFRSF13B) *or* BCMA (TNFRSF17)	B cells: survival, proliferation
Osteoprotegrin (OPG, TNFRSF11B)	Osteoblasts	RANKL	Osteoclast precursor cells: inhibits osteoclast differentiation
IL-1 Family Cytokines			
Interleukin-1α (IL-1α)	Macrophages, dendritic cells, fibroblasts, endothelial cells, keratinocytes, hepatocytes	CD121a (IL-1R1) IL-1RAP *or* CD121b (IL-1R2)	Endothelial cells: activation (inflammation, coagulation) Hypothalamus: fever Liver: synthesis of acute-phase proteins
Interleukin-1β (IL-1β)	Macrophages, dendritic cells, fibroblasts, endothelial cells, keratinocytes, hepatocytes	CD121a (IL-1R1) IL-1RAP *or* CD121b (IL-1R2)	Endothelial cells: activation (inflammation, coagulation) Hypothalamus: fever Liver: synthesis of acute-phase proteins T cells: T_H17 differentiation
Interleukin-1 receptor antagonist (IL-1Ra)	Macrophages	CD121a (IL-1R1) IL-1RAP	Various cells: competitive antagonist of IL-1
Interleukin-18 (IL-18)	Monocytes, macrophages, dendritic cells, Kupffer cells, keratinocytes, chondrocytes, synovial fibroblasts, osteoblasts	CD218a (IL-18Rα) CD218b (IL-18Rβ)	NK cells and T cells: IFN-γ synthesis Monocytes: expression of GM-CSF, TNF, IL-1β Neutrophils: activation, cytokine release
Interleukin-33 (IL-33)	Endothelial cells, smooth muscle cells, keratinocytes, fibroblasts	ST2 (IL1RL1); IL-1 Receptor Accessory Protein (IL1RAP)	T cells: T_H2 development ILCs: activation of group 2 ILCs
Other Cytokines			
Transforming growth factor-β (TGF-β)	T cells (mainly Tregs), macrophages, other cell types	TGF-β R1 TGF-β R2 TGF-β R3	T cells: inhibition of proliferation and effector functions; differentiation of T_H17 and Treg B cells: inhibition of proliferation; IgA production Macrophages: inhibition of activation; stimulation of angiogenic factors Fibroblasts: increased collagen synthesis

APRIL, a proliferation-inducing ligand; *BAFF,* B cell–activating factor belonging to the TNF family; *BCMA,* B cell maturation protein; *CSF,* colony-stimulating factor; *HVEM,* herpesvirus entry mediator; *IFN,* interferon; *MHC,* major histocompatibility complex; *NK* cell, natural killer cell; *OSMR,* oncostatin M receptor; *RANK,* receptor activator for nuclear factor κB ligand; *RANKL,* RANK ligand; *TACI,* transmembrane activator and calcium modulator and cyclophilin ligand interactor; *TNF,* tumor necrosis factor; *TNFSF,* TNF superfamily; *TNFRSF,* TNF receptor superfamily.

[*]Most cytokine receptors are dimers or trimers composed of different polypeptide chains, some of which are shared between receptors for different cytokines. The set of polypeptides that compose a functional receptor (cytokine binding plus signaling) for each cytokine is listed. The functions of each subunit polypeptide are not listed.

[†]All TNF superfamily (TNFSF) members are expressed as cell surface transmembrane proteins, but only the subsets that are predominantly active as proteolytically released soluble cytokines are listed in the table. Other TNFSF members that function predominantly in the membrane-bound form and are not, strictly speaking, cytokines are not listed in the table. These membrane-bound proteins and the TNFRSF receptors they bind to include OX40L (CD252, TNFSF4):OX40 (CD134, TNFRSF4); CD40L (CD154, TNFSF5):CD40 (TNFRSF5); FasL (CD178, TNFSF6):Fas (CD95, TNFRSF6); CD70 (TNFSF7):CD27 (TNFRSF27); CD153 (TNFSF8):CD30 (TNFRSF8); TRAIL (CD253, TNFSF10):TRAIL-R (TNFRSF10A-D); RANKL (TNFSF11):RANK (TNFRSF11); TWEAK (CD257, TNFSF12):TWEAKR (CD266, TNFRSF12); LIGHT (CD258, TNFSF14):HVEM (TNFRSF14); GITRL (TNFSF18):GITR (TNFRSF18); 4-IBBL:4-IBB (CD137).

PRINCIPAL FEATURES OF SELECTED CD MOLECULES

The following list includes selected CD molecules that are referred to in the text. Many cytokines and cytokine receptors have been assigned CD numbers, but we refer to these by the more descriptive cytokine designation. A complete and up-to-date listing of CD molecules may be found at http://www.hcdm.org.

CD Number (Other Names)	Molecular Structure, Family	Main Cellular Expression	Known or Proposed Function(s)
CD1a-d	49 kD; class I MHC-like Ig superfamily; β₂-microglobulin associated	Thymocytes, dendritic cells (including Langerhans cells)	Presentation of non-peptide (lipid and glycolipid) antigens to some T cells
CD1e	28 kD; class I MHC-like; β₂-microglobulin associated	Dendritic cells	Same as CD1a
CD2 (LFA-2)	50 kD; Ig superfamily	T cells, NK cells	Adhesion molecule (binds CD58); T cell activation; CTL- and NK cell–mediated lysis
CD3γ	25-28 kD; associated with CD3δ and CD3ε in TCR complex; Ig superfamily; ITAM in cytoplasmic tail	T cells	Cell surface expression of and signal transduction by the T cell antigen receptor
CD3δ	20 kD; associated with CD3γ and CD3ε in TCR complex; Ig superfamily; ITAM in cytoplasmic tail	T cells	Cell surface expression of and signal transduction by the T cell antigen receptor
CD3ε	20 kD; associated with CD3δ and CD3γ in TCR complex; Ig superfamily; ITAM in cytoplasmic tail	T cells	Cell surface expression of and signal transduction by the T cell antigen receptor
CD4	55 kD; Ig superfamily	Class II MHC–restricted T cells; some macrophages	Coreceptor in class II MHC-restricted antigen-induced T cell activation (binds to class II MHC molecules); thymocyte development; receptor for HIV
CD5	67 kD; scavenger receptor family	T cells; B-1 B cell subset	Signaling molecule; binds CD72
CD8α	34 kD; expressed as a homodimer or heterodimer with CD8β	Class I MHC–restricted T cells; subset of dendritic cells	Coreceptor in class I MHC-restricted antigen-induced T cell activation (binds to class I MHC molecules); thymocyte development
CD8β	34 kD; expressed as a heterodimer with CD8α Ig superfamily	Class I MHC–restricted T cells	Same as CD8α
CD10	100 kD; type II membrane protein	Immature and some mature B cells; lymphoid progenitors, granulocytes	Metalloproteinase; unknown function in the immune system
CD11a (LFA-1 α chain)	180 kD; non-covalently linked to CD18 to form LFA-1 integrin	Leukocytes	Cell-cell adhesion; binds to ICAM-1 (CD54), ICAM-2 (CD102), and ICAM-3 (CD50)
CD11b (Mac-1; CR3)	165 kD; non-covalently linked to CD18 to form Mac-1 integrin	Granulocytes, monocytes, macrophages, dendritic cells, NK cells	Phagocytosis of iC3b-coated particles; neutrophil and monocyte adhesion to endothelium (binds CD54) and extracellular matrix proteins

Continued

CD Number (Other Names)	Molecular Structure, Family	Main Cellular Expression	Known or Proposed Function(s)
CD11c (p150,95; CR4α chain)	145 kD; non-covalently linked to CD18 to form p150,95 integrin	Monocytes, macrophages, granulocytes, NK cells	Similar functions as CD11b
CD14	53 kD; GPI linked	Dendritic cells, monocytes, macrophages, granulocytes	Binds complex of LPS and LPS-binding protein and displays LPS to TLR4; required for LPS-induced macrophage activation
CD16a (FcγRIIIA)	50-70 kD; transmembrane protein; Ig superfamily	NK cells, macrophages	Binds Fc region of IgG; phagocytosis and antibody-dependent cellular cytotoxicity
CD16b (FcγRIIIB)	50-70 kD; GPI linked; Ig superfamily	Neutrophils	Binds Fc region of IgG; synergy with FcγRII in immune complex–mediated neutrophil activation
CD18	95 kD; non-covalently linked to CD11a, CD11b, or CD11c to form γ$_2$ integrins	Leukocytes	See CD11a, CD11b, CD11c
CD19	95 kD; Ig superfamily	Most B cells	B cell activation; forms a coreceptor complex with CD21 and CD81 that delivers signals that synergize with signals from B cell antigen receptor complex
CD20	35-37 kD; tetraspan (TM4SF) family	B cells	? Role in B cell activation or regulation; calcium ion channel
CD21 (CR2; C3d receptor)	145 kD; regulators of complement activation	Mature B cells, follicular dendritic cells	Receptor for complement fragment C3d; forms a coreceptor complex with CD19 and CD81 that delivers activating signals in B cells; receptor for Epstein-Barr virus
CD22	130-140 kD; Ig superfamily; sialoadhesin family; ITIM in cytoplasmic tail	B cells	Regulation of B cell activation; adhesion molecule
CD23 (FcεRIIB)	45 kD; C-type lectin	Activated B cells, monocytes, macrophages	Low-affinity Fcε receptor, induced by IL-4; function is not clear
CD25 (IL-2 receptor α chain)	55 kD; non-covalently associated with IL-2Rβ (CD122) and IL-2Rγ (CD132) chains to form a high-affinity IL-2 receptor	Activated T and B cells, regulatory T cells (Treg)	Binds IL-2 and promotes responses to low concentrations of IL-2
CD28	Homodimer of 44-kD chains; Ig superfamily	T cells (all CD4$^+$ and >50% of CD8$^+$ cells in humans; all mature T cells in mice)	T cell receptor for costimulatory molecules CD80 (B7-1) and CD86 (B7-2)
CD29	130 kD; non-covalently linked to CD49a-d chains to form VLA (β$_1$) integrins	T cells, B cells, monocytes, granulocytes	Leukocyte adhesion to extracellular matrix proteins and endothelium (see CD49)
CD30 (TNFRSF8)	120 kD; TNFR superfamily	Activated T and B cells; NK cells, monocytes, Reed-Sternberg cells in Hodgkin's disease	Not established
CD31 (platelet/ endothelial cell adhesion molecule 1, PECAM-1)	130-140 kD; Ig superfamily	Platelets, monocytes, granulocytes, B cells, endothelial cells	Adhesion molecule involved in leukocyte transmigration through endothelium
CD32 (FcγRII)	40 kD; Ig superfamily; ITIM in cytoplasmic tail; A, B, and C forms are products of different but homologous genes	B cells, macrophages, dendritic cells, granulocytes	Fc receptor for aggregated IgG; acts as inhibitory receptor that blocks activation signals in B cells and other cells
CD34	105-120 kD; sialomucin	Precursors of hematopoietic cells; endothelial cells in high endothelial venules	? Role in cell-cell adhesion
CD35 (type 1 complement receptor, CR1)	190-285 kD (four products of polymorphic alleles); regulator of complement activation family	Granulocytes, monocytes, erythrocytes, B cells, follicular dendritic cells, some T cells	Binds C3b and C4b; promotes phagocytosis of C3b- or C4b-coated particles and immune complexes; regulates complement activation
CD36	85-90 kD	Platelets, monocytes, macrophages, endothelial cells	Scavenger receptor for oxidized low-density lipoprotein; platelet adhesion; phagocytosis of apoptotic cells

CD Number (Other Names)	Molecular Structure, Family	Main Cellular Expression	Known or Proposed Function(s)
CD40	Homodimer of 44- to 48-kD chains; TNFR superfamily	B cells, macrophages, dendritic cells, endothelial cells	Binds CD154 (CD40 ligand); role in T cell–mediated activation of B cells, macrophages, and dendritic cells
CD43	95-135 kD; sialomucin	Leukocytes (except circulating B cells)	?Role in cell-cell adhesion
CD44	80->100 kD, highly glycosylated	Leukocytes, erythrocytes	Binds hyaluronan; involved in leukocyte adhesion to endothelial cells and extracellular matrix
CD45 (Leukocyte common antigen [LCA])	Multiple isoforms, 180-220 kD (see CD45R); protein tyrosine phosphatase receptor family; fibronectin type III family	Hematopoietic cells	Tyrosine phosphatase that regulates T and B cell activation
CD45R	CD45RO:180 kD CD45RA: 220 kD CD45RB: 190-, 205-, and 220-kD isoforms	CD45RO: memory T cells; subset of B cells, monocytes, macrophages CD45RA: naive T cells, B cells, monocytes CD45RB: B cells, subset of T cells	See CD45
CD46 (Membrane cofactor protein (MCP)	52-58 kD; regulators of complement activation family	Leukocytes, epithelial cells, fibroblasts	Regulation of complement activation
CD47	47-52 kD; Ig superfamily	All hematopoietic cells, epithelial cells, endothelial cells, fibroblasts	Leukocyte adhesion, migration, activation; "Don't eat me" signal to phagocytes
CD49d	150 kD; non-covalently linked to CD29 to form VLA-4 ($\alpha_4\beta_1$ integrin)	T cells, monocytes, B cells, NK cells, eosinophils, dendritic cells, thymocytes	Leukocyte adhesion to endothelium and extracellular matrix; binds to VCAM-1 and MadCAM-1; binds fibronectin and collagens
CD54 (ICAM-1)	75-114 kD; Ig superfamily	T cells, B cells, monocytes, endothelial cells (cytokine inducible)	Cell-cell adhesion; ligand for CD11aCD18 (LFA-1) and CD11bCD18 (Mac-1); receptor for rhinovirus
CD55 (Decay-accelerating factor [DAF])	55-70 kD; GPI linked; regulators of complement activation family	Broad	Regulation of complement activation
CD58 (Leukocyte function–associated antigen 3 [LFA-3])	55-70 kD; GPI-linked or integral membrane protein	Broad	Leukocyte adhesion; binds CD2
CD59	18-20 kD; GPI linked	Broad	Binds C9; inhibits formation of complement membrane attack complex
CD62E E-selectin)	115 kD; selectin family	Endothelial cells	Leukocyte-endothelial adhesion
CD62L (L-selectin)	74-95 kD; selectin family	B cells, T cells, monocytes, granulocytes, some NK cells	Leukocyte-endothelial adhesion; homing of naive T cells to peripheral lymph nodes
CD62P (P-selectin)	140 kD; selectin family	Platelets, endothelial cells (present in granules, translocated to cell surface on activation)	Leukocyte adhesion to endothelium, platelets; binds CD162 (PSGL-1)
CD64 (FcγRI)	72 kD; Ig superfamily; non-covalently associated with the FcR common γ chain	Monocytes, macrophages, activated neutrophils	High-affinity Fcγ receptor; role in phagocytosis, ADCC, macrophage activation
CD66e (Carcinoembryonic antigen [CEA])	180-220 kD; Ig superfamily; carcinoembryonic antigen (CEA) family	Colonic and other epithelial cells	? Adhesion; clinical marker of carcinoma burden
CD69	23 kD; C-type lectin	Activated B cells, T cells, NK cells, neutrophils	Binds to and impairs surface expression of S1PR1, thereby promoting retention of recently activated lymphocytes in lymphoid tissues

Continued

CD Number (Other Names)	Molecular Structure, Family	Main Cellular Expression	Known or Proposed Function(s)
CD74 (Class II MHC invariant chain [I$_i$])	33-, 35-, and 41-kD isoforms	B cells, dendritic cells, monocytes, macrophages; other class II MHC–expressing cells	Binds to and directs intracellular sorting of newly synthesized class II MHC molecules
CD79a (Igα)	33, 45 kD; forms dimer with CD79b; Ig superfamily; ITAM in cytoplasmic tail	Mature B cells	Required for cell surface expression of and signal transduction by the B cell antigen receptor complex
CD79b (Igβ)	37-39 kD; forms dimer with CD79α; Ig superfamily; ITAM in cytoplasmic tail	Mature B cells	Required for cell surface expression of and signal transduction by the B cell antigen receptor complex
CD80 (B7-1)	60 kD; Ig superfamily	Dendritic cells, activated B cells and macrophages	Costimulator for T lymphocyte activation; ligand for CD28 and CD152 (CTLA-4)
CD81 (Target for anti-proliferative antigen 1 [TAPA-1])	26 kD; tetraspan (TM4SF)	T cells, B cells, NK cells, dendritic cells, thymocytes, endothelial cells	B cell activation; forms a coreceptor complex with CD19 and CD21 that delivers signals that synergize with signals from the B cell antigen receptor complex
CD86 (B7-2)	80 kD; Ig superfamily	B cells, monocytes; dendritic cells; some T cells	Costimulator for T lymphocyte activation; ligand for CD28 and CD152 (CTLA-4)
CD88 (C5a receptor)	43 kD; G protein–coupled, 7 membrane–spanning receptor family	Granulocytes, monocytes, dendritic cells, mast cells	Receptor for C5a complement fragment; role in complement-induced inflammation
CD89 (Fcα receptor [FcαR])	55-75 kD; Ig superfamily; non-covalently associated with the common FcR γ chain	Granulocytes, monocytes, macrophages, T cell subset, B cell subset	Binds IgA; mediates IgA-dependent cellular cytotoxicity
CD90 (Thy-1)	25-35 kD; GPI linked; Ig superfamily	Thymocytes, peripheral T cells (mice), CD34+ hematopoietic progenitor cells, neurons	Marker for T cells; unknown function
CD94	43 kD; C-type lectin; on NK cells, covalently assembles with other C-type lectin molecules (NKG2)	NK cells; subset of CD8+ T cells	CD94/NKG2 complex functions as an NK cell inhibitory receptor; binds HLA-E class I MHC molecules
CD95 (Fas)	Homotrimer of 45-kD chains; TNFR superfamily	Broad	Binds Fas ligand; delivers signals leading to apoptotic death
CD102 (ICAM-2)	55-65 kD; Ig superfamily	Endothelial cells, lymphocytes, monocytes, platelets	Ligand for CD11aCD18 (LFA-1); cell-cell adhesion
CD103 (α$_E$ integrin subunit)	Dimer of 150- and 25-kD subunits; non-covalently linked to β$_7$ integrin subunit to form α$_E$β$_7$ integrin	Intraepithelial lymphocytes, other cell types	Role in T cell homing to and retention in mucosa; binds E-cadherin
CD106 (Vascular cell adhesion molecule 1 [VCAM-1])	100-110 kD; Ig superfamily	Endothelial cells, macrophages, follicular dendritic cells, marrow stromal cells	Adhesion of cells to endothelium; receptor for CD49dCD29 (VLA-4) integrin; role in lymphocyte trafficking, activation
CD134 (OX40, TNFRSF4)	29 kD; TNFR superfamily	Activated T cells	Receptor for T cell CD252; T cell costimulation
CD150 (Signaling lymphocyte activation molecule [SLAM])	37 kD; Ig superfamily	Thymocytes, activated lymphocytes, dendritic cells, endothelial cells	Regulation of B cell–T cell interactions and lymphocyte activation
CD152 (Cytotoxic T lymphocyte–associated protein 4 [CTLA-4])	33, 50 kD; Ig superfamily	Activated T lymphocytes, regulatory T cells	Mediates suppressive function of regulatory T cells; inhibits T cell responses; binds CD80 (B7-1) and CD86 (B7-2) on antigen-presenting cells
CD154 (CD40 ligand [CD40L])	Homotrimer of 32- to 39-kD chains; TNFR superfamily	Activated CD4+ T cells	Activation of B cells, macrophages, and endothelial cells; ligand for CD40
CD158 (Killer Ig-like receptor [KIR])	50, 58 kD; Ig superfamily; killer Ig-like receptor (KIR) family; ITIMs or ITAMs in cytoplasmic tail	NK cells, T cell subset	Inhibition or activation of NK cells on interaction with appropriate class I HLA molecules

CD Number (Other Names)	Molecular Structure, Family	Main Cellular Expression	Known or Proposed Function(s)
CD159a (NKG2A)	43 kD; C-type lectin; forms heterodimer with CD94	NK cells, T cell subset	Inhibition or activation of NK cells on interaction with class I HLA molecules
CD159c (NKG2C)	40 kD; C-type lectin; forms heterodimer with CD94	NK cells	Activation of NK cells on interaction with the appropriate class I HLA molecules
CD162 (P-selectin glycoprotein ligand 1 [PSGL-1])	Homodimer of 120-kD chains; sialomucin	T cells, monocytes, granulocytes, some B cells	Ligand for selectins (CD62P, CD62L); adhesion of leukocytes to endothelium
CD178 (Fas ligand [FasL])	Homotrimer of 31-kD subunits; TNF superfamily	Activated T cells	Ligand for CD95 (Fas); triggers apoptotic death
CD206 (Mannose receptor)	166 kD; C-type lectin	Macrophages	Binds high-mannose–containing glycoproteins on pathogens; mediates macrophage endocytosis of glycoproteins and phagocytosis of bacteria, fungi, and other pathogens
CD244 (2B4)	41 kD; Ig superfamily; CD2/CD48/CD58 family; SLAM family	NK cells, CD8 T cells, γδ T cells	Receptor for CD148; modulates NK cell cytolytic activity
CD247 (TCR ζ chain)	18 kD; ITAMs in cytoplasmic tail	T cells; NK cells	Signaling chain of TCR- and NK cell–activating receptors
CD252 (OX40 ligand)	21 kD; TNF superfamily	Dendritic cells, macrophages, B cells	Ligand for CD134 (OX40,TNFRSF4); costimulates T cells
CD267 (TACI)	31 kD; TNFR superfamily	B cells	Receptor for cytokines BAFF and APRIL; mediates B cell survival
CD268 (BAFF receptor)	19 kD; TNFR superfamily	B cells	Receptor for BAFF; mediates B cell survival
CD269 (BCMA [B cell maturation antigen])	20 kD; TNFR superfamily	B cells	Receptor for BAFF and APRIL; mediates B cell survival
CD273 (PD-L2)	25 kD; Ig superfamily; structurally homologous to B7	Dendritic cells, monocytes, macrophages	Ligand for PD-1; inhibits T cell activation
CD274 (PD-L1)	33 kD; Ig superfamily; structurally homologous to B7	Leukocytes, other cells	Ligand for PD-1; inhibits T cell activation
CD275 (ICOS ligand)	60 kD; Ig superfamily; structurally homologous to B7	B cells, dendritic cells, monocytes	Binds ICOS (CD278); T cell costimulation
CD278 (ICOS [inducible costimulator])	55-60 kD; Ig superfamily; structurally homologous to CD28	Activated T cells	Binds ICOS-L (CD275); T cell costimulation
CD279 (PD1)	55 kD; Ig superfamily; structurally homologous to CD28	Activated T and B cells	Binds PD-L1 and PD-L2; inhibits T cell activation
CD314 (NKG2D)	42 kD; C-type lectin	NK cells, activated CD8$^+$ T cells, NK-T cells, some myeloid cells	Binds MHC class I, and the class I–like molecules MIC-A, MIC-B, Rae1, and ULBP4; role in NK cell and CTL activation
CD357 (GITR)	26 kD; TNFR superfamily	CD4$^+$ and CD8$^+$ T cells, Treg	? Role in T cell tolerance/Treg function
CD363 (S1PR1 [type 1 sphingosine-1-phosphate receptor 1])	42.8 kD; G protein–coupled, 7 membrane–spanning receptor family	Lymphocytes, endothelial cells	Binds sphingosine 1-phosphate and mediates chemotaxis of lymphocytes out of lymphoid organs

ADCC, antibody-dependent cell-mediated cytotoxicity; *APRIL,* a proliferation-inducing ligand; *BAFF,* B cell–activating factor belonging to the TNF family; *CTL,* cytotoxic T lymphocyte; *gp,* glycoprotein; *GPI,* glycophosphatidylinositol; *ICAM,* intercellular adhesion molecule; *Ig,* immunoglobulin; *IL,* interleukin; *ITAM,* immunoreceptor tyrosine-based activation motif; *ITIM,* immunoreceptor tyrosine-based inhibition motif; *LFA,* lymphocyte function–associated antigen; *LPS,* lipopolysaccharide; *MadCAM,* mucosal addressin cell adhesion molecule; *MHC,* major histocompatibility complex; *NK cells,* natural killer cells; *PAMPs,* pathogen-associated molecular patterns; *TACI,* transmembrane activator and CAML interactor; *TCR,* T cell receptor; *TNF,* tumor necrosis factor; *TNFR,* TNF receptor; *VCAM,* vascular cell adhesion molecule; *VLA,* very late activation.

*The lowercase letters affixed to some CD numbers refer to CD molecules that are encoded by multiple genes or that belong to families of structurally related proteins.

LABORATORY TECHNIQUES COMMONLY USED IN IMMUNOLOGY

Many laboratory techniques that are routine in research and clinical settings are based on the use of antibodies. In addition, many of the techniques of modern molecular biology have provided invaluable information about the immune system. We have mentioned these techniques often throughout the book. In this appendix, we will describe the principles underlying some of the most commonly used laboratory methods in immunology. In addition, we will summarize how B and T lymphocyte responses are studied with use of laboratory techniques. Details of how to carry out various assays may be found in laboratory manuals.

LABORATORY METHODS USING ANTIBODIES

The exquisite specificity of antibodies for particular antigens makes antibodies valuable reagents for detecting, purifying, and quantitating antigens. Because antibodies can be produced against virtually any type of macromolecule and small chemical, antibody-based techniques may be used to study virtually any type of molecule in solution or in cells. The method for producing monoclonal antibodies (see Chapter 5) has greatly increased our ability to generate antibodies of almost any desired specificity. Historically, many of the uses of antibody depended on the ability of antibody and specific antigen to form large immune complexes, either in solution or in gels, that could be detected by various optical methods. These methods were of great importance in early studies but have now been replaced almost entirely by simpler methods based on immobilized antibodies or antigens.

Quantitation of Antigen by Immunoassays

Immunologic methods of quantifying antigen concentration provide exquisite sensitivity and specificity and have become standard techniques for both research and clinical applications. All modern immunochemical methods of quantitation are based on having a pure antigen or antibody whose quantity can be measured by an indicator molecule (or a label). When the antigen or antibody is labeled with a radioisotope, as first introduced by Rosalyn Yalow and colleagues, it may be quantified by instruments that detect radioactive decay events; the assay is called a **radioimmunoassay (RIA)**. When the antigen or antibody is covalently coupled to an enzyme, it may be quantified by determining with a spectrophotometer the rate at which the enzyme converts a clear substrate to a colored product; the assay is called an **enzyme-linked immunosorbent assay (ELISA)**. Several variations of RIA and ELISA exist, but the most commonly used version is the sandwich assay (Fig. A-1). The sandwich assay uses two different antibodies reactive with different epitopes on the antigen whose concentration needs to be determined. A fixed quantity of one antibody is attached to a series of replicate solid supports, such as plastic microtiter wells. Test solutions containing antigen at an unknown concentration or a series

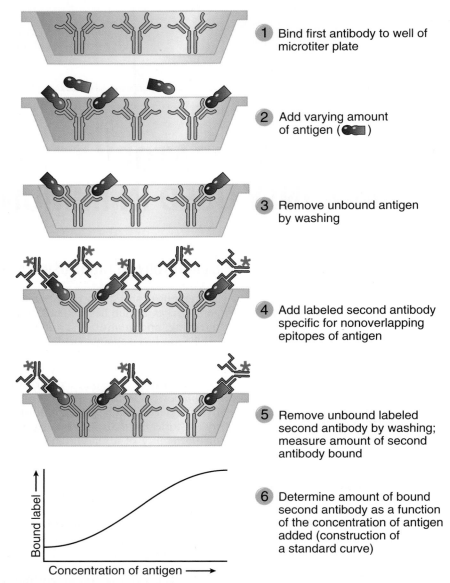

1. Bind first antibody to well of microtiter plate

2. Add varying amount of antigen (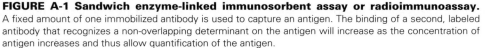)

3. Remove unbound antigen by washing

4. Add labeled second antibody specific for nonoverlapping epitopes of antigen

5. Remove unbound labeled second antibody by washing; measure amount of second antibody bound

6. Determine amount of bound second antibody as a function of the concentration of antigen added (construction of a standard curve)

FIGURE A-1 Sandwich enzyme-linked immunosorbent assay or radioimmunoassay.
A fixed amount of one immobilized antibody is used to capture an antigen. The binding of a second, labeled antibody that recognizes a non-overlapping determinant on the antigen will increase as the concentration of antigen increases and thus allow quantification of the antigen.

of standard solutions with known concentrations of antigen are added to the wells and allowed to bind. Unbound antigen is removed by washing, and the second antibody, which is enzyme linked or radiolabeled, is allowed to bind. The antigen serves as a bridge, so the more antigen in the test or standard solutions, the more enzyme-linked or radiolabeled second antibody will bind. The results from the standard solutions are used to construct a binding curve for the second antibody as a function of antigen concentration, from which the quantities of antigen in the test solutions may be inferred. When this test is performed with two monoclonal antibodies, it is essential that these antibodies see non-overlapping determinants on the antigen; otherwise, the second antibody cannot bind.

In an important clinical variant of immunobinding assays, samples from patients may be tested for the presence of antibodies that are specific for a microbial antigen (e.g., antibodies reactive with proteins from human immunodeficiency virus [HIV] or hepatitis B virus) as indicators of infection. In this case, a saturating quantity of antigen is added to replicate wells containing plate-bound antibody, or the antigen is attached directly to the plate, and serial dilutions of the patient's serum are then allowed to bind. The amount of the patient's antibody bound to the immobilized antigen is determined by use of an enzyme-linked or radiolabeled second antihuman immunoglobulin (Ig) antibody.

Identification and Purification of Proteins

Antibodies can be used to identify and characterize proteins and to purify specific proteins from mixtures. Two

A Immunoprecipitation

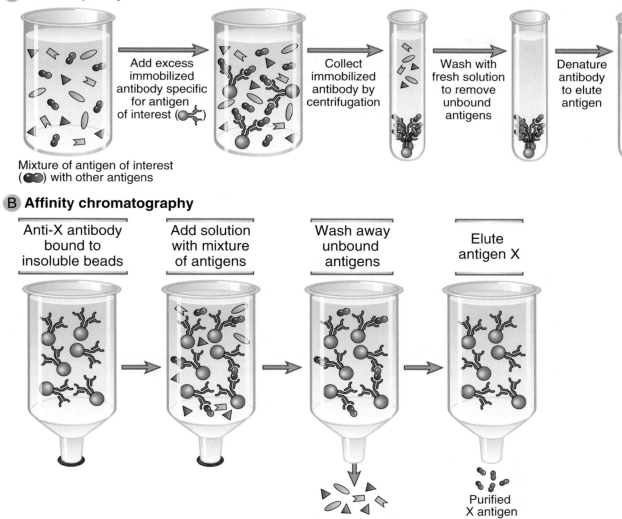

B Affinity chromatography

FIGURE A-2 Isolation of an antigen by immunoprecipitation or affinity chromatography. A, A particular antigen can be purified from a mixture of antigens in serum or other solutions by adding antibodies specific to the antigen that are bound to insoluble beads. Unbound antigens are then washed away, and the desired antigen is recovered by changing the pH or ionic strength of the solution so that the affinity of antibody-antigen binding is lowered. Immunoprecipitation can be used as a means of purification, as a means of quantification, or as a means of identification of an antigen. Antigens purified by immunoprecipitation are often analyzed by sodium dodecyl sulfate–polyacrylamide gel electrophoresis. **B,** Affinity chromatography is based on the same principle as immunoprecipitation, except that the antibody is fixed to an insoluble matrix or beads, usually in a column. The method is often used to isolate soluble antigens (shown) or antibodies specific for an immobilized antigen.

commonly used methods to identify and purify proteins are immunoprecipitation and immuno-affinity chromatography. Western blotting is a widely used technique to determine the presence and size of a protein in a biologic sample.

Immunoprecipitation and Immuno-Affinity Chromatography

Immunoprecipitation is a technique in which an antibody specific for one protein antigen in a mixture of proteins is used to identify this specific antigen (Fig. A-2, *A*). The antibody is typically added to a protein mixture (usually a detergent lysate of specific cells), and staphylococcal protein A (or protein G) covalently attached to agarose beads is added to the mixture. The Fab portions of the

antibody bind to the target protein, and the Fc portion of the antibody is captured by the protein A or protein G on the beads. Unwanted proteins that do not bind to the antibody are then removed by washing the beads (by repeated detergent addition and centrifugation). The specific protein that is recognized by and now bound to the antibody may be eluted from the beads and dissociated from the antibody by use of a harsh denaturant (such as sodium dodecyl sulfate), and the proteins are separated by sodium dodecyl sulfate–polyacrylamide gel electrophoresis (SDS-PAGE). Proteins may be detected after electrophoresis by staining the polyacrylamide gel with a protein stain or by a Western blot analysis (described later). If the original mixture contained radioactively labeled proteins, specific proteins immunoprecipitated by the antibody may be revealed by autofluorography or autoradiography, with protein bands being captured on x-ray film placed on the dried SDS–polyacrylamide gel containing separated proteins.

Immuno-affinity chromatography, a variant of affinity chromatography, is a purification method that relies on antibodies attached to an insoluble support to purify antigens from a solution (Fig. A-2, *B*). Antibodies specific for the desired antigen are typically covalently attached to a solid support, such as agarose beads, and packed into a column. A complex mixture of antigens is passed through the beads to allow the antigen that is recognized by the antibody to bind. Unbound molecules are washed away, and the bound antigen is eluted by changing the pH or by exposure to high salt or other chaotropic conditions that break antigen-antibody interactions. A similar method may be used to purify antibodies from culture supernatants or natural fluids, such as serum, by first attaching the antigen to beads and passing the supernatants or serum through.

Western Blotting

Western blotting (Fig. A-3) is used to identify and determine the relative quantity and molecular weight of a protein within a mixture of proteins or other molecules. The mixture is first subjected to analytical separation, typically by SDS-PAGE, so that the final positions of different proteins in the gel are a function of their molecular size. The array of separated proteins is then transferred from the separating polyacrylamide gel to a support membrane by electrophoresis such that the membrane acquires a replica of the array of separated macromolecules present in the gel. SDS is displaced from the protein during the transfer process, and native antigenic determinants are often regained as the protein refolds. The position of the protein antigen on the membrane can then be detected by binding of an unlabeled antibody specific for that protein (the primary antibody) followed by a labeled second antibody that binds to the primary antibody. This approach provides information about antigen size and quantity. In general, second antibody probes are labeled with enzymes that generate chemiluminescent signals and leave images on photographic film. Near-infrared fluorophores can also be used to label antibodies, and light produced by the excitation of the fluorophore provides more accurate antigen quantitation compared with enzyme-linked second antibodies. The sensitivity and specificity of this technique can be increased by starting with immunoprecipitated proteins instead of crude protein mixtures. This sequential procedure is especially useful for detection of protein-protein interactions. For example, the physical association of two different proteins in the membrane of a lymphocyte can be established by immunoprecipitating a membrane extract by use of an antibody specific for one of the proteins and probing a Western blot of the immunoprecipitate using an antibody specific for the second protein that may have been co-immunoprecipitated along with the first protein.

The technique of transferring proteins from a gel to a membrane is called Western blotting as a biochemist's joke. Southern is the last name of the scientist who first blotted DNA from a separating gel to a membrane by capillary transfer, a technique since called Southern blotting.

By analogy, Northern blotting was the term applied to the technique of transferring RNA from a gel to a membrane, and Western blotting is the term used to describe the transfer of proteins to a membrane.

Labeling and Detection of Antigens in Cells and Tissues

Antibodies specific for antigens expressed on or in particular cell types are commonly used to identify these cells in tissues or cell suspensions and to separate these cells from mixed populations. In these methods, the antibody can be radiolabeled, enzyme linked, or, most commonly, fluorescently labeled, and a detection system is used that can identify the bound antibody. Antibodies attached to magnetic beads can be used to physically isolate cells expressing specific antigens.

Flow Cytometry and Fluorescence-Activated Cell Sorting

The tissue lineage, maturation stage, or activation status of a cell can often be determined by analyzing the cell surface or intracellular expression of different molecules. This technique is commonly done by staining the cell with fluorescently labeled probes that are specific for those molecules and measuring the quantity of fluorescence emitted by the cell (Fig. A-4). The flow cytometer is a specialized instrument that can detect fluorescence on individual cells in a suspension and thereby determine the number of cells expressing the molecule to which a fluorescent probe binds. Suspensions of cells are incubated with fluorescently labeled probes, and the amount of probe bound by each cell in the population is measured by passing the cells one at a time through a fluorimeter with a laser-generated incident beam. The relative amounts of a particular molecule on different cell populations can be compared by staining each population with the same probe and determining the amount of fluorescence emitted. In preparation for flow cytometric analysis, cell suspensions are stained with the fluorescent probes of choice. Most often, these probes are fluorochrome-labeled antibodies specific for a cell surface molecule. Alternatively, cytoplasmic molecules can be stained by temporarily permeabilizing cells and permitting the labeled antibodies to enter through the plasma membrane. In addition to antibodies, various fluorescent indicators of cytoplasmic ion concentrations and reduction-oxidation potential can be detected by flow cytometry. Cell cycle studies can be performed by flow cytometric analysis of cells stained with fluorescent DNA-binding probes such as propidium iodide. Apoptotic cells can be identified with fluorescent probes, such as annexin V, that bind to abnormally exposed phospholipids on the surface of the dying cells. Modern flow cytometers can routinely detect three or more different-colored fluorescent signals, each attached to a different antibody or other probe. This technique permits simultaneous analysis of the expression of many different combinations of molecules by a cell. In addition to detecting fluorescent signals, flow cytometers also measure the forward and side light-scattering properties of cells, which reflect cell size

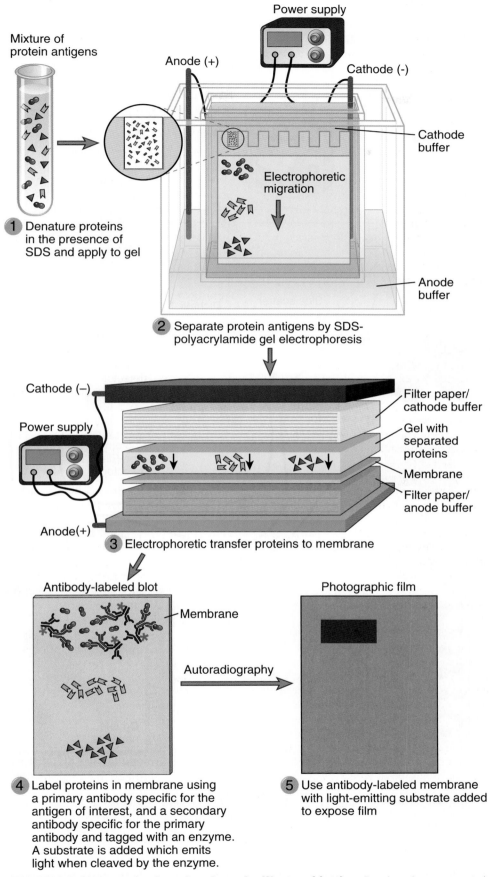

FIGURE A-3 Characterization of antigens by Western blotting. Protein antigens, separated by sodium dodecyl sulfate (SDS)–polyacrylamide gel electrophoresis and transferred to a membrane, can be detected by an antibody that is in turn revealed by a second antibody that may be conjugated to an enzyme such as horseradish peroxidase or to a fluorophore.

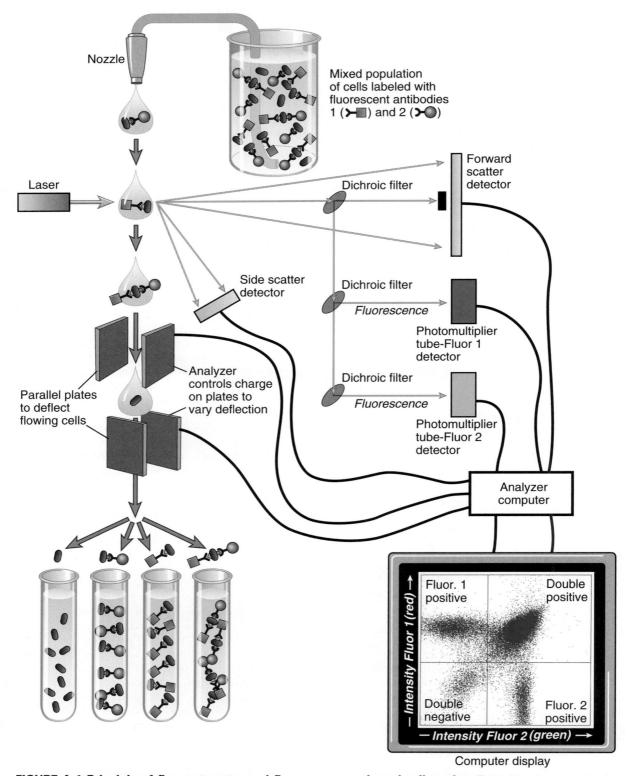

FIGURE A-4 Principle of flow cytometry and fluorescence-activated cell sorting. The incident laser beam is of a designated wavelength, and the light that emerges from the sample is analyzed for forward and side scatter as well as fluorescent light of two or more wavelengths that depend on the fluorochrome labels attached to the antibodies. The separation depicted here is based on two antigenic markers (two-color sorting). Modern instruments can routinely analyze and separate cell populations on the basis of three or more different-colored probes.

and internal complexity, respectively. This information is often used to distinguish different cell types. For example, compared with lymphocytes, neutrophils cause greater side scatter because of their cytoplasmic granules, and monocytes cause greater forward scatter because of their size.

A newly developed antibody-based technology called mass cytometry combines the single-cell flow technology of flow cytometers with mass spectrometry. The commercially available device used for this purpose is called **CyTOF**, with "TOF" indicating that it is a time-of-flight–type of mass cytometer. Antibodies specific for molecules of interest are labeled with any one of a large number of heavy metals, using a different metal for each antibody specificity. These antibodies are incubated with the cell population being studied, and the cells are analyzed by a CyTOF instrument that performs mass spectrometry on individual cells. Unlike fluorescence labels, many different heavy metal labels can be resolved by mass spectrometry without overlap, allowing for the detection of as many as 100 different molecules on a single cell.

Purification of Cells

A fluorescent-activated cell sorter is an adaptation of the flow cytometer that allows one to separate cell populations according to which and how much fluorescent probe they bind. This technique is accomplished by differentially deflecting the cells with electromagnetic fields whose strength and direction are varied according to the measured intensity of the fluorescent signal (see Fig. A-4). The cells may be labeled with fluorescently tagged antibodies ex vivo, or, in the case of experimental animal studies, labeling may be accomplished in vivo by expression of transgenes that encode fluorescent proteins, such as green fluorescent protein. (Transgenic technology is described later in this appendix.)

Another commonly used technique to purify cells with a particular phenotype relies on antibodies that are attached to magnetic beads. These "immunomagnetic reagents" will bind to certain cells, depending on the specificity of the antibody used, and the bound cells can then be pulled out of suspension by a strong magnet.

Immunofluorescence and Immunohistochemistry

Antibodies can be used to identify the anatomic distribution of an antigen within a tissue or within compartments of a cell. To do so, the tissue or cell is incubated with an antibody that is labeled with a fluorochrome or enzyme, and the position of the label, determined with a suitable microscope, is used to infer the position of the antigen. In the earliest version of this method, called immunofluorescence, the antibody was labeled with a fluorescent dye and allowed to bind to a monolayer of cells or to a frozen section of a tissue. The stained cells or tissues were examined with a fluorescence microscope to locate the antibody. Although sensitive, the fluorescence microscope is not an ideal tool to identify the detailed structures of the cell or tissue because of a low signal-to-noise ratio. This problem has been overcome by new technologies including confocal microscopy, which uses optical sectioning technology to filter out unfocused fluorescent light, and two-photon microscopy, which prevents out-of-focus light from forming. Alternatively, antibodies may be coupled to enzymes that convert colorless substrates to colored insoluble substances that precipitate at the position of the enzyme. A conventional light microscope may then be used to localize the antibody in a stained cell or tissue. The most common variant of this method uses the enzyme horseradish peroxidase, and the method is commonly referred to as the immunoperoxidase technique. Another commonly used enzyme is alkaline phosphatase. Different antibodies coupled to different enzymes may be used in conjunction to produce simultaneous two-color localizations of different antigens. In other variations, antibody can be coupled to an electron-dense probe such as colloidal gold, and the location of antibody can be determined subcellularly by means of an electron microscope, a technique called immunoelectron microscopy. Different-sized gold particles have been used for simultaneous localization of different antigens at the ultrastructural level.

In all immunomicroscopic methods, signals may be enhanced by use of sandwich techniques. For example, instead of attaching horseradish peroxidase to a specific mouse antibody directed against the antigen of interest, it can be attached to a second anti-antibody (e.g., rabbit anti-mouse Ig antibody) that is used to bind to the first, unlabeled antibody. When the label is attached directly to the specific, primary antibody, the method is referred to as direct; when the label is attached to a secondary or even tertiary antibody, the method is indirect. In some cases, molecules other than antibody can be used in indirect methods. For example, staphylococcal protein A, which binds to IgG, or avidin, which binds to primary antibodies labeled with biotin, can be coupled to fluorochromes or enzymes.

Measurement of Antigen-Antibody Interactions

In many situations, it is important to know the affinity of an antibody for an antigen. For example, the usefulness of a monoclonal antibody as an experimental or therapeutic reagent depends on its affinity. Antibody affinities for antigen can be measured directly for small antigens (e.g., haptens) by a method called equilibrium dialysis (Fig. A-5). In this method, a solution of antibody is confined within a "semipermeable" membrane of porous cellulose and immersed in a solution containing the antigen. (*Semipermeable* in this context means that small molecules, such as antigen, can pass freely through the membrane pores but that macromolecules, such as antibody, cannot.) If no antibody is present within the membrane-bound compartment, the antigen in the bathing solution enters until the concentration of antigen within the membrane-bound compartment becomes exactly the same as that outside. Another way to view the system is that at dynamic equilibrium, antigen enters and leaves the membrane-bound compartment at exactly the same rate. However, when antibody is present inside the membrane, the net amount of antigen inside the membrane at equilibrium increases by the quantity that is bound to antibody. This phenomenon occurs because only unbound antigen can diffuse across the membrane, and at equilibrium, it is the unbound concentration of

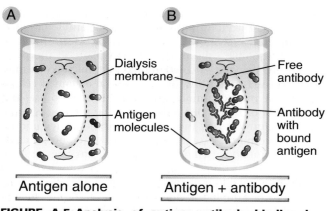

FIGURE A-5 Analysis of antigen-antibody binding by equilibrium dialysis. In the presence of antibody **(B)**, the amount of antigen within the dialysis membrane is increased compared with the absence of antibody **(A)**. As described in the text, this difference, caused by antibody binding of antigen, can be used to measure the affinity of the antibody for the antigen. This experiment can be performed only when the antigen is a small molecule (e.g., a hapten) capable of freely crossing the dialysis membrane.

antigen that must be identical inside and outside the membrane. The extent of the increase in antigen inside the membrane depends on the antigen concentration, on the antibody concentration, and on the dissociation constant (K_d) of the binding interaction. K_d can be calculated by measurement of antigen and antibody concentrations, by spectroscopy, or by other means.

An alternative way to determine K_d is by measurement of the rates of antigen-antibody complex formation and dissociation. These rates depend, in part, on the concentrations of antibody and antigen and on the affinity of the interaction. All parameters except the concentrations can be summarized as rate constants, and both the on-rate constant (K_{on}) and the off-rate constant (K_{off}) can be calculated experimentally by determining the concentrations and the actual rates of association or dissociation, respectively. The ratio of K_{off}/K_{on} allows one to cancel out all the parameters not related to affinity and is exactly equal to the dissociation constant K_d. Thus, one can measure K_d at equilibrium by equilibrium dialysis or calculate K_d from rate constants measured under non-equilibrium conditions.

Another method, more commonly used today, to measure the kinetics of antigen-antibody interactions depends on surface plasmon resonance. In this method, a specialized biosensing instrument (such as the Biacore) uses an optical approach to measure the affinity of an antibody that is passed over an antigen that is immobilized over a metal film. A light source is focused on this film through a prism at a specific angle (resonance), and the reflected light provides a surface plasmon resonance readout. Adsorption of an antibody to the antigen alters the surface plasmon resonance readout, and this alteration can provide information on affinity.

TRANSGENIC MICE AND GENE TARGETING

Three important and related methods for studying the functional effects of specific gene products in vivo are the creation of conventional transgenic mice that ectopically express a particular gene in a defined tissue; the creation of gene "knockout" mice, in which a targeted disruption is used to ablate the function of a particular gene; and the generation of "knockin" mice, in which an existing gene in the germline is replaced with a modified version of the same. A knockin approach could either replace a normal version of a gene with a mutant version or, in principle, "correct" an existing mutant gene with a "normal" version. These techniques involving genetically engineered mice have been widely used to analyze many biologic phenomena, including the development, activation, and tolerance of lymphocytes.

For the creation of conventional transgenic mice, foreign DNA sequences, called transgenes, are introduced into the pronuclei of fertilized mouse eggs, and the eggs are implanted into the oviducts of pseudopregnant females. Usually, if a few hundred copies of a gene are injected into pronuclei, about 25% of the mice that are born are transgenic. One to 50 copies of the transgene insert in tandem into a random site of breakage in a chromosome and are subsequently inherited as a simple Mendelian trait. Because integration usually occurs before DNA replication, most (about 75%) of the transgenic pups carry the transgene in all of their cells, including germ cells. In most cases, integration of the foreign DNA does not disrupt endogenous gene function. Also, each founder mouse carrying the transgene is a heterozygote, from which homozygous lines can be bred.

The great value of transgenic technology is that it can be used to express genes in particular tissues by attaching coding sequences of the gene to regulatory sequences that normally drive the expression of genes selectively in that tissue. For instance, lymphoid promoters and enhancers can be used to overexpress genes, such as rearranged antigen receptor genes, in lymphocytes, and the insulin promoter can be used to express genes in the β cells of pancreatic islets. Examples of the utility of these methods for study of the immune system are mentioned in many chapters of this book. Transgenes can also be expressed under the control of promoter elements that respond to drugs or hormones, such as tetracycline or estrogens. In these cases, transcription of the transgene can be controlled at will by administration of the inducing agent.

A powerful method for development of animal models of single-gene disorders, and the most definitive way to establish the obligatory function of a gene in vivo, is the creation of knockout mice by targeted mutation or disruption of the gene. This technique relies on the phenomenon of homologous recombination. If an exogenous gene is inserted into a cell, for instance, by electroporation, it can integrate randomly into the cell's genome. However, if the gene contains sequences that are homologous to an endogenous gene, it will preferentially recombine with and replace endogenous sequences. To select for cells that have undergone homologous recombination, a drug-based selection strategy is used. The fragment of homologous DNA to be inserted into a cell is placed in a vector typically containing a neomycin resistance gene and a viral thymidine kinase (*tk*) gene (Fig. A-6, *A*). This targeting vector is constructed in such a way that the neomycin resistance gene is always inserted into the chromosomal DNA, but the *tk* gene is lost whenever homologous recombination (as opposed to random insertion) occurs. The vector is introduced into cells, and the cells are grown in neomycin and ganciclovir, a drug that is metabolized by thymidine kinase to generate a lethal product. Cells in which the gene is integrated randomly will be resistant to neomycin but will be killed by ganciclovir, whereas cells in which homologous recombination has occurred will be resistant to both drugs because the *tk* gene will not be incorporated. This positive-negative selection ensures that the inserted gene in surviving cells has undergone homologous recombination with endogenous sequences. The presence of the inserted DNA in the middle of an endogenous gene usually disrupts the coding sequences and ablates the expression or function of that gene. In addition, targeting vectors can be designed such that homologous recombination will lead to the deletion of one or more exons of the endogenous gene.

To generate a mouse carrying a targeted gene disruption or mutation, a targeting vector is used to first disrupt the gene in a murine embryonic stem (ES) cell line. ES cells are pluripotent cells derived from mouse embryos that can be propagated and induced to differentiate in culture or that can be incorporated into a mouse blastocyst, which may be implanted in a pseudopregnant mother and carried to term. Importantly, the progeny of the ES cells develop normally into mature tissues that will express the exogenous genes that have been transfected into the ES cells. Thus, the targeting vector designed to disrupt a particular gene is inserted into ES cells, and colonies in which homologous recombination has occurred (on one chromosome) are selected with drugs, as described earlier (Fig. A-6, *B*). The presence of the desired recombination is verified by analysis of DNA with techniques such as Southern blot hybridization or polymerase chain reaction. The selected ES cells are injected into blastocysts,

which are implanted into pseudopregnant females. Mice that develop will be chimeric for a heterozygous disruption or mutation, that is, some of the tissues will be derived from the ES cells and others from the remainder of the normal blastocyst. The germ cells are also usually chimeric, but because these cells are haploid, only some will contain the chromosome copy with the disrupted (mutated) gene. If chimeric mice are mated with normal (wild-type) animals and either sperm or eggs containing the chromosome with the mutation fuse with the wild-type partner, all cells in the offspring derived from such a zygote will be heterozygous for the mutation (so-called germline transmission). Such heterozygous mice can be mated to yield animals that will be homozygous for the mutation with a frequency that is predictable by simple Mendelian segregation. Such knockout mice are deficient in expression of the targeted gene.

Homologous recombination can also be used to replace a normal gene sequence with a modified version of the same gene (or of another gene), thereby creating a knockin mouse strain. Knockin mice can be used to assess the biologic consequences of a change in a single base, for instance, as opposed to the deletion of a gene. A knockin approach could, in principle, also be used to replace a defective gene with a normal one. In certain circumstances, a different gene may be placed at a defined site in the genome by use of a knockin strategy rather than in a random site as in conventional transgenic mice. Knockin approaches are used when it is desirable to have the expression of the transgene regulated by certain endogenous DNA sequences, such as a particular enhancer or promoter region. In this case, the targeting vector contains an exogenous gene encoding a desired product as well as sequences homologous to an endogenous gene that are needed to target the site of recombination.

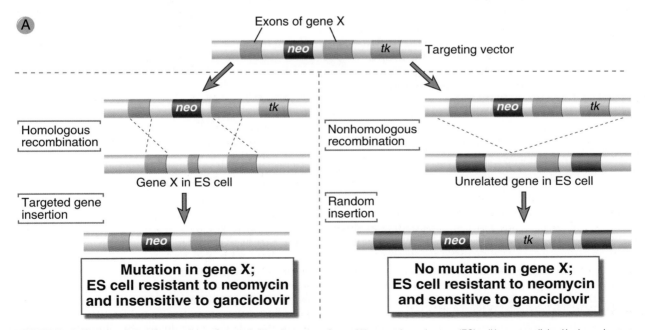

FIGURE A-6 Generation of gene knockout. A, The disruption of gene X in an embryonic stem (ES) cell is accomplished by homologous recombination. A population of ES cells is transfected with a targeting vector that contains sequences homologous to two exons of gene X flanking a neomycin resistance *(neo)* gene. The *neo* gene replaces or disrupts one of the exons of gene X on homologous recombination. The thymidine kinase *(tk)* gene in the vector will be inserted into the genome only if random, non-homologous recombination occurs.

Continued

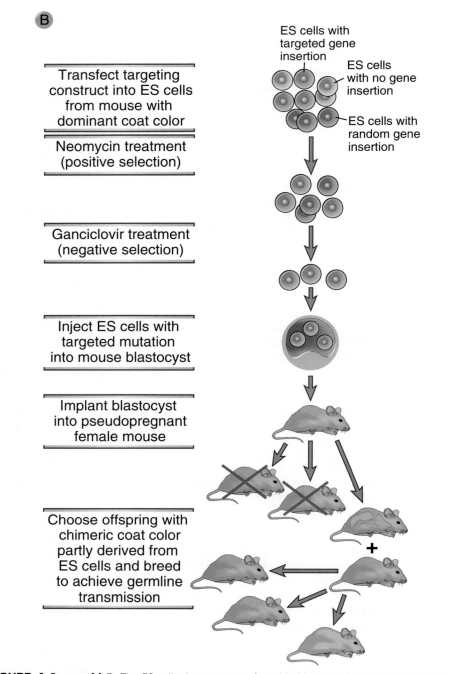

B

Transfect targeting construct into ES cells from mouse with dominant coat color

Neomycin treatment (positive selection)

Ganciclovir treatment (negative selection)

Inject ES cells with targeted mutation into mouse blastocyst

Implant blastocyst into pseudopregnant female mouse

Choose offspring with chimeric coat color partly derived from ES cells and breed to achieve germline transmission

ES cells with targeted gene insertion

ES cells with no gene insertion

ES cells with random gene insertion

FIGURE A-6, cont'd B, The ES cells that were transfected by the targeting vector are selected by neomycin and ganciclovir so that only those cells with targeted insertion (homologous recombination) survive. These cells are then injected into a blastocyst, which is then implanted into the uterus of a pseudopregnant mouse. A chimeric mouse will develop in which some of the tissues are derived from the ES cell carrying the targeted mutation in gene X. These chimeric mice are identified by a mixed-color coat, including the color of the mouse strain from which the ES cells were derived and the color of the mouse strain from which the blastocyst was derived. If the mutation is present in germ cells, it can be propagated by further breeding.

Although the conventional gene-targeting strategy has proved to be of great usefulness in immunology research, the approach has some limitations. First, the mutation of one gene during development may be compensated for by altered expression of other gene products, and therefore the function of the targeted gene may be obscured. Second, in a conventional gene knockout mouse, the importance of a gene in only one tissue or at only one time during development cannot be easily assessed. Third, a functional selection marker gene, such as the neomycin resistance gene, is permanently introduced into the animal genome, and this alteration may have unpredictable results on the phenotype of the animal. An important refinement of gene knockout technology that can overcome many of these drawbacks is a "conditional" targeting approach. A commonly used conditional strategy takes advantage of the bacteriophage-derived Cre/*loxP* recombination system. The Cre enzyme is a DNA recombinase that recognizes a 34-bp sequence motif called ***loxP***, and the enzyme mediates the deletion of gene segments flanked by two *loxP* sites in the same orientation. To generate mice with *loxP*-tagged genes, targeting vectors are constructed with one *loxP* site flanking the neomycin resistance gene at one end and a second *loxP* site flanking the sequences homologous to the target at the other end. These vectors are transfected into ES cells, and mice carrying the *loxP*-flanked but still functional target gene are generated as described for conventional knockout mice. A second strain of mice carrying a *cre* transgene is then bred with the strain carrying the *loxP*-flanked ("floxed") target gene. In the offspring, expression of Cre recombinase will mediate deletion of the target gene. Both the normal gene sequences and the neomycin resistance gene will be deleted. Importantly, expression of the *cre* gene, and therefore deletion of the targeted gene, can be restricted to certain tissues or specified times by the use of *cre* transgene constructs with different promoters. For example, selective deletion of a gene only in macrophages and granulocytes can be accomplished by using a *cre* transgenic mouse in which *cre* is driven by a lysozyme promoter, or the selective loss of a gene only in regulatory T cells can be accomplished using a *foxp3* promoter driving a *cre* transgene. Alternatively, a steroid-inducible promoter can be used so that Cre expression and subsequent gene deletion occur only after mice are given a dose of dexamethasone. Many other variations on this technology have been devised to create conditional mutants. Cre/*loxP* technology can also be used to create knockin mice. In this case, *loxP* sites are placed in the targeting vector to flank the neomycin resistance gene and the homologous sequences, but they do not flank the replacement (knockin) gene sequences. Therefore, after *cre*-mediated deletion, the exogenous gene remains in the genome at the targeted site.

Gene knock in technology has been applied to create "reporter" mice in which cells that would normally express a particular protein will express a fluorescent molecule at the same time as the native protein. This is accomplished by replacing the native gene with a transgene that encodes the fluorescent reporter protein and the native protein, both under the control of the native promoter and enhancer. Reporter mice have been developed that allow the visualization of immune cells of particular subsets in vivo, such as mice in which IL-17–producing Th17 cells also express a fluorescent protein. These cells can be detected using intravital florescence microscopy. The cells expressing the reporter genes can also be isolated alive and subjected to functional studies ex vivo, even if the native gene reported is a nuclear transcription factor whose expression would otherwise only be detectable by methods that kill the cells. For example, live regulatory T cells can be isolated by FACS-sorting lymph nodes from a reporter mouse that expresses green fluorescent protein simultaneously with the transcription factor FoxP3.

A novel approach to generating mutations in cell lines as well as in ES cells utilizes a modification of a bacterial defense system against foreign DNA called the CRISPR (Clustered Regularly Interspaced Short Palindromic Repeats) Cas9 (CRISPR Associated nuclease 9) system. In the gene editing variation of this, a guide RNA hybridizes with a chosen target DNA sequence and allows the Cas9 nuclease to generate a targeted double stranded break. While such a break can disrupt a gene, co-transfecting a plasmid with a mutated version of the target sequence allows efficient homologous recombination and the creation of a targeted knockin mutation. This is the most rapid approach available for the generation of knockout or knockin mutations in cell lines or in the germlines of experimental animals.

METHODS FOR STUDYING T LYMPHOCYTE RESPONSES

Our current knowledge of the cellular events in T cell activation is based on a variety of experimental techniques in which different populations of T cells are activated by defined stimuli, and functional responses are measured. In vitro experiments have provided a great deal of information on the changes that occur in a T cell when it is stimulated by antigen. More recently, several techniques have been developed to study T cell proliferation, cytokine expression, and anatomic redistribution in response to antigen activation in vivo. The new experimental approaches have been particularly useful for the study of naive T cell activation and the localization of antigen-specific memory T cells after an immune response has waned.

Polyclonal Activation of T Cells

Polyclonal activators of T cells bind to many or all T cell receptor (TCR) complexes regardless of specificity and activate the T cells in ways similar to peptide-MHC complexes on antigen-presenting cells (APCs). Polyclonal activators are mostly used in vitro to activate T cells isolated from human blood or the lymphoid tissues of experimental animals. Polyclonal activators can also be used to activate T cells with unknown antigen specificities, and they can evoke a detectable response from mixed populations of naive T cells, even though the frequency of cells specific for any one antigen would be too low to elicit a detectable response. The polymeric carbohydrate-binding plant proteins called lectins, such as concanavalin-A and phytohemagglutinin, are one commonly used group of polyclonal T cell activator. These lectins bind specifically to certain sugar residues on T cell surface glycoproteins, including the TCR and CD3 proteins, and thereby stimulate the T cells. Antibodies specific for invariant framework epitopes on TCR or CD3 proteins also function as polyclonal activators of T cells. Often, these antibodies need to be immobilized on solid surfaces or beads or cross-linked with secondary anti-antibodies to induce optimal activation responses. Because soluble polyclonal activators do not provide costimulatory signals that are normally provided by APCs, they are often used together with stimulatory antibodies to receptors for costimulators, such as anti-CD28 or anti-CD2. Superantigens, another kind of polyclonal stimulus, bind to and activate all T cells that express particular types of TCR β chain (see Chapter 16, Fig. 16-2).

T cells of any antigen specificity can also be stimulated with pharmacologic reagents, such as the combination of the phorbol ester PMA and the calcium ionophore ionomycin, that mimic signals generated by the TCR complex.

Antigen-Induced Activation of Polyclonal T Cell Populations

Polyclonal populations of normal T cells that are enriched for T cells specific for a particular antigen can be derived from the blood and peripheral lymphoid organs of individuals after immunization with the antigen. The immunization serves to expand the number of antigen-specific T cells, which can then be restimulated in vitro by adding antigen and MHC-matched APCs to the T cells. This approach can be used to study antigen-induced activation of a mixed population of previously activated ("primed") T cells expressing many different TCRs, but the method does not permit analysis of responses of naive T cells.

Antigen-Induced Activation of T Cell Populations with a Single Antigen Specificity

Monoclonal populations of T cells, which express identical TCRs, have been useful for functional, biochemical, and molecular analyses. The limitation of these monoclonal populations is that they are maintained as long-term tissue culture lines and therefore may have phenotypically diverged from normal T cells in vivo. One type of monoclonal T cell population that is frequently used in experimental immunology is an antigen-specific T cell clone. Such clones are derived by isolating T cells from immunized individuals, as described for polyclonal T cells, followed by repetitive in vitro stimulation with the immunizing antigen plus MHC-matched APCs and cloning of single antigen–responsive cells in semisolid media or in liquid media by limiting dilution. Antigen-specific responses can easily be measured in these populations because all the cells in a cloned cell line have the same receptors and have been selected for growth in response to a known antigen-MHC complex. Both helper and cytotoxic T lymphocyte clones have been established from mice and humans. Other monoclonal T cell populations used in the study of T cell activation include antigen-specific T cell hybridomas, which are produced like B cell hybridomas (see Fig. 5-9, Chapter 5), and tumor lines derived from T cells have been established in vitro after removal of malignant T cells from animals or humans with T cell leukemias or lymphomas. Although some tumor-derived lines express functional TCR complexes, their antigen specificities are not known, and the cells are usually stimulated with polyclonal activators for experimental purposes. The Jurkat line, derived from a human T cell leukemia cell, is an example of a tumor line that is widely used as a model to study T cell signal transduction.

TCR transgenic mice are a source of homogeneous, phenotypically normal T cells with identical antigen specificities that are widely used for in vitro and in vivo experimental analyses. If the rearranged α and β chain genes of a single TCR of known specificity are expressed as a transgene in mice, a majority of the mature T cells in the mice will express that TCR. If the TCR transgene is crossed onto a RAG-1– or RAG-2–deficient background, no endogenous *TCR* gene expression occurs, and 100% of the T cells will express only the transgenic TCR. TCR transgenic T cells can be activated in vitro or in vivo with a single peptide antigen, and they can be identified by antibodies specific for the transgenic TCR. One of the unique advantages of TCR transgenic mice is that they permit the isolation of sufficient numbers of naive T cells of defined specificity to allow one to study functional responses to the first exposure to antigen. This advantage has allowed investigators to study the in vitro conditions under which antigen activation of naive T cells leads to differentiation into functional subsets such as T_H1 and T_H2 cells (see Chapter 9). Naive T cells from TCR transgenic mice can also be injected into normal syngeneic recipient mice, where they home to lymphoid tissues. The recipient mouse is then exposed to the antigen for which the transgenic TCR is specific. By use of antibodies that label the TCR transgenic T cells, it is possible to follow their expansion and differentiation in vivo and to isolate them for analysis of recall (secondary) responses to antigen ex vivo.

Methods to Enumerate and Study Functional Responses of T Cells

Proliferation assays for T lymphocytes, like those of other cells, are conducted in vitro by determining the amount of ^{3}H-labeled thymidine incorporated into the replicating DNA of cultured cells. Thymidine incorporation provides a quantitative measure of the rate of DNA synthesis, which is usually directly proportional to the rate of cell division. Cellular proliferation in vivo can be measured by injecting the thymidine analogue bromodeoxyuridine (BrdU) into animals and staining cells with anti-BrdU antibody to identify and enumerate nuclei that have incorporated BrdU into their DNA during DNA replication.

Fluorescent dyes can be used to study proliferation of T cells in vivo. T cells are first labeled with chemically reactive lipophilic fluorescent esters and then adoptively transferred into experimental animals. The dyes enter cells, form covalent bonds with cytoplasmic proteins, and then cannot leave the cells. One commonly used dye of this type is 5,6-carboxyfluorescein diacetate succinimidyl ester (CFSE), which can be detected in cells by standard flow cytometric techniques. Every time a T cell divides, its dye content is halved, and therefore it is possible to determine whether the adoptively transferred T cells present in lymphoid tissues of the recipient mouse have divided in vivo and to estimate the number of doublings each T cell has gone through.

Peptide-MHC tetramers are used to enumerate T cells with a single antigen specificity isolated from blood or lymphoid tissues of experimental animals or humans. These tetramers contain four of the peptide-MHC complexes that the T cell would normally recognize on the surface of APCs. The tetramer is made by producing a class I MHC molecule to which is attached a small molecule called biotin by use of recombinant DNA technology. Biotin binds with high affinity to a protein called avidin, and each avidin molecule binds four biotin molecules. Thus, avidin forms a substrate for assembly of four biotin-conjugated MHC proteins. The MHC molecules can be loaded with a peptide of interest and thus stabilized, and the avidin molecule is labeled with a fluorochrome, such as FITC. This tetramer binds to T cells specific for the peptide-MHC complex with high enough avidity to label the T cells, even in suspension. This method is the only feasible approach for identification of antigen-specific T cells in humans. For instance, it is possible to identify and enumerate circulating HLA-A2–restricted T cells specific for an HIV peptide by staining blood cells with a tetramer of HLA-A2 molecules loaded with the peptide. The same technique is being used to enumerate and isolate T cells specific for self antigens in normal individuals and in patients with autoimmune diseases. Peptide-MHC tetramers that bind to a particular transgenic TCR can also be used to quantify the transgenic T cells in different tissues after adoptive transfer and antigen stimulation. The technique is now widely used with class I MHC molecules; in class I molecules, only one polypeptide is polymorphic, and stable molecules can be produced in vitro. This is more difficult for class II molecules because both chains are polymorphic and required for proper assembly, but class II–peptide tetramers are also being produced.

Cytokine secretion assays can be used to quantify cytokine-secreting effector T cells within lymphoid tissues. The most commonly used methods are cytoplasmic staining of cytokines and single-cell enzyme-linked immunosorbent assays (ELISpot). In these types of studies, antigen-induced activation and differentiation of T cells take place in vivo, and then T cells are isolated and tested for cytokine expression in vitro. Cytoplasmic staining of cytokines requires permeabilizing of the cells so that fluorochrome-labeled antibodies specific for a particular cytokine can gain entry into the cell, and the stained cells are analyzed by flow cytometry. Cytokine expression by T cells specific for a particular antigen can be determined by additionally staining T cells with peptide-MHC tetramers or, in the case of TCR transgenic T cells, antibodies specific for the transgenic TCR. By use of a combination of CFSE and anti-cytokine antibodies, it is possible to examine the relationship between cell division and cytokine expression. In the ELISpot assay, T cells freshly isolated from blood or lymphoid tissues are cultured in plastic wells coated with antibody specific for a particular cytokine. As cytokines are secreted from individual T cells, they bind to the antibodies in discrete spots corresponding to the location of individual T cells. The spots are visualized by adding secondary enzyme-linked anti-Ig, as in a standard ELISA (see earlier), and the number of spots is counted to determine the number of cytokine-secreting T cells.

METHODS FOR STUDYING B LYMPHOCYTE RESPONSES

Activation of Polyclonal B Cell Populations

It is technically difficult to study the effects of antigens on normal B cells because, as the clonal selection hypothesis predicted, very few lymphocytes in an individual are specific for any one antigen. An approach to circumventing this problem is to use anti-Ig antibodies as analogues of antigens, with the assumption that anti-Ig will bind to constant (C) regions of membrane Ig molecules on all B cells and will have the same biologic effects as an antigen that binds to the hypervariable regions of membrane Ig molecules on only the antigen-specific B cells. To the extent that precise comparisons are feasible, this assumption appears generally correct, indicating that anti-Ig antibody is a valid model for antigens. Thus, anti-Ig antibody is frequently used as a polyclonal activator of B lymphocytes, similar to the use of anti-CD3 antibodies as polyclonal activators of T lymphocytes, discussed earlier.

Antigen-Induced Activation of B Cell Populations with a Single Antigen Specificity

To examine the effects of antigen binding to B cells, investigators have attempted to isolate antigen-specific B cells from complex populations of normal lymphocytes or to produce cloned B cell lines with defined antigenic specificities. These efforts have met with little success. However, transgenic mice have been developed in which virtually all B cells express a transgenic Ig of known specificity, so that most of the B cells in these mice respond to the same antigen. A somewhat more sophisticated approach has been to generate antigen receptor knockin mice, in which rearranged Ig H and L chain genes have been homologously recombined into their endogenous loci. Such knockin animals have proved particularly useful in the examination of receptor editing.

Assays to Measure B Cell Proliferation and Antibody Production

Much of our knowledge of B cell activation is based on in vitro experiments, in which different stimuli are used to activate B cells and their proliferation and differentiation can be measured accurately. The same assays may be done with B cells recovered from mice exposed to different antigens or with homogeneous B cells expressing transgene-encoded antigen receptors.

B cell proliferation is measured by use of CFSE labeling or ^{3}H-labeled thymidine incorporation in vitro and BrdU labeling in vivo, as described earlier for T cell proliferation.

Antibody production is measured in two different ways: with assays for cumulative Ig secretion, which measure the amount of Ig that accumulates in the supernatant of cultured lymphocytes or in the serum of an immunized individual; and with single-cell assays, which determine the number of cells in an immune population that secrete Ig of a particular specificity or isotype. The most accurate, quantitative, and widely used technique to measure the total amount of Ig in a culture supernatant or serum sample is ELISA. By use of antigens bound to solid supports, it is possible to use ELISA to quantify the amount of antibody in a sample specific for a particular antigen. In addition, the availability of anti-Ig antibodies that detect Igs of different heavy or light chain classes allows measurement of the quantities of different isotypes in a sample. Other techniques to measure antibody levels include hemagglutination for anti-erythrocyte antibodies and complement-dependent lysis for antibodies specific for known cell types. Both assays are based on the demonstration that if the amount of antigen (i.e., cells) is constant, the concentration of antibody determines the amount of antibody bound to cells, and this is reflected in the degree of cell agglutination or subsequent binding of complement and cell lysis. Results from these assays are usually expressed as antibody titers, which are the dilution of the sample giving half-maximal effects or the dilution at which the endpoint of the assay is reached.

A single-cell assay for antibody secretion is the ELISpot assay. In this method, antigen is bound to the bottom of a well, antibody-secreting cells are added, and antibodies that have been secreted and are bound to the antigen are detected by an enzyme-linked anti-Ig antibody, as in an ELISA, in a semisolid medium. Each spot represents the location of an antibody-secreting cell. Single-cell assays provide a measure of the numbers of Ig-secreting cells, but they cannot accurately quantify the amount of Ig secreted by each cell or by the total population. The ELISA and ELISpot techniques can be adapted to assess affinity of antibodies, by the use of antigens with differing numbers of hapten moieties. In this way, affinity maturation can be assessed by testing serum or B cells sampled at different times during an immune response.

Index

Page numbers followed by *f, t,* and *b* indicate figures, tables, and boxes, respectively.

Date Due

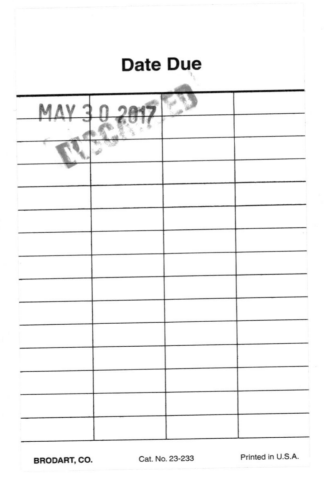

MAY 3 0 2017

BRODART, CO.   Cat. No. 23-233   Printed in U.S.A.